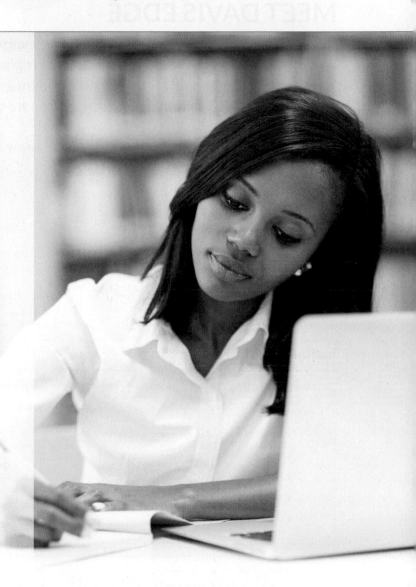
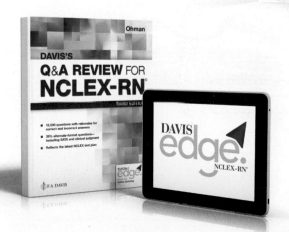

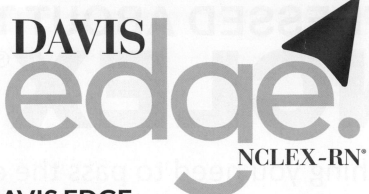

# MEET DAVIS EDGE

Davis Edge helps you master key nursing concepts and prepares you to succeed on the NCLEX®. This online program creates quizzes based on your personal strengths and weaknesses and tracks your progress every step of the way to prepare you for the exam.

Read on for an overview of how Davis Edge works and then go online to redeem your access code.

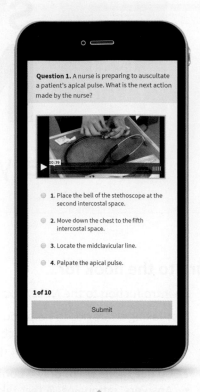

**Practice. Practice. Practice.**
Thousands of NCLEX-style questions make it easy for you to customize quizzes by concept, content area, or client needs category.

**Anytime, anywhere** access lets you quiz yourself on your phone, tablet, or laptop.

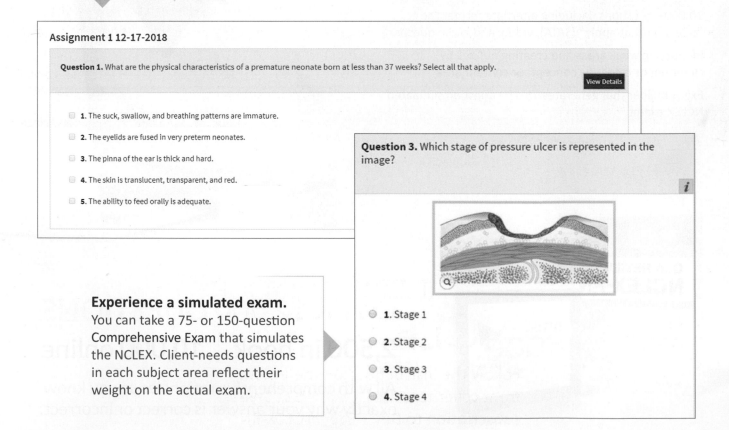

**Experience a simulated exam.**
You can take a 75- or 150-question Comprehensive Exam that simulates the NCLEX. Client-needs questions in each subject area reflect their weight on the actual exam.

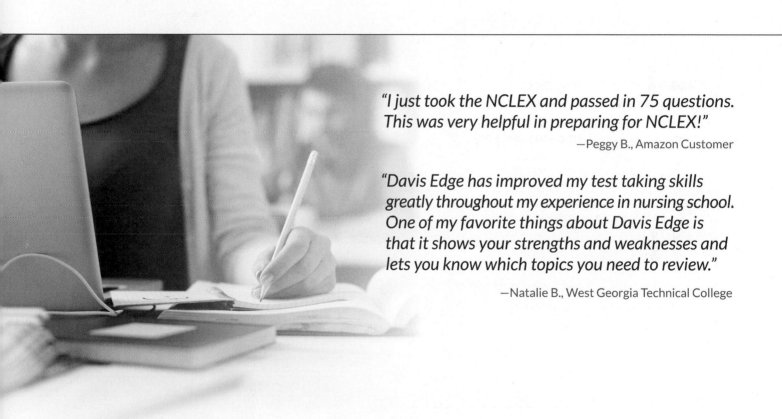

**Question 8.** What should the nurse do to ensure asepsis when caring for a client with a central venous access device (CVAD)?

**Course Topic:** Physiological Adaptation: Fluid and Electrolyte Imbalances | **Concept(s):** Infection; Nursing |
**Cognitive Level:** Knowledge [Remembering]

- ✓ 1. Use sterile gloves, supplies, and mask.
- 2. Scrub catheter hubs with antiseptic for 5 seconds.
- 3. Clean the skin with acetone before insertion of a catheter.
- ✗ 4. Use tincture of iodine to scrub injection ports.

**Rationale**

| | |
|---|---|
| **Option 1:** | The nurse must follow strict aseptic technique by using sterile gloves, supplies, and a mask when caring for the client with a central venous access device (CVAD). |
| **Option 2:** | The nurse should vigorously scrub catheter hubs with an antiseptic for at least 15 seconds before accessing them to minimize contamination. |
| **Option 3:** | The skin should not be cleaned with acetone because it is an organic solvent. |
| **Option 4:** | Injection ports are scrubbed with alcohol or chlorhexidine gluconate. Tincture of iodine is generally not used to scrub injection ports. |

**Test Taking Tip:** Choose the correct answer on the basis of which action ensures protection of the nurse as well as the client.

## Receive immediate feedback.
You'll know immediately how well you've mastered the material through **rationales** for correct and incorrect answers and **test-taking tips** that reduce anxiety and build confidence.

# DAVIS'S
# Q&A REVIEW FOR
# NCLEX-RN®

## THIRD EDITION

## Kathleen A. Ohman, EdD, MS, RN

Professor of Nursing
College of Saint Benedict/Saint John's University
St. Joseph, Minnesota

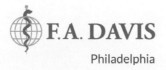

F.A. DAVIS

Philadelphia

F. A. Davis Company
1915 Arch Street
Philadelphia, PA 19103
www.fadavis.com

Printed in the United States of America

Last digit indicates print number: 10 9 8 7 6 5 4 3 2 1

*Publisher, Nursing:* Terri Wood Allen
*Manager of Project and eProject Management:* Catherine H. Carroll
*Senior Content Project Manager:* Christine M. Abshire
*Design/Illustrations Manager:* Carolyn O'Brien
*Electronic Project Editor:* Sandra Glennie

**Library of Congress Cataloging-in-Publication Data**

Names: Ohman, Kathleen A., author.
Title: Davis's Q&A review for NCLEX-RN® / Kathleen A. Ohman.
Other titles: Davis's Q&A review for the NCLEX-RN® examination. | Davis's Q
  and A review for NCLEX-RN® | Q&A review for NCLEX-RN® | Q and A review
  for NCLEX-RN®
Description: Third edition. | Philadelphia : F.A. Davis Company, [2019] |
  Preceded by Davis's Q&A review for the NCLEX-RN® examination / Kathleen
  A. Ohman. Second edition. [2017]. | Includes bibliographical references
  and index.
Identifiers: LCCN 2018055102 (print) | LCCN 2018056571 (ebook) | ISBN
  9780803699144 | ISBN 9780803689855 (pbk.)
Subjects: | MESH: Nursing Care | Licensure, Nursing | Nursing Process |
  Examination Question
Classification: LCC RT55 (ebook) | LCC RT55 (print) | NLM WY 18.2 | DDC
  610.73076—dc23
LC record available at https://lccn.loc.gov/2018055102

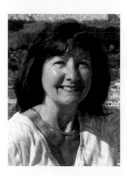

Kathleen Ann Ohman, EdD, MS, RN

## THE STUDY PACKAGE

*Davis's Q&A Review for the NCLEX-RN®* is a study package reflective of the 2019 **NCLEX-RN® Detailed Test Plan** and incorporates the latest information in the NCLEX-RN® Exam. This package provides you with a question and answer (Q&A) review book and access to *Davis Edge NCLEX-RN*, which offers thousands of test items online. As you embark on this study package, you will find numerous pedagogical features to facilitate your learning, whether preparing for course tests or for the NCLEX-RN® Exam.

## KEY FEATURES

To ensure your success on the NCLEX-RN® Exam and to accommodate your own study and preparation style, *key features* are incorporated in this study package.

- *NEW with the third edition!* **Hundreds of new questions that emphasize the key areas on the latest NCLEX-RN® Detailed Test Plan.**
- *NEW with the third edition!* **Sample Next Generation NCLEX Questions similar to those being piloted on the NCLEX-RN® Exam.**
- *NEW!* **More Management of Care questions added! Twenty-nine percent of the questions in the book pertain to Management of Care.**
- *NEW!* **More pharmacology questions have been added to this study package. Twenty-two percent of the questions in the book pertain to pharmacological and parenteral therapies.**
  - This study package has **thousands of questions** like those on the actual NCLEX-RN® Exam.
  - The book contains **2500** questions, with many questions that have been updated with new information.
  - *Davis Edge for NCLEX-RN*, the accompanying online resource, includes **10,000 additional questions**.
- **Concepts are included with each question.** Inclusion of a pertinent concept allows for ease of use in programs that teach conceptually.

- **Each chapter has every alternate item format like those on the exam and include:**
  - Multiple choice
  - Multiple response / Select-all-that-apply
  - Fill-in-the-blank
  - Hot-spot
  - Ordered response (prioritization; drag-and-drop questions)
  - Chart or exhibit
  - Graphic

  There are more alternate format questions in this package than in any other NCLEX-RN® Q&A package.

- **Review tests are organized by content areas.** Organization by content areas facilitates your review for course-specific tests and serves as a means of systematic review in preparation for the NCLEX-RN® Exam.
- **Comprehensive exams are uniquely designed to parallel the percentage of test questions assigned to each *Client Needs* category and subcategory of the NCLEX-RN® Detailed Test Plan.** The Q&A book contains two 75-item comprehensive exams that parallel the NCLEX-RN® categories of *Client Needs* and the respective percentages.
- **All *Client Needs* categories identified in the latest NCLEX-RN® Detailed Test Plan are represented in this study package.** Questions target every component of the test plan including the *Client Needs* categories, subcategories, and outcome statements to ensure a comprehensive coverage of the behaviors expected of an entry-level registered nurse. Each question identifies the *Client Needs* category and a concept.
- **All questions identify the content area and cognitive domain included in the latest NCLEX-RN® Detailed Test Plan.** You can feel secure that the expectations in the latest **NCLEX-RN® Detailed Test Plan** are comprehensively covered in this Q&A package.
- **An answer and rationale section is included with each chapter in the practice tests, and the rationale for each**

**option is provided individually.** You can more easily determine why an option is correct or incorrect. These provide immediate feedback when answering questions and help refresh or build your knowledge base when progressing to the comprehensive tests. This allows you to evaluate your progress in studying for the NCLEX-RN® Exam.

- **Test-taking tips are noted in the answer and rationale section.** Strategies for selecting the correct option are included to assist you when you are unsure of the answer and must guess on a question. Tips for remembering key points are addressed with multiple questions to enhance recalling the information in future questions.
- **All questions are supported by current nursing references. Evidence-based citations (research studies, summaries of research, or evidence-based resources) support the correct option for many questions.** The resources used for question development are included in the bibliography. You can feel confident that every question reflects current nursing practice.

## BOOK ORGANIZATION

This question and answer book is divided into three distinct sections. **Section I** consists of four chapters and provides background and orientation to the NCLEX-RN® Exam as well as chapters on test-taking strategies and guidance for international and repeat test-takers. **Section I** also highlights changes in the exam based on the latest **NCLEX-RN® Detailed Test Plan**.

Section II consists of six units titled by content areas and comprising 50 chapters. The practice tests in these chapters address subject areas within nursing and are organized around the major themes in the latest NCLEX-RN® Detailed Test Plan. Content areas within Section II include various units such as *Management of Care* (ethical, legal, and safety issues in nursing, leadership and management, prioritization and delegation, teaching and learning, communication, cultural diversity, and end-of-life care), *Fundamentals of Nursing* (basic care and comfort, medication administration, disaster preparedness, and infection control), and the more traditional content areas of nursing including *Care of Childbearing Families, Adults, Children and Families,* and *Mental Health Nursing.* Pharmacology is emphasized in four specialized, stand-alone chapters, which are organized by subject area. Additional questions pertaining to pharmacology are integrated in the medication administration tests, other content tests, and the comprehensive tests. Thousands of pharmacology questions are included within the study package. Gerontology and emergency and disaster nursing content is integrated throughout the chapters.

Finally, **Section III** includes two comprehensive exams reflecting all the subject areas covered in the book and on the NCLEX-RN® Exam. Both of these tests are at a higher level of difficulty and include 75 questions, the minimum number included on the NCLEX-RN® Exam itself. A student who performs well on these comprehensive exams should finish the book feeling well prepared for the NCLEX-RN® Exam.

## ONLINE RESOURCE

*Davis Edge NCLEX-RN®* is an adaptive Q&A platform designed to build the critical-thinking, analytical, and decision-making skills essential to NCLEX success. The program includes 10,000 NCLEX questions to create on-the-go practice quizzes by client needs category or content area. Each question provides you with complete rationales for both correct and incorrect answers so you understand why you are answering a question correctly or incorrectly in order to decrease stress and increase comprehension and confidence. Comprehensive exams simulate the NCLEX by pulling 75 or 150 questions in the same proportion you'll see on the NCLEX so you can immediately see your strengths and weaknesses and know where to spend your time studying. Coupled with the text, Davis Edge NCLEX-RN® gives you thousands of practice questions at your fingertips so you can study anytime, anywhere in order to ensure NCLEX success.

## HOW TO USE THIS STUDY PACKAGE

It is important that you read the introductory book chapters, so you become familiar with the NCLEX-RN® Exam and the test plan. Little attention may have been directed at the test plan within your nursing program. It is best to know what is being tested before embarking on a study path. Focus on the test-taking strategies and tips included in the introductory chapters and on how to apply them when answering the questions. The test-taking tips will help you to remember key information.

Once you have read the introductory chapters, you are ready to develop a plan and begin your practice with the test questions. Use the **PQRST APPROACH** presented in Chapter 3. Remember, success begins with a positive mind-set. Focus on your goal, use positive self-talk and self-reassurance as you complete the practice questions, and keep consistent with your study plan.

After you answer the questions, be sure to read the rationales for the correct and incorrect options and the test-taking tips. These provide significant information that will help you to understand the basis for the correct option and the reasons that the other options are incorrect. The test-taking tip provides a method for selecting an option when you are unsure of the answer or a cue for remembering the information.

As you study, use the online resource to select additional questions in a content area, especially if you did poorly on a practice test. Using the online resource intermittently throughout your review will also enhance your proficiency in reading and answering questions from the computer screen and will prepare you to take the NCLEX-RN® Exam on the computer.

# Acknowledgments

My special thanks to:

**Robert G. Martone, Retired Publisher, Nursing, F. A. Davis,** for considering me for the first edition of the book, your faith in me, your enthusiasm, and your encouragement.

**Terri W. Allen, Publisher, Nursing, F. A. Davis,** for your support and recommendations on the third edition.

**Christine M. Abshire, Senior Content Project Manager, F. A. Davis,** for your commitment to this project, and your attention to detail.

**Those who reviewed questions** for your expertise, ideas, and suggestions for enhancement.

## CONTRIBUTORS TO PAST EDITIONS

Nadine M. Aktan, MS, RN, APN-C, Doctoral Candidate

Roberta Basol, MA, RN, CNA, BC

Adrienne Beatty, BA, MS, LPC

Jodi Lisbeth Berndt, RN, BSN, CCRN, PCCN

Matthew D. Byrne, MS, RN, CPAN, PhD-C

Annette J. Caflisch, EdD, MSN, RN

Rachel Choudhury, MSN, MS, RN, CNE

Anne L. Von Fricken Coonrad, JD, MS, RN

Darlene M. Copley, RN, MS, PMHCNS-BC

Michele Crawford, MSN, RN, FNP-BC

Madelyn Danner, MS, RN, CCRN, CEN, CNE

Michele McPhee Davidson, PhD, CNM, CFN, RN

Katherine H. Dimmock, JD, EdD, MSN, RN

Constance Domino, BS Child Psychology

Kimberly Dudas, PhD, RN, ANP-BC, CNE

Heather Evans, PhD, RNC-MNN, CLC

Rhea Faye Felicilda-Reynaldo, EdD, RN

Deb Filer, PhD, RN, CNE

Dorcas C. Fitzgerald, PhD, RN, CNS

Augusta Garbarich, RN, BSN

Denise L. Garee, MSN, RN, CEN, CHSE, PhD

Melissa Garno, EdD, RN

Laura Gerdes, RN, MSN, CPN

Donna Gloe, EdD, RN

Carman Godfrey, MSN, RN

Anne-Marie Goff, PhD, MS, BS, RN

Kay Knox Greenlee, MSN, RN, APRN-BC

Joyce M. Hammer, RN, MSN

Sigrid Hedman-Dennis, RN, MSN, CNS

Debra K. Hoag, RN, MSN, NCSN

Suzanne M. Leson, MS, RD, LD

Lisa S. Lewis, EdD, MSN, RN, CNE

Margaret M. Mahon, PhD, RN, FAAN

Betsy L. Mann, DNP, APRN, CNE, FNP-C

Alice L. March, PhD, RN, FNP, CNE

Maria A. Marconi, RN, MS

Hillary McAlhany, MSN, RN, CEN

Terri D. McCaffrey, MAN, RN, CNS

Denise A. Meijer, DNP, RN, WHNP-BC

Heidi Meyer, MSN, RN, PHN

P. Lea Monahan, BSN, MSN, PhD

Kimberly D. Moss, PhD, RN, CNE, ODCP

Janet Marie Neuwirth, RN, MS

Carol Peterson, PhD, RN, MS, CCRN

Emily Rayman, RN, BSN

Rhoda R. Redulla, PhD, MSN, RN

Leslie Reifel, MSN, RN, CPNP, CNE

Valarie Rumbley, MSN, RN, CFRN, CNL, EMT-P

Rita M. Sarao, MSN, RN, CEN

Elizabeth M. Scarano, MSN, RN

Laree Schoolmeesters, RN, PhD, CNL

Marcia Scott, MSN, RN

Darlene Sredl, PhD, RN

Renotta Stainbrook, BSN, MSN, APRN-BC

Sharon A. Takiguchi, RN, MS, APRN, ABD

Angela Taylor, PhD, MSN, RN

Rita M. Trofino, DNP, MNEd, RN

Linda Turchin, RN, MSN, CNE

Geraldine Tyrell, DNP, RN, CNE

Vanessa V. Uithaler, RN, CCRN

Deborah Uplinger, FNP, MSN

Rose A. Utley, PhD, RN, CNE

Karen Helm Vollen, MA, APRN-BC

Amber Welborn, MSN, RN

Patricia H. White, MSN-Ed, RNC-NIC, CNE

Tonya L. Willingham, MA, MSN, RN, CNE

Bridgette Worlie, RN-BC, BSN

# REVIEWERS OF PAST EDITIONS

Susan Arbogast, RN, MS, CHPN, CNE

Jodi Lisbeth Berndt, PhD, RN, CCRN, PCCN, CNE

Sophia Beydoun, RN, MSN

Jenna L. Boothe, DNP, RN

Donna Bowles, EdD, MSN, RN, CNE

Diana L. Broniec, RN, MSN

Kimberley M. Brownlee, BSN, MSN

Tammy Bryant, RN, MSN

Marlena Bushway, MSNed, RN, CNE

Barbara A. Caton, MSN, RN, CNE

Donna Chapin, MSN, RN, CNOR

Karen Clark, MSN, RN

Elizabeth Cohn, PhD, RN

Margaret D. Cole, RN, DSN

Jessie Daniels, RN, BSN, MA

Lynette H. DeBellis, RN, MA

Aida L. Egues, DNP, RN, APHN-BC, CNE

Joan Eiffe, MSN, RN

Mary Fabick, MSN, MEd, BSN, RN, CEN

Kristen Fenlason, MS, RN

Dawn Ferry, APRN, CNP, CHSE

Ruth Gladen, RN, MS

Susan H. Golden, MSN, RN

Stephanie C. Greer, RN, MSN

Renee Covey Harrison, RN, MS

Karla Haug, MS, RN

Theresa Hoadley, PhD, RN

Stephanie D. Huff, RN, DNP, FNP-BC

Patty Jones, RN, MSN

Dana C. Kemery, MSN, RN, CNE, CEN, CPEN

Anne-Marie Kuchinski, RN, MS, OCN

Nicole Lang, MSN, RN

Dara Lanman, MSN, RN, CNE

Grace G. Lewis, RN, MS, CNS

Susan Malkemes, DNP, RN, CCRN

Cynthia A. McGuire, MS, RN, CNE

June McLachlan, RN, FNP-BC, FNP, DNP

Jacqueline McMahon, RN, MSN, CNE

Denise A. Meijer, DNP, RN, WHNP-BC

Linda Mollino, MSN, RN

Michelle M. Murphy-Rozanski, PhD, MSN, RN, CRNP

Mary Neisen, RN, BSN, MA, APRN - Family Nursing

Judy Nelson, RN, MSN

Katie B. Notch, RN, MSN

Patricia Novak, MSN

Randee Nyman, MSN, RN, CNS, CCRN, CNE

JoAnne M. Pearce, MS, RN

Sharon Ridgeway, PhD, RN

Susan M. Rouse, PhD, RN, CNE

Lara Sheppa, MSN, RN, CNE

Tracey Siegel, EdD, MSN, RN, CWCN, CNE

Brenda Sloan, RN, MA

Jacqueline C. Smith, EdD, RN

Cheryl L. Sorge, MA, RN

Mendy Stanford, BSN, MSN/Ed, CNE

Susan D. Taylor, MSN, RN, CNE

Bethany Tollefson, RN, MSN

Patricia Voelpel, RN, MS, ANP, CCRN

Jo A. Voss, PhD, RN, CNS

Laura J. Wallace, RN, CNM, PhD

Zana Webb, RN, MSN

Julie Willenbrink, MSN, RN

Roxanne Wilson, PhD, RN

Catherine L. Wohletz, BSN, RN

Jean Yockey, PhD, FNP-BC, CNE

Shellah Young, RN

Polly Gerber Zimmermann, RN, MS, MBA, CEN, FAEN

# Contents

# Preparing for the
# NCLEX-RN®

## Chapter One

# The NCLEX-RN® Licensure Exam

To prepare for the NCLEX-RN® licensure exam, you should become familiar with the licensing exam process and the test plan to avoid surprises when taking the exam. Adequate preparation will ease anxiety and instill confidence!

## INFORMATION ABOUT THE LICENSING EXAM

Information about the application process and exam is available from the National Council of State Boards of Nursing (NCSBN; www.ncsbn.org). Faculty at your nursing program usually reviews the application process near graduation. To take the licensure exam, your first step is to submit an application for licensure or registration and the application fee to the board of nursing (BON) or regulatory body (RB) in the state, province, or territory where you wish to be licensed (see Box 1.1). The place where you wish to be licensed may be different from the location of your program. The application can be completed before graduation and is good for a year. Your nursing program official will usually provide the confirmation of program completion to the BON/RB, or the BON/RB may request that you submit a Confirmation of Program Completion form completed by your nursing program official.

In addition to applying to the BON, you will also need to register and pay the fee for writing the NCLEX-RN® with Pearson VUE. Once the BON verifies your eligibility to write the exam, you will receive an authorization to test (ATT). You will receive the ATT about 1 to 2 weeks after you officially graduate from your nursing program. You will need this ATT to schedule an exam time at one of the Pearson VUE centers. Pearson VUE centers are located throughout and outside the United States at multiple national and international sites.

Testing accommodations are available to qualified candidates. You need to make a written request to the BON/RB where you are applying and comply with their requirements. This needs to be completed before submitting your NCLEX registration to Pearson VUE.

The NCLEX Candidate Bulletin, available at the NCSBN Web site (www.ncsbn.org/1213.htm), provides full details regarding the application process, requesting testing accommodations (if applicable), personal identification requirements,

testing centers, and test administration. Candidates are encouraged to carefully review this bulletin.

## COMPUTER ADAPTIVE TESTING (CAT)

The NCLEX-RN® exam is administered exclusively as a computerized test. A tutorial is provided with the exam that includes instructions on using the mouse and recording answers. An on-screen calculator is provided. The tutorial for the NCLEX-RN® exam may be viewed any time before taking the exam at www.pearsonvue.com/nclex. Completing the tutorial and taking practice items on the computer will help ease your nervousness about the exam and provide you with an opportunity to practice the included alternate item formats. The online items available with this book simulate the computer exam.

### Exam Length

CAT allows individualized administration of questions based on your ability and demonstrated competency as you answer questions. Initially you will be given medium-level questions. If you answer these correctly, you are given a more difficult item. The computer adapts to how you answer these questions, giving you either more difficult or easier items. You will be given between 75 and 265 test items. Of these, 15 are pretest items that are not scored but are being tested for use on future exams. It is advisable that you spend only 1 to 2 minutes per item. Each item must be answered before proceeding to the next item. The answer can be changed until the **option** and the <NEXT> button are selected. If an answer is not known, a reasonable attempt should be made to answer the question. Once an item has been answered and the <NEXT> button selected, the computer will not allow a return to previously answered items. Thus you cannot skip items and return to those later. The number of items you receive is based on the difficulty of the items and how well you perform on answering the more difficult items correctly.

### Testing Time

The maximum time limit for the exam is 6 hours. This testing time includes the tutorial and any breaks. Once you correctly answer the minimum number of test items that meets the passing standard, you will have demonstrated competency

## BOX 1.1

### General Steps of the NCLEX-RN® Application Process

- Access the NCSBN Web site at www.ncsbn.org to read about the application process and find the address for the BON/RB where you intend to be licensed.
- Contact the BON/RB and apply for licensure/registration.
- Register with Pearson VUE via the Internet or telephone, and pay the exam fee.
- BON/RB verifies your program completion and makes you eligible to write the exam in the Pearson VUE system.
- Receive the ATT that is e-mailed to you by Pearson VUE.
- Schedule your exam appointment through your Internet account with Pearson VUE or by telephone.

with 95% certainty and the exam will stop. Likewise, if you incorrectly answer a maximum number of test items and have not met the passing standard, the exam will also stop; you will have failed to demonstrate competency. If neither scenario occurs, the exam will end when either the maximum number of test items (265) has been taken or the time limit has expired. The length of the exam should not be interpreted as indicating a pass or fail. A longer exam indicates only that your ability is close to the passing standard and that more questions are needed to determine whether your ability is above or below the passing standard.

### Exam Results

Results of the exam are not released in the testing center. Although the computer scores the exam, the scores are verified by Pearson VUE and then transmitted to the BON or RB where you applied. The exam results are provided by this BON/RB. The NCSBN Web site states that you should receive the results within 6 weeks, or, for a fee, you can obtain unofficial results earlier in some jurisdictions. However, many candidates report getting results much earlier, often within a few days. In many states, you can access your results from the state's BON Web site; this is usually free. The NCSBN Web site (www.ncsbn.org) provides links to the various state BONs for application purposes and for checking exam results.

If a state's BON does not provide access to exam results via its Web site, you may use the *verification of license* option at the state's BON Web site to determine whether a license has been issued by searching for your name. If sufficient time has elapsed since the exam and you have passed it, your name and license will be displayed. If you did not pass the exam or if a license has not yet been issued, your name will not be found. Exam results are not provided when verifying a license.

## NCLEX-RN® EXAM STRUCTURE

Exam content is based on the knowledge, skills, and abilities necessary for a newly licensed, entry-level registered nurse (RN) to provide safe and effective nursing care. The content is determined through using multiple resources including a practice analysis of entry-level RNs in their first year of practice, expert opinions of the NCLEX Exam Committee (NEC), NCSBN content staff, and BONs (NCSBN's member boards). The practice analysis includes nursing activities performed on a regular basis by entry-level nurses. The practice analysis is completed every 3 years through a random survey of newly licensed RNs from a variety of settings and RN education programs. Results of the practice analysis are used by the NEC to evaluate the existing NCLEX-RN® test plan, to make needed revisions, and to present the test plan document for approval to the Delegate Assembly, which is a decision-making body of NCSBN. The test plan for the NCLEX-RN® exam is revised and posted every 3 years and is available at the NCSBN Web site (www.ncsbn.org/testplans.htm).

## THE TEST PLAN

### Client Needs Categories and Subcategories

The NCLEX-RN® test plan is based on a *Client Needs* framework. This framework provides a universal structure for defining nursing actions and competencies and includes clients in all settings. The client refers to the individual, family or group, significant others, or a population. Four major Client Needs categories and six subcategories are identified in the test plan (see Table 1.1).

The percentage distribution of content based on the 2019 test plan is presented in Figure 1.1.

### Integrated Processes

The NCLEX-RN® test plan includes integrated processes foundational to nursing practice. These include nursing

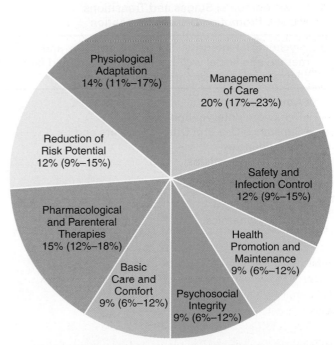

**Figure 1.1:** Distribution of content for the NCLEX-RN®. Adapted from The National Council of State Boards of Nursing. (2018). *2019 NCLEX-RN® Test Plan*. Chicago: Author.

## TABLE 1.1

### Client Needs Categories and Subcategories

**A. Safe Effective Care Environment:** The nurse promotes achievement of client outcomes by providing and directing nursing care that enhances the care delivery setting to protect clients, family/significant others, and other health care personnel.

*1. Management of Care.* Providing and directing nursing care that enhances the care delivery setting to protect clients, family/significant others, and health care personnel.

- Advance Directives/Self-Determination/Life Planning
- Advocacy
- Assignment, Delegation, and Supervision
- Case Management
- Client Rights
- Collaboration With Interdisciplinary Team
- Concepts of Management
- Confidentiality/Information Security

- Continuity of Care
- Establishing Priorities
- Ethical Practice
- Informed Consent
- Information Technology
- Legal Rights and Responsibilities
- Performance Improvement (Quality Improvement)
- Referrals

*2. Safety and Infection Control.* Protecting clients, family/significant others, and health care personnel from health and environment hazards.

- Accident/Error/Injury Prevention
- Emergency Response Plan
- Ergonomic Principles
- Handling Hazardous and Infectious Materials
- Home Safety
- Reporting of Incident/Event/Irregular Occurrence/Variance

- Safe Use of Equipment
- Security Plan
- Standard Precautions/Transmission-based Precautions/Surgical Asepsis
- Use of Restraints/Safety Devices

**B. Health Promotion and Maintenance:** The nurse provides care and directs nursing care of the client and family/significant others that incorporates the knowledge of expected growth and development principles, prevention and/or early detection of health problems, and strategies to achieve optimal health.

- Aging Process
- Antepartum/Intrapartum/Postpartum and Newborn Care
- Developmental Stages and Transitions
- Health Promotion/Disease Prevention

- Health Screening
- High-risk Behaviors
- Lifestyle Choices
- Self-care
- Techniques of Physical Assessment

**C. Psychosocial Integrity:** The nurse provides and directs nursing care that promotes and supports the emotional, mental, and social well-being of the client and family/significant others experiencing stressful events, as well as clients with acute or chronic mental illness.

- Abuse/Neglect
- Behavioral Interventions
- Substance Use and Other Disorders and Dependencies
- Coping Mechanisms
- Crisis Intervention
- Cultural Awareness/Cultural Influences on Health
- End of Life Care
- Family Dynamics

- Grief and Loss
- Mental Health Concepts
- Religious and Spiritual Influences on Health
- Sensory/Perceptual Alterations
- Stress Management
- Support Systems
- Therapeutic Communications
- Therapeutic Environment
- Nutrition and Oral Hydration

## TABLE 1.1

### Client Needs Categories and Subcategories (continued)

**D. Physiological Integrity:** The nurse promotes physical health and wellness by providing care and comfort, reducing client risk potential, and managing health alterations.

*1. Basic Care and Comfort.* Providing comfort and assistance in the performance of activities of daily living.
- Assistive Devices
- Elimination
- Mobility/Immobility
- Nonpharmacological Comfort Interventions
- Personal Hygiene
- Rest and Sleep

*2. Pharmacological and Parenteral Therapies.* Providing care related to the administration of medications and parenteral therapies.
- Adverse Effects/Contradictions/Side Effects/ Interactions
- Blood and Blood Products
- Central Venous Access Devices
- Dosage Calculation
- Expected Actions/Outcomes
- Medication Administration
- Parenteral/Intravenous Therapies
- Pharmacological Pain Management
- Total Parenteral Nutrition

*3. Reduction of Risk Potential.* Reducing the likelihood that clients will develop complications or health problems related to existing conditions, treatments, or procedures.
- Changes/Abnormalities in Vital Signs
- Diagnostic Tests
- Laboratory Values
- Potential for Alterations in Body Systems
- Potential for Complications of Diagnostic Tests/ Treatments/Procedures
- Potential for Complications From Surgical Procedures and Health Alterations
- System-specific Assessments
- Therapeutic Procedures

*4. Physiological Adaptation.* Managing and providing care for clients with acute, chronic, life-threatening physical health conditions
- Alterations in Body Systems
- Fluid and Electrolyte Imbalances
- Hemodynamics
- Illness Management
- Medical Emergencies
- Pathophysiology
- Unexpected Response to Therapies

The National Council of State Boards of Nursing (2019). *2019 NCLEX-RN® Detailed Test Plan.* The National Council of State Boards of Nursing, Inc., Chicago, with permission.

process, caring, communication and documentation, teaching/ learning, and culture and spirituality. *Culture and spirituality* is a newly integrated process included in the 2016 NCLEX-RN® test plan.

- **The Nursing Process.** The nursing process has five phases: (1) assessment, (2) analysis, (3) planning, (4) implementation, and (5) evaluation. An equal number of items on each phase is integrated throughout the NCLEX-RN® exam.
- *Assessment.* Assessment involves collecting information. The nurse collects subjective and objective information about the client, verifies it, gathers additional information if needed, and then communicates relevant assessment findings to other members of the health care team.
- *Analysis.* Analysis involves interpreting the information to identify actual or potential client health care needs and/or problems. Based on the analysis, the nurse collects additional data if needed, establishes nursing diagnoses, and

communicates the analysis findings and nursing diagnoses to relevant members of the health care team.
- *Planning.* Planning involves establishing goals and identifying strategies to meet client needs. The nurse formulates outcome criteria, develops approaches to achieve expected client outcomes, modifies the plan of care, and collaborates with and communicates the plan to relevant members of the health care team.
- *Implementation.* Implementation involves initiating or completing nursing activities to accomplish the identified goals of care. The nurse organizes, manages, and provides care, including teaching and counseling, to accomplish the expected client outcomes. The nurse advocates and collaborates on the client's behalf; supervises, coordinates, and evaluates the delivery of care provided by the nursing staff; and documents information and communicates it to relevant members of the health care team.
- *Evaluation.* Evaluation involves comparing the actual client outcomes/goals with expected outcomes/goals of

care to determine whether these have been achieved. The nurse evaluates adherence to prescribed therapies and knowledge of information. The nurse documents evaluation information, modifies the plan if indicated, and communicates the nursing evaluation and client responses to relevant members of the health care team.

- **Caring.** Caring is the interaction between the nurse and client (individual, family or group, including significant others and population) in an atmosphere of mutual respect and trust. Within a collaborative environment, the nurse encourages and offers support, hope, and compassion to the client and family when providing care and working toward the achievement of desired outcomes.

- **Communication and Documentation.** The verbal and nonverbal interactions between the nurse and the client, the client's significant others, and health care team members are part of communication and documentation. Observations, events, and activities related to client care are documented in the client's electronic and/or paper medical record according to standards of nursing practice and accountability.

- **Teaching/Learning.** Teaching and learning facilitates knowledge acquisition, including skills and attitudes, and disseminates information to others to promote a change in behavior.

- **Culture and Spirituality.** The interaction of the nurse and client identifies and reflects unique individual preferences for client care based on the client's self-report and identification. The interaction and client care include the applicable standard of care and legal instructions.

## THE PASSING STANDARD

The passing standard is the minimum level of ability required for safe and effective entry-level nursing practice. The passing standard for the NCLEX-RN® is reevaluated once every 3 years at the time the test plan is reevaluated. The criteria used to evaluate the passing standard include the results of (1) a standard setting exercise performed by a panel of experts; (2) the historical record of the passing standard and how candidates performed; (3) a standard setting survey sent to educators and employers; and (4) the educational readiness of high school graduates who express an interest in nursing. The passing standard last increased April 1, 2013.

More information about the passing standard can be located at the NCSBN Web site (www.ncsbn.org/4699.htm; www.ncsbn.org/2630.htm).

## STRUCTURE IMPLEMENTATION WITHIN THIS STUDY PACKAGE

To ensure success on the NCLEX-RN® exam, all Client Needs categories and subcategories are extensively represented in this book and in the online items or questions (items and questions are used interchangeably within the NCSBN materials and within this study package). As you begin your study, pay attention to the Client Needs presented. You will have the opportunity to respond to items that test your nursing knowledge and ability for every category and subcategory in the NCLEX-RN® test plan. Focusing on the Client Needs categories will help you confirm your knowledge and identify areas for further study.

You will also have the opportunity to respond to items that incorporate the integrated processes, including all five phases of the nursing process, caring, teaching and learning, communication and documentation, and culture and spirituality. Every chapter in the book has items that include all integrated processes. These processes are used in a variety of care situations, integrating concepts from management of care, fundamentals, childbearing and family nursing, child health nursing, medical-surgical (adult health) nursing, psychiatric/mental health nursing, disaster and emergency nursing, pharmacology, nutrition, and health promotion.

Each chapter in the book includes multiple-choice items and items in alternate formats including multiple response, fill-in-the-blank calculation, ordered response, graphic, and hot spots. Charts, tables, and illustrations are included with many items. Item types that include sound and video are available with the online resources.

One difference between this book and the actual NCLEX-RN® exam is the use of commonly used abbreviations, such as COPD for chronic obstructive pulmonary disease. Although the NCLEX-RN® exam will usually provide you with the unabbreviated terms for diseases or disorders, common abbreviations are used within this book to hone your abilities in interpreting these. You are likely to see common abbreviations used in clinical practice. The list of abbreviated terms with their meanings is included in the appendix.

New alternate item types being trialed and researched by the NCSBN are included in this book. These are more difficult items and will help you in refining your clinical judgment abilities (see Chapter 2). You may have some of these item types on your NCLEX-RN® exam.

An answer section for each chapter test includes the answer (key), the rationale for the answer, the rationales for the incorrect options or distractors, and a test-taking tip. The answer section provides categories with each item that include the content, concept, client needs, integrated processes, and the cognitive level. The references for each chapter are available with the online resources and include evidence-based citations for every chapter.

## Chapter Two

# NCLEX-RN® Items

## COGNITIVE LEVEL OF ITEMS

The NCLEX-RN® exam uses Bloom's taxonomy, and the revised Bloom's taxonomy, of cognitive domains for the writing and coding of items. The lowest level of the taxonomy is **knowledge (remembering),** which includes the ability to recall facts, concepts, principles, terms, or procedures. Knowledge-level items require you to define, identify, or select. The next level of the taxonomy is **comprehension (understanding),** which requires an understanding of information. Comprehension-level items require you to recall, interpret, explain, compare, distinguish, or predict. The third level of the taxonomy is **application (applying).** At this level, you are required to demonstrate, implement, act, intervene, apply, solve, or modify. **Analysis (analyzing)** involves examining relationships between parts. At this level, you are required to question, explore, select, differentiate, interpret, organize, or prioritize. Analysis-type items have complex information or include multiple variables. **Evaluation (evaluating)** includes judging, critiquing, or appraising. **Synthesis (creating)** is the highest level of the cognitive domain. During synthesis, information is combined in new and meaningful ways. At the synthesis level, you are required to develop, organize, create, produce, or generate.

You may find a few lower-cognitive-level items on the NCLEX-RN® exam, such as the one shown in Box 2.1. However, because nursing practice requires application of knowledge, skills, and ability, the majority of items on the NCLEX-RN® exam are written at the **application** and **analysis** levels of cognitive ability. These higher cognitive levels require the use of more complex thought processes.

**Application**-type items require you to prioritize information (see Box 2.2). The nurse needs understanding of the concepts to perform an action. For example, a question may ask which intervention the nurse should implement. All of the options will be viable; you will need to determine which option is appropriate and which requires the most immediate action. Application items may also include key words, such as **best, most appropriate, priority, first, most concerning, exclude,** or **defer.** These key words can also appear in analysis-type items, which would include more variables for you to analyze.

**Analysis**-type items have more complex information and variables in the stem or options for you to consider, and they may be longer (see Box 2.3). For example, rather than

### BOX 2.1

**Sample Comprehension Item**

**MoC** The NA, who usually works on an adult unit, reports to the nurse that the 2-year-old client's blood glucose level is normal at 82 mg/dL. The nurse's response to the NA is based on knowing that the target blood glucose for a toddler is what range?
1. 60–100 mg/dL
2. 80–120 mg/dL
3. 90–150 mg/dL
4. 100–180 mg/dL

**ANSWER: 4**

### BOX 2.2

**Sample Application Item**

The nurse is teaching the client with an ileostomy. Which nutritional information is **most important** for the nurse to emphasize?
1. Avoid foods that are gas forming.
2. Try only one new food at a time.
3. Eat yogurt to help control odor.
4. Drink at least 3000 mL of fluid daily.

**ANSWER: 4**

posing a question that pertains just to the client experiencing acute MI, the item may also include the fact that the client has multiple medications and has abnormal laboratory (lab) values. You will need to apply knowledge from multiple areas and analyze the client's lab findings to answer the question. Analysis-type items may also include groups of clients with various problems, and you will need to determine which client should be seen first by the nurse.

## TYPES OF ITEM FORMATS

A variety of item formats are included in the NCLEX-RN® exam. These include multiple-choice and alternate item formats: multiple response; fill-in-the-blank; ordered response (drag and drop or prioritization); hot spot; chart or exhibit; graphic; audio; and video. Usually the stem of an item ends

## BOX 2.3

### Sample Analysis Item

**PHARM** The HCP prescribes aspirin 75 mg oral daily, lisinopril 10 mg oral daily, furosemide 10 mg oral daily, and potassium chloride 20 mEq oral bid for the client newly diagnosed with acute MI. The client's serum lab report shows a potassium level of 4.2 mEq/L, a creatinine level of 2.3 mg/dL, and platelets of 250,000/mm³. Which intervention is **most** important for the nurse to implement?
1. Ensure that the aspirin is enteric coated.
2. Contact the HCP before giving lisinopril.
3. Time the potassium so it is given with meals.
4. Check the urine output after giving furosemide.

**ANSWER: 2**

## BOX 2.4

### Multiple-Response NCLEX-RN® Screenshot Item

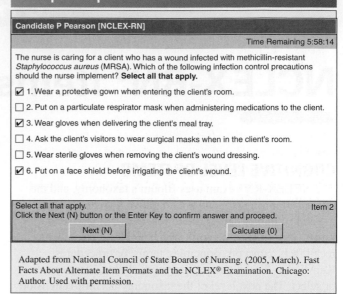

Adapted from National Council of State Boards of Nursing. (2005, March). Fast Facts About Alternate Item Formats and the NCLEX® Examination. Chicago: Author. Used with permission.

with a question or statement. Partial statements ending with a colon usually do not appear on the NCLEX-RN® exam. Each item is a stand-alone item; it is not dependent on a situation presented with a previous item. However, various new alternate format item types are being tested by the NCSBN. If you have time remaining in the 6-hour time limit at the end of your exam, you may be asked if you would like to participate in the testing of some of these new item types.

Information about alternate test item formats is available from the NCSBN Web site (www.ncsbn.org). The Pearson VUE Web site (www.pearsonvue.com/nclex) provides a tutorial for you to practice taking alternate test item formats and an option to pay for taking a practice exam. Any item type can include charts, graphics, illustrations, audio, or video. For example, a fill-in-the-blank item can include a chart that you will need to review to perform the calculation.

**Multiple-choice items** present a situation or scenario and then ask a question. You select *one* option from a list of four options to answer the question. Multiple-choice items at the higher cognitive levels will have more variables in the stem or options for you to consider. Boxes 2.1, 2.2, and 2.3 provide examples of multiple-choice items at the different cognitive levels.

**Multiple-response items** contain a situation or a stem with a question followed by **Select all that apply.** The list of possible answers could have four, five, or six options; it is unusual for an item to have more than six options, but it is possible. You select *one* or more options from the list. The answer could include *all* of the options. These are very difficult items; no partial credit is given. Box 2.4 provides a screenshot of a sample multiple-response item from the NCSBN. On the actual exam, you will be using your mouse to check the boxes in front of the options that you select to answer the question.

For multiple-response practice items in this book, you should either check or circle the number of the options you choose for the answer to the question. Be careful as you read options. You may have a number of these items on the actual exam if you are answering the more difficult items correctly.

This book includes many multiple-response items for you to hone your skills in answering these items. Box 2.5 shows a multiple-response item for practice within this book.

**Fill-in-the-blank items** require typing in a **numerical** answer based on the information presented in the item stem (Box 2.6). This type of format is used to assess your ability to perform a calculation, such as a medication dose for an adult or child, IV infusion rates, or intake and output on the client. Items may include calculations between different units of measure, such as kilograms to pounds or milligrams to grams. The answer box on the actual NCLEX-RN® exam will include the units of measure, such as milliliters, milliliters per hour, milligrams, grams, tablets, and others. It also will identify whether the answer should be rounded and, if so, to how many decimal places. Be sure to read the directions for each item, and do not assume that because you rounded on one item that you should do this on the others.

**Ordered-response** (prioritization or drag and drop) test items require you to place items in the correct order or in the

## BOX 2.5

### Sample Multiple-Response Item

The nurse is caring for the client who has dyspnea associated with HF and COPD. Which interventions should the nurse implement? **Select all that apply.**
1. Weigh each morning after the client voids.
2. Apply 6 liters of oxygen per nasal cannula.
3. Turn and reposition every 1 to 2 hours.
4. Elevate the head of the bed 30 to 40 degrees.
5. Teach use of pursed-lip breathing techniques.

**ANSWER: 1, 4, 5**

## BOX 2.6

### Sample Fill-in-the-Blank Item

The client is to receive cefuroxime sodium 500 mg in 50 mL of NS IVPB. The medication is to be infused over 20 minutes. The nurse should set the infusion pump to deliver how many milliliters per hour?

_____ mL/hr (Record your answer as a whole number.)

**ANSWER: 150**

order of priority. Based on the situation and the information presented, you will need to determine what is first, second, third, and so forth. There may be up to six options to place in a specific order. Items of this type may include client situations and the order that the nurse should assess the clients or intervene. It may also include the sequence for performing a procedure or providing care. When presented with this type of item on the NCLEX-RN® exam, you use the computer mouse to click on an item and drag it from one box on the left-hand side of the page to another box on the right-hand side of the page, placing all items in the correct order or the order of priority (see Box 2.7). All options must be correctly sequenced to receive any credit; no partial credit is given.

When answering ordered-response items in this book, you should use the numbers preceding the options. Place the number of the option you select first, second, and so forth on the answer line below the list of options. Box 2.8 provides an example of an ordered-response item for practice within this book and how it should be answered.

**Hot spot items** are used to demonstrate competence in clinical skills applied in professional nursing practice. An illustration, graph, or diagram is used as part of the stem or question. This type of item requires the identification of *one or more areas*, such as the location of an injection or where

## BOX 2.7

### Ordered Response NCLEX-RN® Sample

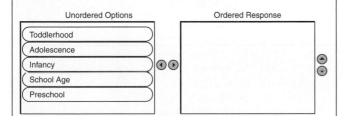

The nurse is preparing a staff education about the stages of childhood development. Place all of the stages listed below in ascending chronological order. Use all the options.

Unordered Options | Ordered Response

- Toddlerhood
- Adolescence
- Infancy
- School Age
- Preschool

Adapted from National Council of State Boards of Nursing. (2005, March). Fast Facts About Alternate Item Formats and the NCLEX® Examination. Chicago: Author. Used with permission.

## BOX 2.8

### Sample Ordered-Response Item

The nurse receives the shift report on four assigned clients. Place the clients in the order that the nurse should plan to assess the clients.

1. The 42-year-old client admitted 2 days ago with a chest wall incision infection, possibly *MRSA*; awaiting culture results
2. The 47-year-old client admitted with chest pain yesterday; monitor shows sinus rhythm; history of 2-pack-per-day cigarette smoker
3. The 54-year-old client admitted with acute exacerbation of HF during previous shift; very anxious 30 minutes prior to shift change
4. The 62-year-old client status post MI 2 days ago; has intermittent chest pain, but pain free at end of previous shift
Answer: _____

**ANSWER: 3, 4, 2, 1**

the nurse should perform an assessment. On the actual exam, you will use your mouse to place the cursor over the desired area and then click the left mouse button to mark an area in the illustration, graph, or diagram. The area can also be deselected with the left mouse button if you wish to change the location. For practice items in this book, you should place an X (or more than one X if directed to do so) on the illustration, graph, or diagram presented. Box 2.9 provides an example of a hot spot item.

## BOX 2.9

### Sample Hot Spot Item

The client who has a history of hepatitis B virus infection is hospitalized with new-onset nausea, vomiting, and jaundice. Place an X in the quadrant where the nurse should palpate for tenderness.

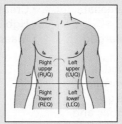

**ANSWER:**

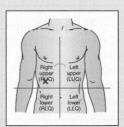

**Chart/exhibit items** require you to examine and analyze a chart or exhibit to answer the question. For example, after analyzing a list of lab values in the client's medical record, you are asked to identify the lab value that indicates that the client is experiencing thrombocytopenia. Some chart/exhibit items on the NCLEX-RN® exam will have three tabs that you need to click on individually to read the information. Each tab should be opened and the information analyzed to answer the question correctly. Box 2.10 provides a chart/exhibit item for practice within this book.

**Graphic items** present you with a question and options that are graphics rather than text. You are required to select the appropriate graphic answer. An example of a graphic item is presented in Box 2.11.

**Audio items** present you with a play button to listen to an audio clip and then select an option based on the audio clip presented. You will use headphones for audio items. The format of an audio item is presented in Box 2.12.

## NEXT GENERATION NCLEX ITEMS

Several different **Clinical Judgment** item types are being trialed and researched by the NCSBN. Some of these new item types include: (1) Enhanced Hot Spots, (2) Extended Drag and Drop, (3) CLOZE, (4) Dynamic Exhibits and Constructed Response, and (5) Rich Media Scenario. These new item types are technology-enhanced items available for computer-generated tests. Multiple questions pertaining to these item types are presented throughout this book for your practice. These have been highlighted **CJ** so that they are easier to locate.

**Enhanced hot spot items** require using the computer mouse to perform a function, such as drawing on an image related to a test item. Box 2.13 shows an example of this item type. Item 551 in Chapter 14 provides an example of how this item appears in this book.

**Extended drag and drop items** require you to "drag" statements or items from one area of the computer screen to "drop" on another area of the same screen. Examples of situations that may be developed into extended drag and drop items include placing items for disposal into the correct receptacle for disposal, or assigning clients to an appropriate hospital room and bed. Box 2.14 shows an example of this item type. Item 113 in Chapter 6 provides an example of how this item appears in this book.

**CLOZE alternate item types** include a case study followed by a question or questions pertaining to the case study. To answer the question, you need to complete a sentence by choosing from a drop-down list of words or statements. Box 2.15 shows how the question and drop-down menu may appear in the exam. Item 761 in Chapter 18 provides an

## BOX 2.10

### Sample Chart/Exhibit Item

The nurse reviews the medical record illustrated for the client hospitalized with cirrhosis.

| Assessment Information | Serum Laboratory and Diagnostic Study Results | Medications Due Now |
|---|---|---|
| • BP 96/55, HR 120 bpm, RR 32 per minute<br>• Extreme dyspnea on exertion<br>• Oxygen at 4L/nasal cannula<br>• Abdomen enlarged from ascites<br>• States divorced, lives alone, and worried about discharge<br>• Former alcoholic and IV drug use<br>• HCV | • AST: 89 units/L (N = 5–40 units/L)<br>• ALT: 101 units/L (N = 7–56 units/L)<br>• Sodium: 136 mEq/L<br>• Potassium, 3.2 mEq/L<br>• Creatinine: 2.5 mg/dL<br>• Hgb 10.9 g/dL<br>• Massive amount of ascites visible on CT scan | • Furosemide 40 mg oral daily<br>• Spironolactone 100 mg oral daily<br>• Folic acid 400 mcg oral daily<br>• Vitamin D 400 units oral daily |

Which action by the nurse is **most important**?
1. Initiate a social worker consult.
2. Notify the HCP.
3. Measure the client's abdominal girth.
4. Administer the medications due now.

**ANSWER: 2**

# BOX 2.11

## Sample Graphic Item

The nurse is assessing the client who is receiving an infusion of IV oxytocin for labor induction at 40 weeks of gestation. Which FHR pattern requires immediate intervention by the nurse due to uteroplacental insufficiency?

1.

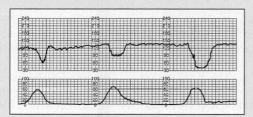

2.

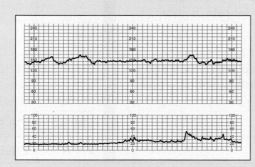

3.

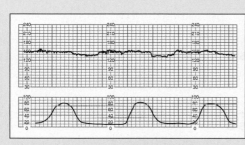

4.

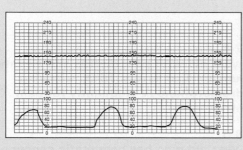

**ANSWER: 3**

# BOX 2.12

## Sample Audio Item

Place your headset on now.

Click the Play button ▶ to listen to the audio clip.

Based on the audio clip, which lung sound is the nurse hearing upon auscultation?

1. Crackles
2. Wheezes
3. Pleural friction rub
4. Rhonchi

# BOX 2.13

## Sample Enhanced Hot Spot Item

The nurse is determining the tube length for the correct placement of the infant's NG tube for gavage feedings. Draw on the infant illustrated where the nurse should measure, from the starting point to the ending point, to determine the correct NG tube length for insertion.

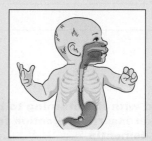

**ANSWER:**

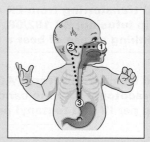

The correct tube length is determined by measuring from the tip of the nose, to the top of the earlobe, then to the midway point between the end of the xiphoid process and the umbilicus.

## BOX 2.14

### Sample Drag and Drop Item

The nurse is planning room assignments/reassignments for six clients. Some clients may require a private room based on the client's diagnosis or current status. Rooms may have one or two clients. Bed A is closest to the doorway. The lowest numbered room is nearest the nurse's station. Which room would result in a safe placement for each client? Select the client and place the client into the assigned room and bed.

| | | | |
|---|---|---|---|
| 55-year old transferring from PACU following right lateral thoracotomy for lung cancer; has type 1 DM. Insulin drip per IV and fentanyl per epidural infusing. | 72-year old transferring from ER and has a PE; heparin drip infusing; BP 182/98, HR 116; reports drinking a case a beer a week. | 275-A | 275-B |
| 65-year old with HF returning to the unit following a pacemaker insertion; ejection fraction 45%; has mid-stage dementia. | 62-year old with pancreatitis and elevated serum amylase levels. NPO; receiving hydro-morphone IV frequently for pain control. | 276-A | 276-B |
| 45-year old who had abdominal hysterectomy 8 hours ago; stable; lots of visitors. | 56-year old who has pancreatic cancer and neutropenia; hx atrial fibrillation that is rate-controlled. | 277-A | 277-B |
| | | 278- A | 278-B |
| | | 279-A | 279-B |

### ANSWER:

| | |
|---|---|
| **275-A**<br>**65-year old with HF returning to the unit following a pacemaker insertion; ejection fraction 45%; has mid-stage dementia.** | **275-B** |
| **276-A**<br>**72-year old transferring from ER and has a PE; heparin drip infusing; BP 182/98, HR 116; reports drinking a case of beer a week.** | **276-B** |
| **277-A**<br>**55-year old transferring from PACU following right lateral thoracotomy for lung cancer; has type 1 DM. Insulin drip per IV and fentanyl per epidural infusing.** | **277-B**<br>**62-year old with pancreatitis and elevated serum amylase levels. NPO; receiving hydromorphone IV frequently for pain control.** |
| **278-A** | **278-B**<br>**56-year old who has pancreatic cancer and neutropenia; hx atrial fibrillation that is rate controlled.** |
| **279-A** | **279-B**<br>**45-year old who had abdominal hysterectomy 8 hours ago; stable; lots of visitors.** |

## BOX 2.15

### CLOZE Item Drop-Down Menu

Based on the case study, which three medications should the nurse bring to the attention of the HCP?

The medication that the nurse should bring to the HCP's attention should be [ Select... ▼ ]

because [ Select... ▼ ]

The medication that the nurse should bring to the HCP's attention should be [ Select... ▼ ]

because [ Select... ▼ ]

The medication that the nurse should bring to the HCP's attention should be [ Select... ▼ ]

because [ Select... ▼ ]

example of a CLOZE item. For this book, instead of drop-down menus for selecting the words or statements, these are presented in two columns where you select the medication from one column and the rationale from another column.

**Dynamic exhibits and constructed response items** may include a scenario that provides information about the client over time points. A radio button is selected to view the information for one time point, for example, 0900. Each radio button must be selected to open information for that time point. After reading the information, there will be a question pertaining to the time points and the information. Additional questions are asked that require typing in a response in the blank box provided. Box 2.16 shows an

example of this item type, with only one time point illustrated. Items 235 and 236 in Chapter 7 provide examples of how the dynamic exhibit and constructed response items appear in this book.

**Rich media scenario** includes a case scenario presented as a video. The video presents a time point, stops, and then a question is asked about information during that time point. The scenario then resumes at a later time point and additional questions are asked. A number of time points may be included in the scenario and the questions related to the scenario. Various scenarios are presented as a case study in this book. Items 1009, 1010, and 1011 in Chapter 23 show a case study and questions related to that case study.

## BOX 2.16

### Sample Dynamic Exhibit and Constructed Response Item

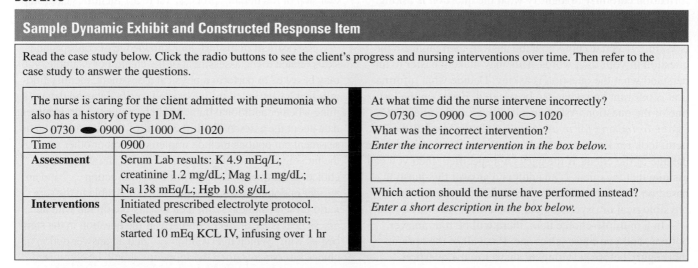

Read the case study below. Click the radio buttons to see the client's progress and nursing interventions over time. Then refer to the case study to answer the questions.

The nurse is caring for the client admitted with pneumonia who also has a history of type 1 DM.
○ 0730 ● 0900 ○ 1000 ○ 1020

| Time | 0900 |
|---|---|
| **Assessment** | Serum Lab results: K 4.9 mEq/L; creatinine 1.2 mg/dL; Mag 1.1 mg/dL; Na 138 mEq/L; Hgb 10.8 g/dL |
| **Interventions** | Initiated prescribed electrolyte protocol. Selected serum potassium replacement; started 10 mEq KCL IV, infusing over 1 hr |

At what time did the nurse intervene incorrectly?
○ 0730 ○ 0900 ○ 1000 ○ 1020
What was the incorrect intervention?
*Enter the incorrect intervention in the box below.*

[ ]

Which action should the nurse have performed instead?
*Enter a short description in the box below.*

[ ]

2 NCLEX-RN® Items

## Chapter Three

# Test-Taking Tips and Strategies

Taking the NCLEX-RN® exam can be a stressful experience. Thus this chapter is designed to help you find ways to read NCLEX-type questions and answer them correctly. Understanding how to take a test using strategies to answer test items is just as important as knowing the content. Some test-taking tips are presented in this chapter to help you improve your testing abilities and to pass the NCLEX-RN® exam. Use these strategies and tips to identify the best option to answer a question or complete an item.

## CAREFULLY READ THE NCLEX-RN® ITEMS AND FOCUS ON THE SUBJECT

NCLEX-RN® exam questions may contain more information than what is specifically needed to answer the question. Most items consist of a clinical situation, the question, and then the options. Therefore make sure to read all of the information carefully to identify what the question is asking.

As you read the question, try to answer it before looking at the options to see if you understand what the question is asking. If you do not know the answer, then rephrase the question in your own words. This may make it easier to understand what the question is asking. Decide what information is relevant and what can be omitted. Focus on the last line of the question. Ask yourself, *"What is the question asking or looking for in an answer?"* In the stem of the item, look for **key words** such as *priority, first,* or *best.* Note the age of the client. If the age is not specified, then you can assume that the client is an adult and answer the question based on principles of adult growth and development or physiological or psychological problems related to adults.

In a multiple-choice item, there will be four answer options, and you must select one. Read all of the options thoroughly before selecting an answer to the question. A multiple-response question has many options, and you must **select all that apply.** In an ordered-response type item, you must list options in order, usually from the highest priority to the lowest priority. These ordered-response items can be diverse and include options such as priority of assessments, interventions, nursing skills, or pathophysiological concepts.

## THE NURSING PROCESS

After carefully reading the question and options, consider whether the nursing process is applied in the question versus the other integrated processes of caring, teaching/learning, communication and documentation, or culture and spirituality. If the nursing process is being applied, decide which step in the process is the focus of the question. The five steps of the nursing process include (1) assessment, (2) analysis, (3) planning, (4) implementation, and (5) evaluation. A complete description of each step in the process is included in Chapter 1, The NCLEX-RN® Licensure Examination.

Because the nursing process incorporates critical thinking, the licensure exam is designed to test your use of this process within the registered nurse role and scope of practice. When a step of the nursing process is applied in a question, examine each option to be sure that the option corresponds to that step of the nursing process. Table 3.1 identifies each step of the nursing process and key words used in test items for the specified step.

**Assessment** items test your knowledge of concepts and skills related to the assessment of the client. For example, you may be asked to perform a physical assessment, identify findings that are expected or unexpected, verify data and determine whether additional data should be collected, or document data about the assessment. If the focus of the question is on assessment but options include implementation or other steps of the nursing process, eliminate those options as an answer choice. If the question begins with "Which action …" and an answer option includes an assessment applicable to the scenario presented in the stem, then usually the option with an assessment is the answer. Similarly, if the question in the stem begins with "Which intervention …" and an answer option includes assessments, then these options should be eliminated.

The nursing process can also be used to prioritize actions. Assessment is the first action and thus is the priority in most situations. In a life-threatening situation, if an initial observation suggests that an immediate intervention is needed, only then is an intervention the priority. Box 3.1 provides a sample assessment question and a test-taking tip to answer the question.

## TABLE 3.1

### Steps of the Nursing Process and Key Words in Test Items

| Nursing Process | Key Words | Key Words | Key Words | Key Words |
|---|---|---|---|---|
| **Assessment** | ascertain<br>assess<br>check<br>collect<br>determine | find<br>gather<br>identify<br>inspect<br>monitor | observe<br>obtain information<br>manifestation<br>perceptions<br>question | signs<br>symptoms<br>sources<br>verify |
| **Analysis** | analyze<br>categorize<br>cluster<br>contribute | deduce<br>diagnose<br>formulate<br>interpret | problem<br>reflect<br>relate<br>relevant | reexamine<br>significant<br>statement<br>validate |
| **Planning** | achieve<br>anticipate<br>arrange<br>collaborate<br>consult | coordinate<br>design<br>desired<br>determine<br>develop | establish<br>expect<br>formulate<br>goal/outcome<br>modify | plan<br>prevent<br>priority<br>select<br>strategy |
| **Implementation** | action<br>apply<br>assist<br>change<br>counsel<br>demonstrate | delegate<br>facilitate<br>give<br>implement<br>inform<br>instruct | method<br>motivate<br>operate<br>perform<br>procedure<br>provide | refer<br>strategize<br>supervise<br>teach<br>technique<br>treatment |
| **Evaluation** | achieved<br>compared<br>defend<br>desired | effective<br>eliminate<br>evaluate<br>expected | failed<br>improve<br>ineffective<br>met | modify<br>reassess<br>review<br>succeeded |

## BOX 3.1

### Sample Nursing Process Assessment Item

`MoC` The nurse is caring for the hospitalized 10-year-old who has chest contusions from an MVA. The pulse oximeter monitor is alarming and is showing an oxygen saturation of 84%. Which action should be taken by the nurse **first?**
1. Check to see if arterial blood gases are being prescribed.
2. Assess the client's level of consciousness and skin color.
3. Replace the machine and probe to obtain a new reading.
4. Administer oxygen through a nasal cannula or by mask.

**ANSWER: 2**

♦ *Test-taking Tip: Use the nursing process. Assessment is the first step in the nursing process. This situation requires additional information before an intervention can be determined; assessment should be the first action in this item. The nurse should be focusing on the client and not the machine. Options pertaining to interventions should be eliminated.*

**Analysis** items involve interpreting information that has been collected to identify actual or potential client health care needs and/or problems. You will need to be able to validate and cluster data to determine their significance and to establish a nursing diagnosis. When analyzing the data, you may determine that additional data need to be collected. When clustering data, you will need a strong foundation in pathophysiology, pharmacology, nursing theory, social sciences, and others to be able to identify commonalities and differences, and how information is related. Box 3.2 provides a sample analysis question and a test-taking tip to answer the question.

**Planning** items involve establishing goals, formulating expected outcomes, setting priorities, anticipating client needs, identifying strategies to meet client needs, developing and modifying the plan of care, communicating the plan of care to others, and collaborating with other health team members. Some planning items may be obvious with the word "plan" or "plan of care" in the stem of the question. However, some items will imply planning in the content of the options rather than the stem of the question. These types of planning questions are more difficult to identify. Box 3.3 provides a sample planning question and a test-taking tip to answer the question.

## BOX 3.2

### Sample Nursing Process Analysis Item

The client is admitted with a tentative diagnosis of acute hepatitis C. The nurse determines that which client statement would be **most** consistent with the diagnosis?
1. "I'm not sleeping well; I have heartburn that wakes me up at night."
2. "Whenever I eat dairy products, I have diarrhea that lasts for hours."
3. "I have dizziness and ringing in my ears when I get up too suddenly."
4. "I've smoked cigarettes for years, but lately I can't tolerate their taste."

### ANSWER: 4

▶ *Test-taking Tip: Analysis questions require understanding of the physiological processes and interpretation of information. In this question, thinking about the signs and symptoms associated with hepatitis is necessary to analyze the client's statements and eliminate options that are inconsistent with the diagnosis. The process of elimination can also be used to eliminate option 3 because it is a sign of activity intolerance often associated with cardiopulmonary problems or with complications associated with hepatitis.*

**Implementation** items will require you to initiate or complete nursing activities safely to accomplish the goals of care. These items can include supervising, organizing, and managing client care; providing client care; counseling, teaching, and motivating clients; and communicating, reporting, and documenting information related to the care provided. Interventions frequently tested include the nurse responding to a life-threatening event, such as initiating cardiopulmonary resuscitation or stopping the administration of blood or an antibiotic in response to the client's allergic

## BOX 3.3

### Sample Nursing Process Planning Item

The client is hospitalized with VRE in a leg wound that is draining but covered by dressings. What is the nurse's **best** plan of action?
1. Assign the client to a private room.
2. Assign only one caregiver to the client.
3. Do not allow pregnant staff to enter the room.
4. Place the client in a room with negative airflow.

### ANSWER: 1

▶ *Test-taking Tip: This question is a nursing process planning item that includes planning care for the client. First determine which options are appropriate and should be included in the nurse's plan for the client. The key words are "best plan of action." Recall that VRE can be transmitted to others but is not airborne. Eliminate option 4. Of the remaining options, determine which is best.*

reaction. The use of critical thinking and clinical judgment is required when responding to these types of events. Box 3.4 provides a sample implementation question and a test-taking tip to answer the question.

**Evaluation** items require a comparison of the actual client outcomes/goals with expected outcomes/goals of care to determine whether these have been achieved. Evaluation items can include any of the steps in the process of evaluation, such as identifying client responses to care, comparing the actual and expected outcomes to determine achievement, analyzing factors that affect the outcomes to draw conclusions about the success or failure of nursing interventions, and determining whether the plan of care should be modified and how. Box 3.5 provides a sample evaluation question and a test-taking tip to answer the question.

## THE ABC'S

The ABC's—*airway, breathing,* and *circulation*—can be very helpful in answering NCLEX-RN® questions. They can be used when determining the order of priority. Priority-type questions can be identified with words such as *first, priority, initial, main concern, most important,* and *primary.* When choosing the correct answer option, if an option pertains to the client's airway and is pertinent to the situation, then this option should be the nurse's first priority. If no option pertains to airway or breathing, then look for an option that pertains to circulation. Remember circulation can include items such as hemorrhage, cardiac output, and BP. You need to be careful with these items. An option may pertain to airway; however, the option that addresses airway may not be appropriate for the situation presented in the stem of the question. You should also evaluate the severity of the condition; a new unstable dysrhythmia or hypotension (circulation) has

## BOX 3.4

### Sample Nursing Process Implementation Item

The nurse checks the blood glucose level of the 6-hour-old full-term infant whose mother has insulin-dependent DM. Which **most** important intervention should the nurse implement when obtaining a reading of 36 mg/dL?
1. Record the result in the newborn's medical record.
2. Bring the infant to the mother to be given a feeding.
3. Report the result to the infant's HCP.
4. Observe the infant closely and repeat the test in 1 hour.

### ANSWER: 2

▶ *Test-taking Tip: This question is a nursing process implementation item that tests your ability to respond to an event. To answer the question, you need to know that the normal glucose level for a newborn is 40 mg/dL. The newborn needs glucose; initiating a feeding should raise the infant's glucose level. If this is unsuccessful, the nurse would notify the HCP so that an IV infusion of glucose could be initiated. The nurse should document the findings, but this is not the most important action.*

# BOX 3.5

## Sample Nursing Process Evaluation Item

The nurse is evaluating teaching for the client who has DM and is beginning insulin therapy using an insulin pen. Which behavior should **best** inform the nurse that teaching about insulin administration was effective?

1. The nurse showing the client a video that explains how to use the insulin pen
2. The nurse demonstrating the correct procedure for preparing the insulin pen
3. The client describing the different types of insulins and how to use an insulin pen
4. The client preparing the insulin pen and self-injecting correctly on the first attempt

**ANSWER: 4**

▶ *Test-taking Tip: Focus on what the question is asking, "teaching ... was effective" and the nursing process step of evaluation. Options that include nursing interventions should be eliminated. "Best" indicates that more than one option may be correct but that one option is better than the others.*

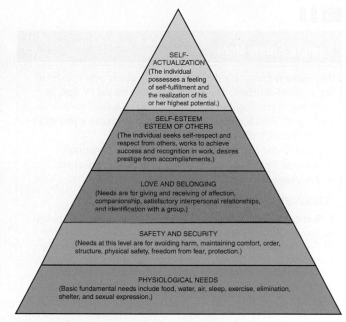

**Figure 3.1:** Applying Maslow's Hierarchy of Needs to establish priorities.

priority over a chronic condition such as a history of asthma (airway). Also, a systemic problem such as sepsis has priority over a local condition. Box 3.6 provides an example of using the ABC's.

# MASLOW'S HIERARCHY OF NEEDS

Maslow's Hierarchy of Needs theory states that physiological needs are the most basic human needs (Figure 3.1); use this theory as another guide to prioritize the options and assist in selecting the correct option. Physiological needs are the priority; therefore physiological needs should be met before psychosocial needs. When a physiological need is not presented in the question or included as one of the answer options, continue using Maslow's Hierarchy of Needs theory

and look for the answer option that addresses safety. Continue to move up the hierarchy ladder to identify the priority if needs at the lower levels are not addressed within the question or options. Remember that a current problem has priority over a potential future problem. Box 3.7 provides an example of applying Maslow's Hierarchy of Needs in a practice item.

# SAFETY

Safety is a high priority in NCLEX-RN® questions. Carefully read each question and answer options. If an item describes a situation that has both a life-threatening safety problem and a non–life-threatening physiological problem, then safety will be the answer rather than the physiological problem. Box 3.8 provides an example of applying the principles of safety to practice items.

# BOX 3.6

## Sample Item Using the ABC's

The 5-year-old is brought to the ED experiencing dyspnea and swelling of the lips and tongue. Audible wheezes, rhinitis, and stridor are also present, and the child is very anxious. What should the nurse do **first?**

1. Administer oxygen therapy.
2. Check the child's vital signs.
3. Give epinephrine as prescribed.
4. Insert an intravenous access device.

**ANSWER: 1**

▶ *Test-taking Tip: Use the ABC's to identify the initial action. Airway is the priority in this situation. In a life-threatening situation, further assessment is not the priority when an observation provides sufficient information to act.*

# BOX 3.7

## Sample Item Using Maslow's Hierarchy of Needs

The nurse is caring for the client who is experiencing diaphoresis during the transition stage of labor. Which is the **most** important nursing intervention?

1. Maintaining adequate hydration
2. Performing frequent linen changes
3. Reassuring the mother and wiping her brow
4. Providing cooling measures, such as fanning

**ANSWER: 1**

▶ *Test-taking Tip: Use the nursing process and Maslow's Hierarchy of Needs theory. Physiological needs are addressed before psychosocial needs.*

## BOX 3.8

### Sample Safety Item

The nurse is caring for the postoperative client who is exhibiting signs of delirium. The client is pulling on the IV line, attempting to climb out of bed, and is talking about "the bugs in this hotel." Which intervention should be the nurse's **priority?**
1. Ask the HCP about prescribing haloperidol.
2. Transfer the client to a room near the nurse's station.
3. Arrange for the nursing assistant to stay with the client.
4. Telephone the client's family to come and sit with the client.

### ANSWER: 3

♦ *Test-taking Tip: Use Maslow's Hierarchy of Needs theory to determine the priority action. Client safety has priority. Determine which option provides for the most thorough, reasonable, and speedy means of addressing the client's safety needs. Safety should be addressed first before addressing the client's physiological problem of delirium.*

multiple-choice–type items, and incorrect options can be eliminated so that just one answer option remains. The nurse should use communication techniques that focus on the client's concerns and facilitate therapeutic communication. Therefore eliminate options that are obviously not therapeutic or those that use barriers to therapeutic communication.

Therapeutic communication includes using techniques such as silence, broad opening statements, focusing, restating, clarifying, validating messages, interpreting body language, sharing observations, exploring issues, and reflecting. Barriers to therapeutic communication include responses such as changing the subject, inattentive listening, giving false reassurance, and giving advice. Tables 3.2 and 3.3 provide a description of common therapeutic communication techniques and barriers to therapeutic communication that you may encounter in practice test items or on the NCLEX-RN® exam. Box 3.9 provides an example of applying therapeutic communication in a practice item.

## THERAPEUTIC COMMUNICATION

Some questions relate to therapeutic communication and the nurse's ability to communicate with the client. Therapeutic communication includes both verbal and nonverbal communication. Normally, communication questions are

## KEY WORDS

Pay attention to key words. There will be questions for which there is more than one correct option; however, based on key words, only one option answers the question correctly. Questions may contain key words such as *most appropriate, best,*

## TABLE 3.2

| Therapeutic Communication Techniques | |
|---|---|
| Acknowledging | Indicating an awareness of a change in the client's behavior |
| Focusing | Collecting additional information, after the client finishes speaking, to help gain further knowledge on a topic that the client addressed |
| Giving information | Providing accurate information that the client did or did not request |
| Offering general leads | Using statements or questions that encourage verbalization, allowing the client to choose the topic of conversation, and facilitating further communication |
| Offering self | Simply being present or asking if the client needs anything without expecting the client to give the nurse anything |
| Reflecting | Directing the topic to an idea or feeling that the client stated, which allows for further exploration of that feeling or idea |
| Seeking clarification | Either stating that what the client said was misunderstood or asking the client to repeat the conversation or basic idea of the message |
| Sharing observations | Verbalizing what is observed or perceived, which allows client recognition of specific behaviors to compare perceptions with the nurse |
| Summarizing and planning | Restating the main ideas of a conversation to clarify the important points; often stated at the end of an interview |
| Using silence | Allowing pauses or silences without interjecting a verbal response and allowing the client an opportunity to collect and organize thoughts |

Adapted from Berman, A., Snyder, S., Kozier, B., & Erb, G. (2008). *Kozier & Erb's fundamentals of nursing: concepts, process, and practice* (8th ed., pp. 469–471). Upper Saddle River, NJ: Pearson Education.

**3 Test-Taking Tips and Strategies**

**TABLE 3.3**

| Barriers to Therapeutic Communication | |
|---|---|
| Asking "why" | Asking why suggests criticism to some and may result in a defensive response from the client. |
| Belittling the feelings | Conveying a lack of empathy and understanding may result in the client's perception that the feelings he expressed are insignificant or unimportant. |
| Changing the subject | Directing the topic into areas of self-interest. This usually indicates that the nurse is unable to handle the topic that is being discussed and avoids listening to what the client is saying and feeling. |
| Giving nonexpert advice | Telling the client what should be done or how to think. Giving advice focuses on the nurse's advice, opinions, and ideas and not on the client's views. This may negate the client's opportunity to participate as a mutual partner in decision-making. |
| Providing false reassurance | Using clichés or making encouraging statements when the situation's outcome is not positive or reassurance is not based on fact. These statements ignore the fears, feelings, and other responses of the client. |
| Interpreting | Telling the client the meaning of his or her experience. |
| Passing judgment | Giving opinions or approving or disapproving the client's values. This may result in the client feeling that he or she must think as the nurse thinks and not have his or her own ideas and opinions. |
| Probing | Asking unnecessary questions; these questions violate the client's rights. |
| Rejecting | Refusing to discuss certain concerns or topics. This may lead the client to believe that the nurse is rejecting not only the client's concerns but also the client himself. |
| Stereotyping | Generalizing about groups of people based on the nurse's previous experiences; categorizes the client and does not look at each client as an individual. |

Adapted from Berman, A., Snyder, S., Kozier, B., & Erb, G. (2008). *Kozier & Erb's fundamentals of nursing: concepts, process, and practice* (8th ed., pp. 469–471). Upper Saddle River, NJ: Pearson Education.

**BOX 3.9**

**Sample Therapeutic Communication Item**

MoC  The observing nurse overhears a conversation between the new nurse and the client. Which statement by the new nurse **best** encourages therapeutic communication?

Client: "I just was told that I might have cancer. I'm having surgery tomorrow morning, and I'm afraid. My mother had cancer and died when I was 7 years old."

1. Nurse: "I see. Why are you afraid? Do you think surgery will reveal that you have cancer?"
2. Nurse: "Are you afraid that it might be cancer?"
3. Nurse: "Having a possible diagnosis of cancer is frightening. Tell me more about how you are feeling about this."
4. Nurse: "This really hits close to you. I'm sorry to hear that your mother died when you were so young."

**ANSWER: 3**

▸ *Test-taking Tip: Read through the written conversation carefully. Choose the option that uses more than one therapeutic communication technique and encourages further communication.*

*first, last, next, most helpful, defer, and ineffective.* These key words bring your attention to a specific point that you need to consider when answering the question. The key words can indicate a priority or negative polarity. Tables 3.4 and 3.5 provide examples of key words.

For priority items, all or most of the options are correct, but you must determine the best option that fits with the key word or phrase to correctly answer the question. Looking for a key word in each of the options that may be a synonym or a related word for a key word in the question is also a technique for selecting the correct option. The previously discussed strategies (ABC's, Maslow's Hierarchy of Needs theory, Nursing Process, and Safety) can be used to determine the best option for items that set a priority with a key word.

Negative polarity items, sometimes called false-response items, are those in which you would select the option that is incorrect. The stem of the item is negatively worded and asks you to identify an exception, detect an error, or identify unacceptable or unsafe nursing actions or actions that are contraindicated by the nurse or client. Negative polarity items may or may not appear on your NCLEX-RN® exam. Although you may have answered exam items that included the words "all except," this type of question does not appear on the NCLEX-RN® exam.

## ELIMINATE ABSOLUTE WORD OPTIONS

Absolute words used in options tend to make those options incorrect. Some absolute words include *must, always, never, all, none, every,* and *only.* Eliminating options containing absolute words can make it easier to answer the question.

## SIMILAR OPTIONS

At times, two or more options may appear to be similar. When you are answering questions, look for these similar options because they can usually be eliminated in multiple-choice items.

### TABLE 3.4

| Key Words That Set a Priority | | |
| --- | --- | --- |
| Best | Last | Most likely |
| Early | Least appropriate | Most suitable |
| Essential | Least helpful | Next |
| First | Least likely | Priority |
| Highest priority | Most appropriate | Primary |
| Immediate | Most important | Safest |
| Initial | Most helpful | Vital |

### TABLE 3.5

| Key Words Indicating Positive and Negative Polarity | |
| --- | --- |
| **Positive Polarity** | **Negative Polarity** |
| Acceptable | Avoid |
| Correct | Contraindicated |
| Effective | Incorrect |
| Indicate | Ineffective |
| Most appropriate | Least appropriate, helpful, or likely |
| Most helpful | Unacceptable |
| Most likely | Unlikely |
| Most suitable | Unrelated |
| Safest | Unsafe |
| | Violate |

For multiple-choice items, there is only *one* correct option, and *usually* the correct option is different from those that are similar. Be careful as you read the stem of the question, however, because the option that may be different may not fit with the question or situation presented. Box 3.10 provides an example of a practice item containing similar options.

In multiple-response items, you should look for similar options that can include similar assessment findings, actions, or concepts. Similar options are most likely the correct options when answering multiple-response type items.

## OPTIONS THAT ARE OPPOSITES

In both multiple-choice and multiple-response items, look for options that are opposites, such as tachycardia and bradycardia. Either one or both of these options may be incorrect. Focus on eliminating one or both of these options before focusing on the other options. Box 3.11 provides an example of a practice item with options that are opposites.

### BOX 3.10

| Sample Similar Options Item |
| --- |

The parents leave the child's hospital room after visiting their 2-year-old. Which finding by the nurse poses the **most** immediate and serious safety threat to the child?
1. Coloring book and crayons left in the crib
2. A doll with movable eyes left in the crib
3. A mobile hanging from the top of the crib
4. The crib rail that was left halfway down

**ANSWER: 4**

▶ *Test-taking Tip: Note the similarities in the risk posed in options 1 and 2, that option 3 may or may not pose a risk, and that option 4 presents a different risk. In a multiple-choice–type question, often the option that is different is the answer.*

### BOX 3.11

| Sample Opposite Options Item |
| --- |

**PHARM** Two hours after initiating TPN, the nurse assesses that the client now has diuresis and a decreased BP. What should the nurse consider when analyzing these findings?
1. The glucose content of the TPN solution is too high.
2. The TPN solution is infusing too slowly.
3. The TPN solution is infusing too rapidly.
4. The protein content of the TPN solution is too low.

**ANSWER: 3**

▶ *Test-taking Tip: You should note that options 2 and 3 are opposites. Examine these options first to determine if one or both can be eliminated. Focus on the time frames of 2 hours and the information that this is the initial infusion of the TPN. Think about the nutrient content of TPN solution and which of those nutrients is metabolized quickly.*

## BOX 3.12

### Sample Global Option Item

The nurse is teaching child-care providers about infectious disease transmission among young children. The nurse should teach about which most common sources for disease transmission?
1. Fecal, oral, and respiratory routes
2. Sharing toys, coughing, and soiled diapers
3. Urinary, oral, and respiratory secretion contact
4. Sneezing, rubbing a runny nose, and then touching others

**ANSWER: 1**

▶ *Test-taking Tip: Note the plural "sources" of infectious disease in the stem and select the option that is most inclusive. Option 1 is the broadest option addressing the various "routes of transmission." The longest option may not be the most global option.*

## GLOBAL OPTIONS

A global or umbrella option is one that will be more comprehensive than the other options and frequently includes information or concepts from one or more of the other options. The three distracter options are usually more specific than the global option. Therefore the global option will be the correct option. Box 3.12 provides an example of a practice item with a global option.

## DUPLICATE INFORMATION AMONG OPTION ITEMS

Some test items are designed so that more than one point or fact is included within each option. For these types of questions, first look for the options with duplicate information and determine if that information is correct or incorrect. If it is incorrect, then you can eliminate all items with the duplicate information. Box 3.13 provides an example of a practice item with duplicate information among answer options.

## BOX 3.13

### Sample Duplicate Information Item

The client is newly admitted with a diagnosis of left-sided HF. Which assessment findings should the nurse expect?
1. Chest tightness and ascites
2. Dyspnea on exertion and ascites
3. Dyspnea on exertion and crackles
4. Neck vein distention and crackles

**ANSWER: 3**

▶ *Test-taking Tip: This item is testing your knowledge of the difference between right and left HF. Duplicate information is presented in the options. If you know one of the findings, such as dyspnea on exertion, you then can eliminate the other options (1 and 4). Now, just examine options 2 and 3. Note that option 3 pertains to just the lungs, whereas option 2 pertains to two different body areas.*

## DELEGATION, ASSIGNMENT, AND MANAGEMENT OF CARE ITEMS

Most likely, there will be questions that ask you to delegate or assign certain clients or tasks to other health care personnel. Read the question thoroughly so that you understand the task or to whom the task is being delegated or assigned. Carefully look at what is being asked and match the skill with the scope of practice of the appropriate caregiver. Use the five rights of delegation: the right task, under the right circumstances, to the right person, with the right direction and communication, and the right supervision and evaluation. Remember that RNs are responsible for assessing, evaluating, teaching, and making decisions about client care and that these tasks cannot be delegated. Note that observations, but not assessments, can be delegated. Because the scope of practice varies by state or regulatory body, you should encounter only the universal tasks that can be delegated. Table 3.6 illustrates examples of tasks that may and may not be delegated to UAPs.

When answering items that pertain to delegation, assignment, and management of care, consider the following: 1) If informed by a caregiver about a concerning situation with the client, the nurse should check the client; 2) If incorrect care is provided that affects the client, such as giving water to the client who is NPO, the nurse would correct the situation immediately and not wait until later; 3) Do not discipline another person in front of others; and 4) If staff is unfamiliar with a procedure, the nurse would accompany the person to teach that person but would not perform the procedure independently or just instruct the person to check the policy and procedure.

When answering items that pertain to making assignments, a new RN graduate would be assigned clients who are stable and do not require specialized care. If a staff member might be impaired (e.g., alcohol on breath), do not let that person care for the client, and report the situation immediately to the charge nurse, nurse manager, or supervisor. Do not assign a staff member who is pregnant to the client who is receiving radiation or has CMV or a communicable disease that could affect the unborn child. Additionally, ensure that only healthy staff are assigned to immunosuppressed clients.

When caring for multiple clients and establishing priorities, determine which client has the greatest risk. In addition to considering alterations in the ABC's, think about the client's comorbidities that may affect the client's main problem, consider whether the client is on immunosuppression, and look at trends in client data and determine any high-risk interventions. These are priority concerns, and clients take priority over paperwork.

NCLEX-RN® questions may also ask you to decide when to notify the health care provider (HCP). On the NCLEX-RN® exam, the option of notifying the HCP may or may not be the correct option. NCLEX-RN® is testing the RN's ability to work safely. Sometimes choosing the option of notifying the HCP or other health care personnel, such as the charge nurse, is relegating your responsibility to someone else when further assessment or an immediate intervention is needed. If you are unable to determine if you must notify the HCP or if another

**TABLE 3.6**

| Tasks That May and May Not Be Delegated to Unlicensed Assistive Personnel (UAP) | |
|---|---|
| **Tasks That *May* Be Delegated to UAP** | **Tasks That *May Not* Be Delegated to UAP** |
| Adding intake and output volumes | Administering enteral feedings through an NG or PEG tube |
| Alerting others if assistance is needed | Administering blood transfusions |
| Ambulating and transferring clients | Administering parenteral medications |
| Clearing the volume on feeding pumps and recording this amount | Assessing clients |
| Delivering meals, snacks, fresh water | Caring for invasive lines |
| Delivering specimens to the laboratory | Clearing the volume of IV infusion pumps with medicated infusions |
| Feeding clients | Creating a nursing care plan |
| Gathering client belongings in preparation for discharge | Documenting client assessments or medication administration |
| Hygiene and linen change | Double-checking medication dosages |
| Obtaining supplies for procedures | Evaluating care effectiveness |
| Maintaining safety; 1:1 monitoring | Educating clients |
| Measuring and recording intake and output (I&O) | Giving telephone advice |
| Performing basic life support (CPR) | Inserting intravenous lines |
| Performing simple dressing changes | Inserting nasogastric or orogastric tubes |
| Postmortem care | Interpreting information and data |
| Preparing the room for an admission | Interpreting the client's cardiac rhythm (ECG) |
| Restocking items for providing care | Making a nursing diagnosis |
| Taking glucometer readings | Performing triage |
| Taking vital signs | Planning client room assignments |
| Toileting clients | Removing tubes or drains |
| Transporting clients | Setting up chest tube suction or patient-controlled or epidural analgesia equipment |
| Weighing clients | Taking prescribed treatment, medication, or other orders from an HCP |

action is indicated, make sure that client safety has been addressed first and that all information necessary to notify the HCP has been obtained. Remember, a person's safety has priority, especially if an unsafe situation can be life-threatening. Box 3.14 provides an example of a delegation practice item.

## PAY ATTENTION TO LABORATORY VALUES

Laboratory (lab) values are included in the NCLEX-RN® exam. The NCLEX-RN® Detailed Test Plan (2019) identifies essential lab values that you need to know. These include arterial blood gases (ABGs [pH, $Po_2$, $Pco_2$, $Sao_2$, $HCO_3$]), serum creatinine (SCr) and blood urea nitrogen (BUN), serum total cholesterol, glucose, hematocrit (Hct), hemoglobin (Hgb), glycosylated hemoglobin (Hgb $A_{1c}$), platelets (Plt), potassium (K), red blood cells (RBCs), sodium (Na), white blood cells (WBCs), and coagulation values. Table 3.7 provides normal adult lab value ranges for the essential lab values on the NCLEX-RN® exam. You

## BOX 3.14

### Sample Delegation Item

**MoC** The nurse, the LPN, and the UAP are caring for a group of clients. Which action indicates appropriate delegation?
1. Directs the LPN to give the client who has incisional pain the first dose of IV analgesic
2. Directs the LPN to assess the client who has itching after receiving an new antibiotic
3. Directs the UAP to assist the client being prepared for surgery onto the surgical cart
4. Directs the UAP to teach the client's family about hand washing before entering the room

**ANSWER: 3**

▸ *Test-taking Tip:* You need to use the scope of practice and the five rights of delegation for appropriate delegation.

---

will find that lab value ranges vary slightly from source to source. However, lab values included on the NCLEX-RN® exam and in the practice items will be either within the typical normal ranges or significantly abnormal.

Besides knowing certain lab values, you should be able to recognize deviations from the normal. Table 3.8 provides normal ranges for the lab values identified in the NCLEX-RN® test plan that you should be able to recognize when taking the NCLEX-RN® exam. Knowing the normal ranges and significance before you start the test will increase your ability to pass the licensure exam. Also, being able to correlate certain lab values with various illnesses will help you answer the more complex questions.

Throughout this book, practice items are presented that will give you an opportunity to improve your skills at analyzing lab values. Box 3.15 provides an example of a practice item with both essential lab values and those you need to recognize for deviations from normal.

## USE MNEMONICS TO REMEMBER KEY INFORMATION

Mnemonics are techniques that help us to remember information. For example, the classic triad for preeclampsia can be remembered by the **pre** in preeclampsia, which refers to **p**roteinuria, **r**ising BP, and **e**dema. To remember the number of vertebrae, just remember the times people typically eat meals: breakfast is at **7** a.m., and there are **7** cervical vertebrae; lunch is at **12** p.m., and there are **12** thoracic vertebrae; and dinner is at **5** p.m., and there are **5** lumbar vertebrae.

An acrostic, a type of mnemonic, uses a phrase, motto, or verse in which a letter (usually the first letter) prompts your memory to retrieve information. An example of an acrostic presented in the test-taking tips is the phrase "**a**ll **p**oints **e**ssential **t**o **m**emorize" to remember the names of the heart valves and auscultation points of the heart: **a**ortic, **p**ulmonic, **E**rb's point, **t**ricuspid, and **m**itral.

## TABLE 3.7

### Laboratory Normal Values for Adults to Know for the NCLEX-RN® Examination

**Laboratory Values and Normal Ranges**
**Arterial Blood Gases (ABGs)**
Arterial pH (7.35–7.45)
$Pco_2$ (32–42 mm Hg)
$HCO_3$ (Bicarb 22–26 mEq/L)
$Pao_2$ (80–100 mm Hg)
$Sao_2$ (95–100 mm Hg)
Base Excess [(–2) – +3] mEq/L]
**Serum Tests of Renal Function**
BUN (10–20 mg/dL)
SCr (0.5–1.5 mg/dL)
**Serum Chemistry**
Glucose, Fasting (70–99 mg/dL)
Hgb $A_{1c}$ (4%–6%)
Sodium (Na: 135–145 mEq/L)
Potassium (K: 3.5–5.0 mEq/L)
**Lipid Profile**
Total Cholesterol (140–200 mg/dL)
**Complete Blood Count (CBC)**
WBC (4–11 K/mm³ or 4–11 × 10³/microL)
RBC (4.5–5.5 mil/mm³ or 4.5–5.5 × 10⁶/microL)
  Male (4.5–6.2 mil/mm³ or 4.5–6.2 × 10⁶/microL)
  Female (4.2–5.4 mil/mm³ or 4.2–5.4 × 10⁶/microL)
Hgb (13.1–17.1 g/dL)
  Male (13.5–18 g/dL)
  Female (12–16 g/dL)
Hct (40%–45%)
  Male (40%–54%)
  Female (38%–47%)
Platelet (Plt: 150–400 K/microL or 150,000–400,000/mm³)
**Coagulation Tests**
Bleeding time (2–7 minutes)
Prothrombin time (PT: 10–14 sec)
International normalized ratio (INR: 0.9–1.1 sec)
Activated partial thromboplastin time (aPTT: 24–36 sec)

Source: Van Leeuwen, A. M., & Bladh, M. L. (2017). *Davis's comprehensive handbook of laboratory and diagnostic tests with nursing implications* (8th ed.). Philadelphia: F. A. Davis.

---

Throughout this book, a variety of mnemonics, acronyms, and acrostics are presented in the test-taking tips to assist you in remembering key information. The practice question in Box 3.15 provides a memory aid to remember the essential lab tests for liver function.

## APPLY MEDICAL TERMINOLOGY

Medical terminology is another easy way to understand questions or answer options. By knowing the meaning of common suffixes and prefixes, it is easier to understand what is being addressed in a question or an option with terms that may be unfamiliar to you. Review common terminology before taking the NCLEX-RN® exam. Some common prefixes and suffixes

## TABLE 3.8

### Deviations From Normal Adult Laboratory Values to Recognize for the NCLEX-RN® Examination

**Laboratory Values and Normal Ranges**
**Other Serum Electrolytes**
Total calcium (9–11 mg/dL)
Magnesium (Mg: 1.5–2.5 mEq/L)
Phosphorus, inorganic (2.8–4.5 mg/dL)
Chloride (Cl: 95–105 mEq/L)
Carbon dioxide ($CO_2$: 20–30 mEq/L)
**Lipid Profile**
Total cholesterol (140–200 mg/dL)
High-density lipoprotein (HDL)
    Male (>45 mg/dL)
    Female (>55 mg/dL)
Low-density lipoprotein (LDL: <130 mg/dL)
Triglycerides (40–150 mg/dL)
**Liver Enzymes**
Albumin (3.5–5.0 g/dL)
Alanine aminotransferase (ALT/SGPT: 5–36 units/L)
Aspartate aminotransferase (AST/SGOT: 7–40 units/L)
Ammonia (30–70 mcg/dL)
Total bilirubin (0.2–1.3 mg/dL)
Alkaline phosphatase (30–120 U/L)
**Nutrition Panel**
Total protein (6–8 g/dL)
**Hematology: WBC Differential**
Neutrophils (43%–70%)
Lymphocytes (20%–40%)
Monocytes (4%–8%)
Eosinophils (EOS: 0–4%)
Basophils (0–2%)
**Hematology: Erythrocyte Sedimentation Rate**
(ESR: 15–30 mm/hr; age and gender dependent)
Male ≤50 yr (<15 mm/hr)
Male >50 yr (<20 mm/hr)
Female ≤50 yr (<20 mm/hr)
Female >50 yr (<30 mm/hr)
**Therapeutic Blood Levels**
Digoxin (0.8–2 ng/mL)
Lithium (0.6–1.2 mEq/L)
**Urine**
pH (4–8)
Albumin (negative)
White blood cells (WBCs: Negative)
**Urine Specific Gravity**
1.003–1.030

Adapted from Van Leeuwen, A. M., & Bladh, M. L. (2017). *Davis's comprehensive handbook of laboratory and diagnostic tests with nursing implications* (8th ed.). Philadelphia: F. A. Davis.

are included in Table 3.9. The test-taking tips within this book will also highlight some other common medical terminology prefixes and suffixes.

## PHARMACOLOGY QUESTIONS

Use medical terminology also to identify unfamiliar medications. Certain classifications of medications will have

## BOX 3.15

### Sample Lab Analysis Item

The nurse is preparing a preoperative client for surgery. Which serum lab values indicate that the client has normal liver function? **Select all that apply.**
1. Hemoglobin 14 g/dL
2. Total bilirubin 1.0 mg/dL
3. White blood cells (WBCs) 8 K/microL
4. Serum creatinine (SCr) 0.7 mg/dL
5. Alanine aminotransferase (ALT) 18 units/L
6. Aspartate aminotransferase (AST) 25 units/L

**ANSWER: 2, 5, 6**

▶ *Test-taking Tip: While all lab values are within the normal ranges, only three of the lab values presented are used to evaluate liver function. A memory cue to remember two of the liver function tests is to associate the liver function tests with AA. You may know the "AA" acronym as Alcoholics Anonymous, but in this situation, it is **A**LT and **A**ST. This tip can also be used to remember the other two lab values that begin with the letter A, albumin and ALP. The letter B follows in the alphabet and can be used to remember bilirubin.*

common suffixes for the generic names of the medications. For example, the generic names of the beta blocker medications end in "-lol." Table 3.10 includes common identifiers for pharmacology questions. Unfortunately, not all medications for treating a certain condition or within a medication classification have common suffixes. Therefore the table of medication suffixes is not inclusive of all medication

## TABLE 3.9

### Common Prefixes and Suffixes in Medical Terminology

| Prefix | Meaning | Suffix | Meaning |
|--------|---------|--------|---------|
| a(n)- | No, not, without | -algia | Pain |
| ab- | Away from | -ase | Enzyme |
| ante- | Before | -ation | Action or process |
| brady- | Slow | -cele | Hernia |
| de- | Down, remove | -cyte | Cell |
| endo- | Inside | -eal | Pertaining to |
| intra- | Within | -ectomy | Excision |
| mal- | Bad | -emia | Blood |
| post- | After, behind | -ia, -iasis | Condition |
| pre- | Before | -itis | Inflammation of |
| tachy- | Fast | -oma | Tumor |

**TABLE 3.10**

## Common Suffixes Pertaining to Pharmacology Questions

| Suffix | Medication Classification | Suffix | Medication Classification |
|---|---|---|---|
| -amide | Sulfonylureas antidiabetics | -lol | Beta-adrenergic antagonists (beta blockers) |
| -ase | Thrombolytic agents | -mycin | Aminoglycoside or macrolide antibiotics |
| -vir | Antivirals | -navir | Protease inhibitors (treatment of HIV and AIDS) |
| -azine | Typical antipsychotics | -pam; -lam | Benzodiazepines; antianxiety; sedative |
| -azole | Antifungal; antiprotozoans or antihelminthics (parasitic infections) | -parin | Anticoagulant |
| -bital | Barbiturates | -pramine or -triptyline | Tricyclic antidepressants |
| -caine | Local anesthetic agents | -pril | Angiotensin-converting enzyme inhibitors (ACE inhibitors) |
| -choline | Cholinergic agonists (direct acting muscarinic agonists) | -profen | Nonsteroidal anti-inflammatory drugs (NSAIDs): Prostaglandin synthetase inhibitors |
| -cillin | Penicillin antibiotics | -sartan | Angiotensin II receptor blockers (ARBs) |
| -curium; -curonium | Neuromuscular blocking agents | -setron | Antiemetics |
| -cycline | Tetracycline antibiotics | -statin | Antihyperlipidemic: Statins |
| -dipine | Calcium channel blockers; antiarrhythmics | -suximide | Antiepileptics |
| -dronate | Antihypercalcemics | -terol | Bronchodilators |
| -floxacin | Quinolone/fluoroquinolone antibiotics | -thiazide | Thiazide diuretics |
| -fungin | Antifungals | -tidine | $H_2$ receptor blockers |
| -glinide | Meglitinide antidiabetics | -triptan | NSAIDs: Serotonin-selective agonists |
| -grastin | Colony-stimulating factors | -urane | Inhalation anesthetic agents |
| -idone | Atypical antipsychotics | -vudine | Nucleoside/nucleotide reverse transcriptase inhibitors (treatment of HIV and AIDS) |
| Interferon | Cytokines (affecting immune response) | -ximab; -zumab | Antibodies affecting immune response |
| -isone; -asone; or -solone | Corticosteroids | -zolamide | Diuretics: Carbonic anhydrase inhibitors |
| -line | Xanthine bronchodilators | -zoline | Topical decongestants |
| | | -zosin; -eride | Alpha-adrenergic antagonists (alpha blockers) |

classifications or medications used in treatment. When answering questions that include medications as an option, the priority is often the medication, especially if it is an antidiabetic agent or antibiotic. However, ensure that the medication is appropriate for the client. Box 3.16 provides an example of a pharmacology practice item.

## VISUALIZATION AND ASSOCIATION

Visualization can be used in answering test items. This can be accomplished by visualizing yourself performing the nursing action in the test item or associating the item to the client for whom you have provided care, for example, when dealing with positions.

Visualization works exceptionally well for prioritization items, for which you will prioritize nursing actions or place items in sequence. These items may include tasks or skills that need to be sequenced in an appropriate order for what should be done first, second, and so forth. First, read the question and understand what is expected of you when completing the item. Then, visualize performing the skill or completing the task addressed. Finally, carefully read the options to prevent missing

essential information and then begin sequencing. Besides visualization, the previously mentioned strategies of using the ABC's, Maslow's Hierarchy of Needs, and the nursing process can also be applied to prioritization items. Box 3.17 provides a practice item for using the skill of visualization.

## THINGS TO AVOID

Avoid answering NCLEX-RN® exam questions according to real-life experiences that may be different from the textbook content. The NCLEX-RN® exam is designed so that the content of the exam is directly related to content in textbooks that you have used during your education and according to national standards of care and best nursing practices. Remember that this exam is supported by information in these sources, and sometimes what you may have experienced in "real-life situations" may not be what is currently being taught; rather, your experiences could be based on time-saving shortcuts, old information, or procedures and practices specific to a health care agency. Studying is the key to success. Study only from current textbooks. In the test item scenarios, remember that the working environment

## BOX 3.16

### Sample Pharmacology Item

**PHARM** The client diagnosed with COPD is hospitalized due to increasing dyspnea. At 1000 the client requests an antianxiety medication. Based on the client's MAR illustrated, which interventions should the nurse implement? **Select all that apply.**

| **Date:** Today | **Medication Administration Record** | | **MRN:** 246810 |
|---|---|---|---|
| **Client:** John Jones | **Sex:** Male | | **Allergies:** Benzodiazepines |
| **Height:** 68 in. | **Weight:** 70 kg | | **Date of Birth:** 01-31-1950 |
| **Medication** | 0001–0730 | 0731–1530 | 1531–2400 |
| Furosemide 20 mg oral bid | | 0800 ABC | 2000 _____ |
| Salmeterol 50 mcg q12h per diskus inhaler | | 1000 _____ | 2200 _____ |
| Alprazolam 0.25–0.5 mg oral tid prn | | | |
| Ondansetron 2–4 mg IV q4–6h prn | 0500 NAN | | |
| Temazepam 15 mg oral HS prn | | | |
| **Nurse Signature and Initials:** Nancy Ann Newton (NAN); Allen Bradley Carlson (ABC) | | | |

1. Administer alprazolam 0.25 mg orally.
2. Administer temazepam 15 mg orally.
3. Give salmeterol, which is due at 1000.
4. Administer ondansetron 4 mg IV push.
5. Contact the client's HCP.

**ANSWER: 3, 5**

▸ *Test-taking Tip: First, carefully review the MAR before answering the question. If unsure of the medications, consider the client's diagnosis of COPD. Use the suffixes "–lam" and "–pam" to determine that both alprazolam (Xanax) and temazepam (Restoril) are benzodiazepines. In carefully reviewing the MAR, you should see that the client is allergic to benzodiazepines. Errors do happen. The client could be prescribed a medication despite having an allergy to it. The nurse needs to notify the HCP.*

## BOX 3.17

### Sample Visualization and Association Item

The nurse is teaching new parents about the best method of bathing their newborn. Prioritize the steps for the newborn's bath in the order that the nurse should teach them to the parents.
1. Wash around the umbilical cord.
2. Wash the face with clear water.
3. Wash the newborn's upper body and then dry.
4. Wipe the newborn's eyes with clear water from the inner canthus outward.
5. Wash and dry the perineal area.
6. Wash the legs and dry.
7. Wash the newborn's hair with a gentle soap.

Answer: _____

### ANSWER: 4, 2, 7, 3, 1, 6, 5

♦ *Test-taking Tip: First, visualize performing the newborn's bath and then visualize teaching the parents. Recall the principle of working from the cleanest to the most soiled areas when performing the newborn's bath.*

## BOX 3.18

### Sample Avoiding Reading Meaning Into a Question Item

**MoC** The monitor of the client's automatic BP machine has the same reading displayed for 8 hours. The nurse documents this reading hourly. The oncoming shift nurse finds that the BP tubing from the machine to the cuff was disconnected. The policy related to automatic BP machine use was reviewed with nurses at a required meeting the previous week. Which intervention by the nurse manager with the involved nurse is **most** appropriate?
1. Terminate the nurse's employment immediately.
2. Review the operation of the BP machine with the nurse.
3. Give the nurse a notice of intent to terminate if further incidents occur.
4. Inform the nurse of the unsafe action and expectations regarding BP assessment.

### ANSWER: 3

♦ *Test-taking Tip: The key words are "most appropriate." Carefully read the situation and question to avoid missing important information. Avoid reading into the question and asking whether or not the nurse attended the department meeting. Even if the meeting had not been attended by the nurse, the meeting was required, and information covered at the meeting would be expected of the employee. Also, avoid thinking as if you were the involved nurse in the situation and about what action you would prefer to be taken. Rather, answer the question focusing on the employee disciplinary process.*

will be ideal and that the nurse will have the time and resources to complete responsibilities, unless otherwise stated.

Avoid reading meaning into the questions. When reading a question and the answer options, simply read what is written. Sometimes, the situation provides more information than needed to answer the specific question. Avoid asking, "What if ... ?" Focus on the information provided and do not add more details. Although you should not read meaning into the question, make sure that you are reading the entire question and not missing pertinent information. You may select the wrong option if an important piece of information is missed in either the situation or the options. Box 3.18 provides an example of avoiding reading meaning into a practice item.

Avoid becoming frustrated or anxious. Use visualization often, seeing yourself as the competent nurse performing professional nursing care. Expect that there may be information that you do not know and use all the strategies that you have learned to arrive at the best option among the items.

## DIFFICULT QUESTIONS ARE A GOOD SIGN

As you are answering questions on the actual NCLEX-RN® exam, if it seems that the test questions are getting increasingly harder, this is a good sign. Answering questions correctly will cue the Computerized Adaptive Testing (CAT) to present more difficult questions. As the number of difficult questions you answer correctly increases, the number of actual test items that you will need to complete decreases. However, do not focus on the difficulty level and the number of items you complete. Items may seem difficult because you do not know the content, but these could actually be easier items. Therefore although the questions may seem to be getting harder, continue to focus on using the test-taking strategies to select the best answer for each item.

This book is designed such that the majority of items are at the more difficult cognitive levels so that you gain

experience with these types of questions. The rationales to both the answers and the incorrect options are sometimes lengthy, providing you with the content necessary to strengthen your knowledge base and prepare you for the actual NCLEX-RN® exam. Like the NCLEX-RN® exam, questions may seem hard initially, but as you progress through this question-and-answer book, you should find that items get easier to answer. Practicing answering the NCLEX-RN®-style questions, understanding the rationales for the answers and the incorrect options, and using a question drill process in which you complete multiple questions during one sitting and analyze your results provide the best opportunity to develop your test-taking skills. At the completion of this book, you should feel confident in your abilities to answer the more complex questions using the test-taking strategies you have learned and should be well prepared for the actual licensure exam.

## NCLEX-RN® PREPARATION: GENERAL TIPS

### PQRST Approach

Use the **PQRST approach** to master studying for the NCLEX-RN® exam and to succeed on your first attempt. Remember that the PQRST mnemonic is used both for assessing pain and for analyzing the rhythm of an electrocardiogram

(ECG) monitor strip. Although the licensure exam can be painful, using strategic interventions can reduce the pain and keep you in a healthy rhythm to achieve your life goal of becoming a registered nurse. The **PQRST approach** includes having a **p**ositive mind-set, **q**uestions to assess and build your knowledge, **r**eview of strengths and weaknesses, **s**tress reduction, and finally **t**aking the NCLEX-RN® test.

### Positive Mind-set

The first step in preparing for the NCLEX-RN® exam is having a positive mind-set. "I can do it! I will pass the NCLEX-RN exam!" Use positive self-talk and self-reassurance. Acknowledge what you already know and use self-congratulation for your success thus far: graduation (or near graduation) from a registered nurse program. You have accomplished much, and you are ready for the final step.

Study with enthusiasm, sincerity, and determination, keeping your goal in mind. Visualizing your goal can keep you motivated. Smile. You know what you are doing! Smiling reduces facial tension and stress, and can help you feel better about yourself.

### Questions

Did you know that mastering test-taking strategies and being ready to take the NCLEX-RN® exam successfully requires completing from 2000 to 4000 practice questions? This book and the online questions provide you with thousands of questions to hone your test-taking skills and review content. Use the strategies from this chapter to answer the questions. Because rationales for all answers are provided with each question in the chapter tests, you will be maximizing your study time by learning new information as well as enhancing your test-taking abilities. Using practice questions improves your testing performance; you become test-wise in learning how to read a question and eliminate incorrect options!

The cognitive level of questions will also boost the likelihood of success on the NCLEX-RN® exam. The majority of questions in this book and online are at the application and analysis level. Practicing with these more difficult questions should make it easier for you to answer the less difficult knowledge- and comprehension-level questions that may appear on the actual NCLEX-RN® exam.

## DEVELOP A PLAN

Before you begin to take the tests in this book, you will need to develop a plan. In addition to example questions provided in the first three chapters of this book, there are 2500 more questions in this book and about 10,000 questions online. The best approach is to start studying as soon as you receive this book and take questions daily. Find the content area you are addressing in class and begin with these questions. You can complete many questions by answering 35 questions daily. Doing this for a year will allow you to complete 12,775 questions, that is, studying 30 to 45 minutes per day.

If you are planning to study less than 3 months, take a couple of comprehensive exams online to determine your weakest areas, then complete the book and online questions in the weaker areas first, and move on to other chapters. Completing all available items will require dedicated time daily. Be sure to allow enough time for taking practice questions! Remember that a high percentage of the exam is on management of care.

Your study plan could include going through each chapter. If you prefer to study by the Client Needs categories of the NCLEX-RN® test plan, refer to Table 3.11 for the location of the content related to the client needs and the

## TABLE 3.11

| NCLEX-RN® Content Areas From the Test Plan and Applicable Tests in the Q&A Book | |
| --- | --- |
| **Content Area** | **Chapters of Primary Focus; Items Integrated in Other Chapters** |
| **Management of Care (17%–23% of the test)** | 5–9 |
| **Safety and Infection Control (9%–15% of the test)** | 12, 13, 41, 45, 47 |
| **Basic Care and Comfort (6%–12% of the test)** | 10, 14 |
| **Health Promotion and Maintenance (6%–12% of the test)** | 18–21, 23, 36 |
| **Reduction of Risk Potential (9%–15% of the test)** | 16, 24–34, 37–45 |
| **Physiological Adaptation (11%–17% of the test)** | 11, 17, 24–33, 37–45 |
| **Psychosocial Integrity (6%–12% of the test)** | 8–9, 47–49 |
| **Pharmacological and Parenteral Therapies (12%–18% of the test)** | 15, 22, 25, 27, 35, 46, 50 |

Adapted from National Council of State Boards of Nursing. (2019). *NCLEX-RN® Detailed Test Plan Effective April 2019*. Candidate Version.

chapters that focus on these areas. Almost all of the Client Needs categories are included in each of the chapters.

## SCHEDULE A CONSISTENT STUDY TIME

After developing a study plan, determine the time of day that works best for you. Some prefer breaking the study period into time blocks of an hour or less to avoid fatigue and boredom. Others prefer longer study periods to allow for greater concentration. Still others prefer to accomplish a certain number of questions once or twice daily rather than setting aside a certain amount of time. Whichever you choose, you should be consistent and diligent. Remember to reward yourself daily for your consistency and accomplishments.

At some point in your schedule, you should plan times to answer 75 questions during one sitting. This is the minimum number of questions on the exam. In addition, you should plan a time to answer 265 items during one sitting. This is the maximum number of items. During these study sessions, time yourself to determine how long it takes you to answer all of the questions.

## STUDY SPACE

Determine your best study space where you can concentrate. Be consistent with this space if possible. Stay focused and do not try to do two things at the same time, such as watching television and studying.

## COMPUTER PRACTICE

Although you should be consistent in your study space, you should allocate time at the computer for completing questions online. You will be taking the NCLEX-RN® exam at the computer from 1 to 6 hours. Thus at some point in your studying, you should practice at the computer from 1 to 6 hours, completing questions on the computer. Do this a few times during your review, varying the time periods. This practice allows acclimating yourself to the rigors of taking the NCLEX-RN® exam at the computer.

In addition, complete some practice questions using headphones. Although not intentional, others can be distracting at the actual NCLEX-RN® exam. If you are easily distracted, you will have the option of using headphones. Your practice using headphones will ease your anxiety if you elect to use these during the actual exam.

Practice taking the chapter and comprehensive tests using a timer so that you can determine how many questions you can correctly answer in a specified amount of time. Practice taking test items at a steady pace so that you do not rush through the test.

### Review of Strengths and Weaknesses

Your goal should be to achieve 75% to 80% correct on the practice and comprehensive tests. If you are unsuccessful, determine if the problem is in a traditional content area, for example, pharmacology, fundamentals, or nursing care of children and families; the integrated processes; or a specific content area on the NCLEX-RN® test plan. Use the unique features of the online format to review questions in the area

that you are weak. For example, the online features will allow you to select a traditional content area, and you will be presented with questions in only the area you select. The unique features also allow you to select areas of the Client Needs categories to ensure your success when taking the NCLEX-RN® exam.

When reviewing your strengths and weaknesses, reflect back on your self-discipline. Consider what has worked for you in studying and staying focused, and what seems to be a deterrent to concentration. If you find that you are lacking motivation to study, consider studying with a friend. Self-discipline is about setting priorities and saying "no" to things that will hinder accomplishment of your developed time plan. For some, using self-rewards can be successful in maintaining motivation.

### Stress Reduction

As you study, focus on using stress reduction strategies. These include but are not limited to positive self-talk, mental rehearsal, progressive muscle relaxation, deep breathing, and repositioning.

### Positive Self-Talk

As you study, continue with positive self-talk. Rather than thinking, "I don't know this information" or "I never learned this," tell yourself, "I can use the test-taking strategies to figure this out." Remember to tell yourself often, "I can do this!" Erase negative thoughts as they come to mind and replace them with positive thoughts. Positive thoughts can help keep you motivated. Avoid frustration that comes with negative thinking; this can sap you of the energy you need to study.

### Mental Rehearsal

Visualize yourself in the room taking the test in a relaxed pose, concentrating on the questions. Focus on sensations of being calm and in control. Do this each time you start a study session. During the study session, if an unfamiliar question appears, visualize yourself reducing your anxiety and rehearse what you will do to control your anxiety. For example, you might take a deep breath or perform positive self-talk: "I can do it; I can use the strategies I've learned." Finally, anticipate the sights and sounds in the actual testing environment. Visualize yourself at the computer, in control of the computer mouse or keyboard arrows, and moving through questions at a steady pace.

### Progressive Muscle Relaxation

Progressive muscle relaxation involves tensing and then relaxing various muscles throughout the body. It can progress from either the face and neck to the toes or vice versa (see Table 3.12). While studying, practice using progressive muscle relaxation. With advance practice you will be ready to use this strategy should you feel tense or experience test-taking anxiety during the exam.

### Deep Breathing

Deep breathing involves taking a deep breath, slowly inhaling to the count of 5, and then slowly exhaling to the count of 10. Performing deep breathing 5 to 10 times increases

**TABLE 3.12**

## Progressive Muscle Relaxation

### Instructions

1. Sit in a quiet, undisturbed place in a comfortable chair.
2. Keep your arms uncrossed and your feet flat on the floor.
3. Close your eyes.
4. Breathe in deeply and slowly for three breaths, inhaling through the nose and exhaling slowly through the mouth.
5. Begin at the feet by pulling the toes forward and upward, and stiffen your calves. Hold 5 to 10 seconds, and become aware of the feeling of tension.
6. Let your muscles relax, letting go of the tension. Become aware of the sensation of relaxation and the warmth as tension flows out of your muscles.
7. Now tense the thigh and buttock muscles and hold 5 to 10 seconds. Become aware of the feeling of tension.
8. Let your muscles relax, letting go of the tension. Become aware of the sensation of relaxation and the warmth as tension flows out of your muscles.
9. Now tense the abdominal muscles and hold for 5 to 10 seconds. Become aware of the feeling of tension.
10. Let your muscles relax, letting go of the tension. Become aware of the sensation of relaxation and the warmth as tension flows out of your muscles. Concentrate on this feeling of relaxation for a few seconds.
11. Next, tense your back muscles and hold for 5 to 10 seconds.
12. Now let your muscles relax. Again, feel the sensation of relaxation. Feel the warmth as the tension flows out of your muscles.
13. Next, clench your hands and tense the biceps and forearm muscles, and hold for 5 to 10 seconds.
14. Now let your muscles relax, and notice the sensations. These may feel light and airy, tingly and warm. Visualize tension leaving your body and your muscles relaxing.
15. Next, tense your shoulder and neck muscles. Bring your shoulders to your ears. Feel the tightness. Hold for 5 to 10 seconds.
16. Now let your muscles relax, and feel the tension as it flows out of your muscles. Feel the sensation of relaxation.
17. Next, tense the face muscles. Frown, wrinkle the forehead, hold your eyes tightly closed, and purse your lips. Hold for 5 to 10 seconds.
18. Now let your muscles relax, and feel the light, warm sensation as the tension flows out of your muscles.
19. Now focus on your whole body and feel the relaxation; you are feeling completely relaxed. All tension is gone.
20. Open your eyes and stretch. Enjoy feeling renewed and reenergized.

Adapted from Townsend, M. (2015). *Psychiatric mental health nursing: Concepts of care in evidence-based practice* (8th ed., p. 5). Philadelphia: F. A. Davis.

oxygen to the brain and can improve thinking. It also helps to relieve tension by refocusing your thoughts on your breathing and not on your concerns.

### Repositioning

Think of how repositioning the client relieves stress on body parts and improves circulation. Use this strategy during studying to improve blood flow to your brain. Change your sitting position, relieving pressure on your bony prominences by leaning from one side to the other. Flex and perform neck circumduction. Move your feet or stand. Repositioning can also relieve the boredom of long study periods.

### Exercise Regularly

Although you usually cannot exercise while studying, do not forget to exercise at least 30 minutes daily. Besides keeping you healthy, walking, running, or other physical exercise will reduce tension and stress by expending nervous energy. Maintaining balance in your life with exercise and healthy eating is just as important to keeping your mind alert and your stress level under control as is studying and using stress reduction strategies. Why not use the natural endorphins produced during exercise to give yourself a boost of energy just before a study session!

### Taking the NCLEX-RN® Test

The day before the test, do something you enjoy and avoid last-minute cramming. Keep your usual routine. Avoid alcoholic beverages and excess amounts of caffeine. Alcohol is a depressant and can reduce your ability to think clearly. Caffeine can reduce your concentration and attention span by overstimulating your body. Plan to get at least 8 hours of sleep, going to bed at your regular time. Use a relaxation strategy that you found successful during your preparation. Give yourself positive affirmation that you are ready and believe that you will be successful!

If driving to the testing site, be sure your gas tank is filled the night before and tires checked. Plan the driving route and know where you can park. Plan to arrive early and allow time for potential events that could cause a delay, such as excessive traffic.

The morning of the test, eat a healthy breakfast that includes a protein. Carbohydrate loading, though recommended by some, should be avoided if this is not your usual routine. Although it may give you an immediate energy boost, it can cause a rebound effect of fatigue once the carbohydrates have been metabolized. Dress for comfort, in layers that can be easily removed or added based on the environmental temperature.

Finally, during the exam remain focused and concentrate on the exam. Use headphones if easily distracted. Do not be concerned if others finish before you. Each person has different test questions. The computer will stop anywhere between 75 and 265 items, depending on your performance. Continue to use positive self-talk during the exam. You have prepared and studied. You can pass the NCLEX-RN® exam!

# NCLEX-RN® PREPARATION: TIPS FOR REPEAT TEST-TAKERS

Individuals who were unsuccessful on the NCLEX-RN® exam must wait a minimum of 45 days before retesting. Some boards of nursing (BON) or regulator bodies (RB) permit the retake of the NCLEX eight times a year, unless otherwise specified by a state BON/RB. If you were unsuccessful, contact your BON/RB to notify them that you plan to retake the exam. You will need to register again with Pearson VUE and pay the exam fee. You will receive a new Authorization to Test. The retake policy is available at the NCSBN Web site (www.ncsbn.org/1224.htm).

If you failed the test, use your 45-day waiting period to enhance your success on the retake exam by applying relaxation skills, focusing your review, and then learning and applying the test-taking strategies presented in this book.

First, establish a positive mind-set: "I can do it! I will pass the NCLEX-RN® exam!" Use positive self-talk and self-reassurance: Acknowledge what you already know and congratulate yourself for this. What you already know has been presented in the Candidate Performance Report (CPR), a report sent to you with your NCLEX-RN® exam results. This individualized two-page document identifies the content areas of the exam, the percentage of the test represented by that content area, a statement of your performance (your ability in that content area), and a description of the content area with a list of topics related to it. Your performance in each content area is described as **Above the Passing Standard, Near the Passing Standard,** or **Below the Passing Standard.** Look at the content areas that are **Above the Passing Standard.** Congratulate yourself because you have mastered this information. Look for the suggestions on how to use the CPR information to develop a study plan specific to the areas that are near or below the passing standard. A sample NCLEX-RN CPR is provided at the NCSBN Web site (www.ncsbn.org/1223.htm).

Now take a deep breath and perform a visualization and self-relaxation exercise. Imagine yourself in a location or in an activity you absolutely love. Incorporate the color blue (a blue sky, a blue lake, a blue room, etc.). With your eyes closed and focusing on your image, begin head-to-toe relaxation. If you have forgotten the steps, refer to Table 3.12. After completing the steps, stay seated for a minute or two, then open your eyes. Stand up and stretch. Congratulate yourself for being able to relax before you begin studying. *Perform this activity each time before starting your review of practice questions.*

Begin your review by identifying your content area or areas of weakness on the NCLEX-RN® CPR so you can focus your review. For example, if the content area on Pharmacological and Parenteral Therapies is **Below the Passing Standard,** then this is a content area on which you should focus first. However, if the content area on Reduction of Risk Potential is **Above the Passing Standard,** this is an area where minimal review is necessary.

Next, review the test-taking strategies in this chapter carefully. Focus on understanding these strategies to select the correct option. Remember to prioritize the options in the following order: actual threats to safety, physiological integrity, psychosocial integrity, and finally health maintenance. When choosing the correct answer for the practice questions, ask yourself, "What part of the nursing process is this question addressing: assessment, analysis, planning, implementation, or evaluation?" Avoid selecting options that include the words *all, always, never,* or *none.* Look for options that are different. If three options state the same information but in different words, choose the option that is different. When given options that are pharmacologically based or nonpharmacologically based, read the question carefully because the nonpharmacological intervention is likely the answer.

After establishing an understanding of the test-taking strategies, go to the tests in the book or online that focus on the content areas in which you were below passing standard. Because the online items can be filtered by Client Needs, using the online resources available with the book may be the best option for you. Table 3.11 identifies the NCLEX-RN® Client Needs categories and content areas included in the CPR and the applicable tests within this book. Although the majority of the questions in the tests will focus on a respective NCLEX-RN® content area, some questions within a test will pertain to other content areas and will help you refresh your knowledge in these other areas. As you answer questions, focus on using the test-taking strategies. Carefully read the rationales to determine why an option is either correct or incorrect.

Finally, complete the comprehensive tests in the book and on the online resource. Once you have achieved a score of 80% correct, you should be well prepared and ready to pass the NCLEX-RN® exam. The night before the exam, use the relaxation strategy that you have been using during your preparation and plan for 8 hours of sleep. Give yourself positive affirmation that you are ready and believe that you will be successful!

## Chapter Four

# Tips for International Test-Takers

## INTRODUCTION

The chapter is intended for individuals who have completed their nursing education outside the United States who are planning to work as a registered nurse (RN) in the United States. Foreign-educated RNs must meet several educational and professional requirements and must pass the NCLEX-RN® licensure exam to obtain RN licensure in the United States. For those who are not citizens of the United States, a work visa is also required.

## GRADUATES OF A CANADIAN NURSING PROGRAM

As of January 2015, graduates of a Canadian nursing program now take the NCLEX-RN® exam. If you are Canadian, you will be applying to take the NCLEX-RN® in the same manner as candidates graduating from a nursing program in the United States (see Chapter 1). However, for French Canadians, the NCLEX-RN® test plan, NCLEX tutorial, and Candidate Bulletin as well as the NCLEX-RN® exam are available in both English and French. Please consult the National Council State Board of Nursing's Web site (NCSBN) for NCLEX FAQs (www.ncsbn.org/4702.htm). If you intend to seek RN licensure to practice in the United States or a province or territory in Canada, it will be important for you to contact the board of nursing (BON)/regulatory body (RB) for the state or jurisdiction where you are seeking RN licensure. Links to the U.S. BONs and most Canadian RBs and contact information are available on the NCSBN Web site (www.ncsbn.org/contact-bon.htm).

## THE LICENSING REQUIREMENTS FOR INTERNATIONALLY EDUCATED NURSES

### The National Council of State Boards of Nursing (NCSBN)

The NCSBN develops and coordinates the administration of the licensure exam (NCLEX-RN®). You will be required to pass the NCLEX-RN® exam to practice as an RN in the United States. However, you will be unable to write the exam until you have met certain requirements. Thus it is important for you to review materials at the NCSBN Web site (www.ncsbn.org). Frequently asked questions and specific information for internationally educated nurses can be found on the NCSBN Web site links (www.ncsbn.org/2362.htm and www.ncsbn.org/171.htm). Additionally, contact information for each state BON where you intend to apply for licensure is accessible on the NCSBN Web site (www.ncsbn.org/contact-bon.htm). Contact information for a specific state BON can also be obtained through writing the National Council of State Boards of Nursing, 111 East Wacker Drive, Suite 2900, Chicago, IL 60601-4277. You can also telephone the NCSBN, if you are within the United States, at 1 (312) 525-3600.

### Individual State Licensure Requirements

Although the NCSBN oversees the development and administration of the NCLEX-RN® exam, each state has its own BON and specific requirements for RN practice within that state. If you are foreign educated, you will need to contact the BON in the state where you are seeking RN licensure to determine the requirements and documents that you will need and where to submit these. Check the NCSBN Web site for the contact information for the state BON where you intend to seek licensure (www.ncsbn.org/contact-bon.htm). If you are using the Internet, once you reach a state BON Web site, search on the term "foreign educated nurses." Requirements will be listed. Additionally, it may be helpful to contact the state BON by e-mail to obtain more information. Examples of how requirements differ between states for foreign-educated nurses can be viewed by accessing the Alabama BON Web site's requirements (Foreign Nursing Program Graduates: www.abn.alabama.gov/apply/#tab-endorse) and the New York BON Web sites (www.op.nysed.gov/prof/nurse/nursing.htm; www.op.nysed.gov/prof/nurse/nurse3f.pdf). When official documents are requested, you will need to contact the licensing authority or agency in your home country and have that agency submit the documents directly to the required U.S. agency.

All state BONs must verify that you graduated from a nursing program that has received accrediting agency or other authority approval in the country where the program is located and that the education is comparable to a Member Board-approved prelicensure program. Additionally, if English is not your native language, classes were not taught in English, and you were not educated with English text-books, you may need to pass an English proficiency exam that includes reading, speaking, writing, and listening. Other documents are also required before you would be eligible to write the NCLEX-RN® exam.

Many states use a credentialing agency to assess and verify your documents. When contacting the state BON, determine whether it uses a credentialing service, obtain the agency's contact information, and complete the required process.

### Commission on Graduates of Foreign Nursing Schools (CGFNS International) Credential Verification and Certification

The Commission on Graduates of Foreign Nursing Schools (CGFNS International) is an official organization qualified to complete the screening process for foreign-educated health care professionals (www.cgfns.org). Many state BONs require credential verification through CGFNS. You can obtain information about the CGFNS credential verification services at the CGFNS Web site (https://cgfns.zendesk.com/hc/en-us/articles/214442266-Choosing-the-Correct-CGFNS-International-Service-for-Nurses). If you are unable to access the Web site, specifics about each of the components of the services may be obtained by writing CGFNS International, 3600 Market Street, Suite 400, Philadelphia, PA 19104-2651, USA or by telephoning 1 (215) 222-8454.

Many states require the CGFNS Credentials Evaluation Service Professional Report. This report includes a review of your nursing education, licensure verification if you were licensed in your home country, and verification of English language proficiency testing.

Some states require the CGFNS Certification Program. This certification includes verification of credentials and a predictor exam (CGFNS exam) to certify your readiness to complete the NCLEX-RN® exam. The CGFNS exam is taken before the NCLEX-RN® exam to test nursing knowl-edge and will provide an indication of your ability to pass the NCLEX-RN® exam. When contacting the state BON where you intend to practice, be sure to determine whether you need to complete the CGFNS Qualifying Exam. This exam is offered at various locations within and outside the United States. These sites are listed at the CGFNS Web site (www.cgfns.org).

### Visa Information

If you are not a U.S. citizen, before you are able to work in the United States, you must obtain a visa. The U.S. Citizen-ship and Immigration Law requires that internationally edu-cated health care professionals, including RNs, successfully complete a screening process and seek a temporary or per-manent occupational visa. This process is separate from the process for obtaining RN licensure in the United States. However, if the state BON where you intend licensure

requires CGFNS VisaScreen verification, then you will re-ceive a CGFNS/International Commission on Healthcare Professions (ICHP) VisaScreen Certificate. This certificate satisfies the federal screening requirements and is required for the visa application. The Department of Homeland Secu-rity, U.S. Citizenship and Immigration Services (USCIS) must receive the CGFNS/ICHP VisaScreen Certificate before you will be issued an occupational visa or Trade NAFTA status to work as an RN in the United States. In some states, a Social Security number is required prior to issuance of an RN license. For information regarding tem-porary or permanent visas, contact the U.S. Department of State and the U.S. Citizenship and Immigration Service at www.uscis.gov/portal/site/uscis. You can also obtain more information about the work visa and application process at Immigration Direct: U.S. Immigration and Citizenship Form Services (www.immigrationdirect.com/). Immigration Direct is an application service and not a government or government-affiliated agency.

## REGISTERING TO TAKE THE NCLEX-RN® EXAM

Once you have successfully met all state and federal require-ments, applied for licensure in the state where you intend to be licensed, paid the fees, and met the eligibility requirements, you will receive an authorization to test (ATT) from the state BON where you applied. You need this ATT to be able to register to take the NCLEX-RN® exam. Be sure to read the NCLEX Candidate Bulletin (www.ncsbn.org/1213.htm) be-fore registering to take the NCLEX. The exam must be taken within the specified time period, usually 90 days. You will need to register and pay for the NCLEX exam with Pearson VUE. Information about registration, fees, and the payment process can be found at the Pearson VUE Web site (www.pearsonvue.com/nclex/).

The NCLEX-RN® exam is administered by Pearson VUE at a number of international Pearson Professional Centers in addition to the Pearson Professional Centers in the United States. International locations include Australia, Canada, England, Hong Kong, India, Japan, Mexico, Philippines, Puerto Rico, and Taiwan. You are encouraged to visit the Pearson VUE Web site for additional information regarding registering for the exam at international testing centers (www.pearsonvue.com/nclex/).

To learn more about the NCLEX-RN® licensure exam and test structure, consult Chapter 1 of this book. The Test Plan can be obtained at the NCSBN Web site (www.ncsbn.org).

## NCLEX-RN® PREPARATION: TIPS FOR FOREIGN-EDUCATED NURSES

The NCLEX-RN® is intended to test basic nursing knowledge required for entry-level RN practice in the United States. How-ever, if you are foreign educated, language and cultural differ-ences may present challenges in passing the NCLEX-RN®. The key to success is in adequate preparation.

It is important that assessment of your English language proficiency be completed early so that you have an understanding of your ability to read and comprehend English. Should you have difficulty in this area, you should consider taking courses in English as a second language (ESL) before completing NCLEX-RN® practice questions. Taking an English medical terminology course may also be helpful. Although the test items on the NCLEX-RN® exam are written at a 10th-grade reading level, the terms used in the exam will be terms used in the health care field.

Once you feel confident in your ability to read and comprehend English and have an understanding of medical terminology, begin taking NCLEX-RN®-type practice questions to assess your knowledge of nursing practice in the United States and to prepare for the NCLEX-RN® exam. Using this book and its online ancillary materials with thousands of questions will provide you with the experience of taking multiple-choice and alternate format items. The more items you complete, the more skillful you will become at deciphering questions, identifying key information in an item, and choosing the best option.

The beginning chapters of this book on the licensure exam, NCLEX-RN® questions, and test-taking strategies will assist you in learning about the structure and content of the exam. Review the included test plan because it will assist you in identifying the RN scope of practice in the United States. Pay particular attention to the test-taking strategies in Chapter 3. These are most helpful when the content of an item may be unfamiliar to you or when you need to eliminate options when some or all seem to be correct.

Begin to review questions from one entire content area before moving to the next content area. If it seems that you are answering many book items incorrectly, answer the questions from the online ancillary test bank in that particular content area before beginning the next content area. Be sure to read the rationales provided, which include the rationale for both the correct and incorrect options.

The rationale should aid you in learning why an option may be correct or incorrect and help to build your knowledge base or enhance recall of content. As you complete the questions, with the assistance of the online ancillary items, you should be able to identify content areas that you may need to study in more depth. The comprehensive tests located in the book and online will serve as an assessment guide to help you determine the need for further study. Your goal is to achieve 80% mastery on questions. The references provided in the appendix will direct you to common nursing textbooks or resources that are used in formulating questions for the NCLEX-RN® exam should additional study be needed.

As you review questions, you should think about your experiences, skills, and knowledge and compare them to those of nursing candidates educated in the United States. In many countries, registered nurses may prescribe medications and treatments. In the United States, however, registered nurses anticipate, plan, and administer medications and treatments that are prescribed by an HCP or other licensed health care providers. Be sure to read the rationales carefully to assist in identifying the scope of registered nursing practice in the United States. The test on prioritization and delegation will be particularly helpful in this area.

The more items that you complete before taking the NCLEX-RN® exam, the better you will be able to identify client needs and responses. You will also become more accustomed to reading questions and selecting options for nursing responses and actions based on nursing practice within the United States and Canada. An electronic copy of the *2019 NCLEX-RN® Detailed Test Plan—Candidate Version* is available free of charge from the NCSBN at www.ncsbn.org.

Finally, use the online test bank associated with the book to assess your knowledge of all the areas identified in the test plan. The features of the online testing will provide you with information about how well you do in each of the content areas and client needs. Once you have achieved 80% mastery, you should be well prepared and ready to pass the NCLEX-RN® exam.

# Practice Tests

*Chapter Five*

# Ethical and Legal Issues in Nursing

1. **MoC**  The hospitalized client diagnosed with end-stage cancer suddenly wants to discontinue treatment including no antibiotics, tube feedings, and mechanical ventilation. When acting as the client's advocate, which **priority** action should be taken by the nurse?

   1. Respect the client's wishes and indicate those wishes on the plan of care.
   2. Notify the client's HCP and have the client tell the family about the decision.
   3. Withhold the treatments and clarify other treatments that the client wishes to withhold.
   4. Decide what to do based on the client's condition when additional treatment is needed.

2. **MoC**  The experienced nurse orienting the new nurse explains that, to advocate for clients, the nurse must be able to identify ethical issues and communicate the clients' wishes to others. Which primary role of the nurse advocate should the experienced nurse also explain to the new nurse?

   1. Safeguard all clients against abuse and violation of their rights.
   2. Make decisions for clients based on the nurse's knowledge and relationship.
   3. Assist clients in openly expressing their rights to other HCPs.
   4. Become knowledgeable of the clients' values to assist the client in decision making.

3. **MoC**  The nurse is completing a variance report after finding an error for the client who is to receive an IV infusion of heparin at 1000 units/hour. Heparin 25,000 units in 500 mL D5W is infusing at 30 mL/hr. At what rate should the nurse record that the heparin should be infusing? _____ mL/hr (Record your answer as a whole number.)

4. **MoC**  The client, who has a recurrence of breast cancer, questions the female nurse about treatment options. Which responses by the nurse would be appropriate? **Select all that apply.**

   1. "You should discuss your concerns with your oncologist; I cannot give any medical advice."
   2. "Tell me about the options that your oncologist told you about so I can clarify them."
   3. "Have you asked for a second opinion yet? There might be other options for treatment."
   4. "I can arrange a conference with the oncologist for you and your family if you would like."
   5. "I know that if I had breast cancer I would have both chemotherapy and radiation."

5. **MoC**  The nurse educator is reviewing the concept of advocacy with new nurses. Which statements by the nurse educator demonstrate examples of advocacy? **Select all that apply.**

   1. "The client expresses concerns regarding surgical intervention for heart disease. The nurse's best action is to listen to the client's concerns."
   2. "The client tells the nurse about no longer wishing to receive chemotherapy and not wanting to discuss it with the HCP for fear that the HCP will disagree. The nurse nods in agreement."
   3. "When a resident HCP fails to respond to an emergency situation, the nurse must step in to seek further assistance."
   4. "The nurse must question inconsistent HCP orders, such as when the client being discharged has been taking clopidogrel following stent placement but it has not been prescribed."
   5. "When the client is being discharged from the ED and hasn't had adequate medical evaluation, the nurse must seek clarification prior to discharging the client."

**6.** MoC The client, postprocedure from an endoscopy in which moderate sedation was used, informs the nurse of having no transportation home and no funds for a taxicab. The charge nurse refuses to approve hospital-paid transportation home. How should the nurse **best** advocate for the client?

1. Because this is a planned procedure and the client is responsible for transportation arrangements, there is no need to advocate in this situation.
2. The nurse should quietly give the client money for a taxicab; no other staff members need to know what the nurse has done.
3. The nurse should document that the charge nurse made the decision that no hospital funds can be used to transport the client home and inform the client it is the client's responsibility.
4. The nurse should consult a social worker to seek an alternative mode of transportation such as state-funded transportation for the poor.

**7.** MoC The client brought to the ED is alert and oriented but has oxygen saturation ($SpO_2$) levels ranging from 88% to 90%. The nurse applies oxygen at 2L per nasal cannula, but there is no improvement in $SpO_2$. Oxygen per mask is initiated at 40% with little improvement. Radiology reports show no obvious injury or fractures. Suddenly the client loses consciousness, has a respiratory arrest, and subsequently dies. During resuscitation efforts, it was determined that the nurse failed to open the oxygen tank valve and the client had not been receiving oxygen. Which key ethical principle is involved in this situation?

1. Nonmaleficence
2. Fidelity
3. Veracity
4. Justice

**8.** MoC The nurse is caring for the female client who is in severe pain, rated at an 8 on a 0 to 10 scale. In her culture, it is tradition for older males to speak for females, and her spouse will not allow the nurse to give analgesics. What is the nurse's **best** action?

1. Administer the analgesic when the client's spouse leaves the room.
2. Educate the spouse on the reason for the pain and the analgesic's action.
3. Respect the client's culture and do not administer the analgesic.
4. Report the issue to the immediate nursing supervisor.

**9.** MoC The nurse gives a medication without checking the client's MAR. When documenting the medication given, the nurse notices that the medication was also given 15 minutes earlier by a relieving nurse. After assessing the client, the nurse who made the error reports this to the charge nurse and HCP. Which additional action should this nurse expect?

1. Assignment of fewer clients at one time for a few shifts
2. Disciplinary action to the first nurse for giving the first dose
3. Disciplinary action, possibly including suspension or termination
4. Told to complete a variance report that would be reviewed by management

**10.** MoC The hospitalized client, who does not have an HCD, consents to a DNR, and an order is placed by the HCP. Which statement by the nurse **most** demonstrates ethical practice when the client has a cardiac arrest and the client's eldest son wants the DNR rescinded and resuscitation attempted?

1. "We must follow your mother's wishes for DNR, and it is much too late to start CPR."
2. "You can rescind the DNR order by speaking to the HCP who discussed this with your mom."
3. "Why would you want to go against your mother's wishes? Hasn't she suffered enough?"
4. "I can see that you are upset about your mother's decision. May I call pastoral care for you?"

**11.** MoC While the nurse is applying restraints to the combative client with a suspected drug overdose, the client spits at staff, and a security officer places a towel across the client's face. Which response by the nurse is **most** appropriate?

1. "Once the client is properly restrained, we will need to remove that towel."
2. "The client is known to be HIV positive; thank you for helping to protect us."
3. "The client must be treated respectfully; please remove that towel from the client's face."
4. "Please leave the room; I can't allow you to treat the client in that manner."

**12.** MoC The graduate nurse notices a distinct odor of alcohol on the precepting nurse's breath. Which action is **most** appropriate and should be taken by the graduate nurse?

1. Immediately inform the charge nurse of the nurse's breath odor.
2. Discuss the situation with another colleague and formulate a plan.
3. Research the state's peer assistance program and discuss the program with the nurse.
4. Ask the impaired nurse to go home, or the incident will be reported to a manager.

**13.** MoC The daughter of the client recently diagnosed with lung cancer informs the nurse that she does not want her mother told of the cancer diagnosis. Which response by the nurse is **best?**

1. "Are you afraid that your mother's condition will worsen more rapidly if she is told?"
2. "Your mother has a right to know; how would you feel if you weren't told?"
3. "We must be honest with your mother. Unfortunately, I will need to inform her."
4. "Let's discuss your concerns with the oncologist and then decide the best approach."

**14.** MoC The client has grown very fond of the nurse. Which items may the nurse accept from the client? **Select all that apply.**

1. A token gift from the client to the individual nurse.
2. The client's permission to be a contact on a social networking site.
3. A position as a private duty nurse for the client upon the client's discharge.
4. A hug from the client upon the client's discharge.
5. A thank-you basket of candy and fruit from the client for the unit staff.

**15.** MoC The client is actively bleeding from the upper GI tract and vomiting bright red blood. The nurse is to administer blood as prescribed, but the client refuses to receive any blood products because of a conflict with religious beliefs. Which statement should be the basis for the nurse's intervention?

1. The client has a right to be involved in decisions about his or her care and treatment.
2. The client has a right to refuse care and treatments regardless of the outcome.
3. The client can be assured of his or her right to privacy and confidentiality.
4. The client cannot expect the HCP to allow spiritual beliefs to influence care decisions.

**16.** MoC The nurse is assigned multiple clients who are being admitted to the ED. Which client would the nurse immediately treat without first obtaining the client's informed consent?

1. The unconscious client who has unequal and sluggish reacting pupils after a MVA.
2. The ill fourth-grade child whose parents cannot be reached and is brought by school personnel.
3. The client who follows the Jehovah's Witness faith and is likely to die without a transfusion of RBCs.
4. The pregnant 15-year-old who arrives in the ED after an episode of food poisoning.

**17.** MoC The client informs the nurse that the HCP is recommending a kidney biopsy. The client fears the result will be cancer and would not want treatment. The client feels it would be better just "not to know." Which action should be taken by the nurse to empower the client to take control of his/her health care needs?

1. Explain to the client that the HCP is doing what is best for the client.
2. Tell the client of his/her right to make decisions based on personal values and beliefs.
3. Encourage the client to talk with family and let the family decide.
4. Talk with the HCP about the client's fear of having the biopsy.

**18.** MoC The competent 90-year-old client admitted to an ED with an MI declines treatment and wishes to be discharged home. Which statement **best** supports the client's right to refuse care?

1. "I have lived a full life; I want to go home to die."
2. "I understand that without treatment, I could die."
3. "It is too expensive to stay in the hospital."
4. "My family wants me to go home; I will be okay."

**19.** MoC The nurse educator is discussing the "Patient's Bill of Rights" with new nurses on an adult medical unit. Which statement by the nurse educator **best** applies the Patient's Bill of Rights?

1. "Our clients have a right to the best care available in our facility."
2. "You may access any client's medical record while caring for clients in the facility."
3. "At time of discharge, the family should be making any needed home care arrangements."
4. "Clients, unless incapacitated, have a right to make decisions about their course of treatment."

**20.** MoC The client reports being in significant pain since surgery earlier in the day. The nurse notes that hydrocodone plus acetaminophen has been documented as being administered at the highest possible dose and at regular intervals since surgery. When the nurse brings the client two hydrocodone plus acetaminophen tablets, the client states, "That isn't what I had before. I only had one pink pill." Which action should be taken by the nurse?

1. Call and ask the pharmacist to send the pink hydrocodone and acetaminophen tablets.
2. Complete a variance report because the client's medication record is incorrect.
3. Report the client's statement and event to the immediate nursing supervisor.
4. Confront the nurse on the previous shift with the suspicion that the nurse took the tablets.

**21.** MoC The nurse is told by the alert and oriented hospitalized client that an unidentified female entered the client's room and searched through the client's personal possessions. After calming the client, which action should be the nurse's **priority**?

1. Notify the police.
2. Complete an incident report.
3. Notify the hospital security officer.
4. Inventory the client's possessions.

**22.** MoC The client is admitted to a surgical unit. The client has multiple rings, a watch, and $65 in cash. What is the **safest** action for the nurse to take regarding the valuables?

1. Allow the client to keep the items so they will be safe-guarded by the client.
2. Collect the items and place them in the client's room closet.
3. Give the cash to the client's spouse; allow the client to keep the jewelry.
4. Collect the items according to hospital policy for safekeeping.

**23.** MoC The adolescent client enters a clinic alone for treatment of a productive cough and low-grade fever. The client discloses being HIV positive. Which is the **best** action by the nurse?

1. Nothing can be done without the consent of the parents.
2. Treat and then educate about birth control, safe sex, and partner disclosure.
3. Draw an HIV titer to confirm the HIV positive status of the client.
4. Obtain a sexual risk history and notify the parents of the clinic visit.

**24.** MoC The nurse is working in a busy ED with multiple admissions. For which clients should the nurse ensure that mandatory reporting is completed? **Select all that apply.**

1. The client who has a gunshot wound
2. The client who has pertussis
3. The child who has cigarette burns
4. The vulnerable adult who is emaciated
5. The adult client who has a broken hip from a fall

**25.** MoC The nurse observes that one of the HCP's sterile gloved hands touches the client's bedspread when placing a central venous catheter. Which intervention by the nurse demonstrates professional conduct?

1. Inform the HCP of the break in sterile procedure and provide new sterile gloves.
2. Inform the HCP of the break in sterile procedure after the procedure is completed.
3. Notify the supervisor of the health care provider's (HCP) break in sterile procedure.
4. Report the event to the infection control nurse; that nurse will follow up with the HCP.

**26.** MoC The client is unable to swallow oral secretions and has gurgling respirations with coughing and choking. The nurse plans to suction the client's oral and nasotracheal airway. The nurse has not performed this task before. Which action should be taken by the nurse?

1. Suction the client immediately before aspiration or a respiratory arrest occurs.
2. Document the findings and contact the respiratory therapist to suction the client.
3. Have the charge nurse come to the room for instruction and supervision in suctioning.
4. Call the HCP to obtain an order to suction the client's secretions.

**27.** MoC The nurse gathers the client's belongings in preparation for the client's hospital discharge. Which statement by the nurse is **most** appropriate regarding the handling of client valuables?

1. "I placed your clothes, glasses, wallet, and cane in this bag; make sure you take them with you when you leave."
2. "Here is your wallet from the hospital safe; please check the contents and sign this form acknowledging its receipt."
3. "Your belongings are awfully heavy. I'll take the bag with your wallet and glasses and give them to your son to carry."
4. "Please make sure you have everything before you leave; the hospital is not responsible for any belongings left behind."

**28.** [MoC] The new nurse is considering employment options and asks a nursing instructor about practice settings in which the legal doctrine of respondeat superior would be **most** applicable. Which practice situations should the nursing instructor describe to the new nurse? **Select all that apply.**

1. Hospital-based home-care setting
2. Critical care
3. A physician's office
4. Private duty
5. Salvation Army volunteer

**29.** [MoC] The mental health nurse is caring for the client diagnosed with a schizoaffective disorder. Which type of malpractice has the nurse committed when telling a coworker, "That client is crazy and may kill someone"?

1. Libel
2. Slander
3. Battery
4. Invasion

**30.** [MoC] The nurse educator is teaching new nurses about whether children may give consent for their own medical treatment. Which statements should the nurse educator use for examples? **Select all that apply.**

1. "A 15-year-old may request a prescription for birth control pills without parental consent."
2. "A lost 10-year-old may consent to treatment for sudden-onset severe headache."
3. "A 13-year-old with leukemia may refuse blood transfusions without parental consent."
4. "A 14-year-old may seek treatment for drug addiction without parental consent."
5. "A 16-year-old with a nondisplaced fractured arm may consent for treatment."

**31.** [MoC] The nurse obtains the form, *Left Without Notifying Staff (Elopement) and Leaving Against Medical Advice (AMA)*, when the client is attempting to leave the facility without being discharged by the HCP. In completing the form, which is the **most** appropriate statement by the nurse?

1. "I will need to have you sign this form under the subsection 'Elopement' before I can let you leave."
2. "I cannot let you leave until you acknowledge in writing that I have informed you of the risks of leaving."
3. "By signing this form, you will be releasing the hospital of any liability should you die from your untreated illness."
4. "You have the right to leave against medical advice at any time, but first I must inform you of the risks of leaving without treatment."

**32.** [MoC] The nurse on a newborn unit is instructed to float to an adult nursing unit. Which response by the nurse to the nurse manager would be appropriate?

1. "I have only cared for newborn clients; I am not qualified to care for adult clients."
2. "I will have to go home if forced to float; I was not hired to work on other units."
3. "I have never worked in an adult unit before, but I would love the opportunity."
4. "I have been to an adult unit before, but I floated last, and it is not my turn to float."

**33.** [MoC] The nurse is mandated to work overtime due to short staffing. The nurse states to the nurse manager, "I am too tired to stay" and leaves the unit. Which action should the nurse expect when returning to work?

1. No action because the nurse acknowledged being too tired to stay for the next shift.
2. The nurse will be told this behavior will not be tolerated again when mandated to stay.
3. Written disciplinary action because leaving the unit constituted abandonment.
4. Termination due to insubordination and potential client harm due to lack of nursing care.

**34.** [MoC] The nurse educator is reviewing the EMTALA with newly hired ED nurses. Which situations should the nurse use to describe EMTALA violations? **Select all that apply.**

1. Paramedics contact the local hospital inbound with an infant in cardiac arrest. The ER nurse advises them to proceed to the next nearest hospital because the pediatric unit is at capacity.
2. After the client receives naloxone in the ED following a heroin overdose, the client leaves the hospital against medical advice (AMA). The client is shot by police the next day.
3. The homeless client, seen in the ED for a swollen and painful leg, is discharged after being told to apply heat and elevate the leg. The client returns a day later with a pulmonary embolus.
4. The client on public assistance presents to the ED experiencing chest pain. The client is treated for pneumonia, and the ECG is never obtained, which goes against protocol.
5. A child with a fever of 104.6°F (40.3°C) is seen in the ED and receives acetaminophen and treatment per protocol. When the fever reduces, the child is discharged home.

**35.** MoC The client arriving at the emergency room following a bar fight has a headache and blurred vision. Upon assisting with undressing the client for an examination, the nurse finds a gun secured under the client's belt. Which actions by the nurse are **most** appropriate given this observation?

1. Confiscate the weapon and call the police.
2. Ask if the client has a permit to carry a gun.
3. Call hospital security personnel for assistance.
4. Care for the client first and ignore the gun for now.

**36.** MoC The 28-year-old uninsured client presents to the emergency room with an asthma attack. Which statements by the nurse comply with the EMTALA? **Select all that apply.**

1. "The client will need to see a health care provider because he needs to have a medical screening before being discharged."
2. "If the hospital is not capable of caring for the client, we can transfer to a facility that provides higher level of care."
3. "The on-call pulmonologist has refused to see the client unless the client agrees to provide payment up front."
4. "A social worker consult will be needed to explore the client's financial situation before we can treat the client."
5. "If a transfer is necessary, the client will be informed of the risks/benefits of a transfer by the attending HCP and documented on the transfer form."

**37.** MoC The nurse has been accused of battery. Which statement by the nurse **best** supports a legal defense to a battery accusation?

1. "The client would not let go of my arm. I was alone, so I elbowed him in the chest to get free."
2. "The client was spitting at us, so I temporarily placed a towel across his face to protect us."
3. "I searched the client's clothes for drugs before placing them in an evidence bag."
4. "To prevent harm, I asked the orderly to restrain the client while I gave the injection."

**38.** MoC PHARM The nurse finds that the client's insulin infusion dose, which was just changed by the previous nurse, is incorrect. The client's prescribed dose is 2 units of insulin per hour. Regular insulin 100 units in 100 mL of NS is infusing at 20 mL/hr. When completing the variance report, how many units per hour should the nurse document that the client had been receiving?

_____ units/hr (Record your answer as a whole number.)

**39.** MoC The nurse manager is discussing situations in which the staff nurse risks disciplinary action related to licensure. Which nurse's actions risk disciplinary action related to licensure? **Select all that apply.**

1. Inserting a central venous catheter under the supervision of the HCP
2. Intentionally documenting incorrect information in the client's medical record
3. Arriving at work with clothing smelling of tobacco smoke
4. Recently convicted of a felony for drug possession
5. Detailing all previous work experience when applying for a nursing position

**40.** MoC The 30-year-old client recently diagnosed with HIV is being counseled by the nurse. Which statement by the nurse is correct?

1. "Unless you give consent, your information will be kept private and your sexual partners will not be informed of your diagnosis."
2. "The Centers for Disease Control must be informed of this HIV diagnosis for epidemiological purposes."
3. "To protect all the nursing staff on this unit, all nurses will be informed of your HIV status."
4. "You may require that each health care provider caring for you obtain your consent to discuss your HIV status with anyone."

**41.** MoC Several family members are present with the client. Wanting to be very helpful, they have been placing the client's oxygen back on when the nasal cannula slips, turning the client's IV pump off when it alarms, and placing the nebulizer tubing back in the mouthpiece of the client's nebulizer. Which action by the nurse is required for the safe care of the client?

1. Inform the family that, for client safety, they are not allowed to touch any medical equipment.
2. Inform the family that they must alert clinical staff when there is an alarm or a need to connect tubing or devices.
3. Thank the family for noticing when tubing is disconnected and getting the client the treatment required.
4. Inform the family that they are only allowed to put the IV pump on hold before alerting the nurse.

**INSTRUCTIONS:** Refer to the information provided in the table to answer Questions 42 and 43.

**42.** `CJ` `MoC` `PHARM` The client is on a heparin protocol preoperatively. Postoperatively a surgeon writes, "Resume heparin at 1600 hours; do not bolus." Then a cardiologist writes an order: "Restart heparin protocol, no bolus previous rate, at 0700 tomorrow if okay with surgeon." Later, an on-call surgeon writes, "Clarification: Resume heparin drip tonight—no bolus, at previous rate." Which intervention should the nurse implement?

### Heparin Protocol

1. aPTT/PT; INR; daily CBC.
2. Initiate IV of 500 mL $D_5W$ with 25,000 units heparin at 25 mL/hr.
3. Give IV bolus of 2500 units heparin (or _____ units heparin).
4. Repeat aPTT/PT in 6 hours from time IV heparin infusion is initiated.
5. Adjust IV rate of heparin and repeat a PTT/PT per protocol.
6. Notify HCP if aPTT >129 sec.

| aPTT/ (sec) | IV Bolus (units) | Hold (minutes) | IV Rate (mL/hr) | Repeat aPTT/ PT |
|---|---|---|---|---|
| <50 | 5000 | 0 | 31 | 6 hr |
| 50–<60 | 0 | 0 | 28 | 6 hr |
| 60–<86 | 0 | 0 | 25 | Next a.m. |
| 86–<96 | 0 | 0 | 23 | Next a.m. |
| 96–120 | 0 | 30 | 21 | 6 hr |
| >120 | 0 | 60 | 17 | 6 hr |

1. Start the heparin at 25 mL/hr because that is the initiation rate on the protocol.
2. Bolus with 5000 units and begin the drip at 31 mL/hr because that is the first line of the protocol.
3. Contact the surgeon to determine the rate at which the heparin drip should be started because the order is not clear.
4. Start the heparin at 28 mL/hr per protocol and obtain an aPTT in 6 hours to reestablish the baseline.

**43.** `CJ` `MoC` The nurse consults another nurse to verify the heparin infusion dose and rate based on the heparin protocol and their interpretation of the HCPs' orders. The heparin infusion is restarted and the client suffers a massive intracranial hemorrhage. What unintentional tort did the nurse commit? Briefly state your answer in the box provided.

**44.** `MoC` The telemetry nurse observes the progression in the heart rhythm of the client hospitalized to rule out MI. At which illustrated point does the nurse **first** risk liability if the nurse fails to notify the HCP of the changes observed in the client's heart rhythm?

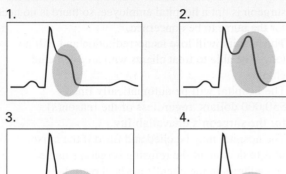

**45.** `MoC` The charge nurse receives a telephone call about the admission of the client with renal failure. The client is confused and restless. Which room should the nurse assign for this client?

1. A semiprivate room 50 feet from the nurses' station
2. A small private room at the end of the hallway
3. A seclusion room that is monitored by a camera for client safety
4. A large private room within view of the nurses' station

**46.** `MoC` `PHARM` The nurse is hanging an IV solution of $D_5NS$ with 20 mEq of KCL. The nurse notices that the label from the pharmacy is correct as indicated; however, the solution is $D_5W$. Which interventions should the nurse implement? **Select all that apply.**

1. Consult the charge nurse.
2. Administer the IV solution.
3. Telephone the pharmacist.
4. Request that the pharmacy send a new label.
5. Check the agency's policy for medication error reporting.

**47.** `MoC` The nurse administers regular insulin 10 units subcutaneously when regular insulin 10 units intravenously had been prescribed as part of a calcium gluconate, insulin, and glucose regimen to lower the client's elevated serum potassium level. Which interventions should the nurse implement? **Select all that apply.**

1. Notify the HCP.
2. Report the error to the charge nurse.
3. Call lab for a STAT serum potassium level.
4. Complete an agency incident/variance report.
5. Place a copy of the incident report in the client's chart.

**48.** The on-call surgeon refuses the nurse's request to treat the Medicaid-eligible client in the ED. Which consequence will the hospital **most** likely face due to this situation?

1. The hospital cannot be held accountable because the surgeon is not a hospital employee, so there is no need for the nurse to be concerned.
2. The hospital will lose its accreditation and will no longer be able to treat clients who are Medicaid eligible.
3. The hospital will be automatically fined $50,000 dollars, regardless of the reason(s) for the surgeon's unavailability.
4. The hospital may be cited and fined if the nurse fails to document the refusing surgeon's name and address in the client's medical record.

**49.** MoC One parent is present with the 14-year-old client who is to have an emergency appendectomy. The nurse has been asked to have the informed consent form signed. Which statement reflects the nurse's best thinking about informed consent?

1. A signed informed consent form ensures client knowledge of the risk and benefits of the procedure.
2. Adolescents have the ability to make decisions for themselves and may sign the informed consent form.
3. Both parents have legal rights regarding medical treatment. Without both parents present, the informed consent form may not be signed.
4. The surgeon is responsible for obtaining informed consent and for explaining the surgical procedure, benefits, and potential risks.

**50.** MoC The nurse is obtaining a urine specimen by catheterization from the 90-year-old female client admitted with fever of unknown origin. The client is somewhat confused and yells out to stop the procedure. Which is the **most** appropriate response by the nurse?

1. The nurse should stop the procedure and discuss the client's wishes not to be touched with the HCP.
2. The nurse should finish the procedure because the urethra is easily identifiable and the specimen can be quickly obtained.
3. The nurse should stop the procedure and calmly talk to the client and explain the importance of the procedure.
4. The nurse should instruct the nursing assistant (NA) to hold the client's legs in the lithotomy position so the specimen can be quickly obtained.

**51.** MoC The 50-year-old client admitted to the emergency room following an MVA has slurred speech, an alcoholic breath odor, and is under police escort after formal arrest. The police officer requests a blood sample be taken for a blood alcohol level. The client verbally declines. Which is the **most** appropriate action by the nurse?

1. Draw the serum sample as directed by the police officer; the client may not decline this procedure.
2. Inform the police officer that the blood alcohol level cannot be drawn at the police officer's request without a warrant for a blood draw.
3. Tell the police officer that the client declined and that the officer needs to draw the blood sample and provide the equipment.
4. Wait until the client loses consciousness, and then draw the blood sample as directed by the police.

**52.** MoC The HCP writes that a written consent must be obtained for the client scheduled for a cholecystectomy in the morning. Which client's statement should indicate to the nurse that follow-up is needed before the client gives written consent?

1. "The doctor told me that he will remove my gallbladder."
2. "My surgeon's name is Dr. Smith, and he will be assisted by Dr. Black."
3. "The doctor told me I don't have anything to worry about; this is routine surgery."
4. "I expect to have pain following surgery, but I know I will be offered pain meds if needed."

**53.** MoC During a multidisciplinary care conference, family members are asked to make a decision regarding long-term care placement for their mother, who is unable to care for herself independently. The family is having difficulty deciding whether to place her in long-term care or to care for her at home. The family asks the nurse, "What should we do?" Which **initial** response by the nurse is **best**?

1. "Because you are undecided, it would be best for your mother to go to a nursing home until you make a decision."
2. "To clarify, you are trying to make a decision about where your mother should go when she leaves the hospital. Is that correct?"
3. "Have you talked to your mother to find out what she would like to do? Maybe she has the resources for in-home help."
4. "I know that if it were my mother, I would not want to place her in a nursing home. I would provide in-home care."

**54.** MoC The client, who is suspected of having cancer, is scheduled for a CT scan. The client's best friend calls on the telephone, and the experienced nurse overhears the new nurse sharing information about the client with the client's friend. Which statement by the experienced nurse is **most** appropriate?

1. "It's a good thing you told him about his friend. The client needs all the support he can get."
2. "I don't believe the client has given permission to share information. He should have been asked first."
3. "The CT scan is canceled for today. We should call the client's friend back to clarify the information."
4. "I heard another nurse talking on the phone yesterday about the client to the client's friend. It's okay to provide information."

**55.** MoC Two staff nurses in an elevator are discussing the client. The new nurse on the same unit, but not assigned to the client, overhears the conversation. Which is the new nurse's **best** course of action?

1. Confront the staff nurses about discussing confidential information.
2. Report the breach of client confidentiality to the agency security officer.
3. Discuss the situation with the client to inform the client of the breach.
4. Ignore the discussion because only hospital staff were on the elevator.

**56.** MoC The client brought to a hospital under police escort after a suicide attempt states to the nurse, "When I get out, my wife is dead meat for calling the police!" Which action should be taken by the nurse?

1. Contact the nursing supervisor and discuss the client's disclosure.
2. Call the police and report the client's threat of harm to his wife.
3. Contact the client's wife directly and notify her of the client's plan.
4. Consult with the psychiatrist to obtain an opinion of the legitimacy of the threat.

**57.** MoC PHARM The nurse is accessing the client's electronic health record to document withholding a medication. What is the correct sequence of steps that the nurse should take?

1. Select the correct client.
2. Enter the user ID and password.
3. Document withholding the medication on the client's electronic MAR.
4. Log out of the client's electronic medical record.
5. Open the electronic medical record computer program.
6. Access the client's electronic MAR.

Answer: _____

**58.** MoC The nurse receives telephone orders from the HCP for ABGs to be drawn STAT. Which is the **most** important safety consideration when obtaining the order?

1. Writing the order down and reading it back to the HCP
2. Calling the respiratory therapist STAT to draw the ABGs
3. Giving the order to the unit coordinator to place in the computer
4. Notifying the charge nurse of the new order for ABGs STAT

**59.** MoC A nursing educator is reviewing the HIPAA with new hospital staff. Which statement should be made by the nurse related to unauthorized access to client information and HIPAA?

1. "Any nurse employed by the organization may access client records."
2. "Unauthorized access of the client record may result in criminal conviction or loss of job."
3. "Audits of medical records are completed to protect clients from unauthorized access."
4. "Consent needs to be given by the client for reimbursement from third-party payers."

**60.** MoC The nurse is reviewing the client's EMR. The nurse allows a colleague who is not caring for the client to view the screen. Place an X on the areas of the computer screen that violate the HIPAA if viewed by a non–care provider.

**Electronic Medical Record:** Maple, John

→ Summary → H&P → Notes → Flowsheets → Imaging → Lab → Surgery → Allergies

| John Maple | MRN | DOB | Age | Gender | Physician |
|---|---|---|---|---|---|
| | 12345 | 11/25/36 | 71 | male | Nelson |

| Date: Today | 0400 | 0800 | 1015 | 1200 | 1400 | 1600 | 1800 | 2000 | 2200 | 2359 |
|---|---|---|---|---|---|---|---|---|---|---|
| BP Systole | 120 | 132 | | 134 | | | | | | |
| BP Diastole | 86 | 80 | | 72 | | | | | | |
| Pulse | 84 | 90 | | 72 | | | | | | |
| Respirations | 16 | 20 | | 16 | | | | | | |
| Temperature | 98.6 | 99.4 | | 98.2 | | | | | | |
| SpO2 | 97 | 98 | | 98 | | | | | | |
| Oxygen | 21 | | | | | | | | | |
| Oxygen Source | NC | | | | | | | | | |
| Pain (0-10) | 2 | 2 | 5 | 1 | 1 | | | | | |

**Notes:**
0400 Awake. Pain rating of 2. Refuses analgesic. Ambulated to bathroom independently.
0800 Increase in temperature of 99.4. Wife called and updated with current status. Will be in mid-morning.
1015 Increase in pain rating to 5. One Vicodin given.
1045 Pain rating 2.
1200 Wife here. Resting comfortably.

**61.** MoC Two clients are in a semiprivate hospital room. The HCP is about to inform client A of a cancer diagnosis. Which statement by the nurse is **best** when attempting to maintain client confidentiality?

1. To client B: "This would be a good time to go for a walk. The doctor needs to tell your roommate something confidential."
2. To the HCP: "For privacy, could you please wait to tell client A about his cancer? His roommate will be going home in a couple of hours."
3. To client B: "The doctor needs to talk to your roommate. Could you please turn on your TV and not listen to what they say?"
4. To client B: "I would like to walk you down to the lounge for 10 or 15 minutes. It's good for your lungs to do some deep breathing with activity."

**62.** MoC The nurse sees the HCP reviewing the client's medical record. After the HCP leaves, the nurse picks up the chart and notices that this HCP is not involved in this client's care. Which professional action should be taken by the nurse?

1. Report the event to the immediate supervisor.
2. Call the HCP and confront him/her with reading the medical record.
3. Report the HCP to the chief of staff.
4. No action is required; all HCPs may look at any client records.

**63.** MoC PHARM The HCP writes the following orders for the client admitted in sickle cell crisis: "Oxygen 2L/NC, MS 4 mg IV now, one unit PRBCs, and hydroxyurea 250 mg oral daily." Which nursing intervention is **most** important?

1. Initiate all orders as prescribed by the HCP.
2. Telephone the HCP to clarify the MS order.
3. Prepare to give 4 mg MS after initiating the oxygen.
4. Telephone the lab to draw blood for a type and crossmatch.

**64.** MoC The older adult client is hospitalized with chest pain. Which interventions should the nurse implement when the client states his religious beliefs prevent him from taking any medications except an unknown supplement for bowel regulation? **Select all that apply.**

1. Document in the client's medical record that the client takes an unknown supplement for bowel regulation.
2. Determine the name of the individual who advised the client about the supplement.
3. Instruct the client that medications not prescribed by the HCP are dangerous and may cause chest pain.
4. Ask the client's family to bring in the supplement, and document the request in the client's medical record.
5. Ask the client the last time the supplement was taken and the amount that was taken.

**65.** MoC The female nurse is to care for the male client who is an Iraqi immigrant. Which approach demonstrates culturally sensitive care?

1. Ask that the client inform the nurse when wishing to pray.
2. Ask interview questions but avoid eye contact with the client.
3. Ask the client if he would prefer to be cared for by the male nurse.
4. Ask the client to identify any cultural preferences while hospitalized.

**66.** MoC The female client and her husband request that only females care for her, citing religious beliefs. Which actions should the nurse manager take in responding to this request? **Select all that apply.**

1. Explain that a hospital treating clients of the Islamic faith employs only female nurses.
2. State that only female nurses and NAs will be assigned to care for the client.
3. Explain that the request will be forwarded to the client advocate representative.
4. Reassure the client and her husband that all cultures and religious beliefs are respected.
5. Post a sign that states only female staff members should enter the client's room.

**67.** **MoC** The hospitalized client, who speaks only Spanish, is diagnosed with a pancreatic tumor. Which is the nurse's **best** plan when preparing for a scheduled conference of the client, surgeon, and family to discuss the client's treatment options?

1. Contact the appropriate hospital department and request a hospital-approved Spanish interpreter to attend the planned meeting.
2. Request that the client's adult son, whom the client named as an advocate, be present to translate for the surgeon.
3. Obtain information from the Internet about the client's treatment options in English and Spanish and give this to the surgeon.
4. Ask that the Spanish-speaking NA working on the unit be available to interpret for the client and the family.

**68.** **MoC** When no interpreter is available, the HCP asks the Spanish-speaking nurse to act as interpreter for the Spanish-speaking client. If the facility does not have a specific policy, which source would **best** help the nurse decide whether it would be appropriate to function as an interpreter?

1. National Council on Interpreting in Health Care
2. American Nurses Association (ANA) Code of Ethics
3. The HCP who is asking the nurse to interpret
4. The nurse manager on the hospital unit

**69.** **MoC** The family brings a sick child to the ED. Upon examination, the nurse sees the markings illustrated on the child's back. Which interpretation of the clinical finding is correct?

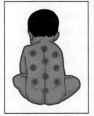

1. Consistent with the practice of coining
2. Insignificant because these are not related to the infant's illness
3. Consistent with findings of abuse and should be reported immediately
4. Consistent with cultural practices but needs to be reported as possible abuse

**70.** **MoC** **PHARM** The nurse is preparing to administer a medication that can only be administered via the subcutaneous route to the 81-year-old client who is intermittently confused and only speaks Chinese. There are no family visiting. Which nursing intervention is **best** after determining that an interpreter is unavailable?

1. Ask another nurse to hold the client's arm while administering the medication promptly; smile while praising the client for cooperating.
2. Use gestures and pictures to explain the medication and administration; if consent is obtained with a head nod, administer the medication.
3. Retime the administration of the medication for that day so that it will be administered when the daughter is present.
4. Notify the HCP that the client will likely be uncooperative, and request that the medication be changed to an intravenous route.

**71.** **MoC** The newly hospitalized client tells the nurse about treating the body and soul with *hanyak*. Based on this information, which statement by the nurse is **most** appropriate?

1. "Tell me more about what is in the herbal remedy that you have been using."
2. "When was the last time a healing ritual was performed by the shaman?"
3. "Have you had any other therapies such as acupressure and moxibustion?"
4. "Show me the site on your body where you were treated with the acupuncture."

**72.** **MoC** The hospitalized client is asking if a voodoo shrine can be set up within the client's room. Which action should be taken by the nurse?

1. Inform the client that this is against hospital policy.
2. Initiate a referral to the pastoral care department.
3. Assist the client in planning where to set up the shrine.
4. Determine the client's reason for requesting the shrine.

**73.** The client who recently emigrated from Somalia is on isolation precautions because of possible active tuberculosis. Which intervention should the nurse implement to **best** improve the client's coping?

1. Allow family members to translate when discussing the treatment plan.
2. Encourage the family to bring traditional foods for the client.
3. Have the client ambulate around the care unit frequently.
4. Contact the chaplain so that the client can receive communion.

**74.** MoC The nurse is caring for the hospitalized female client from Somalia who is a practicing Muslim. Which intervention shows the **greatest** degree of culturally competent nursing care?

1. Informing the client it is unnecessary to fast during Ramadan
2. Bringing a prayer rug for the client to use during prayer time
3. Relaying at shift report that the client's religion prohibits transfusions
4. Arranging for a dietitian to discuss a vegetarian diet with the client

**75.** MoC The student nurse is discussing Lawrence Kohlberg's theory of moral development as it pertains to middle-aged adults with the experienced nurse. Which statement should the experienced nurse correct?

1. "Middle-aged adults are usually concerned about basic individual rights of others."
2. "Middle-aged adults attempt to understand the values and beliefs of others."
3. "Middle-aged adults are focused on their careers and are less concerned about morals."
4. "Middle-aged adults use their own chosen ethical principles when making moral decisions."

**76.** MoC The nurse fails to obtain scheduled VS at 0200 hours for the client who had cardiac surgery 2 days ago. After assessing the client at 0600 hours, the nurse documents the 0600 HR for both the 0200 and 0600 VS. Which conclusion should the supervising charge nurse make about the nurse's actions? **Select all that apply.**

1. The nurse's action was acceptable; neither complications nor harmful effects occurred.
2. The nurse's action is legally concerning; the nurse fraudulently falsified documentation.
3. The nurse's action demonstrates beneficence; the nurse decided what was best for the client.
4. The nurse's action is extremely concerning; it involves the ethical issue of veracity.
5. The nurse's action demonstrates distributive justice; other clients' needs were priority.

**77.** MoC The nurse overhears a UAP reprimanding a resident of the nursing home, stating, "You soiled your underwear again. If you don't call me soon enough next time you need to use the bathroom, I will put a diaper on you." Which tort has the UAP committed?

1. Libel
2. Battery
3. Assault
4. Invasion of privacy

**78.** MoC The adolescent with a history of a renal transplant has not been taking medications as prescribed. The result has been loss of the kidney. The multidisciplinary team, which includes the nurse, is considering whether the client should receive a second transplant. What should be the **next** course of action?

1. Allow the client to decide.
2. Allow the managing HCP to decide.
3. Refer the case to the institution's ethics committee.
4. Perform another transplant only if the bill can be paid.

**79.** MoC A friend brings the older adult client who is homeless to a free health screening clinic. The friend is unable to continue administering the client's morning and evening insulin dose for treating type 1 DM. When advocating for this client, which action by the nurse is **most** appropriate?

1. Notify Adult Protective Services about the client's condition and living situation.
2. Ask where the client lives and whether someone else could administer the insulin.
3. Arrange with a local homeless shelter to have someone give the insulin injections.
4. Have the client return to the screening clinic morning and evening to receive the injections.

**80.** MoC The OR circulating nurse is preparing for a surgical procedure. Which aspects of the Universal Protocol should the nurse verify? **Select all that apply.**

1. The correct type of anesthesia
2. The correct surgical incision site
3. The correct IV infusion rate
4. Two unique client identifiers
5. The correct surgical procedure

**81.** MoC CPR is in progress when the client's wife and teenage son arrive. The nurse intercepts them and tries to move them away from the room, but the wife states, "He needs us there to pray for him!" The son keeps walking and attempts to enter. Which action is **most** appropriate?

1. Call for a member of the clergy to be with the wife and son outside of the client's room.
2. Explain that they will be taken into the room by a designated person who will stay with them.
3. Touch the wife and son to console and detain them and explain what is taking place.
4. Page for security to be available in case the client's wife and son become uncontrollable.

**82.** MoC The nurse is teaching a group of middle-aged, female nurses about middle-aged moral development applicable only to women. Which point should the nurse **most** specifically address?

1. Gilligan's moral development theory includes responsibility and caring for self and others.
2. Kohlberg's moral development theory includes living according to universally agreed-upon principles.
3. Westerhoff's stages of faith include putting faith into personal and social action and standing up for beliefs.
4. Fowler's stages of spiritual development include becoming aware of truth from a variety of viewpoints.

# Answers and Rationales

**1.** MoC **ANSWER: 2**

1. Although the client's wishes should be indicated on the plan of care, this nursing action does not demonstrate advocating for the client.
2. **In advocating for the client, the nurse should contact the HCP and encourage the client to tell the family about the decision. To advocate for someone means to speak on behalf of that person.**
3. An HCP order is required to discontinue treatment.
4. The nurse must act on the client's request when the request is made and not wait until additional treatments are prescribed.

▶ *Test-taking Tip: Note the key word "suddenly," which indicates the decision is new. The nurse should function within the scope of nursing practice.*

Content Area: Management of Care; Concept: Management; Regulations; Integrated Processes: Caring; Client Needs: Safe and Effective Care Environment: Management of Care; Cognitive Level: Application [Applying]

**2.** MoC **ANSWER: 1**

1. **The primary role in advocacy is to keep the client safe—to safeguard clients against abuse and violation of their rights. Clients may not be able to advocate for themselves.**
2. The professional role of the nurse is to defend the client's autonomy in decision making. The nurse must never make a treatment decision for clients.
3. The nurse should keep clients informed about their treatment orders and their rights.
4. Although it is important to know the clients' values, it is not the primary role of the nurse advocate.

▶ *Test-taking Tip: "Primary role" are key words. Recall that advocacy focuses on clients' rights; thus eliminate options 2 and 4. Of the remaining two options, select the option that demonstrates a stronger nursing role.*

Content Area: Management of Care; Concept: Management; Integrated Processes: Nursing Process: Planning; Client Needs: Safe and Effective Care Environment: Management of Care; Cognitive Level: Application [Applying]

**3.** MoC **ANSWER: 20**

**Based on the concentration, the pump should be set at 20 mL/hr. Use a proportion formula to calculate the rate.**
**25,000 : 500 mL :: 1000 : X;**
**Multiply the outside values and then the inside values and solve for X.**
**$25,000X = 500 \times 1000$; $X = 500,000 \div 25,000$; $X = 20$**

▶ *Test-taking Tip: Always calculate infusion rates at the beginning of the shift to identify errors. In this situation, the infusion rate was 10 mL/h faster than prescribed.*

Content Area: Management of Care; Concept: Legal; Integrated Processes: Nursing Process: Analysis; Client Needs: Safe and Effective Care Environment: Management of Care; Cognitive Level: Application [Applying]

**4.** MoC **ANSWER: 2, 4**

1. The nurse may not give medical advice, but the nurse can listen to the client, advocate, and teach where appropriate.
2. **This response provides an opportunity to identify any misunderstandings that the client may have and provide an opportunity to teach.**
3. The client has a right to a second opinion. But when the nurse makes the inquiry in this manner, it may convey a message that a second opinion is necessary rather than optional.
4. **With the client's permission, a meeting with the oncologist, client, and the client's family may assist with the client's decision making regarding treatment options.**
5. It is inappropriate for the nurse to state the treatment options that he or she would choose.

▶ *Test-taking Tip: Focus on the nursing process and choose options that demonstrate that the nurse is advocating for the client. Eliminate the options that would block therapeutic communication.*

Content Area: Management of Care; Concept: Ethics; Integrated Processes: Caring; Client Needs: Safe and Effective Care Environment: Management of Care; Cognitive Level: Application [Applying]

## 5. MoC ANSWER: 3, 4, 5

1. Listening is important, but in this situation the nurse should further act and advocate by assisting the client in a frank discussion with the HCP.
2. Keeping client's confidences is important. The nurse should encourage and assist the client to discuss decisions with the HCP. Only if there is a discussion can the client's wishes be achieved.
3. **The nurse has a duty to act in the client's best interests. If the care the client is receiving is unacceptable, the nurse must advocate.**
4. **The last opportunity to catch errors prior to discharge from the hospital falls to the nurse. If it is clear that the client has not received all the necessary paperwork or a prescription is missing, the nurse must clarify this with the HCP prior to discharging the client. Clopidogrel (Plavix) requires a prescription.**
5. **If the nurse is concerned that the client has not received adequate medical screening or treatment, the nurse must seek clarification from the HCP or the nursing supervisor prior to discharging the client home.**

▶ *Test-taking Tip: Advocacy involves a discussion with another person to protect the health, safety, and the rights of the client. Consider the options that represent the nurse acting in the client's best interest.*

Content Area: Management of Care; Concept: Ethics; Integrated Processes: Teaching/Learning; Client Needs: Safe and Effective Care Environment: Management of Care; Cognitive Level: Application [Applying]

## 6. MoC ANSWER: 4

1. Although it may have been prudent for the client to arrange for transportation, the nurse must protect the client's health and safety, especially after receiving moderate sedation.
2. It is inappropriate to give money to clients.
3. The discharging nurse is responsible for the nurse's own actions. If the nurse follows the advice of the charge nurse, both the charge nurse and the discharging nurse would be held accountable for any untoward client outcome.
4. **The nurse should be familiar with available resources and consult a social worker.**

▶ *Test-taking Tip: You should relate "inability to pay" with option 4 "state funded."*

Content Area: Management of Care; Concept: Ethics; Integrated Processes: Nursing Process: Planning; Client Needs: Safe and Effective Care Environment: Management of Care; Cognitive Level: Analysis [Analyzing]

## 7. MoC ANSWER: 1

1. **Nonmaleficence is doing no harm, either intentionally or unintentionally. The nurse unintentionally harmed the client by failing to open the oxygen tank valve.**
2. Fidelity is the obligation of an individual to be faithful.
3. Veracity is truth-telling.
4. Justice is the obligation to be fair to all people.

▶ *Test-taking Tip: Focus on the nurse's actions. A memory aid is remembering "__non__maleficence" is "__not__ harm."*

Content Area: Management of Care; Concept: Ethics; Integrated Processes: Nursing Process: Analysis; Client Needs: Safe and Effective Care Environment: Management of Care; Cognitive Level: Application [Applying]

## 8. MoC ANSWER: 2

1. In the some cultures, the oldest male traditionally makes health care decisions and may answer questions for female clients. Administering the analgesic without the spouse present would be unethical.
2. **The first stage of ethical decision making is to collect, analyze, and interpret the data. The spouse may not have enough information about pain and pain management. Education may provide the information to assist him in making a decision without compromising his cultural beliefs.**
3. Not treating the pain would be unethical. Promoting comfort is a nursing responsibility.
4. Reporting to the supervisor may result in an action to relieve pain, although it would cause delay.

▶ *Test-taking Tip: The nurse should advocate for the client while still respecting the wishes of all involved. Advocacy involves a discussion with another person to protect the health, safety, and the rights of the client.*

Content Area: Management of Care; Concept: Ethics; Diversity; Integrated Processes: Nursing Process: Assessment; Culture and Spirituality; Client Needs: Safe and Effective Care Environment: Management of Care; Cognitive Level: Application [Applying]

## 9. MoC ANSWER: 4

1. The nurse should not expect a change in the number of client assignments. The nurse did not follow the correct procedure in administering medications.
2. There is no indication that the first nurse did not follow procedure in administering medications correctly.
3. Although disciplinary action varies by organization, generally a pattern of incompetent actions must be demonstrated for suspension or termination.
4. **The nurse who made the error should expect to be told to complete a variance report that would be reviewed by management. A complete review of the situation needs to occur, including the type of medication, dose, outcome of the client, and steps of medication administration, including documentation.**

▶ **Test-taking Tip:** *Focus on the professional responsibility of the nurse and look for the strategic words "variance" and "reviewed."*

**Content Area:** Management of Care; **Concept:** Regulations; Legal; **Integrated Processes:** Communication and Documentation; **Client Needs:** Safe and Effective Care Environment: Management of Care; **Cognitive Level:** Analysis [Analyzing]

## 10. MoC ANSWER: 4

1. This response does not demonstrate therapeutic communication with a family member and does not offer comfort, only information.
2. Generally, a family member may not rescind a DNR order agreed upon by a competent person.
3. This response is judgmental and therefore not therapeutic.
4. **This is the most therapeutic response based on the situation. Generally, a family member may not rescind a DNR order agreed upon by a competent person.**

▶ **Test-taking Tip:** *If a competent individual wishes no heroic measure, this directive should be respected by all HCPs. The nurse should advocate for the client's wishes. Advocacy involves a discussion with another person to protect the health, safety, and the rights of the client. Narrow the options to the only two options that involve other individuals, and then to option 4 because it respects the client's wishes.*

**Content Area:** Management of Care; **Concept:** Ethics; Legal; **Integrated Processes:** Caring; **Client Needs:** Safe and Effective Care Environment: Management of Care; **Cognitive Level:** Analysis [Analyzing]

## 11. MoC ANSWER: 3

1. Although the client's behavior is distasteful, the client retains the right to respectful care. It is unacceptable to leave the towel over the client's face during restraint application.
2. The client's medical history should be on a need-to-know basis. There is no need to disclose the HIV status to nonmedical staff; all staff should be using standard precautions.
3. **The client has a right to respectful care. The nurse should intervene immediately by instructing the security officer to remove the towel from the client's face.**
4. If the security officer fails to follow the nurse's direction, the next step is to instruct the officer to leave the room, but this would not be the most appropriate first response, as the security officer's help is still needed in restraining the client.

▶ **Test-taking Tip:** *You should recognize that clients have a right to respectful care. This should direct you to option 3 as the only logical answer.*

**Content Area:** Management of Care; **Concept:** Ethics; Legal; **Integrated Processes:** Caring; **Client Needs:** Safe and Effective Care Environment: Management of Care; **Cognitive Level:** Application [Applying]

## 12. MoC ANSWER: 1

1. **The graduate nurse should inform the charge nurse or the nurse manager because they have the authority to intervene.**
2. The nurse should not gossip with a peer regarding the situation.
3. While there are state peer assistance programs, it is not the best action for the graduate nurse.
4. Confronting the impaired nurse is not advisable. The graduate nurse does not have the authority to handle the situation.

▶ **Test-taking Tip:** *You should use the chain of command to answer this question correctly.*

**Content Area:** Management of Care; **Concept:** Ethics; Legal; **Integrated Processes:** Nursing Process: Implementation; **Client Needs:** Safe and Effective Care Environment: Management of Care; **Cognitive Level:** Application [Applying]

## 13. MoC ANSWER: 4

1. The nurse is interjecting a possible reason without exploring the daughter's reason for not telling her mother about the cancer diagnosis.
2. It is true that the client has a right to know, but the response is not therapeutic and is challenging.
3. Although this response informs the daughter of the client's right to know her diagnosis, it does not address the daughter's concern. The HCP, and not the nurse, should be discussing the diagnosis with the client.
4. **The best response is to discuss the daughter's concern with the oncologist and then decide the best approach. The client has a right to know the diagnosis, and information would not be withheld from the client unless there is a reason to do so.**

▶ **Test-taking Tip:** *Use the nursing process step of assessment. Additional information is needed, and only one option provides an opportunity to collect additional information.*

**Content Area:** Management of Care; **Concept:** Ethics; **Integrated Processes:** Caring; **Client Needs:** Safe and Effective Care Environment: Management of Care; **Cognitive Level:** Application [Applying]

## 14. MoC ANSWER: 4, 5

1. The nurse client relationship may not exceed certain boundaries. The nurse must avoid becoming emotionally attached to the client, any physical or sexual relationship with the client, financial gain, or accepting gifts or tips from the client. A gift directed at the individual nurse is inappropriate, even if a token, and should be declined.
2. The nurse and client becoming contacts on a social networking site is not advisable; this exceeds professional boundaries.
3. Accepting a position as a private duty nurse may be seen as a financial gain and should be avoided; this exceeds professional boundaries.
4. **Accepting a hug from the client is okay as long as it does not become a physical relationship.**

5. **Often the client or families send food or candy to a nursing unit as a thank you. This type of gesture is long-standing in many facilities and seen as acceptable.**

♦ **Test-taking Tip:** *Think about how to keep your relationship with the client on a professional level and then eliminate the options that do not adhere to appropriate professional relationships.*

**Content Area:** Management of Care; **Concept:** Ethics, Integrated Processes: Caring; **Client Needs:** Safe and Effective Care Environment: Management of Care; **Cognitive Level:** Application [Applying]

15. MoC **ANSWER: 2**
1. This statement is correct in relation to client rights, but it does not directly relate to the refusal of treatment.
2. **When the client is admitted to a health care facility, the client is entitled to specific rights that include the right to make decisions and refuse treatment.**
3. This statement is correct in relation to client rights, but it does not directly relate to the refusal of treatment.
4. The client has the right to refuse treatment based on religious beliefs.

♦ **Test-taking Tip:** *Eliminate options that do not deal with the client's rights and care. Then of the two options, determine which specifically addresses the issue of the client's religious beliefs.*

**Content Area:** Management of Care; **Concept:** Legal; Diversity; **Integrated Processes:** Nursing Process: Analysis; Culture and Spirituality; **Client Needs:** Safe and Effective Care Environment: Management of Care; **Cognitive Level:** Analysis [Analyzing]

16. MoC **ANSWER: 1**
1. **When an unconscious client presents with a life-threatening emergency, treatment may begin without obtaining informed consent.**
2. Informed consent must be obtained for a child who is ill. In most states, if the ED personnel cannot reach the parents, informed consent must be obtained from the school personnel who are acting in place of the parents (*in loco parentis*).
3. Giving blood or blood products without informed consent to someone who is of the Jehovah's Witness faith violates client rights and could result in legal action.
4. The pregnant teen is able to provide consent for treatment. The client's condition is not life-threatening.

♦ **Test-taking Tip:** *Select the option in which the person is most likely unable to provide an informed consent. A reasonable person would want treatment under such circumstances and would give consent, if able; consent is implied.*

**Content Area:** Management of Care; **Concept:** Legal; **Integrated Processes:** Nursing Process: Planning; **Client Needs:** Safe and Effective Care Environment: Management of Care; **Cognitive Level:** Analysis [Analyzing]

17. MoC **ANSWER: 2**
1. The HCP cannot make treatment decisions without the consent of the client.
2. **Clients have the right to make decisions based on personal values and beliefs.**
3. The family cannot make treatment decisions without the consent of the client.
4. It is important to notify the HCP about the client's fear of the biopsy; however, it does not address the client's understanding of client rights.

♦ **Test-taking Tip:** *You should focus on selecting the option that would support client rights.*

**Content Area:** Management of Care; **Concept:** Ethics; **Integrated Processes:** Caring; **Client Needs:** Safe and Effective Care Environment: Management of Care; **Cognitive Level:** Analysis [Analyzing]

18. MoC **ANSWER: 2**
1. This response demonstrates an understanding of what could happen if the client declines treatment, but option 2 is the better option.
2. **This response shows that the client understands that, without treatment, the client could die. As long as the client is competent and has been fully informed of the risks and consequences of declining treatment and makes an informed decision, the client's choice must be respected.**
3. The client should not have to choose between cost and treatment. The client should be Medicare eligible, and financial assistance may be available.
4. If the client has been informed that she or he could die without treatment, a statement about being okay may not be based on reality.

♦ **Test-taking Tip:** *The key word is "best." When deciding between two viable options, look for words in the scenario that are the same as, or similar to, words in an option and decide whether that option will answer the question. Treatment is included in the scenario and in option 2.*

**Content Area:** Management of Care; **Concept:** Legal; **Integrated Processes:** Caring; **Client Needs:** Safe and Effective Care Environment: Management of Care; **Cognitive Level:** Analysis [Analyzing]

19. MoC **ANSWER: 4**
1. The hospital client has a right to high-quality hospital care, not just the best care that would be available.
2. The client's medical record should be accessed only by those directly involved with the client's care.
3. The hospital is responsible for assisting the family with making appropriate discharge planning.
4. **The client has a right to be involved in the discussion of the client's medical condition and the appropriate course of treatment.**

♦ **Test-taking Tip:** *You should be able to narrow the options by eliminating options that violate client confidentiality (option 2) and that are within the responsibilities of health care personnel (option 3). Of the two remaining options, consider which option gives the client control.*

Content Area: Management of Care; Concept: Legal; Integrated Processes: Teaching/Learning; Client Needs: Safe and Effective Care Environment: Management of Care; Cognitive Level: Analysis [Analyzing]

## 20. MoC ANSWER: 3

1. If the formulation prescribed is not available, a medication request to the pharmacy should include the name of the medication, dose, route, and frequency. Requesting a pink hydrocodone plus acetaminophen (Vicodin) is inappropriate; the pharmacy would not change medication suppliers without prior notification.
2. What may have occurred previously is speculation, so completing a variance report is premature.
3. **Reporting the event to the supervisor allows the supervisor to investigate the situation before action is initiated.**
4. Confronting the nurse is premature.

▸ **Test-taking Tip:** You should use the chain of command to answer this question correctly.

Content Area: Management of Care; Concept: Legal; Integrated Processes: Nursing Process: Analysis; Client Needs: Safe and Effective Care Environment: Management of Care; Cognitive Level: Application [Applying]

## 21. MoC ANSWER: 3

1. Agency policy should be followed, and the appropriate person, usually the security officer, will notify the police if a crime has occurred.
2. An incident report should be completed, but it is not the next action.
3. **Because a crime may have occurred, the security officer should be notified immediately.**
4. The inventory of the client's possessions should be completed by or in the presence of the security officer.

▸ **Test-taking Tip:** Focus on the fact that the client is alert and oriented, and that a crime may have occurred. Note the similarities between options 1 and 3.

Content Area: Management of Care; Concept: Legal; Integrated Processes: Nursing Process: Implementation; Client Needs: Safe and Effective Care Environment: Management of Care; Cognitive Level: Application [Applying]

## 22. MoC ANSWER: 4

1. Although the hospital policy may allow the items to stay with the client, the condition of the client may not allow for continuous monitoring of the items to ensure that they are not lost or stolen.
2. The client's room closet can be accessed by others, and items can be lost or stolen.
3. Because the client still has the jewelry, the client may forget that the cash was taken home by the spouse.
4. **Hospital policy will determine whether the items were handled appropriately in the case of loss.**

▸ **Test-taking Tip:** The key word is "safest." Agency policy and procedures for clients are written with the client's safety in mind.

Content Area: Management of Care; Concept: Regulations; Integrated Processes: Communication and Documentation; Client Needs: Safe and Effective Care Environment: Management of Care; Cognitive Level: Application [Applying]

## 23. MoC ANSWER: 2

1. Individuals diagnosed with HIV may receive treatment, including education and counseling, without consent of the parents.
2. **The best action by the nurse is to treat and then educate the client about birth control, safe sex, and partner disclosure.**
3. It is not necessary to redraw the HIV titer to confirm HIV status.
4. Although it is important to obtain an updated sexual risk history, the parents do not need to be notified of the client's clinic visit.

▸ **Test-taking Tip:** Note that options 1 and 4 both involve the parents, so either one or both of these options must be wrong. Of options 2 and 3, select the option that demonstrates the role of the nurse.

Content Area: Management of Care; Concept: Legal; Integrated Processes: Teaching/Learning; Client Needs: Safe and Effective Care Environment: Management of Care; Cognitive Level: Analysis [Analyzing]

## 24. MoC ANSWER: 1, 2, 3, 4

1. **A gunshot wound meets the requirement for mandatory reporting.**
2. **A communicable disease, such as pertussis, meets the requirement for mandatory reporting.**
3. **A child with cigarette burns suggests abuse and meets the requirement for mandatory reporting.**
4. **An emaciated vulnerable adult suggests malnourishment and meets the requirement for mandatory reporting.**
5. An injury from a fall is not a situation for mandatory reporting.

▸ **Test-taking Tip:** Recall that injuries with weapons, communicable diseases, child abuse, and vulnerable adults are reportable. Use this information to select the correct options.

Content Area: Management of Care; Concept: Legal; Integrated Processes: Nursing Process: Implementation; Client Needs: Safe and Effective Care Environment: Management of Care; Cognitive Level: Application [Applying]

## 25. MoC ANSWER: 1

1. **The HCP should be notified immediately of the break in sterile procedure to reduce risk of infection to the client.**
2. Waiting until after the procedure is completed to talk with the HCP will not prevent this client from a hospital-acquired infection.
3. Although the supervisor may be informed, the break in sterile technique should be corrected immediately.
4. Agency policy may or may not indicate that the break in sterile technique be reported to an Infection Control Nurse.

♦ **Test-taking Tip:** *The nurse has a professional responsibility to protect the client from harm in all situations, regardless of who is providing care. Narrow the options to the only option that protects the client from harm immediately.*

**Content Area:** Management of Care; **Concept:** Legal; **Integrated Processes:** Nursing Process: Implementation; **Client Needs:** Safe and Effective Care Environment: Management of Care; **Cognitive Level:** Analysis [Analyzing]

## 26. MoC ANSWER: 3

1. Performing suctioning without instruction may result in client injury for which the nurse could be liable.
2. Delay in taking action by documenting the findings first could result in client injury and nurse liability.
3. **The nurse should seek instruction prior to performing suctioning; this action should prevent negligence and a possible malpractice lawsuit.**
4. The client's airway should be cleared of secretions immediately before aspiration occurs. Telephoning the HCP will delay suctioning.

♦ **Test-taking Tip:** *You should select the one option that allows for a quick intervention but also protects against a negligent action. Negligence can occur when a procedure is performed incorrectly and may result in a malpractice lawsuit.*

**Content Area:** Management of Care; **Concept:** Legal; **Integrated Processes:** Communication and Documentation; **Client Needs:** Safe and Effective Care Environment: Management of Care; **Cognitive Level:** Analysis [Analyzing]

## 27. MoC ANSWER: 2

1. Placing valuables in a bag without the client's acknowledgment is not good practice. Therefore it is not the best option.
2. **The client's valuables may be placed in a safe while the client is hospitalized. The nurse should ensure that these valuables are obtained at discharge and that the client and nurse sign an acknowledgment that the valuables were returned to the client.**
3. Family members may assist with carrying valuables, but the client should be asked if it is acceptable for the son to carry these rather than being informed by the nurse of the person chosen.
4. Although many facilities have disclosures regarding liability for lost personal belongings, it is not the best response by the nurse to the client.

♦ **Test-taking Tip:** *The key word in the stem is "valuables." Most facilities will have a policy on the care of valuables while the client is hospitalized and the manner of returning these to the client.*

**Content Area:** Management of Care; **Concept:** Legal; **Integrated Processes:** Communication and Documentation; **Client Needs:** Safe and Effective Care Environment: Management of Care; **Cognitive Level:** Application [Applying]

## 28. MoC ANSWER: 1, 2, 3

1. *Respondeat superior* **is usually applicable for nurses employed by an organization. The employer shares responsibility for the nurse's practice with the nurse.**

2. *Respondeat superior* **is usually applicable for nurses employed by an organization. The employer shares responsibility for the nurse's practice with the nurse.**
3. *Respondeat superior* **is usually applicable for nurses employed by an individual. The employer shares responsibility for the nurse's practice with the nurse.**
4. In general, private duty nurses are treated as independent contractors with no employing person or organization. They practice under the control of no one but themselves. An agency that connects the private duty nurse with a person or institution would not be liable for the private duty nurse's actions unless the agency had failed to properly establish the nurse's credentials.
5. As a volunteer, the nurse is not employed by the Salvation Army, so *respondeat superior* would not apply.

♦ **Test-taking Tip:** *The words "most applicable" are key words in the stem. Respondeat superior is usually applicable for nurses employed by an individual or an organization.*

**Content Area:** Management of Care; **Concept:** Legal; **Integrated Processes:** Nursing Process: Implementation; **Client Needs:** Safe and Effective Care Environment: Management of Care; **Cognitive Level:** Application [Applying]

## 29. MoC ANSWER: 2

1. Libel refers to written defamation of character.
2. **The nurse has committed slander, which involves making malicious and false spoken statements about the client. Slander is a type of defamation of character.**
3. Battery refers to touching without consent.
4. Invasion refers to invasion of privacy from the client being illegally searched.

♦ **Test-taking Tip:** *You should remember that slander is making malicious and false statements about someone. Use the "s" in the word slander and the "s" in the word statement as a memory aid to remember the meaning of slander.*

**Content Area:** Management of Care; **Concept:** Legal; **Integrated Processes:** Communication and Documentation; **Client Needs:** Safe and Effective Care Environment: Management of Care; **Cognitive Level:** Knowledge [Remembering]

## 30. MoC ANSWER: 1, 4

1. **A 15-year-old may consent to reproductive care without consent of a parent.**
2. Although under the emergency care doctrine the HCP may provide care in the absence of a parent, a headache is not an emergency, and a 10-year-old should be able to telephone a parent.
3. The law recognizes "mature minors" as those children between the ages of 14 to 17. As long as the child understands the "nature and consequences of the proposed therapy," children may make their own independent decision regarding treatments. However, this child is not old enough.

4. **A 14-year-old child may seek treatment for drug addiction without parental consent.**
5. If the fracture is stable, the parent needs to be consulted and consent obtained.

▶ *Test-taking Tip:* You should narrow the options to reproductive or mental health care. A minor is able to obtain reproductive or mental health care without parental consent.

**Content Area:** Management of Care; **Concept:** Legal; **Integrated Processes:** Teaching/Learning; **Client Needs:** Safe and Effective Care Environment: Management of Care; Physiological Integrity: Reduction of Risk Potential; **Cognitive Level:** Analysis [Analyzing]

**31.** MoC **ANSWER: 4**

1. The subsection "Elopement" is used for situations when the client leaves without informing staff.
2. The statement "I cannot let you leave" could be construed as a threat. The client should never be physically restrained when leaving unless the client has been involuntarily admitted to the hospital for a psychiatric condition.
3. The client has the right to leave the hospital and should not be threatened with death.
4. **The nurse should acknowledge the client's right to leave the hospital but should first attempt to inform the client leaving AMA of the risks of leaving without treatment.**

▶ *Test-taking Tip:* Three options include writing, but one option is different. Often the option that is different is the answer.

**Content Area:** Management of Care; **Concept:** Legal; Management; Communication; **Integrated Processes:** Communication and Documentation; **Client Needs:** Safe and Effective Care Environment: Management of Care; **Cognitive Level:** Application [Applying]

**32.** MoC **ANSWER: 1**

1. **Clearly communicating to the nurse manager that the nurse is not qualified, based on experience, to care for the clients on the proposed unit protects the nurse from liability.**
2. This response is inappropriate because it does not reflect a caring attitude toward the clients in the facility.
3. If the nurse knows that she or he is unqualified to care for the clients on that unit, the nurse risks liability if an error occurs.
4. If the nurse has provided care on the particular unit and is qualified, refusing to float based on a rotating basis may not be the best approach.

▶ *Test-taking Tip:* An appropriate response should clearly communicate whether the nurse is qualified to care for clients on another unit.

**Content Area:** Management of Care; **Concept:** Legal; **Integrated Processes:** Communication and Documentation; **Client Needs:** Safe and Effective Care Environment: Management of Care; **Cognitive Level:** Application [Applying]

**33.** MoC **ANSWER: 3**

1. Although the nurse may be tired and unhappy with the situation, the nurse manager has the responsibility to ensure that clients receive safe nursing care. Although being tired is a reasonable concern, refusing to stay and leaving the unit are considered insubordination.
2. Insufficient disciplinary action is being taken by giving only a verbal reminder; expectations should also be in writing.
3. **"Walking out" when staffing is inadequate constitutes abandonment and is grounds for disciplinary action. The disciplinary action should include a written statement of the employee's behavior, a review of the agency policy related to maintaining adequate staffing and the employee's responsibility in short-staffed situations, and the consequences of future acts of abandonment and insubordination.**
4. Termination of the employee is premature. Although disciplinary action varies by organization, generally a pattern of incompetent actions must be demonstrated for termination to occur. There is no indication that this has occurred before.

▶ *Test-taking Tip:* You should eliminate options that are either too lenient or too severe. Of the remaining two options, think about the action that would best ensure employee compliance in future short-staffing incidences.

**Content Area:** Management of Care; **Concept:** Legal; **Integrated Processes:** Communication and Documentation; **Client Needs:** Safe and Effective Care Environment: Management of Care; **Cognitive Level:** Application [Applying]

**34.** MoC **ANSWER: 3, 4**

1. The child was never brought to the facility; therefore, EMTALA is not triggered.
2. If the client receives the proper medical screening and treatment that a similarly situated client would receive, then EMTALA is not violated. The client left the hospital after treatment with naloxone (Narcan) for heroin overdose in stable condition, but AMA.
3. **The medical screening must be adequate. If the medical screening is not sufficient, then EMTALA would be violated.**
4. **If hospital policy requires that an ECG be done on all clients experiencing chest pain, but the HCP deviates from the policy based on the ability to pay, then EMTALA is violated.**
5. When the medical screening follows the same procedure for similarly situated clients, the hospital does not violate EMTALA.

▶ *Test-taking Tip:* The EMTALA was enacted to prevent denial of care to individuals based on the ability to pay. Medical screening and stabilizing treatment should follow the expected standard of care regardless of the ability to pay. Narrow the options to clients who received inadequate medical screening and care.

**Content Area:** Management of Care; **Concept:** Legal; **Integrated Processes:** Teaching/Learning; **Client Needs:** Safe and Effective Care Environment: Management of Care; **Cognitive Level:** Analysis [Analyzing]

## 35. MoC ANSWER: 3

1. It is not advisable for the nurse to handle a weapon. Calling the police should only be done after consultation with hospital administration to avoid a potential HIPAA violation.
2. The issue is not whether the client has the right to possess the gun; it is that a weapon is on hospital property, which poses a danger to staff, visitors, and clients.
3. **The most appropriate action by the nurse would be to seek the assistance of hospital security to protect staff, visitors, and other clients.**
4. Ignoring the weapon is not the best course of action because it can pose a safety hazard.

♦ **Test-taking Tip:** *Thinking about the safest course of action for all involved should lead you to the answer.*

**Content Area:** Management of Care; **Concept:** Safety; **Integrated Processes:** Nursing Process: Planning; **Client Needs:** Safe and Effective Care Environment: Management of Care; **Cognitive Level:** Analysis [Analyzing]

## 36. MoC ANSWER: 1, 2, 5

1. **All clients seeking emergency medical care from a hospital must have an appropriate medical screening.**
2. **The client may be transferred to another facility if the presenting facility is incapable of properly caring for the client. Certain rules must be followed first before a transfer may proceed.**
3. If the on-call HCP refuses to come to the hospital to see an uninsured client, and if the name of the on-call HCP is not included in the transfer form, the facility risks being fined by Centers for Medicare and Medicaid Services.
4. The client has the right to be treated in the ED regardless of ability to pay. A social worker consult would be helpful in exploring the client's financial situation and assisting the client in exploring financial support for medical care.
5. **The risks and benefits must be explained by the HCP and the information discussed with the client documented on the transfer form.**

♦ **Test-taking Tip:** *EMTALA law ensures that the client receives appropriate screening and medical care despite being uninsured. The key word is "comply." Eliminate options that address the client's financial situation before care is provided.*

**Content Area:** Management of Care; **Concept:** Legal; **Integrated Processes:** Communication and Documentation; **Client Needs:** Safe and Effective Care Environment: Management of Care; **Cognitive Level:** Application [Applying]

## 37. MoC ANSWER: 1

1. **Given the information in the option, the nurse's action for self-protection is the most defensible. The nurse is somewhat isolated, the client is holding onto the nurse, and self-defense by elbowing the client may be the only means of getting out of a dangerous situation.**
2. The nurse has other options to avoid contact with the client's body fluids, such as a facemask with a shield.
3. It is not advisable to search the client's clothing for illegal substances.
4. It is not advisable to hold clients during injections unless the client is subject to forced medication administration under a court order.

♦ **Test-taking Tip:** *Read each option and determine which acts by the nurse can be justified based on the interaction between the client and the nurse.*

**Content Area:** Management of Care; **Concept:** Legal; **Integrated Processes:** Communication and Documentation; **Client Needs:** Safe and Effective Care Environment: Management of Care; **Cognitive Level:** Application [Applying]

## 38. MoC PHARM ANSWER: 20

**The ordered dose is 2 units of insulin per hour.**
**One mL of solution contains 1 unit of insulin.**
**Thus, 20 mL per hour is a dose of 20 units of insulin.**

♦ **Test-taking Tip:** *Calculate the units of insulin per mL to arrive at the correct dose. Remember, you are reporting the units of insulin that the client was receiving and not the correct rate.*

**Content Area:** Management of Care; **Concept:** Safety; Legal; **Integrated Processes:** Nursing Process: Evaluation; Communication and Documentation; **Client Needs:** Safe and Effective Care Environment: Management of Care; Physiological Integrity: Pharmacological and Parenteral Therapies; Physiological Integrity: Reduction of Risk Potential; **Cognitive Level:** Evaluation [Evaluating]

## 39. MoC ANSWER: 1, 2, 4

1. **Each individual state's board of nursing develops rules and regulations delineating forbidden conduct. Practicing outside of the nurse's scope of practice is forbidden conduct. The nurse inserting a central venous access device demonstrates an act outside of the nurse's scope of practice.**
2. **Falsifying the medical record is forbidden conduct that can lead to disciplinary action related to licensure.**
3. An employer may discuss with the nurse the clothing odor and the agency policy. Policy violations may result in disciplinary action and loss of employment if agency policy is not followed, but this would not affect the nurse's license.
4. **Criminal convictions may lead to disciplinary action related to licensure including loss of licensure.**
5. Identifying all previous work experience is appropriate. Misleading employers with false information can lead to disciplinary action related to licensure.

▶ *Test-taking Tip: The key phrase is "disciplinary action related to licensure." Some options may lead to disciplinary action by the nurse manager, but not all actions will affect licensure.*

**Content Area:** Management of Care; **Concept:** Legal; Regulations; **Integrated Processes:** Nursing Process: Evaluation; **Client Needs:** Safe and Effective Care Environment: Management of Care; **Cognitive Level:** Evaluation [Evaluating]

### 40. MoC ANSWER: 2

1. Many states have mandatory partner notification of HIV/AIDS status to protect the public at large.
2. **All states require that HIV/AIDS infection be reported to the CDC for epidemiological purposes.**
3. The HIV status of an individual is on a need-to-know basis, and only the nurse providing care for the client might know the client's status, not all nurses on the unit.
4. The HCPs directly involved in the client's care may discuss the client's health issues and HIV status without the client's consent to provide safe, effective care.

▶ *Test-taking Tip: You need to select the option that correctly states the law in regard to mandatory reporting of infectious diseases.*

**Content Area:** Management of Care; **Concept:** Legal; **Integrated Processes:** Teaching/Learning; **Client Needs:** Safe and Effective Care Environment: Management of Care; **Cognitive Level:** Application [Applying]

### 41. MoC ANSWER: 2

1. The family may touch the equipment; however, they should not operate any client care equipment including answering alarms and reconnecting tubing.
2. **The nurse should inform nonclinical staff, clients, and their families that they must get help from clinical staff whenever there is a real or perceived need to connect or disconnect devices or infusions.**
3. The potential for incorrect reconnection exists.
4. Family members can inadvertently make an error when putting the IV pump on hold and cause client harm.

▶ *Test-taking Tip: Options with absolute words such as "any" or "only" are usually incorrect and should be eliminated.*

**Content Area:** Management of Care; **Concept:** Safety; **Integrated Processes:** Teaching/Learning; **Client Needs:** Safe and Effective Care Environment: Management of Care; **Cognitive Level:** Evaluation [Evaluating]

### 42. CJ MoC PHARM ANSWER: 3

1. Although the surgeon indicated to restart the heparin, there is no indication that the previous rate was 25 mL.
2. Although the first line of the protocol is to bolus with 5000 units and administer heparin infusion at a rate of 31 mL/hr, there is no indication that this was the client's previous rate.

3. **The nurse should contact the surgeon because the order is not clear as to what rate to start the heparin.**
4. The nurse cannot assume that the intended rate is 28 mL/hr; the order is unclear.

▶ *Test-taking Tip: Carefully read the directions from the HCPs. Note there is no clear direction. The nurse should never guess or assume what the HCP meant to write. Three options restart heparin, and one option is different. Often the option that is different is the answer.*

**Content Area:** Management of Care; **Concept:** Safety; **Integrated Processes:** Communication and Documentation; **Client Needs:** Safe and Effective Care Environment: Management of Care; Physiological Integrity: Pharmacological and Parenteral Therapies; Physiological Integrity: Reduction of Risk Potential; **Cognitive Level:** Analysis [Analyzing]

### 43. CJ MoC ANSWER:

| Negligence or malpractice. |
|---|

**Negligence is a failure to do what a reasonably prudent person would do in similar circumstances. Malpractice is failure to provide the care based on the standards of nursing practice, in this case, failure to clarify the order with the prescribing surgeon.**

▶ *Test-taking Tip: Focus on the key word, "unintentional tort," which is an unintended accident that leads to injury.*

**Content Area:** Management of Care; **Concept:** Legal; **Integrated Processes:** Nursing Process: Analysis; **Client Needs:** Safe and Effective Care Environment: Management of Care; **Cognitive Level:** Application [Applying]

### 44. MoC ANSWER: 1

1. **ST segment elevation indicates myocardial injury. If the nurse fails to recognize and act on the early symptoms of a possible MI, then the nurse has not fulfilled the duty of care owed to the client.**
2. Although ST segment elevation indicates myocardial injury, this elevation is greater than in option 1. The nurse should have notified the HCP with an earlier change in the ST segment.
3. T wave depression may be indicative of ischemia without infarction, but this illustration shows progression, so the nurse should have notified the HCP sooner.
4. T wave inversion may occur 6 to 24 hours after the ischemic event. If the nurse waits to notify at this point, the nurse would be clearly negligent.

▶ *Test-taking Tip: You must be familiar with the early signs of MI. It is imperative to recognize the ECG changes early on and report accordingly. Thus, the earliest change (option 1) should be selected for the answer.*

**Content Area:** Management of Care; **Concept:** Legal; **Integrated Processes:** Nursing Process: Analysis; **Client Needs:** Safe and Effective Care Environment: Management of Care; Physiological Integrity: Reduction of Risk Potential; **Cognitive Level:** Analysis [Analyzing]

**45.** MoC **ANSWER: 4**

1. A semiprivate room is one that has a roommate. The confused client may be disruptive to the other client.
2. Assigning the client to a small private room at the end of the hallway is too far away for frequent observations.
3. A seclusion room is inappropriate for the confused client unless the client's behavior warrants the seclusion.
4. **Large, uncluttered areas in close proximity to monitor client activity tend to promote safety for most confused clients.**

▶ *Test-taking Tip: The key word is "safety." Note that the client is confused and restless.*

**Content Area:** Management of Care; **Concept:** Safety; **Integrated Processes:** Nursing Process: Assessment; **Client Needs:** Safe and Effective Care Environment: Management of Care; Physiological Integrity: Reduction of Risk Potential; **Cognitive Level:** Application [Applying]

**46.** MoC PHARM **ANSWER: 1, 3, 5**

1. **The charge nurse should be aware that the IV solution was incorrectly labeled.**
2. The IV solution should not be administered because it is not the correct solution.
3. **The pharmacist should be aware that the IV solution was incorrectly labeled and that the correct IV solution needs to be provided.**
4. The solution is incorrect, not the label.
5. **Safe medication practices include knowing the organization's policy for reporting potential medication errors.**

▶ *Test-taking Tip: You should note that the IV solution is incorrect and then identify actions to prevent a medication error.*

**Content Area:** Management of Care; **Concept:** Safety; **Integrated Processes:** Nursing Process: Implementation; **Client Needs:** Safe and Effective Care Environment: Management of Care; Physiological Integrity: Pharmacological and Parenteral Therapies; **Cognitive Level:** Analysis [Analyzing]

**47.** MoC **ANSWER: 1, 2, 4**

1. **The HCP should be notified; new orders may need to be obtained for IV insulin and glucose.**
2. **The charge nurse should be informed of errors for later follow-up. The charge nurse can also provide assistance in implementing new orders and monitoring the client.**
3. An HCP order is needed to obtain a STAT serum potassium level; the level has likely not changed because insulin administered subcutaneously has a slower onset of action.
4. **The medication error must be reported using an incident form or variance, situational or unusual occurrence report form for later follow-up, and root cause analysis to prevent future errors.**

5. A copy of the incident form should never be placed in the client's medical record; it is for agency follow-up and prevention of future errors.

▶ *Test-taking Tip: Narrow the options to include those pertaining to HCP, charge nurse, and facility communication of the error.*

**Content Area:** Management of Care; **Concept:** Nursing Roles; **Integrated Processes:** Nursing Process: Implementation; **Client Needs:** Safe and Effective Care Environment: Safety and Infection Control; **Cognitive Level:** Application [Applying]

**48. ANSWER: 4**

1. It is irrelevant that the surgeon is not employed by the hospital; the hospital may still suffer consequences unless there is a legitimate reason for the surgeon's failure to see and examine the client.
2. Although the hospital may undergo review by on-site surveyors from accrediting or licensing agencies, the hospital will not automatically lose its accreditation due to the surgeon's actions.
3. There is no per se fine for the failure of the on-call surgeon to respond to a call to see the client emergently. If there is a legitimate reason, there may not be a fine.
4. **The hospital could be cited and fined if the name and address of the nonresponding surgeon is not documented in the client's medical record.**

▶ *Test-taking Tip: The question is asking for the consequences to a hospital. You will note that options 1, 2, and 3 contain absolute actions, "will" and "cannot," whereas option 4 contains "may." Often the option that is different is the answer.*

**Content Area:** Management of Care; **Concept:** Legal; **Integrated Processes:** Communication and Documentation; **Client Needs:** Safe and Effective Care Environment: Safety and Infection Control; **Cognitive Level:** Comprehension [Understanding]

**49.** MoC **ANSWER: 4**

1. A signature on the consent form does not ensure client knowledge of risks and benefits.
2. Minor children may not sign informed consent unless emancipated.
3. The consent of both parents is not required for a medical procedure.
4. **Obtaining informed consent should be done after determining that the client's parents have a reasonable understanding of the information presented. The client's parents should understand the procedure, risks, benefits, and alternatives to the recommended procedure. It is the responsibility of the surgeon to obtain informed consent for the medical procedure.**

▶ *Test-taking Tip: The key words are "best thinking." You should look for the statement that is most complete.*

**Content Area:** Management of Care; **Concept:** Regulations; **Integrated Processes:** Nursing Process: Analysis; **Client Needs:** Safe and Effective Care Environment: Management of Care; **Cognitive Level:** Analysis [Analyzing]

**50.** MoC **ANSWER: 1**

1. **If the nurse continues with the procedure, the nurse could be accused of battery (unconsented touching). A discussion is in order with the HCP to determine the best approach.**
2. If the nurse continues to touch the client when the client has clearly indicated that she does not want to be touched, the nurse risks being liable for battery.
3. Attempting to discuss the importance of the procedure to the somewhat confused client is not the best approach.
4. The nurse may not direct staff to use force to hold the client during a procedure.

▶ *Test-taking Tip: Three options are similar, and one is different. Often the option that is different is the answer.*

Content Area: Management of Care; Concept: Legal; Integrated Processes: Caring; Client Needs: Safe and Effective Care Environment: Management of Care; Cognitive Level: Application [Applying]

**51.** MoC **ANSWER: 2**

1. Under some state laws, the client may not be able to refuse having a blood sample taken. However, to avoid liability, five conditions should be met: (1) The client must be under formal arrest; (2) the evidence sought has potential use in a criminal prosecution; (3) if the evidence is not taken, it may be lost; (4) the procedure is reasonable and not AMA; and (5) the procedure is done in a reasonable manner. The best option still is to seek client consent.
2. **A police officer cannot request that blood be drawn for a blood alcohol level. In 2013 the U.S. Supreme Court ruled that blood tests for drunk driving suspects require a warrant, which can readily be obtained electronically.**
3. The police officer is not qualified to perform a procedure in the hospital.
4. This option is dishonest and violates the client's right to be a partner in his health care.

▶ *Test-taking Tip: Identify the option that best respects the client's right to decline care but takes into account potential legal requirements under the law. To prevent injury to the nurse, it is best to have the client's cooperation; the correct option reflects this principle.*

Content Area: Management of Care; Concept: Legal; Regulations; Integrated Processes: Nursing Process: Implementation; Client Needs: Safe and Effective Care Environment: Management of Care; Cognitive Level: Application [Applying]

**52.** MoC **ANSWER: 3**

1. This response indicates that the client understands the proposed procedure.
2. The client has the right to know who will perform the procedure and the name of the assistant.
3. **Even if the surgery is routine, the client needs to be informed of the nature and reason for surgery, and the potential risks and benefits of the proposed surgery.**
4. This response demonstrates that the client is aware that pain is expected and that a plan is in place to address pain management following surgery.

▶ *Test-taking Tip: The key word is "follow-up." Three options are statements that contain precise information, whereas one option is different. Often the option that is different is the answer. The nurse is not responsible for providing information about the risks and benefits of surgery but is responsible for evaluating the client's understanding prior to obtaining informed consent. If there is any question as to sufficiency of the information provided, the nurse must decline to witness the consent and make further inquiry with the HCP.*

Content Area: Management of Care; Concept: Legal; Integrated Processes: Nursing Process: Evaluation; Client Needs: Safe and Effective Care Environment: Management of Care; Physiological Integrity: Physiological Adaptation; Cognitive Level: Evaluation [Evaluating]

**53.** MoC **ANSWER: 2**

1. The nurse is making a recommendation, which is inappropriate. The family should make the decision.
2. **The nurse is clarifying the family's statement to identify the concern. This is the best initial response.**
3. The nurse is offering advice, yet the concerns are not clear.
4. The nurse is making a recommendation, which is inappropriate. The family should make the decision.

▶ *Test-taking Tip: Use the nursing process and therapeutic communication techniques to identify the initial response. The nurse may need to collect more information when assisting families in making ethical decisions.*

Content Area: Management of Care; Concept: Family; Integrated Processes: Communication and Documentation; Client Needs: Safe and Effective Care Environment: Management of Care; Cognitive Level: Analysis [Analyzing]

**54.** MoC **ANSWER: 2**

1. Although it may seem very caring to provide information to the client's best friend for support, it still violates confidentiality.
2. **The client must be asked for consent before sharing any information with anyone. This statement is most appropriate. A breach of confidentiality occurs when the client's trust and confidence are violated by public revelation of confidential or privileged communications without the client's consent.**
3. There is no indication that the CT scan was canceled. Calling the client's friend with this information still violates confidentiality.
4. Overhearing another nurse's conversation about the client to a friend does not indicate that the client's consent was given to provide confidential information.

▶ *Test-taking Tip: You should note similarities between options 1, 3, and 4 in talking about the client's confidential information. Often the option that is different is the correct answer.*

Content Area: Management of Care; Concept: Legal; Integrated Processes: Communication and Documentation; Client Needs: Safe and Effective Care Environment: Management of Care; Cognitive Level: Application [Applying]

**55.** **MoC** **ANSWER: 1**

1. **The new nurse should confront the nurses because a breach of client confidentiality has occurred.**
2. Usually an agency's security officer does not handle breaches of client confidentiality.
3. It is inappropriate for the new nurse, who is not providing care to this client, to approach the client, let alone discuss this matter with the client.
4. The discussion should not be ignored by the new nurse. It is irrelevant that the conversation took place in an elevator and that only staff were privy to the conversation. The client's health care information is on a need-to-know basis, and the new nurse is not caring for the client.

▶ *Test-taking Tip: The key word is "best." You should think about the action that would best stop the discussion of confidential information with those not involved in the care of the client.*

Content Area: Management of Care; Concept: Legal; Integrated Processes: Communication and Documentation; Client Needs: Safe and Effective Care Environment: Management of Care; Cognitive Level: Application [Applying]

**56.** **MoC** **ANSWER: 1**

1. **If the client verbalizes a threat to a known target, there is a duty to warn the target of the threat. Generally a facility will have a written policy stating how, and by whom, the disclosure will be made. Usually it is a hospital administrator who decides whether the client's right to confidentiality will be breached to contact a known target of a threat. Using the chain of command, the nurse can discuss concerns with the nursing supervisor, who in turn can involve the hospital administrator.**
2. This action would breach the client's right to confidentiality.
3. This action would breach the client's right to confidentiality.
4. This action may be helpful, but it is not the best choice. Contacting the nursing supervisor is the best course of action.

▶ *Test-taking Tip: This item requires you to think about balancing the client's right to confidentiality with a target's right to be warned of a threat to bodily harm. There is no indication in the item that the client will be immediately discharged, which eliminates option 2 from consideration.*

Content Area: Management of Care; Concept: Legal; Integrated Processes: Nursing Process: Implementation; Client Needs: Safe and Effective Care Environment: Management of Care; Cognitive Level: Application [Applying]

**57.** **MoC** **PHARM** **ANSWER: 5, 2, 1, 6, 3, 4**

5. **Open the EMR computer program. This EMR is usually one of several programs on the computer.**
2. **Enter the user ID and password. For confidentiality, each person is assigned a unique user ID and password that are entered prior to accessing the client's record.**
1. **Select the correct client. Nurses are often assigned to care for more than one client and will need to select the appropriate client from among those listed.**
6. **Access the client's electronic MAR. The MAR will list all medications the client is receiving.**
3. **Document withholding the medication on the client's electronic MAR. The nurse should select the correct medication after opening the MAR to document that it is being withheld.**
4. **Logging out of the client's EMR is required to maintain client confidentiality.**

▶ *Test-taking Tip: Use visualization to focus on the steps in the process prior to placing items in the correct order.*

Content Area: Management of Care; Concept: Safety; Informatics; Integrated Processes: Communication and Documentation; Client Needs: Safe and Effective Care Environment: Management of Care; Physiological Integrity: Pharmacological and Parenteral Therapies; Cognitive Level: Synthesis [Creating]

**58.** **MoC** **ANSWER: 1**

1. **The Joint Commission National Patient Safety Goals requires telephone orders to be written down and read back. This action will validate the accuracy of the order received.**
2. Although the order is STAT, calling the respiratory therapist is not the most important safety consideration. An order needs to be written before it can be implemented.
3. Although a unit coordinator may notify the respiratory therapist of the need to draw ABGs, only the nurse who takes the order can write it down and read it back to the HCP.
4. Although the nurse may notify the charge nurse, this is not the most important safety consideration.

▶ *Test-taking Tip: The key words are "most important safety consideration." Select the option that would ensure that the nurse's understanding of the order is correct.*

Content Area: Management of Care; Concept: Safety; Integrated Processes: Communication and Documentation; Client Needs: Safe and Effective Care Environment: Management of Care; Cognitive Level: Application [Applying]

**59.** **MoC** **ANSWER: 2**

1. The nurse may access the client record only if it is necessary for performing job duties.
2. **HIPAA was created by the federal government, in part, to guarantee security and privacy of health information. Unauthorized access may result in possible criminal conviction. Many organizations will terminate employees for unauthorized access.**

3. Audits are conducted retrospectively, so they will not protect the client from unauthorized access to the medical record.
4. Access of the record may be done by those who legally need the information including documentation and third-party payers.

▶ **Test-taking Tip:** *Similar words in the stem of the question usually are a clue to the answer. Narrow the options to those using words similar to those in the stem of the question.*

**Content Area:** Management of Care; **Concept:** Legal; **Integrated Processes:** Teaching/Learning; **Client Needs:** Safe and Effective Care Environment: Management of Care; **Cognitive Level:** Analysis [Analyzing]

## 60. MoC ANSWER:

| Electronic Medical Record: Ma~~ple~~ John | | | | | | | |
|---|---|---|---|---|---|---|---|
| ➔ Summary ➔H&P ➔Notes ➔Flowsheets ➔Imaging ➔Lab ➔Surgery ➔Allergies | | | | | | | |

| John ~~Maple~~ | ~~MRN~~ | ~~DOB~~ | Age | Gender | Physician |
|---|---|---|---|---|---|
| | 12345 | 11/25/36 | 71 | male | Nelson |

| Date: Today | 0400 | 0800 | 1015 | 1200 | 1400 | 1600 | 1800 | 2000 | 2200 | 2359 |
|---|---|---|---|---|---|---|---|---|---|---|
| BP Systole | 120 | 132 | | 134 | | | | | | |
| BP Diastole | 86 | 80 | | 72 | | | | | | |
| Pulse | 84 | 90 | | 72 | | | | | | |
| Respirations | 16 | 20 | | 16 | | | | | | |
| Temperature | 98.6 | 99.4 | | 98.2 | | | | | | |
| SpO₂ | 97 | 98 | | 98 | | | | | | |
| Oxygen | 21 | | | | | | | | | |
| Oxygen Source | NC | | | | | | | | | |
| Pain (0-10) | 2 | 2 | 5 | 1 | 1 | | | | | |

**Notes:**
0400 Awake. Pain rating of 2. Refuses analgesic. Ambulated to bathroom independently
0800 Increase in temperature of 99.4. Wife called and updated with current status. Will be in mid-morning.
1015 Increase in pain rating to 5. One Vicodin given.
1045 Pain rating 2.
1200 Wife here. Resting comfortably.

**Client names, medical record numbers, birth dates, and other identifiers cannot be viewable to non-HCPs, according to HIPAA. Room number, age, HCP, and other information displayed cannot be linked to the individual client for identification.**

▶ **Test-taking Tip:** *Apply knowledge of HIPAA. Note that the word "areas" is plural, indicating that more than one X should be placed.*

**Content Area:** Management of Care; **Concept:** Legal; **Integrated Processes:** Communication and Documentation; **Client Needs:** Safe and Effective Care Environment: Management of Care; **Cognitive Level:** Analysis [Analyzing]

## 61. MoC ANSWER: 4

1. Sharing with client B that client A will be receiving confidential information is not appropriate.

2. Asking the HCP to return later may not be realistic for the HCP's schedule, and the client may have another roommate by that time.
3. Expecting client B to turn on his TV and not listen to the conversation will not prevent the client from overhearing confidential information.
4. **Offering to get client B out of bed for the client's benefit completely eliminates the need to share any information about client A.**

▶ **Test-taking Tip:** *The key words are "best" and "maintain confidentiality." The word best indicates that two or more options would be acceptable, but one is better.*

**Content Area:** Management of Care; **Concept:** Legal; **Integrated Processes:** Nursing Process: Planning; **Client Needs:** Safe and Effective Care Environment: Management of Care; **Cognitive Level:** Analysis [Analyzing]

## 62. MoC ANSWER: 1

1. **Breaches of confidentiality are serious offenses. Typically, such issues are handled by management. It would be best to report the event to the nursing supervisor.**
2. Confronting the HCP may not result in appropriate follow-up action related to HIPAA violations.
3. The nurse should always use the chain of command and report to the immediate supervisor, not the chief of staff.
4. This is a potential breach of client confidentiality and must be evaluated. HCPs are also required to be compliant with HIPAA laws.

▶ **Test-taking Tip:** *The key words are "professional action." Use the chain of command when selecting the correct action. Recognize that the HCP's action is illegal.*

**Content Area:** Management of Care; **Concept:** Legal; Informatics; **Integrated Processes:** Communication and Documentation; **Client Needs:** Safe and Effective Care Environment: Management of Care; **Cognitive Level:** Evaluation [Evaluating]

## 63. MoC PHARM ANSWER: 2

1. Initiating all orders as prescribed is unsafe.
2. **It is most important for the nurse to telephone the HCP. The abbreviation MS is on The Joint Commission's "Do Not Use" List. It could be interpreted as morphine sulfate or magnesium sulfate.**
3. Preparing and administering MS is unsafe. The abbreviation could refer to morphine sulfate or magnesium sulfate.
4. Although a type and crossmatch are needed prior to administering a unit of PRBCs, this intervention is not the most important among the options.

▶ **Test-taking Tip:** *Carefully read each prescribed order, noting that all would be appropriate for the client in sickle cell crisis except MS. MS could be either morphine sulfate (which is appropriate) or magnesium sulfate (which would be inappropriate).*

**Content Area:** Management of Care; **Concept:** Medication; Hematologic Regulation; Oxygenation; Legal; **Integrated Processes:** Nursing Process: Analysis; **Client Needs:** Safe and Effective Care Environment: Management of Care; Physiological Integrity: Pharmacological and Parenteral Therapies; **Cognitive Level:** Analysis [Analyzing]

## 64. MoC ANSWER: 1, 4, 5

1. **The nurse should document that an unknown supplement is being taken by the client to ensure that there is follow-up to identify the supplement and in case there is an association between the supplement and the client's chest pain.**
2. Do not assume that anyone advised the client to take the supplement.
3. This instruction would likely block meaningful communication with the client; the supplement is unknown at this time and may not be the cause of the chest pain.
4. **It is appropriate for the nurse to have a family member bring in the supplement because the supplement and its physiological actions should be identified.**
5. **Asking about the time last taken and the amount of the supplement is important because it may affect planned treatment and interact with medications.**

♦ **Test-taking Tip:** *You should focus on selecting options that will improve the treatment of the client. Eliminate option 3 because not all medications need to be prescribed by the HCP. Remember the client's rights to use of alternative therapies.*

**Content Area:** Management of Care; **Concept:** Promoting Health; Diversity; **Integrated Processes:** Nursing Process: Implementation; Culture and Spirituality; **Client Needs:** Safe and Effective Care Environment: Management of Care; **Cognitive Level:** Application [Applying]

## 65. ANSWER: 4

1. The nurse is assuming that the client may have some religious preferences.
2. The nurse is assuming the client may find eye contact a sign of disrespect.
3. The nurse is assuming the client is Muslim and may not want care from a female.
4. **The nurse is using a culturally sensitive approach when asking the client if there are any cultural preferences.**

♦ **Test-taking Tip:** *When providing culturally sensitive care, the nurse should not make assumptions based on the client's nationality or country of origin, but rather ask the client whether the client has any cultural-related preferences that would affect client care.*

**Content Area:** Management of Care; **Concept:** Diversity; Communication; **Integrated Processes:** Nursing Process: Evaluation; Culture and Spirituality; **Client Needs:** Safe and Effective Care Environment: Management of Care; Psychosocial Integrity; **Cognitive Level:** Evaluation [Evaluating]

## 66. MoC ANSWER: 2, 4

1. There is no information about the client and her spouse's faith beliefs. The nurse cannot assume that they are of the Islamic faith. A hospital cannot legally employ only female nurses because hospitals receive federal and state funding and insurance or other reimbursements; the hospital must be an equal opportunity employer and have nondiscrimination policies in place.
2. **The decision to limit caregivers to female nursing staff when caring for the client can be made by nursing management. This is a correct and reasonable statement and respects the client's faith beliefs.**
3. Nursing management controls the assignment of nursing staff; it is inappropriate to forward a request for assigning only female nurses to the client advocate representative.
4. **Reassuring the client and her husband that all cultures and religious beliefs are respected is appropriate and demonstrates the nurse's and hospital's support of people from various cultural or religious backgrounds.**
5. Although posting a sign allowing only female staff members to enter the client's room should prevent male nursing staff from inadvertently entering the room, such a sign would be a breach of confidentiality. A symbol established by the agency would be a better option.

♦ **Test-taking Tip:** *Ascertain that the client's request is reasonable and can be met by the nursing staff. Select the options that fulfill the client's request but maintain client confidentiality.*

**Content Area:** Management of Care; **Concept:** Diversity; Management; **Integrated Processes:** Nursing Process: Implementation; Culture and Spirituality; **Client Needs:** Safe and Effective Care Environment: Management of Care; **Cognitive Level:** Application [Applying]

## 67. MoC ANSWER: 1

1. **The best plan when translating information in another language is to obtain a hospital-approved interpreter who is professionally trained and has knowledge of medical terminology.**
2. The ability of the client's son to translate medical information is not known, and his emotional involvement could interfere with how he interprets the information.
3. Information from the Internet may be unreliable, insufficiently translated, or too content-specific to adequately address treatment options or answer client questions.
4. This request would be outside of the NA's scope of practice and job description. The conference will likely include new information and questions that the NA may be unable to interpret because the NA may have limited medical knowledge.

♦ **Test-taking Tip:** *You should select the option that is most likely to maintain client confidentiality while obtaining an informed consent.*

**Content Area:** Management of Care; **Concept:** Diversity; Management; **Integrated Processes:** Nursing Process: Planning; Culture and Spirituality; **Client Needs:** Safe and Effective Care Environment: Management of Care; Physiological Integrity: Physiological Adaptation; **Cognitive Level:** Application [Applying]

**68.** MoC **ANSWER: 1**

1. **The nurse's best option is to check for best practices such as standards from the National Council on Interpreting in Health Care, which defines the responsibilities of interpreters. Most organizations should have a policy related to staff functioning as interpreters.**
2. The ANA Code of Ethics does not make a statement about the use of nurses as interpreters.
3. The HCP has no authority for determining the standard of practice for the nurse.
4. There is no indication that this client is a hospitalized client. The nurse manager would need to consult another resource to determine if it is appropriate to have the Spanish-speaking nurse interpret for the Spanish-speaking client.

♦ **Test-taking Tip:** *You should think about the use of standards and legal issues related to the use of staff as interpreters. The key term is "best."*

**Content Area:** Management of Care; **Concept:** Diversity; Management; Regulations; **Integrated Processes:** Communication and Documentation; Culture and Spirituality; **Client Needs:** Safe and Effective Care Environment: Management of Care; **Cognitive Level:** Application [Applying]

**69.** MoC **ANSWER: 1**

1. **Members of some cultures practice alternative forms of medicine for illnesses, including coining. Coining involves rubbing heated oil on the skin and then vigorously rubbing a coin over the area until a red mark is seen. Coining is believed to allow a path by which a "bad wind" (cause of the illness) can be released from the body.**
2. The marks are significant because it provides information to the nurse about the use of alternative forms of medicine.
3. Coining has led to false reporting of child abuse because the practice does leave marks.
4. Alternative therapies that do not result in child injuries are not reported as abuse.

♦ **Test-taking Tip:** *Apply knowledge of alternative forms of medicine, and the client's rights pertaining to their use. Use the process of elimination. Options 1 and 2 contain the similar terms "be reported." Eliminate these knowing that this is a cultural practice. Eliminate option 3 because it is a cultural practice related to the infant's illness.*

**Content Area:** Management of Care; **Concept:** Diversity; **Integrated Processes:** Nursing Process: Analysis; Culture and Spirituality; **Client Needs:** Safe and Effective Care Environment: Management of Care; **Cognitive Level:** Application [Applying]

**70.** MoC PHARM **ANSWER: 2**

1. Administering an injection while holding the client's arm without gaining client cooperation could be assault and battery.
2. **The best intervention is one that includes teaching and agreement to receive the medication before administering it; this protects the client's rights.**
3. To maintain therapeutic effectiveness, the medication should be administered in a timely manner.
4. It is inappropriate for the nurse to notify the HCP of an anticipated problem. The drug is administered only by the subcutaneous, not IV, route.

♦ **Test-taking Tip:** *You need to consider that an illegal action should never be performed by the nurse. Also, to maintain the therapeutic effectiveness of medications, they need to be administered by the correct route and in a timely manner.*

**Content Area:** Management of Care; **Concept:** Diversity; Management; Communication; **Integrated Processes:** Nursing Process: Implementation; Culture and Spirituality; **Client Needs:** Safe and Effective Care Environment: Management of Care; Physiological Integrity: Pharmacological and Parenteral Therapies; **Cognitive Level:** Application [Applying]

**71.** MoC **ANSWER: 1**

1. *Hanyak* **is a traditional herbal medicine that can be made from ginseng, berries, roots, stems of trees, flowers, and others. It is most appropriate for the nurse to determine the ingredients of the herbal remedy because these can interact with medications that may be prescribed.**
2. Although the client may also have had a healing ritual performed by a shaman, *hanyak* may or may not have been used as part of the healing ritual. The shaman is usually used to treat illnesses after other means of treatment are exhausted.
3. This statement will elicit a "yes" or "no" response.
4. *Hanyak* is using traditional herbal medicine. There is no indication that the client was treated with acupuncture.

♦ **Test-taking Tip:** *Hanyak is a traditional herbal medicine. Use this information to narrow the options. Remember client's rights to use alternative therapies.*

**Content Area:** Management of Care; **Concept:** Diversity; Medication; **Integrated Processes:** Nursing Process: Assessment; Culture and Spirituality; **Client Needs:** Safe and Effective Care Environment: Management of Care; Physiological Integrity: Basic Care and Comfort; **Cognitive Level:** Analysis [Analyzing]

**72.** MoC **ANSWER: 3**

1. The hospital policy should not prevent the client from practicing cultural beliefs; telling the client that this is against hospital policy would be denying the client's rights.
2. There is no reason to refer this client to the pastoral care department; the nurse should assist the client.

3. **The nurse should assist the client in planning the placement of the voodoo shrine because it supports the client's cultural beliefs and is not contraindicated in the client's care. The client's belief is that supernatural forces such as voodoo can restore health.**

4. The nurse does not need to know the reason that the client is requesting the shrine; the nurse should support the client's request without prejudice.

▶ *Test-taking Tip: The nurse should support the client's cultural beliefs if the practices are not contraindicated in the client's care.*

**Content Area:** Management of Care; **Concept:** Diversity; Management; **Integrated Processes:** Nursing Process: Implementation; Culture and Spirituality; **Client Needs:** Safe and Effective Care Environment: Management of Care; **Cognitive Level:** Application [Applying]

## 73. MoC ANSWER: 2

1. A certified translator should be contacted when the treatment plan is being discussed. Family members may not understand or be able to translate medical terminology.

2. **Encouraging the client's family to bring in traditional foods may help the client preserve a part of his or her identity and autonomy.**

3. Although the client may need to leave the room for procedures and should wear a mask, ambulating around the unit is discouraged to limit infectious disease exposure to other clients. It may also be psychologically difficult for the client to walk through the care unit with a mask on and may in fact hinder coping.

4. The nurse should first identify the client's spiritual and religious beliefs before planning a spiritual intervention.

▶ *Test-taking Tip: Cultural sensitivity can enhance client coping. Only one option demonstrates cultural sensitivity and legal and ethical practice.*

**Content Area:** Management of Care; **Concept:** Diversity; Management; Oxygenation; **Integrated Processes:** Nursing Process: Implementation; Caring; Culture and Spirituality; **Client Needs:** Client Needs: Safe and Effective Care Environment: Management of Care; Physiological Integrity: Physiological Adaptation; **Cognitive Level:** Application [Applying]

## 74. MoC ANSWER: 2

1. Although the sick are not required to fast during Ramadan, some Muslims insist on fasting even when hospitalized.

2. **Providing a prayer rug offers the greatest degree of culturally competent nursing care. Muslims pray using a prayer rug to ensure that the area used for prayer is clean.**

3. Muslims have no prohibition against receiving blood transfusions.

4. Although Muslims are prohibited against the consumption of pork, the client may not be a vegetarian. The client may consume other meats.

▶ *Test-taking Tip: The key phrase is "greatest degree." If no information is noted in the stem about the client's preferences, avoid making assumptions.*

**Content Area:** Management of Care; **Concept:** Diversity; Management; **Integrated Processes:** Nursing Process: Implementation; Culture and Spirituality; **Client Needs:** Safe and Effective Care Environment: Management of Care; Psychosocial Integrity; **Cognitive Level:** Analysis [Analyzing]

## 75. MoC ANSWER: 3

1. Being concerned about basic individual rights of others pertains to stage 5 of Lawrence Kohlberg's theory of moral development, social contract, and legalistic orientation. Kohlberg proposes that middle-aged adults are at either stage 5 or 6 of moral development.

2. Attempting to understand the values and beliefs of others pertains to stage 5 of Lawrence Kohlberg's theory of moral development, social contract, and legalistic orientation. Kohlberg proposes that middle-aged adults are at either stage 5 or 6 of moral development.

3. **The student nurse's statement that middle-aged adults are focused on their careers and are less concerned about morals is not associated with Kohlberg's theory of moral development. The experienced nurse should correct the student nurse's comment.**

4. Using their own chosen ethical principles when making moral decisions pertains to stage 6 of Lawrence Kohlberg's theory of moral development, universal ethical principle orientation.

▶ *Test-taking Tip: In narrowing the options, you should select the option that is unlike the other options.*

**Content Area:** Management of Care; **Concept:** Promoting Health; Diversity; **Integrated Processes:** Nursing Process: Evaluation; Culture and Spirituality; **Client Needs:** Safe and Effective Care Environment: Management of Care; Health Promotion and Maintenance; **Cognitive Level:** Evaluation [Evaluating]

## 76. MoC ANSWER: 2, 4

1. Even if harm had not occurred, the nurse's behavior of falsifying documentation poses an ethical-legal concern and is never the correct action.

2. **Documenting VS that the nurse did not obtain is a legal concern because documents were falsified and the nurse was untruthful regarding obtaining the VS.**

3. Beneficence means doing good. There is no information to indicate the nurse did what was best for the client.

4. **The nurse's actions involve the ethical issue of veracity or telling the truth. The nurse was untruthful regarding obtaining the HR at 0200 hour.**

5. Distributive justice is the distribution of resources to clients. There is no information about the resources available to the nurse.

▶ *Test-taking Tip:* Focus on the nurse's behavior of falsifying documentation. Avoid reading into the question. Despite the unit's being unusually busy, there is no information as to what the nurse was doing during the shift. Eliminate the options that are suggestive of nurse actions other than the behaviors presented.

**Content Area:** Management of Care; **Concept:** Ethics; Perfusion; Management; **Integrated Processes:** Nursing Process: Evaluation; **Client Needs:** Safe and Effective Care Environment: Management of Care; **Cognitive Level:** Evaluation [Evaluating]

## 77. MoC ANSWER: 3

1. Libel is a published statement or photograph that is false and damaging to a person's reputation.
2. Battery is intentional physical contact with another that involves unconsented or offensive contact or injury.
3. **Assault is an intentional attempt or threat that puts the other person in fear of imminent bodily harm.**
4. Invasion of privacy is intruding into another person's private affairs or disclosing private or confidential information.

▶ *Test-taking Tip:* Narrow the options to intentional torts (assault and battery). Then consider which of the two do not require physical contact.

**Content Area:** Management of Care; **Concept:** Legal; **Integrated Processes:** Communication and Documentation; **Client Needs:** Safe and Effective Care Environment: Management of Care; **Cognitive Level:** Application [Applying]

## 78. MoC ANSWER: 3

1. Actions may include discussing the decision with the client, but allowing the client to decide is not the next action.
2. Actions may include discussing the decision with the HCP, but allowing the HCP to decide is not the next action.
3. **Because of a scarcity of donors, expense of the procedure, and costly medications, this case should be referred to the institutional ethics committee.**
4. Performing another transplant only if the bill can be paid is unethical.

▶ *Test-taking Tip:* Three options are similar, and one option is different. Often the option that is different is the answer.

**Content Area:** Management of Care; Child; **Concept:** Ethics; Urinary Elimination; **Integrated Processes:** Nursing Process: Analysis; Caring; **Client Needs:** Safe and Effective Care Environment: Management of Care; **Cognitive Level:** Application [Applying]

## 79. MoC ANSWER: 3

1. Adult Protective Services is an agency that investigates actual or potential abuse.
2. Option 2 is gathering data and not advocacy.
3. **The nurse advocates by ensuring that the client has access to health care services. The nurse should contact a social worker whose role it is to make placement arrangements.**
4. A screening clinic is not a permanent clinic where health care services are provided.

▶ *Test-taking Tip:* Advocacy is speaking on behalf of the rights of others. The client has the right to receive and choose to receive treatment.

**Content Area:** Management of Care; **Concept:** Collaboration; Metabolism; **Integrated Processes:** Nursing Process: Implementation; Caring; **Client Needs:** Safe and Effective Care Environment: Management of Care; **Cognitive Level:** Application [Applying]

## 80. MoC ANSWER: 2, 4, 5

1. The type of anesthesia is not part of the Universal Protocol. The circulating nurse would not make this judgment.
2. **The nurse should verify the correct surgical site as part of the Universal Protocol; the site is marked in indelible ink when possible.**
3. The Universal Protocol does not address intravenous fluids. The rate may vary based on the client's VS and physiological status.
4. **The nurse should verify the correct client by using two unique identifiers, such as name, hospital ID (medical record) number, or birth date, as part of the Universal Protocol.**
5. **The nurse should verify the correct surgical procedure as part of the Universal Protocol, as well as the surgeon to perform the procedure.**

▶ *Test-taking Tip:* You can remember that the Universal Protocol is a legal requirement and is intended to prevent accidental wrong procedures being performed on the wrong client. All elements of the Universal Protocol address this specific issue.

**Content Area:** Management of Care; Fundamentals; **Concept:** Safety; Perioperative; **Integrated Processes:** Nursing Process: Assessment; **Client Needs:** Safe and Effective Care Environment: Management of Care; Safe and Effective Care Environment: Safety and Infection Control; **Cognitive Level:** Knowledge [Remembering]

**81.** **MoC** **ANSWER: 2**

1. Although being outside the room with a member of the clergy is an option, the room door would be closed to protect the client's privacy.
2. **The 2010 CPR guidelines recommend allowing family to be present during CPR with a designated person (clergy, social worker, or nurse) in the room.**
3. Detaining the wife and son is likely to be met with resistance.
4. It is premature to page for security. Explaining that they would be accompanied in the room with a staff member may be sufficient to calm the family members.

▶ *Test-taking Tip: Research has shown that the presence of family during resuscitation assists them in dealing with their grief.*

**Content Area:** Management of Care; Fundamentals; **Concept:** Nursing Roles; Diversity; **Integrated Processes:** Nursing Process: Implementation; Culture and Spirituality; **Client Needs:** Safe and Effective Care Environment: Management of Care; Psychosocial Integrity; **Cognitive Level:** Analysis [Analyzing]

**82.** **MoC** **ANSWER: 1**

1. **Gilligan's theory is specific to women and proposes that women see morality in the integrity of relationships and caring. Women tend to consider what is right to be taking responsibility for others and caring, whereas men tend to consider what is right to be what is just.**
2. Kohlberg's theory is not specific to women. Option 2 describes Kohlberg's postconventional level of moral development for middle-aged or older adults.
3. Westerhoff's stages of faith are spiritual development theories and not moral development theories. These refer in part to the individual's perceptions about the direction and meaning of life.
4. Fowler's stages of spiritual development are spiritual development theories and not moral development theories. These refer in part to the individual's perceptions about the direction and meaning of life.

▶ *Test-taking Tip: Focus on what the question is asking: moral development for women. Eliminate options that pertain to spiritual development.*

**Content Area:** Management of Care; Adult; **Concept:** Promoting Health; Diversity; **Integrated Processes:** Teaching/Learning; Culture and Spirituality; **Client Needs:** Safe and Effective Care Environment: Management of Care; Health Promotion and Maintenance; **Cognitive Level:** Analysis [Analyzing]

# Leadership and Management

**83.** MoC The client who is homeless and uninsured has chest pain and seeks care in the ED. Which action should be taken by the nurse? **Select all that apply.**

1. Ask the HCP to see the client before admission.
2. Provide care according to the standard of care and emergency protocols.
3. Refer the client to the nearest hospital that provides charity care.
4. Treat the client respectfully and honor the client's request to be seen.
5. Initiate a social worker consult after stabilizing and treating the client.

**84.** MoC The older adult client wishes to be discharged home after a kyphoplasty. The client has a history of emphysema requiring oxygen at home. To ensure discharge to home is appropriate, which information is **most important** for the nurse to assess?

1. Home care resources
2. Pain management plan
3. Self-care deficits
4. Medication regime

**85.** MoC The client is admitted for coronary artery bypass surgery (CABG) with an anticipated admission to the coronary care unit (CCU). In preparation for the client's hospital admission, implementation of which component will **best** predict the sequence and timing of care, and direct the course of the client's hospital stay?

1. A clinical pathway
2. A client education plan
3. HCP-initiated interventions
4. Discharge planning at the time of admission

**86.** MoC Which should be the nurse's **most** important safety consideration when receiving a telephone order from a HCP for a blood culture to be drawn STAT?

1. Writing the order down and reading it back to the HCP
2. Calling the laboratory STAT to draw the blood
3. Giving the order STAT to the health unit coordinator to place in the computer
4. Immediately checking the client's chart for a consent for a blood transfusion

**87.** MoC The pediatric client, newly diagnosed with CF, is being discharged home. The client's parents are anxious, asking many questions about the child's nutrition, medication regimen, nebulizer treatments, and chest percussion. They are expressing concerns about the high cost of care and financial hardship. Which health care disciplines should be included in a planned multidisciplinary care conference? **Select all that apply.**

1. Nurse
2. Dietitian
3. Social worker
4. Nursing assistant
5. Respiratory therapist

**88.** MoC The client is hospitalized for GI bleeding. The client's family tells the nurse the client has a history of drinking four to eight beers every day. The client lives alone, is unemployed, and is uninsured. Which collaborative action provides the **best** overall client care?

1. Calling the case manager to obtain a consult for chemical dependency
2. Consulting a multidisciplinary team to review the client's problem list
3. Calling the HCP and recommending orders to treat delirium tremens (DTs)
4. Consulting the social worker to address client finances and placement

**89.** MoC The nurse reviews the plan of care for the client with COPD and limited mobility. The nurse notes that the physical therapist (PT) changed the plan to progress the client's ambulation from 100 to 200 feet twice a day. Which intervention should the nurse implement to ensure that the client's needs are met?

1. Instruct the PT therapist not to ambulate the client without the nurse present
2. Inform the PT of the client's respiratory status prior to ambulation
3. Tell the PT that changes to the plan of care should not be made at this time
4. Inform the HCP about the PT's plan to progress the client's ambulation

**90.** MoC The HCP notifies the nurse that the client will be discharged from the hospital tomorrow. The client is unable to ambulate to the bathroom independently, lives alone, and has a poor appetite. With which discipline is it **most** important for the nurse to collaborate for discharge planning?

1. Dietitian
2. Social worker
3. Pharmacist
4. Physical therapist

**91.** MoC The nurse is caring for the client who has a permanent tracheostomy, is receiving oxygen therapy and oral respiratory medications, and requires chest physiotherapy. Which members of the interdisciplinary team should the nurse **initially** include in the plan of care? **Select all that apply.**

1. Respiratory therapist
2. Physical therapist
3. Speech therapist
4. Social worker
5. Occupational therapist

**92.** MoC The client with CRF is placed on a restricted renal diet that includes limiting protein and dairy intake. After reviewing a list of allowed, limited, and restricted foods, the client tells the nurse, "I don't like any of the acceptable food choices, and some are against my faith beliefs!" Which collaborative action would **best** meet the client's needs?

1. Review the list with the client and compromise on which foods are acceptable
2. Identify the primary meal preparer in the family and review the list with that person
3. Report the client's noncompliance to the HCP so medications may be adjusted
4. Initiate a referral to the dietitian for counseling the client on acceptable foods

**93.** MoC PHARM The client is going home with a new prescription of fluticasone/salmeterol diskus. The client has never used a diskus delivery system before. Which health care team member should the nurse consult to instruct the client in proper use of the diskus?

1. Case coordinator
2. Respiratory therapist
3. Social worker
4. Pharmacist

**94.** MoC Two years ago, the older adult client was diagnosed with CRF requiring dialysis. The client is admitted to a hospital with pneumonia for the third time in the last 9 months. Which health care team member should the nurse consult to enable the client to cope with the chronic disease?

1. Palliative care nurse
2. Social worker
3. Dialysis nurse
4. Charge nurse

**95.** MoC The new nurse reattaches the client's pulse oximeter finger probe after it was off and the machine was alarming. When the alarm is heard again, the nurse finds a reading of 84 with the number quickly changing to 92. The client's pulse oximeter readings continue to vary from 84 to 94, causing the machine to alarm frequently. Which action will help the nurse establish a safe and accurate pulse oximeter reading?

1. Replace the machine with a functioning oximeter machine.
2. Consult with a more experienced nurse about the problem.
3. Turn the alarm off because it is not functioning properly.
4. Notify the HCP of the client's low oximeter readings.

**96.** MoC PHARM The nurse assesses that the client with delirium tremens is becoming increasingly agitated. The nurse notes that IV doses of diazepam, lorazepam, and propofol are prescribed for the client but is unclear regarding which medication would be most effective. Which action by the nurse will **best** improve the client's outcome?

1. Give the same medication given by the previous nurse, knowing it will provide some relief.
2. Contact the HCP for a different medication, knowing these will not reduce agitation.
3. Administer the propofol, because the client's agitation may lead to client self-harm.
4. Consult a pharmacist on the medication actions and ask for advice on which to give.

**97.** MoC The nurse expects the client who returned from surgery performed 2 hours ago to be more alert. The client is difficult to awaken and has intermittent apnea. The client's blood pressure (BP) was in the low 100s but is now 90/54 mm Hg. Place the nurse's actions in the order of importance.

1. Assist in the reassessment of the client.
2. Contact the surgeon.
3. Request the acute response team (ART).
4. Prepare necessary equipment, including an oximeter and noninvasive BP monitor.
5. Communicate using a handoff method such as SBAR.
6. Contact the client's family.

Answer: _____

**98.** MoC The nurse finds the client in respiratory distress with a decreasing level of consciousness and calls the ART. Which action demonstrates that the responding intensive care unit (ICU) nurse is a resource to the nurse on the medical unit?

1. The ICU nurse requests information in the SBAR format.
2. The ICU nurse obtains the client's vital sign measurements.
3. The ICU nurse calls the client's HCP.
4. The ICU nurse reviews assessment findings with the medical nurse.

**99.** MoC The new client is admitted to a facility and requires an initial admission assessment. Which actions should the nurse include in the admission assessment? **Select all that apply.**

1. Ask questions to obtain subjective data.
2. Take the client's vital signs.
3. Develop the client's care plan.
4. Obtain functional ability information.
5. Document the education completed.

**100.** MoC After finding a pressure ulcer on a client's buttock, the nurse documents the following description in a variance (incident) report: *Right buttock area reddened. There is a break in the skin with skin loss involving the dermis and epidermis. It appears crater-like. There is no slough present.* Which illustration **best** identifies the pressure ulcer about which the nurse is documenting in the variance report?

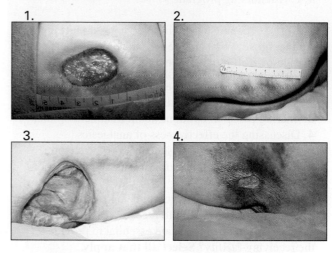

**101.** MoC The client is being transferred to a subacute unit at another facility. The nurse calls the facility to give a verbal report to the nurse assuming the client's care. Which statement **best** ensures that the continuity of care is maintained?

1. "Because I am passing responsibility for care to you, I need to document your name."
2. "I am calling to give you an overview of the client's condition, treatment plan, and needs."
3. "I sent the transfer forms with the client; these provide the information you need for care."
4. "I let the client know about the plans for transfer and the care that the client will receive."

**102.** MoC The client is being referred to the neurosurgeon at another facility. The nurse prepares the client for transfer. Which items should be included in the transfer? **Select all that apply.**

1. Medications supplied by the hospital
2. Clinic records from birth to present time
3. Emergency supplies and medications
4. A copy of the client's medical record
5. Personal belongings brought to the hospital

**103.** MoC The client who is homeless is being discharged from the hospital. The client has no family support or resources. To which service should the nurse refer the client?

1. The Social Security office
2. Homeless shelter facility
3. Public health clinic
4. Parish nursing program

**104.** MoC The nurse is giving a change-of-shift report to another nurse. What are the essential components of a change-of-shift report? **Select all that apply.**

1. Reporting the client's medical diagnosis
2. Sharing new orders, medications, and treatments
3. Sharing personal opinions about treatment options
4. Discussing the effectiveness of analgesics
5. Sharing routine turning schedule for the client
6. Identifying areas for priority focus on the next shift

**105.** MoC The client is urgently being prepared for transfer to another facility to receive a higher level of care. Which documents are essential to provide to the receiving facility? **Select all that apply.**

1. EMTALA form
2. Client teaching record
3. Transfer note
4. History and physical
5. Progress notes
6. Activity flowsheet

**106.** MoC The elderly client, who has been newly diagnosed with end-stage COPD, is to be discharged home. The client is unable to provide self-care and requires continuous assistance. Which service would provide the **greatest** assistance to the client's spouse, who would be the sole caregiver?

1. Skilled nursing care
2. Respite care
3. Hospice care
4. Physical therapy

**107.** MoC The client is scheduled to have a CXR and a pulmonary function test (PFT). The client tires easily. Which action should be taken by the nurse to **best** coordinate the client's care?

1. Send the client for the CXR but have the PFT rescheduled for the next day.
2. Have the CXR changed to a portable CXR and then send the client for the PFT.
3. Escort the client to both tests so the client can be returned to the unit if too tired.
4. Call the radiology department to request that the CXR be taken right before the PFT.

**108.** MoC The nurse on a hospital's performance improvement committee evaluates potential activities that will lead to performance improvement for the department. Which are performance improvement activities? **Select all that apply.**

1. Improve client satisfaction scores
2. Reduce client fall rates
3. Increase client census
4. Reduce anticoagulant medication safety events
5. Increase the number of quality assurance nurse staff
6. Reduce hospital-acquired infections

**109.** MoC The nurse manager is teaching nursing staff about the use of an evidence-based practice (EBP) framework for performance improvement. Which description should the nurse manager include?

1. Utilizing the Cochrane Collaboration Database to find research summaries that have compared and contrasted various research study findings and made recommendations for nursing practice
2. Collecting information on a problem, establishing a clinically focused question, analyzing pertinent research and clinical practice evidence, and identifying implications for practice
3. Accessing guidelines from the National Guideline Clearinghouse to evaluate whether the client's treatments for a particular diagnosis are according to the established guidelines
4. Determining whether the nursing process steps of assessment, analysis, planning, implementation, and evaluation are being implemented when providing nursing care to clients

**110.** MoC The nurse is aware of the American Nurses Association's nursing-sensitive quality indicators regarding the management and prevention of hospital-acquired infections. Which nursing action is most likely to reduce hospital-acquired infection rates?

1. Ensuring appropriate nurse-to-client ratios
2. Improving functioning of the team
3. Monitoring medication safety events
4. Ensuring adequate supplies are available for care delivery

**111.** PHARM MoC The supervising nurse is double-checking the new nurse's heparin dose prior to administration and determines that the dose is incorrect. The nurse has withdrawn 2.5 mL of heparin from a vial labeled 5000 units/mL. The client is to receive 2500 units. How much heparin should the supervising nurse ask the new nurse to expel from the syringe?

_____ mL (Record your answer as a whole number.)

**112.** MoC The new nurse manager on the maternity unit is informed by staff that family members have been unhappy about the policy limiting the number of visitors for the first 24 hours postpartum. Which **initial** action by the nurse manager is most appropriate?

1. Compare policies for the number of allowable visitors in other maternity units in area hospitals.
2. Change the policy to allow an unlimited number of visitors for a 3-month pilot program.
3. Plan to explore this concern in 2 months when the orientation to the new position is finished.
4. Mail surveys to past clients exploring their feelings about the hospital's visiting policies.

**INSTRUCTIONS:** Refer to the information provided in the tables to answer Question 113.

**113.** CJ MoC The nurse is planning room assignments/reassignments for the six clients illustrated. Some clients may require a private room based on their diagnosis or current status. Rooms may have one or two clients. Bed 1 is the closest to the doorway. The lowest numbered room is the nearest to the nursing station. Which room would result in a safe placement for each client?

| Clients | Rooms and Beds | |
|---|---|---|
| Client 1. 55-year-old with possible MI; heparin and nitroglycerin drips; nitroglycerin titrated for pain control | 275-1 | 275-2 |
| Client 2. 65-year-old with heart failure; ejection fraction 25%; confused | 276-1 | 276-2 |
| Client 3. 28-year-old with endocarditis; stable; lots of visitors | 277-1 | 277-2 |
| Client 4. 36-year-old with atrial fibrillation, rate controlled; has pancreatic cancer and neutropenia | 278-1 | 278-2 |
| Client 5. 62-year-old with angina; no chest pain currently; plan for cardiac catheterization in a.m. | 279-1 | 279-2 |
| Client 6. 72-year-old with atrial flutter on a heparin drip; BP 180/98, HR 136; cardioversion in 2 hours | | |

| Rooms and Beds | | | |
|---|---|---|---|
| | Client | | Client |
| 275-1 | | 275-2 | |
| 276-1 | | 276-2 | |
| 277-1 | | 277-2 | |
| 278-1 | | 278-2 | |
| 279-1 | | 279-2 | |

**114.** MoC The table illustrated is presented at a unit's performance improvement committee meeting. Which measure indicates the greatest need for improvement compared to other hospitals?

| Surgical Infection Prevention Measures | Current Rate | Benchmark |
|---|---|---|
| Cardiac surgery clients with controlled 6 a.m. postoperative serum glucose | 90.22% | 85% |
| Colorectal surgery clients with immediate postoperative normothermia | 78.58% | 85% |
| Surgery clients with recommended DVT prophylaxis ordered | 88.72% | 95% |
| Surgery clients who received appropriate DVT prophylaxis within 24 hours prior to surgery to 24 hours after surgery | 84.75% | 95% |
| Prophylactic antibiotic received within 1 hour prior to surgical incision | 90.74% | 100% |
| Prophylactic antibiotics discontinued within 24 hours after surgery end time | 80.57% | 100% |

1. Cardiac surgery clients with controlled 6 a.m. postoperative serum glucose
2. Colorectal surgery clients with immediate postoperative normothermia
3. Surgery clients who received appropriate DVT prophylaxis within 24 hours prior to surgery to 24 hours after surgery
4. Prophylactic antibiotics discontinued within 24 hours after surgery end time

**115.** MoC PHARM The client with hyperglycemia is receiving a continuous IV insulin drip. The nurse checking the client's blood glucose hourly obtains a reading of 32 mg/dL. The client who was alert is now lethargic and does not respond to questions. The nurse administers 25 mL of $D_{50}W$ per protocol. The client begins to respond. Which additional risk-management action should be taken by the nurse?

1. Continue the insulin drip at the same rate.
2. Report the event to the nurse manager.
3. Recheck the blood glucose level in 1 hour.
4. Administer a second dose of 25 mL of $D_{50}W$.

**116.** MoC Prior to medication administration, a hospital policy requires a double-check of two unique client identifiers against the MAR. The nurse manager forms a performance improvement team with the goal of improving nursing compliance with this important safety check. Which activity, related to checking two unique identifiers, should be the responsibility of the performance-improvement team?

1. Hold staff accountable for the practice of checking two unique identifiers.
2. Discipline staff members who fail to comply with checking two unique identifiers.
3. Observe and report the practice of medication administration.
4. Change the practice of two unique identifiers to a more compliant practice.

**117.** MoC A hospital recently formed an ART with the goal of reducing unexpected cardiopulmonary arrests. Which measures should be used to evaluate the performance of the ART? **Select all that apply.**

1. The number of cardiopulmonary arrests
2. The types of supplies used during the ART call
3. Evaluation of the acute response team's actions
4. The outcome of the client following the ART call
5. The types of medications given during the ART call

**118.** MoC The family complains to the oncoming shift nurse about the poor care provided by the previous nurse. They state that discharge instructions including how to perform dressing changes and the client's activity level were confusing and incorrect. After meeting the client and family needs, which action should the oncoming nurse take to prevent this situation from happening again?

1. Ask other nurses if they encountered similar situations while working with that nurse.
2. Review documentation to see if the previous nurse provided the discharge education.
3. Describe the client and family complaint in a report to the risk manager.
4. Report the incident of the nurse's alleged incompetence to the nurse manager.

**119.** MoC The nurse observes the following situations. Which situations would require the nurse to complete a variance (or incident) report? **Select all that apply.**

1. An antibiotic given 2 hours later than scheduled
2. The HCP who is angry with a delayed laboratory report
3. An incomplete laboratory draw ordered for the morning
4. The client falling out of bed and suffering an ankle fracture
5. The new nurse arriving late to work for the third time

**120.** MoC In reviewing an HCP's orders for the client, the oncoming shift nurse finds that an antibiotic was prescribed but is not listed on the client's MAR. Three doses were missed. Which action should minimize the nurse's malpractice risk?

1. Contact the previous nurse to discuss the omission.
2. Complete the agency's incident or variance report.
3. Contact the HCP and request a new antibiotic order.
4. Document the reason for the error in the medical record.

**121.** MoC Two days after the client's admission, the nurse notices an omitted order to implement a venous thromboembolic protocol. Which statement best describes appropriate **initial** follow-up?

1. "I am glad I didn't make that mistake; that other nurse is going to be in trouble."
2. "I am too busy to complete a variance report. I'll do it tomorrow when I work."
3. "I need to contact the HCP and complete a variance report."
4. "I will need to contact the supervisor immediately about this error."

**122.** MoC The nurse plans a medication teaching for the literate, hospitalized client taking multiple new medications. Which actions should be taken by the nurse to ensure that the client understands the newly prescribed medications? **Select all that apply.**

1. Notify the client's HCP that the client needs teaching on the medications.
2. Provide information leaflets to the client on the medications regarding their use and when to take them.
3. Use pictures that illustrate how and when to take the newly prescribed medications.
4. Have the client practice opening the unit dose medication packets before discharge.
5. Ask the client to write the medication information as the nurse presents it to the client.

**123.** MoC The client falls from a bed, and the nurse documents the incident. Based on the following documentation of the client's fall, place an X at the time the nurse would make a risk-management error related to the client's medical record.

| | |
|---|---|
| 2100 | Noise heard from the client's room. Client found lying on the floor. States she hit her head. Alert and oriented X3. PEARLA. No visible injuries, but moaning and holding head. Returned back to bed (see physical findings flowsheet). Will continue to monitor. Client instructed on use of call light for help with getting out of bed. _____ KAO |
| 2115 | Charge nurse A. Smith, RN, and Dr. Brown notified of client fall. Dr. Brown states he will come in to assess the client. _____ KAO |
| 2130 | Dr. Brown here. Client sent for CT of the head with RN monitoring. See physical findings flowsheet. No change in client status. _____ KAO |
| 2145 | Variance form completed and filed in the client's medical record. _____ KAO |
| 2200 | Return from head CT. Voided 300 mL while on bedside commode. Returned to bed with bed exit alarm on. Reminder given on use of call light for help with getting out of bed. Neuro reassessment completed. No change in neuro status. _____ KAO |

**124.** MoC The nurse reviews the admission findings after treating the client who had fallen and determines that a fall assessment was not completed on admission. Which is the **best** action by the nurse?

1. Complete a variance report and place the client on high risk for a fall alert.
2. Complete a variance report and notify the nurse manager regarding the missing assessment.
3. Implement the agency's fall prevention policy.
4. Place wrist restraints on the client to prevent future falls.

**125.** MoC The nurse has a conflict with another staff member regarding a perceived lack of teamwork and negative attitude. Which are common effective conflict-resolution strategies? **Select all that apply.**

1. Avoiding
2. Postponing
3. Opposing
4. Confronting
5. Smoothing

**126.** MoC The nurse manager is planning an orientation program for new graduates. Which strategies should the nurse manager consider to promote retention of these nurses?

1. Implement a self-scheduling system and establish a holiday work schedule based on annual rotation.
2. Plan a party to welcome the new hires and assign a mentor with a ratio of one mentor to four new hires.
3. Involve unit staff in interviewing new hires and initiate a preceptor program using motivated staff nurses.
4. Develop a standardized 6-week orientation for all new hires and celebrate their 1-year anniversary.

**127.** MoC The nurse manager is developing next year's equipment budget. Which factors should be considered when deciding how many oxygen flow meters should be purchased next year? **Select all that apply.**

1. Staff request for more flow meters
2. Cost of nasal cannulas
3. Cost of flow meters
4. Current number of flow meters
5. Predicted client use days for next year

**128.** MoC The nurse manager is evaluating the new nurse's time-management skills. Which statement made by the new nurse may indicate potential concerns with time management?

1. "I am late in giving the eye drops because I needed to assist with a dressing change."
2. "I completed the physical assessment before checking the morning medications to be given."
3. "I admitted the client who came 15 minutes before my shift ended so I didn't get out on time."
4. "I should be leaving, but I am still documenting all of the treatments I performed today."

**129.** MoC At a staff meeting, the nurse manager shares that the unit is over budget by 2% and needs to reduce costs. One of the staff nurses suggests that reports could be shortened so that nurses could finish their shifts on time. How should the nurse manager measure the success of this idea once implemented?

1. Observe the change-of-shift report to determine how many nurses are leaving on time.
2. Delegate monitoring the change-of-shift report to the charge nurses.
3. Review the capital budget expenditures on a monthly basis.
4. Monitor for a reduction in nursing hours per client day.

**130.** MoC The nurse notices a posting on a bulletin board for a continuing education (CE) offering on the prevention of pressure ulcers. Which is the **most** compelling reason for the nurse to attend?

1. The unit has experienced an increase in the number of clients with pressure ulcers.
2. The nurse wants continuing education in order to keep up with current clinical knowledge.
3. The nurse needs one more continuing education unit for state license renewal.
4. The nurse is able to attend by coming in 1 hour earlier than the next scheduled shift.

**131.** MoC The nurse educator is responsible for teaching staff members about a change in a central line dressing change procedure. Which method of education would **best** enhance the staff's retention of this information?

1. In-service education
2. Specialty certification
3. Informal education
4. Providing a contact hour

**132.** MoC The day charge nurse is preparing to report to the oncoming shift nurse. Which action should be taken **first** by the charge nurse when learning that the unit will be short-staffed because two nurses called in ill and the hospital does not have any extra nurses?

1. Ask two off-going nurses to stay and work overtime.
2. Notify the nurse manager of the situation.
3. Ask the ward secretary to call nurses who are off to come in to work.
4. Reallocate responsibilities to better utilize the NAs.

**133.** MoC Several nurses are discussing their unhappiness with some residents of an extended care facility placing increased demands on staff. Which statement, if made by one of the nurses, suggests a unit culture characteristic of transformational leadership?

1. "I discussed this problem with the nurse manager, and the nurse manager will take this concern to the Medical Director."
2. "Because these demands are occurring more at night, the night charge nurse should talk to the residents causing the problems for us."
3. "The nurse manager suggested that I place this concern on the agenda for a weekly staff meeting so we can get staff input."
4. "We made a list of the actual incidents that are concerning to us and now can send these specifics to the nurse manager and Medical Director."

**134.** MoC The nurse manager is mediating a grievance brought by the NA about the nurse after the NA was unsuccessful in resolving the conflict. At the mediation session, the NA repeatedly states that the nurse's delegation is unfair and overloading while the nurse continues to repeat the reasons for the delegated activities. Which is the nurse manager's **best** course of action at this time?

1. Inform the NA that the nurse is delegating appropriately.
2. Tell the two individuals that they need to reach their own resolution.
3. Ask each party to explore if there are other issues surrounding the conflict.
4. Continue to attentively listen as the parties repeat their thoughts and feelings.

**135.** MoC The nurse is obtaining health information from a Web site for the parents of a child diagnosed with sickle cell anemia. Prior to printing information for the parents, the nurse should take which actions? **Select all that apply.**

1. Check the URL domain for the publishing author, such as a Web address ending in ".gov."
2. Determine when the Web page and links were last updated and whether information is current.
3. Evaluate the author's credentials and whether the information is appropriate for the parents.
4. Use a search engine to find blogs for providing facts about the disease to the parents.
5. Provide the Web address for a pharmacy so the parents can check on new medications.
6. Evaluate the content of the document to ascertain whether contents are fact or opinion.

**136.** MoC The nurse is informing clients about the national registry for bone marrow donation. Which nursing interventions might encourage the client to participate? **Select all that apply.**

1. Reassure that there is no risk of acquiring HIV from the donation procedure.
2. Explain that anyone between the ages of 21 and 55 years can donate bone marrow.
3. Focus on the positive aspects that the person is "helping others" through the donation.
4. Explain that recipients must live a healthy lifestyle after receiving the transplant.
5. Inform them that donors are not responsible for costs from the donation procedure.

**137.** MoC The nurse is updating the client's plan of care and asks the client "What is important for us to know about while you are hospitalized?" Which symbol should the nurse include in the client's plan of care when the client identifies the religious beliefs of Islam as being important and shows the nurse this symbol?

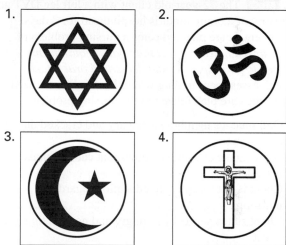

**138.** MoC The nurse educator develops an educational module to assist nursing staff to care for a refugee population new to the community. Which should be the **priority** information that the nurse should include in the module?

1. Include family members in care and learning activities.
2. Treat each client respectfully as an individual.
3. Determine the beliefs that most in the group have in common.
4. Utilize language assistance services available in the hospital.

**139.** MoC The nurse completed an educational program on developing cultural competence. In which order should the nurse place the phases of developing cultural competence? Place the phases in the order of the first to the last phase.

1. Cultural competence
2. Cultural sensitivity
3. Cultural recognition
4. Cultural awareness

Answer: _____

**140.** MoC The medical record of the infant of African descent states that the infant has Mongolian spots. Place an X on the illustration where the nurse should look for Mongolian spots during the admission assessment.

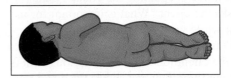

**141.** MoC The 72-year-old client with a left leg DVT and a history of a brain tumor is hospitalized for 3 days. The client's care plan indicates a nursing problem of *Imbalanced nutrition: less than body requirements related to poor appetite and decreased oral intake.* Which assessment finding would **best** indicate a need to revise the care plan related to the nursing problem?

1. Oral mucous membranes are dry and cracked due to dehydration.
2. Daily intake and output shows that caloric intake is inadequate.
3. Client is not receptive to education regarding nutrition.
4. Client states not feeling hungry and not wanting to eat.

**142.** MoC The new nurse is administering an intermittent enteral feeding through an NG tube. Which action demonstrates to the mentor that the new nurse follows proper procedure?

1. Administers the feeding as rapidly as possible
2. Positions the client supine for 1 hour after completing the feeding
3. Confirms tube placement after the feeding has been infused
4. Elevates the head of the client's bed to 45 degrees during the feeding

**143.** MoC A dietary aide shows the nurse the snack options for the client on a clear liquid diet. Which selection should the nurse **eliminate** from the snack choices?

1. Glass of skim milk
2. Small dish of plain gelatin
3. Glass of iced tea
4. Carton of apple juice

**144.** MoC The new nurse, caring for the client with respiratory acidosis, tells the mentor that the client's ABG results show that the client's kidneys have compensated for the imbalance. Which are the values the new nurse identified that indicate compensation?

1. pH 7.43    Paco$_2$ 60 mm Hg    HCO$_3$ 35 mmol/L
2. pH 7.35    Paco$_2$ 50 mm Hg    HCO$_3$ 30 mmol/L
3. pH 7.50    Paco$_2$ 35 mm Hg    HCO$_3$ 30 mmol/L
4. pH 7.44    Paco$_2$ 45 mm Hg    HCO$_3$ 24 mmol/L

**145.** MoC The client with a right femoral arterial line is confused, thrashing about in bed, and picking at the tubing. The HCP prescribes wrist restraints. Based on this information, what should the nurse plan to do?

1. Apply the wrist restraints as prescribed.
2. Request an order for a right ankle restraint also.
3. Request an order for sedation instead of restraints.
4. Question the order; restraints will increase the client's agitation.

**146.** MoC The nurse is developing guidelines to assist personnel in meeting the hygiene needs of clients with dementia. Which guidelines are appropriate for the nurse to include? **Select all that apply.**

1. To limit the client's ability to physically resist, two staff should quickly bathe the client.
2. Include music and dim lighting to create a calm environment when giving a bed bath.
3. Allow clients who are willing and able to participate in some of the hygienic activities.
4. Assess for and treat the client's pain before initiating hygienic cares with the client.
5. Wash the client's hair and body separately if either activity causes the client distress.

**147.** MoC The nurse is orienting the new nurse to a PACU. Which statement by the new nurse indicates further orientation is needed?

1. "Lactated Ringer's (LR) and 5% dextrose with LR are typical IV solutions administered in the PACU."
2. "If the client has an opioid overdose, I should expect to administer naloxone hydrochloride."
3. "I should monitor vital signs and perform a pain assessment every 15 minutes or more often, if necessary."
4. "Once the client responds verbally after a spinal anesthetic, the client can be transferred to the nursing unit."

**148.** **MoC** The nurse is supervising a basic life support class. Which action by the class participants would indicate the need for further instruction?

1. Performing chest compressions at a depth of 1.5 inches on the adult client
2. Implementing use of the head-tilt, chin-lift maneuver to open the airway
3. Applying defibrillator pads to the client's bare chest upon AED arrival
4. Using a bag-valve-mask device to administer ventilations to the client

**149.** **MoC** The 42-year-old client who had a partial hydatidiform molar pregnancy 3 months ago asks the nurse whether she and her husband can try conceiving again. Which response by the nurse is incorrect and warrants follow-up action by the observing nurse manager?

1. "You will need serial levels of beta human chorionic gonadotropin (BHCG) drawn."
2. "You cannot conceive ever again because of your risk of choriocarcinoma."
3. "You should not become pregnant yet for 6 to 12 months."
4. "Your risk of another hydatidiform molar pregnancy is low."

**150.** **MoC** The nurse is educating the postpartum client. Which prevention strategies for postpartum depression should the nurse include? **Select all that apply.**

1. Attend a support group that has other postpartum women.
2. Use the baby's nap time to complete household chores.
3. Keep a journal of feelings during the postpartum period.
4. Call the HCP if feelings of sadness do not subside quickly.
5. Develop a daily schedule of activities, and follow the plan.

**151.** **MoC** The nurse caring for the postpartum client who is 15 years old is concerned about this client's ability to parent a newborn. Which behavior is characteristic of the developmental level of the 15-year-old that justifies the nurse's concern?

1. Developing autonomy
2. Follows rules established by others
3. Career oriented
4. Egocentric

**152.** **MoC** The nurse educator is planning teaching for other nurses after noting that some nurses need additional education on insulin types and how to use the new insulin injection pens. When planning teaching, which question by the educator **best** reflects consideration that the nurses are adult learners?

1. "Does anyone want to volunteer to prepare a poster board and help with handouts?"
2. "What do you need to learn about insulin, and what teaching method would you prefer?"
3. "Can you attend a presentation if I post various times during the day and evening shift?"
4. "What don't you understand about the information in the policy and procedure manual?"

**153.** **MoC** **PHARM** The nurse administers 15 units of glargine insulin at 2100 hours to the client when the client's fingerstick blood glucose reading is 110 mg/dL. At 2300, an NA reports that an evening snack was not given because the client was sleeping. Which instruction by the nurse is **most** appropriate?

1. "You will need to wake the client to check the blood glucose and then give a snack. All diabetics get a snack at bedtime."
2. "It is not necessary for this client to have a snack; glargine insulin is absorbed over 24 hours and doesn't have a peak."
3. "The next time the client wakes up, check a blood glucose level and then give a 15-gram carbohydrate snack."
4. "I will notify the HCP; a snack at this time will affect the next blood glucose level and dose of glargine insulin."

**154.** **MoC** **PHARM** The 18-month-old who has an uncorrected cyanotic heart disease experienced a hypercyanotic spell. The experienced nurse evaluated that the new nurse intervened appropriately. Which actions did the new nurse perform? **Select all that apply.**

1. Placed the child in a knee-chest position
2. Administered 2 L of oxygen via nasal cannula
3. Administered intramuscular morphine sulfate
4. Used a calm and comforting approach
5. Administered oral propranolol if prescribed

**155.** **MoC** The nurse is planning the discharge of the pediatric burn victim to the child's home. The child is able to ambulate with assistance but is cognitively and developmentally unable to function at the age-appropriate milestones due to asphyxiation. Which intervention is **most** important to include in the discharge planning of this child?

1. Identify support groups for the child's parents.
2. Initiate referrals for the child's rehabilitation.
3. Assess the child's home to ensure it is safe.
4. Contact the school regarding the child's needs.

# Answers and Rationales

**83.** MoC **ANSWER: 2, 4, 5**

1. The client should be admitted and then seen by the HCP.
2. **Federal law and many state laws require that hospitals must provide emergency care.**
3. The client can be transferred only after receiving medical screening and stabilization. The client must consent to the transfer, and there must be a facility available to accept the client.
4. **All clients, regardless of ability to pay and living circumstances, should be treated with respect and dignity.**
5. **A social worker consult should be initiated because the social worker's role includes assisting clients with placement and financial issues.**

▸ *Test-taking Tip: The nurse should be aware of the federal, state, and local legal standards under which nursing practice operates. This is an example of a federal legal standard. Remember that the role of a social worker is to assist clients with placement and financial issues.*

**Content Area:** Management of Care; **Concept:** Management; Comfort; **Integrated Processes:** Nursing Process: Implementation; Caring; Culture and Spirituality; **Client Needs:** Safe and Effective Care Environment: Management of Care; Psychosocial Integrity; **Cognitive Level:** Application [Applying]

**84.** MoC **ANSWER: 3**

1. Home care resources may be necessary if the nursing assessment demonstrates that the client has a self-care deficit.
2. The client may have pain related to the surgical procedure, but if the assessment demonstrates no self-care deficits, the client will be able to be discharged safely without further intervention.
3. **The nurse's assessment of the client's self-care deficits will determine if additional resources or education are necessary.**
4. The client may be taking medications, but if the assessment demonstrates no self-care deficits, the client will be able to be discharged safely without further intervention.

▸ *Test-taking Tip: The key phrase is "most important." Clients being discharged to home after hospitalization should either have the ability to care for themselves or have assistance available to meet their care needs.*

**Content Area:** Management of Care; **Concept:** Safety; Oxygenation; **Integrated Processes:** Nursing Process: Assessment; **Client Needs:** Safe and Effective Care Environment: Management of Care; **Cognitive Level:** Application [Applying]

**85.** MoC **ANSWER: 1**

1. **A clinical pathway is a standardized multidisciplinary care plan that projects the client goals, expected course of the client's treatment, and progress over the client's hospital stay.**

2. An education plan will include the information required for the client to understand care and treatment related to the surgical procedure, but it is not a comprehensive plan for the client's care.
3. HCP-initiated intervention is an individual treatment initiated by the HCP related to a medical diagnosis that is then carried out by the nurse.
4. Although discharge planning helps establish client goals and should be started at the time of admission, it will not predict the client's course during the hospital stay.

▸ *Test-taking Tip: The key words are "predict" and "direct." Clinical pathways, care maps, clinical paths, collaborative care plans, or multidisciplinary care plans all provide a timeline with projected client goals, expected course of the client's treatment, and progress over the client's hospital stay.*

**Content Area:** Management of Care; **Concept:** Management; **Integrated Processes:** Nursing Process: Planning; **Client Needs:** Safe and Effective Care Environment: Management of Care; **Cognitive Level:** Synthesis [Creating]

**86.** MoC **ANSWER: 1**

1. **The Joint Commission National Patient Safety Goals requires telephone orders to be written and read back. This action will validate the accuracy of the order received.**
2. Although the order is STAT, calling the laboratory is not the most important safety consideration.
3. Giving the order to the health unit coordinator is not the most important safety consideration.
4. The client is to have blood drawn for a blood culture and not for a culture to receive a blood transfusion.

▸ *Test-taking Tip: The key words are "most important safety consideration." Select the option that would ensure that the nurse's understanding of the order is correct.*

**Content Area:** Management of Care; **Concept:** Safety; **Integrated Processes:** Communication and Documentation; **Client Needs:** Safe and Effective Care Environment: Management of Care; **Cognitive Level:** Application [Applying]

**87.** MoC **ANSWER: 1, 2, 3, 5**

1. **The nurse should coordinate care and provide medication teaching.**
2. **The dietitian should provide diet counseling.**
3. **The social worker should address finances.**
4. There would be no need for a NA to be present for the care conference. If assistance is required in the home, this would be arranged by the social worker or a case coordinator.
5. **The respiratory therapist should instruct on chest percussion and nebulizer treatments.**

▸ *Test-taking Tip: You should recall that care conferences are multidisciplinary and that comprehensive discharge planning involves significant collaboration between disciplines. Consider the roles of the disciplines in managing patient care to determine who should be included in the conference.*

**Content Area:** Management of Care; **Concept:** Collaboration; **Integrated Processes:** Nursing Process: Planning; **Client Needs:** Safe and Effective Care Environment: Management of Care; **Cognitive Level:** Application [Applying]

**88.** MoC **ANSWER: 2**

1. Although the client has a history of alcohol abuse, consulting with chemical dependency is not the most important action at this time for providing the best overall care.
2. **An interdisciplinary team approach incorporating the expertise of the case manager, HCP, social worker, chemical dependency counselor, and other disciplines such as spiritual care will have the most effect on the client's overall plan of care.**
3. Although the client may have DTs and calling the HCP for orders is important, this action alone will not have the same effect in overall care as an interdisciplinary team approach.
4. Consulting the social worker to address client finances and placement will be important for discharge planning; however, consulting with the social worker alone will not have the same effect in overall care as an interdisciplinary team approach.

▶ *Test-taking Tip: Clients with multiple problems require more assistance than that provided by only HCPs and nurses. The key word is "overall." Look for similar words in the options.*

Content Area: Management of Care; Concept: Collaboration; Diversity; Integrated Processes: Nursing Process: Evaluation; Culture and Spirituality; Client Needs: Safe and Effective Care Environment: Management of Care; Cognitive Level: Evaluation [Evaluating]

**89.** MoC **ANSWER: 2**

1. The PT may independently ambulate the client, but the nurse may want to give instructions such as "stop ambulation if the respiratory rate exceeds 30 breaths per minute."
2. **The nurse is responsible for overseeing the client's care. The nurse should inform PT of the client's respiratory status prior to ambulation and give instructions as to when to stop ambulation.**
3. There is no indication that the client would be unable to tolerate the increased activity; the respiratory status of the client should be evaluated prior to and during ambulation.
4. Although it would have been preferable for PT to tell the nurse about the plan to progress ambulation, the plan of care reflects the change; it is unnecessary to notify the HCP.

▶ *Test-taking Tip: To select the correct option, you should focus on the respiratory status of the client and the person responsible for the overall care of the client.*

Content Area: Management of Care; Concept: Collaboration; Mobility; Integrated Processes: Nursing Process: Implementation; Client Needs: Safe and Effective Care Environment: Management of Care; Cognitive Level: Analysis [Analyzing]

**90.** MoC **ANSWER: 2**

1. The dietitian may be consulted regarding the poor appetite; however, consulting with the social worker is more imperative to the discharge plan.

2. **The social worker is most important to consult regarding this client. The social worker's responsibilities include placement issues. The social worker may be able to recommend a nursing home or assisted living facility for discharge placement because the client lives alone and is unable to ambulate independently.**
3. Although the pharmacist may be able to assist with medications should they be affecting the client's appetite, appropriate placement for this client upon discharge is the most pressing need.
4. Although the physical therapist may be able to assist with improving the client's mobility, appropriate placement for this client upon discharge is the most pressing need.

▶ *Test-taking Tip: Key words are "most important." Consider the most pressing need given that the client will be discharged tomorrow.*

Content Area: Management of Care; Concept: Management; Integrated Processes: Nursing Process: Planning; Client Needs: Safe and Effective Care Environment: Management of Care; Cognitive Level: Application [Applying]

**91.** MoC **ANSWER: 1, 3**

1. **A respiratory therapist consult is able to provide assistance with the client's requirements for oxygen and chest physiotherapy.**
2. There is no information to indicate that a physical therapist is needed; the respiratory therapist will provide assistance with chest physiotherapy.
3. **Because the tracheostomy is permanent, a referral for a speech therapist is needed to assist the client in using a speaking valve.**
4. A social worker would be involved if the client needs assistance with financial or placement issues, but there is no indication that this service is needed.
5. No information is available about the client's underlying problem to determine if an occupational therapist should be consulted.

▶ *Test-taking Tip: Focus on the key word "initially." Eliminate options that may be needed if additional information was provided to indicate their need. Use the ABC's.*

Content Area: Management of Care; Concept: Collaboration; Integrated Processes: Nursing Process: Planning; Client Needs: Safe and Effective Care Environment: Management of Care; Cognitive Level: Synthesis [Creating]

**92.** MoC **ANSWER: 4**

1. Renal-failure diets are very specialized, and the nurse should not independently compromise with the client without consulting the dietitian, as this is the dietitian's area of expertise.
2. Working with the primary meal preparer does not involve the client; therefore the outcome may not be successful. The client is not indicating noncompliance.
3. Changing the medication regimen may not be an alternative to following the renal diet.

4. **The nurse should collaborate with the dietitian to assist this client by initiating a referral; a dietician has expertise in diet counseling.**

♦ *Test-taking Tip:* The nurse should collaborate with other health professionals to meet client health needs. Consider which health professional has expertise to give advice on food choices.

**Content Area:** Management of Care; **Concept:** Collaboration; Diversity; **Integrated Processes:** Teaching/Learning; Culture and Spirituality; **Client Needs:** Safe and Effective Care Environment: Management of Care; **Cognitive Level:** Application [Applying]

### 93. MoC PHARM ANSWER: 2

1. The case coordinator's responsibilities do not include individual client teaching on proper use of the diskus.
2. **The respiratory therapist is the most qualified to instruct the client on breathing techniques for proper diskus use and inhalation of medications.**
3. Social workers do not give instruction on the use of medications. Their role includes counseling regarding concerns with finances, living arrangements and placement issues, marital difficulties, and adoption of children.
4. Pharmacists know a great deal about the medication's mechanism of action but may not know the most appropriate teaching method for correct inhalation techniques.

♦ *Test-taking Tip:* Fluticasone/salmeterol (Advair Diskus) is an inhaler. Think about the role of each health care team member and who would be most qualified.

**Content Area:** Management of Care; **Concept:** Collaboration; Oxygenation; **Integrated Processes:** Teaching/Learning; **Client Needs:** Safe and Effective Care Environment: Management of Care; Physiological Integrity: Pharmacological and Parenteral Therapies; **Cognitive Level:** Application [Applying]

### 94. MoC ANSWER: 1

1. **It is most appropriate to consult with a palliative care nurse when the client has a chronic disease. This nurse's role is to provide options to treatment that enhance comfort, control symptoms, and improve the quality of an individual's life, regardless of the stage of the chronic disease or disease prognosis. The palliative care nurse usually counsels clients over an extended period of time.**
2. The social worker's role includes counseling regarding concerns with finances, living arrangements and placement issues, marital difficulties, and adoption of children.
3. The dialysis nurse is a good resource for immediate concerns regarding renal failure and dialysis; however, the dialysis nurse may not be able to address coping with other chronic conditions.
4. The charge nurse is a good resource for immediate concerns but would not be able to address the client's concerns after discharge.

♦ *Test-taking Tip:* Key words are to "cope with a chronic disease." Understand the roles of different health care staff.

**Content Area:** Management of Care; **Concept:** Collaboration; **Integrated Processes:** Nursing Process: Assessment; **Client Needs:** Safe and Effective Care Environment: Management of Care; **Cognitive Level:** Application [Applying]

### 95. MoC ANSWER: 2

1. Alarms from both inaccurate pulse oximeter operation and incorrect sensing of the client's pulse are common; the machine may not need to be replaced.
2. **Consulting with a more experienced nurse may help with establishing safe and accurate readings. The new nurse may not be familiar with techniques to improve the operation of the pulse oximetry machine.**
3. Turning off the alarm is an unsafe practice and should never be done.
4. It would be inappropriate to notify the HCP of the low pulse oximeter reading, as an accurate reading has not been established.

♦ *Test-taking Tip:* Remember that you are working as part of a team and to use resources when necessary; this may include consulting another nurse.

**Content Area:** Management of Care; **Concept:** Collaboration; Oxygenation; **Integrated Processes:** Nursing Process: Analysis; **Client Needs:** Safe and Effective Care Environment: Management of Care; **Cognitive Level:** Application [Applying]

### 96. MoC PHARM ANSWER: 4

1. Continuing to give the same medication as the previous nurse does not demonstrate critical thinking in analyzing the complex needs of managing alcohol withdrawal.
2. Current evidence does not indicate that a particular sedative is most effective in treatment of delirium tremens. Diazepam (Valium), lorazepam (Ativan), and propofol (Diprivan) are recommended as best practice and should be used appropriately until the desired effect is achieved.
3. Propofol is an IV anesthetic and should only be considered if diazepam and lorazepam are ineffective. If propofol is administered, the client should be intubated and mechanically ventilated for safety.
4. **Pharmacists are experts in medication actions and indications, and should be consulted.**

♦ *Test-taking Tip:* Consulting with specialists and experts provides optimal care for each client by helping to solve difficult problems.

**Content Area:** Management of Care; **Concept:** Medication; Critical Thinking; **Integrated Processes:** Nursing Process: Analysis; **Client Needs:** Safe and Effective Care Environment: Management of Care; Physiological Integrity: Pharmacological and Parenteral Therapies; **Cognitive Level:** Analysis [Analyzing]

**97. MoC ANSWER: 3, 4, 5, 1, 2, 6**

3. **To obtain immediate assistance, the nurse should request the ART before the client deteriorates further into respiratory arrest.**
4. **Prepare necessary equipment, including an oximeter and noninvasive BP monitor, so supplies are available for the team.**
5. **Communicate using a handoff method such as SBAR so the team has clear information to treat the client.**
1. **Assist in the reassessment of the client so the team may clearly identify recent changes in the client's condition.**
2. **Contact the surgeon for notification of the presence of the ART.**
6. **Contact the client's family to update them regarding the changes in the client's condition.**

▶ *Test-taking Tip: Use the steps of the nursing process and the ABC's of emergency management to prioritize the nurse's actions. The nurse should be collaborating with other health professionals in emergency situations.*

Content Area: Management of Care; Concept: Management; Integrated Processes: Nursing Process: Evaluation; Client Needs: Safe and Effective Care Environment: Management of Care; Cognitive Level: Synthesis [Creating]

**98. MoC ANSWER: 4**

1. Requesting information in SBAR format indicates that the ICU nurse is independently taking action without involving the medical nurse.
2. Obtaining vital signs indicates that the ICU nurse is independently taking action without involving the medical nurse.
3. Calling the HCP indicates that the ICU nurse is independently taking action without involving the medical nurse.
4. **The resource nurse does not take over the care of the client but teaches and supports the nurse. Reviewing assessment findings may help to identify the underlying cause for the decreased level of consciousness and immediate interventions.**

▶ *Test-taking Tip: The key word is "resource." Carefully read the ICU nurse's action in each of the options; only one option shows collaboration.*

Content Area: Management of Care; Concept: Collaboration; Integrated Processes: Nursing Process: Assessment; Client Needs: Safe and Effective Care Environment: Management of Care; Cognitive Level: Analysis [Analyzing]

**99. MoC ANSWER: 1, 2, 4**

1. **Subjective information can be obtained by asking questions and is part of an admission assessment.**
2. **Vital signs provide information about the client and are part of an admission assessment.**
3. The development of the care plan is completed following the admission assessment and is included in the nursing process step of analysis.

4. **Obtaining functional ability information is an essential component of an admission assessment because it can affect the care needed.**
5. Documentation of any education completed is included in the nursing process step of implementation and is not part of the admission assessment.

▶ *Test-taking Tip: Use the nursing process step of assessment to eliminate options that pertain to the other steps of the nursing process. In assessment, the nurse is collecting information about the client.*

Content Area: Management of Care; Concept: Assessment; Integrated Processes: Nursing Process: Assessment; Client Needs: Safe and Effective Care Environment: Management of Care; Cognitive Level: Application [Applying]

**100. MoC ANSWER: 4**

1. This is a stage III pressure ulcer. There is full-thickness skin loss extending to the subcutaneous fat but not fascia. The ulcer appears crater-like and may have damage of adjacent tissue. Muscle, tendon, and bone are not visible.
2. This is a stage I pressure ulcer. The skin is intact, but the area is nonblanchable. The skin may be red or discolored.
3. This is a stage IV pressure ulcer. There is full-thickness skin loss with exposed tendons. Slough is present. There may be undermining and sinus tracts (tunneling).
4. **There is a break in the skin with partial-thickness skin loss of epidermis and dermis. The ulcer appears as a shallow crater and does not contain slough (yellow fibrous tissue).**

▶ *Test-taking Tip: The nurse is describing a stage II pressure ulcer.*

Content Area: Management of Care; Concept: Management; Skin Integrity; Integrated Processes: Communication and Documentation; Client Needs: Safe and Effective Care Environment: Management of Care; Cognitive Level: Application [Applying]

**101. MoC ANSWER: 2**

1. The report should include transferring responsibility for care to the next nurse whose name is documented in the medical record; however, this will not ensure continuity of care.
2. **Including the client's condition, treatment plan, and needs in the verbal report will ensure the nurse has communicated the client's needs for continuity of care.**
3. All transfer forms should be completed, but communicating key information verbally is a better mechanism for ensuring continuity of care.
4. Informing the client of the plans for transfer is important; however, because the team assuming care is not involved in the discussion, it does not ensure continuity of care.

▶ *Test-taking Tip: Verbal communication is a key element for the continuity of the client's care. Determine which option describes verbal communication with a member of the client's care team.*

Content Area: Management of Care; Concept: Management; Integrated Processes: Communication and Documentation; Client Needs: Safe and Effective Care Environment: Management of Care; Cognitive Level: Analysis [Analyzing]

### 102. MoC ANSWER: 4, 5

1. Medications supplied by the hospital should not be sent to the new facility; only those that are brought to the hospital by the client are sent with the client to another facility.
2. Clinic records are usually not available to the nurse in the hospital.
3. Emergency medications are not sent with transferring clients. If the client is transporting via ambulance, the ambulance is supplied with the necessary emergency medications.
4. **Copies of the client's medical record should be included in transfer documentation to ensure continuity of care. Each facility will have a policy on which documents should be included.**
5. **To prevent items from being lost, personal belongings should be sent with the client to the new facility or should be sent home with the client's family. All items sent with the client or with family members should be documented.**

▶ *Test-taking Tip: Determine if the items are essential for continuity of care. Remember that personal items should stay with the client and should not be left behind.*

Content Area: Management of Care; Concept: Management; Integrated Processes: Nursing Process: Planning; Communication and Documentation; Client Needs: Safe and Effective Care Environment: Management of Care; Cognitive Level: Comprehension [Understanding]

### 103. MoC ANSWER: 2

1. The Social Security office will provide the client with information for obtaining government financial assistance; however, the agency services can take from weeks to months to process and will therefore not meet the immediate needs of the client.
2. **The homeless shelter is most likely to provide the greatest level of service for the homeless client.**
3. The public health clinic is a good resource for follow-up medical care, if necessary.
4. The parish nursing program may be able to provide services; however, the level of service may vary depending on the area.

▶ *Test-taking Tip: Apply knowledge of Maslow's Hierarchy of Needs for basic physiological needs and which service could best meet the client's immediate needs.*

Content Area: Management of Care; Concept: Management; Integrated Processes: Caring; Culture/Spirituality; Client Needs: Safe and Effective Care Environment: Management of Care; Cognitive Level: Analysis [Analyzing]

### 104. MoC ANSWER: 1, 2, 4, 6

1. **The client's diagnosis should be included in the change-of-shift report because this can influence the plan of care.**
2. **New orders, medications, and treatments are important to include because there may be some that the oncoming shift nurse should implement. These also provide information about the client's progression of care.**
3. Personal opinions are not pertinent to providing client care and should be omitted.
4. **The effectiveness of previously administered analgesics may assist the nurse in decision making about the choice of analgesics and the client's pain control.**
5. The turning schedule can be reviewed in documentation and is not necessary in shift report.
6. **Information about areas for priority focus on the next shift will aid in ensuring that essential interventions are not missed.**

▶ *Test-taking Tip: Sufficient information about the client and the client's care should be included in a change-of-shift report so that the nurse can work toward meeting client outcomes safely and efficiently.*

Content Area: Management of Care; Concept: Communication; Integrated Processes: Communication and Documentation; Client Needs: Safe and Effective Care Environment: Management of Care; Cognitive Level: Synthesis [Creating]

### 105. MoC ANSWER: 1, 3, 4, 5

1. **The EMTALA form is required by law from the Health Care Financing Administration. It includes information related to client status prior to transfer.**
2. The client teaching record is a legal part of the medical record but is not required for ongoing urgent care.
3. **The transfer note includes the condition of the client, the reason for and method of transfer, and communications with the receiving facility.**
4. **The history and physical is the HCP's documentation of the client's assessment finding and recommended plan of care.**
5. **The progress notes are a legal part of the medical record and will be required for ongoing urgent care.**
6. The activity flowsheet is a legal part of the medical record but is not required for ongoing urgent care.

▶ *Test-taking Tip: The key word is "essential." Review each option and determine if the document is necessary to continue with care or if the information on that form may be included elsewhere in the documentation.*

Content Area: Management of Care; Concept: Communication; Integrated Processes: Communication and Documentation; Client Needs: Safe and Effective Care Environment: Management of Care; Cognitive Level: Application [Applying]

**106.** MoC **ANSWER: 2**

1. Skilled nursing care would provide direct care for the client but not the client's caregiver.
2. **Respite care is the service that provides relief care for family caregivers.**
3. Hospice care provides end-of-life services for both the client and family.
4. Physical therapy would provide direct care for the client but not the client's caregiver.

▶ *Test-taking Tip: The key words are "greatest assistance to the client's spouse." Review the options to determine which one would be most beneficial to the spouse.*

Content Area: Management of Care; **Concept:** Management; **Integrated Processes:** Caring; **Client Needs:** Safe and Effective Care Environment: Management of Care; **Cognitive Level:** Analysis [Analyzing]

**107.** MoC **ANSWER: 4**

1. Rescheduling the PFT may not be consistent with the HCP's treatment plan and should not be decided by the nurse.
2. A portable CXR may not produce that same quality as a standing CXR in the radiology department. It is the HCP's decision to change to a portable view.
3. It is unrealistic for the nurse to accompany the client to both of these tests, as other clients will need nursing care during this time.
4. **The radiology department may not be aware that the CXR and PFT are scheduled on the same day or that the client tires easily. The client will be most fatigued after the PFT, so the CXR should be completed first.**

▶ *Test-taking Tip: The key words are "to coordinate the client's care." Coordinating care and advocating for the client may include ensuring that two departments work together to provide for the best and most convenient care for the client.*

Content Area: Management of Care; **Concept:** Management; Oxygenation; **Integrated Processes:** Nursing Process: Planning; **Client Needs:** Safe and Effective Care Environment: Management of Care; **Cognitive Level:** Analysis [Analyzing]

**108.** MoC **ANSWER: 1, 2, 4, 6**

1. **Satisfaction scores are a measurable activity that can be changed to improve client care.**
2. **Reducing fall rates is a measurable activity that can be changed to improve client care.**
3. Increasing client census will not result in an improvement in nursing performance.
4. **Reducing medication safety events is a measurable activity that can be changed to improve client care.**
5. Hiring an additional quality assurance nurse may make it possible to have available staff to *measure* performance improvements, but hiring additional staff is not a performance improvement activity.
6. **Reducing hospital-acquired infections is a measurable activity that can be changed to improve client care.**

▶ *Test-taking Tip: Performance improvement activities serve to improve client care through evaluation and subsequent modification of clinical and operational performance measures. Identify the activities that directly affect client care.*

Content Area: Management of Care; **Concept:** Quality Improvement; **Integrated Processes:** Nursing Process: Evaluation; **Client Needs:** Safe and Effective Care Environment: Management of Care; **Cognitive Level:** Evaluation [Evaluating]

**109.** MoC **ANSWER: 2**

1. Utilizing the Cochrane Collaboration Database should be incorporated when compiling and analyzing research, but it is only one step in the process of utilizing an EBP framework.
2. **This option contains all the relevant aspects of utilizing an EBP framework.**
3. Utilizing the National Guideline Clearinghouse should be incorporated when compiling and analyzing research, but it is only one step in the process of utilizing an EBP framework.
4. The nursing process is not utilized within the EBP framework.

▶ *Test-taking Tip: The key phrase is "framework." When you are uncertain, usually the most inclusive option that incorporates other options is the answer.*

Content Area: Management of Care; **Concept:** Quality Improvement; Evidence-based Practice; **Integrated Processes:** Teaching/Learning; **Client Needs:** Safe and Effective Care Environment: Management of Care; **Cognitive Level:** Application [Applying]

**110.** MoC **ANSWER: 1**

1. **The American Nurses Association has identified that the appropriate numbers and mix of nursing personnel (RNs, LPNs, and unlicensed staff) are imperative for the delivery of safe, cost-effective quality care. This includes the reduction of hospital-acquired infections.**
2. Although important for quality client care, improving team functioning has not demonstrated an impact on infection rates.
3. Monitoring medication safety events is not associated with prevention of hospital-acquired infections.
4. Having adequate supplies is important for quality client care in general, but having adequate staff has been shown to have an effect on hospital-acquired infections.

▶ *Test-taking Tip: Although all options address components that may be monitored for quality improvement, look for the same word in the stem of the question (nurse) and in the options to select the correct option.*

Content Area: Management of Care; **Concept:** Quality Improvement; Regulations; **Integrated Processes:** Nursing Process: Evaluation; **Client Needs:** Safe and Effective Care Environment: Management of Care; **Cognitive Level:** Evaluation [Evaluating]

**111.** MoC PHARM **ANSWER: 2**

First determine the correct dose using a proportion formula.

5000 UNITS : 1 mL :: 2500 UNITS : $X$ mL;

$5000X = 2500$; $X = 2500 \div 5000$; $X = 0.5$.

The correct dose is 0.5 mL. Next, subtract the amount in the syringe from the correct dose to determine how much should be removed: $2.5 - 0.5 = 2$ mL.

▶ *Test-taking Tip: Be sure you read the question carefully. Your answer is not what should be administered, but how much should be expelled.*

Content Area: Management of Care; Concept: Management; Medication; Integrated Processes: Nursing Process: Implementation; Client Needs: Safe and Effective Care Environment: Management of Care; Physiological Integrity: Pharmacological and Parenteral Therapies; Cognitive Level: Evaluation [Evaluating]

**112.** MoC **ANSWER: 1**

1. **Comparing visitation policies with area hospitals is an action that the nurse manager should take first because it would be expedient and involve little expense.**
2. Changing the policy is premature.
3. Waiting to explore this concern is inappropriate.
4. Soliciting feedback from key stakeholders (the clients) is a basic tenet of quality improvement programs, but mailing surveys is not cost-effective as an initial action.

▶ *Test-taking Tip: Focus on the key word "initial." Use the nursing process; assessment should be before intervention. The options concerned with collecting information are Options 1 and 4. You should select the most cost-effective approach as an initial action.*

Content Area: Management of Care; Concept: Quality Improvement; Family; Integrated Processes: Nursing Process: Implementation; Client Needs: Safe and Effective Care Environment: Management of Care; Cognitive Level: Application [Applying]

**113.** CJ MoC **ANSWER:**

| Rooms and Beds | | | |
|---|---|---|---|
| | Client | | Client |
| 275-1 | 2 | 275-2 | |
| 276-1 | 6 | 276-2 | |
| 277-1 | 1 | 277-2 | 5 |
| 278-1 | | 278-2 | 4 |
| 279-1 | | 279-2 | 3 |

1. **Client 1 can be safely placed in Room 277-1 and can be placed in the same room as Client 5. Because Client 1 has a nitroglycerin infusion that is being titrated, the client should be as close as possible to the nurse's station and the door, because the nurse will be in and out of the room to titrate the infusion. Because rooms 275-1 and 276-1 are needed for clients who are more unstable and in need of private rooms, 277-1 is the best placement.**

2. **Client 2 can be safely placed in 275-1, nearest the nurse's station. This client is the most unstable and will need close monitoring due to the client's low ejection fraction and confusion.**
3. **Client 3 can be in a room farther from the nurse's station because the client is stable. Room 279-2 is best because it is farthest from the door and will allow space for the visitors without interrupting other clients.**
4. **Client 4 needs to be in a room without a roommate due to neutropenia. Room 278-2 is best and is away from the door and traffic from visitors to room 279-2.**
5. **Client 5 is stable and can share a room; thus 277-2 is the best available placement.**
6. **Client 6 is unstable and should be near the nurse's station for closer observation. Because the client is having a cardioversion, Client 6 should not have a roommate. Room 276-1 is the best placement.**

▶ *Test-taking Tip: You need to consider the safety of the clients. Unstable clients should be nearest the nurse's station. Others should have a room alone.*

Content Area: Management of Care; Concept: Management; Safety; Integrated Processes: Nursing Process: Planning; Client Needs: Safe and Effective Care Environment: Management of Care; Cognitive Level: Analysis [Analyzing]

**114.** MoC **ANSWER: 4**

1. The difference between the benchmark and current rate is 5.22%. The hospital is better able to achieve this measure than the benchmark hospitals.
2. The difference between the benchmark and current rate is 6.42%. There is need for improvement as compared to benchmark hospitals, but Option 4 has the greatest need for improvement.
3. The difference between the benchmark and current rate is 10.25%. There is need for improvement as compared to benchmark hospitals, but Option 4 has the greatest need for improvement.
4. **The difference between the benchmark and current rate is 19.43%. Other hospitals are able to achieve this measure with greater success.**

▶ *Test-taking Tip: Read each option first; then go to the table and calculate the percentage difference between the benchmark and current rate. Review the entire question and table before calculating the percentage. In performance improvement, hospital data are frequently compared to benchmark data from other hospitals and organizations.*

Content Area: Management of Care; Concept: Quality Improvement; Integrated Processes: Nursing Process: Analysis; Client Needs: Safe and Effective Care Environment: Management of Care; Cognitive Level: Analysis [Analyzing]

**115.** MoC PHARM **ANSWER: 2**

1. To continue the insulin drip at the same rate would result in client injury.
2. **Safety events must be reported to the nurse manager. Risk management seeks to identify and eliminate potential safety hazards. The monitoring and medication protocol may need revision based on changes in the client's status and correlating blood glucose results. Reporting the client's hypoglycemia to the nurse manager will result in the monitoring of patterns and trends and possibly regulatory reporting. Some states require reporting of hypoglycemia that leads to client injury or death.**
3. Waiting 1 hour is too long to determine if the client is still hypoglycemic.
4. A second dose of $D_{50}W$ should not be given without first assessing the client's response and taking another blood glucose measurement.

♦ **Test-taking Tip:** *The key words "risk management action" include appropriate follow-up and reporting. Eliminate options that pertain only to the client.*

**Content Area:** Management of Care; **Concept:** Quality Improvement; Medication; Management; **Integrated Processes:** Nursing Process: Evaluation; **Client Needs:** Safe and Effective Care Environment: Management of Care; Physiological Integrity: Pharmacological and Parenteral Therapies; **Cognitive Level:** Evaluation [Evaluating]

**116.** MoC **ANSWER: 3**

1. It is the responsibility of the nurse manager to hold staff members accountable for their practice as well as disciplining staff if appropriate.
2. Performance improvement is focused on education and system changes for client safety, which create a blame-free environment.
3. **The role of a performance improvement team is to observe and report measures within the initiative. Individual clinical units must be active and independent in monitoring their adherence to client safety initiatives.**
4. Evidence-based practice supports improved client safety by checking two unique identifiers; therefore changing this practice would be unsafe.

♦ **Test-taking Tip:** *Note that three options mention two unique identifiers, and one option is different. Often the option that is different is the answer.*

**Content Area:** Management of Care; **Concept:** Quality Improvement; Management; **Integrated Processes:** Nursing Process: Analysis; **Client Needs:** Safe and Effective Care Environment: Management of Care; **Cognitive Level:** Application [Applying]

**117.** MoC **ANSWER: 1, 3, 4**

1. **Performance improvement requires that the process used to deliver services receives close and constant scrutiny. Monitoring the number of cardiopulmonary arrests helps to improve the ART process because the number of arrests should decrease.**
2. Determining the types of supplies and medications used by the ART on each call will not improve the performance of the ART.
3. **Evaluation of the team's actions will help identify where the ART can be more efficient or helpful to prevent the client arrest and improve performance.**
4. **Monitoring the outcome of the client will help to identify if the goal of reducing cardiopulmonary arrests has been met and if not, how to improve the ART's performance.**
5. The types of medications given during the ART call would not measure the effectiveness of the team's response for improving the ART process.

♦ **Test-taking Tip:** *The key word is "performance." You should identify only measures that can be used to evaluate the ART's performance.*

**Content Area:** Management of Care; **Concept:** Quality Improvement; **Integrated Processes:** Nursing Process: Evaluation; **Client Needs:** Safe and Effective Care Environment: Management of Care; **Cognitive Level:** Evaluation [Evaluating]

**118.** MoC **ANSWER: 4**

1. The nurse manager, not the oncoming nurse, is responsible for collecting data regarding the nurse cited by the family and in evaluating competence.
2. Although documentation regarding discharge teaching may be in place, this would not provide information about how completely or clearly the previous nurse provided the instructions.
3. Although it is a client complaint, it is not an issue to be brought forward to the risk manager without first addressing it with the nurse manager.
4. **If care for the client was not complete, the oncoming nurse has a responsibility to report the previous nurse to the nurse manager for follow-up.**

♦ **Test-taking Tip:** *The key phrase is "prevent this situation from happening again." Note the verbs in each of the options. Select an option that ensures follow-up action. **One of the most common reasons for malpractice lawsuits is failing to report another's incompetency or negligence.***

**Content Area:** Management of Care; **Concept:** Quality Improvement; **Integrated Processes:** Nursing Process: Evaluation; **Client Needs:** Safe and Effective Care Environment: Management of Care; **Cognitive Level:** Evaluation [Evaluating]

**119.** MoC **ANSWER: 1, 3, 4**

1. **An antibiotic that is given 2 hours late breaches the standard of care; a variance form should be completed.**
2. The HCP becoming angry does not directly impact failure to provide client care.
3. **Not having all of the ordered laboratory work results can impact care; a variance form should be completed.**
4. **When the client has a fall, a variance form should be completed.**
5. The nurse manager should document the nurse's tardiness in arriving for work, but this is not included on a variance form.

▶ **Test-taking Tip:** *Think about the purpose and requirements of completing a variance report. A variance report is completed when a standard of care is breached or an unusual incident occurs. It is used for quality improvement in the agency and should not be used to discipline staff members or be placed in an employee's file.*

**Content Area:** Management of Care; **Concept:** Regulations; **Integrated Processes:** Nursing Process: Evaluation; **Client Needs:** Safe and Effective Care Environment: Management of Care; Safe and Effective Care Environment: Safety and Infection Control; **Cognitive Level:** Evaluation [Evaluating]

**120.** MoC **ANSWER: 2**

1. It is not the nurse's responsibility to investigate the source of the error.
2. **An incident report, also called an occurrence or variance report, is a formal record of an unusual occurrence or accident. Submitting an incident report will best document the error and minimize the nurse's malpractice risk.**
3. The HCP should be contacted, but requesting a new antibiotic may not minimize the malpractice risk.
4. The report is for the agency and is not a part of the client's record.

▶ **Test-taking Tip:** *The key phrase is "minimize the nurse's malpractice risk." Think about the purpose of the incident report.*

**Content Area:** Management of Care; **Concept:** Safety; Management; **Integrated Processes:** Nursing Process: Evaluation; **Client Needs:** Safe and Effective Care Environment: Management of Care; Safe and Effective Care Environment: Safety and Infection Control; **Cognitive Level:** Evaluation [Evaluating]

**121.** MoC **ANSWER: 3**

1. Emphasis has been placed on making error reporting "blame free" and determining how the system can be used to reduce errors. This statement is inappropriate blaming.
2. Variance reports should be completed right away for appropriate follow-up.
3. **Reporting systems rely on nurses to recognize and report errors when they occur.**

4. It may be appropriate to contact the supervisor, but it is the responsibility of the nurse to initially notify the HCP and document the event in a variance report.

▶ **Test-taking Tip:** *Focus on "appropriate initial follow-up." Eliminate options that do not demonstrate follow-up. Of the remaining options, determine which is best.*

**Content Area:** Management of Care; **Concept:** Regulations; Management; **Integrated Processes:** Nursing Process: Evaluation; Communication and Documentation; **Client Needs:** Safe and Effective Care Environment: Management of Care; Safe and Effective Care Environment: Safety and Infection Control; **Cognitive Level:** Evaluation [Evaluating]

**122.** MoC **ANSWER: 2, 3.**

1. Medication teaching is a nursing responsibility; it is unnecessary to notify the HCP.
2. **The client can use the leaflets containing information about the medications during the teaching and for later reference.**
3. **Visual teaching materials, such as using pictures and illustrations, enhance learning.**
4. Because of costs, prescriptions are ordinarily not filled with unit doses. Bringing packets to have the client practice opening can cause confusion.
5. If the nurse is using patient information leaflets, having the client write information is unnecessary and can be frustrating for the client.

▶ **Test-taking Tip:** *Research comparing various instructional techniques supports the use of integrative instructions, which combine textual, oral, and pictorial communication to promote comprehension and adherence. Eliminate options that could lead to barriers to learning, such as confusion or frustration.*

**Content Area:** Management of Care; **Concept:** Nursing Roles; **Integrated Processes:** Communication and Documentation; Teaching/Learning **Client Needs:** Safe and Effective Care Environment: Management of Care; **Cognitive Level:** Application [Applying]

**123.** MoC **ANSWER:**

| 2145 | Variance form completed and filed in the client's medical record. ___X___ KAO |
|------|---------------------------------------------------------------------------------|

**At 2145 the nurse documented placing a copy of the variance report in the client's medical record. For legal reasons, a copy should not be included in the client's medical record. All other times show correct documentation.**

▶ **Test-taking Tip:** *When an incident occurs, the documentation in the client's medical record should accurately describe what occurred but not highlight any mistakes that could result in litigation or refer to the filing of an incident report.*

**Content Area:** Management of Care; **Concept:** Safety; Legal; Management; **Integrated Processes:** Nursing Process: Evaluation; **Client Needs:** Safe and Effective Care Environment: Management of Care; Safe and Effective Care Environment: Safety and Infection Control; **Cognitive Level:** Evaluation [Evaluating]

**124.** MoC **ANSWER: 1**

1. **A variance report (also called incident or occurrence report) is a tool used by health care facilities to document situations that have caused harm or have the potential to cause harm to clients. The fall should be documented on a variance report, and the client should also be placed on high risk of falls alert to prevent future falls.**
2. Variance reports are reviewed by nurse managers and should include all pertinent information, including the lack of a fall assessment; therefore it is not necessary to report the admission nurse's lack of assessment.
3. Implementation of the fall prevention policy without a variance report is incomplete follow-up.
4. Wrist restraints may not be necessary to prevent another fall and are not an appropriate choice.

♦ *Test-taking Tip: Key words are "best action." Focus on the needs of the client.*

Content Area: Management of Care  Concept: Quality Improvement; Safety; Management; **Integrated Processes:** Nursing Process: Evaluation; **Client Needs:** Safe and Effective Care Environment: Management of Care; Safe and Effective Care Environment: Safety and Infection Control; **Cognitive Level:** Evaluation [Evaluating]

**125.** MoC **ANSWER: 4, 5**

1. In avoiding, involved persons are aware of the conflict but choose not to acknowledge or attempt to resolve it. This is not an effective conflict-resolution strategy.
2. Postponing the conflict is waiting to a later time to deal with the incident either by keeping track of the issues and additional issues and then dumping all the issues at one time on the offender or waiting and using the incident as a threat or blackmail, or until the conflict can be expressed in front of an audience. This is not an effective conflict-resolution strategy.
3. Opposing the conflict is not a strategy that facilitates conflict resolution.
4. **To confront the conflict is either referring the problem to a supervisor or another person for resolution, or setting up a time and place for a one-time meeting to define goals and problem-solve.**
5. **Smoothing occurs when one person attempts to pacify the other or to focus on agreements rather than differences.**

♦ *Test-taking Tip: The key word is "resolution." Eliminate options that would not resolve the conflict.*

Content Area: Management of Care; **Concept:** Management; Communication; **Integrated Processes:** Communication and Documentation; **Client Needs:** Safe and Effective Care Environment: Management of Care; **Cognitive Level:** Knowledge [Remembering]

**126.** MoC **ANSWER: 3**

1. A self-scheduling system is inappropriate for new hires. During orientation they will have a set schedule.
2. The mentor to new staff ratio should be one to one.
3. **Involving unit staff in interviewing new hires and initiating a preceptor program can promote retention of new graduates. The highest turnover in most hospitals is with new graduates, with many leaving during their first year of employment. When implemented effectively, these two programs have been identified as best practices to decrease turnover of new employees.**
4. The typical orientation period for new hires is six weeks, but this may need to be individualized based on the unit of hire. Celebrating a 1-year anniversary may be nice, but the question is focused on the orientation period.

♦ *Test-taking Tip: Use the process of elimination. Make sure both parts of the answer are correct. Focus on those strategies that can be implemented during the orientation period, thus eliminating Option 4.*

Content Area: Management of Care; **Concept:** Health Care System; Evidence-based Practice; **Integrated Processes:** Nursing Process: Planning; **Client Needs:** Safe and Effective Care Environment: Management of Care; **Cognitive Level:** Application [Applying]

**127.** MoC **ANSWER: 1, 3, 4, 5**

1. **Staff request for more flow meters usually indicates that these are in short supply.**
2. Although the cost of nasal cannulas pertains to oxygen therapy, it is not information that will help the nurse manager predict the number of oxygen flow meters needed.
3. **The cost of the flow meters will influence the number that can be purchased.**
4. **The current number of flow meters is needed to determine the number needed.**
5. **The projected need for flow meters based on the predicted client use volume will influence the number requested.**

♦ *Test-taking Tip: Eliminate options that are irrelevant when calculating the total cost of oxygen flow meters. Nurse managers must be able to project and justify supplies and equipment needed and must be able to provide a reasoned argument that quality nursing care is affected by the lack of equipment.*

Content Area: Management of Care; **Concept:** Economics; Management; **Integrated Processes:** Nursing Process: Assessment; **Client Needs:** Safe and Effective Care Environment: Management of Care; **Cognitive Level:** Analysis [Analyzing]

**128.** MoC **ANSWER: 4**

1. Although giving medications on time should be a priority, the nurse should not leave the client in the middle of a procedure.
2. There is no indication that anything was late and that the nurse's time-management skills are a concern.
3. The nurse cannot abandon the newly admitted client.
4. **Documentation should be done as soon as possible and not be completed at the end of a shift.**

▶ *Test-taking Tip: Read the question and answers carefully to make sure that all information is understood before choosing an answer. Note that all options except one provide a rationale for time management.*

**Content Area:** Management of Care; **Concept:** Management; Legal; **Integrated Processes:** Nursing Process: Evaluation; Communication and Documentation; **Client Needs:** Safe and Effective Care Environment: Management of Care; **Cognitive Level:** Evaluation [Evaluating]

**129.** MoC **ANSWER: 4**

1. Observing the shift report will not measure the success in reducing costs.
2. Delegating the monitoring to the charge nurses will not measure the success in reducing costs.
3. The capital budget includes only equipment with a minimum dollar cost and includes no labor costs.
4. **Monitoring nursing hours per client day will allow the nurse manager to determine if staff members are reducing clinical hours by finishing closer to the end of their shift. A reduction in nursing hours per client day may indicate that reducing the duration of the end-of-shift report is effective.**

▶ *Test-taking Tip: Narrow the options by focusing on the goal of reducing costs and the measure that would help to identify if labor costs have indeed been reduced by a shortened change-of-shift report.*

**Content Area:** Management of Care; **Concept:** Economics; **Integrated Processes:** Nursing Process: Evaluation; **Client Needs:** Safe and Effective Care Environment: Management of Care; **Cognitive Level:** Evaluation [Evaluating]

**130.** MoC **ANSWER: 2**

1. An increase in the number of pressure ulcers may motivate the nurse to attend a CE offering about the prevention of pressure ulcers, but this is not the most compelling reason.
2. **This option demonstrates the nurse's desire for professional growth; the desire for professional growth is a strong motivator and is the most compelling reason of the options to attend a CE program.**
3. Meeting requirements for licensure is not a strong motivator for attending an optional CE offering.
4. Ability to attend is not as strong a motivator to attend an optional CE offering as the desire for professional growth.

▶ *Test-taking Tip: The key words are "most compelling reason." Think about what would motivate you to attend a CE offering.*

**Content Area:** Management of Care; **Concept:** Nursing Roles; **Integrated Processes:** Nursing Process: Assessment; **Client Needs:** Safe and Effective Care Environment: Management of Care; **Cognitive Level:** Application [Applying]

**131.** MoC **ANSWER: 1**

1. **In-service education is offered at the work site and should focus on new equipment and the policy change.**
2. Certification is a formal validation of a high level of knowledge in a defined area of practice typically administered by a certifying organization in nursing.
3. Informal education is typically from one person to another to enhance current knowledge.
4. Contact hour is the measure of continuing education credit and would not influence retention of information.

▶ *Test-taking Tip: The key word is "retention." A formalized setting where nurses would have hands-on contact with the supplies and equipment and the ability to receive information about the policy change would best enhance retention of information.*

**Content Area:** Management of Care; **Concept:** Quality Improvement; Management; **Integrated Processes:** Teaching/Learning; **Client Needs:** Safe and Effective Care Environment: Management of Care; **Cognitive Level:** Application [Applying]

**132.** MoC **ANSWER: 2**

1. Asking nurses to stay is an option to ensure adequate staffing, but the nurse manager should be consulted first.
2. **The nurse manager should be informed of the situation because the nurse manager is accountable for adequate staffing to meet client care needs.**
3. Calling to ask the nurse to work is an option to ensure adequate staffing, but the nurse manager should be consulted first.
4. NAs are unable to carry out RN responsibilities, and client needs may not be adequately met.

▶ *Test-taking Tip: The key word is "first," indicating that more than one option is correct, but one option is best. You should consider the nurse manager's responsibility with unit staffing.*

**Content Area:** Management of Care; **Concept:** Management; Regulations; **Integrated Processes:** Nursing Process: Implementation; **Client Needs:** Safe and Effective Care Environment: Management of Care; **Cognitive Level:** Analysis [Analyzing]

**133.** MoC **ANSWER: 3**

1. Taking a concern to the Medical Director without staff input to identify and solve a problem is using the chain of command to solve problems but does not empower staff.
2. Turning over the problem to the night charge nurse uses the chain of command to solve problems but does not empower staff.

3. **Transformational leaders engage all members of the health care team to identify and solve problems. Gaining input from all stakeholders by discussion at a regularly scheduled meeting is an integral step for collaborative problem identification and problem solving. A transformational leader will encourage everyone to speak, build consensus as to what the exact problem is, and determine how the problem should be solved within the organizational unit goals.**

4. Although collecting specifics will help to identify the problem, taking the concerns to the Medical Director is premature and does not empower staff.

▶ *Test-taking Tip: Focus on the statement that empowers the nurses to seek a resolution to the problem. Note that three options have a similar action (using the chain of command) and that one option is different. Often the option that is different is the answer.*

Content Area: Management of Care; Concept: Management; Communication; Integrated Processes: Communication and Documentation; Client Needs: Safe and Effective Care Environment: Management of Care; Cognitive Level: Application [Applying]

## 134. MoC ANSWER: 3

1. There is insufficient information to determine if the nurse is delegating appropriately.

2. The NA has already attempted to resolve the conflict.

3. **The best course of action is to explore if there are other issues contributing to the conflict. It may be that both parties are feeling overloaded. A discussion-based approach to conflict resolution can help prevent difficult situations from escalating.**

4. Continuing to listen will not move the discussion forward to a resolution.

▶ *Test-taking Tip: Identify which option will help move the discussion toward a resolution. Recall that confronting the conflict is often the most effective resolution strategy.*

Content Area: Management of Care; Concept: Management; Integrated Processes: Communication and Documentation; Psychosocial Integrity; Client Needs: Safe and Effective Care Environment: Management of Care; Cognitive Level: Application [Applying]

## 135. MoC ANSWER: 1, 2, 3, 6

1. **The URL domain provides clues as to the author and institution. The URL of .gov indicates a U.S. government Web site and would be an acceptable site if information is appropriate for the client.**

2. **Checking for an updated Web page and links will help ensure that only current information is provided to the parents.**

3. **The credibility of the author should be evaluated to determine if the author has the credentials and qualifications to speak on the topic.**

4. Blogs generally describe a person's experiences and may not contain factually correct information.

5. Information about medications should be obtained from resources developed for teaching clients.

6. **The document should be at the educational and reading level appropriate for the client and based on facts, research, or expert knowledge, not on opinion.**

▶ *Test-taking Tip: Use the steps to evaluate a health information Web site: authority, currency, purpose, availability, content quality, and usability.*

Content Area: Management of Care; Concept: Nursing Roles; Informatics; Integrated Processes: Teaching/Learning; Client Needs: Safe and Effective Care Environment: Management of Care; Cognitive Level: Analysis [Analyzing]

## 136. MoC ANSWER: 1, 3, 5

1. **The nurse should reassure donors that there is no risk of contracting HIV during the donation procedure. Research shows that fear of getting HIV infection was a reason for not registering.**

2. Anyone age 18 to 60 years who meets health guidelines and is willing to donate to any person in need of bone marrow is able to join the registry.

3. **The nurse should focus on the positive aspect of donation in terms of "helping others." Research shows that persons who "wanted to help others" were likely to register.**

4. Recipients are not coerced to live a healthy lifestyle after receiving a transplant. Research revealed that the concern of wasting a bone marrow donation on a noncompliant recipient was a reason cited for not registering as donor.

5. **The nurse should inform donors that they are not responsible for the costs related to donation. Research showed that concern of medical costs involved with the donation limited those willing to become donors.**

▶ *Test-taking Tip: Bone marrow transplants are used to treat persons diagnosed with hematological cancers. Carefully review options with absolute words such as "anyone" and "must."*

Content Area: Management of Care; Concept: Diversity; Evidence-based Practice; Integrated Processes: Communication and Documentation; Culture and Spirituality; Client Needs: Safe and Effective Care Environment: Management of Care; Cognitive Level: Application [Applying]

## 137. MoC ANSWER: 3

1. Option 1 is a hexagram representing the Star of David associated with Judaism, not Islam.

2. Option 2 is the om symbol of Hinduism, not Islam.

3. **The nurse should include in the plan of care that the crescent moon is important to the client and that it is a symbol of the client's religious beliefs of Islam.**

4. Option 4 is the crucifix of the Roman Catholic faith and does not symbolize Islam.

▶ *Test-taking Tip: The key feature in the symbol of Islam is the crescent moon.*

**Content Area:** Management of Care; **Concept:** Diversity; Management; **Integrated Processes:** Nursing Process: Assessment; Culture and Spirituality; **Client Needs:** Safe and Effective Care Environment: Management of Care; **Cognitive Level:** Synthesis [Creating]

**138.** MoC **ANSWER: 2**

1. Inclusion of family members in care is important for culture assimilation and health care but is not the priority.
2. **Treating each client respectfully as an individual is basic to culturally competent care. This is essential to discourage staff from developing stereotypical thinking.**
3. Identifying the common beliefs among the group may promote stereotypical thinking about the group.
4. The use of available language assistance services will promote effective communication but is not a priority.

♦ **Test-taking Tip:** The question calls for the priority. Recognition and respect of the individual client are basic to culturally competent care given to any group.

**Content Area:** Management of Care; **Concept:** Diversity; Communication; Nursing Roles; **Integrated Processes:** Teaching/Learning; Culture and Spirituality; **Client Needs:** Safe and Effective Care Environment: Management of Care; Psychosocial Integrity; **Cognitive Level:** Application [Applying]

**139.** MoC **ANSWER: 4, 2, 3, 1**

4. **Cultural awareness is the first phase. Cultural awareness includes recognizing the values and beliefs of the client and self.**
2. **Cultural sensitivity is the second phase. Cultural sensitivity includes recognizing that there may be different meanings of the client's behavior and looking objectively for possible cues.**
3. **Cultural recognition is the third phase. Cultural recognition is recognizing that clients from different cultures may have different customs and behaviors.**
1. **Cultural competence is the fourth phase. Cultural competence is having sufficient knowledge of c ultural groups that are different from one's own such that a person is able to interact with a member of a different cultural group in a way that makes the other person feel understood and respected.**

♦ **Test-taking Tip:** When placing items in the correct order, start with either the first or the last item. In this situation, common sense should tell you that cultural competence should be the last item.

**Content Area:** Management of Care; **Concept:** Diversity; Nursing Roles; **Integrated Processes:** Teaching/Learning; Culture and Spirituality; **Client Needs:** Safe and Effective Care Environment: Management of Care; **Cognitive Level:** Comprehension [Understanding]

**140.** MoC **ANSWER:**

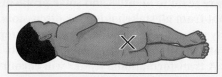

**When assessing for Mongolian spots, the nurse should assess for a bluish-back discoloration of the lower back and buttocks. Mongolian spots are often found in infants of Mediterranean, Latin American, Asian, or African descent.**

♦ **Test-taking Tip:** If unsure, consider that the HCP must be able to differentiate between Mongolian spots and possible signs of abuse.

**Content Area:** Management of Care; **Concept:** Diversity; Assessment; **Integrated Processes:** Nursing Process: Assessment; Culture and Spirituality; **Client Needs:** Safe and Effective Care Environment: Management of Care; Health Promotion and Maintenance; **Cognitive Level:** Application [Applying]

**141.** MoC **ANSWER: 1**

1. **This statement supports an addition to the nursing diagnostic statement ". . . *related to impaired mucous membranes.*" If the client has impaired oral mucous membranes, it may be uncomfortable to chew and swallow food, therefore exacerbating the underlying condition. To help the client achieve the goal of balanced nutrition, including this with the nursing diagnostic statement will alert caregivers and facilitate appropriate interventions.**
2. This statement supports the existing nursing diagnosis.
3. This statement indicates that a new, additional nursing diagnosis should be written.
4. This statement supports the existing nursing diagnosis.

♦ **Test-taking Tip:** The key words are "best indicate." Select an option that would exacerbate the existing condition and require the revision of the nursing diagnostic statement.

**Content Area:** Management of Care; **Concept:** Management; **Integrated Processes:** Nursing Process: Evaluation; **Client Needs:** Safe and Effective Care Environment: Management of Care; **Cognitive Level:** Synthesis [Creating]

**142.** MoC **ANSWER: 4**

1. Rapid administration of a bolus feeding reduces lower esophageal sphincter pressure and increases the risk for aspiration.
2. A supine position after a feeding is completed increases the risk for aspiration.
3. Tube placement should be confirmed before the feeding is started.
4. **Positioning the head of the bed at 45 degrees elevation promotes gravity flow of the formula into the stomach and maintains normal functioning of the lower esophageal sphincter.**

▶ *Test-taking Tip: Focus on the anatomy of the stomach and the way in which food passes into the intestines. The correct intervention is one that decreases the client's risk for aspiration.*

**Content Area:** Management of Care; **Concept:** Nutrition; Safety; **Integrated Processes:** Nursing Process: Evaluation; **Client Needs:** Safe and Effective Care Environment: Management of Care; Physiological Integrity: Basic Care and Comfort; **Cognitive Level:** Evaluation [Evaluating]

### 143. MoC ANSWER: 1

1. **A clear liquid diet contains foods that are clear liquids at room or body temperature. Milk products are not included on a clear liquid diet.**
2. Plain gelatin is considered a clear liquid.
3. Tea is considered a clear liquid.
4. Clear fruit juices such as apple juice are considered clear liquids.

▶ *Test-taking Tip: The question calls for a false response. Look for the option that is different from the other options.*

**Content Area:** Management of Care; **Concept:** Nutrition; Nursing Roles; **Integrated Processes:** Nursing Process: Analysis; **Client Needs:** Safe and Effective Care Environment: Management of Care; Physiological Integrity: Basic Care and Comfort; **Cognitive Level:** Application [Applying]

### 144. MoC ANSWER: 2

1. A normal pH with increased $Paco_2$ and $HCO_3$ indicates metabolic alkalosis with respiratory compensation.
2. **A normal pH with increased $Paco_2$ and $HCO_3$ indicates respiratory acidosis with metabolic compensation. The increased $Paco_2$ results in respiratory acidosis. The kidneys respond slowly by retaining $HCO_3$, which is a base. The normal $HCO_3$ is 20 to 24 mmol/L. Full compensation occurs when the pH returns to the normal range of 7.35 to 7.45.**
3. An increased pH, normal $Paco_2$, and increased $HCO_3$ indicate metabolic alkalosis.
4. A pH of 7.44, $Paco_2$ of 45 mm Hg, and $HCO_3$ of 24 mmol/L are normal blood gas findings.

▶ *Test-taking Tip: Compensated means that the pH returns to normal and that the system that did not initiate the imbalance will respond in the opposite direction (acid or base) of the imbalance.*

**Content Area:** Management of Care; **Concept:** pH Regulation; Oxygenation; **Integrated Processes:** Nursing Process: Evaluation; **Client Needs:** Safe and Effective Care Environment: Management of Care; Physiological Integrity: Reduction of Risk Potential; **Cognitive Level:** Evaluation [Evaluating]

### 145. MoC ANSWER: 2

1. Although applying wrist restraints will prevent side-to-side movement, it will not keep the client's right leg straight to prevent catheter dislodgement.
2. **An ankle restraint will help prevent dislodgement of the arterial catheter and bleeding and injury that could occur from thrashing in bed.**

3. Sedation may be needed in addition to the restraints. Too much sedation can compromise the client's respiratory status.
4. Although restraints can increase agitation, keeping one leg unrestrained may prevent this from occurring. Safety of the client is the priority.

▶ *Test-taking Tip: Focus on the information provided in the scenario and on how to protect the client from injury.*

**Content Area:** Management of Care; **Concept:** Safety; Collaboration; **Integrated Processes:** Nursing Process: Planning; **Client Needs:** Safe and Effective Care Environment: Management of Care; Safe and Effective Care Environment: Safety and Infection Control; **Cognitive Level:** Analysis [Analyzing]

### 146. MoC ANSWER: 2, 3, 4, 5

1. Quick and routine institutional bathing practices, which emphasize efficiency, can add to agitation and lack of cooperation in clients with dementia.
2. **Research findings indicate that hygiene activities can be improved for clients with dementia and their caregivers by providing a calm bathing environment.**
3. **Clients are more likely to cooperate with hygiene activities when they are allowed to participate in the process.**
4. **Clients are more likely to cooperate with hygiene activities when pain is adequately controlled.**
5. **Separating hair washing from bathing limits the stress of activity on the client with dementia.**

▶ *Test-taking Tip: Identify the options that can decrease the client's distress.*

**Content Area:** Management of Care; **Concept:** Management; Evidence-based Practice; Cognition; **Integrated Processes:** Nursing Process: Planning; **Client Needs:** Safe and Effective Care Environment: Management of Care; Physiological Integrity: Basic Care and Comfort; **Cognitive Level:** Synthesis [Creating]

### 147. MoC ANSWER: 4

1. Both LR and dextrose with LR solutions are isotonic and are used for fluid replacement in the PACU. After the client returns to the medical-surgical unit, the type and amount of solution are based on client need.
2. Naloxone hydrochloride (Narcan) is an antagonist for opioids and is used for reversing the respiratory-depressive effects of opioid analgesics.
3. Vital sign observations and pain assessment should be completed every 15 minutes or more frequently based on the client's condition.
4. **Because the client did not receive a general anesthetic that depressed the CNS, the client may be verbally responsive immediately after surgery. The client receiving a spinal anesthetic should remain in the PACU until feeling and voluntary motor movement of the lower extremities has begun to return.**

▶ *Test-taking Tip: Note the key words "further orientation is needed." The answer is an incorrect statement.*

**Content Area:** Management of Care; **Concept:** Management; Safety; **Integrated Processes:** Teaching/Learning; **Client Needs:** Safe and Effective Care Environment: Management of Care; **Cognitive Level:** Evaluation [Evaluating]

## 148. MoC ANSWER: 1

1. **The recommended depth of chest compressions for the adult client is 2 inches.**
2. The head-tilt, chin-lift maneuver is an acceptable technique for opening the client's airway when no cervical spine injury is suspected.
3. It is advised to attach AED pads to the client's bare chest as soon as the AED arrives to the scene.
4. A bag-valve-mask device is one method for ventilating the client.

▶ *Test-taking Tip: Because you are to find the action that indicates further instruction is needed, begin by eliminating the correct actions.*

**Content Area:** Management of Care; **Concept:** Management; Nursing Roles; **Integrated Processes:** Teaching/Learning; **Client Needs:** Safe and Effective Care Environment: Management of Care; Physiological Integrity: Physiological Adaptation; **Cognitive Level:** Evaluation [Evaluating]

## 149. MoC ANSWER: 2

1. Because of the risk of choriocarcinoma, serial serum BHCG testing is completed after a hydatidiform molar pregnancy.
2. **Women who have had a molar pregnancy can conceive again once their BHCG levels are normal and remain normal for a certain time period, usually 6 to 12 months. This response by the nurse is incorrect and should be followed up by the observing nurse manager.**
3. Because the client will undergo serial serum BHCG testing after a hydatidiform molar pregnancy, she should not get pregnant for 6 to 12 months until testing is completed and it is confirmed that she does not have a malignancy.
4. Couples with a past history of molar pregnancy have the same statistical chance of conceiving again and having a normal pregnancy as those without.

▶ *Test-taking Tip: The key word is "incorrect." Note the absolute words in Option 2, "cannot conceive ever again." Options with absolute words are usually the answer for questions asking for an incorrect statement. In a hydatidiform molar pregnancy, instead of normal placental tissue, there is abnormal placental development resulting in fluid-filled grapelike clusters and proliferation of trophoblastic tissue.*

**Content Area:** Management of Care; Childbearing; **Concept:** Female Reproduction; Pregnancy; **Integrated Processes:** Teaching/Learning; **Client Needs:** Safe and Effective Care Environment: Management of Care; Health Promotion and Maintenance; **Cognitive Level:** Analysis [Analyzing]

## 150. MoC ANSWER: 1, 3, 4, 5

1. **A postpartum support group can be a place where realistic information about postpartum depression can be discussed and symptoms recognized.**
2. Fatigue is a major concern for all postpartum women. Clients should be encouraged to nap when their infant is napping rather than using that time for other activities.
3. **Keeping a journal can be emotionally cathartic and can help prevent postpartum depression.**
4. **Postpartum mothers should be encouraged to call their HCPs if symptoms of postpartum depression, such as feelings of sadness, do not subside quickly or if the symptoms become severe.**
5. **Structuring activity with a schedule helps counteract inertia that comes with feeling sad or unsettled.**

▶ *Test-taking Tip: Think about activities that would decrease stress in general. Remember that problem-specific support groups are frequently utilized for psychological support no matter what the client's specific concern.*

**Content Area:** Management of Care; Childbearing; **Concept:** Nursing Roles; Pregnancy; **Integrated Processes:** Teaching/Learning; **Client Needs:** Safe and Effective Care Environment: Management of Care; Health Promotion and Maintenance; **Cognitive Level:** Application [Applying]

## 151. MoC ANSWER: 4

1. The development of autonomy is a developmental task of toddlerhood.
2. School-age children are motivated to follow rules established by others.
3. Adult women are concerned about the effect of childbearing on careers.
4. **Although it is biologically possible for the adolescent female to become a parent, her egocentricity and concrete thinking interfere with her ability to parent effectively. Because of this normal development, the adolescent may inadvertently neglect her child.**

▶ *Test-taking Tip: Read the question carefully. It is asking about developmental tasks of the adolescent.*

**Content Area:** Management of Care; Childbearing; **Concept:** Development; Pregnancy; **Integrated Processes:** Nursing Process: Analysis; **Client Needs:** Safe and Effective Care Environment: Management of Care; Health Promotion and Maintenance; **Cognitive Level:** Application [Applying]

**152.** MoC **ANSWER: 2**

1. Adults learn best by demonstration and hands-on practice. A poster board does not support adult learning styles.
2. **Adults are independent learners. Before deciding what nurses do not know, the nurses themselves should identify their specific learning needs and the methodology for learning.**
3. Adults learn best by demonstration and hands-on practice. A presentation does not support adult learning styles.
4. Asking staff what they don't understand about the policy and procedure is threatening.

▶ *Test-taking Tip: Adult learners are self-directed learners.*

Content Area: Management of Care; Concept: Nursing Roles; Integrated Processes: Teaching/Learning; Client Needs: Safe and Effective Care Environment: Management of Care; Health Promotion and Maintenance; Cognitive Level: Application [Applying]

**153.** PHARM MoC **ANSWER: 2**

1. Waking the client to check the blood glucose and then giving a snack is unnecessary. All diabetics do not need a bedtime snack.
2. **The onset of glargine (Lantus) is 1 hour; it has no peak action, and it lasts for 24 hours. Glargine lowers the blood glucose by increasing transport into cells and promoting the conversion of glucose to glycogen. Because it has no peak action, a bedtime snack is unnecessary.**
3. Checking the blood glucose level and then giving a snack the next time the client wakes up is unnecessary.
4. Glargine is administered once daily, the same time each day, to maintain relatively constant concentrations over 24 hours. It is unnecessary to notify the HCP.

▶ *Test-taking Tip: Insulin glargine has no peak action. Use this information to eliminate options.*

Content Area: Management of Care; Concept: Metabolism; Medication; Integrated Processes: Nursing Process: Evaluation; Client Needs: Safe and Effective Care Environment: Management of Care; Physiological Integrity: Pharmacological and Parenteral Therapies; Cognitive Level: Evaluation [Evaluating]

**154.** MoC PHARM **ANSWER: 1, 3, 4, 5**

1. **During a hypercyanotic episode, the child becomes dyspneic and hypoxic. The knee-chest position reduces cardiac output by decreasing blood return from the lower extremities and increasing the SVR.**
2. The child should receive 100% oxygen via face mask when having a hypercyanotic spell.
3. **Morphine sulfate should be administered to decrease preload and afterload.**
4. **A calm approach helps to settle the child and decrease oxygen demand.**
5. **Propranolol may be given to aid pulmonary artery dilation.**

▶ *Test-taking Tip: In a hypercyanotic episode, the partial pressure of oxygen ($Pao_2$) is lowered, and the partial pressure of carbon dioxide ($Paco_2$) rises. As the respiratory center in the brain overreacts, hypoxemia progressively worsens. The increasing respiratory effort and cardiac output can cause a life-threatening decline unless rapid intervention is successful. You need to consider options that will decrease cardiac output, decrease preload and afterload, and promote pulmonary artery dilation.*

Content Area: Management of Care; Child; Concept: Perfusion; Critical Thinking; Safety; Medication; Integrated Processes: Nursing Process: Implementation; Client Needs: Safe and Effective Care Environment: Management of Care; Physiological Integrity: Pharmacological and Parenteral Therapies; Physiological Integrity: Physiological Adaptation; Cognitive Level: Analysis [Analyzing]

**155.** MoC **ANSWER: 2**

1. The parent will need support systems and support groups, but it is not the most important intervention. The initial focus should be on the child's needs.
2. **Initiating referrals is the most important. This child will require physical, emotional, cognitive, and social assessments post-hospitalization and may need ongoing rehabilitation in the home.**
3. A home safety assessment is included in rehabilitation services.
4. Communication with the school will need to occur but will likely happen postdischarge.

▶ *Test-taking Tip: This is a question for which all options are correct, but you should identify the most important and the most global option.*

Content Area: Management of Care; Child; Concept: Safety; Promoting Health; Skin Integrity; Integrated Processes: Nursing Process: Planning; Client Needs: Safe and Effective Care Environment: Management of Care; Cognitive Level: Analysis [Analyzing]

## Chapter Seven

# Prioritization and Delegation

**156.** MoC  The nurse receives a change-of-shift report on four assigned clients. In what order should the nurse attend to the clients? Prioritize the nurse's actions by placing each client in the correct order.

1. The 57-year-old client who was admitted 24 hours ago after being struck by lightning and has a serum potassium level of 5.5 mEq/L
2. The 33-year-old client with a deep partial-thickness leg burn who has a temperature of 102.8°F (39.3°C), BP 98/66 mm Hg, and P 114 bpm
3. The 25-year-old client admitted 1 week ago with facial and chest burns from a house fire who has been crying since recent visitors left
4. The 58-year-old client who had a skin graft to a leg burn 6 hours ago and is requesting a medication for pain rated at a 6 on a 0 to 10 scale

Answer: _____

**157.** MoC  The RN is leading a team of an NA and an LPN in the care of a group of clients. Which tasks should the nurse assign to the NA and LPN?

1. NA to perform two simple dressing changes; LPN to assess and care for two noncomplex clients
2. NA to empty and record urinary catheter bag drainage; LPN to administer oral and intramuscular medications
3. NA to assist clients with hygiene; LPN to provide postmortem care and meet with a deceased client's family
4. NA to take and document vital signs on all clients; LPN to complete the discharge paperwork to be reviewed with two clients

**158.** MoC  The charge nurse is reviewing documentation completed by the RN and evaluating the RN's delegation abilities to the LPN and NA and appropriate supervision. Which medical record documentation indicates incomplete delegation?

| Client Narrative Notes | | |
|---|---|---|
| 1 | 0800 | BP 150/90 mm Hg (obtained per J. Brown, NA). Rates right shoulder incisional pain at 10/10. Morphine sulfate given IV for pain control. _____ M. Drew, RN |
| 2 | 1000 | Assisted to the bathroom per J. Brown, NA. Voided cloudy, foul-smelling urine. Urine output 20 mL/hr for past 4 hr. Dr. Peters notified. _____ M. Drew, RN |
| 3 | 1200 | Fingerstick blood glucose 55 mg/dL (taken per J. Brown, NA). Given 4 units lispro (Humalog) insulin subcut as ordered before lunch. _____ A. Smith, LPN |
| 4 | 1400 | Ambulated 100 feet in hallway. Assisted with hygiene while sitting in chair per RN direction. Hygienic care refused earlier due to fatigue. _____ J. Brown, NA |

159. **MoC** The nurse is supervising the experienced NA who is new to the unit. Which question is best to evaluate the NA's knowledge and skill in obtaining the client's fingerstick blood glucose, which is a permissible NA-performed skill within the facility?

1. "How many times did you perform a fingerstick blood glucose measurement on the unit in which you previously worked?"
2. "How would you obtain a blood specimen and perform the procedure for measuring the client's blood glucose?"
3. "When was the last time you were observed by a registered nurse (RN) performing a blood glucose measurement on the client?"
4. "When was the last time you obtained a blood glucose measurement that was out of the normal ranges, and what did you do about this?"

160. **MoC** The NA's job responsibilities include totaling the input and output (I&O) records for clients at the end of an 8-hour shift. Near the end of the shift, the LPN reports to the RN that the new NA on the unit has not completed the task. What is the RN's **best** action?

1. Ask the LPN to complete this task because the information is needed to give report.
2. Remind the NA that the task needs to be completed as quickly as possible.
3. Notify the charge nurse that the NA needs more orientation on job responsibilities.
4. Go to the NA to discuss the collection of I&O data and how to total I&O records.

161. **MoC** The RN is informed by the NA that the client, hospitalized last evening with chest pain, plans to leave right now because the pain is gone and "nobody has done anything anyway." Which is the nurse's **best** action?

1. Thank the NA for the information and then call the client's doctor regarding the situation.
2. Tell the NA that the client has the right to leave and send the NA to help the client pack.
3. Talk with the client to discuss the client's concerns and explain the plan of care.
4. Tell the NA to inform the client that it is unsafe to leave; the RN will see the client shortly.

162. **MoC** The nurse determines that the NA did not complete assigned tasks. Which statement is **best**?

1. "All four of the clients' rooms assigned to you today are messy and have a lot of trash. You need to finish your assignment before you leave."
2. "I am concerned that you didn't complete your work assignments today. What interfered with completing the tasks I assigned?"
3. "I checked with the four clients you were assigned to ambulate, and you didn't ambulate anyone. This cannot happen again."
4. "Family members are upset today because you didn't get all the clients bathed yet. Why didn't you let me know you needed help?"

163. **MoC** The new nurse is discussing the organization of client care with the mentor. Which statement made by the new nurse requires **immediate** follow-up by the mentor?

1. "I delegated all the stable vital signs to an unlicensed assistive personnel (UAP) and most of the treatments to the LPN."
2. "I had the LPN bring the urinary catheterization supplies into the room so everything would be available when I got there."
3. "I was taking vitals on one client and having a second client dangle while I had a third client sit on the bedside commode."
4. "I believe my organizational skills are improving and I am able to complete all my client cares myself."

164. **MoC** The RN is working with the UAP and the LPN in providing care to a group of clients. Which tasks should the nurse plan to delegate? **Select all that apply.**

1. LPN to administer oral and intramuscular medications
2. UAP to perform chest tube dressing changes
3. LPN to assess and care for two noncomplex clients
4. UAP to empty and record urinary catheter bag drainage
5. UAP to take and document vital signs on all clients
6. LPN to initiate the discharge paperwork for two clients

**165.** MoC The RN is working with the LPN in providing care to the client. Place the nurse responsibilities associated with delegation, supervision, and evaluation in the order that these should be completed by the nurse.

1. Following an incident, discuss importance of verifying the gag reflex prior to allowing the client who was sedated to have anything by mouth.
2. Intervene when the LPN allows the client who had been sedated for a procedure to have food/drink by mouth prior to verifying gag reflex.
3. Inform the LPN of tasks pertaining to the clients that should be completed.
4. Write a brief anecdotal note regarding appraisal of encounter with the LPN.

Answer: _____

**166.** MoC The client who is hard of hearing and primarily speaks a language other than English is being discharged home. Which action should be the nurse's **priority** when preparing to teach the client about newly prescribed medications?

1. Determine the client's literacy level for both the primary language and English.
2. Obtain literature about the medications written in the primary language and English.
3. Determine if there is another person who should be taught instead of the client.
4. Ask the NA who also speaks the client's primary language to review the information with the client.

**167.** MoC The charge nurse is leading the orientation of new employees. Which statements made by the charge nurse demonstrate appropriate delegation? **Select all that apply.**

1. "The LPN can delegate dressing changes to the unlicensed assistive personnel (UAP)."
2. "The LPN can administer immunizations to a child less than 2 years of age."
3. "The LPN can add a dose of chemotherapy to an existing IV infusion."
4. "The competent UAP can help transfer stable clients using a mechanical lift."
5. "The UAP can assess the client 15 minutes after a blood transfusion begins."

**168.** MoC The new nurse has been oriented to the PACU and is caring for the client who had general anesthesia. The charge nurse determines that the new nurse can correctly position the client in the PACU when making which observation?

1. Assists the client to the prone position when the client is nauseated
2. Places the client in the Trendelenburg position when hypotensive
3. Positions the newly admitted client supine with the head elevated
4. Turns the client side lying when the client arrives in the PACU

**169.** MoC After working with the client, the UAP tells the nurse, "I have had it with that demanding client. I just can't do anything that pleases him. I'm not going in there again." Which should be the nurse's response?

1. "He has a lot of problems. You need to have patience when caring for him."
2. "It is your responsibility to accept your assignment. I will write you up if you don't."
3. "He may be scared and taking it out on you. Let's figure out what to do together."
4. "Ignore him and get the rest of your work done. I can go in and check on him."

**170.** MoC The UAP's job responsibilities include checking vital signs every 4 hours, completing morning care on assigned clients, assisting clients with activity, answering lights, and totaling I&O records for clients at the end of an 8-hour shift. Near the end of the shift, the LPN reports to the RN that the UAP has not completed all of the morning care on assigned clients. Which is the RN's **best** action?

1. Remind the UAP that the morning cares need to be completed as quickly as possible.
2. Notify the charge nurse that the UAP needs additional orientation on job responsibilities.
3. Complete an incident report on the UAP about the inability to complete assigned tasks.
4. Ask the UAP about morning cares completed and the reasons for uncompleted cares.

**171.** MoC The nurse is preparing to supervise the inexperienced LPN inserting a urinary catheter. Which question by the nurse would **best** assess the LPN's knowledge and skill about inserting a urinary catheter?

1. "How many times have you inserted a urinary catheter?"
2. "How would you perform insertion of a urinary catheter?"
3. "When was the last time you were observed inserting a urinary catheter?"
4. "When was the last time you inserted a urinary catheter?"

**172.** MoC The nurse manager is evaluating a new nurse's time management skills. Which statements made by the new nurse would demonstrate acceptable time management? **Select all that apply.**

1. "I am late in getting the client ready for radiology because I had to answer some questions from a family member during a client's discharge."
2. "I did not clock out on time because I needed to wait until the end of the shift to document all nursing care provided today."
3. "I did not clock out on time because I admitted the client who came 30 minutes before the end of my shift."
4. "I made morning rounds on all of my clients today before passing medications and starting treatments to be completed during my shift."
5. "I am late performing a dressing change because my breaks are usually scheduled early, so I eat breakfast after I begin my shift."

**173.** MoC PHARM The LPN reports to the nurse that the client's TPN infusion was inadvertently turned off 1 hour ago. In response to this finding, which statement to the LPN should be the nurse's priority?

1. "Please check the client's respiratory rate."
2. "Please check the client's blood sugar."
3. "Please check the client's BP."
4. "Please check the client's level of consciousness."

**174.** MoC The unlicensed NA is providing care to multiple clients under the supervision of the RN. Which activities are appropriate for the RN to delegate to the NA? **Select all that apply.**

1. Ask if the antiemetic given a half hour ago relieved the client's nausea, and report the finding to the RN.
2. Observe for and report muscle weakness for the client with a serum potassium level of 3.2 mEq/L.
3. Inject air and withdraw medication from a vial after being shown by the RN while the RN administers the client's first prepared medication.
4. Cleanse and redress the client's surgical and wound drain dressing on the client's second postoperative day.
5. Shave the facial hair with an electric razor for the client who needs to lie flat in bed after spinal surgery.

**175.** MoC The new nurse has been on orientation for 2 months. Which client is **best** for the charge nurse to assign to the new nurse?

1. The 2-year-old with a truncus arteriosus receiving digoxin 90 mcg by mouth
2. The 4-year-old who had a balloon dilation procedure as palliative treatment for coarctation of aorta
3. The 6-year-old with endocarditis whose parents need teaching about child care and good hygiene
4. The 8-year-old who is post–heart transplant 2 months ago with a low-grade fever and tachycardia

**176.** MoC The nurse receives shift report on four assigned clients. Prioritize the order that the nurse should assess the assigned clients.

1. The 47-year-old client 2 days postoperative who has pain rated at 2 on a 0 to 10 pain scale
2. The 82-year-old client who was unable to void and has a bladder scan showing 300 mL of urine
3. The 76-year-old client newly admitted with serum blood urea nitrogen (BUN) of 52 mg/dL
4. The 57-year-old client with hypertension who has severe midsternal pain

Answer: _____

**177.** MoC The nurse is assigning tasks to the UAP. Which tasks **best** demonstrate proper delegation?

1. Bathe 10 clients while working the day shift.
2. Insert an NG tube to administer a feeding.
3. Answer the client's question about a medication.
4. Ambulate the client who had a thoracotomy 3 days ago.

**178.** `MoC` The nurse receives a change-of-shift report for four assigned clients. Which clients should the nurse attend to **first**? Place each client in the order of priority.

1. The 44-year-old client who has questions about how to empty the Jackson-Pratt drain at home after being discharged tomorrow
2. The 33-year-old client who has a new order to insert an NG tube and connect to low intermittent suction
3. The usually oriented 76-year-old client diagnosed with thrombophlebitis who has new-onset confusion
4. The 58-year-old client requesting a pain medication for abdominal incision pain rated at a 6 on a 0 to 10 scale

Answer: _____

**179.** `MoC` Prior to delegation, the RN evaluates that the LPN has the ability to correctly obtain urine for a culture from the client who has an indwelling urinary catheter. Place an X at the location on one of the illustrations where the LPN should have obtained the urine for the specimen.

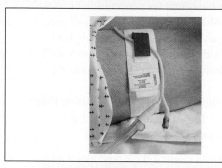

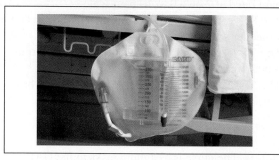

**180.** `MoC` Two hours after admitting the client to a postsurgical unit following a nephrectomy, the client states feeling nauseated. The nurse notes minimal drainage from the NG tube. Which action should the nurse take **first**?

1. Immediately notify the HCP of the reduced nasogastric returns.
2. Give an antiemetic listed on the client's MAR.
3. Withdraw the NG tube an inch to release it from suctioning against the wall of the stomach.
4. Irrigate the NG and check to see if the fluid returns to the collection container.

**181.** `MoC` The new nurse is caring for the client with ARF and hypernatremia. Which tasks should the nurse delegate to the NA? **Select all that apply.**

1. Providing oral care every 3 to 4 hours
2. Checking skin turgor every 8 hours
3. Changing an intravenous bag of saline
4. Evaluating daily weights for trends
5. Calculating the intake and output for the past 8 hours

**182.** `MoC` `PHARM` The nurse notes that the client has dyspnea and red blotches on the face and arms and appears anxious following exposure to latex. The nurse calls the ART, who initiates emergency treatment. Of all the emergency treatments available, which action should be taken **first** by ART?

1. Start oxygen at 1 liter per minute via nasal cannula (NC).
2. Start an intravenous (IV) access with a large-bore IV catheter.
3. Administer diphenhydramine 25 mg intramuscularly (IM).
4. Administer epinephrine hydrochloride 0.4 mL subcutaneously.

**183.** `MoC` The client just returned to the nursing unit following a total laryngectomy. Which observation by the nurse requires the most **immediate** intervention?

1. The client is unable to speak.
2. The client is coughing blood-tinged sputum.
3. Oxygen saturation level is 82%.
4. Jackson-Pratt wound drain is half full.

**184.** MoC While caring for the postoperative client following a total laryngectomy with radical neck dissection, the nurse observes that the client is restless and has a respiratory rate of 28 breaths per minute. Which action is the nurse's **priority?**

1. Suction the client's laryngectomy tube.
2. Apply oxygen by mask at 4 liters per minute.
3. Elevate the head of the client's bed to 45 degrees.
4. Assess the client's oxygen saturation level.

**185.** MoC At 0730, an oncoming shift nurse is planning care for four clients. Which client should the nurse plan to assess **first?**

1. The 23-year-old client with cystic fibrosis who has pulmonary function tests scheduled in 30 minutes
2. The 35-year-old client admitted the previous day with bacterial pneumonia and now has a temperature of 101.2°F (38.4°C)
3. The 46-year-old client who had a chest tube removed an hour ago and now has dyspnea
4. The 77-year-old client with tuberculosis who has four antitubercular medications due at 8:00 a.m.

**186.** MoC The nurse is planning care for the client in the PACU. The client had lengthy abdominal surgery with the general anesthetic agent isoflurane. Which client problem should the nurse plan to attend to **first?**

1. Acute pain
2. Anxiety
3. Altered skin integrity
4. Falls asleep after being stimulated

**187.** MoC The nurse manager is reviewing assignments for an evening shift. The nurse manager should intervene if the experienced LPN is assigned which action?

1. Complete a foot soak for the client who has an infected heel ulcer and is in contact precautions for vancomycin-resistant enterococci (VRE).
2. Assist the client who had a vaginal hysterectomy 6 hours ago to sit at the edge of the bed for a few minutes and then ambulate.
3. Discharge a 34-year-old who had a right mastectomy 4 days ago and needs instruction regarding incision care and a wound drain.
4. Perform intermittent urinary catheterizations for residual urine for the client who had an abdominal hysterectomy 2 days ago.

**188.** MoC The LPN is working with the RN. Which clients should the RN assign to the LPN? **Select all that apply.**

1. The client who needs an intravenous patient-controlled analgesia (PCA) device for pain control
2. The client with a leg cast who needs CMS checks every 4 hours and oral pain medications prn
3. The client who underwent a below-the-knee amputation and is experiencing phantom limb pain
4. The client who was physically abused and now has severe abdominal pain rated at 8 out of 10
5. The client with arthritis who needs routine analgesic medication and heat application to joints

**189.** MoC The client on a telemetry unit has a BP of 88/40 mm Hg, an HR of 44 bpm, feels faint, and is pale and confused. When caring for this client, which tasks should the RN delegate to the NA? **Select all that apply.**

1. Paging for the charge nurse
2. Paging for a respiratory therapist
3. Securing an automatic BP machine
4. Placing an oxygen facemask at 2L/min
5. Obtaining a printed cardiac rhythm strip

**190.** MoC The client recovering from heart failure needs to have diet teaching reinforced prior to being discharged in the afternoon. Which question by the nurse would **best** assess the LPN's knowledge and skill about reinforcing the diet teaching?

1. "How many times have you taught heart failure clients about their diets?"
2. "What information will you reinforce regarding the required diet in heart failure?"
3. "When was the last time you provided diet education to a heart failure client?"
4. "When was the last time you were observed reinforcing teaching about the client's diet?"

**191.** MoC The experienced LPN is caring for the client with acute substernal chest pain. Which actions should the nurse delegate to the LPN? **Select all that apply.**

1. Give a 325-mg chewable aspirin to the client.
2. Give heparin 5000 units intravenously.
3. Administer morphine sulfate 4 mg IV.
4. Apply oxygen at 2–4 liters per nasal cannula.
5. Place leads on the client's chest for cardiac monitoring.

**192.** MoC PHARM The nurse's morning assessment of the client with heart failure reveals bounding peripheral pulses, weight gain of 2 lb, pitting ankle edema, and moist crackles bilaterally. Which prescribed intervention should be the nurse's **priority** at this time?

1. Furosemide 40 mg IV push q8h × 3 doses
2. Enalapril 10 mg orally daily
3. Restrict fluids to 1500 mL per day
4. Echocardiogram as soon as possible

**193.** MoC The nurse is working with the UAP on a telemetry unit caring for the client who had an MI 3 days ago. Which task is appropriate to delegate to the UAP?

1. Administering nitroglycerin if chest discomfort occurs during client activities
2. Monitoring vital signs and oxygen saturation before and after client ambulation
3. Teaching the client energy conservation techniques to decrease myocardial oxygen demand
4. Explaining the rationale for alternating rest periods with exercise to the client and family

**194.** MoC As the nurse and the NA enter the room of the adult client who has undergone cardiac surgery, the client's cardiac monitor begins alarming. Based on the monitor rhythm illustrated, which action is **best** for the nurse to delegate to the NA as soon as the nurse determines that the client has no pulse?

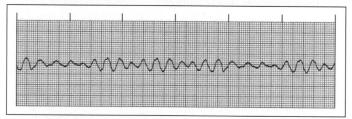

1. Recheck for a pulse.
2. Begin compressions.
3. Prepare to defibrillate the client.
4. Activate the emergency response system (EMS).

**195.** MoC PHARM The hospitalized client with heart failure is receiving dobutamine intravenously. Of the associated responsibilities in the care of the client, which statement is **most appropriate** for the RN when delegating to the experienced NA?

1. "Teach the client about the reasons for remaining on bedrest."
2. "Take the client's vital signs every hour and report these to me."
3. "Turn off the infusion pump if the client becomes hypotensive."
4. "Inform the HCP on rounds that the client's urine output is low."

**196.** MoC The RN and NA are assigned to care for a group of clients. During shift report, the RN learns that a BP taken 1 hour previously for the client was 198/94 mm Hg and that the previous shift RN did not intervene. Prioritize the order that the RN should implement the interventions.

1. Notify the client's HCP about the client's elevated BP.
2. Ask the NA to retake the client's vital signs now and have the NA set an automatic BP machine to retake the BP every 15 minutes.
3. Administer the newly prescribed furosemide and enalapril.
4. Assess the client asking specific questions related to headache, dizziness, and orientation.
5. Inform the charge nurse of the client's critically high BP and the actions taken.

Answer: _____

**197.** The adult client is newly admitted to the PACU from surgery. Which assessment finding should be the nurse's **priority?**

1. The surgical site dressing has a scant amount of blood.
2. The client is sleeping but easily arouses when touched.
3. The client's respirations are 6 to 8 breaths per minute.
4. The client's BP 5 minutes ago was 110/68 mm Hg.

**198.** MoC The UAP reports a sudden increase in temperature of 102.4°F (39°C) in the 48-hour postoperative client. Which instruction should the nurse give to the UAP when the nurse observes a cup of steaming coffee at the client's bedside?

1. "Encourage oral fluids to prevent the client from becoming dehydrated."
2. "Recheck the temperature 15 minutes after the client finishes the coffee."
3. "Ask the client to drink only cold water and juices for the next 24 hours."
4. "Document this temperature elevation on the flowsheet in the client's chart."

**199.** MoC The NA is assisting in the preoperative preparation of the client. Which tasks should the nurse delegate to the NA? **Select all that apply.**

1. Inserting the client's nasogastric tube
2. Obtaining the client's vital signs
3. Recording output after emptying a urinary drainage bag
4. Completing the preoperative checklist
5. Witnessing the client's signature on an operative consent form

**200.** MoC The nurse and the experienced LPN are working together to care for the client who is unconscious. Which tasks should the nurse plan to delegate to the LPN? **Select all that apply.**

1. Listen to the client's lung sounds every 4 hours.
2. Check pupil size and reactivity every 2 hours.
3. Check an axillary temperature every 4 hours.
4. Check enteral feeding residual volumes every 4 hours.
5. Turn and massage the client's back every 2 hours.

**201.** MoC PHARM The older client with osteoarthritis is taking celecoxib. After reviewing the client's laboratory values for the past 3 months, what should be the clinic nurse's **priority** when assessing the client?

| Serum Lab Test | 6 Months Ago | 3 Months Ago | Today |
|---|---|---|---|
| **BUN** | 13 mg/dL | 19 mg/dL | 28 mg/dL |
| **Creatinine** | 0.8 mg/dL | 1.2 mg/dL | 1.8 mg/dL |

1. Review the urinalysis results.
2. Take the client's BP.
3. Auscultate the client's heart sounds.
4. Ask if the client has a loss of appetite.

**202.** MoC The nurse observes the LPN providing care for the client who has contact precautions due to a *Clostridium difficile* infection. Which action by the LPN requires the nurse's immediate correction?

1. Donning medical examination gloves upon entering the client's room
2. Wearing a gown while giving the client a bed bath and changing the bed linen
3. Informing a visitor to wash hands with soap and water upon leaving the client's room
4. Using an alcohol-based hand cleanser for hand hygiene when exiting the client's room

**203.** MoC The nurse is caring for the client with an STI who is immobile. Which task is **most appropriate** to delegate to the UAP?

1. Bathing the client including involved areas to provide local comfort
2. Teaching the client to perform frequent hand washing to prevent secondary infection
3. Encouraging the client to use condoms to help prevent the spread of infection
4. Informing the client about the need for sexual partner(s) to receive treatment

**204.** MoC PHARM The nurse is working with the LPN who is helping care for the client who is HIV-positive with severe esophagitis caused by *Candida albicans*. Which action by the LPN requires the nurse to intervene **immediately?**

1. Suggests that the client might like to order chile con carne for the next meal
2. Places a "No Visitors" sign on the door of the room at the client's request
3. Performs hand hygiene and puts on a mask and gown before entering the client's room
4. Gives the client a glass of water after administering nystatin oral suspension

**205.** MoC The LPN is working under the supervision of the experienced RN. The charge nurse should assign which client to the LPN?

1. The 48-year-old with cystitis who has occasional bladder spasms and is taking oral antibiotics
2. The 52-year-old with pyelonephritis and severe acute flank pain receiving intravenous antibiotics
3. The 64-year-old with kidney stones receiving IV push narcotics and is to have lithotripsy
4. The 72-year-old with urinary incontinence who needs teaching regarding bladder training

**206.** MoC The nurse received change-of-shift report on four clients. Which client should the nurse assess **first?**

1. The 29-year-old client with heart failure who is experiencing anxiety related to scheduling of a valvuloplasty later today
2. The 40-year-old client with restrictive cardiomyopathy who developed severe dyspnea just before the shift change
3. The 48-year-old client who had a coronary angioplasty 1 day ago and has had occasional pain at the right groin puncture site since the procedure
4. The 58-year-old client who transferred from the intensive care unit 1 day ago after coronary artery bypass graft surgery and has a temperature of 100.6°F (38.1°C)

**207.** MoC The experienced UAP is caring for clients on a medical-surgical unit. Which task should the nurse plan to delegate to the UAP?

1. Teaching the client how to administer self-injections
2. Recording intake and output on a group of clients
3. Discontinuing the client's continuous bladder irrigation (CBI)
4. Checking while bathing the client for signs of dehydration

**208.** MoC The nurse is caring for the client admitted with dehydration. Which actions should the nurse delegate to an experienced LPN who is the only individual working with the nurse? **Select all that apply.**

1. Take vital signs every 4 hours.
2. Evaluate the client's hydration status.
3. Consult with the dietitian about the client's swallowing difficulties.
4. Provide mouth care every 2 hours while the client is awake.
5. Remind the client to avoid commercial mouthwashes.

**209.** MoC The UAP is caring for the client with DKA. Which action can the nurse safely delegate to the UAP? **Select all that apply.**

1. Check fingerstick glucose results every hour.
2. Record intake and output every hour.
3. Measure vital signs every 15 minutes.
4. Assess lips, tongue, and mucous membranes every hour.
5. Analyze the client's cardiac rhythm every hour.

**210.** MoC The nurse checks for laboratory results in the electronic medical record of four clients. Based on the results, which client should the nurse assess **first?**

1. The client who has urine that is positive for ketones
2. The client who has a serum T4 of 10 mg/dL
3. The client who has a 2-hour postprandial glucose of 150 mg/dL
4. The client who has a fasting blood glucose of 40 mg/dL

**211.** MoC PHARM The LPN is assisting with care of the client with neutropenia. Which nursing action included in the care plan is appropriate for the RN to delegate to the LPN?

1. Teaching the client the purpose of neutropenic precautions
2. Assessing the client for signs and symptoms of infection
3. Developing a discharge teaching plan for the client and family
4. Giving a prescribed subcutaneous injection of filgrastim

**212.** MoC Six new graduate nurses are hired on a busy oncology unit. What should be the nurse manager's role in orientation? **Select all that apply.**

1. Ensure that each new nurse develops expertise in the client population of the unit.
2. Ensure that each new nurse is socialized into the onco-logical clinical unit.
3. Verify that each new nurse completed the licensure process before starting the position.
4. Verify that each new nurse participates in the unit's orientation program.
5. Verify that each new nurse completes the competency verification process.

**213.** MoC The nurse is caring for the client with esophageal cancer. Which task should the nurse delegate to the UAP?

1. Assist the client with oral hygiene.
2. Observe the client's response to feedings.
3. Facilitate expression of grief or anxiety.
4. Apply viscous lidocaine to mouth sores.

**214.** MoC The nurse is caring for the client who had a squamous cell carcinoma removed from the face. Which task should the nurse delegate to the experienced LPN?

1. Teaching the client about risks for squamous cell carcinoma
2. Demonstrating how to care for the surgical site at home
3. Assessing the surgical site for swelling, bleeding, or pain
4. Reinforcing the rationale for avoiding aspirin use for a week following surgery

**215.** MoC The nurse from the oncology unit was reassigned to a burn unit due to a staffing need. Which client should the charge nurse plan to assign to the nurse from the oncology unit?

1. The 23-year-old newly admitted with burns on 30% of the body from a house fire
2. The 27-year-old recent skin graft recipient needing nutrition and wound care teaching
3. The 29-year-old with partial-thickness back and chest burns needing a sterile dressing change
4. The 30-year-old with full-thickness burns on both arms needing help with positioning

**216.** MoC PHARM The client with heart failure has severe dyspnea and is anxious, tachypneic, and tachycardic. Which intervention should be the nurse's **priority?**

1. Administer diazepam 2.5 mg IV
2. Administer morphine sulfate 2 mg IV
3. Increase dopamine IV infusion by 2 mcg/kg/min
4. Increase nitroglycerin IV infusion by 5 mcg/min

**217.** MoC The nurse initiated an IVPB of cefuroxime sodium for the client. Within 5 minutes, the client is experiencing dyspnea, wheezing, and stridor. Prioritize the nurse's actions in the order that they should be accomplished.

1. Shout for help.
2. Call the HCP.
3. Turn off the antibiotic.
4. Ask another nurse to set up new IV maintenance solution and tubing and to aspirate the IV port before initiating the new solution.
5. Administer the prescribed emergency medications intravenously.
6. Maintain the airway and administer oxygen.

Answer: _____

**218.** MoC A triage nurse working in an ED receives four admissions. Prioritize the order in which the nurse should assess the clients.

1. The 40-year-old client who is diaphoretic and is feeling chest pressure
2. The 18-year-old client who thinks he might have a broken ankle
3. The 35-year-old client who cut her hand with a knife while preparing food
4. The 60-year-old client who is dyspneic and has swollen lips after being stung by a bee

Answer: _____

**219.** MoC The client is in the emergency room with a nail gun injury to the hand incurred while remodeling an old barn. There is a strong odor of alcohol, and the client admits to having three beers during a 3-hour period. Which parameter is **most** important for the nurse to evaluate **first?**

1. Blood type
2. Time of last voiding
3. Current blood alcohol level
4. Date of last tetanus immunization

**220.** MoC The nurse assesses that the client is pale, diaphoretic, dyspneic, and experiencing chest pain. Which nurse actions are **most** appropriate?

1. Stay with the client, call the charge nurse for help, and call the NA to bring an automatic VS machine to the room immediately.
2. Call the NA to take the client's vital signs while the nurse leaves to obtain a narcotic analgesic for administration and to notify the charge nurse.
3. Apply oxygen, call the NA to bring an automatic vital signs machine, call the charge nurse for help, and ask for medications noted on the MAR.
4. Activate the emergency system for a code to get immediate help, apply oxygen, and send responders for needed equipment and medication.

**221.** MoC The ED nurse is supervising the RN who was reassigned from the orthopedic unit to the ED. Which directions should the supervising nurse provide to the RN who is to care for the client admitted with epistaxis? **Select all that apply.**

1. "Apply direct lateral pressure to the client's nose for 5 minutes."
2. "Apply ice or cool compresses to the client's nose."
3. "Instruct the client not to blow the nose for several hours."
4. "Be sure to maintain contact precautions."
5. "Position the client lying laterally."

**222.** MoC The client with primigravida in the active stage of labor with her first pregnancy states, "I just sneezed and think I urinated all over myself; I feel wet." Which action is the nurse's **priority**?

1. Offer the client the bedpan.
2. Inspect the client's perineal area.
3. Change the client's gown and bed linens.
4. Tell the client to begin using her breathing techniques.

**223.** MoC PHARM The nurse assesses that the laboring client receiving an oxytocin infusion has a contraction occurring 1 minute after the previous contraction and has a duration of 95 seconds. Which should be the nurse's **first** action?

1. Notify the HCP.
2. Reassess the fetal heart tones.
3. Stop the oxytocin infusion.
4. Prepare to administer terbutaline sulfate.

**224.** MoC The nurse assesses the postpartum client 2 hours after delivery of a 10-lb infant and finds a blood-soaked pad with large clots. Which action should the nurse take **initially**?

1. Perform fundal massage.
2. Notify the primary HCP.
3. Start a dilute oxytocin infusion intravenously.
4. Assist the woman in ambulating to the bathroom.

**225.** MoC The nurse is caring for the postpartum client experiencing perineal pain and discomfort. Which task is **most** appropriate for the nurse to delegate to the NA?

1. Assessing the perineum for degree of edema
2. Preparing the client for taking a sitz bath
3. Determining relief after applying a perineal ice pack
4. Teaching the client how to apply an anesthetic agent after perineal care

**226.** MoC The RN is speaking to the UAP on the maternal-newborn unit. The charge nurse determines that the RN needs further education regarding appropriate delegation of client care when overhearing the RN make which statement?

1. "I've observed you feeding a newborn; you hold and feed infants safely and accurately."
2. "Prepare a sitz bath for Mrs. Jones, who has a perineal laceration and is uncomfortable."
3. "When checking the infant's temperature, look at the umbilical cord and tell me its color."
4. "Mrs. Smith's baby just died. You need to prepare the baby for the family's viewing."

**227.** MoC The nurse is delegating the task of bottle feeding the 6-hour-old term newborn to the NA. Before delegating, the nurse should evaluate the NA's knowledge of this task by asking the NA which question?

1. "How many times have you fed an infant previously?"
2. "How long have you worked in the newborn nursery?"
3. "How will you position the infant for the feeding?"
4. "Do you have any children who you bottle fed?"

**228.** MoC The LPN on the labor and delivery unit reports to the RN that the client's uterus, shortly after birth, is one finger breadth below the umbilicus and is displaced to the right of the abdomen. Which instruction by the RN to the LPN indicates appropriate delegation?

1. "Assist the client to the bathroom so that she can empty her bladder."
2. "Vigorously massage the client's fundus until her fundus feels more firm."
3. "Set an infusion pump in the room while I prepare oxytocin for infusion."
4. "Obtain her vital signs, and I will come and check her fundus in a few minutes."

**229.** MoC The NA reports to the RN that the client is shivering uncontrollably 1 hour after giving birth. Which is the nurse's **best** response to the NA?

1. "Offer the client a bedpan; a full bladder can cause shivering."
2. "Bring the client additional warm bath blankets and a warm drink."
3. "Check her vital signs; shivering may elevate her BP."
4. "Thank you; I will give chlorpromazine for her shivering."

**230.** MoC The nurse learns from the change-of-shift report that a small-for-gestational-age newborn less than 1 day old has a blood sugar of 39 mg/dL. When beginning care for this infant, which action should the nurse perform **first?**

1. Assess VS and respiratory status.
2. Initiate a feeding for the newborn.
3. Recheck the newborn's blood glucose level.
4. Prepare to administer intravenous glucose.

**231.** MoC The nurse is planning care for four clients on a pediatric unit. Prioritize the order in which the nurse should plan to attend to the clients.

1. The 13-year-old client waiting to be admitted from the emergency department after receiving stitches for facial lacerations from a dog bite
2. The 9-year-old client whose mother is present to receive teaching about wound care for her child's left leg skin graft in anticipation of discharge tomorrow
3. The 5-year-old client with an infected leg wound who is scheduled for a dressing change now
4. The 2-year-old client whose temperature has risen to 103.8°F (39.9°C)

Answer: _____

**232.** MoC The newly oriented patient care assistant (PCA), working under the supervision of the RN, is providing care to clients at a family birthing center. Which tasks should the nurse delegate to the PCA? **Select all that apply.**

1. Transporting the client who is 2 days postcesarean section suspected of having a pulmonary embolus to radiology for a chest x-ray
2. Supporting the active-labor client, whose spouse has not yet arrived, by having her focus on breathing and relaxation
3. Catheterizing the pregnant client to obtain urine for culture and sensitivity and sending this to the laboratory
4. Removing meal trays from client rooms and documenting the amount of intake and percent of meal eaten
5. Obtaining and double-checking a unit of blood with another RN who is preparing the blood for transfusion
6. Recording the 8-hour volume infused intravenously from intravenous (IV) pumps and clearing the volume infused for all clients

**233.** MoC The nurse has medications to administer at 10:00 a.m. to four pediatric clients. Which child should be the nurse's priority for administering medications?

1. The child with a frequent, productive cough who has an antitussive medication due
2. The child with burns who has a debridement at 10:45 a.m. and needs an oral analgesic
3. The child with aspiration pneumonia who has a scheduled intravenous antibiotic that is due
4. The child with an infection who has a fever of 102°F (38.9°C) and is receiving acetaminophen

**234.** MoC The nurse delegated to the NA to calculate the 8-month-old's output for the past 8 hours. The child had three wet diapers during the 8-hour shift weighing 45 g, 40 g, and 50 g. The weight of a dry diaper is 15 g. The child also had a 100-mL emesis and 50-mL diarrheal stool. What amount in milliliters (mL) should the NA report for the infant's total output for the 8 hours?

_____ mL (Record your answer as a whole number.)

**INSTRUCTIONS:** Read the case study, noting the times and the nurse's assessment and intervention. Refer to the case study to answer Questions 235 and 236.

| The Nurse Is Caring for a Client Admitted with Pneumonia Who also Has a History of Type 1 DM. | | |
| --- | --- | --- |
| **Time** | **Assessment** | **Interventions** |
| 0730 | Alert and oriented; BP 110/68, P. 100, RR 22, Oral temp. 102.2°F (39°C); Fingerstick glucose 140 mg/dL | Gave scheduled 4 units insulin aspart; 5 minutes after insulin aspart, meal given<br>Gave prescribed acetaminophen 325 mg (o) |
| 0900 | Serum lab results: K 4.9 mEq/L; Creatinine 1.2 mg/dL; Mag 1.1 mg/dL; Na 138 mEq/L; Hgb 10.8 g/dL | Initiated prescribed electrolyte protocol; Selected serum potassium replacement; started 10 mEq KCL IV, infusing over 1 hr |
| 1000 | Diaphoretic; States not feeling well. BP: 97/51, P. 118, RR 28, Oxygen saturation at 89%. | Performed fingerstick blood glucose; Requested STAT serum glucose per protocol<br>Initiated oxygen at 2 L/NC per emergency protocol; Notified HCP who was in surgery and would return the call; Asked LPN to retake client temperature |
| 1020 | Diaphoretic; Chest pain 6 on scale 0–10. BP: 96/50, P. 122, RR 30, Oral temp. 101°F (38.3°C); Oxygen saturation at 86%.; *Lab result*: Serum glucose: 72 mg/dL; | Administered 2 mg morphine sulfate IV prescribed on MAR; Increased oxygen to 4 L/NC; Telephoned HCP again to come see client |

**235.** CJ MoC At which time did the nurse intervene incorrectly?

1. 0730
2. 0900
3. 1000
4. 1020

**236.** CJ MoC Which actions should the nurse have performed instead? Enter the information in the text box provided.

[ ]

**237.** MoC The nurse is admitting the child diagnosed with MRSA. Which sign should the nurse direct the NA to place on the door of the child's room?

1.

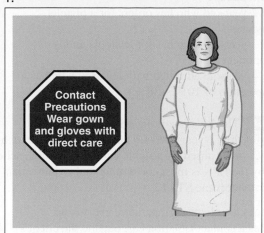

2.

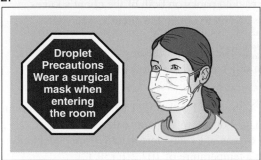

3.

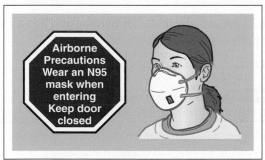

4.

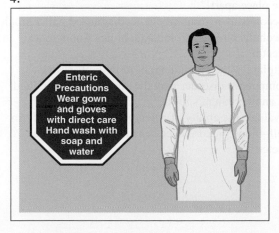

**238.** MoC The 4-month-old infant with no previous health problems is seen for a routine well-child appointment. The senior student nurse, working with the RN, completes the infant's physical assessment and reports to the RN that the baby's pulse rate is 165 bpm and that the infant is awake and calm. Which action should the nurse take **first** in evaluating the accuracy of this measurement?

1. Immediately retake the infant's vital signs and perform a complete assessment.
2. Notify the HCP of the abnormal heart rate finding and infant status.
3. Advise the student to ask the parent if there is a family history of cardiovascular disease.
4. Direct the student to compare the heart rate value with those obtained at previous clinic visits.

**239.** MoC The RN's assessment findings of the 2-year-old with meningitis include an altered level of consciousness, decreased urine output, and temperature of 103.4°F (39.7°C). The LPN who works on an adult oncology unit arrives to assist in "any way possible." Which task should the RN delegate to the LPN?

1. Notifying the HCP
2. Checking the size of the child's pupils
3. Administering an acetaminophen suppository
4. Removing the child's extra blankets and clothing

**240.** MoC The RN is the preceptor for the new graduate nurse during the new nurse's second week of orientation. Which clients should the charge nurse assign to the graduate nurse under the supervision of the preceptor? **Select all that apply.**

1. The 16-year-old client with moderate chronic asthma to be discharged in 24 hours
2. The 5-year-old client with a tracheostomy needing tracheostomy care every shift
3. The 12-year-old client who had surgery for a ruptured appendix with a temperature of 99°F (37.2°C)
4. The 8-year-old client just admitted with a new diagnosis of leukemia
5. The 4-year-old client diagnosed with hemophilia and admitted for a blood transfusion

**241.** MoC The parent brings the 2-year-old child into an urgent care setting with blistering burns due to sun exposure. Following an initial assessment, which action should be the nurse's priority?

1. Determine the percent of burn injury.
2. Administer an analgesic medication.
3. Open the blisters for débridement.
4. Apply cool compresses for 20 minutes.

**242.** MoC The nurse completes an initial assessment of an adolescent weighing 88 pounds who was injured in an MVA. What should be the priority order for the nurse's follow-up of the assessment findings? Place items in the order of priority.

1. The client states, "I was given pain medication in the ambulance."
2. Blood is noted at an abdominal wound site.
3. Client is responsive, but based on previous documentation is less responsive.
4. Urinary output is less than 30 mL in the last 2 hours.

Answer: _____

**243.** MoC The 15-month-old toddler with acute laryngotracheobronchitis (croup) is placed in a prescribed mist oxygen tent. When assessing the toddler 2 hours later, the RN obtains an increased HR of 122 bpm and a respiratory rate of 58 breaths per minute. Which action should the nurse take **next?**

1. Notify the HCP immediately of the child's vital signs.
2. Ask the PCA to obtain a BP while calling the charge nurse.
3. With the assistance of the PCA, remove the child from the oxygen tent.
4. Ask the PCA to obtain an oximeter to check the toddler's oxygen saturation level.

**244.** MoC The NA is caring for the 10-year-old child who has just completed chemotherapy treatments. Which action by the NA requires the RN to intervene?

1. Applies unscented body lotion to the child's dry skin and performs a back and foot massage
2. Assists the child to put on a freshly laundered hand-sewn hat that a parent brought from home
3. Offers a soft toothbrush with toothpaste for oral care and helps the child rinse with water
4. Applies nystatin oral suspension that was left at the bedside to mouth sores

**245.** MoC The nurse has received change-of-shift report. Which client should the nurse plan to assess **first?**

1. The 1-year-old with tetralogy of Fallot who has signs of cyanosis
2. The 3-year-old with rheumatic fever who is experiencing severe knee pain
3. The 5-year-old with endocarditis who has crackles bilaterally in all lung lobes
4. The 7-year-old with measles who has a temperature of 101.2°F (38°C)

**246.** MoC The RN is working with the experienced LPN. Which client should the RN assign to the LPN?

1. The 1-year-old who is scheduled to receive chemotherapy
2. The 2-year-old who has orders for a platelet transfusion
3. The 3-year-old who has loose stools and is incontinent
4. The 4-year-old admitted with lethargy who has a temperature of 101°F (38°C)

**247.** MoC The RN is working with the LPN who is caring for the 12-year-old who has severe abdominal, hip, and knee pain caused by a sickle cell crisis. Which action taken by the LPN is most concerning and requires that the nurse intervene **STAT?**

1. Checks the client's temperature every hour
2. Places a contact isolation cart outside the client's room
3. Places cold packs on both of the client's knees
4. Asks an NA to obtain the client's vital signs

**248.** MoC The nurse has been assigned four clients. In what order should the nurse plan to assess the clients?

1. The 14-year-old with a UTI who reports urinary burning at a 2 on a 0 to 10 pain scale
2. The 6-year-old 1 day postoperative appendectomy with a temperature of 102.2°F (39°C)
3. The 5-year-old newly admitted with pharyngitis and drooling
4. The 2-year-old admitted with diarrhea who had three loose stools on the previous shift

Answer: _____

**249.** MoC The RN is managing a mental health unit. Which activity should the RN delegate to the UAP?

1. Implement physical restraints prescribed as needed (prn) on the 35-year-old client with a history of aggressive behavior who is threatening to "tear the place apart!"
2. Accompany a group of clients diagnosed with chronic alcoholism to an off-unit Alcoholics Anonymous meeting.
3. Explain to the client diagnosed with obsessive-compulsive disorder why the client is not permitted in another client's room.
4. Evaluate the ability of a depressed client to perform self–blood glucose checks using a blood glucose meter.

**250.** MoC The client is returning to a unit after ECT treatment. Which intervention should the nurse delegate to the UAP?

1. Assessing the client's level of consciousness every 15 minutes
2. Observing the client for restlessness or agitation and reporting it to the nurse
3. Assisting with the client's first food and beverage intake after the treatment
4. Informing the client's family that the client's memory loss is generally temporary

**251.** MoC The RN is working with the ancillary staff member on a mental health unit. The RN recognizes the need to provide further education regarding the scope of practice when the staff member offers to take which action?

1. Facilitate the smoking breaks earned by the various clients on the mental health unit.
2. Accompany the 25-year-old client with schizophrenia to an off-site eye appointment.
3. Provide visual observation every 15 minutes for the client who expresses suicidal ideations.
4. Determine whether restraints may be removed from the client who was acting aggressively.

**252.** MoC The RN caring for the elderly client with dementia as a result of metastatic brain cancer is delegating actions to the NA. Which action is **inappropriately** delegated to the NA?

1. Toileting the client prior to settling the client in bed for the night
2. Informing the family that the client will need a follow-up brain scan
3. Accompanying the client on a walk in the gardens on the hospital grounds
4. Reinforcing the client's orientation by frequently stating the year, month, and day

**253.** MoC The nurse is admitting the client with OCD who has ritualistic behavior. Which intervention should the nurse **best** delegate to ancillary staff?

1. Assisting the client to store personal belongings to minimize the client's anxiety
2. Asking the client to identify someone who can be notified regarding the client's admission
3. Providing the client with the general "unit rules" that the client will be expected to follow
4. Encouraging the client to "talk to someone" if feeling anxious, excited, or out of control

**254.** MoC The nurse is assessing the appropriateness of a self-help group for the 20-year-old client recently diagnosed with an eating disorder. The nurse should **initially** obtain which information?

1. The average age of the self-help group's membership
2. The ratio of clients to involved health care professionals
3. How compatible the group's meeting schedule is with the client's expectations
4. The composition of the self-help group's membership and similarity with the client

**255.** MoC The client is being treated for severe depression and is receiving information regarding self-help groups. Which statement made by the client best reflects understanding of the **priority** goal for crisis intervention?

1. "I'm going to attend a self-help group to learn how to best cope with stress."
2. "Stress causes my depression, and I must learn to deal with it effectively."
3. "I know to take my medication regularly as prescribed by my provider."
4. "I really think I can learn how to cope so that I can get my old life back."

**256.** MoC The client being treated for exacerbation of depression states, "Caring for all my children is just too hard!" Which intervention should the nurse implement **initially** when providing crisis intervention?

1. Ask the grandparents to assume temporary responsibility for the children's care.
2. Provide one-on-one nurse-client time to reinforce the nurse's commitment to help.
3. Arrange for the client to attend a self-help group that addresses parenting stressors.
4. Have the client identify the stressors that immediately preceded this crisis situation.

**257.** MoC The client on the mental health unit is displaying manic symptoms. Which intervention should be the nurse's **priority** for this client?

1. Applying restraints to protect the client from self-inflicted injury
2. Administering tranquilizing medication as prescribed by the HCP
3. Monitoring the client for signs and symptoms of physical exhaustion
4. Reducing all forms of stimulation in the client's environment

**258.** MoC Two hours after taking a regular morning dose of regular insulin, the client presents to a clinic with diaphoresis, tremors, palpitations, and tachycardia. Which nursing action has **priority**?

1. Check pulse oximetry; if 94% or less, start oxygen at 2 L per nasal cannula.
2. Give a baby aspirin and one nitroglycerin tablet; obtain an electrocardiogram.
3. Check blood glucose level; provide carbohydrates if less than 70 mg/dL (3.8 mmol/L).
4. Check heart rate; if the HR is above 120 beats per minute, give atenolol 25 mg orally.

**259.** MoC The home health nurse is providing care to the child with HF. Which action should be the nurse's **priority** when thinking that the child may have developed a dysrhythmia?

1. Compare apical and radial pulse rates.
2. Arrange for Holter monitor placement.
3. Administer the daily dose of digoxin.
4. Immediately apply ice to the face.

**260.** MoC The child is hospitalized following renal trauma. The nurse should assess for signs of which complication **first**?

1. Anuria
2. Hypertension
3. Internal bleeding
4. Electrolyte imbalance

# Answers and Rationales

**156.** MoC **ANSWER: 2, 4, 1, 3**
2. **The 33-year-old client with a deep partial-thickness leg burn who has a temperature of 102.8°F (39.3°C), BP 98/66 mm Hg, and P 114 bpm should be attended to first. The elevated temperature, low BP, and tachycardia are signs that indicate septic shock or sepsis may be developing.**
4. **The 58-year-old client who had a skin graft to a leg burn 6 hours ago and is requesting a medication for pain rated at a 6 on a 0 to 10 scale should be attended to next. Postoperative pain control is needed to keep on top of the pain and enable the client to be involved in postoperative activities, such as coughing and deep breathing, to prevent complications of bedrest.**
1. **The 57-year-old client who was admitted 24 hours ago after being struck by lightning and has a serum potassium level of 5.5 mEq/L should be attended to third. The serum potassium level is borderline high (normal 3.5 to 5.5 mEq/L).**
3. **The 25-year-old client admitted 1 week ago with facial and chest burns from a house fire who has been crying since recent visitors left can be attended to last among the clients. The client needs emotional support, which is important to recovery, but clients with physiological needs are priority.**

▶ *Test-taking Tip: Use the ABC's and Maslow's Hierarchy of Needs to establish priority. Physiological needs are priority over psychosocial needs.*

Content Area: Management of Care; Concept: Critical Thinking; Nursing Roles; Management; Integrated Processes: Nursing Process: Planning; Client Needs: Safe and Effective Care Environment: Management of Care; Cognitive Level: Synthesis [Creating]

**157.** MoC **ANSWER: 2**
1. The NA is able in some facilities to perform a simple dressing change, but if the RN changes it, the RN would be able to assess the incision. The RN may not delegate assessment of the client.
2. **The scope of practice for the NA includes measuring and recording I&O and for the LPN includes administering oral and IM medications.**
3. The NA is able to assist with hygiene, but meeting with the family of the deceased client should be completed by the RN and not the LPN.
4. The NA is able to take and document vital signs, but the RN should be completing discharge paperwork to be reviewed with the clients. The discharge paperwork often includes a review of the care plan and addressing unmet needs of the client.

▶ *Test-taking Tip: Eliminate options that include aspects of the RN role that should not be delegated, including assessment, evaluation, and education.*

Content Area: Management of Care; Concept: Management; Regulations; Integrated Processes: Nursing Process: Planning; Client Needs: Safe and Effective Care Environment: Management of Care; Safe and Effective Care Environment: Safety and Infection Control; Cognitive Level: Synthesis [Creating]

## 158. MoC ANSWER: 3

1. Taking a BP and reporting the findings to the RN is evident, and administering IV medications is within the RN scope of practice.
2. Assisting the client to the bathroom is an appropriate task for the NA, reporting to the RN the findings is evident, and the RN's role in calling the HCP is appropriate.
3. **Delegation includes assessing the abilities of the delegate. The glucose level of 55 mg/dL is low (normal = 70–110 mg/dL), and rapid-acting lispro (Humalog) insulin should not have been administered. There is no indication that the RN assessed the LPN's knowledge about the normal glucose levels and when to withhold insulin. Also, there is no indication that the LPN notified the RN of the abnormal findings.**
4. Assisting the client with activity and offering hygienic care are appropriate NA tasks, and reporting of refused hygienic care is evident. Documenting completion of tasks is appropriate for the NA. The location of documentation of task completion may vary by facility and may include only a flowsheet or narrative documentation.

▶ **Test-taking Tip:** Consider the RN's responsibility in assessing the knowledge and skills of the delegate.

Content Area: Management of Care; Concept: Management; Integrated Processes: Communication and Documentation; Client Needs: Safe and Effective Care Environment: Management of Care; Cognitive Level: Analysis [Analyzing]

## 159. MoC ANSWER: 2

1. Asking the NA the number of times the skill has been performed does not evaluate knowledge and abilities; the NA could be performing the procedure incorrectly.
2. **The NA describing the procedure is one method of evaluating the NA's knowledge and skill. Using an open-ended question elicits conversation and details.**
3. Asking the NA when last observed by the RN does not evaluate knowledge and abilities.
4. Asking what the NA did when obtaining abnormal results may provide information about the NA's ability to follow through with information, but it does not evaluate the procedure.

▶ **Test-taking Tip:** Select an option with an open-ended question.

Content Area: Management of Care; Concept: Management; Integrated Processes: Communication and Documentation; Client Needs: Safe and Effective Care Environment: Management of Care; Cognitive Level: Evaluation [Evaluating]

## 160. MoC ANSWER: 4

1. Delegation of the NA-assigned job responsibilities is inappropriate and can create tension between team members.
2. Reminding the NA may be insufficient if the NA does not know how to total I&O records.
3. Notifying the charge nurse may be premature. Additional information is needed regarding the reason the NA is not performing the task.
4. **Delegation of assigned tasks includes determining the delegate's knowledge and ability to perform the task correctly. Discussing the task with the NA may clarify what the NA knows and where additional teaching is needed regarding the task.**

▶ **Test-taking Tip:** Focus on the tasks of delegation, ensuring that the delegate has the knowledge to perform the task.

Content Area: Management of Care; Concept: Management; Regulations; Integrated Processes: Nursing Process: Implementation; Client Needs: Safe and Effective Care Environment: Management of Care; Cognitive Level: Application [Applying]

## 161. MoC ANSWER: 3

1. Unjustifiable detention is false imprisonment. The client has a right to leave.
2. Sending the NA to help the client to pack or to speak to the client is inappropriate delegation of the nurse's responsibilities.
3. **Seeing the client provides an opportunity for further assessment and client teaching. The nurse's responsibility is to inform clients of the status of their care.**
4. Telling the client it is unsafe to leave does not explain why the client should remain in the hospital.

▶ **Test-taking Tip:** Focus on the option that uses therapeutic communication techniques and correct decision making regarding the RN's responsibility.

Content Area: Management of Care; Concept: Communication; Nursing Roles; Management; Integrated Processes: Communication and Documentation; Client Needs: Safe and Effective Care Environment: Management of Care; Physiological Integrity: Reduction of Risk Potential; Cognitive Level: Synthesis [Creating]

## 162. MoC ANSWER: 2

1. Not allowing the person an opportunity for any explanation does not foster team communication.
2. **This statement is best. Giving the NA an opportunity to provide a rationale fosters team communication.**
3. The nurse's comment is intimidating. It does not allow the NA an opportunity for any explanation and does not foster team communication.
4. Asking a why question is nontherapeutic and can precipitate a defensive response. It does not foster team communication.

▶ *Test-taking Tip: Focus on selecting the option that uses therapeutic communication and principles of teamwork. You should be able to identify the statement that treats the NA respectfully.*

**Content Area:** Management of Care; **Concept:** Management; **Integrated Processes:** Communication and Documentation; **Client Needs:** Safe and Effective Care Environment: Management of Care; **Cognitive Level:** Application [Applying]

### 163. MoC ANSWER: 3

1. This statement shows appropriate delegation that will promote organization and does not require immediate follow-up.
2. This statement shows appropriate delegation that will promote organization and does not require immediate follow-up.
3. **This statement may appear that the new nurse is organized. However, leaving the client dangling and another on a bedside commode while taking vital signs on another client is unsafe and indicates that the new nurse is not properly delegating tasks. This statement would require immediate follow-up by the mentor because these actions increase the client's risk for falls.**
4. By being organized, the nurse maximizes the number of tasks that can be accomplished throughout the shift. This statement does not require follow-up.

▶ *Test-taking Tip: You should be able to recognize the statement that indicates that the nurse has not delegated tasks appropriately and has put the clients at risk for falls.*

**Content Area:** Management of Care; **Concept:** Management; Safety; **Integrated Processes:** Nursing Process: Evaluation; **Client Needs:** Safe and Effective Care Environment: Management of Care; **Cognitive Level:** Evaluation [ᴱvaluati ɪg]

### 164. MoC ANSWER: 1, 4, 5

1. **It is within the LPN's scope of practice to administer oral and IM medications.**
2. It is not acceptabˡᵉ practice for the UAP to complete complex dressing changes.
3. It is not within the LPN's scope of practice to assess clients.
4. **It is acceptable practice for the UAP to empty and record urinary catheter bag drainage.**
5. **It is acceptable practice for the UAP to check and document vital signs on all clients.**
6. It is not within the LPN's scope of practice to initiate discharge paperwork. The LPN can reinforce discharge instructions but not initiate the discharge instructions.

▶ *Test-taking Tip: Focus on the scope of practice for the RN and LPN and on acceptable practices for UAP. Aspects of the RN scope of practice that include assessment, evaluation, and teaching should not be delegated.*

**Content Area:** Management of Care; **Concept:** Management; Regulations; **Integrated Processes:** Nursing Process: Planning; **Client Needs:** Safe and Effective Care Environment: Management of Care; **Cognitive Level:** Application [Applying]

### 165. MoC ANSWER: 3, 2, 1, 4

3. **Informing the LPN of tasks pertaining to the clients that should be completed should be the first action after giving or receiving report on the clients. The RN is delegating tasks to the LPN.**
2. **Intervene when the LPN allows the client who had been sedated for a procedure to have food/drink by mouth prior to verifying gag reflex is the second action. This involves supervision.**
1. **Following an incident, discuss the importance of verifying the gag reflex prior to allowing the client who was sedated to have anything by mouth is third. Supervision includes providing feedback.**
4. **Write a brief anecdotal note regarding appraisal of the encounter with the LPN is next. Appraisal involves evaluation.**

▶ *Test-taking Tip: You should be able to use the cues in the stem—delegation, supervision, and evaluation—to place the actions in the correct sequence. Remember that accountability and documentation are very important when supervising another.*

**Content Area:** Management of Care; **Concept:** Management; Regulations; **Integrated Processes:** Communication and Documentation; **Client Needs:** Safe and Effective Care Environment: Management of Care; **Cognitive Level:** Synthesis [Creating]

### 166. MoC ANSWER: 1

1. **For the client who primarily speaks a language other than English, the nurse should first determine the client's literacy level in both the primary language and English so that the nurse can select the appropriate printed materials for client teaching.**
2. The nurse should provide literature in the language that will best assist the client in learning about the medications; providing literature in both languages could confuse the client.
3. The nurse should ask about contacts willing to learn about the medications in addition to the client, not instead of the client. Teaching another person in addition to the client could ensure that the client is appropriately taking the medications.
4. It is not within the scope of practice for the NA to complete teaching even though the NA may know the client's primary language.

▶ *Test-taking Tip: When caring for the culturally diverse client, be sure to take measures to teach the client using linguistically appropriate materials and resources.*

**Content Area:** Management of Care; **Concept:** Diversity; **Integrated Processes:** Teaching/Learning; Culture and Spirituality; **Client Needs:** Safe and Effective Care Environment: Management of Care; **Cognitive Level:** Application [Applying]

**167.** MoC **ANSWER: 2, 4**

1. It is inappropriate for the LPN to delegate dressing changes; the RN should be determining the skills and abilities of the delegate and following agency policy and state laws regarding appropriate responsibilities of the UAP.
2. **The LPN can administer most medications; this would be appropriate delegation.**
3. The LPN should not add chemotherapy to an existing IV infusion. In some agencies, only chemotherapy-certified RNs administer chemotherapy.
4. **Once competency is demonstrated, it is appropriate to delegate transfer of the client using a mechanical lift to the UAP.**
5. Once a blood transfusion has been started, the nurse should assess the client for the first 15 minutes to ensure a reaction is not occurring. It is not appropriate for the UAP to assess.

▶ *Test-taking Tip: Focus on the tasks of delegation, ensuring that the delegate has the knowledge to perform the task. Focus on the LPN's and UAP's scope of practice.*

**Content Area:** Management of Care; **Concept:** Management; Regulations; **Integrated Processes:** Nursing Process: Implementation; **Client Needs:** Safe and Effective Care Environment: Management of Care; **Cognitive Level:** Application [Applying]

**168.** MoC **ANSWER: 4**

1. The prone position is not usually used and would make it difficult to assess the client's respiratory effort and cardiovascular status.
2. The Trendelenburg position is avoided because it increases the work of breathing.
3. The client is placed supine with the head elevated after regaining consciousness.
4. **The client should initially be placed in the lateral side-lying position to keep the client's airway open and avoid aspiration.**

▶ *Test-taking Tip: Utilize the ABC's.*

**Content Area:** Management of Care; **Concept:** Management; **Integrated Processes:** Nursing Process: Evaluation; **Client Needs:** Safe and Effective Care Environment: Management of Care; **Cognitive Level:** Evaluation [Evaluating]

**169.** MoC **ANSWER: 3**

1. Telling the UAP to be patient does not foster team communication.
2. Making a threatening statement does not foster team communication.
3. **Offering to "figure out what to do together" uses problem-solving, fosters team communication, and facilitates teamwork.**
4. Ignoring the problem does not foster team communication.

▶ *Test-taking Tip: Focus on selecting the option that uses therapeutic communication and principles of teamwork.*

**Content Area:** Management of Care; **Concept:** Management; **Integrated Processes:** Communication and Documentation; Caring; **Client Needs:** Safe and Effective Care Environment: Management of Care; **Cognitive Level:** Application [Applying]

**170.** MoC **ANSWER: 4**

1. Prior to reminding the UAP that the task needs to be completed, the nurse should assess to ensure that the UAP understands the job responsibilities and to explore the reason for uncompleted cares.
2. The nurse should attempt to handle the situation prior to notifying management.
3. Prior to completing an incident report, the nurse should assess the UAP's knowledge of responsibilities and the reason for uncompleted cares.
4. **Asking the UAP about cares completed and the reason for uncompleted a.m. cares will help determine the UAP's understanding of job responsibilities and any impeding factors, and is the most appropriate action to be taken by the nurse. The UAP's workload may have been too heavy.**

▶ *Test-taking Tip: Focus on the tasks of delegation, ensuring that the delegate has the knowledge, skills, and abilities to perform the task. Utilize assessment, the first step of the nursing process, to collect additional information.*

**Content Area:** Management of Care; **Concept:** Management; Regulations; **Integrated Processes:** Nursing Process: Implementation; **Client Needs:** Safe and Effective Care Environment: Management of Care; **Cognitive Level:** Application [Applying]

**171.** MoC **ANSWER: 2**

1. Asking how many times the skill has been performed does not evaluate knowledge and skill.
2. **Having the LPN describe the procedure is one method of evaluating the LPN's knowledge and skill. Using an open-ended question elicits conversation and details.**
3. Asking when the LPN was last observed performing a catheterization does not evaluate knowledge and skill.
4. Asking when the LPN last performed the skill does not evaluate knowledge and skill.

▶ *Test-taking Tip: Select an option with an open-ended question. Option 2 is different from the other options, which focus on time. Often the option that is different is the answer.*

**Content Area:** Management of Care; **Concept:** Management; Nursing Roles; **Integrated Processes:** Nursing Process: Evaluation; Communication and Documentation; **Client Needs:** Safe and Effective Care Environment: Management of Care; **Cognitive Level:** Evaluation [Evaluating]

**172.** MoC **ANSWER: 1, 3, 4**

1. **Due to factors of a constantly changing client care environment, individual components of care may be delayed.**
2. Documentation should be completed as soon as possible.

3. **Due to factors of a constantly changing client care environment, nurses may not finish their assigned shift on time.**

4. **Making rounds on all clients is acceptable as long as treatments and medications are not late due to this practice. There is no indication that treatments and medications were late.**

5. This statement does not provide a rationale for adequate time management. Breakfast should be eaten before the shift begins.

▶ *Test-taking Tip: Read the question and options carefully to make sure that all information is understood before choosing the answers. Avoid reading into Option 4. There is no indication that medications or treatments are late, and it does not identify how many clients were assigned to the nurse.*

**Content Area:** Management of Care; **Concept:** Management; Nursing Roles **Integrated Processes:** Nursing Process: Evaluation; Communication and Documentation; **Client Needs:** Safe and Effective Care Environment: Management of Care; **Cognitive Level:** Evaluation [Evaluating]

## 173. MoC PHARM ANSWER: 2

1. Lack of TPN infusion for 1 hour will not alter respiratory rate.

2. **Because TPN solution is high in glucose, discontinuing the infusion quickly may result in hypoglycemia. The nurse should ask the LPN to check the client's blood glucose level.**

3. BP will not alter respiratory rate.

4. Level of consciousness, unless the client is extremely hypoglycemic, will not alter respiratory rate.

▶ *Test-taking Tip: The key focus is the time (1 hour). Think about the nutrients in the TPN solution and determine which one, if withdrawn, would cause an immediate body reaction.*

**Content Area:** Management of Care; **Concept:** Metabolism; Management; **Integrated Processes:** Nursing Process: Analysis; **Client Needs:** Safe and Effective Care Environment: Management of Care; Physiological Integrity: Pharmacological and Parenteral Therapies; **Cognitive Level:** Analysis [Analyzing]

## 174. MoC ANSWER: 1, 2, 5

1. **The nurse can inform the NA of intended therapeutic effects of an antiemetic and direct the NA to report specific client observations to the nurse for follow-up.**

2. **The nurse can inform the NA of the client's laboratory value alterations and direct the NA to report specific client observations to the nurse for follow-up.**

3. Preparing medications from a vial involves knowledge and use of sterile technique and should not be delegated.

4. The nurse can ask the NA to report soiled dressings, but the nurse should change the dressing because it involves knowledge, problem solving, and aseptic technique.

5. **Hygienic care can be safely performed by the NA and delegated unless the condition of the client would warrant otherwise.**

▶ *Test-taking Tip: Consider the role of the NA and the aspects of care in the options that do not involve knowledge of sterile technique or complex procedures. The nurse should not administer a medication prepared by another.*

**Content Area:** Management of Care; **Concept:** Management; **Integrated Processes:** Nursing Process: Implementation; **Client Needs:** Safe and Effective Care Environment: Management of Care; Safe and Effective Care Environment: Safety and Infection Control; **Cognitive Level:** Application [Applying]

## 175. MoC ANSWER: 1

1. **The client with truncus arteriosus receiving digoxin (Lanoxin) is the most stable client of the options and is best for a new nurse's assignment.**

2. This client had balloon dilation as palliative treatment and will require careful monitoring and quick response to complications, making this assignment quite complex.

3. Therapeutic communication, along with knowledge of the disease process, will be required to do teaching about child care and hygiene, making this assignment more complex.

4. This client who had a heart transplant and is now admitted with low-grade fever and tachycardia suggests the client could have possible complications. An experienced nurse should be caring for this client.

▶ *Test-taking Tip: A new nurse should be assigned more stable clients who require routine care.*

**Content Area:** Management of Care; **Concept:** Management; Regulations; **Integrated Processes:** Nursing Process: Planning; **Client Needs:** Safe and Effective Care Environment: Management of Care; **Cognitive Level:** Analysis [Analyzing]

## 176. MoC ANSWER: 4, 3, 2, 1

4. **The 57-year-old client with hypertension who has severe midsternal pain should be assessed first. The client may be experiencing angina and needs immediate intervention.**

3. **The 76-year-old client newly admitted with serum BUN of 52 mg/dL should be assessed second. The elevated BUN could indicate dehydration.**

2. **The 82-year-old client who was unable to void and has a bladder scan showing 300 mL of urine should be the third client assessed; if the client is unable to void, the nurse should assess the client, initiate other measures to promote voiding, and, if unsuccessful, contact the HCP; the client may need intermittent urinary catheterization for bladder emptying.**

1. **The 47-year-old client 2 days postoperative who has pain rated at 2 on a 0 to 10 pain scale should be assessed last of the four clients. A pain level of 2 may be acceptable to the client.**

▶ *Test-taking Tip: Use the ABC's to establish priority and select the client who needs immediate assessment due to a worsening condition. The client who is the most stable should be assessed last.*

Content Area: Management of Care; Concept: Critical Thinking; Management; Regulations; Integrated Processes: Nursing Process: Planning; Client Needs: Safe and Effective Care Environment: Management of Care; Cognitive Level: Synthesis [Creating]

## 177. MoC ANSWER: 4

1. Delegating hygiene assistance is appropriate, but it may be unreasonable to expect the UAP to sufficiently bathe 10 clients during a shift.
2. The UAP in some facilities may assist with feeding the client through a gastric tube but not inserting the gastric tube.
3. The nurse may not delegate teaching to the UAP, as teaching is within the scope of practice of the RN.
4. **Generally, by the third day following a thoracotomy, the client may be safely ambulated with the assistance of the UAP.**

▶ *Test-taking Tip: You will need to be aware of what tasks may be delegated. Be sure when delegating to unlicensed individuals, delegate the right task, under the right circumstances, and to the right person.*

Content Area: Management of Care; Concept: Management; Regulations; Integrated Processes: Nursing Process: Planning; Client Needs: Safe and Effective Care Environment: Management of Care; Cognitive Level: Application [Applying]

## 178. MoC ANSWER: 3, 4, 2, 1

3. **The usually oriented 76-year-old client diagnosed with thrombophlebitis who has new-onset confusion needs immediate assessment because confusion may be a sign of a complication, such as a stroke or pulmonary embolism.**
4. **The 58-year-old client requesting a pain medication for abdominal incision pain rated at a 6 on a 0 to 10 scale should be attended to next because pain can interfere with necessary postoperative activities, such as deep breathing, coughing, and ambulating.**
2. **The 33-year-old client who has a new order to insert an NG tube and connect to low intermittent suction should be attended to third. There is no indication that this client is nauseated or that the placement of the NG has priority.**
1. **The 44-year-old client who has questions about how to empty the Jackson-Pratt drain at home after being discharged tomorrow should be the last client to be seen. Teaching is a lower priority than interventions for physiological integrity.**

▶ *Test-taking Tip: Use the ABC's to establish the priority client who should be attended to first. Confusion can indicate a breathing or circulatory problem. Then follow Maslow's Hierarchy of Needs to address comfort and psychosocial concerns.*

Content Area: Management of Care; Concept: Critical Thinking; Integrated Processes: Nursing Process: Planning; Client Needs: Safe and Effective Care Environment: Management of Care; Cognitive Level: Synthesis [Creating]

## 179. MoC ANSWER:

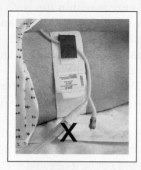

**The sampling port on the urinary catheter should be used to collect a sterile urine specimen. The tubing should be first clamped below the sampling port, located on the side of the catheter tubing, to allow sterile urine to collect. Once collected, the urine should be obtained through the sampling port.**

▶ *Test-taking Tip: Read the item carefully. Because the urine needs to be sterile to obtain a sterile culture, eliminate the second illustration and focus on the first illustration. Differentiate the balloon inflation port from the sampling port. If unsure, look carefully at the drainage system and select the port on the drainage tubing.*

Content Area: Management of Care; Concept: Management; Integrated Processes: Nursing Process: Evaluation; Client Needs: Safe and Effective Care Environment: Management of Care; Cognitive Level: Comprehension [Understanding]

## 180. MoC ANSWER: 4

1. It is unnecessary to notify the HCP as the first action; nurses are responsible for maintaining the patency of the NG tube.
2. Administering an antiemetic is important with nausea, but it is not the first action because a functioning NG should relieve the nausea by decompressing the stomach contents.
3. In a Salem sump–type NG with a vent lumen, air may need to be injected to release the tube from suctioning against the wall of the stomach, but the tube should not be partially withdrawn unless it has been determined that intestinal and not gastric drainage is returning.
4. **Nausea and minimal returns from the NG tube suggest possible occlusion of the tube. The tube should be irrigated per agency policy, or HCP's order, especially if the surgical area involved the GI system.**

▶ *Test-taking Tip: Focus on the situation and the type of surgery to determine the appropriate action. Use the process of elimination. When there is minimal drainage, the initial focus should be determining the patency of the NG tube. Thus eliminate Options 1 and 2. Withdrawing the NG tube could cause displacement. Eliminate Option 3.*

Content Area: Management of Care; Concept: Nursing Roles; Medication; Integrated Processes: Nursing Process: Implementation; Client Needs: Safe and Effective Care Environment: Management of Care; Cognitive Level: Analysis [Analyzing]

**181.** MoC **ANSWER: 1, 5**

1. **Providing oral care is within the NA's scope of practice and does not require advanced knowledge and critical thinking.**
2. Checking skin turgor is an assessment and not within the NA's scope of practice.
3. Administering IV fluids should be performed by a licensed nurse and is not within the NA's scope of practice.
4. Evaluating daily weights for trends requires critical thinking; evaluation is a component of the nursing process and should not be delegated.
5. **Calculating total intake and output is within the NA's scope of practice; it requires the ability to add, which is usually a job requirement.**

▶ **Test-taking Tip:** Focus on the tasks of delegation and the NA's scope of practice. Consider that the NA should have the knowledge and abilities to perform the delegated task. You should remember that assessments, medication administration, and evaluation are not tasks that should be delegated to the NA.

Content Area: Management of Care; Concept: Management; Regulations; Integrated Processes: Nursing Process: Planning; Client Needs: Safe and Effective Care Environment: Management of Care; Cognitive Level: Analysis [Analyzing]

**182.** MoC PHARM **ANSWER: 4**

1. Oxygen should be initiated at the onset, but 1 liter per NC is too low. Generally in an emergency, oxygen is administered using a nonrebreather mask at 90% to 100% oxygen concentration.
2. Obtaining IV access will take longer than administering a medication subcutaneously, so it should not be the first action.
3. Diphenhydramine (Benadryl) administered by IM injection has an onset of 20 to 30 minutes.
4. **Epinephrine hydrochloride (Adrenalin) is a sympathomimetic that acts rapidly to prevent or reverse cardiovascular collapse, airway narrowing from bronchospasm, and inflammation. It is rapidly absorbed when administered subcutaneously.**

▶ **Test-taking Tip:** Consider the amount of time it takes for each action to have an effect.

Content Area: Management of Care; Concept: Oxygenation; Management; Integrated Processes: Nursing Process: Implementation; Client Needs: Safe and Effective Care Environment: Management of Care; Physiological Integrity: Pharmacological and Parenteral Therapies; Cognitive Level: Application [Applying]

**183.** MoC **ANSWER: 3**

1. Inability to speak is expected immediately following a total laryngectomy.
2. Blood-tinged sputum is expected following a total laryngectomy.
3. **Oxygen saturation should be above 92%; immediate intervention is needed to increase the client's oxygen saturation level, which may include increasing the oxygen concentration, elevating the client's head of the bed, and/or suctioning the client's tracheostomy.**
4. A Jackson-Pratt wound drainage bulb should be emptied and compressed but is not the most immediate need.

▶ **Test-taking Tip:** Use the ABC's (airway, breathing, and circulation) to determine the assessment finding that has priority.

Content Area: Management of Care; Concept: Critical Thinking; Oxygenation; Management; Integrated Processes: Nursing Process: Planning; Client Needs: Safe and Effective Care Environment: Management of Care; Cognitive Level: Application [Applying]

**184.** MoC **ANSWER: 4**

1. Suctioning removes secretions and clears the client's airway, but assessment of the client has priority; restlessness and an increased respiratory rate may not indicate that the client needs suctioning. These findings are also associated with pain.
2. Applying oxygen is appropriate, but assessment has priority to determine if oxygen is necessary.
3. Elevation of the head of the bed would be appropriate, but assessment of the client has priority.
4. **Assessment has priority to determine the cause of the client's symptoms.**

▶ **Test-taking Tip:** Following the steps of the nursing process will assist you in answering this question. Assessment is the first step of the nursing process. Key words such as "priority" indicate that there is more than one option that may be correct, but one should be performed before another.

Content Area: Management of Care; Concept: Critical Thinking; Management; Integrated Processes: Nursing Process: Assessment; Client Needs: Safe and Effective Care Environment: Management of Care; Cognitive Level: Application [Applying]

**185.** MoC **ANSWER: 3**

1. The client with CF should be assessed prior to pulmonary function tests, but this is not the priority client.
2. An increased temperature is expected in the client with bacterial pneumonia.
3. **The client with dyspnea who had a chest tube removed 1 hour ago has the priority because dyspnea could indicate a pneumothorax.**
4. Medications may be given 30 minutes before or after the scheduled time, but this is not urgent.

▶ **Test-taking Tip:** Use the ABC's to establish priority and select the client who needs immediate airway protection, especially with the recent onset of dyspnea.

Content Area: Management of Care; Concept: Critical Thinking; Oxygenation; Management; Integrated Processes: Nursing Process: Planning; Client Needs: Safe and Effective Care Environment: Management of Care; Cognitive Level: Analysis [Analyzing]

**186.** MoC **ANSWER: 1**
1. **After managing the ABC's (airway, breathing, circulation) in the immediate postoperative period, the focus is on managing pain. General anesthetic agents such as isoflurane (Forane) are removed quickly through lung exhalation, and, as the client wakens, the need for postoperative analgesia increases.**
2. Anxiety is important but does not have priority in the immediate postoperative period. If pain is controlled, anxiety may decrease.
3. The client would have an abdominal incision that the nurse should assess, but this can be accomplished after treating the client's acute pain.
4. Although general anesthetics may be removed quickly through lung exhalation, the client will still be sleepy until the full effects of the medication have worn off.

♦ **Test-taking Tip:** Note the key word "first." Use Maslow's Hierarchy of Needs to identify the priority.

Content Area: Management of Care; Concept: Comfort; Management; Integrated Processes: Nursing Process: Planning; Client Needs: Safe and Effective Care Environment: Management of Care; Cognitive Level: Application [Applying]

**187.** MoC **ANSWER: 3**
1. The LPN should have the skill and ability to care for the client needing a foot soak who is in contact precautions.
2. The LPN should have the skill and ability to provide general postoperative care for the client following a vaginal hysterectomy.
3. **The 34-year-old client preparing for discharge will need teaching related to the care of the incision and wound drain and will have other psychosocial and physical needs. The nurse manager should intervene because the RN should assess the client's readiness for discharge and complete the teaching.**
4. The LPN should have the skill and ability to perform urinary catheterizations.

♦ **Test-taking Tip:** Focus on the role of the RN and on abilities that should not be delegated. Nursing tasks for stable clients with expected outcomes should be assigned to the LPN.

Content Area: Management of Care; Concept: Management; Regulations; Integrated Processes: Nursing Process: Analysis; Client Needs: Safe and Effective Care Environment: Management of Care; Cognitive Level: Analysis [Analyzing]

**188.** MoC **ANSWER: 2, 3, 5**
1. The RN should be preparing a PCA device that delivers medications intravenously because it is a complex skill with a high risk for error. To avoid an error, the RN will likely have the settings double-checked by another nurse. In some agencies, this could be the LPN.

2. Focused assessments such as CMS checks and administering pain medications by mouth are within the LPN's scope of practice.
3. The LPN can assist the client with phantom limb pain on measures to control the pain.
4. This client would require more extensive physical and psychological assessment. Due to the complexity of the situation, it would not be appropriate to delegate the client's care to the LPN.
5. **Administering oral pain medications and heat applications are within the LPN's scope of practice.**

♦ **Test-taking Tip:** Focus on the tasks of delegation, ensuring that the delegate has the knowledge to perform the task. Focus on the LPN's scope of practice.

Content Area: Management of Care; Concept: Management; Regulations; Integrated Processes: Nursing Process: Planning; Client Needs: Safe and Effective Care Environment: Management of Care; Cognitive Level: Analysis [Analyzing]

**189.** MoC **ANSWER: 1, 3, 5**
1. **Because the client's condition is deteriorating, additional assistance is needed. The PCA should be able to page for the charge nurse.**
2. There is no indication of respiratory distress, so it is unnecessary to page for a respiratory therapist.
3. **The client should have frequent BP measurements because the BP is low. Securing an automatic BP machine is appropriate delegation.**
4. There is no indication that the client needs oxygen. If oxygen is indicated, a nasal cannula should be applied at 2–4 L/min.
5. **Obtaining a printed rhythm strip is appropriate delegation.**

♦ **Test-taking Tip:** Focus on the client's symptoms to eliminate options that do not pertain, such as paging a respiratory therapist. RN-only responsibilities, including assessment and evaluation of information, should not be delegated to the PCA.

Content Area: Management of Care; Concept: Management; Regulations; Integrated Processes: Nursing Process: Planning; Client Needs: Safe and Effective Care Environment: Management of Care; Cognitive Level: Application [Applying]

**190.** MoC **ANSWER: 2**
1. Asking how many times the skill has been performed does not evaluate knowledge and skill.
2. **Having the LPN describe the information that will be provided is one method of evaluating the LPN's knowledge and skill. Using an open-ended question elicits conversation and details.**
3. Asking when the LPN last provided diet education does not evaluate knowledge and skill.
4. Asking when the LPN was last observed reinforcing diet teaching does not evaluate skill and knowledge.

▶ *Test-taking Tip: Select an option with an open-ended question. Option 2 is different from the other options, which focus on time. Often the option that is different is the answer.*

**Content Area:** Management of Care; **Concept:** Management; Nursing Roles; **Integrated Processes:** Teaching/Learning; **Client Needs:** Safe and Effective Care Environment: Management of Care; **Cognitive Level:** Evaluation [Evaluating]

### 191. MoC ANSWER: 1, 4, 5

1. **It is within the LPN's scope of practice to administer oral medication.**
2. It is not within the LPN's scope of practice to administer IV push medications.
3. It is not within the LPN's scope of practice to administer IV push medications.
4. **It is within the LPN's scope of practice to administer oxygen.**
5. **It is within the scope of the practice of the LPN to attach cardiac monitor leads.**

▶ *Test-taking Tip: Use the five rights of delegation: the right task, under the right circumstances, to the right person, with the right direction and communication, and the right supervision and evaluation. Remember that the RN must delegate within the LPN's scope of practice and that person must have the knowledge and ability to perform the task.*

**Content Area:** Management of Care; **Concept:** Management; Regulations; **Integrated Processes:** Nursing Process: Implementation; **Client Needs:** Safe and Effective Care Environment: Management of Care; **Cognitive Level:** Analysis [Analyzing]

### 192. MoC PHARM ANSWER: 1

1. **Findings suggest fluid volume overload. Diuretics such as furosemide (Lasix) are the first-line treatment for fluid volume overload in the client with heart failure and should be the priority.**
2. Ace inhibitors such as enalapril (Vasotec) are utilized to treat heart failure by decreasing cardiac output, but the priority for this client is to treat excess fluid volume.
3. Fluid restriction is important, but the priority is to eliminate excessive fluid.
4. An echocardiogram will evaluate the heart's function and is important, but beginning the diuretic to help eliminate excessive fluid has priority.

▶ *Test-taking Tip: The key word "priority" indicates that there may be more than one right option, but one option should be done prior to the others. You should recognize that an IV medication will have a more rapid onset than one administered orally.*

**Content Area:** Management of Care; **Concept:** Critical Thinking; Management; **Integrated Processes:** Nursing Process: Implementation; **Client Needs:** Safe and Effective Care Environment: Management of Care; Physiological Integrity: Pharmacological and Parenteral Therapies; **Cognitive Level:** Analysis [Analyzing]

### 193. MoC ANSWER: 2

1. Administering medication is not within the UAP's scope of practice.
2. **Monitoring vital signs and oxygen saturation is within the UAP's scope of practice.**
3. Teaching is not within the UAP's scope of practice.
4. Explaining the rationale for rest and exercise involves teaching and is not within the UAP's scope of practice.

▶ *Test-taking Tip: Use the five rights of delegation: the right task, under the right circumstances, to the right person, with the right direction and communication, and the right supervision and evaluation. Remember that the RN must delegate within the UAP's scope of practice. The UAP's scope of practice does not include medication administration or teaching.*

**Content Area:** Management of Care; **Concept:** Management; Regulations; **Integrated Processes:** Nursing Process: Implementation; **Client Needs:** Safe and Effective Care Environment: Management of Care; Physiological Integrity: Reduction of Risk Potential; **Cognitive Level:** Application [Applying]

### 194. MoC ANSWER: 4

1. The first action for the client in ventricular fibrillation is to assess for a pulse. Once pulselessness is established, the pulse is not rechecked until after a full minute of CPR or 5 cycles of 30 compressions.
2. Compressions should begin once pulselessness has been established. Because the client had cardiac surgery, the nurse should perform compressions rather than the NA due to the potential for harm to the client.
3. Defibrillation is performed as soon as the defibrillator is available. It is premature to tell the NA to prepare the client for defibrillation.
4. **The nurse should tell the NA to activate the EMS. In the hospital setting, it may be pushing a code blue button or calling a designated number.**

▶ *Test-taking Tip: Apply basic life support protocol and consider which action would be safest to delegate to the NA. Only actions that are within the NA scope of practice should be delegated.*

**Content Area:** Management of Care; **Concept:** Management; Regulations; **Integrated Processes:** Nursing Process: Implementation; **Client Needs:** Safe and Effective Care Environment: Management of Care; **Cognitive Level:** Analysis [Analyzing]

### 195. MoC PHARM ANSWER: 2

1. Teaching the client the reasons for bedrest should be completed by the RN because it would involve providing information about the client's condition.
2. **An experienced NA would be able to monitor the client's vital signs and should know to report significant changes to the RN.**
3. If the client's infusion pump needs to be turned off due to hypotension, the nurse should be making this judgment and not the NA.

4. The RN should call the HCP about the decreased urine output and not wait until the HCP is rounding. The RN will need to provide additional information about the client's status to the HCP and may receive orders for prescribed medications.

▶ **Test-taking Tip:** *Assessment, teaching, and evaluation cannot be delegated. Focus on the tasks of delegation, the scope of practice for the NA, and the knowledge and skills needed to perform the identified responsibilities.*

**Content Area:** Management of Care; **Concept:** Management; Regulations; **Integrated Processes:** Nursing Process: Planning; **Client Needs:** Safe and Effective Care Environment: Management of Care; Physiological Integrity: Physiological Adaptation; **Cognitive Level:** Application [Applying]

**196.** MoC **ANSWER: 2, 4, 1, 3, 5**

2. **Asking the NA to retake the client's vital signs now and having the NA set an automatic BP machine to retake the BP every 15 minutes should be first. Current values are needed prior to notifying the HCP.**

4. **Assess the client asking specific questions related to headache, dizziness, and orientation after the NA obtains the BP. A stroke can result from uncontrolled hypertension.**

1. **Notifying the client's HCP about the client's elevated BP is next. Essential information is needed before calling.**

3. **Administer the newly prescribed furosemide (Lasix) and enalapril (Vasotec). Interventions are needed to quickly lower the client's BP.**

5. **Inform the charge nurse of the client's critically high BP and the actions taken. If the situation is under control and the charge nurse's assistance is not needed, then the charge nurse can be informed of the situation after actions are taken.**

▶ **Test-taking Tip:** *Use the nursing process to establish priority interventions. Assessment should be first. The nurse must have sufficient information about the client prior to notifying the HCP.*

**Content Area:** Management of Care; **Concept:** Critical Thinking; Management; **Integrated Processes:** Nursing Process: Implementation; **Client Needs:** Safe and Effective Care Environment: Management of Care; **Cognitive Level:** Synthesis [Creating]

**197.** MoC **ANSWER: 3**

1. Assessing the dressing is important but not the priority because there is only a scant amount of blood.

2. If the client is sleepy but easily aroused, this would be an expected finding following surgery when an anesthetic or sedative-hypnotic agent is used.

3. **A low respiratory rate has the priority because anesthetic agents decrease respirations. Adult respirations should be 12–20 breaths per minute.**

4. The BP is within the normal limits.

▶ **Test-taking Tip:** *ABC's (airway, breathing, circulation) have the priority in the PACU.*

**Content Area:** Management of Care; **Concept:** Critical Thinking; Management; **Integrated Processes:** Nursing Process: Analysis; **Client Needs:** Safe and Effective Care Environment: Management of Care; Physiological Integrity: Physiological Adaptation; **Cognitive Level:** Application [Applying]

**198.** MoC **ANSWER: 2**

1. The client's temperature is elevated from improper procedure and not the client's illness.

2. **Assessment of any previous activity that would alter temperature should be made (e.g., smoking or oral intake) and avoided prior to taking the temperature. Asking the UAP to recheck the temperature in 15 minutes is most appropriate.**

3. The client's temperature is elevated from improper procedure and not the client's illness; increasing fluids is unnecessary.

4. Charting an inaccurate temperature is inappropriate; the temperature recorded should be one that avoids anything that would affect it for a period of time before taking the temperature.

▶ **Test-taking Tip:** *Focus on the situation and the important information provided in the stem. You should associate "steaming" in the stem with the temperature obtained and realize that if the client consumed any coffee, then the temperature of the coffee would affect the oral temperature reading.*

**Content Area:** Management of Care; **Concept:** Management; **Integrated Processes:** Communication and Documentation; **Client Needs:** Safe and Effective Care Environment: Management of Care; Physiological Integrity: Basic Care and Comfort; **Cognitive Level:** Application [Applying]

**199.** MoC **ANSWER: 2, 3**

1. Inserting the client's NG tube is a complex skill that involves assessment of the client's ability to swallow and evaluation of correct placement.

2. **Obtaining vital signs is within the NA's scope of practice. The nurse should consider the knowledge and skills of the person receiving the delegation.**

3. **Emptying a urinary drainage bag and recording output are within the NA's scope of practice.**

4. Completion of the preoperative checklist involves evaluation of client information and readiness for surgery.

5. Witnessing the operative consent involves evaluation of the client's understanding of the surgical procedure, its associated complications, and whether the client is giving voluntary, informed consent.

▶ **Test-taking Tip:** *The nurse should never delegate tasks that require assessments, analysis, teaching, or evaluation.*

**Content Area:** Management of Care; **Concept:** Management; Regulations; **Integrated Processes:** Nursing Process: Planning; **Client Needs:** Safe and Effective Care Environment: Management of Care; Physiological Integrity: Reduction of Risk Potential; **Cognitive Level:** Application [Applying]

**200.** MoC **ANSWER: 3, 4, 5**

1. Listening to lung sounds is an assessment; assessment is not within the LPN's scope of practice.
2. Checking pupil size and reactivity is an assessment and should not be delegated.
3. **The experienced LPN is able to check axillary temperatures every 4 hours and should know to report significant changes to the RN.**
4. **The experienced LPN should be able to check enteral feeding residual volumes every 4 hours and should know to report significant findings to the RN.**
5. **Turning and rubbing the client is necessary to prevent skin breakdown and is appropriate to delegate to the LPN.**

▶ *Test-taking Tip: You should focus on the LPN's scope of practice. The nurse should not delegate assessments; thus Options 1 and 2 should be eliminated as choices.*

**Content Area:** Management of Care; **Concept:** Management; Regulations; **Integrated Processes:** Nursing Process: Planning; **Client Needs:** Safe and Effective Care Environment: Management of Care; Physiological Integrity: Reduction of Risk Potential; **Cognitive Level:** Analysis [Analyzing]

**201.** MoC PHARM **ANSWER: 2**

1. The urinalysis provides information about the renal system but does not have the priority.
2. **Adverse effects of long-term use of Cox-2 inhibitors such as celecoxib (Celebrex) include renal impairment, which can be manifested by an elevated BP. The progressive elevation of serum creatinine and BUN suggests renal impairment.**
3. Auscultation of the heart is included in a health assessment but does not have the priority based on the findings.
4. Asking about a loss of appetite is important because it is a side effect of medications, but does not have the priority.

▶ *Test-taking Tip: Note the key word "priority." Think about the adverse effects of celecoxib.*

**Content Area:** Management of Care; **Concept:** Medication; Management; **Integrated Processes:** Nursing Process: Assessment; **Client Needs:** Safe and Effective Care Environment: Management of Care; Physiological Integrity: Pharmacological and Parenteral Therapies; **Cognitive Level:** Analysis [Analyzing]

**202.** MoC **ANSWER: 4**

1. Wearing gloves is part of contact precautions.
2. Wearing a gown is part of contact precautions.
3. Family members should be informed about hand washing with soap and water to prevent transmission of *Clostridium difficile.*
4. **Alcohol-based hand cleansers should not be used for hand hygiene with the organism *Clostridium difficile.* The organism forms spores, and alcohol-based antiseptic agents have poor activity against spores.**

▶ *Test-taking Tip: Read the stem carefully and determine that the question calls for a false answer. All the options are consistent with contact precautions. Recall that Clostridium difficile forms spores and requires hand hygiene with use of soap and water.*

**Content Area:** Management of Care; **Concept:** Infection; Management; **Integrated Processes:** Nursing Process: Evaluation; **Client Needs:** Safe and Effective Care Environment: Management of Care; Physiological Integrity: Reduction of Risk Potential; **Cognitive Level:** Evaluation [Evaluating]

**203.** MoC **ANSWER: 1**

1. **It is best to delegate bathing because it is within the UAP's scope of practice.**
2. Emphasizing frequent hand washing should be carried out by the nurse because it involves teaching.
3. Encouraging the client to use condoms should be carried out by the nurse because it involves teaching.
4. Teaching is not within the UAP's scope of practice and should not be delegated.

▶ *Test-taking Tip: Focus on the tasks of delegation, ensuring that the delegate has the knowledge to perform the task. All options except one include teaching.*

**Content Area:** Management of Care; **Concept:** Management; Regulations; **Integrated Processes:** Nursing Process: Implementation; **Client Needs:** Safe and Effective Care Environment: Management of Care; **Cognitive Level:** Application [Applying]

**204.** MoC PHARM **ANSWER: 4**

1. Spicy foods should not be consumed by the client with esophagitis. This should be addressed but does not require immediate intervention because of the amount of time between ordering and receiving the meal.
2. The client's reason for requesting a "No Visitors" sign should be addressed with the client; the LPN is following the client's wishes.
3. Because this client does not require contact precautions, this should be addressed but does not require immediate intervention.
4. **The nurse should immediately intervene because nystatin (Mycostatin) should be administered by having the client swish the medication in the mouth and then swallow it; it should not be followed with anything to drink.**

▶ *Test-taking Tip: The key word is "immediately." You should avoid selecting the first option that is an incorrect action because another incorrect action may be more important. Consider the implications of each action and determine if intervening immediately is necessary or if it can be delayed.*

**Content Area:** Management of Care; **Concept:** Critical Thinking; Regulations; Management; **Integrated Processes:** Nursing Process: Evaluation; **Client Needs:** Safe and Effective Care Environment: Management of Care; Physiological Integrity: Pharmacological and Parenteral Therapies; **Cognitive Level:** Evaluation [Evaluating]

**205.** MoC **ANSWER: 1**

1. **This 48-year-old client is the most stable client. The LPN should be able to treat the client's bladder spasms with medication and administer the oral antibiotics.**
2. This 52-year-old client has severe flank pain, which could indicate complications. The client should be assessed and monitored by an experienced nurse.
3. Administering IV push narcotics is not within the LPN's scope of practice; this client will also require teaching for the lithotripsy.
4. Teaching bladder training should be completed by the RN.

▶ *Test-taking Tip: Focus on the tasks of delegation, ensuring that the LPN has the knowledge to perform the tasks for the assigned client. You should assign the client with the cares within the LPN's scope of practice.*

Content Area: Management of Care; Concept: Management; Regulations; Integrated Processes: Nursing Process: Planning; Client Needs: Safe and Effective Care Environment: Management of Care; Cognitive Level: Analysis [Analyzing]

**206.** MoC **ANSWER: 2**

1. Anxiety is expected. This will require urgent attention, but this client is not the priority client.
2. **This client has priority because new-onset dyspnea could indicate worsening of the client's condition.**
3. Groin pain is expected after an angioplasty, but the area should be assessed for hematoma development.
4. This client is stable. Low-grade temperature is to be expected and should be closely monitored but does not require immediate attention.

▶ *Test-taking Tip: Use the ABC's (airway, breathing, circulation) to establish priority and select the client who needs immediate airway protection, especially with the recent onset of dyspnea.*

Content Area: Management of Care; Concept: Critical Thinking; Management; Integrated Processes: Nursing Process: Planning; Client Needs: Safe and Effective Care Environment: Management of Care; Physiological Integrity: Reduction of Risk Potential; Cognitive Level: Analysis [Analyzing]

**207.** MoC **ANSWER: 2**

1. Teaching is not within the UAP's scope of practice; this requires abilities that the UAP is not expected to possess and should not be delegated.
2. **The UAP should be able to record I&O on a group of clients; recording does not require clinical judgment.**
3. Discontinuing a CBI requires nursing judgment to evaluate whether the amount delivered is accounted for in the total output. Evaluation should not be delegated.
4. Checking for dehydration involves assessment and is not within the UAP's scope of practice; this should not be delegated.

▶ *Test-taking Tip: The nurse cannot delegate teaching, assessment, evaluation, or any action that requires nursing judgment to the UAP.*

Content Area: Management of Care; Concept: Management; Regulations; Integrated Processes: Nursing Process: Planning; Client Needs: Safe and Effective Care Environment: Management of Care; Cognitive Level: Analysis [Analyzing]

**208.** MoC **ANSWER: 1, 4, 5**

1. **Taking vital signs is within the LPN's scope of practice.**
2. Evaluation requires clinical judgment and is not within the LPN's scope of practice.
3. Consultation about the client's swallowing difficulties requires clinical judgment and is not within the LPN's scope of practice.
4. **Providing mouth care is within the LPN's scope of practice.**
5. **Reminding the client regarding previously taught instruction is within the LPN's scope of practice.**

▶ *Test-taking Tip: Focus on the tasks of delegation, ensuring that the delegate has the knowledge to perform the task. Focus on the LPN's scope of practice. Eliminate options that require clinical judgment.*

Content Area: Management of Care; Concept: Management; Regulations; Integrated Processes: Nursing Process: Implementation; Client Needs: Safe and Effective Care Environment: Management of Care; Cognitive Level: Application [Applying]

**209.** MoC **ANSWER: 2, 3**

1. Checking fingerstick glucose is an invasive procedure and is not within the UAP's scope of practice.
2. **Recording I&O is within the UAP's scope of practice.**
3. **Measuring vital signs is within the UAP's scope of practice.**
4. Assessment is not within the UAP's scope of practice because it requires clinical judgment.
5. Analyzing is not within the scope of practice of the UAP because it requires clinical judgment.

▶ *Test-taking Tip: Focus on the tasks of delegation, ensuring that the delegate has the knowledge to perform the task. Focus on the UAP's scope of practice.*

Content Area: Management of Care; Concept: Critical Thinking; Management; Regulations; Integrated Processes: Nursing Process: Planning; Client Needs: Safe and Effective Care Environment: Management of Care; Cognitive Level: Application [Applying]

**210.** MoC **ANSWER: 4**

1. Urine that is positive for ketones is an abnormal finding; the client should be assessed soon. However, the client with a blood glucose of 40 mg/dL has priority.
2. A serum T4 of 10 mg/dL is a normal finding.
3. A 2-hour postprandial glucose of 150 mg/dL is abnormal, and the client should be assessed soon, but the client with a blood glucose of 40 mg/dL has priority.

4. **Because a fasting blood glucose of 40 mg/dL is life-threatening, the nurse should assess this client first.**

▶ *Test-taking Tip: The client who has a potential life-threatening problem should be assessed first. Key words such as "priority" mean there is more than one option that could be the answer, but one should be done before another.*

Content Area: Management of Care; Concept: Critical Thinking; Management; Integrated Processes: Nursing Process: Analysis; Client Needs: Safe and Effective Care Environment: Management of Care; Physiological Integrity: Reduction of Risk Potential; Cognitive Level: Analysis [Analyzing]

### 211. MoC PHARM ANSWER: 4

1. Teaching is not within the LPN's scope of practice.
2. Assessment is not within the LPN's scope of practice.
3. Developing a discharge teaching plan is not within the LPN's scope of practice.
4. **Administration of medications, such as filgrastim (Neupogen), is included in LPN education and scope of practice. Filgrastim is a synthetic granulocyte-colony stimulating factor that stimulates the production of neutrophils.**

▶ *Test-taking Tip: Focus on the scope of practice for the LPN. Each state's board of nursing defines the scope of practice for licensed nurses.*

Content Area: Management of Care; Concept: Management; Regulations; Integrated Processes: Nursing Process: Planning; Client Needs: Safe and Effective Care Environment: Management of Care; Physiological Integrity: Pharmacological and Parenteral Therapies; Cognitive Level: Synthesis [Creating]

### 212. MoC ANSWERS: 2, 4, 5

1. Expertise will not be developed during the orientation period.
2. **The nurse manager's role is management of the unit, which includes ensuring that new nurses are socialized into the clinical unit.**
3. Responsibilities for ensuring licensure registration are not the responsibility of a unit-based manager but rather those of a centralized department, such as human resources, because this is a condition of employment.
4. **The nurse manager's role is management of the unit, which includes verifying that the new nurses are participating in the unit orientation.**
5. **The nurse manager's role is management of the unit, which includes ensuring that the new nurses are completing the competency verification process.**

▶ *Test-taking Tip: Focus on just the orientation period. Eliminate any options that would be a condition of employment.*

Content Area: Management of Care; Concept: Management; Integrated Processes: Nursing Process: Evaluation; Client Needs: Safe and Effective Care Environment: Management of Care; Cognitive Level: Evaluation [Evaluating]

### 213. MoC ANSWER: 1

1. **Providing oral care is within the UAP's scope of practice. Providing oral care does not require advanced nursing skills. Orientation to the unit would include oral care needs of clients with cancer who have undergone radiation or chemotherapy.**
2. Observing the client's response to feedings is not within the UAP's scope of practice; this is client assessment and evaluation.
3. Facilitating expression of grief or anxiety is not within the UAP's scope of practice because it requires advanced education in therapeutic communication skills.
4. Viscous lidocaine is a medication; the UAP can assist with oral care, but medications are to be administered by licensed personnel.

▶ *Test-taking Tip: Focus on the tasks of delegation, ensuring that the delegate has the knowledge to perform the task. You should remember that assessments, therapeutic communication, and medication administration should not be delegated to the UAP.*

Content Area: Management of Care; Concept: Management; Regulations; Integrated Processes: Nursing Process: Planning; Client Needs: Safe and Effective Care Environment: Management of Care; Cognitive Level: Application [Applying]

### 214. MoC ANSWER: 4

1. Teaching is not within the LPN's scope of practice.
2. Demonstrating is one method of teaching and is not within the LPN's scope of practice.
3. Assessing is not within the scope of practice of the LPN.
4. **Reinforcing information previously taught is within the LPN's scope of practice.**

▶ *Test-taking Tip: Focus on the LPN's scope of practice. The RN should not delegate assessment and teaching.*

Content Area: Management of Care; Concept: Management; Regulations; Integrated Processes: Nursing Process: Implementation; Client Needs: Safe and Effective Care Environment: Management of Care; Cognitive Level: Application [Applying]

### 215. MoC ANSWER: 3

1. An experienced nurse in the burn unit should care for the newly admitted client due to complex needs of the client.
2. An experienced nurse in the burn unit should complete the nutrition and wound teaching because the client is likely to have questions that may be unfamiliar to an oncology nurse.
3. **The 29-year-old client is the most stable. The nurse from the oncology unit should be able to complete a sterile dressing change.**
4. An experienced nurse in the burn unit should care for the client who requires assistance with positioning in hand splints; the nurse from the oncology unit may be unfamiliar with the splints.

▶ *Test-taking Tip:* Eliminate clients who have complex care issues. The nurse inexperienced in caring for clients on a burn unit should have the most stable client.

**Content Area:** Management of Care; **Concept:** Management; Regulations; **Integrated Processes:** Nursing Process: Planning; **Client Needs:** Safe and Effective Care Environment: Management of Care; **Cognitive Level:** Analysis [Analyzing]

## 216. MoC PHARM ANSWER: 2

1. Diazepam (Valium) may decrease the client's anxiety, but it will not improve the cardiac output or gas exchange.
2. **The nurse's priority should be giving morphine sulfate. This medication improves alveolar gas exchange, improves cardiac output by reducing ventricular preload and afterload, decreases anxiety, and assists in reducing the subjective feeling of dyspnea.**
3. Increasing the dopamine may improve cardiac output but will also increase the heart rate and myocardial oxygen consumption.
4. Nitroglycerin will improve cardiac output and may be appropriate for this client, but it will not directly reduce anxiety and will not act as quickly as morphine to decrease dyspnea.

▶ *Test-taking Tip:* You need to focus on giving a medication that will both reduce the client's anxiety and improve cardiac output.

**Content Area:** Management of Care; **Concept:** Critical Thinking; Management; **Integrated Processes:** Nursing Process: Implementation; **Client Needs:** Safe and Effective Care Environment: Management of Care; Physiological Integrity: Pharmacological and Parenteral Therapies; **Cognitive Level:** Application [Applying]

## 217. MoC ANSWER: 3, 1, 6, 4, 2, 5

3. **Turn off the antibiotic cefuroxime sodium (Zinacef) immediately because it is the cause of the problem.**
1. **Shout for help; extra people will be needed for interventions to stabilize the client.**
6. **Maintain the airway and administer oxygen to treat the client's dyspnea, wheezing, and stridor.**
4. **Ask another nurse to set up new IV maintenance solution and tubing and aspirate the IV port before initiating the new solution. Aspirating the IV port will remove any remaining antibiotic in the port. It is necessary to keep the IV open for the administration of emergency medications.**
2. **Call the HCP to report the client's reaction and status and receive orders. In some settings, the call for help may be to an emergency response team, and an HCP often responds as part of this team. The client's primary HCP should also be notified.**
5. **Administer the prescribed emergency medications intravenously.**

▶ *Test-taking Tip:* Visualize the steps in responding to an emergency: remove from immediate danger (stopping the IV in this situation), call for help, and maintain the airway. Prioritizing is placing items in the correct sequence.

**Content Area:** Management of Care; **Concept:** Collaboration; Management; **Integrated Processes:** Nursing Process: Implementation; **Client Needs:** Safe and Effective Care Environment: Management of Care; **Cognitive Level:** Synthesis [Creating]

## 218. MoC ANSWER: 4, 1, 3, 2

4. **The 60-year-old client who is dyspneic and has swollen lips after being stung by a bee should be assessed first; the client is likely experiencing an anaphylactic reaction. Airway maintenance and medication administration are required to prevent death.**
1. **The 40-year-old client who is diaphoretic and is feeling chest pressure should be assessed next. The client could be experiencing an MI, and "time is muscle." Ideally, the nurse should be able to delegate actions for this client while assessing the first client.**
3. **The 35-year-old client who cut her hand with a knife while preparing food is a priority because of the potential blood loss. However, this client should be assessed third because it is not as life-threatening as either the client with a possible anaphylactic reaction or the client with a possible MI.**
2. **The 18-year-old client who thinks he might have a broken ankle is the last client to be assessed. An x-ray is needed to confirm a fracture, but the client is stable and does not have a life-threatening problem.**

▶ *Test-taking Tip:* Use the ABC's (airway, breathing, circulation) to establish priority and select the client who needs immediate airway protection as the first client to be assessed.

**Content Area:** Management of Care; **Concept:** Critical Thinking; Management; **Integrated Processes:** Nursing Process: Analysis; **Client Needs:** Safe and Effective Care Environment: Management of Care; **Cognitive Level:** Analysis [Analyzing]

## 219. MoC ANSWER: 4

1. There usually is not a large blood loss from a hand injury.
2. A urinal should be provided for the client to void.
3. A level may be drawn; however, alcohol is metabolized at a constant rate of approximately one drink (or 12 oz. beer) per hour.
4. **There is a strong risk of infection with *Clostridium tetani*. The spores are present in soil, garden mold, and manure, and enter the body through a traumatic or suppurative wound. Tetanus immune globulin is recommended when the client's history of tetanus immunization is not known.**

▶ *Test-taking Tip:* Focus on the situation and note the key words "hand injury," "barn," and "most important." Select Option 4 using knowledge of infectious diseases.

Content Area: Management of Care; **Concept:** Infection; Management; **Integrated Processes:** Nursing Process: Assessment; **Client Needs:** Safe and Effective Care Environment: Management of Care; Safe and Effective Care Environment: Safety and Infection Control; **Cognitive Level:** Analysis [Analyzing]

### 220. MoC ANSWER: 3

1. The charge nurse is responding, but then either the nurse or the charge nurse would need to leave the room to obtain needed medication, causing a loss of time in treating the client's pain.
2. The nurse leaves the room but should have stayed, as the client is in distress.
3. **Because the client is in distress, the nurse should stay with the client, apply oxygen, and obtain help from other members of the health care team.**
4. The code system should only be activated if the client's pulse or respirations are absent because activation will bring members from multiple departments. Some facilities have an ART, which has a different composition of personnel who can respond in emergency situations.

▶ **Test-taking Tip:** Read each option carefully and systematically. Eliminate any options that allow the nurse to leave the room. Use the ABC's to establish the priority intervention for the nurse.

Content Area: Management of Care; **Concept:** Collaboration; Management; **Integrated Processes:** Nursing Process: Implementation; **Client Needs:** Safe and Effective Care Environment: Management of Care; **Cognitive Level:** Application [Applying]

### 221. MoC ANSWER: 1, 2, 3

1. **The nurse should instruct the nurse in appropriate care, which includes applying direct lateral pressure to the client's nose for 5 minutes.**
2. **The nurse should instruct the nurse in appropriate care, which includes applying ice or cool compresses to constrict vessels and control bleeding.**
3. **The nurse should instruct the nurse in appropriate care, which includes instructing the client not to blow the nose to prevent another episode of epistaxis.**
4. Universal and not contact precautions should be used with this client; the nurse working on another unit should already have this knowledge.
5. The client should be positioned upright and not lying laterally.

▶ **Test-taking Tip:** When delegating and supervising care, it is important to determine the knowledge and abilities of the delegate. If the delegate lacks knowledge of how to care for the client, the supervising nurse should inform the nurse of the appropriate care. Thus you should be selecting interventions appropriate for the client with epistaxis.

Content Area: Management of Care; **Concept:** Management; **Integrated Processes:** Nursing Process: Implementation; **Client Needs:** Safe and Effective Care Environment: Management of Care; Safe and Effective Care Environment: Safety and Infection Control; **Cognitive Level:** Application [Applying]

### 222. MoC ANSWER: 2

1. Placing the client on the bedpan does not have priority; membrane rupture should first be determined.
2. **The nurse's priority should be to assess the perineum to determine if rupture of the membranes has occurred. A nitrazine strip test can be done to check fluid leaking from the vaginal introitus, but contamination of the strip with urine could result in false-positive test results.**
3. Changing the gown and linens should be done after ruling out ruptured membranes.
4. Although breathing may be helpful during contractions, the woman is already in the active phase of labor, and typically breathing techniques are addressed in the latent phase.

▶ **Test-taking Tip:** Focus on the phase of the labor. Use the nursing process; assessment should be first.

Content Area: Management of Care; **Concept:** Assessment; Critical Thinking; **Integrated Processes:** Nursing Process: Assessment; **Client Needs:** Safe and Effective Care Environment: Management of Care; **Cognitive Level:** Application [Applying]

### 223. MoC PHARM ANSWER: 3

1. Only after stopping the infusion and reassessing FHT should the nurse notify the HCP.
2. Only after stopping the infusion should the nurse reassess the FHT.
3. **Because oxytocin (Pitocin) stimulates contractions, the nurse should first stop the infusion. A contraction that occurs more frequently than every 2 minutes and has a prolonged duration suggests hyperstimulation and approaching tetany. This could lead to uterine rupture.**
4. Terbutaline sulfate (Brethine), a beta-adrenergic receptor medication, stops the hyperstimulation and may be ordered to decrease myometrial activity, but this requires a call to the HCP.

▶ **Test-taking Tip:** Note that all options suggest an unsafe situation; this should cue you to the correct option.

Content Area: Management of Care; **Concept:** Pregnancy; Management; **Integrated Processes:** Nursing Process: Implementation; **Client Needs:** Safe and Effective Care Environment: Management of Care; Physiological Integrity: Pharmacological and Parenteral Therapies; **Cognitive Level:** Analysis [Analyzing]

### 224. MoC ANSWER: 1

1. **Because uterine atony is the most frequent cause of postpartum hemorrhage, initial management is fundal massage.**
2. If the uterus does not remain contracted with fundal massage, the primary HCP should be notified.
3. Although a dilute IV infusion of oxytocin helps the uterus maintain tone, the fundus should be first massaged because the infusion may not be necessary.

4. There is no indication that the client has a full bladder; the concern is heavy bleeding. The bladder should be kept empty to prevent a full bladder from pushing an uncontracted uterus into an even more uncontracted state.

▸ *Test-taking Tip: The key word is "initially." Because the client is hemorrhaging, use the ABC's (airway, breathing, circulation) to identify the correct option to control bleeding.*

Content Area: Management of Care; **Concept:** Pregnancy; Management; **Integrated Processes:** Nursing Process: Implementation; **Client Needs:** Safe and Effective Care Environment: Management of Care; **Cognitive Level:** Analysis [Analyzing]

## 225. MoC **ANSWER: 2**

1. Checking the perineum for edema is assessment and cannot be delegated to the NA.
2. **The NA is able to assist the client with hygiene and should be aware of safety and comfort concerns with a sitz bath.**
3. Evaluation is a component of the nursing process and cannot be delegated to the NA.
4. Teaching is an RN responsibility and cannot be delegated to the NA.

▸ *Test-taking Tip: Consider the role of the NA and the aspects of care in the options that do not involve assessment, teaching, or evaluation.*

Content Area: Management of Care; **Concept:** Management; Regulations; **Integrated Processes:** Nursing Process: Implementation; Caring; **Client Needs:** Safe and Effective Care Environment: Management of Care; **Cognitive Level:** Application [Applying]

## 226. MoC **ANSWER: 3**

1. Observing a skill and providing feedback indicate appropriate evaluation of the UAP's skill prior to delegation.
2. Hygienic care is a responsibility that can be safely delegated to ancillary staff.
3. **The scope of practice for ancillary staff does not include assessment. Assessing the umbilical cord is not a responsibility that the RN can delegate to the ancillary staff.**
4. Postmortem care is a responsibility that can be safely delegated to ancillary staff.

▸ *Test-taking Tip: The key phrase "needs further education" indicates that this is a false-response item. Select the option that indicates incorrect delegation. Assessment, planning, evaluation, or teaching are responsibilities that the RN cannot delegate.*

Content Area: Management of Care; **Concept:** Management; Regulations; **Integrated Processes:** Nursing Process: Evaluation; **Client Needs:** Safe and Effective Care Environment: Management of Care; **Cognitive Level:** Evaluation [Evaluating]

## 227. MoC **ANSWER: 3**

1. Knowing how many times the assistant has performed the task previously does not tell the nurse about the assistant's actual abilities in bottle feeding.

2. Knowing the length of time the NA worked in the nursery does not tell the nurse about the assistant's actual abilities in bottle feeding.
3. **Asking open-ended questions about the specific task to be delegated will help the nurse to determine if the NA has the knowledge to perform the assigned task.**
4. Knowing the number of children the assistant has would not necessarily provide any information about the assistant's ability to bottle-feed a newborn.

▸ *Test-taking Tip: Review each option individually, and select the option that would provide the most information about the specific activity to be delegated.*

Content Area: Management of Care; **Concept:** Communication; Management; **Integrated Processes:** Nursing Process: Evaluation; Communication and Documentation; **Client Needs:** Safe and Effective Care Environment: Management of Care; **Cognitive Level:** Evaluation [Evaluating]

## 228. MoC **ANSWER: 1**

1. **A full bladder causes displacement of the fundus to the right. Having the LPN assist the client to the bathroom will help promote elimination and is appropriate delegation. A full bladder is a concern because the bladder of a postpartum client rapidly fills as the body attempts to rid itself of the extra fluid volume returned from the uteroplacental circulation and from any IV fluids administered. There is also a decreased sensation to void and decreased bladder tone caused by the trauma to the urethra and bladder during childbirth.**
2. Vigorous massaging can cause unnecessary discomfort.
3. Oxytocin (Pitocin) should only be initiated if the uterus becomes boggy and is unable to contract.
4. Obtaining the vital signs will only delay emptying a full bladder.

▸ *Test-taking Tip: Focus on the location of the uterus and possible causes to select the option. Note that three options pertain to the fundus and that one option is different; often the option that is different is the answer.*

Content Area: Management of Care; **Concept:** Pregnancy; Regulations; **Integrated Processes:** Communication and Documentation; **Client Needs:** Safe and Effective Care Environment: Management of Care; **Cognitive Level:** Application [Applying]

## 229. MoC **ANSWER: 2**

1. Shivering is not a response to a full bladder, so a bedpan is unnecessary.
2. **A heated bath blanket next to the client and a warm drink help alleviate the shivering; this is the best response. Shivering is common in the fourth stage of labor and is thought to be caused by exhaustion, a difference in internal and external body temperatures, or a reaction to the fetal cells that have entered the maternal circulation at the placental site.**

3. BP should already be monitored every 15 minutes for the first 1 to 2 hours, along with fundal checks.

4. Chlorpromazine (Thorazine) is used to control shivering, but it is not used in the fourth stage of labor.

▶ **Test-taking Tip:** *The key words are "best response." Think about the role of the NA and tasks that can be delegated.*

**Content Area:** Management of Care; **Concept:** Pregnancy; Regulations; Management; **Integrated Processes:** Communication and Documentation; **Client Needs:** Safe and Effective Care Environment: Management of Care; Physiological Integrity: Basic Care and Comfort; **Cognitive Level:** Application [Applying]

**230. MoC ANSWER: 1**

1. **Assessment is the initial step in the nursing process and should be performed by the nurse before decisions are made about necessary interventions. Normal serum glucose for an infant less than 1 day old is 40 to 60 mg/dL.**

2. After the respiratory and VS assessment is completed, the nurse can determine if the infant should be fed immediately.

3. After the respiratory and VS assessment is completed, the nurse can determine if there is a need to recheck the blood sugar.

4. If the respiratory and VS assessment reveals that the infant is unable to feed, then IV glucose may be needed.

▶ **Test-taking Tip:** *Apply the steps of the nursing process. The assessment should be completed unless initial observations suggest a life-threatening condition.*

**Content Area:** Management of Care; **Concept:** Assessment; Management; **Integrated Processes:** Nursing Process: Planning; **Client Needs:** Safe and Effective Care Environment: Management of Care; **Cognitive Level:** Analysis [Analyzing]

**231. MoC ANSWER: 4, 3, 1, 2**

4. **The 2-year-old client whose temperature has risen to 103.8°F (39.9°C) should have priority. This child should be assessed first because the child's situation is the most life-threatening.**

3. **The 5-year-old client with an infected leg wound who is scheduled for a dressing change should be next. Delaying the dressing change increases the risk of sepsis.**

1. **The 13-year-old client waiting to be admitted from the ED after receiving stitches for facial lacerations from a dog bite is next. The child should still be monitored while in the emergency room, and it is appropriate to delay admission to the unit if other interventions are priority.**

2. **The 9-year-old client whose mother is present to receive teaching about wound care for her child's left leg skin graft in anticipation of discharge tomorrow is the last client. The client is being discharged tomorrow, which means that the wound care teaching, although important, can be delayed.**

▶ **Test-taking Tip:** *Immediate physiological needs should be attended to first.*

**Content Area:** Management of Care; **Concept:** Nursing Roles; Management; **Integrated Processes:** Nursing Process: Planning; **Client Needs:** Safe and Effective Care Environment: Management of Care; **Cognitive Level:** Synthesis [Creating]

**232. MoC ANSWER: 1, 2, 4**

1. **The tasks that the PCA could assume include transporting clients.**

2. **The tasks that the PCA could assume would include supporting a woman's breathing techniques.**

3. Sterile procedures, such as a catheterization, should be performed only by the nurse because of the risk to both the woman and the fetus.

4. **The tasks that the PCA could assume include removing meal trays and documenting percent eaten and total intake.**

5. In some facilities, only RNs are able to double-check blood products for transfusion.

6. Complex abilities that have high potential for error should be performed by licensed personnel, such as RNs or LPNs. Some clients may be on medicated infusions, and there is high potential for error if the PCA is also clearing these pumps of the volume infused.

▶ **Test-taking Tip:** *Eliminate complex abilities that require a high level of critical thinking and analysis of information and thus have a high potential for error.*

**Content Area:** Management of Care; **Concept:** Management; Regulations; **Integrated Processes:** Nursing Process: Planning; **Client Needs:** Safe and Effective Care Environment: Management of Care; **Cognitive Level:** Application [Applying]

**233. MoC ANSWER: 2**

1. Treating the child's cough is important for the child's comfort, but it is of lesser importance than treating pain.

2. **The nurse should administer the analgesic first. This child will be undergoing a débridement in 45 minutes. The medication, given orally, will take approximately 30 to 45 minutes for analgesic effects to occur.**

3. The IV antibiotic can be given after the pain medication because there is a half-hour window for medication administration.

4. Although giving acetaminophen does not have priority, it should be administered in a timely manner.

▶ **Test-taking Tip:** *Identify the child most at risk for negative outcomes if the medication is not given in a timely manner.*

**Content Area:** Management of Care; **Concept:** Critical Thinking; Management; **Integrated Processes:** Nursing Process: Planning; **Client Needs:** Safe and Effective Care Environment: Management of Care; **Cognitive Level:** Analysis [Analyzing]

**234.** MoC **ANSWER: 240**

One milliliter of urine output equals 1 g of body weight. First add the total weight of each diaper: 45 + 40 + 50 = 135. Next determine the dry diaper weight for 3 diapers: 15 × 3 = 45. Finally, subtract the dry weight from the total weight of the diapers to determine the total urine output for 8 hours: 135 − 45 = 90. The 90 g of fluid loss equals 90 mL of urine output. Next, add the urine output and the output from the emesis and diarrhea: 90 + 100 + 50 = 240 mL.

▶ *Test-taking Tip: Use the equivalent of 1 mL of urine output equals 1 g of body weight to calculate the amount of urine output.*

**Content Area:** Management of Care; **Concept:** Urinary Elimination; Nursing Roles; **Integrated Processes:** Communication and Documentation; **Client Needs:** Safe and Effective Care Environment: Management of Care; **Cognitive Level:** Application [Applying]

**235.** CJ MoC **ANSWER: 2**

1. Interventions are correct. Insulin aspart should be administered 5 to 15 minutes before a meal. The glucose level of 140 mg/dL is elevated above the expected range of 70-110 mg/dL.
2. **The nurse provided incorrect interventions because the client's serum potassium level of 4.9 mEq/L is WNL of 3.5–5.3 mEq/L. The nurse incorrectly selected the potassium replacement from the protocol.**
3. Interventions were correctly performed. An oxygen saturation at 89% is below the expected range of 92–100%; oxygen administration is an appropriate intervention.
4. Interventions are correct. Although the client has a low BP, the mean arterial pressure (MAP) is adequate to support administration of morphine sulfate (MAP is [(96 + 50 +50) ÷ 3] = 65.3). A MAP of greater than 65 indicates adequate perfusion.

▶ *Test-taking Tip: To answer this question, you need to determine if the intervention is appropriate based on the assessment information. The normal serum potassium level is 3.5–5.3 mEq/L.*

**Content Area:** Management of Care; **Concept:** Nursing Roles; Safety; Regulations; **Integrated Processes:** Nursing Process: Evaluation; **Client Needs:** Safe and Effective Care Environment: Management of Care; **Cognitive Level:** Analysis [Analyzing]

**236.** CJ MoC **ANSWER:**

The serum magnesium of 1.1 mg/dL is low (normal: 1.7–2.2 mg/dL). The nurse should have selected replacing magnesium from the protocol. If the magnesium was not on the protocol, the nurse should have telephoned the results to the HCP.

▶ *Test-taking Tip: To answer this question, you need to determine the appropriate intervention based on the assessment information. The normal serum magnesium level is 1.7–2.2 mg/dL.*

**Content Area:** Management of Care; **Concept:** Nursing Roles; Safety; Regulations; **Integrated Processes:** Nursing Process: Evaluation; **Client Needs:** Safe and Effective Care Environment: Management of Care; **Cognitive Level:** Analysis [Analyzing]

**237.** MoC **ANSWER: 1**

1. **The nurse should direct the NA to post a contact isolation sign for the client with MRSA. It is appropriate to use either soap and water or an alcohol-based hand sanitizer when entering and leaving the room.**
2. The droplet precaution sign is appropriate for airborne diseases, not MRSA.
3. The airborne precaution sign is designated for negative pressure rooms such as for the client with tuberculosis, not MRSA.
4. The enteric precautions sign is appropriate for the client with *Clostridium difficile*, not MRSA. Only soap and water should be used for hand washing. Alcohol-based hand sanitizers should not be used.

▶ *Test-taking Tip: MRSA is the leading cause of skin and soft tissue infections. Use this information to eliminate options pertaining to the respiratory and GI system.*

**Content Area:** Management of Care; **Concept:** Nursing Roles; Management; Regulations; **Integrated Processes:** Nursing Process: Implementation; **Client Needs:** Safe and Effective Care Environment: Management of Care; Safe and Effective Care Environment: Safety and Infection Control; **Cognitive Level:** Knowledge [Remembering]

**238.** MoC **ANSWER: 4**

1. Because the HR is near the normal range, an immediate reassessment of the infant is unnecessary.
2. Notifying the HCP is premature; further information needs to be collected. The HCP would not be notified if findings are normal.
3. Infants rarely have hereditary cardiac problems; cardiovascular diseases commonly seen in adults are atypical of this young age group.
4. **The first action is to compare the value both to the norms for the infant's age group and to the infant's previous readings. A normal HR for an infant 1 to 11 months is 80 to 160 bpm. Environmental changes and stressors can cause temporary increases in HR.**

▶ *Test-taking Tip: Use the nursing process to narrow the options to those pertaining to assessment. Then focus on the term "evaluating" in the stem and on an action that would evaluate the significance of the HR.*

**Content Area:** Management of Care; **Concept:** Assessment; Management; **Integrated Processes:** Nursing Process: Assessment; **Client Needs:** Safe and Effective Care Environment: Management of Care; Health Promotion and Maintenance; **Cognitive Level:** Analysis [Analyzing]

**239. MoC ANSWER: 4**

1. The RN should be communicating with HCPs. In most health care facilities, only RNs can accept HCP verbal orders.
2. Assessment of the child, including pupils, is the responsibility of the RN and should not be delegated. The LPN would not have a frame of reference for the normal size of a 2-year-old child's pupils.
3. Although the LPN may be experienced on an oncology unit, the LPN may not have the experience of administering a suppository to the 2-year-old child, which would include the use of a smaller finger and shorter depth, and the RN would not have the time to assess the LPN's ability.
4. **Measures should be taken to lower the child's temperature, including removing extra blankets and clothing; this can be appropriately delegated to this LPN.**

▶ *Test-taking Tip: Focus on the child's health problem, the unit where the LPN usually works, and the immediacy of the situation to determine appropriate delegation.*

Content Area: Management of Care; Concept: Management; Regulations; Integrated Processes: Nursing Process: Planning; Client Needs: Safe and Effective Care Environment: Management of Care; Physiological Integrity: Basic Care and Comfort; Cognitive Level: Analysis [Analyzing]

**240. MoC ANSWER: 1, 3**

1. **The new nurse may be assigned to older children who have stable conditions.**
2. Although tracheostomy care may be a routine skill, a more experienced nurse should perform this care due to the age of the child.
3. **An elevated temperature would be expected following a ruptured appendix. This client would have routine care needs and can be assigned to the new graduate nurse.**
4. The child with a new diagnosis of leukemia should have an experienced nurse because the parents will likely have multiple questions, and a comprehensive admission assessment will be required.
5. A blood transfusion has a high potential for error and should be performed by an experienced nurse.

▶ *Test-taking Tip: When a new nurse is at an early point in orientation, the new nurse should be assigned to clients who are stable and have routine care needs.*

Content Area: Management of Care; Concept: Management; Regulations; Integrated Processes: Nursing Process: Planning; Client Needs: Safe and Effective Care Environment: Management of Care; Cognitive Level: Application [Applying]

**241. MoC ANSWER: 4**

1. Percent of burn injury would be determined with the overall assessment.
2. Pain medications should be administered as soon as the toddler's pain level is determined and would be the next priority.
3. Blisters should be left intact, not opened. After the blister has burst, only devitalized tissues would be débrided.
4. **The first priority is to stop the burning process and relieve the pain. Cool compresses will accomplish both. Epidural burns, such as sunburns, are painful.**

▶ *Test-taking Tip: The main priority is to stop the burning process and relieve the pain. You should consider what action would be the fastest.*

Content Area: Management of Care; Concept: Comfort; Management; Integrated Processes: Nursing Process: Implementation; Client Needs: Safe and Effective Care Environment: Management of Care; Cognitive Level: Application [Applying]

**242. MoC ANSWER: 3, 2, 4, 1**

3. **Client is responsive, but based on previous documentation is less responsive; this finding should be the first for follow-up because a change in level of consciousness can be due to hypoxia, hypoglycemia, hypovolemia, abnormal lab values, and other conditions.**
2. **Blood noted at an abdominal wound site is the second priority. The amount needs to be determined because it could potentially put the child at risk for hypovolemia.**
4. **Urinary output is less than 30 mL in the last 2 hours should be followed up next. Urine output should be 0.5 to 1 mL/kg/hr or 20 to 40 mL/hr (88 lb/2.2 kg/lb = 40 kg). Low urine output could result from inadequate fluids or blood loss.**
1. **The client states, "I was given pain medication in the ambulance." The nurse should follow up to determine when the pain medication was last given, but if the client is comfortable, this can be followed up after addressing the other findings that are more critical.**

▶ *Test-taking Tip: You need to consider from a physiological perspective the potential complications that would be most critical for this adolescent.*

Content Area: Management of Care; Concept: Critical Thinking; Management; Integrated Processes: Nursing Process: Planning; Client Needs: Safe and Effective Care Environment: Management of Care; Cognitive Level: Synthesis [Creating]

**243. MoC ANSWER: 4**

1. Notifying the HCP is premature because additional assessment information is needed.
2. A BP should be taken after obtaining the oxygen saturation level.
3. Oxygen is being delivered into the tent. Removal decreases oxygen delivery.
4. **The increased respiratory rate and HR could be signs of progressive airway obstruction. The RN should stay with the toddler to assess the respiratory status and ask the PCA to retrieve an oximeter to determine the saturation level and degree of respiratory impairment.**

## 244. MoC ANSWER: 4

1. Lotions, powders, and soaps are avoided on target skin areas during radiation treatments but can be used on dry skin while receiving chemotherapy.
2. Despite the child's immune system being depressed, a freshly laundered hat would not increase the risk for infection.
3. Toothpaste can be used unless it causes discomfort.
4. **Even though nystatin (Mycostatin) is an oral suspension applied to the mouth after oral care, medication administration is not within the scope of practice of the NA. The medication should not be left at the client's bedside even if oral care has not yet been performed.**

▸ **Test-taking Tip:** Focus on the scope of practice of the NA to select the correct option.

**Content Area:** Management of Care; **Concept:** Management; Medication; Regulations; **Integrated Processes:** Nursing Process: Evaluation; **Client Needs:** Safe and Effective Care Environment: Management of Care; Physiological Integrity: Basic Care and Comfort; **Cognitive Level:** Evaluation [Evaluating]

## 245. MoC ANSWER: 3

1. Cyanosis is expected in a child with tetralogy of Fallot. Although it is important to assess the client soon, this child is not the nurse's priority.
2. The child's knee pain should be evaluated as soon as possible, but this child is not the nurse's priority.
3. **Because bilateral crackles in a child with endocarditis indicate a complication, this child should be the nurse's priority.**
4. The child with an elevated temperature is stable. Although the child's temperature should be closely monitored, the child does not require immediate attention.

▸ **Test-taking Tip:** Use the ABC's (airway, breathing, circulation) to establish priority and select the child that needs immediate airway protection, especially with crackles bilaterally.

**Content Area:** Management of Care; **Concept:** Critical Thinking; Management; **Integrated Processes:** Nursing Process: Planning; **Client Needs:** Safe and Effective Care Environment: Management of Care; Physiological Integrity: Basic Care and Comfort; **Cognitive Level:** Analysis [Analyzing]

## 246. MoC ANSWER: 3

1. It is not within the LPN's scope of practice to administer chemotherapy.
2. It is not within the LPN's scope of practice to administer blood products.

3. **The nurse should delegate the care of the client with loose stools because the client is most stable of the options, and skin and toilet care is within the LPN's scope of practice.**
4. The client who is lethargic requires assessment and frequent monitoring, so it would not be appropriate to delegate the client's care to the LPN.

▸ **Test-taking Tip:** Focus on the tasks of delegation. The LPN should have the knowledge and skills to care for the client within the LPN's scope of practice. Focus on the least complex client.

**Content Area:** Management of Care; **Concept:** Management; Regulations; **Integrated Processes:** Nursing Process: Implementation; **Client Needs:** Safe and Effective Care Environment: Management of Care; **Cognitive Level:** Application [Applying]

## 247. MoC ANSWER: 3

1. Monitoring the client's temperature hourly is unnecessary; the nurse should discuss this with the LPN soon, but this does not require immediate intervention.
2. Although infection control is important in sickle cell crisis, there is no need for contact isolation precautions; the nurse should discuss this with the LPN soon, but this does not require immediate intervention.
3. **Applying cold packs to the client's knees is most concerning and requires immediate intervention and removal of the packs. Pain in sickle cell crisis is caused from obstruction of blood flow by sickled RBCs. Cold packs would further decrease blood flow to the client's knees and increase sickling.**
4. The NA can be directed by the LPN to take vital signs. The LPN is not delegating because this is usually included in the NA's assignment and job responsibility.

▸ **Test-taking Tip:** The key phrase "most concerning" suggests that more than one option is correct but that one is more concerning than the others. Safety has priority.

**Content Area:** Management of Care; **Concept:** Management; Safety; **Integrated Processes:** Nursing Process: Implementation; Physiological Integrity: Basic Care and Comfort; **Client Needs:** Safe and Effective Care Environment: Management of Care; **Cognitive Level:** Analysis [Analyzing]

## 248. MoC ANSWER: 3, 2, 4, 1

3. **The 5-year-old who is newly admitted with pharyngitis and drooling should be the first to be assessed. These are symptoms of epiglottitis and a medical emergency.**
2. **The 6-year-old 1 day postoperative appendectomy with a temperature of 102.2°F (39°C) should be the second client to be assessed. An elevated temperature suggests an infection. Additional information should be obtained to R/O developing sepsis.**

4. **The 2-year-old admitted with diarrhea who had three loose stools on the previous shift should be the third child to be assessed. Additional information should be obtained to rule out fluid and electrolyte imbalances.**

1. **The 14-year-old with a UTI who reports urinary burning at a 2 on a 0 to 10 pain scale should be assessed last. Additional information needs to be obtained to determine if treatment is effective. The pain rating of a 2 may be at an acceptable level for the client.**

▶ *Test-taking Tip: Use the ABC's (airway, breathing, circulation) to establish priority and select the client who needs immediate airway protection as the first client to be assessed. The client who does not have a potential life-threatening problem should be assessed last.*

Content Area: Management of Care; Concept: Critical Thinking; Management; Integrated Processes: Nursing Process: Planning; Client Needs: Safe and Effective Care Environment: Management of Care; Cognitive Level: Synthesis [Creating]

## 249. MoC ANSWER: 2

1. Implementing restraints involves evaluation of client behaviors and should not be delegated.

2. **Accompanying clients to off-site treatments is within the scope of practice for the UAP and is appropriate delegation. This involves a noninvasive action.**

3. Explaining unit requirements is within the RN scope of practice and should not be delegated.

4. Evaluation of a skill being performed by the client requires clinical judgment and is within the RN scope of practice.

▶ *Test-taking Tip: Look at the verb in each of the options: implement, accompany, explain, and evaluate, respectively. Select the option that would require the least amount of critical thinking.*

Content Area: Management of Care; Concept: Management; Regulations; Integrated Processes: Nursing Process: Planning; Client Needs: Safe and Effective Care Environment: Management of Care; Psychosocial Integrity; Cognitive Level: Application [Applying]

## 250. MoC ANSWER: 2

1. Assessing the level of consciousness is a nursing responsibility that may not be delegated.

2. **Asking the UAP to observe the client's behavior and report any changes is appropriate.**

3. Being present when the client eats or drinks for the first time after the treatment is not a task that the nurse should delegate because the client is at risk for aspiration due to an absent gag reflex.

4. Informing the family about a temporary memory loss involves teaching and answering the family's questions and should not be delegated.

▶ *Test-taking Tip: Although all of the options are appropriate when implementing post-ECT care, the nurse should only delegate care that is noninvasive and does not require nursing judgment. The five rights of delegation include the right situation. Ask yourself if assisting the client to eat after ECT is the right situation for delegation.*

Content Area: Management of Care; Concept: Management; Regulations; Integrated Processes: Nursing Process: Planning; Client Needs: Safe and Effective Care Environment: Management of Care; Cognitive Level: Application [Applying]

## 251. MoC ANSWER: 4

1. Facilitating smoking breaks does not involve clinical judgment and can be delegated to ancillary staff.

2. Accompanying the client to an off-site appointment is appropriate delegation. The RN should have already evaluated whether this client is stable.

3. Observing the client involves appropriate delegation.

4. **The scope of practice for ancillary staff does not include evaluation of client status/condition/ behavior. Determining whether the removal of physical restraints is appropriate is not within the scope of ancillary staff.**

▶ *Test-taking Tip: Focus on the information presented in the item's stem and in the options. You should eliminate actions that are physically invasive or that involve client assessment, planning, evaluation, or teaching.*

Content Area: Management of Care; Concept: Management; Regulations; Integrated Processes: Nursing Process: Planning; Client Needs: Safe and Effective Care Environment: Management of Care; Psychosocial Integrity; Cognitive Level: Application [Applying]

## 252. MoC ANSWER: 2

1. Assisting with basic cares, such as toileting, is an appropriate action to delegate.

2. **The scope of practice for ancillary staff does not include the management of client care. Discussing the client's diagnostic needs is not a responsibility that the RN can delegate to the ancillary staff.**

3. Ambulation is an appropriate action to delegate; this does not involve clinical judgment because the client is stable.

4. Assisting to reorient the client is an appropriate action to delegate; this does not involve clinical judgment.

▶ *Test-taking Tip: The key word in the stem is "inappropriately." You should eliminate options of appropriate delegation to unlicensed ancillary staff to narrow the options.*

Content Area: Management of Care; Concept: Management; Regulations; Integrated Processes: Nursing Process: Planning; Client Needs: Safe and Effective Care Environment: Management of Care; Psychosocial Integrity; Cognitive Level: Application [Applying]

## 253. MoC ANSWER: 1

1. **The client with OCD who has ritualistic behavior may find storing belongings stressful if not done in a particular manner. Facilitating the client in storing belongings in a fashion that does not produce stress is an intervention that the RN can delegate to the ancillary staff.**

2. Although the ancillary staff could obtain contact information from the client, Option 1 is best to delegate because the nurse may need additional information from the client, or the client may have questions.

3. Providing the unit rules involves teaching; this should not be delegated.

4. Communicating with the client about seeking someone to talk with when anxious, excited, or out of control involves teaching and should not be delegated.

▶ *Test-taking Tip: Focus on the tasks presented in the options. Note that Options 2, 3, and 4 involve communicating with the client, whereas Option 1 is different in that it involves helping the client.*

**Content Area:** Management of Care; **Concept:** Management; Regulations; **Integrated Processes:** Nursing Process: Planning; **Client Needs:** Safe and Effective Care Environment: Management of Care; Psychosocial Integrity; **Cognitive Level:** Application [Applying]

**254.** MoC **ANSWER: 4**

1. The average age of members may affect the client's comfort with the group, but it is not the initial consideration.

2. This statement reflects a consideration that may affect the client's comfort with the group as well as its management of clients, but it is not the initial consideration.

3. This statement reflects a consideration that may affect the client's comfort with the group and ultimate attendance, but it is not the initial consideration.

4. **A group that has clients who are similar is more likely to promote positive adaptive responses among its clients.**

▶ *Test-taking Tip: Use your understanding of the goals of a self-help group and the variables that naturally exist between similar group members.*

**Content Area:** Management of Care; **Concept:** Nursing Roles; **Integrated Processes:** Nursing Process: Planning; **Client Needs:** Safe and Effective Care Environment: Management of Care; Psychosocial Integrity; **Cognitive Level:** Analysis [Analyzing]

**255.** MoC **ANSWER: 4**

1. This statement reflects an outcome of crisis intervention, but it is not the initial goal of crisis intervention.

2. This statement reflects an understanding of the role of stress in the development and management of depression, but it is not the initial goal of crisis intervention.

3. This statement reflects an understanding of the role medication compliance plays in the prevention of relapse, but it is not the initial goal of crisis intervention.

4. **The priority goal for crisis intervention should be the client's return to a precrisis level of functioning.**

▶ *Test-taking Tip: Focus on the information presented in the item's stem while noting the key word "priority." Use your understanding of crisis intervention, focusing on the goal and being able to identify outcomes as well as teaching topics.*

**Content Area:** Management of Care; **Concept:** Stress; Management; **Integrated Processes:** Nursing Process: Evaluation; **Client Needs:** Safe and Effective Care Environment: Management of Care; Psychosocial Integrity; **Cognitive Level:** Evaluation [Evaluating]

**256.** MoC **ANSWER: 1**

1. **Arranging for appropriate alternative child care would be considered the initial intervention. This is changing environmental factors, which is the first level of crisis intervention.**

2. One-on-one nurse-client time reflects an intervention that is more appropriately implemented during Level 2 (General Support).

3. A self-help group reflects an intervention that is more appropriately implemented during Level 4 (Individual Approach).

4. Identifying stressors reflects an intervention that is more appropriately implemented during Level 3 (Generic Approach).

▶ *Test-taking Tip: There are four levels of crisis intervention: environmental manipulation, general support, generic approach, and individual approach.*

**Content Area:** Management of Care; **Concept:** Mood; Management; **Integrated Processes:** Nursing Process: Implementation; **Client Needs:** Safe and Effective Care Environment: Management of Care; Psychosocial Integrity; **Cognitive Level:** Analysis [Analyzing]

**257.** MoC **ANSWER: 4**

1. Applying restraints may cause an overreaction; less-invasive methods should be implemented first.

2. Administering tranquilizers should be implemented as a last resort when other less-invasive interventions have proved ineffective.

3. Monitoring the client should be implemented after steps have been taken to ensure the client's safety through manipulation of stimuli and removal of hazardous objects.

4. **The client is in a highly distractible state and is likely to overreact to even the slightest stimuli. Manipulating the external environment will have the most therapeutic initial impact on the client's hyperactivity.**

▶ *Test-taking Tip: Focus on the information presented in the item's stem while noting the key word "priority." Use your understanding of crisis intervention for the manic client, and note the priority given to manipulation of the environment.*

**Content Area:** Management of Care; **Concept:** Safety; Management; **Integrated Processes:** Nursing Process: Planning; Psychosocial Integrity; **Client Needs:** Safe and Effective Care Environment: Management of Care; **Cognitive Level:** Analysis [Analyzing]

**258.** MoC **ANSWER: 3**

1. The symptoms do not suggest a respiratory problem; giving oxygen when saturations are 94% is unnecessary.
2. Although diaphoresis, palpitations, and tachycardia are symptoms of both hypoglycemia and cardiac problems, the client had taken insulin 2 hours earlier. Treating the low blood sugar first rather than giving aspirin and nitroglycerin will likely resolve the client's symptoms.
3. **Regular insulin (Humulin R) peaks in 2 to 4 hours after administration. The client's symptoms suggest hypoglycemia, so a blood glucose level should be checked and carbohydrates given if low.**
4. Atenolol (Tenormin) should never be given without also knowing the BP.

▶ *Test-taking Tip: When selecting an answer, consider that regular insulin peaks in 2 to 4 hours after administration.*

**Content Area:** Management of Care; **Concept:** Metabolism; Medication; **Integrated Processes:** Nursing Process: Implementation; **Client Needs:** Safe and Effective Care Environment: Management of Care; Physiological Integrity: Physiological Adaptation; **Cognitive Level:** Analysis [Analyzing]

**259.** MoC **ANSWER: 1**

1. **Counting the apical rate for 1 minute and comparing it to the radial rate can help to determine if the child has an irregular or fast or slow heartbeat.**
2. A Holter monitor may be used to help diagnose whether an arrhythmia is occurring but is not the priority.
3. The dysrhythmia may be a bradycardia (slow HR); administering digoxin may slow the heart further.
4. Applying ice may be prescribed if SVT is diagnosed, but this action would not be taken if the dysrhythmia is not known.

▶ *Test-taking Tip: Use the nursing process to answer the question. Assessment should be the priority, and only one option pertains to assessment.*

**Content Area:** Management of Care; Child; **Concept:** Perfusion; **Integrated Processes:** Nursing Process: Implementation; **Client Needs:** Safe and Effective Care Environment: Management of Care; **Cognitive Level:** Application [Applying]

**260.** MoC **ANSWER: 3**

1. Assessing for absence of urine is important but is not the first consideration.
2. Hypertension may occur due to loss of kidney function but is not the first consideration.
3. **Following renal trauma, the client is at risk for internal bleeding. This assessment should be first because the blood supply to the kidney constitutes approximately one-fifth of the total cardiac output.**
4. Electrolyte imbalances can occur due to alteration in kidney function, but this is not the first consideration.

▶ *Test-taking Tip: Use the ABC's to determine which assessment should be made first.*

**Content Area:** Management of Care; Child; **Concept:** Urinary Elimination; Perfusion; Assessment; **Integrated Processes:** Nursing Process: Implementation; **Client Needs:** Safe and Effective Care Environment: Management of Care; **Cognitive Level:** Application [Applying]

## Chapter Eight

# Communication and Teaching and Learning

**261.** The nurse is establishing a therapeutic nurse-client relationship. In what order will the nurse progress through initiating and ending the therapeutic relationship?

1. Termination phase
2. Working phase
3. Preinteraction phase
4. Conclusion of relationship
5. Orientation phase

Answer: _____

**262.** While collecting information from the 16-year-old who is in the first trimester of pregnancy, the nurse learns that the client drinks four to six alcoholic beverages three to four times a week. Based on the client's current developmental stage, what should be the nurse's **initial** focus of care?

1. Establish a trusting relationship with the client.
2. Educate the client about the risk for developing fetal alcohol syndrome (FAS).
3. Inform the client about the personal health risks of continuing with excessive drinking.
4. Seek clarification about her home life and the friends with whom she spends time.

**263.** **MoC** The adult client is being transferred from a hospital to a rehabilitation facility. Which information should the nurse include in the transfer note documentation? **Select all that apply.**

1. Reason for the transfer
2. Name of person receiving a verbal report
3. Condition of the client
4. Medication and food allergies
5. Client's ability to pay for expenses

**264.** **MoC** When the nurse is completing the history of the 16-year-old client at a clinic, the client says, "I think that I might be pregnant." What is the nurse's **best** response?

1. "How long have you been sexually active?"
2. "Why do you think you are pregnant?"
3. "Who have you spoken to about this?"
4. "When was your last menstrual cycle?"

**265.** The nurse is to obtain a medical history for the client who has a tracheostomy. The client's spouse states that the client does not use a speaking valve. Which actions should be taken by the nurse to communicate with the client? **Select all that apply.**

1. Make eye contact and speak to the client directly.
2. Ask only the spouse for information about the client.
3. Provide the client with a writing board and pen.
4. Place a speaking valve over the client's tracheostomy.
5. Assess the client's preferred communication method.
6. Ask the client only "yes" and "no" questions.

**266.** The nurse is teaching the client who is hard of hearing and wears bilateral hearing aids. Which action by the nurse would **best** evaluate the teaching on how to change a urinary drainage bag?

1. Have the client demonstrate how to change the bag.
2. Ask during teaching if the client has any questions.
3. Ask the client to state the steps for changing the bag.
4. Provide a handout with instructions of the procedure.

**INSTRUCTIONS:** Refer to the information provided in the table to answer Questions 267 and 268.

**267.** CJ The nurse is having a conversation with the client who is beginning hemodialysis. How many different therapeutic communication techniques does the nurse use in conversing with the client?

| Interaction Number | Interaction |
|---|---|
| 1 | Nurse: "Tell me what I can teach you about your dialysis treatments." <br> Client: "I don't know much about it except what my doctor told me." |
| 2 | Nurse: "Tell me what the doctor told you so I can be more helpful." <br> Client: "Because my kidneys aren't working, I will need dialysis treatments three times weekly." |
| 3 | Nurse: "What will it be like for you going for the treatments?" <br> Client: "I don't know. My husband can't drive anymore with his failing eyesight." |
| 4 | Nurse: "Your husband can't drive anymore because of his failing eyesight?" <br> Client: "That's right." |
| 5 | Nurse: "Oh." *Sits quietly.* <br> Client: "I don't know how I'm going to get to the center for my treatments." |
| 6 | Nurse: "You should have one of your children drive you for treatments. You told me they live nearby." <br> Client: "Both of my children work during the day." |
| 7 | Nurse: "Well, don't worry. I'll have a social worker make transportation arrangements." <br> Client: "You are so kind." |

1. One technique
2. Two techniques
3. Three techniques
4. Four techniques

**268.** CJ Which statement did the nurse make that belittled the client's feeling during the conversation? Briefly state your answer in the box provided.

---

**269.** The clinic nurse is caring for four clients. Which interaction demonstrates the use of the communication technique of reflection?

1. Child: "Don't turn out the light. I don't like the dark." Nurse: "I will have your mommy hold you while I turn out the light to check your eye."
2. Adolescent: "My mom won't let me pierce my tongue." Nurse: "What would it be like to have a pierced tongue?"
3. Adult: "My blood sugar was really out of control yesterday." Nurse: "Was your blood sugar high or low yesterday?"
4. Older Adult: "My life means nothing anymore." Nurse: "Socializing more allows you to reflect back on good times and will help you feel better about your life."

**270.** The nurse is completing the final visit with the client being discharged from home-care services. Each time that the nurse attempts to leave, the client offers a new subject and attempts to delay the nurse's departure. Which is the **best** action by the nurse?

1. Abruptly tell the client that the session has ended and that the nurse must leave.
2. Set up another appointment for an additional home-care visit.
3. Plan to meet the client for coffee at a time that the client would like.
4. Be firm and clear about the relationship terminating and seek feedback from the client.

**271.** An adult daughter is sitting at the bedside of her mother, a devoutly religious person, who developed a serious postoperative infection. Which statement by the nurse to the daughter demonstrates empathy?

1. "I know how you feel. We also prayed at my grandmother's bedside when she was sick."
2. "You've been here a long time and look exhausted. Tell me how things are going for you."
3. "You might as well go home because your mother is sleepy. Maybe tomorrow will go better."
4. "The new antibiotic was started this morning. We will pray that your mother gets well."

**272.** The nurse is setting up supplies to complete a dressing change at 2000 hours on the client's stump following a right leg BKA. The client looks away and angrily says, "I don't want to look at that thing. Can't you come back later?" Which is the nurse's **best** action?

1. Put the supplies away and reattempt the dressing change in 1 hour.
2. Complete the dressing change because it is prescribed for 2000.
3. Ask the client, "Why don't you want your dressing changed now?"
4. Restate, "You don't want to look at your leg?" and allow time for a response.

**273.** The nurse and the client are engaged in a conversation. The client states, "I just learned I might have cancer and I am having surgery tomorrow morning." Which statement made by the nurse best encourages therapeutic communication?

| | |
|---|---|
| 1. | Nurse: "I see. Why are you afraid? Do you think surgery will reveal that you have cancer?"<br>Client: "I am afraid because I don't want to have cancer." |
| 2. | Nurse: "Are you afraid that it might be cancer?"<br>Client: "I guess." |
| 3. | Nurse: "Having a possible diagnosis of cancer is fearful. Tell me more about how you are feeling about this."<br>Client: "I'm afraid I will die. My mother died of cancer when I was 10, and I have a 10-year-old." |
| 4. | Nurse: "This really hits close to you."<br>Client: "Yes. I don't want my 10-year-old to grow up alone." |

1. Response 1
2. Response 2
3. Response 3
4. Response 4

**274.** The hospitalized infant had five wet diapers during an 8-hour period that weighed 22 g, 24 g, 38 g, 34 g, and 21 g. The weight of a dry diaper is 15 g. What amount in milliliters (mL) should the nurse document for the infant's total urine output for the 8 hours?

_____ mL (Record your answer as a whole number.)

**275.** The nurse is caring for the client with Alzheimer's disease who is yelling obscenities at the staff. The client's spouse tearfully states to the nurse, "Never would you have heard those things before the Alzheimer's. I wish that you would have known my spouse before the sickness." Which is the **best** response by the nurse?

1. "Why do you think that your spouse is acting like this?"
2. "How long has your spouse had Alzheimer's disease?"
3. "I can see that it is difficult for you to see your spouse like this."
4. "Tell me about the things your spouse did before the Alzheimer's was diagnosed."

**276.** MoC After falling at home, the 84-year-old client is brought to the ED by the client's adult child. Upon assessing the client, the nurse discovers that the client is aphasic and unable to answer any of the nurse's questions. Which intervention should be taken by the nurse **initially?**

1. Ask the client to nod his or her head "yes" or "no" to questions.
2. Consult a speech therapist.
3. Give the client a writing board.
4. Direct questions to the client's adult child.

**277.** The newly hospitalized 90-year-old client has difficulty answering the nurse's questions and reports progressive hearing loss. Which nursing action would **best** aid in communication between the nurse and client?

1. Overexaggerating facial expressions
2. Using simple sentences
3. Overenunciating longer words
4. Speaking quickly in a higher-pitched voice

**278.** MoC The nurse is leading a team to develop an evidence-based practice guideline for preventing skin breakdown in the hospitalized client. To fully use the databases available to the nurse, which should be the nurse's **first** step in the process for developing the guidelines?

1. Critically appraise the resources for their use in clinical decision making.
2. Formulate the issue into a searchable, answerable question.
3. Critically appraise the quantitative and qualitative evidence.
4. Determine the model and strategies for the evidence-based practice.

**279.** MoC The new nurse is told by experienced unit nurses that the nurse manager is an empowering manager. Which statements made by the nurse manager should lead the new nurse to agree with the experienced nurses' opinions? **Select all that apply.**

1. "You hardly ever complete your documentation during work hours. I'll have the charge nurse work on making better assignments for you."
2. "The team worked well together on the pain documentation project. Through your efforts, there were improvements in client satisfaction scores for pain control on client surveys."
3. "Today you were timely in your clients' care, but most days you stay overtime to complete documentation. Is there something we can do to help you complete all duties within the scheduled work time?"
4. "The charge nurse told me that you didn't complete some of your client care today. What was the problem?"
5. "We are at peak census. For the next shift, I need one more nurse than usual. Our options include a volunteer, calling in an off-duty staff, or mandating someone. Is there a volunteer?"
6. "I've arranged for a new staffing schedule because no one working part-time will volunteer for extra shifts and administration won't allow me to pay nurses overtime anymore."

**280.** MoC The RN is discharged for jeopardizing client safety by consistently failing to notify the HCP of changes in clients' health status. Which statement by the nurse manager is most appropriate when another health care facility telephones for a reference check on the RN?

1. "The RN resigned due to safety concerns such as failure to notify the provider when the health status of clients changed."
2. "The RN is uncomfortable communicating with providers. Otherwise, the nurse's work meets standards of care."
3. "I need to consult with the hospital attorney to determine if any information can be provided about the nurse previously employed here."
4. "The nurse worked at this facility on the telemetry unit but was discharged after 2 years of employment."

**281.** MoC The nurse is providing a change-of-shift report to the oncoming shift nurse for the client. Besides the client's name and room number, which information should the nurse include in a typical shift report? **Select all that apply.**

1. Brief medical history of the client's current problem
2. Client's satisfaction with the nursing care provided
3. Client-family dynamics and client psychosocial concerns
4. Surgery, tests, or procedures for the next 24 hours
5. The status of tubes and intravenous (IV) infusions
6. The telephone number of the nurse giving report if questions arise

**282.** MoC The nurse is notifying the HCP of the client's change in status using the SBAR format. In which order should the nurse place the statements?

1. "I suggest that the client be transferred to the critical care unit, and I would like you to come evaluate the client."
2. "The client is deteriorating, and I'm afraid the client is going to arrest."
3. "I am calling about {client name and location}. Vital signs are BP=100/50, P=120, RR=30, T=100.4°F (38°C)."
4. "The client is becoming confused and agitated. The skin is pale, mottled, and diaphoretic. The client is very dyspneic with an oxygen saturation of 85% despite placing a nonrebreather mask."

Answer: _____

**283.** MoC The client is scheduled for an MRI scan. Which is **most** important for the nurse to include prior to the client's MRI scan?

1. SBAR-format report to the receiving unit
2. Accurate documentation of the client's vital signs
3. Accurate documentation of the client's intake and output
4. Inclusion of a discharge planning report

**284.** MoC A hospital implemented computerized provider order entry (CPOE). Which additional task related to CPOE is required for the nurse to provide safe care?

1. Checking the computer periodically for new orders
2. Checking the computer every hour for medications due
3. The HCP telephoning the nurse about the new computer orders
4. Documenting blood sugars in the computer for HCP viewing

**285.** MoC The experienced nurse is reviewing a new nurse's documentation in the client's EMR. Which abbreviation should be corrected by the new nurse because it appears on The Joint Commission's published list of "Do Not Use" abbreviations? Place an X on the abbreviation that should be corrected.

| Progress Notes | | |
|---|---|---|
| **Date** | **Time** | **Entry** |
| 6-15-17 | 1600 | At 1530 given M.S., 2.0 mg IV for chest incisional pain rated 5 on a 0 to 10 scale; 30 minutes later pain rated at a 1. Will plan to give analgesic again at H.S. Remains on q6h blood glucose checks for NPO status; covered elevated blood glucose with 2 units regular insulin subcut. at 1800. ———————— J. Peters, RN |

**286.** MoC The nurse hears a thud and, upon entering a room finds the client on the floor beside a wheelchair. Which notations are **most** appropriate for the nurse to make in the client's EMR regarding the incident? **Select all that apply.**

1. The client stated, "I was trying to reach for my water and fell from the wheelchair."
2. The client refused to lock the wheelchair when told to do so.
3. A loud noise was heard from the client's room, and the client was found on the floor.
4. The client stated, "Nothing hurts. I don't think I have any injuries."
5. An incident report has been completed and filed; a copy is in the client's chart.

**287.** MoC The new nurse is working in an agency that uses only narrative documentation. Which entries made by the new nurse in multiple clients' medical records would earn praise from the charge nurse? **Select all that apply.**

1. "Client being difficult, refusing suggestions for improving appetite."
2. "Alert, oriented ×3, responds to verbal stimuli. See assessment flowsheet."
3. "Furosemide 40 mg IV given over 4 minutes through NS maintenance infusion."
4. "On commode to void after first attempting to use the bedpan."
5. "Client up, out of bed, walked down hallway with assistance, tolerated well."

**288.** MoC At 1000, the client states, "I can't get enough air," and the nurse assesses fine crackles in the client's bilateral lung bases. At 1010 the nurse increases the client's oxygen from 2 liters per nasal cannula (NC) to 4 liters per protocol. Which is the **most** appropriate nursing documentation?

1. 1010: Increased oxygen to 4 L/NC.
2. 1010: Client dyspneic. Lung sounds bilat crackles in bases. Incr. $O_2$ to 4L/NC per protocol.
3. 1000: Client dyspneic. Left message for HCP to return call; will wait for orders.
4. 1020: Client dyspneic. Oxygen to 4L/mask. $O_2$ saturation improved, and client denies dyspnea.

**289.** MoC The nurse manager learns that the LPN employed by the agency documented and signed the client's EMR with the nurse's name and credentials of LPN when the LPN was providing care as a student in an RN program. Based on this information, which action should be taken by the nurse manager?

1. Report the incident to the student's clinical instructor and request that the clinical instructor assist the LPN in correcting the documentation.
2. Discuss the incident with the LPN and advise the LPN to leave the medical record untouched because it is a legal document.
3. Advise the LPN to delete the incorrect entry and use the registered student nurse log-in ID to reenter the information.
4. Make a notation in the client's medical record that the LPN was functioning in the registered nurse student role.

**290.** `MoC` The new nurse is being oriented to the EMR on a nursing unit. Which points should be included in the new nurse's orientation session? **Select all that apply.**

1. Any entries into the computer will be credited to the person who is logged in to the computer.
2. Leaving a computer without first logging off can be a breach of client confidentiality.
3. For the experienced EMR user, the EMR enhances time efficiency and accuracy of data.
4. An incorrect entry can be opened and edited, thus keeping the original date and time.
5. Most agencies using EMR incorporate a system for tracking computer printouts.

**291.** `MoC` The experienced nurse is orienting the new nurse to essential documentation when caring for clients through a home health care agency. Which statement should be made by the experienced nurse regarding home health documentation?

1. "During each visit, an assessment is performed and then documented similarly to hospital documentation."
2. "Your documentation must show the need for professional medical services."
3. "Reimbursements for visits are directly related to the accuracy and wording of documentation."
4. "The assistance you provide with activities of daily living (ADLs) can be documented on a flowsheet."

**292.** `MoC` The nurse makes an error by documenting the wrong VS in the client's written medical record. Which action would be **best** to correct the error?

1. Draw a line through the error, initial and date the line, and then document a corrected entry.
2. Circle the incorrect entry, write "error" above the entry, and then date and initial the entry.
3. Highlight the error in yellow, write the correct VS on the line, and date and initial the line.
4. Cover the incorrect VS with the correct VS in such a manner that these are clearly readable.

**293.** `MoC` The client is admitted with a suspected stroke. What information should the nurse document about the client's admission? **Select all that apply.**

1. Orientation to the room including use of the call light
2. Admitting medical diagnosis of possible ischemic stroke
3. Nurse's physical and other assessment findings
4. Allergies to foods, medications, and other substances
5. That the client is wearing a 1-carat diamond ring

**294.** The nurse is planning prenatal classes for pregnant adolescents intending to keep their babies. Which teaching strategy would be most effective for the adolescents?

1. Inviting mothers and daughters for one-to-one teaching sessions
2. Preparing group sessions for teaching the pregnant adolescents together
3. Offering open sessions for the pregnant adolescents and anyone else who wants to attend
4. Designing poster boards that may be viewed individually in the school nurse's office

**295.** `PHARM` The nurse is instructing parents who emigrated from another country about administering their toddler's oral medication. What method is **best** to ensure that the toddler will get the prescribed amount of medicine at the appropriate times?

1. Have an interpreter available to translate information to the parents.
2. Have a parent demonstrate the medication administration process prior to discharge.
3. Initiate a referral to a home health care agency for a follow-up visit.
4. Provide written instructions to the parents on how to administer the medication.

**296.** When preparing a class to teach children, the nurse reviews Piaget's stages of development. With which age group do concrete operations roughly correspond?

1. Toddlerhood
2. Preschool-age children
3. School-age children
4. Adolescence

**297.** The nurse is preparing a campaign for seventh- and eighth-grade teachers. The purpose of the campaign is to decrease and subsequently eliminate bullying at school. Which strategy should the nurse utilize to most effectively present this information to the teachers?

1. Panel presentation with small-group discussion
2. Case studies with time for discussion of the cases
3. Lecture presentation with assignments before classes
4. Educational videos that students can view independently

**298.** MoC The nurse is preparing to educate parents who are extremely anxious because their infant has a physical disability. What is the **initial** purpose of this education?

1. Ensure that the parents who are being educated can perform a repeat demonstration.
2. Assist the parent to understand that there are multiple causes for their infant's disability.
3. Reduce the parents' anxiety to effect change in the parents' knowledge, attitudes, and skills.
4. Understand family factors that may influence their ability to live with their infant's disability.

**299.** MoC The pediatric nurse is planning time for teaching. The nurse assesses that which parent and child should be **most** ready to learn?

1. The mother sitting with her 4-year-old daughter who has just learned that the child has leukemia
2. The father who is sitting with his 10-year-old daughter who just returned from physical therapy
3. The father with his 2-year-old son who received an analgesic prior to a wound dressing change
4. The mother and her 3-year-old son who are reading a story about being sick in the hospital

**300.** PHARM The nurse completes teaching on insulin self-administration for the client newly diagnosed with diabetes. The nurse will document that the teaching is effective if the client demonstrates which injection technique for insulin administration?

1.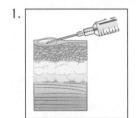
2.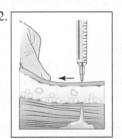
3.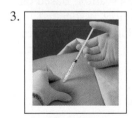
4.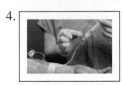

**301.** MoC The nurse is completing discharge teaching for the older adult client who is fully dressed and watching a television program. The nurse sits in a chair facing the client and shows the client a handout. The client squints while reading the paper and periodically looks at the television. Nearing completion of the teaching, the family arrives. The nurse should determine that the client may need additional teaching due to which barriers to learning? **Select all that apply.**

1. The client is watching a television program.
2. The client is an older adult.
3. The client is fully dressed.
4. The client squints to read the handout.
5. The family arrives during teaching.

**302.** When attempting to teach the client about medications, the client states, "Just tell my wife. She gives me all my pills." Which is the nurse's **best** response?

1. "You need to learn about your medications. What will you do if your wife isn't around?"
2. "I will write out a list for her with instructions about how and when they should be given."
3. "When will your wife be visiting next? I can go over the medications with both of you then."
4. "Having your wife set up your medications is a good plan; this avoids making mistakes."

**303.** The nurse is providing discharge teaching to the client newly diagnosed with type 2 DM. Prioritize the nurse's actions by placing each step of the teaching process in the correct order.

1. Implement the teaching plan.
2. Collect and analyze information about the client's knowledge of type 2 DM.
3. Formulate an educational nursing diagnosis and client outcomes for teaching.
4. Develop a teaching plan for the client, including content and teaching strategies.
5. Evaluate client learning based on the established outcomes.
6. Identify the client's learning needs.

Answer: _____

**304.** MoC The nurse teaches the postoperative adult client how to perform incision care. Prior to discharge, how should the nurse best evaluate the client's learning?

1. Ask the client questions and discuss the steps for performing incision care.
2. Have the client return-demonstrate cleansing and dressing the incision.
3. Reinforce the teaching with a handout at the time of the client's discharge.
4. Ask a family member to be present when the client is being discharged.

**305.** MoC The 78-year-old client who has arthritis is being discharged from the hospital with a Jackson-Pratt (JP) wound drainage system. To teach the client, the nurse should plan to take which action? **Select all that apply.**

1. Assess the client's manual dexterity in compressing the device and replacing the stopper.
2. Provide a group teaching session with younger and older adults who have JP drains.
3. Provide Web-based references for additional reading on emptying and caring for JP drains.
4. Provide sufficient opportunities for the client to return-demonstrate emptying the reservoir.
5. Evaluate the client's learning, and if unable to manage the drain, initiate a home care referral.

**306.** The new nurse is planning to change a central-line dressing. Which statement by the new nurse to the experienced nurse indicates that further teaching is needed?

1. "I will wash my hands immediately before and right after the dressing change."
2. "I will put on a pair of clean gloves only before I start to remove the dressing."
3. "I will ask that the client face away from the dressing while I am changing it."
4. "I will cleanse the site with an antiseptic solution before applying the new dressing."

**307.** MoC The nurse is preparing teaching materials for highly educated, self-directed adult clients on a cardiac step-down unit. Which methods of instruction should the nurse consider when preparing the instruction materials? **Select all that apply.**

1. Computer-assisted instruction
2. Closed-circuit television programs
3. Group sessions presented by hospitalized clients
4. Printed materials for handouts
5. Poster boards strategically placed on the unit

**308.** MoC The hospitalized client, who smokes two packs of cigarettes per day, voices concerns about not being able to smoke. Which actions should be taken by the nurse to educate the client about the effects of cigarette smoking and smoking cessation? **Select all that apply.**

1. Obtain smoking-cessation information for client education on the hospital's Web site.
2. Find the latest evidence on the Internet about smoking cessation during hospitalization.
3. Inform the client that cigarette smoking during hospitalization is prohibited by hospital policy.
4. Check the American Lung Association Web site for current guidelines on smoking cessation.
5. Go to the hospital library, conduct a literature search, and write a policy on smoking cessation.

**309.** MoC The nurse is using an interpreter when teaching the non–English-speaking client. Which action by the nurse would be **most** inappropriate?

1. Arrange the seating in a triangle.
2. Keep statements and questions short.
3. Maintain eye contact with the interpreter.
4. Ask the client to explain back the information.

**310.** MoC The hospitalized client, who speaks a foreign language and has minimal English, suddenly begins crying and shouting in his or her native language. Which nursing intervention would act as a barrier to the nurse-client relationship?

1. Speak loudly and instruct the client to calm down immediately.
2. Use a simple phrase in the client's native language to ask what is bothering the client.
3. Contact the hospital's interpreter to see the client immediately.
4. Remain at the client's bedside to be calmly present with the client.

**311.** MoC An elderly female client, who is Japanese and does not speak or understand English, is hospitalized. Which interventions should the nurse utilize to promote effective communication? **Select all that apply.**

1. Place a picture communication board at the bedside for client and family use.
2. Work with family to write a list of common client requests in English and Japanese.
3. Ask that a family member always be present so that the client will have a translator.
4. Explain that several nurses who are Eastern Asian can be available to help the client.
5. Inform the family that all nursing staff are required to have cultural sensitivity training.

**312.** MoC The nurse is planning an educational session for clients living on a Navajo reservation. Based on the major health risks and conditions associated with the Native American population, which topics should the nurse consider for the program? **Select all that apply.**

1. Proper use of seat belts
2. Risks of alcohol abuse
3. Symptoms of lactose intolerance
4. Reduction of sports injuries
5. Prevention of heart disease

**313.** MoC Which intervention should the nurse implement when overhearing the client and a relative speaking loudly, repeating phrases often, and using hand gestures?

1. Ask the relative to leave because it may be upsetting to the client.
2. Close the client's door to allow the client and relative privacy.
3. Ask the client and relative to speak softer and lower their tone of voice.
4. Observe the interaction to determine whether the relative is being abusive.

**314.** MoC The nurse manager in a hospital setting is developing culturally sensitive printed discharge instructions for Spanish-speaking clients. Which strategies should the nurse manager utilize? **Select all that apply.**

1. Create a brochure that has minimal text but humorous cartoons and illustrations.
2. Telephone the parish nurse from the clients' neighborhood to obtain input.
3. Translate the current brochure into Spanish and then have a Spanish-speaking client edit it.
4. Obtain feedback from previously hospitalized clients on a sample brochure written in Spanish.
5. Plan for a blank area within the brochure for clients and families to write specific instructions.

**315.** MoC The 19-year-old client is being discharged from the hospital following surgery. The client's primary language is French, but the client also speaks English fluently. Which action by the nurse would be **most** appropriate?

1. Provide written instructions in the client's primary language obtained from the Internet.
2. Provide written instructions in English but have a trained interpreter available.
3. Provide oral instructions in English; give choice of written instructions in French or English.
4. Provide written instructions in both English and French.

**316.** MoC The nurse at the community mental health center conducts an intake interview with the client from Africa. Which question from the nurse demonstrates a lack of cultural sensitivity?

1. "To what cultural group do you belong?"
2. "What languages do you speak in a typical day?"
3. "Are there cultural rules that guide your life?"
4. "How is your lifestyle different from an American lifestyle?"

**317.** MoC The nurse is educating multiple African American clients about their risk for developing ESRD. Which diseases associated with being African American place the clients at **greater** risk for ESRD? **Select all that apply.**

1. Hypertension
2. Skin cancer
3. Lactose intolerance
4. Diabetes mellitus
5. Polycystic kidney disease (PKD)
6. Systemic lupus erythematosus (SLE)

**318.** MoC The nurse is giving another nurse shift report on four clients. How many stereotypical statements did the nurse make?

| Client A | "Mrs. Yang requires an informed consent for an angiogram tomorrow, but wait until her husband arrives." |
| Client B | "Mr. Chen doesn't express his pain verbally and doesn't ask for pain meds. He needs to be carefully assessed for nonverbal signs of pain." |
| Client C | "Mr. Beliveau has type 2 DM. He recently emigrated from France. When completing diabetic education, he wanted to know which foods he should avoid. I placed a consult for a dietitian to see him." |
| Client D | "Mrs. Garcia is soon to be discharged after her gastric bypass surgery. It will be important to assess her knowledge of acceptable Hispanic foods and amounts that she can eat after her gastric bypass surgery." |

_____ Stereotypical statements (Record your answer as a whole number.)

**319.** MoC Two days after hospital discharge, the nurse is assessing the mother and her newborn twins in their home. Which statement or question made by the nurse **best** demonstrates empathy?

1. "You may be feeling overwhelmed. This is normal."
2. "I can't imagine how tired you must be with twins."
3. "How are you feeling about being the mother of twins?"
4. "I saw that laundry is piling up. Do you want a home aide?"

**320.** MoC The nurse teaches the 18-year-old diabetic client to perform self-administration of insulin. Each time the client makes even a small mistake, the client apologizes for getting it wrong. The client also profusely apologizes when making a minimal mistake in other activities. Based on Erikson's developmental stages, the nurse concludes that the client may have an unresolved developmental task of which age period?

1. Infancy
2. Early childhood
3. School-aged childhood
4. Adolescence

**321.** MoC The client diagnosed with ESRD states to the nurse, "I don't think I want to be on dialysis anymore; it's just too painful for me." What is the **most** appropriate response by the nurse?

1. "Why do you think staying on dialysis is so painful for you?"
2. "You feel that dialysis is painful for you. Tell me more about that."
3. "It really isn't hard to stay on dialysis. You can sleep during these."
4. "You should stay on dialysis so you won't get worse or even die."

**322.** MoC The 10-year-old with precocious puberty is being teased by classmates. Which approach should the school nurse use to assist the child in communicating with peers?

1. Use role-playing to show the child how to handle teasing from other children.
2. Tell the child to ignore the comments from peers because then the teasing will stop.
3. Provide a book about a child being teased and the child's humorous responses.
4. Instruct the child to inform an adult when a peer makes teasing comments.

**323.** MoC The experienced nurse overhears a conversation between the mother of the 12-year-old newly diagnosed with Crohn's disease and the new nurse (see exhibit). The mother has just been told by the HCP, in the presence of the new nurse, that her child does not require surgery but will need long-term therapy. Which is the **most** important conclusion that the experienced nurse should make about this conversation?

| New Nurse | "The doctor was just in the room. Do you have any questions?" |
|---|---|
| Client | "No. Andy will be well again in a short time. I am so thankful." |
| New Nurse | "You seem relieved that your son is improving. Tell me what you understand about your child's treatment plan." |
| Client | "Andy's intestines are healing just fine; I just need to take Andy for frequent checkups." |
| New Nurse | "Do you mean that your son doesn't need parenteral nutrition anymore?" |
| Client | "He doesn't need anything. Not even surgery. This will soon be over." |
| New Nurse | "That's wonderful. Your son is very lucky." |

1. The new nurse used appropriate therapeutic communication skills.
2. The new nurse acknowledged the client's feelings and offered support.
3. The new nurse failed to address the son by name in the conversation.
4. The new nurse failed to provide the client with accurate information.

**324.** MoC The nurse is developing the plan of care for the 4-year-old who is to have eye surgery. Which intervention should the nurse **most definitely** include in the plan to prepare the child for surgery?

1. Discuss the impending surgery with parents, who should then discuss it with their child.
2. Provide a doll with an eye patch in place and allow time for the child to play with the doll.
3. Introduce the child to others on the unit who have had eye or other types of face surgery.
4. Show the child a 30-minute animated movie featuring a child being prepared for surgery.

**325.** MoC The nurse is discharging the 10-year-old who was hospitalized for RF with signs of CHF. What should be the nurse's **priority** with discharge teaching?

1. Allow time for the parents to talk about their feelings regarding their child's illness.
2. Inform the parents of the child's increased risk for infection when on a corticosteroid.
3. Ensure that the child is aware of the activity restrictions and the need for adherence.
4. Emphasize to the child that the rash on the trunk and the swollen joints will go away.

**326.** MoC The parents are visiting their newborn, who is in the neonatal intensive care unit (NICU) after being diagnosed with a terminal cardiac condition. Which statement **best** reflects the nurse's judgment about interventions to promote parental attachment?

1. Interventions should be delayed until it is certain that the newborn will live.
2. The parents should be encouraged to provide as much care as possible.
3. The parents should only be encouraged to touch and name their newborn.
4. The parents should be assured that they did not do anything to cause this condition.

# Answers and Rationales

**261. ANSWER: 3, 5, 2, 1, 4**

3. **The preinteraction phase is the first phase, before the nurse meets the client. In the phase the nurse gathers information about the client.**
5. **The orientation phase is next. Introductions are made during an initial meeting, the relationship is defined, and the purpose of the visit is established.**
2. **The working phase occurs next, which is the active part of the relationship in which techniques of therapeutic communication are used to discuss the issues of importance.**
1. **Next is the termination phase. After the working phase is completed, the termination phase begins, and the relationship is reviewed and summarized.**
4. **The conclusion of relationship is the final phase in which the relationship with the client comes to an end.**

♦ *Test-taking Tip: Pre- should be a clue to you that this option should be first. Conclusion is the only option that does not include phase and should be a clue that this option should be last.*

Content Area: Management of Care; Concept: Communication; Integrated Processes: Communication and Documentation; Client Needs: Psychosocial Integrity; Cognitive Level: Synthesis [Creating]

**262. ANSWER: 1**

1. **The nurse should first establish a trusting relationship with the client to be able to counsel the client about the effects of alcohol on the developing fetus and the client's health. According to Erikson's theory of development, adolescents are very egocentric, and peers are a strong influence. Because it is very important to be a part of a group, many will do whatever is necessary, believing that "nothing bad will ever happen" to them.**

2. Teaching about FAS is premature; the client may not be ready to hear the information. The nurse first needs to establish a trusting relationship.
3. The nurse must first establish a trusting relationship. The short-term effects of drinking with friends may far outweigh concerns about the physiological effects of alcohol.
4. Only with a trusting relationship will the nurse be able to gather more information about the client's home life and friends.

♦ *Test-taking Tip: The key word is "initial." Be cognizant of the client's developmental stage and the need for the client to be a part of a group.*

Content Area: Management of Care; Concept: Development; Integrated Processes: Nursing Process: Analysis; Caring; Client Needs: Psychosocial Integrity; Cognitive Level: Analysis [Analyzing]

**263.** MoC **ANSWER: 1, 2, 3, 4**

1. **The reason for the transfer is needed to provide continuity of the client's care and to protect the client from injury.**
2. **Verbal report should be given to the transferring facility, and the name of the person receiving the report should be documented for legal protection of both nurses and for follow-up if needed.**
3. **The condition of the client is important so that the receiving nurse can anticipate the type of care the client will need and any immediate needs.**
4. **Medication, food, and environmental allergies should be included in the transfer note to protect the client from injury.**
5. Insurance information is included in records that are prepared for transfer, but not the financial status or client's ability to pay for expenses. If a social worker has been assigned for follow-up due to financial concerns, this should be noted in the transfer note.

▶ **Test-taking Tip:** *Eliminate any options that should not impact the continuity of care. The client cannot be denied care, regardless of ability to pay.*

**Content Area:** Management of Care; **Concept:** Management; **Integrated Processes:** Communication and Documentation; **Client Needs:** Safe and Effective Care Environment: Management of Care; Safe and Effective Care Environment: Safety and Infection Control; **Cognitive Level:** Knowledge [Remembering]

### 264. ANSWER: 4

1. Although determining sexual activity of a teenager is important for client teaching, the nurse's best response should be obtaining information pertaining to the pregnancy.
2. Asking a "why" question may make the client defensive.
3. This is an acceptable question, but the nurse needs to begin with the facts.
4. **A direct question related to the client's menstrual cycle is best and is necessary prior to obtaining other information.**

▶ **Test-taking Tip:** *When communicating with a teenager, ensure that the tone of the conversation is nonjudgmental. Select the option that focuses on the facts and does not risk making the client defensive.*

**Content Area:** Management of Care; **Concept:** Communication; **Integrated Processes:** Communication and Documentation; Caring; **Client Needs:** Psychosocial Integrity; **Cognitive Level:** Application [Applying]

### 265. ANSWER: 1, 3, 5

1. **Making eye contact and speaking to the client directly convey an interest in the client and are essential to facilitate communication.**
2. Asking only the spouse information excludes the client from the conversation and does not facilitate trust between the nurse and client.
3. **Supplying the client with a writing board allows the client to answer and ask questions about care.**
4. Placing a speaking valve over the tracheostomy should not occur until the client has been assessed for the ability to tolerate cuff deflation without aspiration or respiratory distress.
5. **Assessing the client's preferred communication method allows the client to participate in care and shows that the client's needs are valued.**
6. Asking the client only "yes" and "no" questions does not allow the client to provide any descriptions, can be frustrating for the client, and does not allow the client to ask any questions.

▶ **Test-taking Tip:** *Eliminate the responses that do not encourage communication between the client and nurse. Eliminate Option 4 because assessment of the ability to tolerate cuff deflation is not evident.*

**Content Area:** Management of Care; **Concept:** Communication; **Integrated Processes:** Communication and Documentation; **Client Needs:** Psychosocial Integrity; **Cognitive Level:** Application [Applying]

### 266. ANSWER: 1

1. **Having the client demonstrate how to change a urinary drainage bag is the best way to assess that the client understands the teaching. If the client is unable to return the demonstration, the client will need further teaching, possibly with a different nonverbal method if the client's hearing loss is a barrier to understanding.**
2. Asking if the client has any questions about the procedure does not evaluate whether learning has occurred. The client may state that he or she has no questions, especially if the client is unable to hear the information or is embarrassed by the hearing loss or subject matter.
3. Although having the client state the procedure may be one method of evaluating information, for a psychomotor skill the best method of evaluation is having the client perform the skill.
4. Providing a handout with instructions would be helpful and is a teaching strategy, but it does not aid in evaluating the client's understanding of the teaching.

▶ **Test-taking Tip:** *Read the question carefully. When teaching a psychomotor skill, the best method for evaluating performance of the skill is through demonstration.*

**Content Area:** Management of Care; **Concept:** Nursing Roles; Sensory Perception; **Integrated Processes:** Nursing Process: Evaluation; **Client Needs:** Psychosocial Integrity; **Cognitive Level:** Evaluation [Evaluating]

### 267. CJ ANSWER: 4

1. There is more than one therapeutic communication technique being used by the nurse.
2. There are more than two therapeutic communication techniques being used by the nurse.
3. There are more than three therapeutic communication techniques being used by the nurse.
4. **There are four therapeutic communication techniques being used by the nurse. In Interaction 1, the nurse uses a broad opening. In Interaction 2, the nurse is asking for clarification. In Interaction 3, the nurse is reflecting. In Interaction 5, the nurse is using silence to allow time to think about what to say next or to allow the client to further express concerns. The nurse uses nontherapeutic techniques in the remaining interaction. In Interaction 4, the nurse is "parroting." If it were restating, the nurse would paraphrase the message back to the client. In Interaction 6, the nurse is advising. In Interaction 7, the nurse is belittling the client's feelings by telling the client not to worry.**

▶ **Test-taking Tip:** *The key word is "therapeutic." Eliminate the interactions in which the nurse uses nontherapeutic techniques, and count the remaining options to determine the answer.*

**Content Area:** Management of Care; **Concept:** Communication; **Integrated Processes:** Communication and Documentation; **Client Needs:** Psychosocial Integrity; **Cognitive Level:** Analysis [Analyzing]

**268.** `CJ` **ANSWER:**

> "Well, don't worry."

▶ **Test-taking Tip:** *Eliminate all therapeutic statements and then the nontherapeutic statements that are parroting or advising.*

**Content Area:** Management of Care; **Concept:** Communication; **Integrated Processes:** Nursing Process: Evaluation; **Client Needs:** Psychosocial Integrity; **Cognitive Level:** Evaluation [Evaluating]

**269. ANSWER: 2**

1. Option 1 is presenting reality but offering support to the child to boost confidence in handling the dark.
2. **When using reflection as a communication technique, the nurse selects one or two of the client's words to reflect back to the client for consideration. This technique strengthens client confidence.**
3. Option 3 seeks clarification.
4. Option 4 demonstrates advising, a nontherapeutic communication technique.

▶ **Test-taking Tip:** *Reflection is a therapeutic communication technique in which one or two of the client's words are reflected back to the client for consideration.*

**Content Area:** Management of Care; **Concept:** Communication; **Integrated Processes:** Communication and Documentation; **Client Needs:** Psychosocial Integrity; **Cognitive Level:** Analysis [Analyzing]

**270. ANSWER: 4**

1. Abruptly telling the client that the session has ended does not leave room for feedback from the client and may also leave the client with negative feelings about the interaction. The client may feel as though he or she did or said something wrong to cause the nurse to leave abruptly.
2. Setting up an additional home-care visit only prolongs the termination phase and may allow the client to become manipulating.
3. Planning to meet the client for a social visit is inappropriate and may violate professional and ethical codes of conduct.
4. **Being firm and clear about the termination of the relationship maintains professional boundaries, while soliciting feedback helps the client maintain a positive attitude about the interaction.**

▶ **Test-taking Tip:** *Read each response carefully and select the response that allows for termination of the interaction while maintaining a positive interaction.*

**Content Area:** Management of Care; **Concept:** Communication; **Integrated Processes:** Nursing Process: Implementation; **Client Needs:** Psychosocial Integrity; **Cognitive Level:** Analysis [Analyzing]

**271. ANSWER: 2**

1. This statement focuses on the nurse's feelings, not the daughter's.
2. **The statement focuses on the daughter's feelings and demonstrates the nurse's concern.**
3. This statement reinforces the powerlessness of the daughter in the situation and blocks therapeutic communication.
4. This response offers information and hope but not empathy.

▶ **Test-taking Tip:** *Recall that empathy is identifying the way another feels; thus select the option that focuses on the daughter's feelings.*

**Content Area:** Management of Care; **Concept:** Communication; Diversity; **Integrated Processes:** Communication and Documentation; Caring; Culture and Spirituality; **Client Needs:** Psychosocial Integrity; **Cognitive Level:** Application [Applying]

**272. ANSWER: 4**

1. Putting the supplies away and reattempting in 1 hour avoids discussing the client's feelings about the amputation when the client is clearly upset and the opportunity is there for establishing a relationship.
2. Completing the dressing change despite the client's request, because it is prescribed for 2000, takes the control away from the client and violates any trust between the nurse and client.
3. Asking the client a question can be interrogating and does not address the client's feelings about the amputation.
4. **Restating provides an opportunity for the client to clarify further and encourages discussion of the client's feelings about having an amputation.**

▶ **Test-taking Tip:** *Select the option that best addresses the client's emotional reaction. Using therapeutic communication techniques will allow the client to express feelings.*

**Content Area:** Management of Care; **Concept:** Communication; **Integrated Processes:** Communication and Documentation; Nursing Process: Implementation; **Client Needs:** Psychosocial Integrity; **Cognitive Level:** Evaluation [Evaluating]

**273. ANSWER: 3**

1. Asking the client "why" questions belittles the client's feelings and may cause the client to withdraw from the interaction.
2. Response 2 is an example of restating and clarifying the client's response, but it does not further stimulate conversation. Asking the client a "yes/no" question, as in Response 2, ends the conversation and does not allow for further opportunity to build a relationship.
3. **Response 3 uses therapeutic communication techniques of sharing observations and using an open-ended statement. The statement allows the client to elaborate further about the client's feelings and fears while building a trusting nurse-client relationship.**

4. Response 4 is an example of restatement. Although the statement allows the client to further elaborate and is therapeutic, Response 3 is the best statement because it uses two therapeutic communication techniques, whereas Response 4 uses one.

▶ **Test-taking Tip:** *Read through the written conversation carefully. Choose the option that uses more than one therapeutic communication technique and encourages further communication.*

**Content Area:** Management of Care; **Concept:** Communication; **Integrated Processes:** Communication and Documentation; **Client Needs:** Psychosocial Integrity; **Cognitive Level:** Analysis [Analyzing]

## 274. ANSWER: 64

**First, add the five wet diaper weights: 22 g + 24 g + 38 g + 34 g+ 21 g = 139 g. Next determine the weight of 5 dry diapers (15 g × 5 = 75 g). Next, subtract the weight of the 5 dry diapers from the weight of the wet diapers to determine the urine output (139 g – 75 g = 64 g). Finally, convert grams to milliliters. One milliliter of urine output equals 1 g of body weight. Thus 64 g equals 64 mL of urine output.**

▶ **Test-taking Tip:** *Use the equivalent of 1 mL of urine output equals 1 g of body weight to calculate the amount of urine output.*

**Content Area:** Management of Care; **Concept:** Communication; Urinary Elimination; **Integrated Processes:** Communication and Documentation; **Client Needs:** Physiological Integrity: Basic Care and Comfort; **Cognitive Level:** Application [Applying]

## 275. ANSWER: 3

1. Asking the "why" questions may suggest criticism of the client's actions, and the spouse may become defensive.
2. Asking "How long has your spouse had Alzheimer's disease?" is a closed-ended question.
3. **Response 3 is a statement that uses the therapeutic technique of sharing observations. This statement validates the spouse's feelings and allows the client to elaborate further.**
4. The statement "Tell me about the things your spouse did before being diagnosed with Alzheimer's disease" is inappropriate at this time because the spouse is crying, and these emotions should be addressed first.

▶ **Test-taking Tip:** *Eliminate the responses that would be considered blocks to therapeutic communication and would not encourage communication.*

**Content Area:** Management of Care; **Concept:** Communication; **Integrated Processes:** Communication and Documentation; Caring; **Client Needs:** Psychosocial Integrity; **Cognitive Level:** Analysis [Analyzing]

## 276. MoC ANSWER: 1

1. **Asking the client to nod his or her head "yes" or "no" to questions is the best initial intervention to assess further if the aphasia is expressive (Broca's aphasia) or also receptive (Wernicke's aphasia). If the client is able to communicate by head nodding, the nurse should continue to include the client in the plan of care and preserve any communication ability that the client retains to prevent the client from becoming withdrawn.**
2. Consulting a speech therapist may be helpful at a later stage, but this is not the best initial intervention.
3. Giving the client a writing board may only discourage the client, as written deficits usually parallel speech deficits in clients with Broca's aphasia.
4. Directing questions to the client's adult child excludes the client from the conversation and forces the client to become withdrawn.

▶ **Test-taking Tip:** *When communicating with the client, the focus should be on the client, even if the client is impaired.*

**Content Area:** Management of Care; **Concept:** Communication; **Integrated Processes:** Nursing Process: Implementation; **Client Needs:** Safe and Effective Care Environment: Management of Care; **Cognitive Level:** Analysis [Analyzing]

## 277. ANSWER: 2

1. Overexaggerating should be avoided because it will not increase the client's ability to hear and may be insulting to the client.
2. **Using simple sentences will assist in communicating with the client. There will be fewer words to decipher and less room for error in interpreting the meaning of the sentences.**
3. Overenunciating should be avoided because this will not increase the client's ability to hear and may be insulting to the client.
4. Speaking quickly, in a higher-pitched voice, should be avoided because older adult clients with presbycusis often lose the ability to hear higher-pitched sounds first and are able to hear lower-pitched sounds better when they are spoken slowly.

▶ **Test-taking Tip:** *Age-related physiological changes can affect hearing loss. Select the option that takes into account the hearing loss while maintaining respectful communication.*

**Content Area:** Management of Care; **Concept:** Communication; **Integrated Processes:** Communication and Documentation; **Client Needs:** Psychosocial Integrity; **Cognitive Level:** Analysis [Analyzing]

## 278. MoC ANSWER: 2

1. Critically appraising the resource is the second step in the process of looking for evidence-based research.
2. **Formulating a well-built question will help determine the resources to access for the best available evidence.**

3. Once the research methods have been identified, there should be criteria and a process for evaluating the quantitative and qualitative evidence. This is the third step.

4. Evidence-based practice is the utilization of research knowledge that takes into consideration factors such as best evidence from a thorough search and critical appraisal of the research, context, health care resources, practitioner skills, client status and circumstance, and client references and values. But, this is the fourth step in the process.

▶ **Test-taking Tip:** The key word is "first." Look at each of the options to determine which options are dependent upon another option. The word "searchable" in Option 2 should draw you to this option because other options are dependent on first completing a search. In questions asking for the first step, the more specific option should be the answer.

**Content Area:** Management of Care; **Concept:** Informatics; Evidence-based Practice; **Integrated Processes:** Teaching/Learning; **Client Needs:** Safe and Effective Care Environment: Management of Care; **Cognitive Level:** Application [Applying]

### 279. MoC ANSWER: 2, 3, 5

1. This statement uses a variation of "you didn't," which is not empowering the nurses.

2. **This statement is empowering because the nurse manager's statements indicate personal ownership of beliefs, values, and needs while communicating expectations about values and goals. The nurse manager uses a variation of "I want" or "I need" rather than "you must" or "you didn't."**

3. **This statement is empowering because the nurse manager's statements indicate personal ownership of beliefs, values, and needs while communicating expectations about values and goals. The nurse manager uses a variation of "I want" or "I need" rather than "you must" or "you didn't."**

4. This statement uses a variation of "you didn't," which is not empowering the nurses.

5. **This statement is empowering because the nurse manager's statements indicate personal ownership of beliefs, values, and needs while communicating expectations about values and goals. The nurse manager uses a variation of "I want" or "I need" rather than "you must" or "you didn't."**

6. This statement uses a variation of "you didn't," which is not empowering the nurses.

▶ **Test-taking Tip:** Recall that empowering means giving power to another person. Read each option carefully to determine if the nurse manager's statements give power to the nurse or staff.

**Content Area:** Management of Care; **Concept:** Management; **Integrated Processes:** Nursing Process: Evaluation; **Client Needs:** Safe and Effective Care Environment: Management of Care; **Cognitive Level:** Evaluation [Evaluating]

### 280. MoC ANSWER: 4

1. Option 1 is incorrect information. The RN was discharged.

2. Option 2 suggests that the employee's failure to notify is related to discomfort with communication, which could be an incorrect conclusion.

3. Option 3 is inappropriate. The nurse manager should know the policies of the agency.

4. **Only factual information should be provided. The former employee has not consented to provide additional information.**

▶ **Test-taking Tip:** Select the option that provides the most factual information.

**Content Area:** Management of Care; **Concept:** Management; **Integrated Processes:** Communication and Documentation; **Client Needs:** Safe and Effective Care Environment: Management of Care; **Cognitive Level:** Analysis [Analyzing]

### 281. MoC ANSWER: 1, 3, 4, 5

1. **A brief medical history of the client's current problem should be provided at the shift report so the oncoming shift nurse can provide focused care.**

2. A typical end-of-shift report does not include the client's satisfaction with the nurse's care. This information is unnecessary to providing quality care and meeting the client's needs.

3. **Client-family dynamics and client psychosocial concerns are important to include because family is part of the client's support system.**

4. **Surgery, tests, or procedures scheduled for the next 24 hours should be included in the report so the nurse can teach and prepare the client for these.**

5. **Tube and equipment status, including IVs, should be reported so that the nurse can determine priorities.**

6. A typical end-of-shift report does not include the telephone number of the nurse giving report. If the report is complete, there should be no reason to consult the nurse whose shift has ended.

▶ **Test-taking Tip:** You should focus on providing information about the client that is needed to meet client care needs and protect the client from injury.

**Content Area:** Management of Care; **Concept:** Communication; Management; **Integrated Processes:** Communication and Documentation; **Client Needs:** Safe and Effective Care Environment: Management of Care; Safe and Effective Care Environment: Safety and Infection Control; **Cognitive Level:** Evaluation [Evaluating]

### 282. MoC ANSWER: 3, 4, 2, 1

3. **"I am calling about {client name and location}. Vital signs are BP=100/50, P=120, RR=30, T=100.4°F (38°C)" describes the situation and what is happening at the present time. This represents the S of SBAR.**

4. "The client is becoming confused and agitated. The skin is pale, mottled, and diaphoretic. The client is very dyspneic with an oxygen saturation of 85% despite placing a nonrebreather mask" describes the background of what has occurred leading up to the situation. This represents the B of SBAR.

2. "The client is deteriorating, and I'm afraid the client is going to arrest" is an assessment of the primary problem and represents the A of SBAR.

1. "I suggest that the client be transferred to the critical care unit, and I would like you to come evaluate the client" describes the recommendations for correcting the problem, which is the R of SBAR.

▶ *Test-taking Tip: Be familiar with reporting formats. The SBAR format (Situation-Background-Assessment-Recommendation) is approved and recommended by the Centers for Medicare and Medicaid Services as well as The Joint Commission.*

**Content Area:** Management of Care; **Concept:** Safety; Management; Communication; **Integrated Processes:** Communication and Documentation; **Client Needs:** Safe and Effective Care Environment: Management of Care; Safe and Effective Care Environment: Safety and Infection Control; **Cognitive Level:** Synthesis [Creating]

### 283. MoC ANSWER: 1

1. **For the safety of the client and continuity of care, the nurse should communicate with the receiving department (radiology) using the SBAR-formatted report (situation, background, assessment, and recommendation). SBAR is a standardized, widely adopted reporting format.**

2. Vital signs, if pertinent, should be included in the SBAR report.

3. I&O or fluid status, if pertinent, should be included in the SBAR report.

4. Because the client is not being discharged, this information is not pertinent to the radiology department.

▶ *Test-taking Tip: Concentrate on selecting the most global option. Options 2 and 3, if pertinent, should be a part of the SBAR-formatted report and should be eliminated as option choices.*

**Content Area:** Management of Care; **Concept:** Critical Thinking; Communication; Management; **Integrated Processes:** Nursing Process: Planning; **Client Needs:** Safe and Effective Care Environment: Management of Care; Safe and Effective Care Environment: Safety and Infection Control; **Cognitive Level:** Application [Applying]

### 284. MoC ANSWER: 1

1. **With CPOE, the HCP can enter orders from any location, and the nurse must check for these periodically (usually every half hour).**

2. The nurse may check the computer at the beginning of the shift and note the medications due during the shift; this does not require hourly checking.

3. When new orders are placed in the computer, it is the responsibility of the nurse to check the computer for the new orders. Usually the HCP does not telephone the nurse about these unless it is a STAT order.

4. Documentation of blood sugars is unrelated to checking for new orders.

▶ *Test-taking Tip: The key words are "related to CPOE." The nurse must check the computer for new orders because the client's chart is no longer on paper.*

**Content Area:** Management of Care; **Concept:** Informatics; Management; **Integrated Processes:** Nursing Process: Implementation; **Client Needs:** Safe and Effective Care Environment: Management of Care; Safe and Effective Care Environment: Safety and Infection Control; **Cognitive Level:** Application [Applying]

### 285. MoC ANSWER:

| Progress Notes | | |
| --- | --- | --- |
| **Date** | **Time** | **Entry** |
| 6-15-17 | 1600 | At 1530 given ~~M.S.~~, 2.0 mg IV for chest incisional pain rated 5 on a 0 to 10 scale; 30 minutes later pain rated at a 1. Will plan to give analgesic again at H.S. Remains on q6h blood glucose checks for NPO status; covered elevated blood glucose with 2 units regular insulin subcut. at 1800. ———— J. Peters, RN |

**M.S. should be corrected. It appears on The Joint Commission's published list of "Do Not Use" abbreviations. M.S. could mean either morphine sulfate or magnesium sulfate.**

▶ *Test-taking Tip: The abbreviation for morphine sulfate can be confused with magnesium sulfate.*

**Content Area:** Management of Care; **Concept:** Informatics; Management; **Integrated Processes:** Communication and Documentation; **Client Needs:** Safe and Effective Care Environment: Management of Care; **Cognitive Level:** Application [Applying]

### 286. MoC ANSWER: 1, 3, 4

1. **The documentation should be factual and objective. Quoting the client's statements of how the fall happened is appropriate.**

2. This notation lays blame on the client. If prior to the fall the nurse had repeatedly instructed the client to leave the wheelchair locked, and the nurse found the wheelchair in the unlocked position, a notation as to the observations and interventions would be appropriate. But the notation must be in a nonaccusatory manner and not as a result of the incident.

3. **This is a factual statement based on what the nurse observed.**
4. **The nurse's assessment and client's statements may be placed in the medical record.**
5. An incident report should be completed. However, stating it has been completed is never documented in the medical record because it then becomes discoverable evidence if litigation ensues.

▶ *Test-taking Tip: When documenting a fall, only factual and objective information should be included. It is important to include client statements of the incident as well as assessment findings. An incident report form is for agency use only, and the form or the reference to it is never included in a medical record.*

Content Area: Management of Care; Concept: Safety; Informatics; Legal; Communication; Integrated Processes: Communication and Documentation; Client Needs: Safe and Effective Care Environment: Management of Care; Cognitive Level: Application [Applying]

## 287. MoC ANSWER: 2, 3

1. Documentation should include objective data unless directly quoted from the client.
2. **Specific information was included in the documentation.**
3. **The documentation is specific and detailed identifying the medication, dose, route, and administration rate.**
4. Documentation is incomplete; it does not indicate whether or not the client was able to void.
5. Documentation is incomplete and does not describe the distance ambulated. The phrase "tolerated well" is vague and does not describe what the nurse had been observing to make this determination.

▶ *Test-taking Tip: Narrative documentation should be specific and as detailed as possible unless an agency has a documentation policy that includes the use of flowsheets and documentation by exception. Eliminate options that are subjective and not specific.*

Content Area: Management of Care; Concept: Legal; Communication; Informatics; Integrated Processes: Communication and Documentation; Client Needs: Safe and Effective Care Environment: Management of Care; Cognitive Level: Evaluation [Evaluating]

## 288. MoC ANSWER: 2

1. This is incomplete documentation of the events; there is no reason provided for the increase of oxygen administration.
2. **The documentation is complete and reflects that the nurse identified the problem (client reports), sought a solution (reviewed protocol), and implemented the solution to the problem (action taken).**
3. The nurse did not document any action taken with the client. The nurse should have checked the orders and intervened accordingly. This would be viewed as a failure to rescue.
4. There is no indication that oxygen was administered via mask or that the oxygen saturation was improved.

▶ *Test-taking Tip: Focus on selecting the option with the most complete information. Documentation should reflect identifying the problem, checking the orders or a protocol to see if an intervention is already prescribed, and acting on those orders or protocol.*

Content Area: Management of Care; Concept: Critical Thinking; Communication; Integrated Processes: Communication and Documentation; Client Needs: Safe and Effective Care Environment: Management of Care; Cognitive Level: Evaluation [Evaluating]

## 289. MoC ANSWER: 1

1. **While in the student nurse role, the LPN is not considered an employee of the agency. The nurse manager should inform the clinical instructor who is responsible for clinical supervision.**
2. The nurse's credentials are in error on the day of care. A notation and correction should be made in the client's medical record.
3. Although the LPN should be instructed to make a correction entry, the person discussing the incident with the LPN should be the clinical instructor.
4. The nurse manager should not make a notation in the client's medical record but should ensure that an incident (unusual occurrence) report is completed by the nurse who found the documentation error.

▶ *Test-taking Tip: Think carefully about who was providing supervision when the documentation error occurred.*

Content Area: Management of Care; Concept: Management; Informatics; Integrated Processes: Communication and Documentation; Client Needs: Safe and Effective Care Environment: Management of Care; Cognitive Level: Analysis [Analyzing]

## 290. MoC ANSWER: 1, 2, 3, 5

1. **The log-in access includes an electronic signature with the name of the person to whom the log-in access is assigned.**
2. **Information displayed on the monitor can be viewed by others. This may lead to a breach in client confidentiality.**
3. **Studies have shown that EMR enhances time efficiency, direct client care time, user satisfaction, accuracy of data, and completeness of the medical record.**
4. If a correction is made in an incorrect entry, the current date and time are entered. An incorrect entry should be corrected by making a new entry. The date of the entry will be the log-in date at the time of the correction entry.
5. **Both computer printouts and log-ins are tracked by most agencies. Computer printouts are tracked to prevent indiscriminate duplication or distribution.**

▶ *Test-taking Tip: Read each option carefully and think about whether these could be features on an EMR.*

Content Area: Management of Care; Concept: Informatics; Management; Integrated Processes: Communication and Documentation; Client Needs: Safe and Effective Care Environment: Management of Care; Cognitive Level: Analysis [Analyzing]

**291.** MoC **ANSWER: 3**

1. This statement is very broad. Only a focused physical assessment may be completed during a home care visit, and documentation usually will not include a complete physical assessment. Assessment of the home environment may be included if it impacts the client's ability to care for himself or herself.
2. Nurses justify the need for nursing, not medical services.
3. **With each visit, the need for a professional nurse must be noted. Reimbursement for a visit is directly related to the documentation showing a need for professional assistance.**
4. The professional nurse would not be performing ADLs during a visit. These are completed by a home health aide.

▶ *Test-taking Tip: Think about how home health nursing differs from acute-care nursing. Documentation of a home care visit should justify the need of a professional nurse.*

**Content Area:** Management of Care; **Concept:** Communication; **Integrated Processes:** Communication and Documentation; **Client Needs:** Safe and Effective Care Environment: Management of Care; **Cognitive Level:** Application [Applying]

**292.** MoC **ANSWER: 1**

1. **Common agency policy includes drawing a single line through the error, adding the date, and then initialing the entry. Writing "void" in the space above the entry is sometimes included in agency policy. The vital signs should be documented in the correct client's medical record.**
2. Although agency policy may include circling the error, writing "error" in a medical record should be avoided. This option does not include entering the correct vital signs.
3. If medical records are copied for any reason, the highlighted information may not show up as being highlighted.
4. Writing over (covering) an existing entry is not permitted because of the implication of covering up an error or mistake.

▶ *Test-taking Tip: Agency policy should be followed for correcting a documentation error. Correction of the error would include documentation of the correct information. Select the option that corrects the error and includes the correct information in the clearest and most unambiguous manner.*

**Content Area:** Management of Care; **Concept:** Communication; Legal; **Integrated Processes:** Communication and Documentation; **Client Needs:** Safe and Effective Care Environment: Management of Care; **Cognitive Level:** Comprehension [Understanding]

**293.** MoC **ANSWER: 1, 3, 4**

1. **The client should be oriented to the room and use of the call light for the client's safety. This information should be documented.**

2. There is no information indicating that the client had an ischemic stroke.
3. **Physical assessment findings should be documented on admission for baseline information and for comparison if the condition of the client changes.**
4. **All allergies should be documented on admission to protect the client from harm.**
5. Valuables such as jewelry should be described in general terms, such as a "yellow ring with a clear stone."

▶ *Test-taking Tip: An admit note is the first note acknowledging the arrival of a new client. It should be one of the most complete documentations to ensure continuity of care. Select the options relevant to the client's immediate safety and care.*

**Content Area:** Management of Care; **Concept:** Communication; **Integrated Processes:** Communication and Documentation; **Client Needs:** Safe and Effective Care Environment: Management of Care; Safe and Effective Care Environment: Safety and Infection Control; **Cognitive Level:** Application [Applying]

**294. ANSWER: 2**

1. Inviting mothers and daughters for individual teaching sessions may be effective for teaching the adolescent mothers but less effective for the pregnant adolescents.
2. **Peer groups are important for adolescents, so utilizing group teaching sessions is the most effective teaching strategy.**
3. Prenatal teaching, especially the topic of body changes with pregnancy, could threaten the adolescent's self-esteem and body image if it is discussed in open sessions where anyone could attend.
4. Poster boards could be an effective strategy for young adults, but not adolescents.

▶ *Test-taking Tip: Focus on the issue: teaching strategies appropriate for adolescents.*

**Content Area:** Management of Care; **Concept:** Nursing Roles; **Integrated Processes:** Nursing Process: Planning; **Client Needs:** Health Promotion and Maintenance; **Cognitive Level:** Application [Applying]

**295.** PHARM **ANSWER: 2**

1. Having an interpreter may be warranted, but there is no indication that the parents are unable to speak English.
2. **In adult learning theory, return demonstration or demonstrating ability to do the task is the most effective means of evaluating performance.**
3. Initiating a referral would not be warranted unless there are other health care or parenting concerns.
4. Providing written instructions is a supplemental resource for the parents but would require evaluation of reading and comprehension skills.

▶ *Test-taking Tip: The key word is "best." Consider adult learning theory as it relates to parent education.*

**Content Area:** Management of Care; **Concept:** Nursing Roles; Diversity; **Integrated Processes:** Teaching/Learning; Culture and Spirituality; **Client Needs:** Physiological Integrity: Pharmacological and Parenteral Therapies; **Cognitive Level:** Application [Applying]

## 296. ANSWER: 3

1. Toddlers, 12 to 24 months, are in the sensorimotor phase of cognitive development.
2. Preschool children, 2 to 4 years, are in the preconceptual phase, where everything is significant and relates to "me."
3. **Concrete operations occur between the ages of 7 and 11 years.**
4. Adolescents are in the formal operations phase and are able to use rational thinking and deductive and futuristic reasoning.

▶ *Test-taking Tip: Preoperational roughly corresponds with preschool; operations follow.*

Content Area: Management of Care; Concept: Development; Integrated Processes: Teaching/Learning; Client Needs: Health Promotion and Maintenance; Cognitive Level: Knowledge [Remembering]

## 297. ANSWER: 1

1. **Adults see themselves as doers; therefore interactive sessions are most effective when dealing with issues in which the targeted audience has variable knowledge and/or experience. Panel presentation with small-group discussion would be most effective.**
2. Case studies may be useful, but they are not as interactive as a panel presentation and small-group discussion.
3. A lecture may be useful, but it is not as interactive as a panel presentation and small-group discussion.
4. Educational videos may be useful, but they are not as interactive as a panel presentation and small-group discussion.

▶ *Test-taking Tip: This is a session for the teachers (not the junior high students). Apply concepts of adult learning theory to identify the method that would be the most interactive and provide the most discussion.*

Content Area: Management of Care; Concept: Informatics; Integrated Processes: Teaching/Learning; Client Needs: Health Promotion and Maintenance; Cognitive Level: Analysis [Analyzing]

## 298. MoC ANSWER: 3

1. Repeat demonstrations are good for skills; however, they do not necessarily indicate a change in the cognitive or affective domains of learning.
2. Knowing the causes of their infant's disease may increase, not decrease, the parents' anxiety and may be a barrier to learning.
3. **The purpose of education with extremely anxious parents is to reduce the parents' anxiety and provide information to prepare the family to live with the child.**
4. Understanding causes and how to live with the condition are the products of education; however, they are not the *purpose* of education.

▶ *Test-taking Tip: Anxiety is a barrier to learning. Select the option that will reduce this barrier so the teaching will be more effective.*

Content Area: Management of Care; Concept: Nursing Roles; Integrated Processes: Caring; Teaching/Learning; Nursing Process: Planning; Client Needs: Safe and Effective Care Environment: Management of Care; Psychosocial Integrity; Cognitive Level: Application [Applying]

## 299. MoC ANSWER: 4

1. Preoccupation with the illness or grieving as in Option 1 is a barrier to learning.
2. Child fatigue and pain are barriers to learning.
3. Analgesics are a barrier to learning.
4. **Clients most ready to learn are those who are experiencing the least amount of stress and would be the least preoccupied with other concerns. Reading a book, seeking out information, and asking questions are indicators of readiness to learn.**

▶ *Test-taking Tip: Select the option in which the clients face the smallest barrier to learning.*

Content Area: Management of Care; Concept: Nursing Roles; Integrated Processes: Nursing Process: Assessment; Client Needs: Safe and Effective Care Environment: Management of Care; Cognitive Level: Analysis [Analyzing]

## 300. PHARM ANSWER: 3

1. Insulin is administered as a subcutaneous injection. This illustration shows an intradermal administration technique.
2. Insulin is administered as a subcutaneous injection. This illustration shows an intramuscular Z-track administration technique.
3. **Insulin is administered as a subcutaneous injection, which is shown in this illustration.**
4. Insulin is administered as a subcutaneous injection. This illustration shows an intravenous administration technique.

▶ *Test-taking Tip: Insulin for self-administration is only administered via subcutaneous injection. Regular insulin may be administered during hospitalization via an infusion, not via an IV push.*

Content Area: Management of Care; Concept: Medication; Nursing Roles; Integrated Processes: Teaching/Learning; Nursing Process: Evaluation; Client Needs: Physiological Integrity: Pharmacological and Parenteral Therapies; Cognitive Level: Application [Applying]

## 301. MoC ANSWER: 1, 4, 5

1. **The television is a distracter and can affect learning.**
2. Just because the client is elderly does not mean that the client cannot comprehend the information being taught. There is no indication that the client may have a cognitive dysfunction.
3. Just because the client is fully dressed does not mean that the client cannot comprehend the information being taught.
4. **The client squinting suggests that the lettering is too small or that the client does not understand the information in the handout.**

5. **The family entering the room is a distraction and can affect learning.**

▶ *Test-taking Tip: When completing teaching, distracters should be eliminated because these can affect learning. Identify the options that could be distractions.*

Content Area: Management of Care; Concept: Nursing Roles; Integrated Processes: Nursing Process: Evaluation; Client Needs: Safe and Effective Care Environment: Management of Care; Cognitive Level: Evaluation [Evaluating]

### 302. ANSWER: 3

1. The statement in Option 1 is nontherapeutic and challenging.
2. Although the nurse may also write out a list of medications, the list of medications should be reviewed with the client and his wife and not given to the wife.
3. **If the wife will be administering the medications, then both the husband and wife should be included in the teaching. Psychological and situational stressors can interfere with concentration and learning.**
4. Option 4 addresses only setting up the medications and does not reflect the client's comment regarding the wife giving the client the pills.

▶ *Test-taking Tip: Focus on using both therapeutic communication techniques and principles of teaching and learning. Note the key word "best."*

Content Area: Management of Care; Concept: Nursing Roles; Integrated Processes: Communication and Documentation; Client Needs: Health Promotion and Maintenance; Cognitive Level: Application [Applying]

### 303. ANSWER: 2, 6, 3, 4, 1, 5

2. **Collect and analyze information about the client's knowledge of type 2 DM to identify learning needs.**
6. **Identify the client's learning needs.**
3. **Formulate an educational nursing diagnosis and client outcomes for teaching.**
4. **Develop a teaching plan for the client, including content and teaching strategies.**
1. **Implement the teaching plan.**
5. **Evaluate client learning based on the established outcomes.**

▶ *Test-taking Tip: The teaching process is similar to the nursing process. Use the steps of the nursing process to guide correct sequencing of the options.*

Content Area: Management of Care; Concept: Nursing Roles; Integrated Processes: Teaching/Learning; Client Needs: Health Promotion and Maintenance; Cognitive Level: Synthesis [Creating]

### 304. MoC ANSWER: 2

1. Discussion encourages active participation, but it is not the best method for teaching motor skills involved in incision care.

2. **Demonstration is the best method for teaching motor skills. Learning can be exhibited and reinforced by having the client return-demonstrate the incision care.**
3. Reinforcing teaching is not evaluating whether the client has learned.
4. A family member's presence does not ensure that client learning has occurred.

▶ *Test-taking Tip: Use the process of elimination, and eliminate options that do not relate to evaluation. Then select the option that would be best to evaluate the motor skill of incision care.*

Content Area: Management of Care; Concept: Nursing Roles; Integrated Processes: Teaching/Learning; Client Needs: Safe and Effective Care Environment: Management of Care; Cognitive Level: Application [Applying]

### 305. MoC ANSWER: 1, 4, 5

1. **Arthritis can affect manual dexterity, preventing the client from being able to empty and care for the JP drain.**
2. The teaching strategies for younger adults may vary from those of older adults; a mixed-age-group teaching session is not advised. Older adults may need large-print materials, aids to manual dexterity, and repeated opportunities for practice, whereas younger adults may learn more quickly.
3. Providing Web-based references is an unnecessary detail that can lead to confusion with irrelevant information.
4. **An older person may need more time to process information and perform psychomotor skills.**
5. **Regardless of age, if a person is unable to perform a task related to self-care such as managing the drain, a referral should be initiated.**

▶ *Test-taking Tip: Apply principles of teaching and learning for older adults.*

Content Area: Management of Care; Concept: Nursing Roles; Integrated Processes: Nursing Process: Planning; Client Needs: Safe and Effective Care Environment: Management of Care; Cognitive Level: Analysis [Analyzing]

### 306. ANSWER: 2

1. Washing hands before and after the dressing change limits the spread of microorganisms.
2. **The nurse should put on sterile gloves prior to removing the dressing on a central line to prevent contamination of the catheter and site. Once the dressing is removed, the nurse should don a new set of sterile gloves to complete the dressing change. This statement indicates that further teaching is needed.**
3. Asking the client to face away from the site helps prevent catheter-related bloodstream infections from the client's expired air.
4. Cleaning the site with an antiseptic solution helps prevent microorganisms on the client's skin from entering the catheter insertion site.

▶ *Test-taking Tip: The key words are "further teaching needed." Choose the statement that is incorrect.*

Content Area: Management of Care; Concept: Infection; Nursing Roles; Integrated Processes: Nursing Process: Evaluation; Client Needs: Safe and Effective Care Environment: Safety and Infection Control; Physiological Integrity: Reduction of Risk Potential; Cognitive Level: Evaluation [Evaluating]

**307.** MoC **ANSWER: 1, 2, 4, 5**
1. **Computer-assisted instruction is an appropriate learning strategy. The nurse will need to consider whether the client would have access to a hospital-based computer.**
2. **Closed-circuit television programs allow for individual or group learning.**
3. Professionals should lead group sessions and not hospitalized clients, who are in the hospital for health reasons.
4. **Handouts allow learners to learn at their own pace and can be reviewed at a later time.**
5. **Poster boards allow visual learning and can be read at the learner's own pace.**

▶ *Test-taking Tip: The teaching methods depend on the subject matter and the client's background, personality, and needs. Select the options that are most appropriate for the clients who are described in the question, and eliminate Option 3 because it is inappropriate.*

Content Area: Management of Care; Concept: Nursing Roles; Informatics; Integrated Processes: Communication and Documentation; Client Needs: Safe and Effective Care Environment: Management of Care; Cognitive Level: Application [Applying]

**308.** MoC **ANSWER: 1, 2, 4**
1. **The hospital Web site should provide information that is in a format and at a reading level appropriate for educating the client.**
2. **Latest evidence found on the Internet may provide strategies to assist the client in smoking cessation.**
3. Discouraging the client from smoking by citing agency policy is not a supported strategy for smoking cessation.
4. **The American Lung Association is a reputable source for obtaining smoking cessation information.**
5. Conducting a literature search and writing a policy will not be done in time to assist this client.

▶ *Test-taking Tip: Focus on client education and eliminate options that would not educate the client.*

Content Area: Management of Care; Concept: Informatics; Integrated Processes: Caring; Teaching/Learning; Client Needs: Safe and Effective Care Environment: Management of Care; Cognitive Level: Application [Applying]

**309.** MoC **ANSWER: 3**
1. Seating in a triangle would allow the nurse to look directly at the client while communicating but allow the client to see both the nurse and the interpreter.

2. Short statements and questions will allow time for interpretation.
3. **The nurse should maintain eye contact with the client, not the interpreter.**
4. Asking the client to explain back the information will help to ensure that the client understands what is being said.

▶ *Test-taking Tip: The key word is "inappropriate." You should be selecting the incorrect option.*

Content Area: Management of Care; Concept: Diversity; Communication; Integrated Processes: Communication and Documentation; Culture and Spirituality; Client Needs: Safe and Effective Care Environment: Management of Care; Cognitive Level: Application [Applying]

**310.** MoC **ANSWER: 1**
1. **Speaking loudly and instructing the client to calm down immediately when the client is crying and shouting is inappropriate; the nurse should use a normal tone to calmly explore the situation.**
2. Using a simple phrase in the client's native language is appropriate when the client is crying and shouting and may assist the client to communicate what is bothering the client.
3. Calling an interpreter is appropriate because an interpreter may be able to have the client explain what is bothering the client.
4. Being present with the client will enhance security when the client is crying and shouting and is appropriate.

▶ *Test-taking Tip: The key word is "barrier." Eliminate options that promote communication and enhance security.*

Content Area: Management of Care; Concept: Diversity; Communication; Integrated Processes: Nursing Process: Implementation; Culture and Spirituality; Client Needs: Safe and Effective Care Environment: Management of Care; Psychosocial Integrity; Cognitive Level: Application [Applying]

**311.** MoC **ANSWER: 1, 2**
1. **The nurse should utilize a communication picture board to facilitate communication.**
2. **Writing a list of common communication needs in English and Japanese will limit frustration for the client and nurses and facilitate communication.**
3. Having a family member present for translation at all times is unrealistic, and family members are not the best means of translating medical information.
4. There is diversity within specific cultural groups; all Asians do not communicate with the same language.
5. Being culturally sensitive is not the same as being able to communicate effectively with the non-English-speaking client.

▶ *Test-taking Tip: Focus on the goal of the question: effective communication with the non-English-speaking client. Option 4 incorrectly assumes that persons from Asia speak and understand the same language. The stem of the question asks for interventions that promote communication, not cultural sensitivity.*

Content Area: Management of Care; **Concept:** Communication; Diversity; **Integrated Processes:** Nursing Process: Implementation; Culture and Spirituality; **Client Needs:** Safe and Effective Care Environment: Management of Care; **Cognitive Level:** Application [Applying]

### 312. MoC ANSWER: 1, 2, 3, 5

1. The nurse should consider proper use of seat belts because noncompliance with their use is high among Native Americans.
2. The nurse should consider risks of alcohol abuse because alcoholism is a major health concern among Native Americans.
3. The nurse should consider symptoms of lactose intolerance because lactose intolerance is a major health concern among Native Americans.
4. Sports injuries are not a major health concern associated with Native Americans.
5. The nurse should consider prevention of heart disease because heart disease is a major health concern among Native Americans.

▶ **Test-taking Tip:** The key phrase is "major health risks and conditions." In a multiple-response question, there could be more than one correct option. Thus you should focus on the descriptive key words or phrases.

Content Area: Management of Care; **Concept:** Diversity; Nursing Roles; **Integrated Processes:** Teaching/Learning; Culture and Spirituality; **Client Needs:** Safe and Effective Care Environment: Management of Care; **Cognitive Level:** Application [Applying]

### 313. MoC ANSWER: 2

1. Asking the relative to leave is an inappropriate intervention; there is no indication that the client is upset.
2. When the client is speaking loudly, using hand gestures, and repeating phrases, the nurse should close the client's door and allow for privacy.
3. Asking the client and relative to speak softer and lower their tone of voice is an inappropriate intervention because it does not show respect for their communication style.
4. Observing the interaction is inappropriate because it does not respect the client's right to privacy.

▶ **Test-taking Tip:** Do not assume that a person speaking loudly, repeating phrases, and using hand gestures is being argumentative, confrontational, or aggressive.

Content Area: Management of Care; **Concept:** Diversity; Communication; **Integrated Processes:** Nursing Process: Implementation; Culture and Spirituality; **Client Needs:** Safe and Effective Care Environment: Management of Care; **Cognitive Level:** Application [Applying]

### 314. MoC ANSWER: 2, 3, 4, 5

1. The discharge instructions should be written clearly with sufficient text so that clients will take the instructions seriously and follow these; avoid humorous illustrations because what may be perceived as humorous in one culture may be offensive to another.

2. When developing handouts that are culturally sensitive, the nurse manager should utilize available resources such as the parish nurse working with the Spanish-speaking clients in their neighborhood; the nurse would have knowledge and insight into client needs upon discharge.
3. Translating words from English to Spanish would be important, and having the Spanish-speaking client edit it would aid in using language to address the postoperative needs of these specific Spanish-speaking clients.
4. Feedback from Spanish-speaking clients, especially those who have already experienced hospitalization, will help ensure that the instructions are clear and culturally sensitive.
5. Nursing interventions always need to be individualized; the client or family can make note of specific instructions if there is space allocated on the handout.

▶ **Test-taking Tip:** Remember that what may seem humorous to one cultural group may be offensive to another. Merely translating from one language to another does not demonstrate cultural sensitivity. Consider if each option promotes accurate and effective communication of instructions.

Content Area: Management of Care; **Concept:** Diversity; Management; Nursing Roles; **Integrated Processes:** Teaching/Learning; Culture and Spirituality; **Client Needs:** Safe and Effective Care Environment: Management of Care; **Cognitive Level:** Application [Applying]

### 315. MoC ANSWER: 3

1. Using instructions obtained from the Internet is not advisable. The nurse would not know for sure that the appropriate information was being provided.
2. The client is fluent in English; an interpreter is not necessary.
3. The client understands English fluently; therefore the nurse could verbally provide discharge instructions. The client should be given the choice of written instructions in French or English.
4. Providing written instructions in English and French is redundant.

▶ **Test-taking Tip:** When making a selection, don't forget your common sense. If the client is fluent in English, the best option gives the client the choice of the written material that will best suit the client's needs.

Content Area: Management of Care; **Concept:** Diversity; Communication; Informatics; **Integrated Processes:** Teaching/Learning; Culture and Spirituality; **Client Needs:** Safe and Effective Care Environment: Management of Care; **Cognitive Level:** Application [Applying]

### 316. MoC ANSWER: 4

1. Asking the client to identify one's culture demonstrates the nurse's willingness to provide culturally sensitive care.
2. Identifying the client's linguistic competence will promote communication.

3. Asking about life rules can assist the nurse in providing culturally sensitive care.

4. **Asking how the client's lifestyle is different implies a difference and devalues the client's culture. It demonstrates a preference for the American culture.**

▶ **Test-taking Tip:** *This is a false-response question and calls for selecting an incorrect response. When examining options, focus on what is different about the options. Only Option 4 introduces another ethnic group.*

**Content Area:** Management of Care; **Concept:** Communication; Diversity; **Integrated Processes:** Nursing Process: Implementation; Culture and Spirituality; **Client Needs:** Safe and Effective Care Environment: Management of Care; Psychosocial Integrity; **Cognitive Level:** Analysis [Analyzing]

## 317. MoC **ANSWER: 1, 4, 6**

1. **Increased incidence of hypertension in African Americans results in vascular changes, kidney damage, and ESRD.**

2. Skin cancer is not associated with ESRD in African American clients; clients with lighter skin and lower levels of melanin are at increased risk to develop skin cancer.

3. African Americans are at increased risk for lactose intolerance, but this is not a factor for ESRD.

4. **The increased incidence of DM in African Americans leads to vascular complications predisposing the clients to ESRD.**

5. Clients with PKD usually develop ESRD after middle age, but this genetic condition occurs mainly in white clients.

6. **African Americans have an increased incidence of SLE, which may result in lupus nephritis and ESRD.**

▶ **Test-taking Tip:** *Evaluate each option and decide whether the disease occurs more frequently in African Americans, and then decide if the disease results in kidney complications including ESRD. Select the options that meet both criteria.*

**Content Area:** Management of Care; **Concept:** Diversity; Urinary Elimination; Metabolism; **Integrated Processes:** Teaching/Learning; Culture and Spirituality; **Client Needs:** Safe and Effective Care Environment: Management of Care; Physiological Integrity: Reduction of Risk Potential; **Cognitive Level:** Application [Applying]

## 318. MoC **ANSWER: 2**

**The statement about Client A is stereotyping. There is no indication that Client A asked for her husband to be present prior to giving informed consent; the nurse should first ask the client's preference. The statement about Client D is stereotyping. Although Client D may have a common Hispanic last name, there is no indication that the client is Hispanic.**

▶ **Test-taking Tip:** *Stereotyping is assuming that all people with a particular characteristic are the same or have the same beliefs.*

**Content Area:** Management of Care; **Concept:** Diversity; Communication; **Integrated Processes:** Nursing Process: Analysis; Culture and Spirituality; **Client Needs:** Safe and Effective Care Environment: Management of Care; **Cognitive Level:** Analysis [Analyzing]

## 319. MoC **ANSWER: 3**

1. Projecting feelings onto the client does not demonstrate empathy.

2. This statement imposes a personal assumption and does not demonstrate empathy.

3. **This question demonstrates empathy. The nurse is asking a question to allow the client to explain her situation and feelings while the nurse listens. The nurse is attempting to understand the experience as lived by the client.**

4. Acknowledging that laundry is piling up and offering home aide services do not demonstrate empathy. Commenting on the laundry on the first visit may suggest to the client that she lacks support, and she may be defensive or hurt by the acknowledgment.

▶ **Test-taking Tip:** *Empathy is understanding and sharing the thoughts, feelings, or emotions of another.*

**Content Area:** Management of Care; Childbearing; **Concept:** Pregnancy; Communication; **Integrated Processes:** Communication and Documentation; Caring; **Client Needs:** Safe and Effective Care Environment: Management of Care; Health Promotion and Maintenance; **Cognitive Level:** Application [Applying]

## 320. MoC **ANSWER: 2**

1. The central task of infancy is determining trust versus mistrust. Unresolved conflict manifests itself in withdrawal, mistrust, or estrangement.

2. **The behavior indicates an unresolved conflict of "autonomy versus shame and doubt" associated with the 18-month to 3-year-old age group. When parents are overly critical and controlling, the child may develop an overly critical superego. As an adult, it manifests in constantly apologizing for small mistakes.**

3. The central task of the school-aged child is "industry versus inferiority." Unresolved conflict of this stage manifests itself in withdrawal from school and peers, loss of hope, or sense of being mediocre.

4. The central task of adolescence is "identity versus role confusion." If unresolved, it manifests itself in indecisiveness, antisocial behavior, or feelings of confusion.

▶ **Test-taking Tip:** *Focus on the behaviors exhibited by the client. Relate these to behaviors associated with shame and doubt. In doing so, this should lead you to the answer.*

**Content Area:** Management of Care; **Concept:** Promoting Health; Stress; **Integrated Processes:** Nursing Process: Analysis; **Client Needs:** Safe and Effective Care Environment: Management of Care; Health Promotion and Maintenance; **Cognitive Level:** Analysis [Analyzing]

**321.** MoC **ANSWER: 2**

1. Asking a "why" question is asking for information that the client may not be able to express.
2. **Paraphrasing the client's statement encourages the client to verbalize feelings and conveys that the message is understood. An open-ended response allows for a more lengthy response from the client.**
3. Telling the client that dialysis treatment "isn't really hard" devaluates the client's feelings.
4. Telling the client what to do, giving advice, and threatening the client blocks therapeutic communication.

▶ **Test-taking Tip:** *Use therapeutic communication techniques, focusing on the client's statements in the stem. Only one response uses a therapeutic communication technique (paraphrasing).*

**Content Area:** Management of Care; **Concept:** Grief and Loss; Communication; Urinary Elimination; **Integrated Processes:** Caring; Communication and Documentation; **Client Needs:** Safe and Effective Care Environment: Management of Care; Psychosocial Integrity; **Cognitive Level:** Application [Applying]

**322.** MoC **ANSWER: 1**

1. **Using role-playing will allow the child to practice responses so that when teasing occurs, the child should be able to respond appropriately.**
2. Ignoring teasing comments may provoke children to tease more and does not stop the behavior.
3. Although a book about a child being teased and how the child in the book responded to the teasing may be helpful, using humor may not be the most appropriate response.
4. An adult may not always be present when teasing occurs; the child needs to know how to respond to teasing comments.

▶ **Test-taking Tip:** *Use key words in the stem to narrow the options. The key words are "communicating with peers." Only Option 1 pertains to communicating with peers.*

**Content Area:** Management of Care; Child; **Concept:** Development; Metabolism; **Integrated Processes:** Communication and Documentation; **Client Needs:** Safe and Effective Care Environment: Management of Care; Health Promotion and Maintenance; **Cognitive Level:** Application [Applying]

**323.** MoC **ANSWER: 4**

1. The new nurse used therapeutic communication skills of reflecting in the nurse's first question, restating, and an open-ended question in the nurse's second interaction, but this is not the most significant conclusion.
2. The nurse acknowledged the client's feeling in the second interaction, but the final statement by the nurse provided unwarranted and inaccurate reassurance.

3. Even though the nurse should address the son by name, this is not the most significant conclusion.
4. **Persons under stress often do not hear information well and focus on the information that they want to hear. Even though the new nurse explored what the parent did hear, the nurse failed to correct the parent misinformation, "He doesn't need anything," and provide accurate information regarding the treatment plan.**

▶ **Test-taking Tip:** *Read all the options first before trying to analyze each option. Focus on selecting "the most important" option.*

**Content Area:** Management of Care; Child; **Concept:** Bowel Elimination; Communication; Stress; **Integrated Processes:** Communication and Documentation; Caring; **Client Needs:** Safe and Effective Care Environment: Management of Care; Physiological Integrity: Physiological Adaptation; **Cognitive Level:** Analysis [Analyzing]

**324.** MoC **ANSWER: 2**

1. Explanations should be provided by both the nurse and parents to the child using neutral words.
2. **Allowing the child to play with a doll with an eye patch provides the opportunity to play out fears and concerns, and allows clarification of misconceptions. The child should have the opportunity for rehearsing and handling items that will be used in providing care.**
3. A preschooler is egocentric and needs information on how surgery will affect him or her and not on how it affects other children.
4. A 30-minute movie is too long, even if it is animated. A child has a limited concept of time, and a teaching session should be no more than 10 to 15 minutes.

▶ **Test-taking Tip:** *The key phrase is "most definitely," indicating that more than one option may be correct but that one is better than the others.*

**Content Area:** Management of Care; Child; **Concept:** Sensory Perception; Promoting Health; Nursing Roles; **Integrated Processes:** Nursing Process: Planning; **Client Needs:** Safe and Effective Care Environment: Management of Care; Psychosocial Integrity; **Cognitive Level:** Synthesis [Creating]

**325.** MoC **ANSWER: 3**

1. Allowing time for the parents to talk about their feelings is important and should have happened prior to discharge. If the parents need to verbalize, time should be allowed at discharge, but this is not priority.
2. A corticosteroid may be prescribed to reduce joint pain. If on a corticosteroid, the parent and child should be aware of the increased risk for infection, but it is more important to address activity restrictions because this is where the child is likely to be injured.

3. **RF is a serious illness lasting about 6-8 weeks and has many major and minor characteristics and sequelae. This child is at the developmental age and stage at which it is difficult to ensure compliance with activity level, and the child will want to be very active.**

4. Although the child may be concerned about the rash and swollen joints, this is not priority.

▸ *Test-taking Tip: You need to consider the age of the child and the greatest concern upon the child's return to home after being hospitalized.*

**Content Area:** Management of Care; Child; **Concept:** Infection; Nursing Roles; **Integrated Processes:** Teaching/Learning; **Client Needs:** Safe and Effective Care Environment: Management of Care; Physiological Integrity: Physiological Adaptation; **Cognitive Level:** Evaluation [Evaluating]

### 326. MoC ANSWER: 2

1. Interventions to promote parental attachment should be implemented, even if the newborn is very sick and likely to die.

2. **The parents should be encouraged to provide care for their newborn, even if the newborn is very sick and likely to die. If the infant should die, detachment is easier if attachment has been established because the parents will be comforted by the knowledge that they did all they could for their infant while he or she was alive.**

3. Parents may be hesitant to bond with a sick infant; however, attachment should be encouraged, not limited to touching and naming their baby.

4. There is not enough information in the question stem to determine the cause of the cardiac condition, but feelings of guilt and failure often plague parents of sick newborns. Rather than assuring the parents that they did nothing wrong, the nurse should allow the parents to express their feelings.

▸ *Test-taking Tip: Options with absolute words such as "only" are usually incorrect. You should consider which option is most global in promoting parental attachment.*

**Content Area:** Management of Care; Childbearing; **Concept:** Stress; Pregnancy; Nursing Roles; **Integrated Processes:** Nursing Process: Implementation; Caring; **Client Needs:** Safe and Effective Care Environment: Management of Care; Health Promotion and Maintenance; **Cognitive Level:** Application [Applying]

## Chapter Nine

# Advanced Directives and End-of-Life Care

**327.** [MoC] The nurse is assisting the client to complete an HCD. Which information should the nurse discuss? **Select all that apply.**

1. Preference for health care treatment
2. Preference for hospitalization
3. Actions if client confidentiality is violated
4. Wishes for cardiopulmonary resuscitation
5. Names and addresses of all family members
6. Durable power of attorney for health care

**328.** [MoC] The client with end-stage cardiomyopathy states, "I do not want to be resuscitated if I stop breathing." Full resuscitation is noted on the client's medical record under code status. Based on this information, which action should the nurse take **first?**

1. Inform the client's HCP of the client's request.
2. Ask if the client wishes to complete an advance health care directive.
3. Document the client's statements in quotes in the client's medical record.
4. Advise the client to discuss these wishes with the surrogate decision maker.

**329.** [MoC] The unresponsive client is unable to give consent for surgery. The client has an advance health care directive that identifies a friend as the legal health care agent. Who should the nurse contact for obtaining consent for this client?

1. The client's spouse
2. The client's oldest adult child
3. No one; surgery cannot be performed without client consent
4. The client's friend who is identified as the legal health care agent

**330.** The male client newly diagnosed with stage II prostate cancer states to the nurse, "With this diagnosis, I want the doctor to write a *Do not resuscitate* order." Which is the nurse's best **initial** action?

1. Contact the HCP to discuss the client's wishes.
2. Ask the client to share his feelings related to the new diagnosis.
3. Make a referral for the hospital chaplain to come see the client.
4. Ask the client if he knows anyone else who has had prostate cancer.

**331.** The client tells the nurse, "I wish my family would let me die in peace. I'm angry that they keep hovering as if I've given up. I have terminal lung cancer, and there is no cure!" Which is the nurse's **best** therapeutic response?

1. "Your family is hovering over you? I can ask them not to hover and leave if you wish."
2. "You are angry because your family thinks that you have given up hope for a cure?"
3. "Have you talked to your family about your feelings; maybe they will stop hovering?"
4. "You shouldn't feel angry. Your family is just trying to show that they love and care for you."

**332.** The terminally ill client of the Catholic faith is to be weaned from a ventilator. The family requests that the client receive the Anointing of the Sick. Which intervention should be implemented **first** by the nurse?

1. Consult with the charge nurse whether the client is able to receive Anointing of the Sick.
2. Explain to the family that the client must be off the ventilator before anointing can occur.
3. Offer to pray with the family until the client is weaned and removed from the ventilator.
4. Contact a priest and delay discontinuing the ventilator until the priest arrives to see the client.

**333.** The nurse is caring for the client illustrated, who just learned that he has a terminal condition. The client responds as illustrated to the nurse's presence and greeting. Which action should be taken by the nurse?

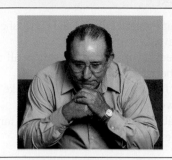

1. Inform the client that you will notify the available hospital chaplain.
2. Ask if the client would like to receive hospice care when discharged.
3. Touch and rub the client's arm and ask him to please make eye contact.
4. State, "You have a lot to think about"; then sit silently with the client.

**334.** **MoC** The client with terminal lung cancer is considering hospice care. Which statement made by the client indicates that the client needs further clarification about hospice care?

1. "Hospice care will shorten the time that I have left to live."
2. "Hospice care will help with keeping my pain under control."
3. "I could go home with hospice care if I had somebody to care for me."
4. "The cost for hospice care will be covered by my Medicare insurance."

**335.** A hospice nurse educator is planning an educational program for employees caring for Islamic clients. Which information should the nurse include in the program? **Select all that apply.**

1. Extended family members usually stay and pray throughout the client's dying process.
2. Female clients of the Islamic faith usually wear loose-fitting, nonrevealing clothing.
3. Fluids are usually refused, so these should be withheld during the dying process.
4. Examination gloves cannot be worn while caring for the deceased client's body.
5. Persons of the same sex and faith as the deceased will perform a cleansing ritual.
6. Anyone providing care should not touch family members when showing support.

**336.** The client of the Orthodox Jewish faith dies after being on hospice care for a month. The hospice nurse and the client's wife and daughter are with the deceased. Which practice by the family should the nurse consider?

1. Prayer five times per day on a prayer rug while facing toward Mecca
2. Mourning for 7 days after burial including no wearing of cosmetics or working
3. The client's body remains unattended while the family prepares for the client's burial
4. No discussion of death because the family members believe it will bring bad luck

**337.** An elderly widow learns she has a terminal condition and tells the nurse, "I am afraid to die." Which is the nurse's **best** response?

1. "I understand that you are frightened. Tell me more about your fears."
2. "What about getting a second opinion? Perhaps there is a new treatment."
3. "You are anxious and need to relax. I'll get the chaplain here to talk with you."
4. "Have you talked to the hospice nurse who could explain about all their services?"

**338.** The client of the Islamic faith suffers a massive stroke and is to receive end-of-life care. Which statement made by the nurse to a coworker is correct in describing Islamic beliefs and end-of-life care?

1. "Mechanical ventilation should be continued until the client's heart stops beating."
2. "A Do Not Resuscitate (DNR) order is allowed if approved by the family and HCP."
3. "Assisted suicide is allowed if the Islamic religious leader knows the client's wishes."
4. "Withdrawal of hydration and nourishment is allowed if there is no hope of recovery."

**339.** The nurse learns that the Muslim female client is a recent widow. In addition to praying, which behavior should the nurse anticipate from the client in dealing with the loss of a loved one?

1. Seeking psychiatric care
2. Utilizing family support
3. Receiving hugs from caregivers
4. Joining a bereavement support group

**340.** The adult daughter of the terminally ill client tells the nurse, "I'll never get to talk to my mom again" and begins to sob. Which is the nurse's **best** response?

1. Suggest to the daughter that she must be very tired and needs to take a break.
2. Tell the daughter that she has been fortunate to have her mom for so many years.
3. State to the daughter that she will always be able to talk to her mother.
4. Pat the daughter's hand, remain silent, and wait for the daughter to speak.

**341.** **MoC** The nurse is assessing the hospitalized client who has ESRD. The client states, "I told Dr. Nelson yesterday that I do not want CPR or drugs if my heart stops beating. Also, I am allergic to Claforan." In reviewing the client's medical record illustrated, which information is most important for the nurse to address with the HCP? Place an X over the most important information.

| EMR | MRN | DOB | HCP |
|---|---|---|---|
| Jung, Jack | 14579 | 12/19/1935 | Dr. Xie |

| Diagnosis | HCD | Code Status | Allergies |
|---|---|---|---|
| ESRD | On File | Full | Cefotaxime |

**342.** A parish nurse leads a bereavement support group for clients whose spouses died over a year ago. Which client should the nurse identify as displaying signs of dysfunctional grieving?

1. The client who states talking to the deceased spouse out loud when making a decision
2. The client who prevents a daughter from donating the clothes of a deceased spouse
3. The client who started a new habit of reading verses from the Bible on a daily basis
4. The client who cries daily and is unable to attend the church where the funeral was held

**343.** The woman who is a Roman Catholic gives birth to an infant who is unlikely to survive. Which should be the nurse's **priority?**

1. Perform Anointing of the Sick.
2. Ensure that the infant is baptized.
3. Notify the woman's husband.
4. Offer to pray the rosary.

**344.** The nurse is caring for the client who is dying. A family member states that burning tobacco leaves during the dying process is a cultural belief, and asks if the family can do this. Which response by the nurse is **best?**

1. Suggest that the family bring the cold ashes of burned tobacco leaves.
2. Tell the client the door must be shut at all times while the leaves burn.
3. Inform the family that the scent will make the client's condition worse.
4. Explain that the hospital does not allow any burning due to risk of a fire.

**345.** **MoC** The hospitalized client practicing the Jewish faith is grieving after being told that the client's condition is terminal. Which is the nurse's **best** intervention to assist in meeting the client's spiritual needs?

1. Bring a crucifix to hang on the wall in the client's room.
2. Call a rabbi at the local synagogue to visit the client.
3. Notify the agency's spiritual care department.
4. Prepare the client for Anointing of the Sick.

**346.** The client's spouse states to a hospice nurse that she regrets that her husband remained agnostic even unto death. Which response by the nurse is **best?**

1. "You tried and it was your husband's choice. You should not blame yourself."
2. "Tell me more about the reason you feel regret about your husband's agnosticism."
3. "Were his parents religious, or did they also not believe that there is a God?"
4. "Would you like me to contact a pastor who will conduct a funeral service?"

**347.** The home health nurse assesses that the client is in need of hospice care. Which should be the nurse's **initial** response when the daughter tells the nurse that she will never agree to hospice care for her father?

1. Immediately notify the client's HCP that the daughter is refusing needed hospice care.
2. Assure the daughter that she has tried her best to provide care, but the client is just too sick.
3. Explain that hospice care can be given in the client's home or in a separate hospice facility.
4. Acknowledge that the daughter is in charge of her parent's care and explore her concerns.

**348.** MoC  The client who is Muslim dies unexpectedly in the hospital ED. Which interventions should the nurse implement? **Select all that apply.**

1. Obtain the family's consent to perform an autopsy.
2. Notify the hospital chaplain to anoint the body.
3. Offer to assist the family with notifying the local Islamic center.
4. Wear examination gloves if needing to touch the deceased person.
5. Allow family members to perform a cleansing ritual.
6. Prepare paperwork for prompt release of the body.

**349.** The client who is Buddhist dies. What should the nurse consider when notifying the client's family about the death?

1. The family may want to bury the client before sundown.
2. The family may want to donate all of the client's organs.
3. The family may want to move the client's body when it is still warm.
4. The family may want to wait for a full year to complete their funeral rites.

**350.** The nurse observes that a parent of a child who just died is rocking the child back and forth and sobbing; the other parent is sitting quietly nearby. Which response by the nurse is most appropriate?

1. "I will certainly remember your child. What things will you recall when you think of him?"
2. "I know this is hard; why don't you go spend some time alone while I prepare his body."
3. "Let me contact the health care provider for a prescribed medication to help calm you."
4. "Tell me what I can do to help you say goodbye to your child who just died."

**351.** PHARM  The terminally ill client is prescribed morphine sulfate 2 to 6 mg IV q2h prn for pain. The nurse administers 2 mg for the first dose, but after 20 minutes the client has no pain relief. Which prescribed medication should the nurse give **now?**

1.
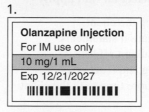

2.
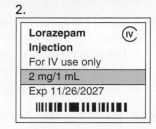

3.
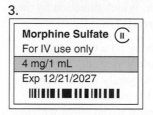

4.
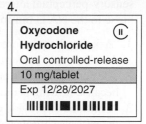

**352.** The nurse calls the family of the terminally ill client to come to the hospital because the client's death is imminent. Which assessment findings indicated that the client's death is near? **Select all that apply.**

1. Rattling sounds with breathing
2. Reports seeing persons who died
3. States that he or she is dying
4. Extremities feel warm to touch
5. BP is 80/55 mm Hg
6. Body held in a fixed, rigid position

**353.** MoC  The client with a terminal illness is hospitalized for palliative care. Which conclusion by the nurse about palliative care is correct?

1. The client will require minimal nursing care because a cure is no longer a treatment option.
2. The client is expected to expire within a short period of time, usually 5 to 7 days.
3. The client is unable to make decisions independently regarding medical treatment.
4. The client will receive care that relieves symptoms without hastening or postponing death.

**354.** The client states to the nurse, "I'm dying from AIDS and I am nothing but a bag of bones. All these sores make my family uncomfortable, and they won't come near me." Which interventions should the nurse implement to assist the client to cope with the disturbed body image? **Select all that apply.**

1. Spend extra time grooming the client.
2. Limit the client's self-negation statements.
3. Initiate a psychiatric consultant referral.
4. Assess the family's coping and reaction.
5. Tell the family to spend more time with the client.

**355.** **MoC** The NA is caring for the dying client who has sensory-perceptual alteration. Which direction by the nurse to the NA is **inappropriate?**

1. "Ask the client before turning on a bright light; the client may prefer a darkened room."
2. "Be sure to whisper or talk quietly to the client because hearing is the last sense to be lost."
3. "Continue to provide comfort to the client with touch; the pressure of touch can still be felt."
4. "Reposition the client slowly; quick repositioning causes dizziness and a sensation of falling."

**356.** The hospitalized client, who is of a different faith than the nurse, states to the nurse, "Would you pray with me?" Which action by the nurse is best?

1. Explain that the nurses are not allowed to pray with clients.
2. Suggest that they pray together the "Our Father" prayer.
3. Offer to sit with the client while the client initiates a prayer.
4. Suggest that the nurse could read from the client's Bible.

**357.** The nurse is caring for four clients of varying religious beliefs who are near death or have died. Which action should the nurse plan?

1. Reposition the bed so it is turned toward Mecca for the client of the Jewish faith.
2. Call a priest to anoint the sick and hear the confession of the client of the Methodist faith.
3. Allow male family members of the Muslim faith to wash the body of a male who just died.
4. Speak to the family of the client of the Buddhist faith about having cremation within 24 hours.

**358.** The parents of a 10-year-old were just told that their child is dying. What is the nurse's **priority?**

1. Support the child's and family's anticipatory grieving.
2. Provide end-of-life comfort care to the child.
3. Teach the family about caring for their child.
4. Allow the client as much independence as possible.

**359.** The nurse is present with the family of the Catholic client who just died. Which statements are therapeutic when the nurse is communicating with the grieving family? **Select all that apply.**

1. "It's all right for you to grieve over the loss of your father."
2. "God has called your loved one home to be with Him."
3. "Everyone has to die sometime. It was your father's time."
4. "I know how you feel. I lost my dad this time last year."
5. "I will be thinking of and praying for you and your family."

**360.** The nurse is counseling a mother who has had prolonged grief after the death of her child. Which statement would assist the nurse in assessing whether the mother is experiencing guilt?

1. "Are you especially troubled by a certain memory or thought?"
2. "Tell me about your favorite memories with your child."
3. "Writing your feelings in a journal helps overcome guilt."
4. "Are there things you are having trouble doing now?"

**361.** The 5-year-old tells the nurse, "If I wish hard enough, I know my mom will come back from the dead." Which should the nurse conclude about the child's statement?

1. The child's statement is characteristic of the child's developmental age.
2. The child's statement is expressing magical thinking.
3. The child is ineffectively coping with the loss of her mother.
4. The child is denying the reality that her mother has died.

**362.** **MoC** The nurse is caring for the adult client who was told an illness is terminal and is offered hospice care. Which statement by the nurse is appropriate?

1. "I know this is not what you wanted to hear."
2. "There is nothing more we can do for you."
3. "We will focus on your comfort and pain control."
4. "Hospice care will help you have a peaceful death."

**363.** The nurse determines that five clients are in five different stages of grief according to Kübler-Ross's stages. Place the five clients in the order of these stages from the first to the last stage.

1. The 45-year-old client who is terminal with breast cancer says to the nurse, "If only God would let me live until I see my son graduate, then I will be ready to die."
2. The 20-year-old client who was just told that his mother and father were killed in an automobile accident says to the nurse, "Check the name again; you must be wrong."
3. The parent whose child died 6 months previously says to the nurse, "I have begun to remove items from my baby's room and given them to my sister, who is having a baby."
4. The 75-year-old woman receiving palliative care for throat cancer refuses tube feedings and refuses to look at herself in the mirror.
5. The parent of the brain-injured child says to the nurse, "You keep disturbing my child with your incessant checking; he isn't getting better because you keep trying to wake him."

Answer: _____

**364.** **MoC** The nurse overhears the client tell his family, "I can't go on with chemotherapy treatments. I want to go home to die." The wife begins crying and responds, "You are giving up!" The son responds, "Dad can get over this if he just tries." The client becomes withdrawn and avoids eye contact with his family. Which nursing diagnosis would be **best** to add to the client's plan of care?

1. Defensive coping
2. Compromised family coping
3. Situational anxiety
4. Dysfunctional grieving

**365.** The 85-year-old spouse of the client, who passed away 2 months ago, states to the nurse, "Thankfully, my friends and family have been driving me places; I don't have a driver's license anymore." How should the nurse interpret the client's statements?

1. Total dependency on others
2. Positive adaptation to the loss
3. An exaggerated grief response
4. Inhibited grief response

**366.** The nurse is counseling the parents of an adolescent with a terminal illness. Which statement is appropriate when helping the parents with decisions about their child's care?

1. "Adolescents should be expected to handle feelings about death in the same way as adults."
2. "Adolescents have the right to make all their own decisions related to their health care."
3. "The Self-Determination Act lets those 16 and older make their own health care decisions."
4. "Adolescents often become angry with treatment changes and loss of independence."

**367.** The nurse is performing postmortem care for the client who died. Which action should be taken by the nurse?

1. Remove the client's dentures and give them to a family member to take home.
2. Wash soiled areas of the client's body and place absorbent pads around the rectal area.
3. Remove all rings, including the wedding band if worn, and give them to security.
4. Turn the client's body side-lying to allow secretions to drain from the oral cavity.

**368.** The client who is dying is talking to her deceased spouse, "I see you at the end of the tunnel in the garden." The family thinks the client is hallucinating and expresses concern to the nurse. Which nursing actions are appropriate? **Select all that apply.**

1. Gently touch the client to reorient the client to time, place, and person.
2. Affirm to the client and family that this is part of a transition from this life.
3. Encourage the family to talk with and reassure the client who is dying.
4. Allow privacy for the family to express their feelings and say their goodbyes.
5. Treat the client's hallucinations by medicating the client with haloperidol.

**369.** MoC The hospice nurse shares with the supervisor that dealing with the death of a specific client has been particularly hard. Which response by the nursing supervisor is **best**?

1. "Take time away from work; I can offer you a temporary management position."
2. "These are commonly felt emotions, and they will lessen with time and experience."
3. "Discussing the situation with a grief counselor may help you overcome these feelings."
4. "Hospice care is not a good fit for you because you would be caring for other dying clients."

**370.** The family of the terminally ill client has decided to withdraw life support. A family member states, "I don't want to be there when he dies. I want to remember him as he was." What is the nurse's **best** response?

1. "I understand completely; I would feel the same way as well."
2. "Your family will understand that you need to do what is best for you."
3. "It's healthy to want to preserve good memories; I'll support you in your decision."
4. "I appreciate how you feel, but be sure so that you won't regret your decision later."

**371.** The nurse is caring for the terminally ill client. Which interventions should the nurse implement to help minimize the stress and frustration experienced by the client and his or her family? **Select all that apply.**

1. Clarifying the rationale for giving pain medication as prescribed
2. Explaining the reason why a diagnostic procedure has been delayed
3. Limiting interactions with them to maximize their private family time
4. Allowing them unlimited access to the staff in order to meet their needs
5. Asking that they repeat information they were given to check for accuracy

**372.** The nurse is caring for the terminally ill client. Which planned intervention will provide the family of the client with the **greatest** sense of both control and satisfaction with the end-of-life care their loved one is receiving?

1. Taking a proactive approach to identifying their concerns
2. Keeping them informed of the client's condition frequently
3. Promptly attending to any care-related problems they identify
4. Respectfully listening to them express their anticipatory grief

**373.** The nurse is communicating with the client receiving hospice care. Which statement is **ineffective** because it displays the nurse's personal beliefs?

1. "Good morning. What would you like me to help you with today?"
2. "You said you were frightened yesterday. Tell me how you feel now."
3. "I feel you made the right choice to go ahead with the tube feedings."
4. "You keep squinting your eyes. Are you having difficulty seeing?"

**374.** MoC After the death of her spouse, the woman confides to the nurse that she feels inadequate to meet the physical and emotional needs of her 1-year-old child. Which **initial** intervention should the nurse implement?

1. Provide information to the woman on normal feelings after the death of a spouse.
2. Contact social services to remove the child from the home to be placed in foster care.
3. Have the woman identify family and friends and ask permission to contact them for care.
4. Assist the client to identify personal needs and develop a plan to meet these needs at home.

**375.** MoC The client requests to die at home in a familiar setting, and hospice care is initiated. Which **initial** action by a hospice nurse would best support family coping?

1. Explaining the roles of all interdisciplinary team members involved in hospice
2. Providing 24-hour home care for meeting the daily basic care needs of the client
3. Telling the family about the bereavement visits made after the death of the client
4. Coordinating care when and if the client needs to be readmitted to the hospital

**INSTRUCTIONS:** Use the information presented in the table below to answer Questions 376 and 377.

| PRN Medications | 0000–0759 | 0800–1559 | 1600–2359 |
|---|---|---|---|
| Hydromorphone 0.5–2 mg IV q30 min prn | 0500 NNN 0.5 mg<br>0640 PRD 0.5 mg<br>0725 NNN 1 mg<br>0745 PRD 1 mg | 0815 KAO 1.5 mg<br>0850 KAO 0.5 mg<br>0920 JJR 2 mg | |

**376.** CJ PHARM The terminally ill client is receiving comfort care. At 9:45 a.m., the nurse checks the client's MAR to determine the dose of hydromorphone to administer. How many mg of hydromorphone did the client receive in the last 4 hours?

_____ mg (Record your answer rounded to the nearest tenth.)

**377.** CJ PHARM What is the nurse's legal responsibility after reviewing the information on the MAR? Enter the information into the box below.

[   ]

## Answers and Rationales

**327.** MoC **ANSWER: 1, 2, 4, 6**
1. **The nurse should discuss the client's preferences for health care treatment in the future, when the client may be unable to make personal treatment choices.**
2. **Preference for hospitalization may be included on the advance HCD.**
3. Actions to be taken if client confidentiality is violated do not pertain to directions for future health care.
4. **Wishes for CPR pertain to directions for future health care and should be discussed.**
5. It would be inappropriate to include the names and addresses of all family members on the health care directive; include only those who are named as the durable power of attorney for health care.
6. **Durable power of attorney for health care is the person or persons who will be making health care decisions when the client is unable to make these decisions.**

♦ *Test-taking Tip: An advance health care directive is a written document that provides direction for health care in the future, when the client may be unable to make personal decisions. Consider which options relate specifically to health care.*

**Content Area:** Management of Care; **Concept:** Legal; Management; **Integrated Processes:** Nursing Process: Assessment; **Client Needs:** Safe and Effective Care Environment: Management of Care; **Cognitive Level:** Application [Applying]

**328.** MoC **ANSWER: 1**
1. **The HCP must prescribe "Do not resuscitate" to act on the client's wishes. The nurse should notify the HCP immediately.**
2. The client can complete an HCD to make wishes known, but this is not the first action.
3. The nurse should document the client's statements in quotes as they are stated to the nurse.
4. Advising the client to discuss wishes with the surrogate decision maker is important so that the client's wishes are followed when the client is unable to make decisions, but this is not first.

▶ *Test-taking Tip:* The key word is "first." DNR status needs to be prescribed by the HCP before it can be implemented.

**Content Area:** Management of Care; **Concept:** Management; Legal; **Integrated Processes:** Nursing Process: Implementation; **Client Needs:** Safe and Effective Care Environment: Management of Care; **Cognitive Level:** Application [Applying]

### 329. MoC ANSWER: 4

1. The client's spouse is not named as the legal health care agent to make decisions on the client's behalf when the client is unable to do so.
2. The client's oldest adult child is not named as the legal health care agent to make decisions on the client's behalf when the client is unable to do so.
3. The legal health care agent can provide consent.
4. **Because the client has named a friend as the durable power of attorney for health care (health care agent), that person should be contacted to make health care decisions when the client is unable to do so.**

▶ *Test-taking Tip:* The health care directive specifies the wishes of the client when the client is unable to make decisions related to health care.

**Content Area:** Management of Care; **Concept:** Legal; Management; **Integrated Processes:** Nursing Process: Analysis; **Client Needs:** Safe and Effective Care Environment: Management of Care; **Cognitive Level:** Analysis [Analyzing]

### 330. ANSWER: 2

1. Contacting the HCP would be a priority but not the best initial action; the client may be asking for the order as a reaction to fear generated by the new diagnosis.
2. **Asking the client to share his feelings related to the new diagnosis would be the best initial action to determine why the client desires this new DNR order and would encourage communication between the nurse and client.**
3. Making a referral for the hospital chaplain may be helpful if the client desires it, but the nurse should assess the client's feelings first.
4. Asking the client if he knows anyone else who has had prostate cancer may be helpful in the working phase of the relationship, when the nurse and client are exploring alternatives together, but it would not be the best initial action.

▶ *Test-taking Tip:* Use the nursing process of assessment to gather additional information from the client.

**Content Area:** Management of Care; **Concept:** Stress; Cellular Regulation; Legal; **Integrated Processes:** Nursing Process: Implementation; **Client Needs:** Psychosocial Integrity; **Cognitive Level:** Analysis [Analyzing]

### 331. ANSWER: 2

1. The nurse is repeating what the client has stated as a closed statement and offers a solution. It does not promote a therapeutic interaction.
2. **The nurse is restating what the client says to ensure understanding and to review what the client has said. Restating is a therapeutic communication technique.**
3. The nurse is attempting to assess the client's ability to discuss feelings openly with family members, which is premature. It can also be misconstrued as offering advice, which hinders therapeutic communication.
4. The nurse is belittling the client's feelings, which hinders therapeutic communication.

▶ *Test-taking Tip:* Focus on the only option that uses a therapeutic communication technique.

**Content Area:** Management of Care; **Concept:** Communication; Grief and Loss; **Integrated Processes:** Communication and Documentation; **Client Needs:** Psychosocial Integrity; **Cognitive Level:** Analysis [Analyzing]

### 332. ANSWER: 4

1. Consulting the charge nurse will delay contacting the priest and prolong the time the client is on the ventilator. The nurse caring for the client should know that Anointing of the Sick is a practice within the Catholic faith.
2. The client may receive Anointing of the Sick while on the ventilator.
3. The nurse should first notify a Catholic priest and then offer to pray with the family. Praying is not a substitute for the Anointing of the Sick.
4. **Roman Catholics believe the Anointing of the Sick should be given prior to death, and the nurse should respect the family's wishes and delay the terminal weaning. The client may or may not survive long after the ventilator has been discontinued.**

▶ *Test-taking Tip:* The word "sick" implies that the person is alive. Select the option that allows the client to receive the anointing and sacrament while still alive.

**Content Area:** Management of Care; **Concept:** Grief and Loss; Diversity; **Integrated Processes:** Nursing Process: Implementation; Culture and Spirituality; **Client Needs:** Psychosocial Integrity; **Cognitive Level:** Application [Applying]

### 333. ANSWER: 4

1. Suggesting the presence of a chaplain is an appropriate intervention but should occur after the client has had time to deal with the news.
2. The client is not ready to deal with future decisions such as hospice care.
3. It would be insensitive to "intrude" when the client is drawn inward with his own thoughts.
4. **The nurse makes an empathic statement and then is present and supportive of the client.**

▶ *Test-taking Tip:* The illustration and question should help you determine that the client is likely in a state of shock and disbelief from learning he has a terminal condition. Option 4 offers the client the needed support and the nurse's presence.

Content Area: Management of Care; Concept: Communication; Grief and Loss; Integrated Processes: Communication and Documentation; Client Needs: Psychosocial Integrity; Cognitive Level: Analysis [Analyzing]

**334. MoC ANSWER: 1**

1. **Hospice care neither hastens nor extends the life of the client; this statement indicates the client needs further education.**
2. Hospice maintains the quality of life with pain and symptom control during the dying process.
3. Hospice care can be delivered in a home setting, nursing home, or a specific hospice unit.
4. Medicare insurance covers the cost of hospice care.

▶ **Test-taking Tip:** Note that the question calls for the incorrect response. Eliminate Options 2, 3, and 4, which are correct about hospice care.

Content Area: Management of Care; Concept: Grief and Loss; Nursing Roles; Integrated Processes: Nursing Process: Evaluation; Client Needs: Safe and Effective Care Environment: Management of Care; Psychosocial Integrity; Physiological Integrity: Physiological Adaptation; Cognitive Level: Evaluation [Evaluating]

**335. ANSWER: 1, 2, 5, 6**

1. **It is a common practice for members of the Islamic faith to gather around the bedside of a dying person and pray because they feel closer to God.**
2. **A female of the Islamic faith will wear traditional clothing (hijab) even during the dying process to maintain modesty.**
3. The Islamic faith prohibits discontinuing hydration and nourishment, and fluids should continue to be offered.
4. Gloves should be worn by caregivers if handling the body; however, caregivers should avoid touching the body of the deceased.
5. **A cleansing ritual is performed by members of the Islamic center and the family.**
6. **Typically, family members of the Islamic faith do not appreciate being hugged or touched by caregivers who may want to show support or sympathy.**

▶ **Test-taking Tip:** Recall that the Islamic faith contains precepts respecting life and limiting contact with persons outside of the Islamic faith. Select options that respect Islam and limit outsider contact.

Content Area: Management of Care; Concept: Diversity; Grief and Loss; Integrated Processes: Teaching/Learning; Culture and Spirituality; Client Needs: Psychosocial Integrity; Physiological Integrity: Basic Care and Comfort; Cognitive Level: Application [Applying]

**336. ANSWER: 2**

1. Muslims, not Orthodox Jews, pray five times per day and face Mecca.
2. **Shiva occurs during the first 7 days of mourning after burial, and the nurse can expect during Shiva that the client's wife and daughter will not be working, wearing cosmetics, cutting their hair, or changing their clothes.**

3. Orthodox Jews do not leave the body of the deceased unattended.
4. In some Southeast Asian cultures, discussing death is thought to bring bad luck; this is not a belief of Orthodox Jews.

▶ **Test-taking Tip:** Recall that in Judaism there is a strong belief in the sacredness of life.

Content Area: Management of Care; Concept: Diversity; Grief and Loss; Integrated Processes: Nursing Process: Evaluation; Culture and Spirituality; Client Needs: Psychosocial Integrity; Cognitive Level: Evaluation [Evaluating]

**337. ANSWER: 1**

1. **The best response when the client expresses fear about dying should be to respond with empathy, clarify that the client is fearful, and encourage further expression.**
2. The nurse is ignoring the client's concern about dying and changing the subject to obtaining a second opinion.
3. The nurse is incorrectly making a judgment about the client's comment and blaming the client for not relaxing.
4. The nurse is ignoring the client's statement about not wanting to die and supporting the hospice option.

▶ **Test-taking Tip:** In communication questions, select the option that demonstrates therapeutic communication and eliminate those that utilize blocks to therapeutic communication.

Content Area: Management of Care; Concept: Communication; Grief and Loss; Integrated Processes: Communication and Documentation; Client Needs: Psychosocial Integrity; Cognitive Level: Application [Applying]

**338. MoC ANSWER: 2**

1. Prolonging life with the use of machines for an extended amount of time is not encouraged in the Islamic faith.
2. **Under appropriate circumstances, the HCP may issue a DNR order with the approval of the family; this is the correct nurse's statement.**
3. Islam prohibits assisted suicide.
4. Islam prohibits the withdrawal of hydration and nourishment.

▶ **Test-taking Tip:** Life is considered sacred for those of the Islamic faith. Eliminate Options 3 and 4.

Content Area: Management of Care; Concept: Diversity; Grief and Loss; Integrated Processes: Communication and Documentation; Culture and Spirituality; Client Needs: Safe and Effective Care Environment: Management of Care; Cognitive Level: Application [Applying]

**339. ANSWER: 2**

1. Muslims are reluctant to seek psychiatric care.
2. **The nurse should anticipate that family members of the Muslim client will be present as a source of support while the client is grieving the loss of a loved one.**

3. Generally Muslims do not want to be touched by persons outside of specific family members.
4. Generally Muslims do not utilize community bereavement services.

▶ *Test-taking Tip: Recall that Muslim culture finds its Islamic faith and family to be major sources of support.*

**Content Area:** Management of Care; **Concept:** Nursing Roles; Diversity; Grief and Loss; **Integrated Processes:** Nursing Process: Planning; Culture and Spirituality; **Client Needs:** Psychosocial Integrity; **Cognitive Level:** Application [Applying]

## 340. ANSWER: 4

1. The nurse is changing the subject and not addressing the daughter's loss.
2. The nurse is giving the daughter false reassurance and not addressing her concern.
3. The nurse is answering the daughter with a cliché and not addressing the daughter's concern.
4. **The nurse is using touch and nonverbal communication to convey understanding to the daughter; this is the nurse's best response.**

▶ *Test-taking Tip: Identify therapeutic communication techniques and select the nonverbal technique that demonstrates the nurse is listening and is present for the daughter. Eliminate Options 1, 2, and 3, which are blocks to therapeutic communication.*

**Content Area:** Management of Care; **Concept:** Communication; Grief and Loss; **Integrated Processes:** Communication and Documentation; **Client Needs:** Psychosocial Integrity; **Cognitive Level:** Analysis [Analyzing]

## 341. MoC ANSWER:

| EMR | MRN | DOB | HCP |
|---|---|---|---|
| Jung, Jack | 14579 | 12/19/1935 | Dr. Xie |

| Diagnosis | HCD | ~~Code Status~~ | Allergies |
|---|---|---|---|
| ESRD | On File | ~~Full~~ | Cefotaxime |

**The most important information to address with the HCP is the client's code status. The client requested no CPR or drugs. The code status needs to be changed to "No Code." This must be prescribed by the HCP. The EMR indicates that Dr. Peterson is the HCP; another HCP covers for the primary HCP when not working. Claforan is the trade name for cefotaxime.**

▶ *Test-taking Tip: The key words are "most important." You need to consider the safety of the client and the client's expressed wishes.*

**Content Area:** Management of Care; **Concept:** Nursing Roles; Informatics; Management; **Integrated Processes:** Nursing Process: Analysis; **Client Needs:** Safe and Effective Care Environment: Management of Care; **Cognitive Level:** Analysis [Analyzing]

## 342. ANSWER: 4

1. The client talking with a deceased spouse is using an appropriate coping strategy because the client acknowledges that the spouse is deceased.

2. The client is dealing with the loss but is not ready to depart with treasured possessions; this does not indicate dysfunctional grieving.
3. The client is using an appropriate coping strategy for the loss of a loved one by becoming more spiritual and insightful.
4. **The nurse should identify that the client who cries daily and is unable to attend church where the funeral was held is displaying dysfunctional grieving.**

▶ *Test-taking Tip: The key words are "dysfunctional grieving." You should select the client who is unable to cope with daily life beyond a year following a spouse's death.*

**Content Area:** Management of Care; **Concept:** Nursing Roles; Grief and Loss; **Integrated Processes:** Nursing Process: Assessment; **Client Needs:** Psychosocial Integrity; **Cognitive Level:** Analysis [Analyzing]

## 343. ANSWER: 2

1. Although the woman may wish for Anointing of the Sick, this is completed by a priest and not the nurse.
2. **Ensuring that the infant is baptized should be the nurse's priority; Catholics may believe infant baptism is necessary for salvation.**
3. There is no indication that the woman giving birth to the seriously ill infant is married.
4. Although the woman may wish to pray the rosary, the nurse's priority would be to ensure that the infant is baptized.

▶ *Test-taking Tip: A mother who is Catholic may want baptism performed at birth for a seriously ill infant. This may be performed by the nurse or HCP if a priest is not present.*

**Content Area:** Management of Care; **Concept:** Diversity; Grief and Loss; **Integrated Processes:** Nursing Process: Implementation; Culture and Spirituality; **Client Needs:** Psychosocial Integrity; **Cognitive Level:** Application [Applying]

## 344. ANSWER: 1

1. **The nurse's best response to the family's request to burn tobacco leaves is to suggest bringing the cold ashes of burned tobacco leaves. This is a compromise that shows support of the cultural beliefs; if this suggestion is not acceptable, the client's family will inform the nurse, and additional options can be explored.**
2. Open flames are not allowed in any health care facility; closing the door would violate agency policy.
3. Informing the family that the scent will make the client's condition worse is not necessarily true; the client is dying.
4. Although the hospital should not allow any burning, the nurse should support the cultural beliefs of the dying client and family; this response is not the best.

▶ *Test-taking Tip: The nurse should support the client's cultural beliefs as long as their practice is not contraindicated in the client's care. The key word is "best." If more than one answer seems correct, select the one that best supports the client's cultural beliefs.*

Content Area: Management of Care; Concept: Diversity; Grief and Loss; Integrated Processes: Nursing Process: Implementation; Culture and Spirituality; Client Needs: Psychosocial Integrity; Cognitive Level: Analysis [Analyzing]

## 345. MoC ANSWER: 3

1. A crucifix is a representation of Jesus Christ on the cross and is associated with the Catholic faith, not Judaism.
2. Although calling a rabbi would be appropriate, this does not keep other disciplines involved in the care of the client informed.
3. **The nurse's best intervention to provide spiritual support to the client who is Jewish is to contact the agency's spiritual care department if desired by the client. The nurse should relay a request for a rabbi so that all disciplines remain informed throughout the care delivery process.**
4. Anointing of the Sick is a practice in Catholicism and some other religions, but it is not a Jewish religious practice.

▶ *Test-taking Tip: The key word "best" indicates that two or more options may be correct, but one is better than the other option. The nurse should be collaborating and keeping other disciplines informed about the care of the client.*

Content Area: Management of Care; Concept: Diversity; Grief and Loss; Integrated Processes: Nursing Process: Implementation; Culture and Spirituality; Client Needs: Safe and Effective Care Environment: Management of Care; Cognitive Level: Application [Applying]

## 346. ANSWER: 2

1. The nurse is giving advice and not addressing the wife's concern.
2. **The nurse is using an open-ended response to clarify the meaning of the wife's comment so that the wife's real concerns can be addressed.**
3. The nurse is asking questions and not focusing on the wife's present concern. It also defines atheism, rejection of belief in the existence of deities including God, and not agnosticism.
4. The nurse is changing the subject, moving on to a memorial service, and not addressing the wife's present concern.

▶ *Test-taking Tip: Agnostics believe that it is impossible to know for certain the existence or nonexistence of deities including God and thus may not practice any faith. Focus on selecting an option that includes therapeutic communication, and eliminate options that block communication.*

Content Area: Management of Care; Concept: Communication; Grief and Loss; Diversity; Integrated Processes: Communication and Documentation; Culture and Spirituality; Client Needs: Psychosocial Integrity; Cognitive Level: Application [Applying]

## 347. ANSWER: 4

1. Ignoring the daughter's statement blocks communication and does not address the daughter's present concerns and possible misunderstanding about hospice.

2. The nurse is belittling the daughter by not acknowledging her concerns.
3. The nurse is giving information but is not addressing the daughter's present concerns.
4. **The nurse's initial response should be to confirm that the daughter is in control and address the daughter's immediate concerns. The daughter may be feeling powerless and unsupported.**

▶ *Test-taking Tip: Your initial response should be to address and explore the daughter's immediate concern using techniques of therapeutic communication.*

Content Area: Management of Care; Concept: Grief and Loss; Communication; Integrated Processes: Communication and Documentation; Client Needs: Psychosocial Integrity; Cognitive Level: Analysis [Analyzing]

## 348. MoC ANSWER: 1, 3, 4, 5, 6

1. **The nurse should obtain consent for an autopsy. Although these are discouraged, they are allowed for legal circumstances under Islamic law.**
2. A minister of another faith would not be permitted to anoint the body of the deceased.
3. **The nurse should offer to assist family members with making contacts because the death was unexpected.**
4. **Although the body of the deceased should not be touched by persons who are not of the Islamic faith, in cases where it is necessary the nurse should wear examination gloves.**
5. **The nurse should allow for a cleansing ritual that is performed by family members of the Islamic faith.**
6. **The nurse should prepare paperwork and ensure a prompt release of the body because Islamic law requires death rites and burial be completed within 24 hours.**

▶ *Test-taking Tip: A Muslim is of the Islamic faith and believes in respecting life and limiting contact with persons outside of the Islamic faith. Select options that respect Islam and limit outsider contact.*

Content Area: Management of Care; Concept: Diversity; Grief and Loss; Integrated Processes: Caring; Culture and Spirituality; Client Needs: Safe and Effective Care Environment: Management of Care; Cognitive Level: Analysis [Analyzing]

## 349. ANSWER: 2

1. Orthodox Jews generally bury the body before sundown.
2. **Buddhists consider it an act of mercy to donate organs and encourage it.**
3. Buddhists may refuse to move the body after death until it is cold, believing that time is needed for the spirit of the dead to leave the body.
4. Hindus will want to wait for a full year to complete their funeral rites. Buddhists have elaborate rituals so that the soul of the deceased has unhindered passage to its next destination, but the rituals do not take a full year.

▶ **Test-taking Tip:** Narrow the options by eliminating statements associated with Orthodox Jews and Hindus.

**Content Area:** Management of Care; **Concept:** Diversity; Grief and Loss; **Integrated Processes:** Nursing Process: Planning; Culture and Spirituality; **Client Needs:** Psychosocial Integrity; **Cognitive Level:** Analysis [Analyzing]

### 350. ANSWER: 1

1. **Allowing reminiscence can facilitate parental coping and provide the parents with an opportunity to say goodbye. The parents should be provided adequate time to understand that their child has died.**
2. When attempting to move the parents out of the room, the nurse is not considering where the parents are in the process of saying goodbye.
3. Offering to obtain a prescribed medication for the parents is inappropriate; the parents' grief is real.
4. Although the nurse is offering support to the parents, grieving parents typically are unable to articulate what they need.

▶ **Test-taking Tip:** Select the option that responds to the parents' grief and provides support. Eliminate Options 2 and 3 because the parents would be separated from the nurse. Eliminate Option 4 because the focus is on the nurse rather than on the deceased child and his parents.

**Content Area:** Management of Care; **Concept:** Grief and Loss; Communication; **Integrated Processes:** Communication and Documentation; Caring; **Client Needs:** Psychosocial Integrity; **Cognitive Level:** Analysis [Analyzing]

### 351. PHARM ANSWER: 3

1. Olanzapine (Zyprexa) is an atypical antipsychotic; it would not be effective for pain control.
2. Lorazepam (Ativan) is an antianxiety medication; it would not be effective for pain control.
3. **The nurse should give 4 mg of morphine sulfate IV. The client's total dose of morphine sulfate is 6 mg in a 2-hour period. Because the client had no relief after 20 minutes and no side effects, 4 mg should be administered to maximize pain control. The peak time for morphine sulfate administered IV is 20 minutes.**
4. Oxycodone hydrochloride (Oxycontin) is a narcotic analgesic, but because it is controlled-release and given orally, it would have a slower onset of action for pain control.

▶ **Test-taking Tip:** Select the option that maximizes immediate pain control.

**Content Area:** Management of Care; **Concept:** Comfort; Medication; Grief and Loss; **Integrated Processes:** Nursing Process: Implementation; **Client Needs:** Physiological Integrity: Pharmacological and Parenteral Therapies; Physiological Integrity: Basic Care and Comfort; **Cognitive Level:** Analysis [Analyzing]

### 352. ANSWER: 1, 2, 3, 6

1. **The inability to swallow saliva leads to its accumulation in the back of the throat, causing a rattling sound with breathing, or a death rattle.**
2. **Altered brain function may cause hallucinations of seeing persons who have died.**
3. **Some people report knowing that he or she is dying.**
4. Extremities will feel cold to touch, not warm, due to a lowering of the BP and its compensatory mechanism to shunt blood to vital organs.
5. A BP of 80/55 mm Hg has an MAP of 63, indicating that organs are adequately perfused. The systolic BP would be below 70 mm Hg and the diastolic BP below 50 mm Hg when death is imminent.
6. **Loss of muscle tone may cause diminished movement.**

▶ **Test-taking Tip:** Besides physical signs of imminent death, the client may express feelings of impending death. Eliminate Option 4 because it is opposite of expected findings. You need to calculate the mean arterial pressure to evaluate Option 5 as an answer.

**Content Area:** Management of Care; **Concept:** Grief and Loss; **Integrated Processes:** Nursing Process: Evaluation; **Client Needs:** Physiological Integrity: Physiological Adaptation; **Cognitive Level:** Evaluation [Evaluating]

### 353. MoC ANSWER: 4

1. The client and family will require more than minimal care; palliative care is complex.
2. There is not a specific timetable involved with the client's life expectancy.
3. Clients participate in deciding symptom control options until actively dying.
4. **Palliative care is supportive and compassionate care given to clients who opt not to seek curative treatment for a terminal illness. Treatment focuses on symptom control and assisting the client and family through preparation for and through the dying process.**

▶ **Test-taking Tip:** Palliative care is often complex; it includes support for clients and their families while controlling the client's symptoms such as pain.

**Content Area:** Management of Care; **Concept:** Grief and Loss; Nursing Roles; **Integrated Processes:** Nursing Process: Analysis; **Client Needs:** Safe and Effective Care Environment: Management of Care; **Cognitive Level:** Analysis [Analyzing]

### 354. ANSWER: 1, 2, 3, 4

1. **Spending extra time with the client may promote the client's verbalization of feelings and aid in the client's coping. Appearance-enhancing measures can promote the client's sense of control and enhance self-esteem.**

2. **Self-negating statements can prolong the issue of a disturbed self-image and can interfere with maintaining the highest quality of life possible at the end of life.**
3. **Collaboration promotes a holistic care plan and can hasten problem solving.**
4. **Additional information about the family responses can aid in planning interventions for the client and family. The family's reaction could be related to anticipatory grieving and not to the client's appearance or illness.**
5. The family may feel uncomfortable, and telling them to spend more time may increase their discomfort and result in less time with the client.

▶ *Test-taking Tip: Use the process of elimination to eliminate the one option that could increase the client's feelings of a disturbed body image.*

Content Area: Management of Care; Concept: Stress; Grief and Loss; Integrated Processes: Nursing Process: Implementation; Client Needs: Psychosocial Integrity; Cognitive Level: Synthesis [Creating]

**355. MoC ANSWER: 2**
1. Preferences when dying may include a dark or light room. Light sensitivity may occur, yet shadows may result in confusion or hallucinations.
2. **The nurse should not direct the NA to whisper or talk quietly. Although hearing is the last sense to be lost when dying, speech should be clear and not whispering.**
3. The NA should continue to touch the client. Even though the sensation of touch is diminished when dying, the pressure of touch is still felt.
4. A dying person's physiological alterations such as hypotension can cause dizziness and altered sensations. The NA should reposition the client slowly.

▶ *Test-taking Tip: The key word is "inappropriate." Select the option that is not correct.*

Content Area: Management of Care; Concept: Cognition; Grief and Loss; Integrated Processes: Nursing Process: Implementation; Client Needs: Safe and Effective Care Environment: Management of Care; Physiological Integrity: Physiological Adaptation; Cognitive Level: Analysis [Analyzing]

**356. ANSWER: 3**
1. It is appropriate for the nurse to pray with a client who initiated the request.
2. The nurse's suggestion limits the type and purpose of the prayer.
3. **The nurse should allow the client to choose the prayer that meets the client's spiritual needs. The nurse should not be expected to pray with the client, but to be present for the client.**
4. The nurse changes the subject and refuses to meet the client's expressed request.

▶ *Test-taking Tip: Select the option that addresses the client's immediate request and respects the religious preferences of the client and the nurse.*

Content Area: Management of Care; Concept: Diversity; Integrated Processes: Cultural and Spirituality; Client Needs: Psychosocial Integrity; Cognitive Level: Application [Applying]

**357. ANSWER: 3**
1. Muslims, not Jews, who are dying want their body or heads turned toward Mecca.
2. A priest would anoint the sick for a person of the Catholic, not Methodist, faith.
3. **Persons of the Islamic faith believe in special procedures for care of the body after death, including a ritual bath with male family members washing male bodies or females washing female bodies.**
4. Hindus cremate the body within 24 hours to release the soul from any earthly attachment.

▶ *Test-taking Tip: Focus on both the action and the faith of the client to narrow the options.*

Content Area: Management of Care; Concept: Nursing Roles; Diversity; Grief and Loss; Integrated Processes: Nursing Process: Planning; Culture and Spirituality; Client Needs: Psychosocial Integrity; Cognitive Level: Analysis [Analyzing]

**358. ANSWER: 1**
1. **Anticipatory grieving consists of psychological and physiological responses to an impending real or imagined loss of a significant person, object, belief, or relationship. Because the child and family will be overwhelmed with the news, this is priority.**
2. Providing comfort cares may be pertinent, but this is not a priority.
3. Teaching may be pertinent, but this is not a priority.
4. Allowing independence may be pertinent depending on the child's state, but this is not a priority.

▶ *Test-taking Tip: The key word is "priority." Use steps of the grieving process to answer this question. The first grief response is shock. The nurse's focus should be on the client and the family.*

Content Area: Management of Care; Concept: Nursing Roles; Grief and Loss; Integrated Processes: Caring; Client Needs: Psychosocial Integrity; Physiological Integrity: Basic Care and Comfort; Cognitive Level: Analysis [Analyzing]

**359. ANSWER: 1, 5**
1. **This statement conveys nonjudgmental acceptance of grief.**
2. This statement minimizes the client's death and is a block to therapeutic communication.
3. Telling the family that everyone has to die and that it was their father's time is minimizing the family's grief and a block to therapeutic communication.
4. Stating that the nurse knows how the family feels is not helpful and a block to therapeutic communication. The focus is on the nurse and not the client's family.
5. **The nurse is conveying nonjudgmental acceptance and offering support through prayer.**

▶ *Test-taking Tip:* Focus on therapeutic communication techniques and eliminate options that would be a barrier to communication or grieving.

**Content Area:** Management of Care; **Concept:** Communication; Grief and Loss; **Integrated Processes:** Communication and Documentation; **Client Needs:** Psychosocial Integrity; **Cognitive Level:** Analysis [Analyzing]

### 360. ANSWER: 1

1. **Asking the mother if she is especially troubled by a certain memory or thought is an assessment-type question that should elicit additional information. Feelings of guilt or regret can delay the normal grieving process.**
2. This is an open-ended statement that supports the mother's expression of positive memories, and is an intervention.
3. Encouraging journaling is an intervention.
4. This is a question to assess coping skills.

▶ *Test-taking Tip:* Use the nursing process and eliminate options that do not relate to assessment but rather interventions. Of the two remaining options, determine which would be best.

**Content Area:** Management of Care; **Concept:** Communication; Grief and Loss; Assessment; **Integrated Processes:** Nursing Process: Assessment; **Client Needs:** Psychosocial Integrity; **Cognitive Level:** Application [Applying]

### 361. ANSWER: 1

1. **Children ages 5 to 6 years believe in the power of wishes and perceive death as unnatural, reversible, and avoidable.**
2. Magical thinking is expressed by children younger than 5 years.
3. There is no indication that the child is coping ineffectively.
4. There is no indication that the child is denying the reality of the mother's death.

▶ *Test-taking Tip:* Think about the developmental level of a 5- to 6-year-old and his or her experience with death.

**Content Area:** Management of Care; **Concept:** Grief and Loss; Communication; **Integrated Processes:** Nursing Process: Evaluation; **Client Needs:** Psychosocial Integrity; **Cognitive Level:** Evaluation [Evaluating]

### 362. MoC ANSWER: 3

1. This statement does not offer the client realistic hope.
2. This statement does not offer the client realistic hope.
3. **This statement focuses on the needs of the client and offers realistic hope for symptom and pain control.**
4. This statement focuses on what hospice care can do and not on the immediate needs of the client.

▶ *Test-taking Tip:* Focus on an option that meets the immediate needs of the client.

**Content Area:** Management of Care; **Concept:** Communication; Grief and Loss; **Integrated Processes:** Communication and Documentation; **Client Needs:** Safe and Effective Care Environment: Management of Care; **Cognitive Level:** Analysis [Analyzing]

### 363. ANSWER: 2, 5, 1, 4, 3

2. **The 20-year-old client who was just told that his mother, father, and two younger siblings were killed in an automobile accident is in denial.**
5. **The parent of a brain-injured child who says to the nurse, "You keep disturbing my child with your incessant checking; he isn't getting better because you keep trying to wake him" is in the anger phase.**
1. **The 45-year-old client who is terminal with breast cancer and says to the nurse, "If only God would let me live until I see my son graduate, then I will be ready to die" is bargaining.**
4. **The 75-year-old woman receiving palliative care for throat cancer who refuses tube feedings and refuses to look at herself in the mirror is exhibiting signs of depression.**
3. **The parent whose child died 6 months previously and says to the nurse, "I have begun to remove items from my baby's room and given them to my sister, who is having a baby" is displaying signs of acceptance.**

▶ *Test-taking Tip:* The five stages of grief according to Kübler-Ross are denial, anger, bargaining, depression, and acceptance.

**Content Area:** Management of Care; **Concept:** Grief and Loss; Management; **Integrated Processes:** Nursing Process: Analysis; **Client Needs:** Psychosocial Integrity; **Cognitive Level:** Synthesis [Creating]

### 364. MoC ANSWER: 2

1. Defensive coping is repeated projection of a falsely positive self-evaluation that defends against perceived threats to positive self-regard.
2. **Compromised family coping occurs when a supportive person provides insufficient support or encouragement that may be needed by the client to manage adaptive tasks related to the health challenge.**
3. Anxiety is a vague, uneasy feeling of discomfort or dread accompanied by an autonomic response.
4. Dysfunctional grieving is extended, unsuccessful use of intellectual and emotional responses to work through modifying the self-concept based on the perceptions of the loss.

▶ *Test-taking Tip:* Read the situation carefully. Family is noted in the scenario, and only one option includes the word "family."

**Content Area:** Management of Care; **Concept:** Family; Grief and Loss; **Integrated Processes:** Nursing Process: Analysis; **Client Needs:** Safe and Effective Care Environment: Management of Care; **Cognitive Level:** Synthesis [Creating]

### 365. ANSWER: 2

1. If the client had identified only one person, it could be interpreted as dependence on a particular person. Assistance is provided only for driving, and the client is not totally dependent.

2. **The client is adjusting to changes that have occurred because of the loss.**
3. An exaggerated grief response would be exhibiting feelings of sadness, helplessness, hopelessness, powerlessness, anger, and guilt as well as somatic symptoms that render the individual dysfunctional with daily living.
4. Inhibited grief is absence of grief when ordinarily it would be expected. It may or may not be expected 2 months after the death of a spouse.

▶ **Test-taking Tip:** *Three options are similar, and one is different. Often the option that is different is the answer.*

Content Area: Management of Care; **Concept:** Stress; Grief and Loss; **Integrated Processes:** Nursing Process: Analysis; **Client Needs:** Psychosocial Integrity; **Cognitive Level:** Application [Applying]

## 366. ANSWER: 4
1. Adolescents handle feelings about death according to their developmental level.
2. Unless the adolescents are emancipated adults, parents are the decision makers related to the health care of children under the age of 18 years.
3. An emancipated minor has the same right as a competent adult to consent to or refuse medical treatment. In some states, an unemancipated minor has the right to refuse life-sustaining treatment pursuant to the conditions and procedures of that state. These rights are unrelated to the Self-Determination Act.
4. **Adolescents may become angry when changes occur or when they are not involved in decisions. They want to feel independent and be informed of their medical treatment plan.**

▶ **Test-taking Tip:** *Options with absolute words such as "all" are usually incorrect statements. Focus on an option that you can associate with the developmental needs of the adolescent.*

Content Area: Management of Care; **Concept:** Stress; Grief and Loss; **Integrated Processes:** Communication and Documentation; **Client Needs:** Psychosocial Integrity; **Cognitive Level:** Evaluation [Evaluating]

## 367. ANSWER: 2
1. Dentures are placed in the mouth to give the client's face a more natural appearance for viewing.
2. **Postmortem care includes washing soiled areas of the client's body and presenting the body according to religious custom. Absorbent pads can be used to absorb feces or urine released as the sphincter muscles relax after death.**
3. Rings, if removed, should be given to a family member. If left in place, they should be secured with a bandage (to avoid damage to a stone) or taped.
4. The client's body should be placed in a supine position, with the arms either at the sides, palms down, or on the abdomen.

▶ **Test-taking Tip:** *Postmortem care should demonstrate respect for the client's body and family. Recognize that Options 1 and 3 both have the same action "remove," and so they are most likely incorrect.*

Content Area: Management of Care; **Concept:** Nursing Roles; Grief and Loss; **Integrated Processes:** Nursing Process: Implementation; Caring; **Client Needs:** Physiological Integrity: Basic Care and Comfort; **Cognitive Level:** Application [Applying]

## 368. ANSWER: 2, 3, 4
1. Reorienting the dying client can be perceived as noncaring because vision-like experiences sometimes occur at the end of life.
2. **Vision-like experiences assist the dying person in coming to terms with meaning in life and transition from this life.**
3. **The family should be supported, reassured, and made aware that the client is dying.**
4. **Allowing family privacy with the client is appropriate, especially when the client is dying.**
5. Haloperidol (Haldol) is useful in managing delirium, acute and chronic psychotic disorders, or aggressive or agitated clients; its use is inappropriate in this situation.

▶ **Test-taking Tip:** *Recall that vision-like experiences may be a normal part of the dying process.*

Content Area: Management of Care; **Concept:** Nursing Roles; Grief and Loss; **Integrated Processes:** Nursing Process: Implementation; **Client Needs:** Psychosocial Integrity; **Cognitive Level:** Analysis [Analyzing]

## 369. MoC ANSWER: 3
1. Although transferring to another area of nursing practice either temporarily or permanently is an option, it should not be considered initially because there are other methods to help manage the nurse's situation.
2. Such feelings seldom self-resolve and require professional assistance.
3. **Working with grieving clients and families can be stressful, and one means of managing the stress is to discuss the situation with a grief counselor.**
4. This statement would increase the nurse's stress.

▶ **Test-taking Tip:** *Stress management is a need that occurs on a regular basis. Review the options for the one that provides such an opportunity in the most effective way.*

Content Area: Management of Care; **Concept:** Grief and Loss; Management; Stress; **Integrated Processes:** Nursing Process: Implementation; **Client Needs:** Safe and Effective Care Environment: Management of Care; **Cognitive Level:** Application [Applying]

## 370. ANSWER: 3
1. It is not appropriate to provide personal opinions. This blocks therapeutic communication.
2. The family may or may not understand the decision, but it is the individual family member's decision to make.

3. **It is not uncommon for a family member to choose not to be present when a loved one dies. The nurse's responsibility is to support that individual.**
4. It is not appropriate to either support or disagree with a family member's decision. This blocks therapeutic communication.

▶ *Test-taking Tip: The nurse is responsible for facilitating the individual's right to make well-informed decisions and for supporting that individual. Eliminate options that may appear to support the individual but that use statements that block therapeutic communication.*

**Content Area:** Management of Care; **Concept:** Grief and Loss; Communication; **Integrated Processes:** Nursing Process: Implementation; **Client Needs:** Psychosocial Integrity; **Cognitive Level:** Application [Applying]

## 371. ANSWER: 1, 2, 5

1. **Frustration and stress are magnified when communication is not clear and fully understood.**
2. **Explaining why procedures and treatments are provided in a certain manner will help minimize the chance of misinterpretation of events.**
3. Limiting time with the client and family will likely add to the chances that information and actions will be misunderstood because the opportunity to clarify will be limited.
4. Allowing the client and family to monopolize nursing staff is not acceptable. The nurse should set reasonable limits with the family and establish times to check on the client and family.
5. **Information can be misunderstood; having the facts restated helps eliminate miscommunication.**

▶ *Test-taking Tip: Frustration and stress are often a result of poor communication. Review the options and select those that promote effective communication between all involved parties.*

**Content Area:** Management of Care; **Concept:** Management; Grief and Loss; **Integrated Processes:** Nursing Process: Implementation; **Client Needs:** Psychosocial Integrity; **Cognitive Level:** Application [Applying]

## 372. ANSWER: 1

1. **Taking a proactive approach to identifying family concerns encompasses all of the other options and will provide the family with the greatest sense of control and satisfaction.**
2. Keeping the client and family informed is important, but this option addresses only the client's condition.
3. Attending to care needs is important, but this option addresses only these needs and no other concerns.
4. Listening is important, but this option addresses only anticipatory grief and no other concerns.

▶ *Test-taking Tip: One option is more global than the other options. The more global option is often the answer.*

**Content Area:** Management of Care; **Concept:** Grief and Loss; **Integrated Processes:** Nursing Process: Planning; **Client Needs:** Psychosocial Integrity; **Cognitive Level:** Application [Applying]

## 373. ANSWER: 3

1. Asking what the client would like today is providing a general lead that encourages the client to verbalize.
2. Asking the client to tell how he or she feels is using an open-ended statement that invites the client to explore thoughts or feelings.
3. **Stating that the client has made the right choice is giving unwarranted reassurance and blocks the fears, feelings, and other thoughts of the client.**
4. Noting that the client is squinting the eyes and asking a related question is acknowledging or recognizing a change in behavior and provides the client an opportunity to expand on this.

▶ *Test-taking Tip: The key word is "ineffective." Select the option that would be a barrier to communication.*

**Content Area:** Management of Care; **Concept:** Communication; Grief and Loss; **Integrated Processes:** Communication and Documentation; **Client Needs:** Psychosocial Integrity; **Cognitive Level:** Application [Applying]

## 374. MoC ANSWER: 3

1. Feelings vary from person to person. Information should be provided on the stages of grief.
2. Removing the child from the home can increase the woman's distress.
3. **The safety of the child is priority, but support systems may be available to provide child care in the home and support for the woman.**
4. Personal needs may be unmet, and it is important to identify these and develop a plan to meet these, but this is not priority.

▶ *Test-taking Tip: The key word is "initial." Use Maslow's Hierarchy of Needs theory and identify that safety is priority. Eliminate options that do not pertain to safety. Then select the best option.*

**Content Area:** Management of Care; **Concept:** Management; Grief and Loss; **Integrated Processes:** Nursing Process: Implementation; **Client Needs:** Safe and Effective Care Environment: Management of Care; **Cognitive Level:** Application [Applying]

## 375. MoC ANSWER: 1

1. **The hospice care philosophy uses an interdisciplinary team approach. Explaining roles can provide support to the family and aid coping.**
2. Hospice team members are accessible 24 hours but do not provide 24-hour home-care services.
3. Making bereavement visits is important to aid family coping after death, but this is not the initial action.
4. Coordinating care is important to facilitate family coping, but this statement includes coordination should the client be readmitted to the hospital.

▶ *Test-taking Tip: The key words are "initial." Eliminate options that occur after the client has been receiving hospice care.*

**Content Area:** Management of Care; **Concept:** Stress; Grief and Loss; **Integrated Processes:** Nursing Process: Implementation; **Client Needs:** Safe and Effective Care Environment: Management of Care; **Cognitive Level:** Analysis [Analyzing]

**376.** CJ PHARM **ANSWER: 6.5**

The past 4 hours would be from 0545 to 0945. Add the doses starting with 0600 and ending with 0915: 0.5 mg + 1 mg + 1 mg + 1.5 mg + 0.5 mg + 2 mg = 6.5 mg

▶ **Test-taking Tip:** Focus on what the question is asking: the past 4 hours and not the start of the nurse's shift.

**Content Area:** Management of Care; **Concept:** Comfort; Medication; **Integrated Processes:** Nursing Process: Planning; Caring; **Client Needs:** Physiological Integrity: Pharmacological and Parenteral Therapies; **Cognitive Level:** Application [Applying]

**377.** CJ PHARM **ANSWER:**

The nurse should complete a variance report. The hydromorphone was to be administered every 30 minutes PRN, but the night nurse PRD gave 1 mg of hydromorphone 10 minutes after it was given by nurse NNN.

▶ **Test-taking Tip:** Carefully read the PRN medication and its frequency to identify that a medication error has occurred.

**Content Area:** Management of Care; **Concept:** Safety; Medication; **Integrated Processes:** Nursing Process: Implementation; Caring; **Client Needs:** Physiological Integrity: Pharmacological and Parenteral Therapies; **Cognitive Level:** Application [Applying]

# Nutrition

378. The nurse determines that the nutrient intake of the 19-year-old female is **inadequate** according to the U.S. Department of Agriculture *MyPlate* food group recommendations. Which finding of the client's intake prompted this conclusion?

1. Eats 6 ounces of whole grain bread, cereal, or pasta daily
2. Eats 3 cups of a variety of fruits, juices, and vegetables daily
3. Eats 5½ oz of protein daily with seafood eaten 4 of the 7 days
4. Eats 1 cup of yogurt, 1½ cups skim milk, and ½ ounce cheddar cheese daily

379. The client with a BMI of 30 is attending a health promotion program at a clinic. Which outcome is best for the nurse to document in the client's plan of care?

1. The client will lose 2 lb per week for the next 4 weeks.
2. The client will gain 2 lb per week for the next 4 weeks.
3. Teach the client to increase intake of fruits and vegetables.
4. Inform the client to call the clinic weekly with weight results.

380. The nurse is planning a nutrition session during a health fair. Which food choices should the nurse include when teaching about omega-3 fatty acids?

1. Fatty fish at least twice weekly
2. Leafy green vegetables daily
3. Low-fat mozzarella cheese weekly
4. Cholesterol-free margarine once daily

381. The client is told to consume high protein foods for wound healing. Of the food choices, which should the nurse recommend?

1. 1 hard-boiled egg
2. 1 cup of cooked broccoli
3. ½ cup 1% cottage cheese
4. 1 ounce cheddar cheese

382. The nurse is ensuring that an adolescent diagnosed with type 1 DM knows about foods that are high in carbohydrates and those that contain little or no carbohydrates. Which foods should the adolescent identify as those that contain approximately 15 g of carbohydrate per serving? **Select all that apply.**

1. Pancake
2. Green beans
3. Corn
4. Taco shells
5. Carrots
6. Cottage cheese

383. The nurse taught the client who has type 2 DM about carbohydrate counting and the fact that 15 g of carbohydrate equals one carbohydrate choice. When consuming the following meal, the client should calculate that the meal contains how many carbohydrate choices?

1 small banana
2 slices bread with 1 slice turkey breast
1 cup milk
2 tomato slices

_____ Carbohydrate choices (Record your answer as a whole number.)

384. The nurse is caring for the client with a history of chronic alcoholism. Which observation should prompt the nurse to assess for a magnesium deficiency?

1. Flickerlike movements under the skin
2. Absent reaction when kneecap is tapped
3. Falling from having flaccid muscles
4. Rumbling bowel sounds after eating

**385.** MoC The new nurse is caring for the client experiencing CRF. The experienced nurse determines that the new nurse is able to list acceptable foods for the client when the list contains which low-potassium foods (less than 400 mg of potassium per serving)?

1. Cranberry juice, grapes, fresh string beans, and fortified puffed rice cereal
2. Prune juice, dried fruit, tomatoes, and all-bran cereal
3. Milk, cantaloupe, peas, and granola cereal
4. Orange juice, raisins, spinach, and dried beans

**386.** The client with early-stage iron-deficiency anemia is on a high-iron diet. An increase in the level of which specific serum laboratory test should indicate to the nurse that the diet has been effective?

1. Hemoglobin
2. Folate
3. Ferritin
4. Vitamin $B_{12}$

**387.** The nurse teaches the client with iron-deficiency anemia to eat high-iron foods and those containing vitamin C at the same meal to increase iron absorption. Which foods included in the meal indicate that teaching has been effective?

1. Yogurt and oranges
2. Shrimp and potatoes
3. Lean beefsteak and broccoli
4. Chicken and leafy green vegetables

**388.** The nurse plans to discuss ways to prevent food poisoning. What information should the nurse plan to address?

1. Keep all meat together during the preparation, cooking, and serving processes.
2. Drink natural unpasteurized milk because it contains less harmful chemicals.
3. Wash fruits and vegetables thoroughly, especially those that will be eaten raw.
4. Ensure that ground beef patties are cooked to a temperature of 125°F (51.7°C).

**389.** The nurse is caring for the malnourished adolescent consuming a vegan diet. The nurse should assess for signs of which vitamin deficiency in the client?

1. Vitamin A
2. Vitamin C
3. Vitamin K
4. Vitamin $B_{12}$

**390.** The nurse educates the client recovering from acute diverticulitis about the need to increase the amount of dietary fiber in the diet. The nurse evaluates that teaching has been effective when the client makes which menu selection for lunch?

1. A chicken sandwich on whole wheat bread with raw carrots and celery sticks
2. Baked chicken, mashed potatoes, and herbal tea
3. Chicken noodle soup with soda crackers and chocolate pudding
4. Cooked acorn squash, fried chicken, and pasta

**391.** The client prescribed a high-protein, high-calorie diet is not meeting protein or caloric intake goals. The client states, "I feel full quickly after eating three meals daily." Which interventions should the nurse recommend? **Select all that apply.**

1. Include more fresh fruits and vegetables in the diet.
2. Eat six smaller meals instead of three meals daily.
3. Include protein bars and whole milk yogurt as snacks.
4. Drink regular instead of diet carbonated beverages.
5. Add protein supplements to cooked cereals.

**392.** The nurse evaluates that the client placed on a DASH diet can correctly identify the salt content per serving on a food label. Place an X on the food label illustrated where the client should have identified the salt content per serving.

| Nutrition Facts | | |
| --- | --- | --- |
| Serving Size 1/2 cup (114g) | | |
| Servings Per Container 4 | | |
| **Amount Per Serving** | | |
| **Calories** 90 | Calories from Fat 30 | |
| | | **% Daily Value \*** |
| **Total Fat** 3g | | 5% |
| Saturated Fat 0g | | 0% |
| Trans Fat 0g | | 0% |
| **Cholesterol** 0mg | | 0% |
| **Sodium** 300mg | | 13% |
| **Total Carbohydrate** 13g | | 4% |
| Dietary Fiber 3g | | 12% |
| Sugars 3g | | |
| **Protein** 3g | | |

| | | | |
| --- | --- | --- | --- |
| Vitamin A | 80% | Vitamin C | 60% |
| Calcium | 4% | Iron | 4% |

\* Percent Daily Values are based on a 2,000 calorie diet. Your daily values may be higher or lower depending on your calorie needs:

| | | Calories | 2,000 | 2,500 |
| --- | --- | --- | --- | --- |
| Total Fat | Less than | | 65g | 80g |
| Sat Fat | Less than | | 20g | 25g |
| Cholesterol | Less than | | 300mg | 300mg |
| Sodium | Less than | | 2,400mg | 2,400mg |
| Total Carbohydrate | | | 300g | 375g |
| Dietary Fiber | | | 25g | 30g |

Calories per gram:
Fat 9   •   Carbohydrate 4   •   Protein 4

**393.** The client tells the nurse, "My mother has celiac disease, and I might also have the disease." The nurse agrees that this may be possible when the client states having diarrhea after eating which food?

1. Eggs
2. Peanut butter
3. Whole wheat bread
4. Dark leafy green vegetables

**394.** The client is recovering from an exacerbation of ulcerative colitis. The nurse evaluates that the client understands the dietary teaching for disease management when the client selects which foods?

1. Fried Cajun chicken, French fries, steamed pea pods, and a glass of fruit juice
2. Cream of tomato soup, mixed green salad with oil, and a glass of whole milk
3. Baked fish, steamed green beans, buttered mashed potatoes, and herbal tea
4. Chili con carne, whole wheat bread with butter, and a half glass of red wine

**395.** The clinic nurse is planning to measure the skinfold of an underweight older adult client to estimate the amount of total body fat. Prioritize the nurse's steps when measuring the triceps skinfold on the client.

1. Mark the midpoint of the client's arm with a pen.
2. Place the calipers at the midpoint mark and read the measurement to nearest milliliter (mL).
3. Grasp the skin and subcutaneous tissue between thumb and forefinger, pulling away from the muscle.
4. Measure the distance between the acromion and olecranon processes and divide by 2.
5. Ask the client to bend his or her arm at the elbow and lay the arm across his or her stomach.
6. Ask the client to hang his or her arm loosely at the side.

Answer: _____

**396.** The nurse reads in the HCP's history and physical note that the hospitalized child has a pica eating disorder. Which conclusions by the nurse are correct? **Select all that apply.**

1. The child consistently eats nonfood substances such as dirt, crayons, and paper.
2. The child regurgitates, chews, and then reswallows previously ingested food.
3. A primary safety concern for the child is the possibility of accidental poisoning.
4. The child's greatest risk, aspiration, should be monitored for at all times.
5. Complications of the disorder can include malabsorption and fecal impaction.
6. Usually children with a pica disorder are intellectually bright and precocious.

**397.** Which nutrients should the nurse encourage the client to consume to protect against cataract development?

1. Minerals
2. Lecithins
3. Antioxidants
4. Amino acids

**398.** The nurse is caring for the older adult client who has experienced unintended weight loss. Which energy-dense protein foods should the nurse offer when the client requests a snack?

1. Carrot sticks or apple wedges with dip
2. Peanut butter on celery or a hard-boiled egg
3. Whole wheat toast with grape jelly or a bagel
4. Yogurt or cottage cheese with blueberries

**399.** A mother is concerned about achieving a nutritious intake for her 14-month-old child. Which advice by the nurse would be **best**?

1. Feed the child before the rest of the family and then let the child play while the family eats.
2. Because the child's stomach holds only ½ cup, select food from one food group for each meal.
3. Offer 1 ½ tablespoons of food from each food group with every meal; offer nutritious snacks.
4. Avoid retrying foods that the child pushes away because these are foods the child dislikes.

**400.** The nurse is caring for the 2-year-old with iron-deficiency anemia. Which should the nurse recommend? **Select all that apply.**

1. Limit the toddler's milk intake to 24 ounces per day.
2. Limit the toddler's juice intake to 4 to 6 ounces per day.
3. Offer iron-rich foods such as beef, lentils, broccoli, and raisins.
4. Even if vegan, avoid feeding the toddler a vegan diet.
5. Feed the toddler to ensure an adequate intake.

**401.** The 6-year-old with chronic constipation is prescribed a high-fiber diet and increased fluid intake. Which foods should the nurse teach the parents as having the highest amount of fiber per serving?

1. Whole wheat or rye breads
2. Raw or cooked vegetables
3. Fresh, frozen, or dried fruits
4. Baked beans or black-eyed peas

**402.** The hospitalized child has lactose intolerance and is placed on a lactose-restricted diet. Which dietary supplement should the nurse anticipate being added to the child's diet?

1. Protein
2. Calcium
3. Vitamin $B_{12}$
4. Beta-carotene

**403.** The home health nurse is evaluating the parents' dietary management of the child with celiac disease. Which foods, or products that contain those foods, should the parents eliminate from their child's diet? **Select all that apply.**

1. Rice
2. Barley
3. Wheat
4. Corn
5. Oats

**404.** The clinic nurse is teaching the mother about child-hood nutrition. Which statements is the clinic nurse likely to include? **Select all that apply.**

1. Infants and children need all the vitamins that adults need but in different amounts.
2. Forcing a toddler to eat a distasteful food imprints a permanent avoidance behavior.
3. Calculate the recommended grams of fiber for the child by taking the child's age in years.
4. Children ages 1 to 2 years should be drinking whole milk rather than skim milk.
5. Preschoolers are able to meet their nutritional needs by eating three healthy meals a day.
6. Preschoolers tend to eat more and stay at the table longer when eating with their peers.

**405.** The child is found to be deficient in iron. To increase the child's absorption of iron, which vitamin should the nurse encourage the parents to supplement?

1. Vitamin A
2. Vitamin C
3. Vitamin D
4. Vitamin E

**406.** The nurse is obtaining nutrition information from four 20-year-old female clients. All have a BMI of 20 to 23. Which client requires the most immediate follow-up?

1. The client eats three nutritious meals a day with no snacks.
2. The client limits her intake to 2500 calories per day.
3. The client eats only fruits, vegetables, seeds, and nuts.
4. The client eats three 350-calorie meals per day.

**407.** The nurse is caring for four children. Which child should the nurse further assess for a vitamin C deficiency (scurvy)?

1.

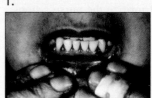

2.

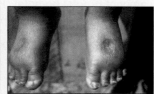

3.

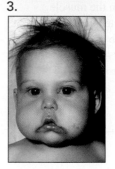

4.

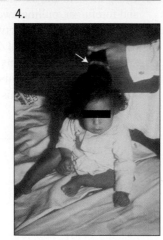

**408.** The child recovering from surgery is advanced from a clear liquid to a full liquid diet. The child is requesting something to eat. Which full liquid food item should the nurse offer to the child?

1. Pudding
2. Chicken noodle soup
3. Applesauce
4. Plain gelatin

**409.** The nurse is caring for the client with agoraphobia who has an inadequate milk intake. For which vitamin deficiency should the nurse specifically assess when caring for the client?

1. Vitamin $B_6$
2. Vitamin A
3. Vitamin D
4. Vitamin C

**410.** **MoC** The NA plans to deliver the meal tray to the client experiencing dysphagia. Which food item should the nurse ask that the NA remove from the client's meal tray?

1. Corn
2. Custard
3. Pureed meat
4. Moist pasta

**411.** The older adult client is asking the nurse about nutritional information. Which response gives good nutrition advice for the older adult?

1. "Maintain an appropriate weight for your height, and include high-nutrient foods."
2. "Increase vitamin E intake, and do muscle strengthening exercises 20 minutes daily."
3. "Avoid high-fiber and gas-forming foods, and take a multivitamin supplement daily."
4. "A vegan diet and drinking at least 2 quarts of water daily are recommended as we age."

**412.** **PHARM** An experienced nurse is observing a new nurse teaching the client about TPN. Which statement indicates that the new nurse needs additional orientation regarding the administration of TPN?

1. "A gastrostomy tube will be inserted through the abdominal wall into your stomach to administer your TPN."
2. "Your blood glucose will be monitored frequently because the TPN has a high concentration of dextrose."
3. "Although an infusion pump will be used to administer the TPN solution, you can still ambulate with assistance."
4. "The TPN provides nutrients of proteins, carbohydrates, fats, electrolytes, vitamins, and trace minerals."

**413.** **PHARM** The client's infusion pump delivering TPN malfunctions. The nurse determines that, based on the amount still in the bag, the client did not receive any TPN for the last 6 hours. The nurse should monitor the client for which immediate complication?

1. Air embolism
2. Rebound hypoglycemia
3. Rebound hyperglycemia
4. Low serum albumin level

**414.** **PHARM** The client taking lithium to treat a bipolar disorder is concerned that the medication is becoming less effective. It is **most** important for the nurse to question the client's intake of which nutrient?

1. Salt
2. Protein
3. Potassium
4. Carbohydrates

**415.** The nurse is presenting a nutritional teaching session in a rural community. Which statement should the nurse exclude?

1. "Iron is needed for energy; fish and poultry are significant sources of iron."
2. "Fluoride is needed for bone and teeth health; well water is a good source of fluoride."
3. "Iodine deficiency can cause intellectual disability; seafood is a good source of iodine."
4. "Potassium is essential to heart function; bananas are a good source of potassium."

**416.** The client with hypertension is prescribed a low sodium diet. Which meal represents the best choice for this client?

1. Roast beef, rice, salad, banana, and 2% milk
2. Bowl of chicken noodle soup, potato chips, small apple, and iced tea with lemon
3. Wiener with bun with ketchup and mustard, 2% milk, carrot sticks, and a diet cookie
4. Grilled American cheese sandwich on rye bread, celery and carrot sticks, and 8 oz skim milk

**417.** Which menu item should the adolescent client be offered after having a tonsillectomy?

1.

2.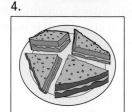

3.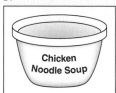

4.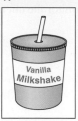

## Answers and Rationales

### 378. ANSWER: 2

1. Eating 6 ounces of whole grains daily exceeds the recommendation for grains. The recommendation is 5 ounces, with 3 of these ounces being whole grains.
2. **According to the *MyPlate* recommendation, the 19-year-old should consume 2 cups of fruits or juices and 2 ½ cups of vegetables every day. Vegetables and fruits are two separate food groups.**
3. Eating 5 ½ oz of protein daily meets the *MyPlate* recommendation. It exceeds the recommendation for seafood, which is at least 8 ounces per week.
4. The intake of dairy products exceeds the *MyPlate* recommendation by ½ cup.

▶ *Test-taking Tip: The key word is "inadequate." When reviewing the options, consider that food groups should not be combined.*

Content Area: Fundamentals; Concept: Nutrition; Integrated Processes: Nursing Process: Analysis; Client Needs: Physiological Integrity: Basic Care and Comfort; Cognitive Level: Analysis [Analyzing]

### 379. ANSWER: 1

1. **A BMI of 30 indicates the client is overweight. Losing 2 lb per week is the client-centered, realistic, and measurable outcome.**
2. Weight gain is an inappropriate outcome. A BMI of 30 indicates the client is overweight, not underweight.
3. Teaching is an intervention, not an outcome.
4. Informing the client is an intervention, not an outcome.

▶ *Test-taking Tip: A correctly stated outcome should be client centered, realistic, and measurable. Recognize that the question asks for an outcome, and Options 3 and 4 are interventions.*

Content Area: Fundamentals; Concept: Nutrition; Communication; Integrated Processes: Communication and Documentation; Client Needs: Health Promotion and Maintenance; Physiological Integrity: Basic Care and Comfort; Cognitive Level: Synthesis [Creating]

### 380. ANSWER: 1

1. **Fatty fishes, such as mackerel, salmon, bluefish, mullet, sablefish, menhaden, anchovy, herring, lake trout, sardines, and tuna, are high in omega-3 fatty acids. All except tuna provide at least 1 g of omega-3 fatty acids in 100 g or 3.5 ounces of fish.**
2. Leafy green vegetables do not include omega-3 fatty acids.
3. Low-fat mozzarella cheese does not include omega-3 fatty acids.
4. Cholesterol-free margarine does not include omega-3 fatty acids.

▶ *Test-taking Tip: Consider which option involves a fatty food. If uncertain, think about fish oil capsules that contain omega-3 fatty acids to answer this question.*

Content Area: Fundamentals; Concept: Nutrition; Promoting Health; Integrated Processes: Nursing Process: Planning; Client Needs: Physiological Integrity: Basic Care and Comfort; Cognitive Level: Application [Applying]

### 381. ANSWER: 3

1. There are 6 g of protein in one egg.
2. There are 4 g of protein in 1 cup of cooked broccoli.

3. A half-cup of cottage cheese supplies 16 g of protein.
4. There are 7 g of protein in 1 ounce of cheddar cheese.

▶ *Test-taking Tip:* Determine the protein content of each food to answer this question.

Content Area: Fundamentals; Concept: Nutrition; Nursing Roles; Integrated Processes: Nursing Process: Implementation; Client Needs: Physiological Integrity: Basic Care and Comfort; Cognitive Level: Application [Applying]

**382. ANSWER: 1, 3, 4**

1. A serving is one 4-inch pancake. Each serving has 15 g of carbohydrates or is equivalent to 1 carbohydrate choice.
2. Green beans contain little carbohydrates and are considered "free" foods.
3. One half-cup of corn. Each serving has 15 g of carbohydrates or is equivalent to 1 carbohydrate choice.
4. Two taco shells. Each serving has 15 g of carbohydrates or is equivalent to 1 carbohydrate choice.
5. Carrots contain little carbohydrates and are considered "free" foods.
6. Cottage cheese has zero grams of carbohydrate.

▶ *Test-taking Tip:* Focus on selecting starchy foods.

Content Area: Fundamentals; Concept: Nutrition; Promoting Health; Integrated Processes: Nursing Process: Evaluation; Caring; Client Needs: Physiological Integrity: Basic Care and Comfort; Physiological Integrity: Reduction of Risk Potential; Cognitive Level: Evaluation [Evaluating]

**383. ANSWER: 4**

One small banana, two breads, and milk each contain about 15 g of carbohydrates. This equals four carbohydrate food choices. Turkey breast is a non-carbohydrate-containing food, and diced raw tomato is a nonstarchy vegetable. Nonstarchy vegetables can be disregarded in carbohydrate counting if less than three servings are eaten.

▶ *Test-taking Tip:* Be sure to calculate the carbohydrate choices and not the total number of carbohydrates for the answer.

Content Area: Fundamentals; Concept: Nutrition; Metabolism; Integrated Processes: Teaching/Learning; Client Needs: Health Promotion and Maintenance; Cognitive Level: Analysis [Analyzing]

**384. ANSWER: 1**

1. A neuromuscular sign of hypomagnesemia includes fasciculation, or flickerlike movements under the skin from spontaneous contractions of muscle fibers. Other signs include tetany, twitches, hyperreflexia, and seizures.
2. Hyperreflexia, not an absent reaction to a kneecap tap, occurs with hypomagnesemia.

3. Hyperreflexia, not muscle flaccidity, occurs with a magnesium deficiency.
4. GI effects of hypomagnesemia include decreased bowel motility; rumbling sounds indicate increased motility.

▶ *Test-taking Tip:* Use the process of elimination, eliminating Options 2 and 3 because they are similar. Select Option 1, knowing that magnesium normally inhibits nerve impulse transmission at synapses and that the lack of magnesium will increase nerve impulse transmission and muscle excitability.

Content Area: Fundamentals; Concept: Nutrition; Addiction; Fluid and Electrolyte Balance; Integrated Processes: Nursing Process: Assessment; Client Needs: Physiological Integrity: Basic Care and Comfort; Physiological Integrity: Physiological Adaptation; Cognitive Level: Application [Applying]

**385.** MoC **ANSWER: 1**

1. Cranberry juice, grapes, fresh string beans, and fortified puffed rice cereal are all low-potassium foods.
2. Prune juice, dried fruit, tomatoes, and all-bran cereal are high-potassium, not low-potassium, foods.
3. Milk, cantaloupe, and peas are high-potassium, not low-potassium, foods.
4. Orange juice, raisins, spinach, and dried beans are high-potassium, not low-potassium, foods.

▶ *Test-taking Tip:* Identify key high-potassium foods in each option (tomatoes, cantaloupe, and orange juice) and use the process of elimination.

Content Area: Fundamentals; Concept: Nutrition; Urinary Elimination; Integrated Processes: Nursing Process: Planning; Client Needs: Safe and Effective Care Environment: Management of Care; Physiological Integrity: Basic Care and Comfort; Cognitive Level: Application [Applying]

**386. ANSWER: 3**

1. In iron deficiency, the body cannot synthesize Hgb, but Hgb levels drop fairly late in the development of iron-deficiency anemia. Other nutrient deficiencies and medical conditions can affect Hgb levels.
2. Serum folate is specific to folate-deficiency, and not iron-deficiency, anemia.
3. Ferritin levels reflect the available iron stores in the body and are specific to iron-deficiency anemia. A level less than 10 ng/mL is diagnostic of iron-deficiency anemia. As the condition improves, ferritin levels rise.
4. Vitamin $B_{12}$ deficiency is one cause of anemia and may be associated with iron deficiency, but a rise in vitamin $B_{12}$ levels does not indicate that the iron-deficiency anemia is resolved.

▶ *Test-taking Tip:* Note the key words "specific" and "iron deficiency." Use knowledge of terminology to answer this question (ferritin is an iron-phosphorus-protein complex).

Content Area: Fundamentals; Concept: Nutrition; Hematologic Regulation; Integrated Processes: Nursing Process: Evaluation; Client Needs: Physiological Integrity: Reduction of Risk Potential; Cognitive Level: Evaluation [Evaluating]

## 387. ANSWER: 3

1. Yogurt contains less iron than lean beefsteak.
2. Shrimp contains less iron than lean beefsteak.
3. **Good sources of iron include lean beefsteak; dark green vegetables such as broccoli have significant sources of vitamin C.**
4. Chicken contains less iron than does lean beefsteak.

▶ *Test-taking Tip:* The option must have foods high in vitamin C and iron to answer this question.

Content Area: Fundamentals; Concept: Nutrition; Hematologic Regulation; Nursing Roles; Integrated Processes: Nursing Process: Evaluation; Client Needs: Physiological Integrity: Basic Care and Comfort; Cognitive Level: Evaluation [Evaluating]

## 388. ANSWER: 3

1. Different types of meat should be separated when preparing and cooking these, not kept together. Raw meat should be kept separated from cooked meat.
2. Only pasteurized, not unpasteurized, milk should be consumed.
3. **Bacteria from improper handling can remain on raw fruits and vegetables. Therefore these should all be carefully washed before eating.**
4. Because *E. coli* is killed at 160°F (71.1 °C), the USDA sets the minimum safe internal temperature for ground beef at 160°F (71.1°C).

▶ *Test-taking Tip:* Foods can become contaminated with microorganisms when being handled.

Content Area: Management of Care; Concept: Infection; Integrated Processes: Nursing Process: Planning; Client Needs: Safe and Effective Care Environment: Safety and Infection Control; Health Promotion and Maintenance; Cognitive Level: Application [Applying]

## 389. ANSWER: 4

1. Fruits and vegetables that are eaten by vegans contain vitamin A.
2. Fruits and vegetables that are eaten by vegans contain vitamin C.
3. Fruits and vegetables that are eaten by vegans contain vitamin K.
4. **Vegans abstain from eating animal products, which provide vitamin B$_{12}$.**

▶ *Test-taking Tip:* Think about the vitamins in fruits and vegetables consumed by those on a vegan diet and about the deficiency that can occur from not eating meat.

Content Area: Fundamentals; Concept: Nutrition; Assessment; Integrated Processes: Nursing Process: Assessment; Culture and Spirituality; Client Needs: Physiological Integrity: Basic Care and Comfort; Cognitive Level: Application [Applying]

## 390. ANSWER: 1

1. **Whole wheat bread and raw fruits and vegetables are foods that are high in fiber content.**
2. There is very little fiber in baked chicken, mashed potatoes, and herbal tea.

3. There is very little fiber in chicken noodle soup with soda crackers and chocolate pudding.
4. There is less fiber in cooked acorn squash, fried chicken, and pasta than in Option 1.

▶ *Test-taking Tip:* Cooking food will cause breakdown of the dietary fiber content. Eliminate Options 2 and 4.

Content Area: Fundamentals; Concept: Nutrition; Nursing Roles; Inflammation; Integrated Processes: Nursing Process: Evaluation; Client Needs: Physiological Integrity: Basic Care and Comfort; Physiological Integrity: Reduction of Risk Potential; Cognitive Level: Evaluation [Evaluating]

## 391. ANSWER: 2, 3, 5

1. Although fresh fruits and vegetables contain needed vitamins, these foods are not good sources of needed calories or protein.
2. **The client is likely to increase caloric intake by eating more frequently.**
3. **Eating protein bars and whole milk yogurt as snacks will increase both protein and calorie intake.**
4. Regular carbonated beverages supply calories as simple sugars, are not a source of protein, and lack other nutrients.
5. **Protein supplements add calories and protein to the diet.**

▶ *Test-taking Tip:* Narrow the options to those that include like words from the scenario.

Content Area: Fundamentals; Concept: Nutrition; Nursing Roles; Integrated Processes: Nursing Process: Implementation; Caring; Client Needs: Physiological Integrity: Basic Care and Comfort; Cognitive Level: Analysis [Analyzing]

## 392. ANSWER:

| Cholesterol 0mg | | 0% |
|---|---|---|
| Sodium 300mg | X | 13% |
| Total Carbohydrate 13g | | 4% |

**The salt content of one serving is sodium 300 mg.**

▶ *Test-taking Tip:* The DASH diet includes limiting the intake of sodium.

Content Area: Fundamentals; Concept: Nutrition; Nursing Roles; Promoting Health; Integrated Processes: Nursing Process: Evaluation; Client Needs: Health Promotion and Maintenance; Cognitive Level: Comprehension [Understanding]

## 393. ANSWER: 3

1. Eggs do not contain gluten.
2. Peanut butter does not contain gluten.
3. **Celiac disease is an autoimmune disease that results in chronic intestinal inflammation after ingesting gluten. Whole wheat bread contains gluten.**
4. Dark leafy green vegetables do not contain gluten.

▶ *Test-taking Tip:* Gluten precipitates bowel inflammation in clients with celiac disease.

Content Area: Fundamentals; **Concept:** Nutrition; Bowel Elimination; **Integrated Processes:** Nursing Process: Analysis; **Client Needs:** Physiological Integrity: Basic Care and Comfort; **Cognitive Level:** Application [Applying]

## 394. ANSWER: 3

1. Spicy and high-residue foods should be avoided because these stimulate the bowels.
2. Milk products should be avoided because lactose intolerance is common in those with ulcerative colitis.
3. **A low-residue diet that is high in calories and protein should be gradually introduced as the client's tolerance for solid food increases.**
4. Alcohol and spicy foods are intestinal stimulants and should be avoided.

▶ *Test-taking Tip: Three of the options contain foods that are intestinal stimulants and should be eliminated.*

Content Area: Fundamentals; **Concept:** Nutrition; Bowel Elimination; **Integrated Processes:** Nursing Process: Evaluation; **Client Needs:** Physiological Integrity: Basic Care and Comfort; **Cognitive Level:** Evaluation [Evaluating]

## 395. ANSWER: 5, 4, 1, 6, 3, 2

5. **Ask the client to bend his or her arm at the elbow and lay the arm across his or her stomach. This is performed first so that a correct measurement of the distance between the acromion process and olecranon can be obtained.**
4. **Measure the distance between the acromion and olecranon processes and divide by 2. This measurement is needed to determine the midpoint.**
1. **Mark the midpoint of the client's arm with a pen. The midpoint will be the location where the calipers are applied to obtain the measurement.**
6. **Ask the client to hang his or her arm loosely at the side. This position relaxes the arm.**
3. **Grasp the skin and subcutaneous tissue between thumb and forefinger, pulling away from the muscle. Only the skin and subcutaneous tissue are used to measure the skinfold thickness.**
2. **Place the calipers at the midpoint mark and read the measurement to the nearest milliliter (mL). This step is performed last.**

▶ *Test-taking Tip: Visualize the steps of the procedure before attempting to place the actions in the correct sequence.*

Content Area: Fundamentals; **Concept:** Nutrition; Promoting Health; **Integrated Processes:** Nursing Process: Planning; **Client Needs:** Health Promotion and Maintenance; **Cognitive Level:** Synthesis [Creating]

## 396. ANSWER: 1, 3, 5

1. **Pica is an eating disorder of young children who persistently eat nonfood substances such as dirt, clay, paint chips, crayons, yarn, or paper.**
2. The act of regurgitating, chewing, and then reswallowing previously ingested food is a rumination disorder.
3. **Accidental poisoning can occur from toxic substances in nonfood items that are ingested.**
4. Accidental poisoning, not aspiration, is the greatest risk associated with a pica disorder. Regurgitating can increase the risk for aspiration.
5. **Malabsorption, fecal impaction, constipation, and intestinal obstruction are complications associated with eating nonfood substances.**
6. The incidence of a pica disorder increases with children who are cognitively challenged, possibly because of their inability to distinguish edible from inedible substances as early as other children can.

▶ *Test-taking Tip: Apply knowledge of medical terminology. Pica is the Latin word for magpie (a bird that is an indiscriminate eater).*

Content Area: Fundamentals; **Concept:** Nutrition; Nursing Roles; **Integrated Processes:** Nursing Process: Analysis; **Client Needs:** Physiological Integrity: Basic Care and Comfort; Physiological Integrity: Physiological Adaptation; **Cognitive Level:** Analysis [Analyzing]

## 397. ANSWER: 3

1. Minerals generally do not have an antioxidant function.
2. Lecithins are emulsifiers, not antioxidants, and do not protect against vision problems.
3. **Oxidative stress plays a role in cataract formation. Antioxidants such as vitamin E and vitamin C may reduce the likelihood of developing cataracts.**
4. Amino acids are building blocks of protein.

▶ *Test-taking Tip: If unsure, think about the protective effect of vitamins and then identify the appropriate nutrient from the options listed.*

Content Area: Fundamentals; **Concept:** Nutrition; Sensory Perception; **Integrated Processes:** Nursing Process: Implementation; **Client Needs:** Physiological Integrity: Basic Care and Comfort; **Cognitive Level:** Knowledge [Remembering]

## 398. ANSWER: 2

1. Fruit and vegetables are not good sources of protein and are generally low in calories per serving. Dip can be high in fat content.
2. **Peanut butter and eggs are good sources of complete proteins and are energy and nutrient dense.**
3. Grain products, such as whole wheat toast, are not good sources of protein and are not energy dense.
4. Yogurt and cottage cheese are good sources of protein but are not energy dense even with blueberries, which are low in calories.

▶ *Test-taking Tip: Select the best sources of complete proteins providing the most calories per serving.*

Content Area: Fundamentals; **Concept:** Nutrition; Promoting Health; **Integrated Processes:** Nursing Process: Implementation; **Client Needs:** Physiological Integrity: Basic Care and Comfort; **Cognitive Level:** Application [Applying]

**399. ANSWER: 3**

1. To develop healthy eating habits, the child should eat with the rest of the family and, if not hungry, should remain at the table.
2. The 14-month-old child's stomach holds a little more than 1 cup.
3. **The 14-month-old child's serving size should be about a tablespoonful for each year of age. Offering a variety of foods from the food groups will help ensure a nutritious diet and avoid consuming too much or too little food from any one food group. Offering three meals and three nutritious snacks a day increases the likelihood that the toddler will obtain sufficient nourishment.**
4. If foods are pushed away, they should be retried later. It takes 8 to 15 exposures to a food to effect behavior change.

♦ *Test-taking Tip: Focus on the issue of achieving a nutritious intake for the toddler. The serving size for a toddler is about one-fifth the size of an adult's serving.*

**Content Area:** Fundamentals; **Concept:** Nutrition; Promoting Health; **Integrated Processes:** Teaching/Learning; **Client Needs:** Physiological Integrity: Basic Care and Comfort; **Cognitive Level:** Analysis [Analyzing]

**400. ANSWER: 1, 2, 3**

1. **Milk should be limited to 24 ounces per day to maintain an appetite for iron-enriched cereals, meats, fruits, and vegetables.**
2. **Juice should be limited to 4 to 6 ounces per day for children ages 1 to 5 years.**
3. **Beef, lentils, broccoli, and raisins are some of the iron-rich foods.**
4. A toddler can consume a vegan diet if the diet is well planned to include iron-rich foods.
5. Toddlers are developing independence and will want to feed themselves. Parental feeding can delay the child's mastering of developmental stages and cause the child to dislike the foods if the parent attempts to force-feed the child.

♦ *Test-taking Tip: Focus on iron-rich foods, the size of the child's stomach, and child and parental behaviors that could limit the child's intake of iron-rich foods.*

**Content Area:** Fundamentals; **Concept:** Nutrition; Hematologic Regulation; **Integrated Processes:** Nursing Process: Implementation; **Client Needs:** Physiological Integrity: Basic Care and Comfort; **Cognitive Level:** Analysis [Analyzing]

**401. ANSWER: 4**

1. Whole wheat or rye breads provide 1 g of fiber per serving.
2. Raw or cooked vegetables provide 2 to 3 g of fiber per serving.
3. Fresh, frozen, or dried fruits have about 2 g of fiber per serving.
4. **Legumes such as baked beans, navy beans, or black-eyed peas provide about 8 g of fiber per serving.**

♦ *Test-taking Tip: The key phrase is "highest amount."*

**Content Area:** Fundamentals; **Concept:** Nutrition; Bowel Elimination; **Integrated Processes:** Teaching/Learning; **Client Needs:** Physiological Integrity: Basic Care and Comfort; **Cognitive Level:** Analysis [Analyzing]

**402. ANSWER: 2**

1. The ability to ingest protein is unaffected in persons with lactose intolerance.
2. **A deficiency of the enzyme lactase results in an inability to digest lactose, the sugar found in dairy products. A lactose-restricted diet, which removes milk and other dairy products from the diet, can result in a calcium, riboflavin, and vitamin D deficiency.**
3. The ability to ingest vitamin $B_{12}$ is unaffected in persons with lactose intolerance.
4. The ability to ingest beta-carotene from foods in the meat and bean, grain, vegetable, and fruit food groups is unaffected in persons with lactose intolerance.

♦ *Test-taking Tip: Recall that lactose is found in milk and other dairy products. You should think about the other nutrients in milk.*

**Content Area:** Fundamentals; **Concept:** Nutrition; Nursing Roles; **Integrated Processes:** Nursing Process: Planning; **Client Needs:** Physiological Integrity: Basic Care and Comfort; **Cognitive Level:** Analysis [Analyzing]

**403. ANSWER: 2, 3, 5**

1. Rice does not contain gluten and can be eaten by someone with celiac disease.
2. **Barley contains gluten and should be eliminated if celiac disease is present.**
3. **Wheat contains gluten and should be eliminated if celiac disease is present.**
4. Corn does not contain gluten and can be eaten by someone with celiac disease.
5. **Oats contain gluten and should be eliminated if celiac disease is present.**

♦ *Test-taking Tip: Select the gluten-containing grains because these should be eliminated in the diet of someone with celiac disease.*

**Content Area:** Fundamentals; **Concept:** Nutrition; Nursing Roles; **Integrated Processes:** Nursing Process: Evaluation; **Client Needs:** Physiological Integrity: Basic Care and Comfort; Physiological Integrity: Reduction of Risk Potential; **Cognitive Level:** Evaluation [Evaluating]

**404. ANSWER: 1, 2, 4, 6**

1. **Infants, children, and adults do require the same vitamins but in different amounts.**
2. **Permanent avoidance behaviors can be imprinted by forcing distasteful foods onto a toddler. Foods should be introduced and if refused reintroduced at a later time.**

3. The grams of fiber recommended for the child are calculated by taking the child's age in years plus 5. Considering only the child's age in determining the amount of fiber will result in an insufficient amount of fiber.
4. **Whole milk provides adequate fat for the still-growing child's brain.**
5. Preschoolers and toddlers need to eat three meals a day and wholesome snacks between meals to meet their nutritional needs.
6. **Preschoolers are developing socially and mimic behavior, so they will tend to eat more and stay at the table longer when eating with peers.**

▸ *Test-taking Tip: Before answering the question, think about childhood development and children's nutritional needs.*

Content Area: Fundamentals; Concept: Nutrition; Promoting Health; Integrated Processes: Teaching/Learning; Client Needs: Physiological Integrity: Basic Care and Comfort; Cognitive Level: Analysis [Analyzing]

## 405. ANSWER: 2

1. Vitamin A does not affect iron absorption. It is essential to night vision, the health of epithelial tissue, normal bone growth, and energy regulation.
2. **Vitamin C (ascorbic acid) facilitates iron absorption by acting on hydrochloric acid to keep iron in the more absorbable ferrous form.**
3. Vitamin D does not affect iron absorption. It is essential for absorption and use of calcium for bone and tooth growth.
4. Vitamin E does not affect iron absorption. It is an antioxidant that stimulates the immune system.

▸ *Test-taking Tip: If unsure, look for similarities and differences: vitamins A, D, and E are fat-soluble vitamins, whereas vitamin C is a water-soluble vitamin. An option that is different is likely to be the answer.*

Content Area: Fundamentals; Concept: Nutrition; Nursing Roles; Integrated Processes: Nursing Process: Implementation; Client Needs: Physiological Integrity: Basic Care and Comfort; Cognitive Level: Application [Applying]

## 406. ANSWER: 4

1. The meals are nutritious and may contain enough calories whereby snacks are not required.
2. This is an appropriate caloric intake for an average young adult female.
3. The client is eating a vegetarian diet. The nurse should further assess for protein sources, but the diet would not cause immediate concern because beans and nuts contain protein.
4. **By limiting meals to only 350 calories at a time, the client is only consuming 1050 calories per day. This does not meet the basic energy needs for a sedentary female. Further follow-up is required immediately.**

▸ *Test-taking Tip: Clients aged 20 to 30 years old need 25 kcalories/kg body weight/day. The energy needs of a sedentary 20-year-old are 1800 calories per day. Normal BMI is 18.5–24.9.*

Content Area: Adult; Concept: Nutrition; Integrated Processes: Nursing Process: Analysis; Client Needs: Physiological Integrity: Basic Care and Comfort; Physiological Integrity: Physiological Adaptation; Cognitive Level: Analysis [Analyzing]

## 407. ANSWER: 1

1. **Inflamed, spongy, and bleeding gums are associated with a vitamin C deficiency; this child should be further assessed for scurvy.**
2. The child with the swollen feet is experiencing kwashiorkor due to a severe dietary protein deficiency.
3. The infant presented in this illustration has swollen, red cracks at the corners of the mouth, indicative of a vitamin B deficiency.
4. This child is displaying "flag sign" hair, involving alternating light and dark bands of color along individual hair fibers, and thinning hair, also due to a severe dietary protein deficiency.

▸ *Test-taking Tip: Vitamin C is essential to tissue growth and repair. Narrow the options to 1 and 4, which show impaired tissues.*

Content Area: Fundamentals; Concept: Nutrition; Assessment; Integrated Processes: Nursing Process: Assessment; Client Needs: Physiological Integrity: Basic Care and Comfort; Cognitive Level: Analysis [Analyzing]

## 408. ANSWER: 1

1. **Full liquid foods include nontransparent foods that turn liquid at room temperature. Food items include pudding, custard, ice cream, sherbet, breakfast drinks, milk, and strained soups or vegetable juices.**
2. Unstrained chicken noodle soup is a food item on a regular diet.
3. Applesauce does not turn liquid at room temperature; it would be on a regular diet.
4. Plain gelatin is a clear liquid food item.

▸ *Test-taking Tip: Think about foods that turn liquid at room temperature but are not normally clear.*

Content Area: Fundamentals; Concept: Nutrition; Perioperative; Integrated Processes: Nursing Process: Implementation; Client Needs: Physiological Integrity: Basic Care and Comfort; Cognitive Level: Application [Applying]

## 409. ANSWER: 3

1. Vitamin $B_6$ is primarily found in meat, fish, and poultry, and it is not associated with sunshine.
2. Vitamin A is not synthesized with exposure to sunlight.
3. **Agoraphobia is a fear of the outdoors, crowds, or uncontrolled social conditions. Milk is a major source of vitamin D, and vitamin D can be synthesized in the body by exposure to sunlight.**
4. Vitamin C is not synthesized with exposure to sunlight.

▸ *Test-taking Tip: The key word is "milk." If unfamiliar with agoraphobia, focus on the nutrients found in milk to answer this question.*

Content Area: Fundamentals; **Concept:** Nutrition; Assessment; **Integrated Processes:** Nursing Process: Assessment; **Client Needs:** Physiological Integrity: Basic Care and Comfort; Physiological Integrity: Reduction of Risk Potential; **Cognitive Level:** Application [Applying]

### 410. MoC ANSWER: 1

1. **The nurse should ask the NA to remove the corn from the meal tray of the client with dysphagia (swallowing difficulties). Chunky vegetables, such as corn, should be avoided due to the risk of choking.**
2. Custard that is flavorful or well chilled will stimulate the swallowing reflex.
3. Pureed foods, such as pureed meats, are easier to swallow and prevent choking.
4. Moist pasta will stimulate the swallowing reflex.

▶ **Test-taking Tip:** Use the process of elimination, noting key words "remove" and "dysphagia." Select Option 1 because corn is chunky and could cause choking.

Content Area: Fundamentals; **Concept:** Nutrition; Safety; **Integrated Processes:** Nursing Process: Implementation; **Client Needs:** Safe and Effective Care Environment: Management of Care; Physiological Integrity: Basic Care and Comfort; **Cognitive Level:** Application [Applying]

### 411. ANSWER: 1

1. **Overall weight control and consumption of foods high in nutrients will promote healthy aging.**
2. Supplements, such as vitamin E, are not substitutes for food.
3. Fiber is needed by the older adult because bowel motility decreases with aging.
4. A vegan diet does not ensure a nutrient-dense diet.

▶ **Test-taking Tip:** Consider the broad picture of healthy aging before selecting an option.

Content Area: Fundamentals; **Concept:** Nutrition; Promoting Health; **Integrated Processes:** Teaching/Learning; **Client Needs:** Physiological Integrity: Basic Care and Comfort; **Cognitive Level:** Application [Applying]

### 412. PHARM ANSWER: 1

1. **Parenteral nutrition provides nutrients by the IV route, not through a gastrostomy tube.**
2. Because TPN solutions are 10% to 50% dextrose in water, blood glucose is monitored frequently for signs of hyperglycemia.
3. The TPN solution is delivered via a pump at a controlled rate to prevent glucose and volume overload. The pump is attached to a mobile IV stand for ambulation.
4. The composition of the TPN solution includes proteins, carbohydrates, fats, electrolytes, vitamins, and trace minerals. It also contains sterile water.

▶ **Test-taking Tip:** The key words in the stem are "needs additional orientation." Choose the statement by the nurse that is incorrect.

Content Area: Fundamentals; **Concept:** Nutrition; Management; **Integrated Processes:** Nursing Process: Evaluation; **Client Needs:** Physiological Integrity: Pharmacological and Parenteral Therapies; **Cognitive Level:** Application [Applying]

### 413. PHARM ANSWER: 2

1. There is no indication that air has been allowed to enter the infusion line.
2. **Because the TPN solution is high in dextrose, rebound hypoglycemia can occur from the delayed pancreatic reaction to a change in insulin requirements.**
3. Dextrose is no longer being given; thus hyperglycemia is unlikely to occur.
4. Although TPN contains protein, not receiving TPN for 6 hours would not affect the serum albumin level immediately, or at all.

▶ **Test-taking Tip:** The key word is "immediate." Avoid reading into the question.

Content Area: Fundamentals; **Concept:** Nutrition; Metabolism; **Integrated Processes:** Nursing Process: Implementation; **Client Needs:** Physiological Integrity: Pharmacological and Parenteral Therapies; **Cognitive Level:** Application [Applying]

### 414. PHARM ANSWER: 1

1. **A high-salt diet increases urinary excretion of lithium, limiting the drug's effectiveness.**
2. Lithium is unaffected by high protein.
3. Lithium is unaffected by potassium.
4. Lithium is unaffected by carbohydrate diets.

▶ **Test-taking Tip:** Knowing that lithium is excreted 95% in the urine should lead you to Option 1.

Content Area: Fundamentals; **Concept:** Nutrition; Medication; **Integrated Processes:** Nursing Process: Evaluation; **Client Needs:** Physiological Integrity: Basic Care and Comfort; Physiological Integrity: Pharmacological and Parenteral Therapies; **Cognitive Level:** Evaluation [Evaluating]

### 415. ANSWER: 2

1. This statement is correct.
2. **Well water usually does not contain fluoride. City water is fluoridated.**
3. This statement is correct.
4. This statement is correct.

▶ **Test-taking Tip:** Note the key word "exclude." Select the option with the incorrect statement.

Content Area: Fundamentals; **Concept:** Nutrition; Nursing Roles; **Integrated Processes:** Teaching/Learning; **Client Needs:** Physiological Integrity: Basic Care and Comfort; **Cognitive Level:** Analysis [Analyzing]

### 416. ANSWER: 1

1. **The meal contains foods with the lowest amount of sodium. Roast beef has 60 mg of sodium per 4 oz serving.**
2. Chicken noodle soup that contains broth and potato chips are high in sodium.
3. Wiener, ketchup, and mustard are high in sodium.
4. American cheese is high in sodium.

▶ *Test-taking Tip: Consider that foods that are processed, contain broth, are salted snack foods, and contain cheeses are high in sodium content. Evaluate each option for these foods and use the process of elimination.*

Content Area: Fundamentals; Concept: Nutrition; Perfusion; Integrated Processes: Nursing Process: Analysis; Client Needs: Physiological Integrity: Basic Care and Comfort; Cognitive Level: Analysis [Analyzing]

### 417. ANSWER 1

1. **Although the vanilla milk shake would be cold, straws should not be used after a tonsillectomy.**
2. The best option is the white grape juice. It will be cold and soothing, and provide liquid and calories. If an emesis occurs, blood can be detected.
3. The chicken noodle soup will be hot and can increase swelling and discomfort.
4. The sharp edges from a grilled cheese sandwich will irritate the throat and be more difficult to swallow.

▶ *Test-taking Tip: Focus on the food item that will provide the most comfort without causing harm.*

Content Area: Fundamentals; Concept: Nutrition; Caring; Integrated Processes: Nursing Process: Implementation; Client Needs: Physiological Integrity: Basic Care and Comfort; Cognitive Level: Application [Applying]

## Chapter Eleven

# Fluid, Electrolytes, and Acid-Base Imbalances

**418.** The nurse is caring for the child with hydronephrosis. Which assessment should the nurse perform to obtain the **most** accurate determination of fluid balance?

1. Measuring the child's intake and output
2. Weighing the child on the same scale
3. Assessing for the presence of edema
4. Evaluating serum electrolyte results

**419.** The nurse is calculating the client's weight loss from vomiting and diarrhea. The client's weight prior to the illness was 135 lb, and current weight is 55 kg. The nurse should calculate that the client lost how many pounds?

_____ lb (Record your answer as a whole number.)

**420.** The nurse is caring for the client admitted with dehydration. Which factors should the nurse explore as contributing to the client's dehydration? **Select all that apply.**

1. Diarrhea
2. Hemorrhage
3. Diabetic ketoacidosis
4. Hypoventilation
5. Decreased urination

**421.** The child is prescribed oral rehydration therapy to treat dehydration from vomiting and diarrhea. Which intervention should the nurse implement?

1. Give 50 to 100 mL/kg of sterile water every 4 hours.
2. Give 40 to 50 mL/kg of rehydration solution every hour.
3. Give 40 to 50 mL/kg of rehydration solution over 4 hours.
4. Give 50 to 100 mL/kg of tap water every hour for 4 hours.

**422.** Fluid replacement is prescribed for the child hospitalized after an electrical burn. Which indicators should the nurse use to determine adequacy of fluid resuscitation? **Select all that apply.**

1. Capillary refill time
2. Sensorium
3. Urine output
4. Blood pressure
5. Skin turgor

**423.** **PHARM** The client is to receive lactated Ringer's 1000 mL IV to be delivered over 8 hours. At how many mL/hr should the nurse set the infusion rate?

_____ mL/hr (Record your answer as a whole number.)

**424.** The nurse is caring for the comatose client receiving IV fluids at the amount that equals urine output. The client is losing weight. Which should be the nurse's reasoning for the client's weight loss?

1. About 500 mL/day of fluid is lost through the GI tract.
2. Insensible fluid loss accounts for about 400 mL/day.
3. About 200 mL/day of fluid is lost through perspiration.
4. Total fluid loss other than urine can equal 1000 mL/day.

**425.** The client with ESRD has 2+ pitting edema, and a total serum protein of 5.8 g/dL. The client's height is 6 feet and weight is 180 lb. Which physiological process should the nurse consider as the cause of the edema?

1. Decreased capillary hydrostatic pressure
2. Decreased plasma oncotic pressure
3. Increased capillary permeability
4. Decreased serum electrolytes

**426.** The client with renal insufficiency is prescribed to have a 1500-mL fluid restriction and strict monitoring of I&O. Which interventions should the nurse include in the client's plan of care? **Select all that apply.**

1. Discuss the plan of care and fluid restriction with the client and family.
2. Document any pureed foods as part of the client's liquid intake.
3. Record as intake the amount of water after subtracting for the ice chips.
4. Provide a collection device for measuring the client's urine output.
5. Tell the family to record fluids they give on the facility intake record.
6. Encourage the family to bring the client's favorite food items.

**427.** MoC The client being admitted to the ED reports feeling weak and having "almost passed out." The client was gardening in an outside temperature of 100°F (41.3°C). Assessment findings reveal poor skin turgor, dry and dull mucous membranes, HR 120 bpm, and BP 92/54 mm Hg. Which problem is the nurse's **priority**?

1. Impaired mucous membranes
2. High risk for falls
3. Decreased cardiac output
4. Fluid volume deficit

**428.** The nurse is assessing the 10-year-old client with ARF. Which electrolyte imbalance should be the nurse's **priority** concern?

1. Hypercalcemia
2. Hyperphosphatemia
3. Hyperkalemia
4. Hypernatremia

**429.** MoC The client is placed on strict I&O. The nurse is instructing the NA on items on a food tray that should be recorded as liquid intake. Place an X on the items on the food tray that should be recorded as liquid intake.

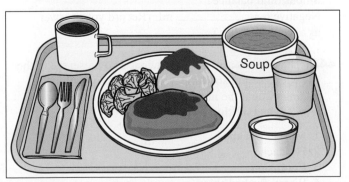

**430.** The nurse is caring for the client with hypotension. Which electrolytes should be closely monitored by the nurse?

1. Sodium, potassium, and chloride
2. Sodium, chloride, and calcium
3. Calcium, phosphate, and magnesium
4. Magnesium, potassium, and sodium

**431.** The client is placed on a 2000-mL fluid restriction. Which plan for fluid distribution over 24 hours should the nurse establish?

| Shift/Time | 0700–1500 | 1500–2300 | 2300–0700 |
|---|---|---|---|
| 1. | 1000 mL | 1000 mL | 0 mL |
| 2. | 900 mL | 900 mL | 200 mL |
| 3. | 1000 mL | 700 mL | 300 mL |
| 4. | 900 mL | 400 mL | 200 mL |

**432.** The daughter of the 82-year-old client with Alzheimer's disease contacts a clinic because her father has been unwilling to drink any fluids for more than 24 hours. Which statement by the nurse is **most** appropriate?

1. "Take your father to the hospital for intravenous fluid replacement."
2. "Bring your father to the clinic to have blood drawn for electrolytes."
3. "Tell me about other symptoms your father has been experiencing."
4. "Offer popsicles and ice cream and call the clinic again tomorrow."

**433.** The 1-day-old infant exhibits jitteriness, apnea, cyanotic episodes, abdominal distention, and a high-pitched cry. The mother is diabetic. Which electrolyte imbalance pertaining to the infant should the nurse further explore?

1. Early-onset hypocalcemia
2. Late-onset hypocalcemia
3. Hyperglycemia
4. Hypoglycemia

**434.** **MoC** The client admitted with fluid volume overload is being treated with a loop diuretic. Serum potassium levels are being monitored as illustrated. Which day is **best** for the nurse to consult with the HCP regarding initiating potassium replacement?

| Day 1 | Day 2 | Day 3 | Day 4 |
|-------|-------|-------|-------|
| 5.6 mEq/L | 4.4 mEq/L | 3.5 mEq/L | 3.1 mEq/L |

1. Day 1
2. Day 2
3. Day 3
4. Day 4

**435.** The nurse obtains the response illustrated when assessing the client who has hypocalcemia. How should the nurse document the client's response to this assessment?

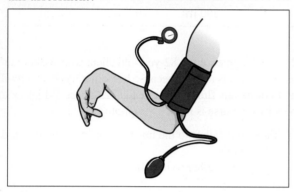

1. Positive Trousseau's sign
2. Positive Homan's sign
3. Positive Chvostek's sign
4. Positive Weber test

**436.** The client admitted to the ED has a serum potassium level of 3.0 mEq/L. The nurse should assess for which finding?

1. Hypotension
2. Bounding pulses
3. Weak, irregular pulses
4. Increased GI motility

**437.** The nurse is caring for the client who has an NG tube that is attached to intermittent suction. The nurse should monitor for which **most** important electrolyte imbalances?

1. Hyponatremia and hypocalcemia
2. Hypokalemia and hypophosphatemia
3. Hypomagnesemia and hypochloremia
4. Hypokalemia and hyponatremia

**438.** The client is hyponatremic as a result of fluid volume overload. A fluid restriction of 800 mL/24 hours is prescribed. Which action by the nurse is **most** appropriate?

1. Provide ice chips and refill the client's glass every 4 hours.
2. Have the client perform mouth care when feeling thirsty.
3. Offer sugary lozenges for the client to hold in the mouth.
4. Allow the client to salt foods to increase the sodium level.

**439.** The nurse is caring for the client who is 1-day postthyroidectomy. Which assessment findings should prompt the nurse to check the client's serum calcium level?

1. Fatigue, decreased cardiac function, and tetany
2. Weakness, tachycardia, and disorientation
3. Muscle cramps, paresthesia, and Chvostek's sign
4. Weakness, edema, and orthostatic hypotension

**440.** **MoC** The nurse reviews the serum laboratory results of four clients. Based on the findings, which client should the nurse assess **first**?

1. The client with heart failure whose ionized serum calcium level is 3.8 mg/dL
2. The client admitted with nausea and vomiting whose sodium level is 145 mg/dL
3. The client admitted with SIADH whose potassium level is 3.5 mEq/L
4. The client admitted with GI bleed whose phosphorus level is 2.4 mg/dL

**441.** The nurse is calculating the fluid balance for the client with DI. The client's I&O for 8 hours is as follows:

**Intake:** PO: 2000 mL water, 350 mL juice, ½ cup gelatin (110 mL), 360 mL milk, and IV fluid of D₅W at 125 mL/hour.
**Output:** 5000 mL urine
What amount should the nurse document for the 8-hour fluid balance?
Negative (−) _____ mL (Record your answer as a whole number.)

**442.** The nurse is assessing the client who presented to the ED with a serum sodium level of 114 mEq/L. Which findings would the nurse relate to the serum sodium level? **Select all that apply.**

1. Muscle weakness
2. Headache
3. Confusion
4. Warm, flushed skin
5. Abdominal cramping

**443.** **PHARM** The nurse is caring for the client with cardiac and renal disease. The client now has a serum potassium level of 6.0 mEq/L. Which medications, if prescribed, should the nurse administer? **Select all that apply.**

1. Sodium polystyrene 15 grams orally now
2. Regular insulin 4 units intravenously (IV) now
3. Dextrose 50% injection (50 mL) IV push now
4. Calcium gluconate 1.5 grams IV now
5. Potassium chloride 20 mEq orally now
6. Albuterol inhaler with spacer 2 puffs now

**444.** The nurse is caring for the 90-year-old client with hypernatremia. Which assessment findings should prompt the nurse to conclude that interventions have been **ineffective?**

1. Lethargy and paresthesias
2. Muscle cramps and spasms
3. Restlessness and agitation
4. Hypothermia and shivering

**445.** The nurse is teaching the client with hypoparathyroidism. Which recommendation should the nurse make knowing that the client is of the Orthodox Jewish faith?

1. Have milk or a dairy product with each meal.
2. Avoid carbonated and caffeinated beverages.
3. Ensure a calcium intake of 1 to 1.5 g daily.
4. Eat foods high in iodine, such as shellfish.

**446.** **MoC** The nurse is assessing the client who has a possible magnesium deficiency. Which assessment should be the nurse's **priority?**

1.
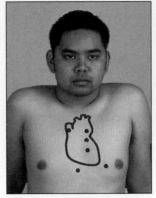

2.
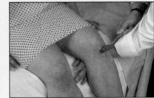

3.
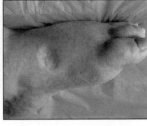

4.
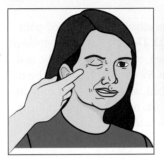

**447.** **MoC** The hospitalized client has a serum magnesium level of 0.9 mg/dL. Which plan is the nurse's **priority?**

1. Contact the HCP about stopping a prescribed loop diuretic.
2. Encourage the client to consume foods high in magnesium.
3. Check for a protocol to give oral magnesium supplements.
4. Contact the HCP about giving a bolus IV dose of magnesium.

**448.** The emaciated client is admitted with a total serum protein level of 4 g/dL. When assessing the client, the nurse should check for which alteration due to the low serum protein level?

1. Confusion
2. Restlessness
3. Edema
4. Pallor

11 Fluid, Electrolytes, and Acid-Base Imbalances

**449.** MoC The nurse assesses the client who presents to the ED with a panic attack. Which findings should prompt the nurse to confer with the HCP about obtaining ABGs? **Select all that apply.**

1. Respirations 40 bpm
2. Tingling in the fingers
3. Muscle twitching
4. Salivation
5. Increased urination

**450.** The client is hospitalized with a history of chronic emesis from purging. Based on the client's history, the nurse should monitor for which complication?

1. Hyperkalemia
2. Hyperchloremia
3. Metabolic alkalosis
4. Metabolic acidosis

**451.** The child has an asthma attack and is treated with epinephrine while in the ED. Despite receiving epinephrine, the child is still agitated, sweating profusely, and has an oxygen saturation of 89% and a RR of 30 bpm. Breath sounds are diminished, and wheezing is absent. Based on this information, the nurse should anticipate interventions to treat which acid-base imbalance?

1. Respiratory acidosis
2. Respiratory alkalosis
3. Metabolic alkalosis
4. Metabolic acidosis

**452.** The client has arterial blood results of pH 7.50, $Paco_2$ 35 mm Hg, and $HCO_3$ 30 mmol/L. Which nursing interpretation of the client's acid-base imbalance is correct?

1. Respiratory alkalosis
2. Metabolic alkalosis
3. Respiratory acidosis
4. Metabolic acidosis

**453.** The client with DKA has a blood sugar of 320 mg/dL, a RR of 32 breaths/min, and a deep, regular respiratory effort. The nurse should implement interventions for which acid-base imbalance?

1. Respiratory acidosis
2. Respiratory alkalosis
3. Metabolic acidosis
4. Metabolic alkalosis

**454.** The nurse is monitoring for complications when caring for the client with a pulmonary embolism. Which ABG findings should indicate to the nurse that the client has respiratory alkalosis?

1. pH 7.54    $Paco_2$ 25 mm Hg    $HCO_3$ 24 mEq/L
2. pH 7.35    $Paco_2$ 35 mm Hg    $HCO_3$ 22 mEq/L
3. pH 7.50    $Paco_2$ 40 mm Hg    $HCO_3$ 28 mEq/L
4. pH 7.32    $Paco_2$ 48 mm Hg    $HCO_3$ 24 mEq/L

**455.** MoC The nurse assigned to care for multiple clients is reviewing the laboratory reports. Based on the information provided, in which sequence should the nurse assess the clients? Prioritize the order in which the nurse should plan to assess the clients.

1. The client with renal insufficiency whose serum potassium level is 5.2 mEq/L
2. The client with hyperemesis whose serum sodium level is 122 mEq/L
3. The client recovering following head trauma whose serum osmolality is 290 mOsm/kg
4. The client with DM whose ABG results are pH = 7.22, $Paco_2$ = 35 mm Hg, $HCO_3$ = 15 mEq/L

Answer: _____

**456.** The nurse analyzed the ABG results for the newly admitted client with ethylene glycol toxicity (see exhibit). Which interventions should the nurse plan to implement? **Select all that apply.**

| Client's ABG Results | |
|---|---|
| pH | 7.18 |
| $Paco_2$ | 25 mm Hg |
| $HCO_3$ | 9 mEq/L |
| $Pao_2$ | 60% |

1. Initiating mechanical hyperventilation
2. Giving sodium bicarbonate
3. Initiating hemodialysis
4. Giving an intravenous (IV) colloid
5. Giving IV potassium replacement
6. Starting supplemental oxygen

**457.** MoC The nurse is evaluating assessment information gathered for four assigned clients. Based on the information illustrated, which client requires **priority** interventions for excess fluid volume?

| | Client A | Client B | Client C | Client D |
|---|---|---|---|---|
| **Medical Diagnosis** | COPD | Renal failure | Heart failure | Abdominal aortic aneurysm (AAA) repair (postoperative day 1) |
| **Physical Exam** | Crackles<br>1+ edema<br>Dyspnea | Crackles<br>No edema<br>No dyspnea | Crackles<br>1+ edema<br>Dyspnea | Inspiratory crackles<br>3+ edema<br>Dyspnea, cough |
| **Intake/Output** | 2250/1125 | 2250/200 | 2250/4250 | 6500/1000 |
| **Weight** | Up 2 lb | No change | Down 3 lb | Up 10 lb |
| **Laboratory:**<br>BUN<br>Hct | 15 mg/dL<br>46% | 25 mg/dL<br>40% | 15 mg/dL<br>32% | 20 mg/dL<br>32% |

1. Client A
2. Client B
3. Client C
4. Client D

# Answers and Rationales

## 418. ANSWER: 2

1. I&O provides data, but there is additional fluid lost through skin, lungs, and the GI tract that cannot be measured.
2. **Obtaining the child's weight using the same scale is most accurate.**
3. Edema is an indication of fluid retention but is not accurate.
4. Electrolyte levels are not measures of fluid balance, although some are affected by fluid excess or deficit.

▶ *Test-taking Tip: Note the key phrase "most accurate." Think critically about each option, using the process of elimination to rule out incorrect options. Remember that an increase of 1 kg (2.2 lb) is equal to 1000 mL of fluid.*

**Content Area:** Fundamentals; **Concept:** Fluid and Electrolyte Balance; Urinary Elimination; **Integrated Processes:** Nursing Process: Assessment; **Client Needs:** Physiological Integrity: Reduction of Risk Potential; **Cognitive Level:** Comprehension [Understanding]

## 419. ANSWER: 14

**Using a proportion formula:**
**First convert the 55 kg to pounds by setting up a proportion formula (1 kg = 2.2 lb)**
**1 kg : 2.2 kg :: 55 lb : $X$ lb (Multiply the outside values and then the inside values.)**
$X = 2.2 \times 55$; $X = 121$ lb
**Next subtract the preadmission weight from the admission weight:**
**135 − 121 = 14 lb**
**Using dimensional analysis:**

$$X = \frac{2.2\ \text{lb}}{1\ \text{kg}} \times 55\ \text{kg} \qquad X = \frac{2.2\ \text{lb}}{1} \times 55 \qquad X = 121\ \text{lb}$$

**Next subtract the preadmission weight from the admission weight:**
**135 − 121 = 14 lb**

▶ *Test-taking Tip: Recall that 1 kg is equal to 2.2 lb.*

**Content Area:** Fundamentals; **Concept:** Fluid and Electrolyte Balance; Nursing Roles; Assessment; **Integrated Processes:** Nursing Process: Assessment; **Client Needs:** Physiological Integrity: Basic Care and Comfort; **Cognitive Level:** Application [Applying]

## 420. ANSWER: 1, 2, 3

1. **Fluid volume deficit occurs with abnormal loss of body fluids, including diarrhea.**
2. **Hemorrhage can result in fluid volume deficit from a large loss of volume.**
3. **DKA is a risk factor or cause of dehydration because increased blood glucose levels cause diuresis.**
4. Hyperventilation and not hypoventilation is a risk factor or cause of dehydration.
5. Decreased urine output is a clinical manifestation of volume deficit, not a cause or contributing factor.

♦ **Test-taking Tip:** *Dehydration occurs when there is insufficient water to replace fluid loss throughout the day. Dehydration can occur from not drinking enough fluids.*

**Content Area:** Fundamentals; **Concept:** Fluid and Electrolyte Balance; Assessment; **Integrated Processes:** Nursing Process: Assessment; **Client Needs:** Physiological Integrity: Physiological Adaptation; **Cognitive Level:** Application [Applying]

## 421. ANSWER: 3

1. Water is not indicated as a fluid for rehydration because it lacks glucose, sodium, potassium, and a base solution to equal an osmolality of 200 to 310 mOsm/L.
2. Giving 40 to 50 mL/kg of rehydration solution every hour could increase nausea and vomiting from fullness.
3. **The nurse should start with small sips of rehydration solution and increase it so the child receives 40 to 50 mL/kg over 4 hours.**
4. Tap water is not indicated as a fluid for rehydration because it lacks glucose, sodium, potassium, and a base solution to equal an osmolality of 200 to 310 mOsm/L.

♦ **Test-taking Tip:** *Look for key terms in the options: "water," "every," "over," and "as much," respectively. Think about what method would be best for rehydration and eliminate options that would not provide for continuous hydration with electrolytes.*

**Content Area:** Child; **Concept:** Fluid and Electrolyte Balance; Nursing Roles; **Integrated Processes:** Nursing Process: Implementation; **Client Needs:** Physiological Integrity: Basic Care and Comfort; Physiological Integrity: Reduction of Risk Potential; **Cognitive Level:** Application [Applying]

## 422. ANSWER: 1, 2, 3, 5

1. **The capillary refill time is useful in evaluating peripheral tissue perfusion.**
2. **Changes in sensorium are useful in evaluating cerebral tissue perfusion.**
3. **Urine output is useful in evaluating perfusion to the kidneys.**
4. The child's BP can remain normotensive even with a state of hypovolemia.
5. **Skin turgor is useful in evaluating tissue hydration.**

♦ **Test-taking Tip:** *The child will lose 20% of fluid volume before the volume loss has an impact on BP.*

**Content Area:** Child; Fundamentals; **Concept:** Fluid and Electrolyte Balance; Nursing Roles; **Integrated Processes:** Nursing Process: Evaluation; **Client Needs:** Physiological Integrity: Physiological Adaptation; **Cognitive Level:** Evaluation [Evaluating]

## 423. PHARM ANSWER: 125

**1000 mL divided by 8 hours equals 125 mL/hour.**

♦ **Test-taking Tip:** *To determine the mL/hr, divide the volume to be infused by the number of hours over which it should be infused.*

**Content Area:** Fundamentals; **Concept:** Fluid and Electrolyte Balance; Medication; **Integrated Processes:** Nursing Process: Implementation; **Client Needs:** Physiological Integrity: Pharmacological and Parenteral Therapies; **Cognitive Level:** Application [Applying]

## 424. ANSWER: 4

1. Fluid lost through the GI tract is 100 to 200 mL/day, not 500 mL.
2. Insensible fluid loss refers to the fluid lost through the lungs and skin and is 700 to 800 mL/day.
3. Perspiration, under normal conditions, results in the loss of about 100 mL/day of fluid.
4. **Besides urine, body fluid is lost through perspiration, the GI tract, skin, and lungs. This can account for over 1000 mL/day, which is equal to approximately 1 kg, or 2.2 lb.**

♦ **Test-taking Tip:** *Examine each option, noting the amount of fluid lost. Two options excrete too much fluid, and one option excretes too little.*

**Content Area:** Fundamentals; **Concept:** Fluid and Electrolyte Balance; Nursing Roles; **Integrated Processes:** Nursing Process: Analysis; **Client Needs:** Physiological Integrity: Physiological Adaptation; **Cognitive Level:** Application [Applying]

## 425. ANSWER: 2

1. Increased, not decreased, capillary hydrostatic pressure can result in edema.
2. **The total serum protein of 5.8 g/dL is low (normal serum protein total is 6.0 to 8.0 g/dL). ESRD clients often have low plasma protein from malnutrition and protein restriction. These reduce plasma oncotic pressure and result in fluid remaining in the interstitial space because pressure is not great enough to pull fluid into the capillaries.**
3. Although edema can result from increased capillary permeability, the low serum protein suggests decreased oncotic pressure is the most likely cause of the edema.
4. Because the client's kidneys in ESRD are unable to excrete electrolytes, an increased (not decreased) level of serum electrolytes is present.

♦ **Test-taking Tip:** *Focus on the client's diagnosis of ESRD and the dietary restriction of protein that influences fluid shifting between the vascular compartment and the tissues. This information should lead you to select Option 2.*

Content Area: Adult; **Concept:** Fluid and Electrolyte Balance; Urinary Elimination; **Integrated Processes:** Nursing Process: Evaluation; **Client Needs:** Physiological Integrity: Physiological Adaptation; **Cognitive Level:** Evaluation [Evaluating]

## 426. ANSWER: 1, 4

1. **Informing the client and family of the plan of care helps to provide reinforcement for the client and to ensure compliance with the fluid restriction and plan.**
2. Pureed foods are not counted as liquid because they are considered solid in a different form.
3. Ice chips are considered fluid; a 200-mL cup of ice is equal to 100 mL of water.
4. **Measurement and collection devices are necessary when strict monitoring is required.**
5. Only health care personnel should document on official agency records. The family should be informed not to provide the client with additional liquid intake.
6. Bringing favorite food items from home should be discouraged to ensure that the client follows the plan of care for fluid, protein, and electrolyte restrictions.

▶ *Test-taking Tip: Think about the food and fluid restrictions that are likely with renal insufficiency and about measures that the nurse can use to ensure that the client adheres to the plan of care.*

Content Area: Adult; **Concept:** Fluid and Electrolyte Balance; Urinary Elimination; **Integrated Processes:** Nursing Process: Planning; Teaching/ Learning; **Client Needs:** Physiological Integrity: Basic Care and Comfort; Physiological Integrity: Reduction of Risk Potential; **Cognitive Level:** Synthesis [Creating]

## 427. MoC ANSWER: 4

1. Although the nurse should moisturize the client's dry, dull mucous membranes, this is not priority.
2. Falling is a concern, especially after feeling weak and faint, but the client is talking now.
3. There are no symptoms of decreased cardiac output. The client's MAP is 67, suggesting adequate cardiac output for tissue perfusion ([systolic BP + 2 diastolic BP] ÷ 3).
4. **The priority problem is fluid volume deficit. Signs of dehydration and hypovolemia are evident (weakness, syncope, poor skin turgor, dry and dull mucous membranes, hypotension).**

▶ *Test-taking Tip: Focus on the client's symptoms to establish the priority problem.*

Content Area: Adult; **Concept:** Fluid and Electrolyte Balance; Nursing Roles; Caring; **Integrated Processes:** Nursing Process: Analysis; **Client Needs:** Safe and Effective Care Environment: Management of Care; Physiological Integrity: Reduction of Risk Potential; **Cognitive Level:** Analysis [Analyzing]

## 428. ANSWER: 3

1. Hypercalcemia may result in changes in the neuromuscular system and bradycardia.
2. Hyperphosphatemia may result in the presence of hypocalcemia.
3. **Hyperkalemia can lead to life-threatening cardiac arrhythmias and is priority. ARF in children often results from acute glomerulonephritis with retention of potassium.**
4. Hypernatremia may result in disorientation and lethargy.

▶ *Test-taking Tip: Use the ABC's to determine which electrolyte imbalance would be the most life-threatening.*

Content Area: Child; Fundamental; **Concept:** Fluid and Electrolyte Balance; Urinary Elimination; **Integrated Processes:** Nursing Process: Assessment; **Client Needs:** Physiological Integrity: Physiological Adaptation; **Cognitive Level:** Analysis [Analyzing]

## 429. MoC ANSWER:

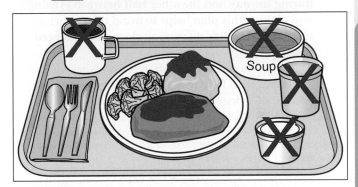

**Juice, ice cream, soup, and coffee are considered liquids and should be recorded as fluid intake.**

▶ *Test-taking Tip: Only foods that turn liquid at room temperature should be recorded as fluid intake.*

Content Area: Fundamentals; **Concept:** Fluid and Electrolyte Balance; Nutrition; Management; **Integrated Processes:** Nursing Process: Analysis; **Client Needs:** Safe and Effective Care Environment: Management of Care; **Cognitive Level:** Comprehension [Understanding]

## 430. ANSWER: 1

1. **The nurse should closely monitor sodium, potassium, and chloride levels. Renin secretion increases plasma levels of angiotensin II, increases serum potassium, and decreases serum sodium. Aldosterone is also released in response to renin. Aldosterone increases sodium reabsorption and potassium excretion, resulting in an increase in chloride.**
2. Calcium balance is controlled by the parathyroid hormone, calcitonin, and vitamin D.
3. Calcium balance is controlled by the parathyroid hormone, calcitonin, and vitamin D. Phosphorus and magnesium are regulated by the kidneys and influenced by calcium balance, and not regulated by the renin-angiotensin system.

4. Magnesium is regulated by the kidneys and influenced by calcium balance, and not regulated by the renin-angiotensin system.

▶ *Test-taking Tip: Look for the same electrolytes in the options. Sodium is in Options 1, 2, and 4; thus eliminate Option 3. Potassium is in Options 1 and 4; thus eliminate Option 2. Sodium affects the chloride level; thus eliminate Option 4.*

**Content Area:** Fundamentals; **Concept:** Fluid and Electrolyte Balance; Perfusion; **Integrated Processes:** Nursing Process: Assessment; **Client Needs:** Physiological Integrity: Physiological Adaptation; **Cognitive Level:** Application [Applying]

## 431. ANSWER: 3

1. This plan is incorrect because fluids should be available during the night.
2. A large amount of fluid intake is planned from 1500 to 2300; this should be avoided because it disrupts sleep if taken just before bedtime.
3. **Generally, half of the total restriction is provided during the day and the other half between evening and nights. This plan helps to avoid thirst during the day and avoids disrupting sleep with the need to urinate.**
4. This total amount is 1500 mL, less than what was prescribed for a fluid restriction. The client may become dehydrated.

▶ *Test-taking Tip: Think about your own fluid intake and when you likely consume the most amount of fluid. Two meals are provided between 0700 and 1500 hours, which may increase your need for fluids during this time.*

**Content Area:** Adult; **Concept:** Fluid and Electrolyte Balance; Urinary Elimination; **Integrated Processes:** Nursing Process: Planning; **Client Needs:** Physiological Integrity: Basic Care and Comfort; **Cognitive Level:** Application [Applying]

## 432. ANSWER: 3

1. There is insufficient information regarding hydration status to suggest hospital admission for IV fluid replacement.
2. Laboratory tests, such as electrolytes, would not be indicated without first knowing the client's symptoms and hydration status.
3. **The nurse should ask about signs and symptoms of dehydration (change in speech, weakness, dry mucous membranes, decreased urine output). The treatments for dehydration will depend on whether or not the client is symptomatic.**
4. Popsicles and ice cream, though sources of fluids, would be insufficient to replace fluid and electrolyte needs if the client is severely dehydrated.

▶ *Test-taking Tip: Use the nursing process to determine the most appropriate statement. Additional assessment is needed before recommending an intervention.*

**Content Area:** Fundamentals; **Concept:** Fluid and Electrolyte Balance; Cognition; **Integrated Processes:** Nursing Process: Implementation; **Client Needs:** Physiological Integrity: Physiological Adaptation; Safe and Effective Care Environment: Safety and Infection Control; **Cognitive Level:** Analysis [Analyzing]

## 433. ANSWER: 1

1. **Early-onset hypocalcemia (first 34 to 48 hours) tends to accompany the hypoglycemia that occurs shortly after birth in the infant of a diabetic mother.**
2. Late-onset hypocalcemia occurs 3 to 4 days following birth in infants fed modified cow's milk.
3. Hyperglycemia in infants is usually asymptomatic; this infant has symptoms not associated with hyperglycemia.
4. Hypoglycemia may occur with newborns of diabetic mothers, but signs would not include abdominal distention or apnea with cyanosis.

▶ *Test-taking Tip: Focus on the symptoms of abdominal distention, apnea, and cyanosis to narrow the options.*

**Content Area:** Child; **Concept:** Fluid and Electrolyte Balance; Metabolism; Pregnancy; **Integrated Processes:** Nursing Process: Evaluation; **Client Needs:** Physiological Integrity: Physiological Adaptation; **Cognitive Level:** Evaluation [Evaluating]

## 434. MoC ANSWER: 3

1. The serum potassium of 5.6 mEq/L on day 1 is high and would not require replacement.
2. The serum potassium of 4.4 mEq/L on day 2 is in the midrange of normal.
3. **The nurse should consult the HCP on day 3, when the client's level is at the low end of normal. The client's serum potassium level is decreasing, and the client is taking a diuretic. Supplementation is needed to prevent a reduction of serum potassium level below normal.**
4. The serum potassium of 3.1 mEq/L on day 4 is low; replacement should have started a day earlier to prevent a reduction of the serum potassium level below normal.

▶ *Test-taking Tip: The normal serum potassium level is 3.5 to 5.0 mEq/L. A loop diuretic will decrease serum potassium levels.*

**Content Area:** Adult; **Concept:** Fluid and Electrolyte Balance; Medication; **Integrated Processes:** Nursing Process: Implementation; Communication and Documentation; **Client Needs:** Safe and Effective Care Environment: Management of Care; Physiological Integrity: Physiological Adaptation; **Cognitive Level:** Analysis [Analyzing]

## 435. ANSWER: 1

1. **Trousseau's sign is an indicator of tetany associated with hypocalcemia. In hypocalcemia, carpal spasms can be seen when a BP cuff is inflated on the client's arm.**
2. The Homan's sign is a possible indicator of thrombophlebitis; it is elicited by sharp dorsiflexion of the foot and is not associated with the facial nerve in front of the ear.
3. Chvostek's sign is an indicator of tetany associated with hypocalcemia. Chvostek's sign is a contraction of facial muscles in response to a tap over the facial nerve in front of the ear.

4. The Weber test is a screening test for hearing. A vibrating tuning fork is placed on the midline of the head to ascertain in which ear the sound is heard by bone conduction.

▶ *Test-taking Tip: You can remember Trousseau's sign by associating the beginning letter "T" in both Trousseau and thumb. You should be able to eliminate Options 2 and 4, as they are not related to electrolytes.*

**Content Area:** Fundamentals; **Concept:** Fluid and Electrolyte Balance; Communication; **Integrated Processes:** Communication and Documentation; **Client Needs:** Physiological Integrity: Reduction of Risk Potential; **Cognitive Level:** Analysis [Analyzing]

## 436. ANSWER: 3

1. Hypotension is a sign of hyperkalemia, not hypokalemia.
2. Bounding pulses are a sign of hyponatremia, not hypokalemia.
3. **A serum potassium level of 3.0 mEq/L is low (hypokalemia). The nurse should assess for a weak, irregular pulse.**
4. With hypokalemia smooth muscle function is altered; this may cause a decrease in GI motility, not an increase in GI motility, as well as a decrease in peristalsis.

▶ *Test-taking Tip: Normal serum potassium is 3.5–5.0 mEq/L. Focus on clinical manifestations of hypokalemia and eliminate those associated with hyperkalemia.*

**Content Area:** Fundamentals; **Concept:** Fluid and Electrolyte Balance; Perfusion; Assessment; **Integrated Processes:** Nursing Process: Assessment; **Client Needs:** Physiological Integrity: Physiological Adaptation; **Cognitive Level:** Analysis [Analyzing]

## 437. ANSWER: 4

1. Although sodium is lost through NG fluids, calcium is not.
2. Although potassium is lost through NG fluids, phosphorus is not.
3. Magnesium and chloride may be lost with NG suctioning, but sodium and potassium are the important electrolytes lost.
4. **The nurse should monitor for hypokalemia and hyponatremia. NG losses contain both sodium and potassium. These are most important because abnormalities can increase the risk of life-threatening dysrhythmias.**

▶ *Test-taking Tip: Use the ABC's to determine which electrolyte losses would be most important. The options that include electrolytes that are essential for cardiac function are the most important.*

**Content Area:** Fundamentals; **Concept:** Fluid and Electrolyte Balance; Nursing Roles; **Integrated Processes:** Nursing Process: Assessment; **Client Needs:** Physiological Integrity: Reduction of Risk Potential; **Cognitive Level:** Application [Applying]

## 438. ANSWER: 2

1. Ice chips are considered fluid and should be included in the intake volume. A full glass of ice chips is equivalent to 120 mL of fluid. If replaced every 2 hours, ice chips alone would equal 1440 mL of fluid.
2. **Frequent mouth care can help to reduce the sensation of thirst.**
3. Lozenges, especially if high in sugar content, can produce the sensation of thirst.
4. Salt will increase fluid retention and may worsen the client's condition.

▶ *Test-taking Tip: The key phrase is "most appropriate." Consider the nurse's action in maintaining the fluid restriction and alleviating the client's thirst.*

**Content Area:** Adult; **Concept:** Fluid and Electrolyte Balance; Comfort; **Integrated Processes:** Nursing Process: Implementation; **Client Needs:** Physiological Integrity: Physiological Adaptation; **Cognitive Level:** Analysis [Analyzing]

## 439. ANSWER: 3

1. Fatigue is associated with sodium, potassium, and phosphorus imbalances.
2. Tachycardia is most often associated with abnormal serum magnesium levels.
3. **Muscle cramps, paresthesia, and a positive Chvostek's sign are common manifestations of hypo- or hypercalcemia because of the irritation to the neuromuscular system.**
4. Hypotension relates most often to volume changes rather than electrolyte imbalances.

▶ *Test-taking Tip: Calcium affects the neuromuscular system. You can remember Chvostek's sign as pertaining to calcium because they both begin with the letter c.*

**Content Area:** Adult; **Concept:** Fluid and Electrolyte Balance; Metabolism; **Integrated Processes:** Nursing Process: Assessment; **Client Needs:** Physiological Integrity: Physiological Adaptation; **Cognitive Level:** Analysis [Analyzing]

## 440. MoC ANSWER: 1

1. **The client's ionized serum calcium level of 3.8 mg/dL is low (normal is 4.64 to 5.28 mg/dL). The nurse should assess this client first because calcium is essential to cardiac function.**
2. The client's serum sodium level of 142 mg/dL is within the normal range of 135 to 145 mEq/L.
3. The client's serum potassium level of 3.7 mEq/L is within the normal range of 3.5 to 5.0 mEq/L.
4. The client's serum phosphorus level of 2.4 mg/dL is slightly below the normal range of 2.5 to 4.5 mg/dL. Although it is important to assess this client, the client with the low ionized serum calcium is priority.

▶ *Test-taking Tip: Use the ABC's to establish the priority client.*

**Content Area:** Fundamentals; **Concept:** Fluid and Electrolyte Balance; Management; Assessment; **Integrated Processes:** Nursing Process: Assessment; **Client Needs:** Safe and Effective Care Environment: Management of Care; **Cognitive Level:** Analysis [Analyzing]

**441. ANSWER: 1180**

**First determine the IV fluid intake. 125 mL/hr ×
8 hrs = 1000 mL**
**Next, add this total to the other fluid intake.**
**1000 mL + 2000 mL + 350 mL + 110 mL +
360 mL = 3820 mL**
**Next subtract the intake from the output:**
**5000 mL – 3820 mL = 1180 mL**
**Because the client's output is greater than the
intake, the nurse would record the 1180 as a
negative fluid balance.**

▶ *Test-taking Tip: Intake includes total IV fluid for 8 hours
as well as fluid and foods that become liquid at room
temperature.*

Content Area: Fundamentals; Concept: Fluid and Electrolyte Balance;
Neurologic Regulation; Metabolism; Integrated Processes: Nursing
Process: Implementation; Client Needs: Physiological Integrity:
Physiological Adaptation; Cognitive Level: Analysis [Analyzing]

**442. ANSWER: 1, 2, 3, 5**

1. **The serum sodium level is low. Hyponatremia
results in weakness and muscle cramps from
cellular changes. In hyponatremia, sodium
outside cells decreases and water moves into
the cells, causing the cells to swell with water.**
2. **Water excess in hyponatremia lowers plasma
osmolality, shifting fluid into brain cells causing
headache.**
3. **Water excess in hyponatremia lowers plasma
osmolality, shifting fluid into brain cells causing
confusion.**
4. Cold, clammy skin, not warm, flushed skin, is
associated with hyponatremia.
5. **Increased GI motility occurs in hyponatremia,
resulting in abdominal cramping.**

▶ *Test-taking Tip: Focus on clinical manifestations
of hyponatremia. The normal serum sodium level is
135–145 mEq/L.*

Content Area: Fundamentals; Concept: Fluid and Electrolyte Balance;
Nursing Roles; Integrated Processes: Nursing Process: Analysis;
Client Needs: Physiological Integrity: Physiological Adaptation;
Cognitive Level: Analysis [Analyzing]

**443. PHARM ANSWER: 1, 2, 3, 4, 6**

1. **Sodium polystyrene (Kayexalate) is a cation
exchange resin that exchanges sodium ions for
potassium ions in the intestine, helping to lower the
serum potassium level.**
2. **Regular insulin temporarily shifts potassium
into the cell; it is given with IV glucose to prevent
hypoglycemia.**
3. **Dextrose 50% injection is given with regular
insulin IV to temporarily shift potassium into the
cells.**
4. **Calcium gluconate (Kalcinate) is administered to
stabilize the cardiac cell membrane in the presence
of hyperkalemia.**

5. Potassium supplements are contraindicated in clients
with hyperkalemia because a further increase in serum
potassium concentration in hyperkalemia can produce
cardiac arrest.
6. **Beta-2 adrenergic agonists, such as albuterol
(Proventil), promote cellular reuptake of potassium,
possibly via the cyclic guanosine monophosphate
(gAMP) receptor cascade.**

▶ *Test-taking Tip: Normal serum potassium level is 3.5 to
5.0 mEq/L. Memorization of common laboratory values,
such as potassium, is required to answer questions on the
NCLEX-RN® examination.*

Content Area: Adult; Concept: Fluid and Electrolyte Balance;
Medications; Integrated Processes: Nursing Process: Planning;
Client Needs: Physiological Integrity: Pharmacological and Parenteral
Therapies; Physiological Integrity: Physiological Adaptation;
Cognitive Level: Analysis [Analyzing]

**444. ANSWER: 3**

1. Paresthesias are associated with hyperkalemia
and not hypernatremia.
2. Muscle cramps and spasms are symptoms of
hyponatremia, not hypernatremia.
3. **Hypernatremia (serum sodium greater than
145 mEq/L) results in water shifting out of
cells into the extracellular fluid with resultant
dehydration and shrinkage of cells. Dehydration of
brain cells results in neurological manifestations
such as restlessness, agitation, lethargy, seizures,
and even coma.**
4. Increased body temperature can be a cause of the hypernatremia; a decrease might suggest improvement,
but the client should not be hypothermic.

▶ *Test-taking Tip: Hypernatremia is increased serum sodium.*

Content Area: Adult; Concept: Fluid and Electrolyte Balance; Nursing
Roles; Integrated Processes: Nursing Process: Evaluation; Client
Needs: Physiological Integrity: Physiological Adaptation; Cognitive
Level: Evaluation [Evaluating]

**445. ANSWER: 3**

1. Dairy products are the primary source of calcium and
should be increased in the presence of hypoparathyroidism. However, persons of the Orthodox Jewish
faith do not eat meat and dairy products at the same
meal. Two meals contain dairy products, and one meal
contains meat.
2. Carbonated beverages do not impact calcium, but
caffeinated beverages inhibit calcium absorption.
3. **The client should be taught to ensure an adequate
calcium intake, or supplements may be required. In
hypoparathyroidism, decreased function of the
parathyroid glands leads to decreased levels of
parathyroid hormone (PTH). In the absence of
adequate PTH activity, the ionized calcium concentration in the extracellular fluid falls.**

4. Those of the Orthodox Jewish faith do not eat shellfish or other fish without fins. Iodine intake is unrelated to hypoparathyroidism. Iodine deficiency may result in an enlarged thyroid gland.

▶ *Test-taking Tip: Hypoparathyroidism may result in hypocalcemia. You need to consider cultural differences when answering this question.*

**Content Area:** Adult; **Concept:** Fluid and Electrolyte Balance; Diversity; Metabolism; Caring; **Integrated Processes:** Teaching/Learning; Culture and Spirituality; Caring; **Client Needs:** Health Promotion and Maintenance; Psychosocial Integrity; **Cognitive Level:** Analysis [Analyzing]

## 446. MoC ANSWER: 1

1. **The nurse's priority should be to assess the heart. Hypomagnesemia can cause life-threatening dysrhythmias, resulting in cardiovascular failure and arrest.**
2. Hypomagnesemia causes neuromuscular irritability, but assessment of the reflexes is not the nurse's priority.
3. The nurse would stroke the cheek to assess for a Chvostek's sign seen with hypocalcemia, not hypomagnesemia.
4. It is important to assess for pitting edema with any condition, but it is not the priority assessment in hypomagnesemia.

▶ *Test-taking Tip: The key phrase is "priority." Use the ABC's to eliminate options.*

**Content Area:** Fundamentals; **Concept:** Fluid and Electrolyte Balance; Assessment; Management; **Integrated Processes:** Nursing Process: Assessment; **Client Needs:** Safe and Effective Care Environment: Management of Care; Physiological Integrity: Physiological Adaptation; **Cognitive Level:** Application [Applying]

## 447. MoC ANSWER: 1

1. **Some drugs cause increased renal losses of magnesium, including loop and thiazide diuretics. Stopping these is priority.**
2. Encouraging foods high in magnesium will take longer to increase the level of magnesium than holding or discontinuing medications that promote magnesium loss.
3. The route of magnesium replacement is dependent on the severity of the condition. Parenteral replacement is needed because the level is very low. Oral supplements will take longer to be effective.
4. IV magnesium is not given as a bolus. It is important to use caution to prevent hypermagnesemia.

▶ *Test-taking Tip: The key word is "priority." Normal serum magnesium is 1.6 to 2.6 mg/dL. You should think about causes of magnesium loss and interventions that would correct it.*

**Content Area:** Fundamentals; **Concept:** Fluid and Electrolyte Balance; Management; **Integrated Processes:** Nursing Process: Implementation; **Client Needs:** Safe and Effective Care Environment: Management of Care; **Cognitive Level:** Analysis [Analyzing]

## 448. ANSWER: 3

1. Confusion is not associated with low serum protein levels.
2. Restlessness is not associated with low serum protein levels.
3. **Low serum protein decreases plasma oncotic pressure, allowing fluid to remain in interstitial tissues. This results in edema.**
4. Pallor is not associated with low serum protein levels.

▶ *Test-taking Tip: One of the most common consequences of low total serum protein is fluid retention. The normal total serum protein level is 6 to 8 g/dL.*

**Content Area:** Fundamentals; **Concept:** Fluid and Electrolyte Balance; Assessment; **Integrated Processes:** Nursing Process: Assessment; **Client Needs:** Physiological Integrity: Physiological Adaptation; **Cognitive Level:** Knowledge [Remembering]

## 449. MoC ANSWER: 1, 2, 3

1. **Respiratory alkalosis may occur with a panic attack due to blowing off of carbon dioxide with hyperventilation.**
2. **Tingling occurs in respiratory alkalosis due to the increase in neuromuscular excitability associated with hyperventilation.**
3. **Muscle twitching occurs from neuromuscular excitability associated with hyperventilation.**
4. Excess salivation is not associated with respiratory alkalosis that may result from a panic attack.
5. Increased urination can occur from the stress response but is not associated with respiratory alkalosis.

▶ *Test-taking Tip: The most common reason for respiratory alkalosis is mechanical or spontaneous hyperventilation. In respiratory alkalosis, the amount of carbon dioxide in the blood decreases to below normal. This condition produces a shift in the body's pH balance and causes the body's system to become more alkaline (basic).*

**Content Area:** Fundamentals; **Concept:** pH Regulation; Management; **Integrated Processes:** Nursing Process: Analysis; Communication and Documentation; **Client Needs:** Safe and Effective Care Environment: Management of Care; **Cognitive Level:** Analysis [Analyzing]

## 450. ANSWER: 3

1. Hypokalemia, not hyperkalemia, is caused by diarrhea and vomiting.
2. Hypochloremia, not hyperchloremia, is associated with volume depletion due to vomiting.
3. **The nurse should monitor for metabolic alkalosis, which occurs when there is a loss of acid such as with prolonged vomiting.**
4. Metabolic alkalosis, not metabolic acidosis, occurs with prolonged vomiting.

▶ *Test-taking Tip: You can remember that acid and not base is lost through emesis by noting that both words begin with vowels.*

**Content Area:** Fundamentals; **Concept:** Fluid and Electrolyte Balance; Assessment; **Integrated Processes:** Nursing Process: Assessment; **Client Needs:** Physiological Integrity: Physiological Adaptation; **Cognitive Level:** Application [Applying]

## 451. ANSWER: 1

1. **The nurse should anticipate interventions to treat respiratory acidosis. This child is most likely in status asthmaticus with continued respiratory distress despite treatment. Even though the child has a high RR, there is hypoventilation from bronchoconstriction. This results in carbon dioxide retention, increased $Paco_2$ (greater than 45 mm Hg), and a lowering of pH or an acidotic state.**
2. Respiratory alkalosis would occur if excess carbon dioxide is blown off with hyperventilation.
3. The client's symptoms are associated with a respiratory and not a metabolic problem; thus metabolic alkalosis is not correct.
4. The client's symptoms are associated with a respiratory and not a metabolic problem; thus metabolic acidosis is not correct.

▶ **Test-taking Tip:** Diminished ventilation increases $Paco_2$, which is the respiratory component of acid-base balance. Thus eliminate Options 3 and 4.

Content Area: Child; Concept: pH Regulation; Integrated Processes: Nursing Process: Analysis; Client Needs: Physiological Integrity: Physiological Adaptation; Cognitive Level: Analysis [Analyzing]

## 452. ANSWER: 2

1. Respiratory alkalosis would result in a $Paco_2$ lower than the normal range of 35 to 45 mm Hg.
2. **A pH of 7.50 indicates alkalosis. The $HCO_3$ of 30 mmol/L is above the normal range of 20 to 24 mmol/L, indicating the primary acid-base imbalance is metabolic alkalosis.**
3. Respiratory acidosis would result in a pH less than 7.35 and an increased $Paco_2$.
4. Metabolic acidosis would result in a pH less than 7.35 and an increased $HCO_3$.

▶ **Test-taking Tip:** Label the pH, the $Paco_2$, and $HCO_3$ as either acid or base. The $Paco_2$ is the respiratory component and $HCO_3$ the metabolic component of acid-base balance. The component that matches the pH as acid or base is the system (respiratory or metabolic) initiating the acid-base imbalance.

Content Area: Adult; Concept: pH Regulation; Metabolism; Integrated Processes: Nursing Process: Analysis; Client Needs: Physiological Integrity: Reduction of Risk Potential; Cognitive Level: Analysis [Analyzing]

## 453. ANSWER: 3

1. DKA is a metabolic, not a respiratory, acid-base imbalance.
2. DKA is a metabolic, not a respiratory, acid-base imbalance.
3. **The nurse should implement interventions for treating metabolic acidosis. In DKA, the elevated blood sugar results in polyuria with a resultant decrease in the pH and $HCO_3$ levels. Kussmaul respirations allow the body to "blow off" excess carbon dioxide to compensate for the acidotic state and the decreased $HCO_3$.**

4. As DKA implies, it is an acidotic, not an alkalotic, imbalance.

▶ **Test-taking Tip:** DKA is a metabolic acid-base imbalance; thus eliminate options that pertain to the respiratory system.

Content Area: Adult; Concept: pH Regulation; Metabolism; Integrated Processes: Nursing Process: Implementation; Client Needs: Physiological Integrity: Reduction of Risk Potential; Cognitive Level: Analysis [Analyzing]

## 454. ANSWER: 1

1. **In respiratory alkalosis the pH is greater than 7.45 (normal is 7.35 to 7.45). The $Paco_2$ is less than 35 mm Hg (the normal is 35 to 45 mm Hg). The $HCO_3$ is normal (22–26 mEq/L). Because pulmonary emboli interfere with gas exchange, the respiratory center is stimulated to meet oxygenation demands. The tachypnea produces respiratory alkalosis.**
2. The blood gas findings of pH 7.35, $Paco_2$ 35 mm Hg, and $HCO_3$ 22 mEq/L are all normal.
3. The elevated pH of 7.50 and increased $HCO_3$ of 28 mEq/L indicate metabolic alkalosis.
4. The decreased pH of 7.32 and increased $Paco_2$ of 48 mm Hg indicate respiratory acidosis.

▶ **Test-taking Tip:** First look at the pH and eliminate the option with a decreased pH because this indicates acidosis. Of the remaining options, look at the $Paco_2$ because it is the respiratory component for ABG analysis. Select the option with the decreased $Paco_2$ because a low $Paco_2$ is present in respiratory alkalosis.

Content Area: Adult; Concept: pH Regulation; Oxygenation; Integrated Processes: Nursing Process: Assessment; Client Needs: Physiological Integrity: Physiological Adaptation; Cognitive Level: Analysis [Analyzing]

## 455. MoC ANSWER: 4, 2, 1, 3

4. **The client with DM whose ABG results are pH = 7.22, $Paco_2$ = 35 mm Hg, $HCO_3$ = 15 mEq/L. The ABG results indicate metabolic acidosis. A compensatory mechanism will include Kussmaul respirations to eliminate excess acid. Airway assessment is priority, and further assessment is needed to determine the underlying cause for the metabolic acidosis.**
2. **The client with hyperemesis whose serum sodium level is 122 mEq/L. This client is experiencing severe hyponatremia with serum sodium below the normal range of 135 to 145 mEq/L and is at risk of seizures. Safety is a major concern.**
1. **The client with renal insufficiency whose serum potassium level is 5.2 mEq/L. This client's serum potassium level is slightly above the normal of 3.5 to 5.0 mEq/L and should be assessed for signs of hyperkalemia.**
3. **The client recovering following head trauma whose serum osmolality is 290 mOsm/kg. The serum osmolality level is normal (normal is 285 to 295 mOsm/kg). This client is the most stable.**

▶ **Test-taking Tip:** *Use the ABC's and Maslow's Hierarchy of Needs theory to establish priority.*

**Content Area:** Adult; **Concept:** Fluid and Electrolyte Balance; Management; Assessment; **Integrated Processes:** Nursing Process: Assessment; **Client Needs:** Safe and Effective Care Environment: Management of Care; **Cognitive Level:** Synthesis [Creating]

### 456. ANSWER: 2, 3, 5, 6

1. Mechanical ventilation may be needed to support the client but not with hyperventilation. The $Paco_2$ is below normal. This occurred because the client would initially hyperventilate as a compensatory mechanism to return the acid-base balance back to normal by increasing the loss of $Paco_2$ through the lungs. At this time, mechanical hyperventilation will increase the loss of carbonic acid and further lower the $Paco_2$ level without correcting the problem.

2. **The nurse should plan to give sodium bicarbonate. The ABGs reveal partially compensated metabolic acidosis with the pH below the normal of 7.35 to 7.45, the $Paco_2$ below the normal of 35 to 45 mm Hg, and the $HCO_3$ below the normal of 22 to 26 mEq/L. Ethylene glycol toxicity can produce metabolic acidosis. Half of the total bicarbonate deficit should be replaced during the first few hours of therapy with sodium bicarbonate.**

3. **Hemodialysis is an option for correcting a severe metabolic acidosis associated with ethylene glycol toxicity.**

4. Crystalloids, not colloids, would be used for fluid replacement.

5. **The nurse should plan to give an IV potassium replacement. Initially, as a compensatory mechanism in metabolic acidosis, potassium shifts out of the vascular compartment and into the cell in exchange for hydrogen ion to reestablish acid-base balance. Until full compensation occurs, potassium replacement is needed.**

6. **The $Pao_2$ is low, so supplemental oxygen is needed.**

▶ **Test-taking Tip:** *You need to identify the acid-base imbalance before selecting interventions. Label the pH, the $Paco_2$, and $HCO_3$ as either acid or base. $Paco_2$ is the respiratory component and $HCO_3$ the metabolic component of acid-base balance. The component that matches the pH as acid or base is the system (respiratory or metabolic) initiating the acid-base imbalance. The component that is abnormal but does not match the direction of the pH as acid or base is the system that is compensating for the imbalance.*

**Content Area:** Adult; **Concept:** pH Regulation; Medication; **Integrated Processes:** Nursing Process: Implementation; **Client Needs:** Physiological Integrity: Physiological Adaptation; **Cognitive Level:** Synthesis [Creating]

### 457. MoC ANSWER: 4

1. Client A has edema, dyspnea, and a weight increased by 2 lb supporting fluid volume excess, but these findings are not as extreme as those with Client D.

2. Client B has crackles, an intake that exceeds output, and an elevated BUN supporting fluid volume excess, but these findings are not as extreme as those with Client D.

3. Client C has crackles, 1+ edema, and dyspnea. However, the output exceeds input, and the client's weight is down 3 lb. This client is not a priority.

4. **Client D needs priority interventions for excess fluid volume because the client has a greater degree of fluid volume excess than the other clients. Clients with excess fluid volume may have crackles and report dyspnea. Edema varies from trace to 4+ and can be dependent to generalized edema. Excess fluid volume will most often result in an increased weight and BUN and decreased Hct because of dilution.**

▶ **Test-taking Tip:** *Carefully review the information about the clients. Recall that weight and I&O are key findings when considering fluid volume, so analyze these first for each client.*

**Content Area:** Adult; **Concept:** Fluid and Electrolyte Balance; Management; **Integrated Processes:** Nursing Process: Analysis; Caring; **Client Needs:** Safe and Effective Care Environment: Management of Care; **Cognitive Level:** Analysis [Analyzing]

## Chapter Twelve

# Safety: Accident, Injury, and Error Prevention

**458.** **MoC** The charge nurse is observing nursing staff. In which activity illustrated should the charge nurse intervene because it places the nurse **most** at risk for back injury?

1.

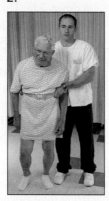

2.

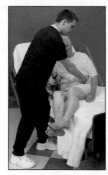

3.

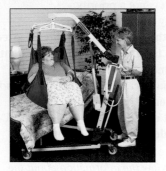

4.

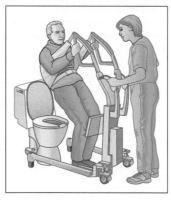

**459.** **MoC** A power outage occurs at a hospital, and a backup generator supplying power to a telemetry unit fails. After obtaining a flashlight, what is the nurse's **next** best action?

1. Call the nursing supervisor.
2. Assess the most critically ill clients.
3. Obtain oxygen tanks for clients on oxygen.
4. Delegate which clients the NA should monitor.

**460.** The client with a left-sided weakness is to be discharged to home, where the client has an electrical bed. In preparation for discharge, the nurse assesses the client's ability to get out of bed independently. Which client actions indicate that further instruction is needed? **Select all that apply.**

1. Places the bed in the lowest position
2. Raises the head of the bed (HOB)
3. Rolls onto the left side
4. Pushes against the mattress with the weak elbow and stronger hand to rise to a sitting position
5. Slides legs off the bed while pushing against the mattress to raise the body off the bed
6. Once in a sitting position, sits at the edge of the bed for a few minutes before standing

**461.** Pressure is being exerted to the client's foot ulcer from the bottom bed guard, and the client needs to be pulled up in bed. The client weighs 130 lb. Which action by the nurse is **best** when no one is available to assist the nurse?

1. Wait until sufficient help is available to pull up and reposition the client in bed.
2. Place pillows over the bed guard and elevate both of the client's legs on the pillows.
3. Place the bed in Trendelenburg position to relieve the pressure and then wait for help.
4. Use a slight Trendelenburg position, have the client lift the heels, and pull the client up in bed.

**462.** MoC The new NA is caring for the client who is at risk for a fall. Which statement by the nurse to the new NA is **most** important?

1. "Remind the client to call for assistance before getting out of bed."
2. "Clip the call light to the bedcovers so the client can find it easily."
3. "Be sure the bed is in the lowest position when you leave the room."
4. "Check that you have all four siderails up after you provide care."

**463.** MoC The experienced nurse is observing the new nurse providing care to the hospitalized client. Which action requires the experienced nurse to intervene to ensure client safety?

1. Turns on the client's bathroom light and turns out the room lights after settling the client for sleep
2. Checks the room number and name band to verify the client's identity before giving a medication
3. Stirs thickening powder into the glass of juice and cup of milk before giving these to the client who has dysphagia
4. Delays the HCP from performing a thoracentesis by calling "a timeout" to verify the client's identity, consent, procedure, and site

**464.** The client that the nurse is ambulating becomes dizzy and feels faint. Place the nurse's actions in the correct order to prevent the client from falling.

1. Support and ease the client to the floor by sliding the client down the forward leg.
2. Call for help.
3. Bend at the knees and pull the client toward the forward leg.
4. Assess the client for injuries.
5. Protect the client's head from hitting objects on the floor.
6. Assume a broad stance with the stronger leg somewhat behind the other leg.

Answer: _____

**465.** The client states, "I can't wait for anyone to take me to the bathroom, or I will wet my pants." What should the nurse plan to do? **Select all that apply.**

1. Assess the client's risk for a fall using a rating scale.
2. Document that the client is frequently incontinent.
3. Ensure an immediate response to the client's call light.
4. Educate the client regarding fall prevention strategies.
5. Place a note on the door stating, "Bathroom every 2 hours."
6. Request that the HCP prescribe placement of a urinary catheter.

**466.** The nurse documents in the client's medical record: "Client uses a three-point gait correctly to maintain non–weight-bearing on left foot when ambulating with crutches. Maintains steady balance and keeps eyes focused ahead." On the illustration, place an X in the tripod position box in the column that **most** accurately illustrates the gait documented by the nurse.

**467.** MoC The client with dementia and confusion is transferred from the hospital to the nursing home. The client's family has not yet arrived at the nursing home. Which direction is appropriate for the RN to provide to the LPN?

1. "Take a photograph of the new resident; it is needed to administer medications."
2. "Place the resident in a wheelchair near the nurse's station until the family arrives."
3. "Help the new resident change into clothing with Velcro closures for easy removal."
4. "Perform a full-body assessment and document this in the resident's medical record."

**468.** MoC The nurse asks the NA to apply a mitten restraint for the client seated in the wheelchair next to the bed. Which observation by the nurse indicates that the NA needs further instructions on applying restraints?

1. Restraint strap is tied to the bed frame next to the client.
2. Restraint straps are secured using a half-bow slipknot.
3. Two fingers can be inserted between the restraint and client's skin.
4. Mesh portion of the mitten restraint is on the back of the hand.

**469.** MoC The UAP is caring for the client who has been placed in bilateral wrist restraints. Which direction should the nurse give to the UAP?

1. "The wrist restraint must remain on at all times but can be loosened if needed."
2. "The client attempted to harm staff; only enter the room with another person."
3. "Ask the client about the need for toileting and offer liquids every 2 hours."
4. "Assess the client's skin condition and provide hand exercises every 2 hours."

**470.** MoC The client with DM is receiving care in the home for a foot ulcer. The home health nurse documents the narrative note illustrated below. Which problem should be the nurse's **priority** on the return visit?

| Progress Notes | |
| --- | --- |
| **Time** | **Entry** |
| 0900 | Client visited in home. Left foot ulcer showing signs of healing with granulation tissue. Wet-to-dry dressing change completed. Instructed on wearing nonskid slipper on left foot and shoe on right after noting client wearing white socks for ambulation. BP 140/86 mm Hg; states has not yet taken morning dose of medication: "Can't stomach breakfast if eaten before the dressing change." Plan to return in a.m. for further assessment. ———————— B. Green, RN |

1. Impaired skin integrity related to left foot ulcer
2. Potential for injury related to improper footwear
3. Potential altered nutrition: less than body requirements related to nausea
4. Ineffective therapeutic regimen management related to not taking medications as prescribed

**471.** The client had a THR. The nurse is discussing home modifications with the client's son. Which modifications should the nurse recommend? **Select all that apply.**

1. Pad bedside rails.
2. Install safety bars around the toilet and shower.
3. Install an elevated toilet seat in the bathroom.
4. Plan for the client's bed to be in a main floor room.
5. Use a nonskid bathmat in the bathtub for the client's daily bath.
6. Remove scatter rugs and secure electrical cords against baseboards.

**472.** The client makes the following statements to the home health nurse. Which statement requires the nurse to intervene **immediately**?

1. "I can't lift pans from the back burners, but I can manage by using the front burners of my stove."
2. "I almost fell down the stairs, so I bought myself a pair of slippers with nonskid soles."
3. "The grass near the sidewalk will be dead; my son insists on putting salt on the icy sidewalk."
4. "Heating my home costs less when I keep the gas stove's oven door open to heat just my living areas."

**473.** The home health nurse is using the home Safety Assessment Scale to evaluate the dangers that may exist in the home of the client who is mildly cognitively impaired. Which finding on the scale should be **most** concerning to the nurse?

1. Lives alone and has no spouse or living children
2. Places hot pads on stove when burners are on
3. Is unable to recognize when food is spoiled
4. Has poor vision and doesn't wear glasses

**474.** The nurse is teaching the client with a latex allergy about home and personal safety. Which information should the nurse emphasize? **Select all that apply.**

1. Remove items in the home made from synthetic materials.
2. Keep emergency telephone numbers readily accessible.
3. Have someone remove any latex balloons and rubber bands.
4. Avoid foods such as kiwi, bananas, avocados, and chestnuts.
5. Certain plants, such as poinsettia plants, help remove allergens.

**475.** When entering the client's room, the nurse sees that the client is standing on the far side of the room with clothing on fire. Which action should be taken by the nurse **immediately?**

1. Go find the nearest fire alarm box.
2. Grab a blanket to smother the fire.
3. Obtain water to douse the clothes.
4. Tell the client to drop and roll on the floor.

**476.** The nurse realizes that a fire has started in the client's room. Which action should be taken by the nurse **first?**

1. Find the nearest fire alarm to activate.
2. Extinguish the fire with a blanket.
3. Remove the client from the room.
4. Telephone the operator to announce a fire.

**477.** The nurse is demonstrating the use of a fire extinguisher during a fire drill. Place the steps for using a fire extinguisher in the correct order.

1. Squeeze the handle.
2. Sweep from side to side.
3. Pull the pin.
4. Aim at the base of the fire.

Answer: _____

**478.** The hospitalized client tells the nurse about feeling a strong shock when turning on an electric hair dryer. What should the nurse do **first?**

1. Assess the client's heart rhythm and apical pulse.
2. Disconnect the hair dryer from the electrical outlet.
3. Assess the client's skin for signs of electrical burn.
4. Tag and send the hair dryer for inspection.

**479.** The nurse is caring for clients in a hospital setting. Which observations made by the nurse require intervention? **Select all that apply.**

1. The client's infusion pump is noted to have a cut in the center of the cord.
2. The client's bed is in the high position after a NA left the room.
3. The client's battery-operated CD player does not have an agency inspection tag.
4. The client's bed exit alarm is beeping, and another nurse just left the room.
5. The client's bedside table is placed in front of the chair where the client is sitting.

**480.** MoC The nurse is evaluating the performance of the UAP. The nurse should provide feedback to the UAP about which unsafe action?

1. Cleanses and returns a wheelchair to a storage area after being used by the client.
2. Ties the confused client's wrist restraint ties to the bed frame using a quick-release knot.
3. Grasps the cord to unplug an intravenous infusion pump for the client's transport to x-ray.
4. Turns on a bed exit alarm for the confused client who was talking incoherently to the UAP.

**481.** The expectant mother asks the nurse, "With all the babies in the nursery, how will I know that the nurse is bringing me my baby?" What is the nurse's **best** response?

1. "The baby has a plastic bracelet with permanent locks that must be cut for removal."
2. "If taken from the unit, your baby's security band will set off an alarm and lock exits."
3. "Your identification number and full name are printed on your baby's ID band."
4. "An ID band is applied to your infant, and footprints are taken and kept on record."

**482.** The mother calls the nurse to ask when her newborn will be brought back to her room to finish feeding. The mother states that a doctor came about 30 minutes ago to take the baby for an examination and has not returned with her baby. Which action should be taken by the nurse **first**?

1. Check the unit for the infant.
2. Initiate procedures for possible newborn abduction.
3. Ask other staff if they saw any physicians on the unit.
4. Check to see if the doctor is still examining the infant.

**483.** The nurse is discussing with the parents their full-term newborn's transportation in a vehicle. Which information should the nurse provide? **Select all that apply.**

1. The infant should be restrained in a car seat located in the backseat facing the rear of the car.
2. The infant should be restrained in a car seat located in the backseat facing the front of the car.
3. An infant car seat may be designed only for infants; if so, obtain another one when the infant reaches the weight limit for that model.
4. Some states and provinces in the United States and Canada have mandated the use of infant and child restraints.
5. A car seat should have a certification label stating that it complies with federal motor vehicle safety standards.

**484.** **PHARM** A child is admitted to the ED after ingesting oxycodone tablets that had been prescribed for the parent. The prescription bottle provided by the parent originally had 15 tablets of 5 mg oxycodone. The parent stated taking 3 tablets. There are 9 tablets remaining. If the child ingested the missing tablets, how many mg of oxycodone did the child ingest?

_____ mg (Record your answer as a whole number.)

**485.** The nurse is planning an educational session for a group of parents with toddlers. Based on the two leading causes of death in toddlers, the nurse should make which topics **priority? Select all that apply.**

1. Water safety and methods to prevent drowning
2. Use of age- and weight-appropriate car seats
3. Nutrition guidelines and age-appropriate foods
4. Use of labels to identify poisonous substances
5. Safety when outdoors and crossing the street

**486.** The nurse is teaching parents measures to prevent scald and burn injuries to toddlers in the home. Due to toddlers' inquisitiveness, which recommendation by the nurse is **most** important?

1. Turn pot handles toward the back of the stove.
2. Use the microwave cautiously when cooking.
3. Ensure that the smoke detector is on and working.
4. Verify that the bathwater temperature is tepid.

**487.** The non–English-speaking hospitalized client begins to enter a room with the sign illustrated. Which intervention should the observing nurse implement?

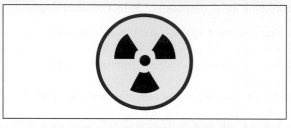

1. Inform the client's assigned nurse that the client is back in his or her room.
2. Intercept the client and check the client's name band for a room number.
3. Stop the client and ask for his or her name and the assigned room number.
4. Ask the nearby UAP to help the client back into the room with the sign posted.

**488.** **MoC** The nurse is caring for the client who received afterload internal radiotherapy (brachytherapy) for treatment of uterine cancer. The nurse manager evaluates that the nurse uses correct hazardous material precautions when noting that the nurse takes which action?

1. Double-bags linens before removing them from the client's room
2. Minimizes the amount of time spent in contact with the client
3. Maintains a distance of 1 foot away from the client
4. Wears lead gloves and apron and a dosimetry badge with client contact

**INSTRUCTIONS:** Use the information provided to answer Question 489.

**489.** `CJ` A health care agency has different receptacles for the various categories of institutional waste. Into which container should the nurse dispose of the soiled items illustrated? Place the items into the correct receptacle.

| Soiled Items | Receptacles |
|---|---|
| A. | 1. Wastebasket in the client's bathroom |
| B. | 2. Injurious waste receptacle |
| C. | 3. Hazardous waste receptacle |
| D. | 4. Infectious waste receptacle |

Answer:

| Receptacles and Items | |
|---|---|
| **Receptacles** | **Item Letter** |
| 1. Wastebasket | |
| 2. Injurious waste | |
| 3. Hazardous waste | |
| 4. Infectious waste | |

**490.** `MoC` The nurse manager is reviewing a list of serious reportable events that occurred in a hospital setting before submitting the list to an external agency. Which event should the nurse manager remove from the list before it is submitted?

1. The nurse is seriously injured when touching the client during a cardioversion procedure.
2. The client obtains a skin tear and abrasion while transferring from the bed to a wheelchair.
3. The client has a hip fracture after wandering off the unit and falling down the stairs.
4. The client has a cardiac arrest; the serum potassium level was low and not reported to the HCP.

**491.** Prior to checking a fingerstick blood glucose level, the nurse checks the identification band of the newly admitted client transferred from another facility. The nurse notes that the name and birth date are correct but that the band has the logo from another facility. Which is the **best** action by the nurse?

1. Ask the UAP to obtain a new band while the nurse performs the planned procedure.
2. Stop and replace the band with the current facility band that has the client identifiers.
3. Ask the client to state his or her name and birth date and to verify them against the band.
4. Leave the band in place; a name band from one facility can be used in another facility.

**492.** `MoC` The nurse confides to a coworker that when reporting a change in the client's condition to the HCP, the HCP stated, "It seems that every time you work, there is some catastrophe. Can't you problem-solve earlier so this doesn't happen?" What is the coworker's **best** response?

1. "This HCP responds to everyone the same. You did everything right; don't feel bad."
2. "You should obtain our hospital policy and initiate the steps to report the HCP."
3. "Let the nurse manager know; I think our manager is already dealing with the HCP."
4. "Let's go to the medical director, who should be told about this HCP's angry response."

**493.** MoC The nurse is preparing a presentation on workplace incivility. Which incivility behaviors should the nurse plan to include in the presentation? **Select all that apply.**

1. Verbal intimidation of nurses and invasion of personal space by HCPs
2. Personal insults, then ignoring a person as if that person is not present
3. Discussion between the nurse and HCPs about the client's condition
4. Teasing that occurs between nurses, HCPs, or other employees
5. Reporting the behaviors using the facility's incivility report form

**494.** MoC The nurse manager overhears multiple conversations on a hospital unit. Based on the statement made, the nurse manager should initiate the process for reporting incivility with which person?

1. Charge nurse to the nurse, "I need to discuss the medication error you made yesterday."
2. HCP to the nurse, "Tell me again what the client's vital signs were before he collapsed."
3. Nurse to a coworker, "You forgot to document the client's noon glucometer reading."
4. HCP to the client, "I can't do anything more for you; you don't follow my advice anyway."

## Answers and Rationales

**458.** MoC **ANSWER: 4**

1. The nurse is using a mechanical lift to move the client. Because another person is not present to assist, there is a perceived increased risk for injury to the client.
2. Ambulating the client with a transfer belt increases the nurse's risk for a back injury should the client fall, but it is less of a risk than the twisting and bending illustrated in activity D.
3. The nurse is using a standing assist device to help the client move from a sitting to a standing position and vice versa. Using assistive devices minimizes the risk for injury to the client and nurse.
4. **Bending and twisting the torso can cause back injury if the nurse does not use correct body mechanics. The nurse has reduced the risk by using a transfer belt and proper body mechanics, but the risk for injury exists because the client could easily grab the nurse's shoulder or arm with his left hand, altering the nurse's stance.**

♦ *Test-taking Tip: Examine each illustration carefully and focus on the position of the client and nurse to determine the nurse's risk for injury.*

**Content Area:** Fundamentals; **Concept:** Safety; **Integrated Processes:** Nursing Process: Evaluation; **Client Needs:** Safe and Effective Care Environment: Management of Care; Safe and Effective Care Environment: Safety and Infection Control; Physiological Integrity: Basic Care and Comfort; **Cognitive Level:** Evaluation [Evaluating]

**459.** MoC **ANSWER: 3**

1. A call to the nursing supervisor may be necessary for assistance on the unit but is not the next action.
2. Assessment of the most critical clients is also important, but those in need of oxygen have priority.

3. **When power is interrupted, the oxygen sources in the room will also fail. Oxygen will need to be delivered by oxygen tanks.**
4. The nurse should delegate activities, but rather than monitoring clients, the nurse should delegate retrieving oxygen tanks.

♦ *Test-taking Tip: Use the ABC's to determine the priority action. In emergency situations, an intervention (oxygen) has priority over assessment.*

**Content Area:** Fundamentals; **Concept:** Critical Thinking; Oxygenation; Management; **Integrated Processes:** Nursing Process: Implementation; **Client Needs:** Safe and Effective Care Environment: Management of Care; **Cognitive Level:** Analysis [Analyzing]

**460. ANSWER: 3, 4**

1. A low bed position prevents a fall from the feet not touching the floor.
2. Raising the HOB decreases the distance to a sitting position.
3. **With a left-sided weakness, the client should turn onto the stronger side, which would be the right and not the left side. Further instruction is needed.**
4. **The stronger (not weaker) elbow, hand, and leg should be used to push off from the bed into a sitting position. Further instruction is needed.**
5. The weight of the legs dangling will decrease the effort required to push into a sitting position.
6. Sudden position changes can cause orthostatic hypotension. Sitting awhile ensures that the client is not dizzy prior to standing.

♦ *Test-taking Tip: Note that the client has a left-sided weakness. Visualizing the steps that the client should use to transfer when the left side is weak should direct you to the correct actions. Note the similarities in Options 3 and 4 of using the weaker side to rise from the bed.*

## 461. ANSWER: 4

1. Waiting for help delays relieving the pressure and can increase pain and tissue damage.
2. Placing pillows over the bed guard and elevating the client's legs increases the risk of the client sliding off of the bed when unattended.
3. Leaving the client in the Trendelenburg's position can compromise the client's respiratory status.
4. **The force of gravity, created by the slight Trendelenburg's position, increases the ability to move a lightweight client up in bed safely while alone. Lifting the heels prevents friction injury.**

▶ *Test-taking Tip: Select the option that applies ergonomic principles and maintains the safety of the client.*

## 462. MoC ANSWER: 3

1. Reminding the client to call for assistance is an important statement, but a more serious injury can occur from a fall from a bed that is too high.
2. An easily accessible call light will be a reminder to the client to call for assistance, but this is not the most important statement.
3. **Reminding a new NA to be sure that the bed is in the lowest position before leaving the room is the most important statement to prevent the client from falling out of bed.**
4. Having all four siderails up is considered a restraint. Other measures to prevent a fall should be implemented first.

▶ *Test-taking Tip: To determine the most important statement, you need to evaluate the risk for injury if the action in the option is not performed. The option that poses the greatest risk for injury if not performed is the answer.*

## 463. MoC ANSWER: 2

1. Keeping a light on can prevent confusion about the surroundings if the client should waken during the night.
2. **The experienced nurse should intervene when the nurse incorrectly verifies the client's identity prior to medication administration. The client's room number is not one of the two unique client identifiers. The usual identifiers are the client's name and medical record number on the name band.**

3. The client with dysphagia has difficulty swallowing. Thickening liquids will help aid in swallowing to prevent aspiration.
4. A final verification process to confirm the correct client, procedure, and site should be conducted prior to the start of any invasive procedure.

▶ *Test-taking Tip: The key phrase is "ensure client safety." Read each option carefully to identify the situation that increases the risk for the nurse to cause an error.*

## 464. ANSWER: 2, 6, 3, 1, 5, 4

2. **First, call for help. Extra staff will be needed to support the client and obtain a wheelchair or stretcher to accompanying the client back to bed.**
6. **Assume a broad stance with the stronger leg somewhat behind the other leg. This position forms a solid base of support for bearing the weight on the stronger leg.**
3. **Bend at the knees and pull the client toward the forward leg.**
1. **Support and ease the client to the floor by sliding the client down the forward leg.**
5. **Protect the client's head from hitting objects on the floor.**
4. **Assess the client for injuries.**

▶ *Test-taking Tip: Visualize the steps prior to placing them in the correct order.*

## 465. ANSWER: 1, 3, 4

1. **The nurse should assess the client for factors in addition to voiding urgency that may increase the client's fall risk.**
2. The nurse cannot infer from the client's statement that the client is incontinent and should not document that the client is frequently incontinent.
3. **The nurse should ensure an immediate response to the client's call light and inform other caregivers of the client's statement.**
4. **The nurse should educate the client about strategies to prevent a fall, such as calling for help, wearing nonskid slippers, and ensuring appropriate lighting.**
5. A note placed on the client's door stating bathroom every 2 hours violates the client's right to privacy and should not be completed.
6. Requesting urinary catheter placement is unnecessary and increases the client's risk for an infection.

▶ *Test-taking Tip: Implementing safety measures to prevent a fall when the client has voiding urgency should not disclose the client's confidential information or increase the client's risk for injury.*

**Content Area:** Fundamentals; **Concept:** Safety; **Integrated Processes:** Nursing Process: Planning; **Client Needs:** Safe and Effective Care Environment: Safety and Infection Control; **Cognitive Level:** Analysis [Analyzing]

## 466. ANSWER:

A three-point gait should be used for non–weight-bearing ambulation. Both the crutches and the weaker leg move forward first. Then, the stronger leg advances. Column 1 illustrates a two-point gait. This is a partial weight-bearing gait. Column 3 illustrates a four-point gait. This is a partial weight-bearing gait. Column 4 illustrates a swing-to gait, a weight-bearing gait.

▶ *Test-taking Tip: If unsure of the types of gaits, focus on the illustration and try to determine which illustration shows a non-weight-bearing gait.*

**Content Area:** Fundamentals; **Concept:** Mobility; **Integrated Processes:** Communication and Documentation; **Client Needs:** Safe and Effective Care Environment: Safety and Infection Control; Physiological Integrity: Basic Care and Comfort; **Cognitive Level:** Comprehension [Understanding]

## 467. MoC ANSWER: 2

1. The permission to take a picture, even for medication administration purposes, must be obtained from the person's legal guardian.

2. **The client with dementia and confusion is cognitively impaired and is at risk for falling if left alone. Placing the resident near the nurse's station until the family arrives will allow for supervision and may help to keep the person safe.**

3. Although clothing with Velcro closures will be easier to don and remove, there is no indication that a change of clothing is needed. The client will likely arrive in the clothing worn to the hospital.

4. Performing a physical assessment is not within the LPN's scope of practice.

▶ *Test-taking Tip: Use Maslow's Hierarchy of Needs theory to determine the priority. The client's safety should be priority, and only one option addresses the client's immediate safety need.*

**Content Area:** Fundamentals; **Concept:** Safety, Regulations; **Integrated Processes:** Communication and Documentation; **Client Needs:** Safe and Effective Care Environment: Management of Care; **Cognitive Level:** Analysis [Analyzing]

## 468. MoC ANSWER: 1

1. **When the client is seated in the wheelchair, the mitten restraint should be secured to the frame of the wheelchair. Client injury can occur if the wheelchair is pulled away from the bed.**

2. A half-bow slipknot should be used for quick release.

3. Allowing room for two fingerbreadths between the restraint and client's skin prevents circulatory constriction.

4. The mesh portion of the mitten restraint should be on the back of the hand to observe hand and finger color while the mitten restraint is in place.

▶ *Test-taking Tip: Focus on client safety. Select the option that could result in client injury if the wheelchair is moved.*

**Content Area:** Fundamentals; **Concept:** Safety; **Integrated Processes:** Nursing Process: Evaluation; **Client Needs:** Safe and Effective Care Environment: Management of Care; Safe and Effective Care Environment: Safety and Infection Control; **Cognitive Level:** Evaluation [Evaluating]

## 469. MoC ANSWER: 3

1. Wrist restraints should be removed every 2 hours and ROM performed.

2. A violent/self-destructive restraint such as a four-point leather restraint would be used if the client is at risk of harming others. The cloth ties can be broken by a violent client.

3. **The need for toileting and liquids should be determined every 2 hours. Because the client is restrained, the client is unable to meet these needs independently. This is an appropriate direction for the nurse to give to the UAP.**

4. Although the UAP can perform hand exercises, performing an assessment of the client's skin condition is not within the scope of practice of the UAP.

▶ *Test-taking Tip: You should use the type of restraint, wrist restraints, as a clue to narrow the options. Assessments are within the RN scope of practice and cannot be delegated to the UAP.*

**Content Area:** Fundamentals; **Concept:** Safety, Regulations; Management; **Integrated Processes:** Communication and Documentation; **Client Needs:** Safe and Effective Care Environment: Management of Care; Safe and Effective Care Environment: Safety and Infection Control; **Cognitive Level:** Application [Applying]

### 470. ANSWER: 2

1. The impaired skin integrity is not currently health-threatening because the wound is showing signs of healing.
2. **The risk for injury should be the nurse's priority. The client with diabetes may have decreased sensation to the feet. Trauma to the foot can result in injury that may not be felt by the client. Falling is also a concern because the client's mobility is impaired due to the foot ulcer. A fall could be life-threatening.**
3. Nutrition is not currently health-threatening, but it could be if it persists.
4. Although the BP is slightly elevated, there is no indication that the client does not plan to take the medication.

▶ *Test-taking Tip: Use Maslow's Hierarchy of Needs theory to establish priority. Actual or potential life-threatening situations have priority, Option 2.*

**Content Area:** Fundamentals; **Concept:** Safety; **Integrated Processes:** Nursing Process: Analysis; **Client Needs:** Safe and Effective Care Environment: Safety and Infection Control; **Cognitive Level:** Analysis [Analyzing]

### 471. ANSWER: 2, 3, 4, 6

1. Padded siderails are unnecessary; these are used for injury prevention with seizure activity or agitation.
2. **Safety bars around the toilet and shower are useful for support and fall prevention.**
3. **An elevated toilet seat is necessary. The client should avoid greater than a 90-degree hip flexion for 4 to 6 weeks postoperatively.**
4. **A main floor bedroom will prevent unnecessary stair climbing that could cause a fall.**
5. The client should shower rather than bathe. Tub baths are generally not allowed for 4 to 6 weeks to avoid greater than a 90-degree hip flexion.
6. **Scatter rugs and stray electrical cords can cause tripping and falls.**

▶ *Test-taking Tip: Focus on client safety and the type of surgery when selecting the answer options. Generally, greater than a 90-degree hip flexion should be avoided for 4 to 6 weeks after a total hip arthroplasty.*

**Content Area:** Fundamentals; **Concept:** Safety; **Integrated Processes:** Teaching/Learning; **Client Needs:** Safe and Effective Care Environment: Safety and Infection Control; Health Promotion and Maintenance; Physiological Integrity: Reduction of Risk Potential; **Cognitive Level:** Application [Applying]

### 472. ANSWER: 4

1. Inability to lift pans from the back burners poses a safety concern for burns and scalds, but the client states using front burners. Although further assessment is required, this does not require immediate intervention.
2. Wearing nonskid slippers promotes client safety.
3. Applying salt to icy sidewalks promotes client safety.
4. **Using a gas oven or range to heat the home can result in carbon monoxide accumulation and poisoning. The nurse should intervene immediately.**

▶ *Test-taking Tip: Eliminate the statements that promote client safety, Options 2 and 3. Of the remaining options, determine which needs further assessment and which needs immediate intervention.*

**Content Area:** Fundamentals; **Concept:** Safety; Management; **Integrated Processes:** Communication and Documentation; **Client Needs:** Safe and Effective Care Environment: Safety and Infection Control; Physiological Integrity: Reduction of Risk Potential; **Cognitive Level:** Analysis [Analyzing]

### 473. ANSWER: 2

1. Living alone is a concern for safety, but the risk of fire is most concerning.
2. **If cloth items are placed on a hot stove, the risk of fire is the most concerning.**
3. Inability to recognize spoiled foods is a safety concern, but the risk of fire is the most concerning.
4. Poor vision is a concern regarding safety in the home, but the risk of fire is the most concerning.

▶ *Test-taking Tip: Select the option that puts the client in immediate danger.*

**Content Area:** Fundamentals; **Concept:** Safety; **Integrated Processes:** Nursing Process: Analysis; **Client Needs:** Safe and Effective Care Environment: Safety and Infection Control; **Cognitive Level:** Application [Applying]

### 474. ANSWER: 2, 3, 4

1. Persons with a latex allergy react to either contact with or aerosolized particles of natural latex rubber, not synthetic materials.
2. **Emergency telephone numbers should be available because an anaphylactic reaction can occur.**
3. **Latex balloons and rubber bands should be removed from the home by someone other than the person with a latex allergy.**
4. **Foods such as kiwi, bananas, avocados, and chestnuts should be avoided because these increase the risk of an allergic reaction.**
5. Plants such as poinsettia can initiate an allergic reaction and should be removed from the house.

▶ *Test-taking Tip: Recall that foods, plants, and many other items in the home can initiate an allergic response.*

Content Area: Fundamentals; Concept: Safety; **Integrated Processes:** Teaching/Learning; **Client Needs:** Safe and Effective Care Environment: Safety and Infection Control; Physiological Integrity: Reduction of Risk Potential; **Cognitive Level:** Analysis [Analyzing]

## 475. ANSWER: 4

1. The client has priority. Those responding can locate and activate the alarm box.
2. Smothering the fire with a blanket would occur after the client is told to roll on the floor.
3. Finding and obtaining water is too time-consuming, and the fire will continue to burn.
4. **The nurse should tell the client to drop and roll on the floor. Rolling on the ground will smother the flames and help put the fire out.**

▶ *Test-taking Tip: Remember the key phrase when on fire, "Stop, drop, and roll."*

Content Area: Fundamentals; Concept: Safety; **Integrated Processes:** Nursing Process: Implementation; **Client Needs:** Safe and Effective Care Environment: Safety and Infection Control; **Cognitive Level:** Application [Applying]

## 476. ANSWER: 3

1. Finding the nearest fire alarm leaves the client unattended and susceptible to injury from the fire.
2. Trying to extinguish the fire with a blanket increases the risk for injury to both the client and the nurse if the fire is not able to be extinguished and the blanket catches fire.
3. **The nurse should remove the client from the room; rescuing the client is the first action because it reduces the risk of harm to the client.**
4. Taking time to telephone the operator increases the risk for harm to the client because the fire can rapidly spread.

▶ *Test-taking Tip: The nurse's first action should focus on promoting client safety.*

Content Area: Fundamentals; Concept: Safety; **Integrated Processes:** Nursing Process: Implementation; **Client Needs:** Safe and Effective Care Environment: Safety and Infection Control; **Cognitive Level:** Application [Applying]

## 477. ANSWER: 3, 4, 1, 2

3. **Pull the pin; the safety chain must be released to activate the extinguisher.**
4. **Aim at the base of the fire; the fuel for the fire is at the base of the fire.**
1. **Squeeze the handle; the contents of the extinguisher need to be released.**
2. **Sweep from side to side; a side-to-side motion will help to distribute the extinguisher contents across the base of the fire.**

▶ *Test-taking Tip: Use the memory cue of PASS to place the items in the correct order.*

Content Area: Fundamentals; Concept: Safety; **Integrated Processes:** Teaching/Learning; **Client Needs:** Safe and Effective Care Environment: Safety and Infection Control; Health Promotion and Maintenance; **Cognitive Level:** Knowledge [Remembering]

## 478. ANSWER: 1

1. **The nurse should first assess the client's heart rhythm and apical pulse after the client feels an electrical shock. Because body fluids (consisting of sodium chloride) are an excellent conductor of electricity, an electrical shock can be transmitted through the body. The electrical charge may interfere with the heart's electrical conduction system, causing a dysrhythmia.**
2. Disconnecting the hair dryer is contraindicated because it may place the nurse at risk.
3. Assessing the client's skin is not the priority; depending on the voltage, electrical burns may or may not be evident.
4. Although sending the hair dryer for inspection should be completed, it does not have priority.

▶ *Test-taking Tip: Use the nursing process and the ABC's to establish priority. Assessment is the first step and should have priority.*

Content Area: Fundamentals; Concept: Critical Thinking; Safety; Assessment; **Integrated Processes:** Nursing Process: Assessment; **Client Needs:** Safe and Effective Care Environment: Safety and Infection Control; **Cognitive Level:** Analysis [Analyzing]

## 479. ANSWER: 1, 2, 4

1. **A frayed or cut cord increases the risk for an electrical shock. The nurse should intervene and replace the infusion pump.**
2. **A bed in a high position increases the risk for the client falling if left unattended. The nurse should intervene by lowering the bed.**
3. Personal electrical equipment, not battery-operated equipment, should be inspected for safety.
4. **The nurse should immediately respond to a beeping alarm device even if another nurse just left the client's room. The client may be attempting to get out of the bed and may fall.**
5. Placing a bedside table in front of a chair where the client is sitting makes items on the table easily accessible to the client and may prevent the client from falling if attempting to reach these.

▶ *Test-taking Tip: The nurse should intervene whenever there is a safety risk to the client, such as the risk for falling or electrical injuries.*

Content Area: Fundamentals; Concept: Safety; **Integrated Processes:** Nursing Process: Planning; **Client Needs:** Safe and Effective Care Environment: Safety and Infection Control; **Cognitive Level:** Application [Applying]

## 480. MoC ANSWER: 3

1. The UAP is appropriately cleansing the wheelchair prior to returning it to storage.
2. The ties for restraints should be applied to the bed frame using a quick-release knot.
3. **The nurse should provide feedback to the UAP who grasped the cord to unplug the infusion pump. This can loosen the cord from the plug, increasing the risk of an electrical shock.**

4. The UAP's actions are appropriate in activating a bed exit alarm for the confused client; the bed exit alarm is a safety device to prevent a fall.

▶ *Test-taking Tip: In review of the options, you should consider which action could harm either the client or the UAP.*

Content Area: Fundamentals; Concept: Safety; Regulations; Management; Integrated Processes: Nursing Process: Evaluation; Client Needs: Safe and Effective Care Environment: Management of Care; Cognitive Level: Evaluation [Evaluating]

### 481. ANSWER: 3

1. Although the plastic band must be cut for removal, this is an extra security measure and not the main means for identifying the infant.
2. A security band may be in place, but this is an extra security measure and not the main means for identifying the infant.
3. **Identification numbers and the mother's full name on both the mother's and infant's ID bands must match. Some agencies require the application of two ID bands, one on the wrist and another on an ankle in the event that one slides off. Some agencies also have bands that can be scanned for proper identification.**
4. The infant's footprints are on file, but this is an extra security measure and not the main means for infant identification.

▶ *Test-taking Tip: The nurse's best response answers the mother's question directly. Focus on the issue, the method for identifying newborns.*

Content Area: Fundamentals; Childbearing; Concept: Safety; Pregnancy; Integrated Processes: Communication and Documentation; Caring; Client Needs: Safe and Effective Care Environment: Safety and Infection Control; Cognitive Level: Application [Applying]

### 482. ANSWER: 2

1. Checking the unit would be included in the procedure for possible newborn abduction.
2. **The circumstances are suspicious enough to warrant initiating procedures for possible newborn abduction to retrieve the newborn immediately.**
3. Checking with other staff will delay getting the help needed to search the hospital and notify authorities.
4. The HCP would usually examine the infant while in the mother's room and not take the infant to another location.

▶ *Test-taking Tip: Read the situation carefully to ascertain whether a pediatrician is likely to retrieve a newborn in the middle of a feeding for an examination when the baby could be examined while with the mother.*

Content Area: Fundamentals; Childbearing; Concept: Safety; Pregnancy; Integrated Processes: Nursing Process: Implementation; Client Needs: Safe and Effective Care Environment: Safety and Infection Control; Cognitive Level: Application [Applying]

### 483. ANSWER: 1, 3, 5

1. **The infant should be restrained in a car seat located in the backseat, facing the rear of the car to provide protection should an accident occur.**
2. If an accident should occur when the infant is facing forward, the force of the crash would whip the infant's head forward, causing tremendous neck stress.
3. Some models are for infants only; others convert for toddler use. Infants and toddlers should be in the child restraint device (car seat) appropriate for the infant's weight and size.
4. In the United States and Canada, all states and provinces have mandated the use of child restraints while traveling in a car.
5. **Parents should only purchase a car seat that has a certification label stating that it complies with federal motor vehicle safety standards.**

▶ *Test-taking Tip: Consider the disproportionally heavy head and weak neck muscles of the infant and then select the options that are safest for the infant.*

Content Area: Fundamentals; Childbearing; Concept: Safety; Pregnancy; Integrated Processes: Teaching/Learning; Caring; Client Needs: Safe and Effective Care Environment: Safety and Infection Control; Health Promotion and Maintenance; Cognitive Level: Application [Applying]

### 484. PHARM ANSWER: 15

**$15 - 3 = 12$; $12 - 9 = 3$; the child ingested 3 tablets. Each tablet contains 5 mg. $5 \times 3 = 15$. The child ingested 15 mg of oxycodone (OxyContin).**

▶ *Test-taking Tip: Your answer should be the amount in milligrams and not the number of tablets ingested.*

Content Area: Fundamentals; Child; Concept: Safety; Medication; Integrated Processes: Nursing Process: Analysis; Client Needs: Safe and Effective Care Environment: Safety and Infection Control; Physiological Integrity: Pharmacological and Parenteral Therapies; Cognitive Level: Analysis [Analyzing]

### 485. ANSWER: 1, 2

1. **Drowning is the major cause of death in toddlers. Water safety and methods to prevent drowning should be addressed.**
2. **Motor vehicle accidents are the second leading cause of death in toddlers. Use of age- and weight-appropriate car seats should be the nurse's priority topic when teaching a group of parents with toddlers.**
3. Although toddlers are picky eaters and choking is one of the major causes of death in toddlers, more toddlers die in drowning accidents and in MVAs than from choking.
4. Although poisoning is a major cause of death in toddlers, more toddlers die in drowning accidents and MVAs.

5. Unintentional pedestrian accidents are a major cause of death, but more toddlers die in drowning accidents and in MVAs than in pedestrian accidents.

▶ **Test-taking Tip:** *The word "two" in the stem should be a clue that only two of the options are correct.*

**Content Area:** Fundamentals; **Concept:** Safety; **Integrated Processes:** Nursing Process: Planning; Teaching/Learning **Client Needs:** Safe and Effective Care Environment: Safety and Infection Control; Health Promotion and Maintenance; **Cognitive Level:** Application [Applying]

### 486. ANSWER: 1

1. **Toddlers are curious, and if a pot handle is easily accessible to a toddler, the toddler may grasp it and experience a scald and burn injury. This is the most important recommendation among the options.**
2. One cause of a burn injury may be providing food that is too hot to a toddler, and this can result in a burn injury. But this option does not address the inquisitiveness of toddlers.
3. The parent should ensure that smoke detectors are working properly to prevent burn injuries from a fire, but this option does not address the toddlers' inquisitiveness.
4. Tepid bathwater is only lukewarm and would be uncomfortable for bathing a toddler and is unnecessary. Warm water that is not too hot is appropriate for bathing.

▶ **Test-taking Tip:** *Most options are plausible for preventing a burn injury, but only one option pertains to the toddlers' curiosity.*

**Content Area:** Fundamentals; **Concept:** Safety; **Integrated Processes:** Teaching/Learning; **Client Needs:** Safe and Effective Care Environment: Safety and Infection Control; Health Promotion and Maintenance; **Cognitive Level:** Application [Applying]

### 487. ANSWER: 2

1. The client with a radiation sign posted on the client's door would not be leaving the room.
2. **The nurse should intercept the client before entering the room. The sign indicates that the client is receiving radiation therapy. If this were the client's room, the client should not have left the room. The name band may provide the client's room number.**
3. Although stopping the client is appropriate, the client is non–English-speaking and may not know what the nurse is asking.
4. UAP should not accompany the client into a room with a radiation sign; if this were the client's room, the client would not have left the room.

▶ **Test-taking Tip:** *Not knowing the meaning of various signs increases the risk for injury. The black trefoil on a yellow background is a universal sign for radiation. If unsure of the answer, consider which would best protect the client and others.*

**Content Area:** Fundamentals; **Concept:** Safety; Diversity; Caring; **Integrated Processes:** Nursing Process: Implementation; Culture and Spirituality; **Client Needs:** Safe and Effective Care Environment: Safety and Infection Control; **Cognitive Level:** Analysis [Analyzing]

### 488. MoC ANSWER: 2

1. Linens should be kept in the room until the radioactive source is removed and the room is swept with a radiation detector to assess for spills or contamination. After clearance, the linens may be sent to the laundry.
2. **In afterload radiation therapy, the radioactive substance is inserted into the client in the client's private hospital room after prepared applicators have been placed in surgery. Exposure to radiation is controlled by minimizing the time spent with the client.**
3. A 1-foot distance increases the nurse's chance of exposure to the radiation. The nurse standing 2 feet away from the source of radiation receives only one-quarter as much exposure as when standing only 1 foot away.
4. Lead gloves and aprons are insufficient to block gamma rays during brachytherapy. Dosimetry badges measure the amount of radiation exposure and are not a precaution.

▶ **Test-taking Tip:** *The key phrase is "hazardous material precautions." Read each option carefully and eliminate options that would not protect the nurse from radiation exposure.*

**Content Area:** Fundamentals; **Concept:** Safety; Management; **Integrated Processes:** Nursing Process: Evaluation; **Client Needs:** Safe and Effective Care Environment: Management of Care; Physiological Integrity: Physiological Adaptation; **Cognitive Level:** Evaluation [Evaluating]

### 489. CJ ANSWER:

| Receptacles and Items | |
|---|---|
| **Receptacles** | **Item Letter** |
| 1. Wastebasket | D |
| 2. Injurious waste | A |
| 3. Hazardous waste | |
| 4. Infectious waste | B and C |

1. **Injurious wastes would include items such as needles, scalpel blades, lancets, or other objects that could injure another person.**
2. Hazardous waste includes radioactive material, chemotherapy agents, or caustic chemicals.
3. **Blood and body fluids are considered infectious waste. Therefore the suction canister and the blood sponges should be placed in the infectious waste receptacle.**

4. **Regular waste that does not pose a health hazard to others can be placed in a regular wastebasket.**

▶ *Test-taking Tip: Not every receptacle is being used. Visualize the different types of containers and this may help you to dispose of the items correctly.*

Content Area: Fundamentals; **Concept:** Safety; **Integrated Processes:** Nursing Process: Implementation; **Client Needs:** Safe and Effective Care Environment: Safety and Infection Control; **Cognitive Level:** Analysis [Analyzing]

## 490. MoC ANSWER: 2

1. A serious injury to staff associated with an electrical shock during the course of care in a health care setting is a serious reportable event.
2. **A skin tear, although concerning and usually reported internally, is not a serious reportable event to be reported to an external agency. Any Stage 3, Stage 4, and unstageable pressure ulcer acquired after admission to a health care setting is a serious reportable event.**
3. Serious injury, such as a hip fracture, that is associated with a fall while being cared for in a health care setting is a reportable event.
4. Death or serious injury resulting from failure to follow up on or communicate laboratory test results, such as a low serum potassium level, is a reportable event.

▶ *Test-taking Tip: Serious injury or death of the client or staff member is a serious reportable event. You should select the option that is the least serious.*

Content Area: Fundamentals; **Concept:** Safety; Management; Legal; **Integrated Processes:** Nursing Process: Analysis; **Client Needs:** Safe and Effective Care Environment: Management of Care; Safe and Effective Care Environment: Safety and Infection Control; **Cognitive Level:** Application [Applying]

## 491. ANSWER: 2

1. Having the UAP obtain a new band while the nurse performs the procedure is not the best action because the medical record number usually is not the same from one facility to the next.
2. **The best action is to replace the name band before performing a procedure to ensure that the procedure is being performed on the correct client. The medical record number usually is not the same from one facility to the next. Unique identifiers must match between the client's name band and medical record before proceeding with any procedure.**
3. Although the client's name and birth date may match the name band, the medical record number will usually not be the same between facilities. There is still the potential for performing a procedure on the wrong client.
4. Name bands from one facility should not be used in another facility because the medical record number for the client is usually different between facilities.

▶ *Test-taking Tip: The key words are "best action." When selecting the best action consider what is safest and prevents performing a procedure on the wrong client.*

Content Area: Fundamentals; **Concept:** Safety; Legal; **Integrated Processes:** Nursing Process: Implementation; **Client Needs:** Safe and Effective Care Environment: Safety and Infection Control; **Cognitive Level:** Analysis [Analyzing]

## 492. MoC ANSWER: 2

1. The coworker's response that the HCP responds to everyone the same does not assist in solving the problem and is not the best response.
2. **Obtaining the hospital policy and initiating steps to report the HCP is the coworker's best response. The HCP is displaying incivility. Behavior can escalate to harassment, aggression, and physical assault.**
3. Although the nurse manager should be informed of the behavior, the best response is to follow the agency policy for reporting the behavior. Even if the manager is already dealing with the HCP's behavior, there is no indication as to whether the steps in the policy have been implemented.
4. Although the steps may include reporting the behavior to the medical director, the first step is usually filing a written report so that the facts are in writing.

▶ *Test-taking Tip: The key words are "best response." A global option such as following the agency policy is usually the correct option.*

Content Area: Fundamentals; **Concept:** Safety; Management; Legal; Nursing Roles; **Integrated Processes:** Communication and Documentation; **Client Needs:** Safe and Effective Care Environment: Management of Care; Psychosocial Integrity; **Cognitive Level:** Analysis [Analyzing]

## 493. MoC ANSWER: 1, 2, 4

1. **Both verbal intimidation and invasion of personal space are behaviors characteristic of incivility and should be included as planned topics in a presentation about incivility.**
2. **Both personal insults and ignoring a person are behaviors characteristic of incivility and should be included as planned topics in a presentation about incivility.**
3. Discussion between the nurse and HCPs about the client's condition does not characterize incivility unless the HCPs or nurse exhibit behaviors that are threatening, insulting, or others that characterize incivility.
4. **Teasing can be hurtful and not respectful of the other person and is characteristic of incivility and should be included as a planned topic in a presentation about incivility.**
5. Although reporting incivility should be included in the presentation, the question is asking for incivility behaviors.

▶ *Test-taking Tip: Be sure to read the question and options carefully. Only select options that address incivility behaviors and not the other topics that may be included in the presentation.*

**Content Area:** Fundamentals; **Concept:** Safety; Nursing Roles; Legal; **Integrated Processes:** Teaching/Learning; **Client Needs:** Safe and Effective Care Environment: Management of Care; Psychosocial Integrity; **Cognitive Level:** Application [Applying]

**494.** **MoC** **ANSWER: 4**

1. Although a statement from the charge nurse to the nurse about a medication error made by the nurse may be alarming to the nurse, the statement as made should be nonthreatening and is an appropriate request for follow-up on an error.

2. Asking the nurse to repeat information such as the vital signs is an appropriate request. The statements should be nonthreatening.

3. Telling the coworker of missing documentation, such as a glucometer reading, is an appropriate request and should be nonthreatening.

4. The HCP's statement of not being able to do anything more for the client and stating that the client does not follow the HCP's advice does not demonstrate respect for the client. The statement is demeaning, humiliating, and intimidating and demonstrates incivility.

▶ *Test-taking Tip: Incivility can include such actions as personal insults, uninvited physical contact, invading personal space, threats, intimidation, sarcastic jokes, teasing, humiliation, abusive e-mails, rude interruptions, public shaming, verbal attacks, ignoring a person as if that person is not present, nonverbal threats, and others. What these actions have in common is disrespect for the person being addressed. Select the option that demonstrates disrespect.*

**Content Area:** Fundamentals; **Concept:** Safety; Legal; Ethics; **Integrated Processes:** Communication and Documentation; **Client Needs:** Safe and Effective Care Environment: Management of Care; Psychosocial Integrity; **Cognitive Level:** Analysis [Analyzing]

## Chapter Thirteen

# Infection Control

**495.** The nurse surveys the client's hospital room. Which findings require the nurse's immediate attention to remove possible sources of infection? **Select all that apply.**

1. A capped bottle of saline with the notation "opened 10 hours ago"
2. The bed has bloody drainage from the saturated abdominal dressing
3. An infusing IV tubing has no notation of the date when it was last changed
4. An empty container in the bathroom that is labeled *urine* and has the client's initials
5. Opened packages of gauze and abdominal pads sitting on the windowsill
6. An uncovered cup of figs on the bedside table brought by a family member

**496.** The nurse is preparing for a dressing change using surgical aseptic technique. Which action by the nurse is correct when setting up the sterile field?

1. Dons exam gloves to open the package that contains the sterile drape
2. Uses alcohol to cleanse a solution bottle before placing it on the sterile drape
3. Opens a sterile package of gloves away from the field before donning them
4. Leaves the sterile field unattended to obtain a package of sterile scissors

**497.** The client is placed on contact precautions. When should the nurse plan to put on disposable examination gloves?

1. As soon as the nurse enters the client's room
2. Only if anticipating contact with the client's wound
3. Only if anticipating contact with blood or body fluids
4. Only if providing care within 3 feet of the client

**498.** The nurse sees multiple items on the client's bedside table. Which items should the nurse remove because they pose a risk of infection for the client? **Select all that apply.**

1. The menu from the client's last meal
2. A glass of water without a cover
3. An empty urinal that had been rinsed
4. A sealed package of soda crackers
5. A pitcher of water covered with a lid
6. A bloody alcohol swab from an injection

**499.** The clinic nurse encounters the client who has a congested cough and rhinorrhea. The nurse follows droplet precautions/cough protocol by taking which action? **Select all that apply.**

1. Offering the client sterile disposable tissues
2. Wearing a mask while examining the client
3. Offering the client water to drink while waiting
4. Teaching how to cover the mouth when coughing
5. Performing hand hygiene before and after client contact
6. Separating the client by at least 3 feet from others in the area

**500.** The nurse is caring for hospitalized clients. Which nursing actions require the nurse to use sterile gloves? **Select all that apply.**

1. Inserting a nasogastric tube
2. Administering an enema
3. Giving a subcutaneous injection
4. Inserting a urinary catheter
5. Suctioning a tracheostomy tube

**501.** The nurse is caring for the client with DM who has an open wound on the left heel. Which assessment findings should the nurse associate with a wound infection? **Select all that apply.**

1. Oral temperature 100.6°F (38°C)
2. Heel feels warm when touched
3. Yellow and purulent drainage
4. Reduced sensation in the left foot
5. Elevated white blood cell count

**502.** PHARM The client with an infected leg wound receives treatment and a prescription for amoxicillin during a clinic visit. Which information should the nurse emphasize when completing discharge teaching?

1. Return to the clinic in 1 week for a repeat tetanus injection.
2. Avoid disturbing the dressing until next week's clinic visit.
3. If your temperature is over 101°F (38.3°C), call the HCP.
4. Do not take cold medicines while taking amoxicillin.

**503.** MoC The nurse and NA are caring for the client with hepatitis A. The nurse determines that the NA understands correct infectious precautions for this client when observing what action?

1. Wears a mask, gown, and gloves when taking the client's vital signs
2. Wears a gown and gloves when changing the client's incontinent briefs
3. Wears gloves when providing urinary catheter and perineal care
4. Wears a gown and gloves when asking the client about snack food options

**504.** The nurse learns that the hospitalized client has a history of chronic hepatitis C. Which precaution should the nurse plan to implement?

1. Airborne
2. Contact
3. Droplet
4. Standard

**505.** The client is admitted with a tentative diagnosis of hepatitis. The nurse determines that which client statement would be consistent with hepatitis?

1. "I've not been sleeping well; I have heartburn at night that wakes me."
2. "Whenever I eat dairy products, I have diarrhea for a few days."
3. "Lately I've been short of breath when walking short distances."
4. "I am a smoker, but lately I can't tolerate the taste of cigarettes."

**506.** PHARM The client who is receiving TPN through a subclavian triple-lumen catheter expresses concern to the nurse about bacteria entering the blood through the catheter. The nurse explains that the risk of catheter-related infections can be decreased by taking which action?

1. Applying an antibiotic ointment at the catheter insertion site daily
2. Changing the dressing over the catheter insertion site every day
3. Designating one port of the catheter exclusively for the TPN solution
4. Instilling an antibiotic solution daily into each port of the catheter

**507.** MoC The hospitalized client has protective precautions (reverse isolation) in place because of severe neutropenia. Which statement by the nurse to the NA is correct regarding the use of protective precautions?

1. "You should don gloves as soon as you enter the client's room."
2. "Minimize the amount of time the client spends outside the room."
3. "The client needs to be moved to a private room with negative air pressure."
4. "Everyone entering the client's room should be sure to put on a mask."

**508.** The client has protective precautions (reverse isolation) in place due to a severely depressed neutrophil count. Which statement by the client demonstrates a good understanding of the precautions?

1. "Persons entering the room with colds should stay at least 3 feet from me."
2. "My family plans to bring flowers from my garden to help me feel better."
3. "The precautions will protect me and help my blood count recover faster."
4. "Persons entering my room should perform hand hygiene before entering."

**509.** MoC The NA is preparing to provide care for four clients. The nurse should direct the NA to utilize contact precautions for which client?

1. The client with influenza
2. The client with mumps
3. The client with gonorrhea
4. The client with a draining abscess

**510.** MoC The charge nurse is planning hospital bed placements for the five male clients identified in the exhibit below. Two double rooms and one private room are available. Which room assignments should be made by the charge nurse?

| Client | Diagnosis/Medical Information |
|--------|------------------------------|
| A | Has infected abdominal wound, cultured positive for methicillin-resistant *Staphylococcus aureus* |
| B | Admitted with ketoacidosis, history of chronic hepatitis C |
| C | Has history of bloody sputum, night sweats; airborne precautions currently in place |
| D | Had vascular surgery; leg ulcers cultured positive for methicillin-resistant *Staphylococcus aureus* |
| E | 1 day postoperative small bowel resection; had postoperative hypotension |

1. Client B: private room; clients C and E in same room; clients A and D in same room
2. Client C: private room; clients A and D in same room; clients B and E in same room
3. Client E: private room; clients B and C in same room; clients A and D in same room
4. Client C: private room; clients A and B in same room; clients D and E in same room

**511.** The client who has airborne precautions states, "Please do not shut my door." Which response is **most** appropriate?

1. "If I open the door, you will need to always wear a mask."
2. "The door must be kept closed, but I can open the curtains."
3. "Don't worry; I can leave the door open if it's bothering you."
4. "I'm sorry, but I can only leave the door partially open."

**512.** PHARM The nurse is to administer cefazolin sodium 1 g in 100 mL 0.9% NaCl over 30 minutes. At what rate in mL/hour should the nurse plan to set the infusion pump?

_____ mL/hr (Record your answer as a whole number.)

**513.** MoC Following morning shift report the nurse plans to assess clients who had surgery 2 days ago. Which client should the nurse assess **first?**

1. The 30-year-old who had a splenectomy and has an oral temperature of 102.2°F (39°C)
2. The 69-year-old who had a right total hip arthroplasty and has a WBC count of 12,100/mm$^3$
3. The 55-year-old who had a lumbar discectomy and was given 30 mg oral oxycodone at 0700
4. The 40-year-old with external traction for a tibia fracture and has a platelet count of 100 K/mm$^3$

**514.** While the nurse transfers the client who has *Clostridium difficile* from the bed to the commode, the client has loose stool that falls on the floor. After wiping up the stool, how should the nurse proceed to cleanse the floor?

1. Clean the area with soap and water.
2. Clean the area with a 1:10 bleach-water solution.
3. Ask the housekeeper to use the unit's mop and bucket.
4. Clean the area with alcohol-based hand wash.

**515.** MoC The nurse asks the UAP to change the soiled bed linens of the client with acute diarrhea of unknown origin. Which interventions should the nurse direct the UAP to implement? **Select all that apply.**

1. Wear a mask while changing the soiled linens.
2. Wear gown and gloves while in the room.
3. Use alcohol-based hand wash before and after care.
4. Request that the HCP prescribe a stool culture.
5. Post an enteric precaution sign outside the room.

**516.** The nurse is using contact precautions to change the soiled bed sheet of the client with *Clostridium difficile*. In the process, the nurse's right glove and skin on a finger is torn. After removing the soiled gloves, which action is **priority**?

1. Hold pressure to stop any bleeding.
2. Use a bleach wipe to clean the hands.
3. Wash the hands with soap and water.
4. Cleanse hands using alcohol-based hand rub.

**517.** The client is admitted with a positive culture for methicillin-resistant *Staphylococcus aureus* (MRSA). Which precaution should be implemented to prevent spreading the infection to health care workers and other clients?

1. Wearing a mask within 3 feet of the client
2. Placing the client in a private room
3. Wearing an N95 respirator mask
4. Ensuring a negative-air-pressure room

**518.** The nurse is caring for the client with a urinary catheter. Which interventions should the nurse implement to prevent a catheter-acquired UTI? **Select all that apply.**

1. Rubbing for 10 seconds when using alcohol-based hand rubs
2. Changing urinary catheters and drainage bags once a week
3. Using the smallest numbered catheter with intermittent catheterizations
4. Properly securing the catheter on the client's thigh to prevent movement
5. Keeping a urinary drainage bag below the level of the client's bladder

**519.** MoC The nurse observes that the NA enters the client room, provides direct care, and then exits without performing any hand hygiene. Which is the appropriate **initial** action of the nurse?

1. Inform the nurse manager about the NA's performance.
2. File a facility incident or variance report immediately.
3. Talk to the NA immediately about performing hand hygiene.
4. Tell the client to remind all staff to perform hand hygiene.

**520.** MoC The nurse is instructing the client who is to have surgery. According to Medicare's Surgical Care Improvement Project, what instruction is important for the client to receive prior to arrival at the hospital to prevent postoperative infection?

1. Arrive in time to receive an antibiotic before surgery.
2. Notify the nurse of any antibiotic and food allergies.
3. Be sure to wash your hands before the surgery.
4. Do not shave hair from the surgical incision site.

**521.** The nurse gives the client a container to collect sputum for culture and sensitivity. Which interventions should the nurse implement? **Select all that apply.**

1. Tell the client to spit into the container two to three times during the day.
2. Wear gloves and protective eyewear when handling the specimen.
3. After collection, place the sealed container in a clean plastic bag.
4. Place a biohazard alert symbol on the bag containing the specimen container.
5. Send the specimen to the laboratory within 30 minutes of collection.

**522.** MoC Newly admitted clients are being screened for possible undiagnosed or unsuspected TB. Which questions should the nurse ask? **Select all that apply.**

1. "Have you been exposed to someone with TB?"
2. "What was the date of your last TB skin test?"
3. "Have you had a cough that lasted more than 3 weeks?"
4. "Have you experienced blood in your urine or stools?"
5. "Have you had a recent weight gain or night sweats?"

**523.** The nurse is completing a variance report after finding a plastic bag at the nurse's station with contents and the sticker illustrated. The nurse should document finding a plastic bag with a symbol indicating that the contents of the bag include which type of item?

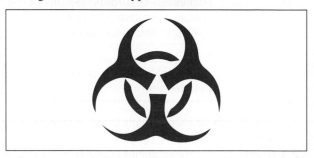

1. Potentially infectious specimen
2. Radioactive medication
3. Flammable substance
4. Poisonous substance

**524.** The client who has sutures in place after a skin biopsy receives discharge instructions. Which client statements indicate an understanding of the teaching? **Select all that apply.**

1. "The incision should be clean, dry, and not separated."
2. "I will return in 2 to 3 days to have the stitches removed."
3. "If I have an elevated temperature, I'll contact my provider."
4. "I'll keep the bandage on for a week before I check the incision."
5. "Excessive redness, pain, or drainage may mean it is infected."

**525.** A clinic nurse is teaching parents with young children. Which sources of infectious disease transmission should the nurse teach the parents?

1. Stool and oral and respiratory secretions
2. Sharing dirty toys and used utensils
3. Contact with blood from scrapes and sores
4. Touching others after rubbing a runny nose

**526.** MoC Staff are being assigned to care for the client with disseminated herpes zoster. Which staff member should the charge nurse exclude from being assigned?

1. The 7-month pregnant nurse who had confirmed chickenpox in childhood
2. The 32-year-old nurse with unknown disease or vaccination history for chickenpox
3. The 28-year-old nurse with a history of varicella vaccine and 2 small children at home
4. The 60-year-old nurse with a history of having the live herpes zoster vaccine

**527.** MoC The nurse is supervising the NA caring for a group of clients with antibiotic-resistant organisms. Which observation of the NA's performance should prompt the supervising nurse to intervene?

1. Uses an alcohol-based hand hygiene after emptying the urinary drainage bag of the client with vancomycin-resistant enterococci (VRE)
2. Performs hand hygiene, then dons gloves to perform oral care for the client with β-lactamase–producing *Klebsiella pneumoniae*
3. Uses an alcohol-based hand rub and wears gloves before and after taking the temperature of the client with penicillin G–resistant *Streptococcus pneumoniae*
4. Tells visitors to use the alcohol-based hand wash when entering and leaving the room of the client with methicillin-resistant *Staphylococcus aureus* (MRSA)

**528.** PHARM The nurse is using contact precautions when caring for the client. When changing the client's IV solution bag, the nurse inadvertently touches the end of the exposed spike of the tubing. Which is the **most** appropriate action by the nurse?

1. Insert the spike into the new IV solution bag.
2. Remove the gloves and obtain another pair.
3. Discard the tubing and obtain another sterile tubing.
4. Use alcohol to cleanse the spike of the tubing.

**529.** The client's total WBC count is 20,000/mm³ 2 days after surgery. Which assessment finding should the nurse **most** associate with this laboratory result?

1. Respiratory rate slow and shallow
2. Skin incision pink, crusty, and intact
3. Dark amber urine per urinary catheter
4. Diminished lung sounds with crackles

**530.** The HCP documents that the client has a generalized infection. Which specific assessment finding should the nurse expect?

1. Redness and warmth at the site
2. Swelling and pain at the site
3. Hypertension and bradycardia
4. Fever and widespread muscle aches

**531.** PHARM The nurse is caring for the client with an IV. Which findings should prompt the nurse to conclude that the client is experiencing inflammation (phlebitis) at the IV insertion site? **Select all that apply.**

1. Pain
2. Redness
3. Warmth
4. Drainage
5. Mottling
6. Swelling

**532.** The nurse is wearing PPE. Place the steps to removing the PPE in the correct sequence.

1. Remove gown
2. Remove gloves and perform hand hygiene
3. Remove mask
4. Remove eye protection
5. Perform hand hygiene

Answer: _____

**533.** The nurse is preparing to care for the client diagnosed with TB who has been coughing up blood. Which illustration **best** shows the PPE that the nurse should plan to wear?

1.
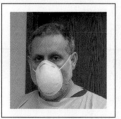
2.
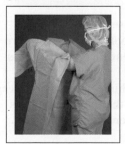

3.
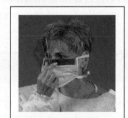
4.
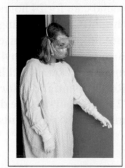

**534.** MoC The charge nurse is planning a room assignment for the client with meningococcal meningitis. Which room and precautions should the nurse plan for this client?

1. A private room with droplet precautions
2. A private room with airborne precautions
3. A semiprivate room with a roommate who has a similar diagnosis and standard precautions
4. A semiprivate room with a roommate who has a similar diagnosis and contact precautions

**535.** MoC A college student is hospitalized with meningococcal meningitis after being seen in the campus clinic. What is the nurse's responsibility to the campus community regarding this diagnosis?

1. Quarantine all students and faculty remaining on the campus.
2. E-mail school administrators with the names of infected students.
3. Identify all individuals who have had close contact with the student.
4. Ensure that everyone on campus receives prophylactic antibiotics.

**536.** MoC The new nurse is caring for the client with a VRE infection. Which statement to the client indicates the new nurse needs additional orientation when caring for clients with a VRE infection?

1. "All hospital staff should be wearing gown and gloves when they enter your room."
2. "Visitors should use soap and water for hand washing when entering and leaving your room."
3. "You are in a private room because VRE is transmitted by direct and indirect contact."
4. "VRE is a new strain of enterococci bacteria normally found in a person's GI tract."

**537.** MoC The infection control nurse receives hospital laboratory confirmation that the client has positive sputum cultures for *Mycobacterium tuberculosis*. Which action should be taken by the nurse?

1. Prepare a statement for the hospital spokesperson to release to the news agencies.
2. Recommend that only staff with recent negative tuberculin skin tests provide care.
3. Implement measures to notify the local or state health department about the case.
4. Notify the nearest infectious disease facility and prepare the client for transfer.

**538.** The nursing student approaches the instructor after being stuck by a bloody needle. Which instructor statement is **most** accurate knowing that the client was HIV-positive?

1. "Wash with soap and water and see the doctor now; treatment should begin within 1 to 2 hours."
2. "The first HIV antibody testing is completed in 6 weeks and then repeated in 3 months."
3. "Wash with soap and water now. At the end of the clinical shift, notify your physician."
4. "Flush immediately with water for 10 minutes and then cover with a bandage and glove."

**539.** MoC The HCP is about to examine the client on contact precautions for MRSA without donning PPE. Which is the **best** action by the nurse?

1. Hand the provider a gown and gloves.
2. Not say anything; it is the HCP's decision.
3. Notify the charge nurse and unit manager.
4. Monitor for increased infections on the unit.

## Answers and Rationales

**495. ANSWER: 2, 3, 5, 6**

1. Open bottles of solutions for wound care are considered aseptic and suitable for use with wound care for 24 hours.
2. **The saturated dressing represents a risk for contamination because microorganisms can move through the moist environment through the dressing to the wound and back.**
3. **Recommendations for IV tubing changes are every 72 to 96 hours. If the date of the tubing change is unknown, it represents a potential infection risk.**

4. Care equipment, especially items contaminated with body fluids, should be labeled and used for just one client.
5. **Opened packages of dressings are considered contaminated and should not be used for dressing changes. These should be removed.**
6. **Although figs may have special meaning in some cultures, leaving them uncovered increases the risk for infection because they can harbor microorganisms. This finding requires the immediate attention of the nurse.**

▶ *Test-taking Tip: As you read the options, think about the items that potentially could be contaminated with microorganisms.*

Content Area: Fundamentals; Concept: Infection; Diversity; Integrated Processes: Nursing Process: Assessment; Client Needs: Safe and Effective Care Environment: Safety and Infection Control; Cognitive Level: Analysis [Analyzing]

## 496. ANSWER: 3

1. Wearing exam gloves to open a sterile drape is not necessary. The package is opened by just touching the outer portion.
2. The irrigation solution should be poured into a sterile container on the field. Only sterile items should be placed on the sterile field.
3. **Sterile gloves should be donned away from the sterile field before touching items in the sterile field. This is correct.**
4. A sterile field should be considered contaminated if not visualized.

▸ *Test-taking Tip: Visualize performing each option to set up a sterile field.*

Content Area: Fundamentals; Concept: Infection; Integrated Processes: Nursing Process: Implementation; Client Needs: Safe and Effective Care Environment: Safety and Infection Control; Cognitive Level: Analysis [Analyzing]

## 497. ANSWER: 1

1. **Gloves should be donned by the nurse upon entry into the room of the client requiring contact precautions.**
2. Gloves should be donned upon entering the room, not just if anticipating contact with the client's wound.
3. Gloves should be donned upon entering the room, not just if anticipating contact with blood or body fluids.
4. Gloves should be donned upon entering the room, not just if providing care within 3 feet of the client.

▸ *Test-taking Tip: An option that is more comprehensive than the other options is usually the answer.*

Content Area: Fundamentals; Concept: Infection; Integrated Processes: Nursing Process: Planning; Client Needs: Safe and Effective Care Environment: Safety and Infection Control; Cognitive Level: Application [Applying]

## 498. ANSWER: 2, 3, 6

1. A menu does not pose a risk for infection.
2. **Fluid containers should be covered because prolonged exposure leads to contamination and promotes microbial growth.**
3. **The urinal on the bedside table is a vehicle for microorganism transmission and a potential source for nosocomial infection.**
4. The soda crackers are sealed and still edible without transmitting microorganisms.
5. The container is covered, preventing environmental contamination.
6. **A bloody alcohol swab can harbor microorganisms.**

▸ *Test-taking Tip: You should think about which items could be contaminated from the environment or from blood and body fluids.*

Content Area: Fundamentals; Concept: Infection; Integrated Processes: Nursing Process: Implementation; Client Needs: Safe and Effective Care Environment: Safety and Infection Control; Cognitive Level: Analysis [Analyzing]

## 499. ANSWER: 2, 4, 5, 6

1. Sterile disposable tissues are unnecessary; unsterile tissues are sufficient.
2. **Droplet precautions are a component of respiratory hygiene; this includes wearing a mask when caring for the client.**
3. Clients with URIs should increase their fluid intake, but this will not limit transmission of pathogens.
4. **Droplet precautions/cough protocol measures include educating clients about source control measures including how to cover the mouth when coughing.**
5. **Hand hygiene should be performed before and after client contact to prevent the transmission of microorganisms.**
6. **Separating ill persons by 3 feet will prevent transmission of microorganisms.**

▸ *Test-taking Tip: You should select options that are consistent with standard and droplet precautions.*

Content Area: Fundamentals; Concept: Infection; Integrated Processes: Nursing Process: Implementation; Client Needs: Safe and Effective Care Environment: Safety and Infection Control; Physiological Integrity: Basic Care and Comfort; Cognitive Level: Analysis [Analyzing]

## 500. ANSWER: 4, 5

1. The nurse uses nonsterile, not sterile, examination gloves when inserting an NG tube for self-protection from blood and body fluids. The GI tract contacts microorganisms and is not sterile.
2. The nurse uses nonsterile, not sterile, examination gloves when administering an enema for self-protection from blood and body fluids.
3. The nurse maintains sterility of the needle with a subcutaneous injection by not touching the needle and disinfecting the client's skin prior to the injection. Sterile gloves are not needed. Nonsterile gloves are worn for self-protection against the client's blood.
4. **The urinary tract is at great risk for nosocomial infection. Therefore use of sterile gloves and sterile technique during insertion of a urinary catheter decreases the risk of introducing microorganisms.**
5. **The respiratory tract is at great risk for nosocomial infection. Use of sterile gloves and sterile technique while suctioning a tracheostomy decreases the risk of introducing microorganisms.**

▶ *Test-taking Tip: Think about the normal flora of each system involved in the procedures and the potential for introducing microorganisms.*

**Content Area:** Fundamentals; **Concept:** Infection; **Integrated Processes:** Nursing Process: Planning; **Client Needs:** Safe and Effective Care Environment: Safety and Infection Control; **Cognitive Level:** Analysis [Analyzing]

## 501. ANSWER: 1, 2, 3, 5

1. **Signs of wound infection include fever; even a low-grade fever would be concerning.**
2. **If there is an infection, the area around the wound may be warm to the touch.**
3. **Yellow-, green-, or blue-colored drainage may indicate a wound infection.**
4. The inflammation from an infection would make the foot more sensitive. Reduced sensation may be due to diabetic neuropathy.
5. **An elevated WBC count may indicate that the client's immune system is fighting infection.**

▶ *Test-taking Tip: Focus on signs and symptoms of infection only and eliminate an option associated with the disease processes.*

**Content Area:** Fundamentals; **Concept:** Infection; **Integrated Processes:** Nursing Process: Assessment; **Client Needs:** Physiological Integrity: Physiological Adaptation; **Cognitive Level:** Application [Applying]

## 502. PHARM ANSWER: 3

1. The client with a tetanus-prone wound should have received tetanus immunoglobulin (TIG) when seen in the clinic. The injection is not repeated.
2. Frequent dressing changes would have been prescribed for an infected wound, especially if the client is not being seen again for a week.
3. **Having an elevated temperature may indicate that the antibiotics are not effective.**
4. Cold medicines usually treat symptoms and usually are not contraindicated with amoxicillin (Amoxil), an antibiotic. However, the client should check with the pharmacist or HCP before taking cold medicines when antibiotics are prescribed.

▶ *Test-taking Tip: Focus on the one option that indicates a worsening of the client's condition.*

**Content Area:** Fundamentals; **Concept:** Infection; **Integrated Processes:** Teaching/Learning; **Client Needs:** Safe and Effective Care Environment: Safety and Infection Control; **Cognitive Level:** Application [Applying]

## 503. MoC ANSWER: 2

1. There is no need to wear a mask at any time during client care because the virus is not airborne.
2. **Contact precautions should be taken with gown and gloves worn when changing the incontinent briefs. Hepatitis A virus is present in the feces for 2 weeks after symptoms appear and can live for several months outside the body.**

3. Wearing gloves when providing urinary catheter and perineal care is correct but is not enough protection; gowns should also be worn to protect clothing from contamination and transmission.
4. There is no need to wear a gown when talking with the client as long as there is no physical contact with the client or anything in the environment.

▶ *Test-taking Tip: Think about how hepatitis A is transmitted. A memory aid to remember the mode of transmission for hepatitis A would be the letter "A," which is for anus. This should enable elimination of Options 1 and 4.*

**Content Area:** Fundamentals; **Concept:** Infection; Management; Nursing Roles; **Integrated Processes:** Nursing Process: Evaluation; **Client Needs:** Safe and Effective Care Environment: Management of Care; **Cognitive Level:** Evaluation [Evaluating]

## 504. ANSWER: 4

1. Hepatitis C is not transmitted via the respiratory tract, so airborne precautions are unnecessary.
2. Contact precautions are not necessary because hepatitis C is transmitted primarily through infected blood and body fluids.
3. Hepatitis C is not transmitted via the respiratory tract, so droplet precautions are unnecessary.
4. **Standard precautions protect against infectious agents present in body fluids, including the blood. Hepatitis C is transmitted through body fluids, principally the blood.**

▶ *Test-taking Tip: Hepatitis C is transmitted primarily through infected blood and body fluids.*

**Content Area:** Fundamentals; **Concept:** Infection; **Integrated Processes:** Nursing Process: Planning; **Client Needs:** Safe and Effective Care Environment: Safety and Infection Control; **Cognitive Level:** Knowledge [Remembering]

## 505. ANSWER: 4

1. Heartburn at night is a symptom of GERD, not hepatitis.
2. Diarrhea after eating dairy products can be a symptom of lactose intolerance, not hepatitis.
3. Shortness of breath can be related to circulatory or respiratory problems, usually not hepatitis.
4. **Anorexia can be severe in the acute phase of hepatitis. Distaste for cigarettes in smokers is characteristic of early profound anorexia.**

▶ *Test-taking Tip: Anorexia is a symptom associated with hepatitis. Of the options, consider the one most associated with taste.*

**Content Area:** Fundamentals; **Concept:** Infection; **Integrated Processes:** Nursing Process: Analysis; **Client Needs:** Physiological Integrity: Reduction of Risk Potential; **Cognitive Level:** Application [Applying]

## 506. PHARM ANSWER: 3

1. Using antibiotic ointment daily to the site may predispose the client to developing antibiotic-resistant bacteria.

2. Unless loose, soiled, or bloody, the dressing should be changed weekly or every 10 days depending on the cleansing solution used.
3. **Consistently utilizing one port for TPN solution minimizes the risk of infection. The high glucose concentration of the TPN solution is a good culture media for bacteria.**
4. Instilling antibiotic solution may predispose the client to developing antibiotic-resistant bacteria.

▶ **Test-taking Tip:** *Focus on the nutrient content of the TPN, which is high in dextrose, and the relationship to increased infection risk.*

Content Area: Fundamentals; Concept: Infection; Medication; Integrated Processes: Nursing Process: Implementation; Caring; Client Needs: Safe and Effective Care Environment: Safety and Infection Control; Physiological Integrity: Pharmacological and Parenteral Therapies; Cognitive Level: Application [Applying]

## 507. MoC ANSWER: 2

1. Barrier precautions including gloves are not necessary if the client does not have a suspected or actual infection.
2. **The client should remain in the room as much as possible to minimize exposure to pathogens.**
3. The client should be in a private room with positive, not negative, air pressure. Negative pressure in the room would draw air from the hospital environment (possibly containing pathogens) into the client's room.
4. Masks are not necessary if the client does not have a suspected or actual infection.

▶ **Test-taking Tip:** *Key words in the stem are "protective precautions" and "neutropenia." Neutropenia is a low neutrophil count. The client has a decreased resistance against infection and is being protected from pathogens.*

Content Area: Fundamentals; Concept: Infection; Management; Integrated Processes: Nursing Process: Implementation; Client Needs: Safe and Effective Care Environment: Management of Care; Physiological Integrity: Reduction of Risk Potential; Cognitive Level: Analysis [Analyzing]

## 508. ANSWER: 4

1. Those with colds should not be entering the client's room.
2. Fresh flowers are prohibited in the client area to prevent introducing microorganisms.
3. The precautions limit client contact with potential pathogens while in the neutropenic state, but they will not improve the client's neutrophil count.
4. **Hand hygiene is of utmost importance for persons entering the room or caring for the client because the client's ability to ward off an infection is reduced.**

▶ **Test-taking Tip:** *The client with a depressed neutrophil count has a decreased resistance against infection and is being protected from pathogens.*

Content Area: Fundamentals; Concept: Infection; Integrated Processes: Nursing Process: Evaluation; Client Needs: Safe and Effective Care Environment: Safety and Infection Control; Physiological Integrity: Reduction of Risk Potential; Cognitive Level: Evaluation [Evaluating]

## 509. MoC ANSWER: 4

1. Influenza requires droplet precautions for 5 days from onset of symptoms.
2. Mumps requires droplet precautions for 9 days after treatment begins.
3. Gonorrhea requires standard precautions.
4. **Contact precautions should be used when caring for the client with a draining abscess because there is the potential for transmission of infectious organisms.**

▶ **Test-taking Tip:** *Transmission-based precautions help prevent organisms from being transmitted to other clients or health care personnel.*

Content Area: Fundamentals; Concept: Infection; Management; Integrated Processes: Nursing Process: Planning; Client Needs: Safe and Effective Care Environment: Management of Care; Cognitive Level: Application [Applying]

## 510. MoC ANSWER: 2

1. Client C requires a private room with airborne precautions and cannot be in the same room as client E.
2. **Client C has airborne precautions and requires a private room. Clients A and D have the same organism, may be roomed together, and require contact precautions. Clients B and E may be roomed together because both require only the standard precautions. Transmission of hepatitis C occurs mainly with blood, and this is addressed with the standard precautions.**
3. Client C requires a private room with airborne precautions and cannot be in the same room as Client B.
4. Client A requires contact precautions and should be with Client D, who also has contact precautions, and not with Client B.

▶ **Test-taking Tip:** *Read the chart carefully. Client C with airborne precautions may have infectious TB and definitely requires a private room. This eliminates Options 1 and 3. Determine that Clients A and D require contact precautions for the same organism and that Clients B and E both require standard precautions; then select Option 2.*

Content Area: Fundamentals; Concept: Infection; Management; Integrated Processes: Nursing Process: Planning; Client Needs: Safe and Effective Care Environment: Management of Care; Physiological Integrity: Reduction of Risk Potential; Cognitive Level: Analysis [Analyzing]

## 511. ANSWER: 2

1. Leaving the door open allows airborne pathogens to escape the room.

2. **The door must remain closed to contain the infectious pathogens. Opening the curtains will help the client feel less closed in while still preventing the spread of the airborne agent.**

3. Opening the door allows airborne organisms to escape and defeats the purpose if in a negative-air-pressure room. Stating "Don't worry" belittles the client's feelings.

4. Leaving the door partially open still allows for escape of the airborne pathogens and defeats the purpose if in a negative-air-pressure room.

▶ *Test-taking Tip: Use Maslow's Hierarchy of Needs to determine an alternative option to this client's request.*

Content Area: Fundamentals; Concept: Infection; Integrated Processes: Communication and Documentation; Caring; Client Needs: Safe and Effective Care Environment: Safety and Infection Control; Psychosocial Integrity; Cognitive Level: Application [Applying]

### 512. PHARM ANSWER: 200
**Using dimensional analysis:**

$$mL/hr = \frac{100 \text{ mL}}{30 \text{ min}} \times \frac{60 \text{ min}}{1 \text{ hr}} = \frac{6,000}{30} = 200 \text{ mL/hr}$$

▶ *Test-taking Tip: Do not be confused with the dose of the medication. Focus only on the amount to be infused over 60 minutes or 1 hour.*

Content Area: Fundamentals; Concept: Safety; Infection; Medication; Integrated Processes: Nursing Process: Planning; Client Needs: Physiological Integrity: Pharmacological and Parenteral Therapies; Cognitive Level: Application [Applying]

### 513. MoC ANSWER: 1
1. **The nurse should first assess the client with the high temperature of 102.2°F (39°C). This client does not have the normal filter of the spleen and could be septic. Fluids and antibiotics may be required.**

2. A WBC count of 12,100/mm$^3$ is slightly elevated (normal WBC is 3900 to 11,900/mm$^3$ or mcL). This is expected due to inflammation from surgery. An immediate assessment is not required.

3. Assessing the client's response to the analgesic is important, but the client is not priority.

4. A platelet count of 100K/mm$^3$ is low (normal Plt is 150 to 450 K/mm$^3$ or mcL), but this client is not at a significant risk of bleeding.

▶ *Test-taking Tip: Three of the clients have orthopedic conditions, and one is different. Often the option that is different is the answer. Consider which client is most at risk for a bloodstream infection.*

Content Area: Fundamentals; Concept: Infection; Management; Integrated Processes: Nursing Process: Planning; Client Needs: Safe and Effective Care Environment: Management of Care; Physiological Integrity: Reduction of Risk Potential; Cognitive Level: Analysis [Analyzing]

### 514. ANSWER: 2
1. Soap and water will not adequately disinfect the area.

2. **The nurse should wipe up the stool and clean the area with a bleach solution to adequately disinfect the area and prevent transmission of the microorganism.**

3. To maintain the dignity of the client, the nurse should stay with the client and avoid having housekeeping personnel present while the client is using the commode. Using the unit's mop and bucket could cause transmission to other areas of the unit.

4. Alcohol-based hand wash is ineffective against the spores of *C. difficile*.

▶ *Test-taking Tip: Recall that C. difficile is a spore-forming microbe and is relatively resistant to disinfectants.*

Content Area: Fundamentals; Concept: Infection; Integrated Processes: Nursing Process: Implementation; Client Needs: Safe and Effective Care Environment: Safety and Infection Control; Cognitive Level: Application [Applying]

### 515. MoC ANSWER: 2, 5
1. Intestinal bacteria are not airborne, so a mask is not necessary.

2. **Gown and gloves should be worn because the diarrheal stool could be infectious.**

3. Hand washing should be carried out before and after the task, but soap and water should be used for hand washing. The stool could be infected with *Clostridium difficile*, and its spores are not killed by the alcohol hand wash.

4. Acute diarrhea of unknown origin could be caused by *Clostridium difficile*. A stool culture is needed to rule this out. However, the nurse and not the NA needs to request the stool culture.

5. **Enteric precautions should be used to prevent possible transmission of *Clostridium difficile*. If the culture results are negative, the sign can be removed.**

▶ *Test-taking Tip: All cases of acute diarrhea should be considered infectious until the cause is known. Bacteria in the loose stool of infected persons can be passed from one person to another through direct contact and through contact with soiled surfaces. Rule out options that are only within the nurse's scope of practice and should not be delegated to the UAP.*

Content Area: Fundamentals; Management of Care; Concept: Infection; Management; Legal; Integrated Processes: Nursing Process: Implementation; Client Needs: Safe and Effective Care Environment: Management of Care; Safe and Effective Care Environment: Safety and Infection Control; Cognitive Level: Application [Applying]

### 516. ANSWER: 3
1. Bleeding will help flush the wound, and pressure should not be applied to stop bleeding.

2. Bleach should be used on contaminated objects but not on the skin. It damages tissues.

3. **Hand washing with soap and water is the most effective way of removing potentially infectious material.**
4. Because alcohol does not kill *Clostridium difficile* spores, use of soap and water is more efficacious than alcohol-based hand rubs.

▶ *Test-taking Tip: Think about the best action to prevent the spread of an infection.*

**Content Area:** Fundamentals; **Concept:** Infection; **Integrated Processes:** Nursing Process: Implementation; **Client Needs:** Safe and Effective Care Environment: Safety and Infection Control; **Cognitive Level:** Application [Applying]

## 517. ANSWER: 2

1. A mask is not necessary for contact precautions.
2. **The client should be placed in a private room or in a room with the client with an active infection caused by the same organism and no other infections.**
3. The N95 respirator is not necessary for contact precautions.
4. Negative-air-pressure rooms are included in airborne precautions and are not necessary for contact precautions.

▶ *Test-taking Tip: Note the similarities in Options 1, 3, and 4 related to air, whereas Option 2 is related to placing the client in a private room. When an option is different, it is usually correct.*

**Content Area:** Fundamentals; **Concept:** Infection; **Integrated Processes:** Nursing Process: Implementation; **Client Needs:** Safe and Effective Care Environment: Safety and Infection Control; **Cognitive Level:** Application [Applying]

## 518. ANSWER: 4, 5

1. Although hand hygiene is a key component of infection prevention, when using alcohol-based hand rubs the hands should be rubbed for 15 to 30 seconds for effective disinfection.
2. Routine changing of catheters and drainage bags can be associated with increased risk of infection. Institutional guidelines should be followed.
3. The smallest-sized catheter that will adequately drain the bladder should be used. Using the French system, the larger the number, the larger the diameter of the catheter.
4. **Proper securement should prevent irritation of the urethra and bladder. Irritation and inflammation increase the risk for a UTI.**
5. **The urinary drainage bag should be kept below the level of the client's bladder to prevent reflux of contaminated urine.**

▶ *Test-taking Tip: You should carefully read the options; specific details within the options can make an option incorrect.*

**Content Area:** Fundamentals; **Concept:** Infection; **Urinary Elimination; Integrated Processes:** Nursing Process: Implementation; **Client Needs:** Safe and Effective Care Environment: Safety and Infection Control; **Cognitive Level:** Application [Applying]

## 519. MoC ANSWER: 3

1. The nurse manager should be notified of deviations from standards of practice, but this does not address the NA's behavior immediately.
2. An incident or variance report does not provide immediate feedback to the individual.
3. **The nurse should immediately talk to the NA about performing hand hygiene upon exiting the client's room.**
4. Telling the client to remind staff to perform hygiene does not address the NA's lack of performing hand hygiene.

▶ *Test-taking Tip: Although other options may be considered, the word "initial" in the stem should prompt you to select the only option that provides immediate feedback to the NA.*

**Content Area:** Fundamentals; **Concept:** Infection; Management; Communication; **Integrated Processes:** Communication and Documentation; **Client Needs:** Safe and Effective Care Environment: Management of Care; **Cognitive Level:** Application [Applying]

## 520. MoC ANSWER: 4

1. It is important that clients receive an antibiotic within 1 hour of the incision time; however, preoperative preparations will easily allow the 1-hour time frame to be met.
2. Notifying the nurse of allergies is important information for the team but will not prevent infection.
3. Having the client wash hands before arrival to the hospital will not prevent infection.
4. **Shaving the surgical site with a razor induces small skin lacerations, creating a potential site of infection. Shaving disturbs hair follicles, which are often colonized with *Staphylococcus aureus*. The greatest threat for infection occurs when shaving is performed the night before surgery.**

▶ *Test-taking Tip: Focus on the key phrase "prevent postoperative infection" to narrow the options.*

**Content Area:** Fundamentals; **Concept:** Infection; Management; **Integrated Processes:** Teaching/Learning; **Client Needs:** Safe and Effective Care Environment: Management of Care; **Cognitive Level:** Application [Applying]

## 521. ANSWER: 3, 4, 5

1. The client should expectorate once into the container. The specimen is best collected early in the morning when sputum has collected in the lungs during the night.
2. Only gloves are needed when handling the specimen; splashing is not expected.
3. **A bag that is clean on the outside is required to prevent transmission of microorganisms from the potentially infectious material.**
4. **A biohazard alert symbol on the bag holding the specimen container indicates that the specimen is potentially infectious.**

5. **The specimen should reach the laboratory within 30 minutes of collection.**

▶ *Test-taking Tip: Apply standard precaution principles to select the correct options.*

Content Area: Fundamentals; Concept: Infection; Integrated Processes: Nursing Process: Implementation; Client Needs: Safe and Effective Care Environment: Safety and Infection Control; Cognitive Level: Analysis [Analyzing]

## 522. MoC ANSWER: 1, 2, 3

1. **Screening questions include asking about client history of exposure to TB.**
2. **The tuberculin skin test is used for TB screening. If not recent, one should be completed.**
3. **Common symptoms associated with TB include a cough lasting more than 3 weeks.**
4. Blood in the sputum, not blood in the urine or stools, is associated with TB.
5. Fever and night sweats are common symptoms of TB, but weight loss, and not weight gain, occurs.

▶ *Test-taking Tip: Narrow the options by associating TB addressed in the stem with the word TB in the option. Weight gain is often not associated with a debilitating disease.*

Content Area: Fundamentals; Concept: Assessment; Infection; Integrated Processes: Nursing Process: Assessment; Client Needs: Safe and Effective Care Environment: Safety and Infection Control; Cognitive Level: Analysis [Analyzing]

## 523. ANSWER: 1

1. **The universal biohazard symbol indicating a potentially infectious specimen is fluorescent orange or orange-red with a background of any color that provides sufficient contrast for the symbol to be clearly defined.**
2. The "trefoil" is the international symbol for radiation. The symbol on a yellow background can be magenta or black.
3. A flammable substance should have the National Fire Protection Association's (NFPA) diamond label and coding system. A red square within the diamond indicates flammability.
4. A poisonous substance should have the National Fire Protection Association's (NFPA) diamond label and coding system. A blue square within the diamond indicates a health hazard.

▶ *Test-taking Tip: Think about the color of a biohazard bag when discarding infectious wastes.*

Content Area: Fundamentals; Concept: Safety; Infection; Integrated Processes: Communication and Documentation; Client Needs: Safe and Effective Care Environment: Safety and Infection Control; Cognitive Level: Comprehension [Understanding]

## 524. ANSWER: 1, 3, 5

1. **The incision should be clean, dry, and intact. This statement indicates understanding.**
2. If sutures are in place, the client should return to the HCP in 7 to 10 days, not 2 to 3 days, to have them removed.

3. **Fever is a sign of infection and should be reported to the HCP. This statement indicates understanding.**
4. The client should check the incision daily and place a new bandage on the incision if directed.
5. **Redness, bleeding, pain, and drainage are signs of possible infection. This statement indicates understanding.**

▶ *Test-taking Tip: You should pay attention to the time frame when reading the options.*

Content Area: Fundamentals; Concept: Infection; Integrated Processes: Nursing Process: Evaluation; Client Needs: Safe and Effective Care Environment: Safety and Infection Control; Health Promotion and Maintenance; Cognitive Level: Evaluation [Evaluating]

## 525. ANSWER: 1

1. **Young children have not fully developed good hygiene behaviors and transmit infectious diseases from their stool or oral or respiratory secretions to other children in their play or school group.**
2. Although dirty toys and used utensils are a source of disease transmission, it is not as inclusive as Option 1.
3. Although infectious diseases can be transmitted through blood, few children are carrying these infectious diseases. Stool and oral and respiratory secretions are more common sources.
4. A runny nose is only concerned with disease transmission from the respiratory route.

▶ *Test-taking Tip: Note the plural "sources" of infectious disease in the stem and select the option that is most inclusive. A global option that encompasses other options is usually the answer.*

Content Area: Fundamentals; Concept: Infection; Integrated Processes: Teaching/Learning; Client Needs: Safe and Effective Care Environment: Safety and Infection Control; Health Promotion and Maintenance; Cognitive Level: Application [Applying]

## 526. MoC ANSWER: 2

1. The nurse has had confirmed chickenpox and would have some immunity against the virus causing the herpes zoster.
2. **The nurse who has not had the chickenpox or received the vaccine is at an increased risk of contraction of the varicella virus that causes chickenpox.**
3. Having the varicella vaccine provides immunity against reinfection.
4. The 60-year-old may have had exposure to chickenpox; this nurse also received the live herpes zoster vaccine (Zostavax) and would not be at an increased risk.

▶ *Test-taking Tip: Disseminated herpes zoster (shingles) is caused by the reactivation of the varicella-zoster virus, the same virus that causes varicella (chickenpox). The nurse at greatest risk should be excluded.*

Content Area: Fundamentals; Concept: Infection; Medication; Integrated Processes: Nursing Process: Analysis; Client Needs: Safe and Effective Care Environment: Management of Care; Cognitive Level: Analysis [Analyzing]

**527.** MoC **ANSWER: 1**
1. **With VRE, hands should be washed with soap and water and not an alcohol-based hand wash when visibly soiled or in contact with equipment or environmental surfaces that could be soiled. VRE can remain on equipment and environmental surfaces for weeks. Spores may not be killed with alcohol-based hand hygiene.**
2. Hand hygiene and wearing gloves when providing oral care are appropriate for the client with β-lactamase–producing *Klebsiella pneumoniae*.
3. Hand hygiene with an alcohol-based hand wash and wearing gloves when obtaining the temperature are appropriate for the client with penicillin G–resistant *Streptococcus pneumoniae*.
4. Visitors should use the alcohol-based hand wash provided when entering and leaving the room of the client with MRSA. It is appropriate for the NA to direct visitors to do this.

♦ *Test-taking Tip: Focus on the situation "antibiotic-resistant organisms" and note that one option has the greatest potential for hand contamination.*

Content Area: Fundamentals; Concept: Infection; Management; Nursing Roles; Integrated Processes: Nursing Process: Evaluation; Client Needs: Safe and Effective Care Environment: Management of Care; Cognitive Level: Evaluation [Evaluating]

**528.** PHARM **ANSWER: 3**
1. The nurse wears nonsterile gloves with contact precautions. The spike of the tubing is contaminated and will contaminate the solution if inserted into the new IV solution bag.
2. There is no need to remove the gloves. The gloves are not sterile; nor do they risk contamination from the IV tubing spike.
3. **The nurse contaminated the spike end of the tubing. This requires replacement of the tubing to prevent the risk of an infection for the client.**
4. Cleansing the IV tubing spike with alcohol is not an appropriate action for preventing possible infection.

♦ *Test-taking Tip: Remember to read responses carefully. Eliminate options that do not focus on client safety and reduction of risk of infection.*

Content Area: Fundamentals; Concept: Infection; Integrated Processes: Nursing Process: Analysis; Client Needs: Physiological Integrity: Pharmacological and Parenteral Therapies; Cognitive Level: Application [Applying]

**529. ANSWER: 4**
1. An infection would increase the respiratory rate.
2. The normal appearance of a healing incision is pink and crusty. It should be intact.

3. Dark amber urine may indicate that the client is dehydrated. Dehydration can result from an infection if the temperature is elevated, but this is not the finding that should be most associated with the elevated WBC.
4. **The WBC count is elevated, suggesting an infection. Clients with a respiratory tract infection may have lung sounds that include crackles, rhonchi, or wheezes.**

♦ *Test-taking Tip: A WBC of 20,000/mm³ is elevated and indicates an infection.*

Content Area: Fundamentals; Concept: Infection; Integrated Processes: Nursing Process: Assessment; Client Needs: Physiological Integrity: Reduction of Risk Potential; Cognitive Level: Application [Applying]

**530. ANSWER: 4**
1. Redness and warmth at the site are signs of a localized infection.
2. Swelling and pain at the site are signs of a localized infection.
3. Hypotension (not hypertension) and tachycardia (not bradycardia) occur with a generalized infection.
4. **Generalized infections occur when there is systemic or whole body involvement. Symptoms include muscle aches, fever, headache, malaise, anorexia, elevated WBC count, hypotension, tachycardia, and mental confusion.**

♦ *Test-taking Tip: Note the terms "generalized" in the stem and "widespread" in Option 4.*

Content Area: Fundamentals; Concept: Infection; Integrated Processes: Nursing Process: Assessment; Client Needs: Physiological Integrity: Reduction of Risk Potential; Cognitive Level: Knowledge [Remembering]

**531.** PHARM **ANSWER: 1, 2, 3, 6.**
1. **Pain results from the capillaries leaking blood plasma into the tissues.**
2. **Redness is caused by the release of histamine, serotonin, and kinins that produce small vein constriction and arteriole dilation at the insertion site.**
3. **Warmth is caused by the release of histamine, serotonin, and kinins that produce small vein constriction and arteriole dilation at the insertion site.**
4. Drainage indicates an infection and not inflammation.
5. A mottling or a discolored or blotchy appearance does not indicate inflammation. It could be extravasation from drugs.
6. **Swelling results from the capillaries leaking blood plasma into the tissues.**

♦ *Test-taking Tip: Visualize the signs of an inflammation (not infection) to answer this question.*

Content Area: Fundamentals; **Concept:** Infection; **Integrated Processes:** Nursing Process: Assessment; **Client Needs:** Physiological Integrity: Pharmacological and Parenteral Therapies; **Cognitive Level:** Application [Applying]

**532. ANSWER: 2, 4, 1, 3, 5**

2. **Remove gloves and perform hand hygiene. The gloves would harbor the most microorganisms from contact with the client. Hand hygiene is performed because contact with microorganisms can occur while removing the gloves.**
4. **Remove eye protection. Protective eyewear is no longer needed and can be removed prior to removing the gown.**
1. **Remove gown. The gown is removed when preparing to leave the room.**
3. **Remove mask. The mask is removed last, at the doorway to the client's room.**
5. **Perform hand hygiene. Hand hygiene should be performed again because contact with microorganisms can occur while removing the remaining PPE.**

▶ **Test-taking Tip:** Visualize the steps of removing PPE before attempting to place the items in the correct sequence.

Content Area: Fundamentals; **Concept:** Infection; **Integrated Processes:** Nursing Process: Evaluation; **Client Needs:** Safe and Effective Care Environment: Safety and Infection Control; **Cognitive Level:** Synthesis [Creating]

**533. ANSWER: 4**

1. The N95 respirator and a gown are insufficient protection when the client is coughing up blood.
2. A surgical mask with a shield and a gown is insufficient protection for an airborne infection.
3. A surgical mask and gown are insufficient protection for an airborne infection. A cap is not necessary.
4. **TB requires airborne precautions with use of N95 respirator. Because the client has been coughing up blood, the nurse should also plan to wear a face shield.**

▶ **Test-taking Tip:** Airborne precautions require the use of an N95 respirator. A face shield provides protection against contact with blood.

Content Area: Fundamentals; **Concept:** Infection; Oxygenation; **Integrated Processes:** Nursing Process: Planning; **Client Needs:** Safe and Effective Care Environment: Safety and Infection Control; **Cognitive Level:** Application [Applying]

**534. MoC ANSWER: 2**

1. Droplet precautions alone are insufficient precautions for the client with meningococcal meningitis.
2. **A private room with airborne precautions should be planned for the client. Meningococcal meningitis is transmitted by contact with pharyngeal secretions and may be airborne.**
3. Standard precautions alone are insufficient precautions for the client with meningococcal meningitis.

4. Contact precautions alone are insufficient precautions for the client with meningococcal meningitis.

▶ **Test-taking Tip:** Meningococcal meningitis is a highly infectious disease. Thus eliminate Options 3 and 4. Of the remaining options, select the option that would provide the most protection.

Content Area: Fundamentals; **Concept:** Infection; Neurologic Regulation; Management; **Integrated Processes:** Nursing Process: Planning; **Client Needs:** Safe and Effective Care Environment: Management of Care; **Cognitive Level:** Analysis [Analyzing]

**535. MoC ANSWER: 3**

1. Quarantine is unnecessary because only those who have had close contact with the infected student are at risk.
2. Administrators may need to be informed of an outbreak, but student names should not be disclosed. Disclosing names is a violation of protected health information.
3. **The nurse should identify all individuals who have had close contact with the student. Meningococcal meningitis, caused by *Neisseria meningitidis*, can spread to those who have had close or prolonged contact with an infected person. This includes those having direct contact with the person's oral secretions.**
4. Only persons who have had close contact need to receive antibiotics. Vaccination against *Neisseria meningitidis* should be recommended for everyone, not prophylactic antibiotics.

▶ **Test-taking Tip:** Meningitis is spread to those who have had close or prolonged contact with the person infected with *Neisseria meningitidis*.

Content Area: Fundamentals; **Concept:** Infection; Nursing Roles; Management; **Integrated Processes:** Nursing Process: Analysis; Caring; **Client Needs:** Safe and Effective Care Environment: Safety and Infection Control; Safe and Effective Care Environment: Management of Care; **Cognitive Level:** Analysis [Analyzing]

**536. MoC ANSWER: 1**

1. **Gowns are required only if contamination of clothing is likely.**
2. Hand washing with soap and water is the first line of defense in preventing VRE transmission.
3. A private room is required for infection control. VRE can remain viable on environmental surfaces for weeks.
4. Enterococci normally found in the GI tract genetically mutate and develop antibiotic resistance by producing enzymes that destroy or inactivate vancomycin-type antibiotics.

▶ **Test-taking Tip:** "Needs additional orientation" is a false-response item. Select the incorrect statement.

Content Area: Fundamentals; **Concept:** Infection; Management; **Integrated Processes:** Teaching/Learning; **Client Needs:** Safe and Effective Care Environment: Management of Care; Psychosocial Integrity; **Cognitive Level:** Analysis [Analyzing]

**537. MoC ANSWER: 3**

1. An official report does not involve the local news media.
2. Staff receive annual tuberculin skin tests or a CXR. Anyone who does not have TB can care for the client. Airborne precautions should be in place, controlling the risk for transmission.
3. **The infection control nurse must notify the local or state health department of the case. States mandate which diseases are reportable, and surveillance is managed through local and state health departments.**
4. Clients with respiratory TB receive treatment in hospitals, clinics, and at home with specific antibiotic and antitubercular medications. Specific tertiary facilities for treatment of clients with TB are no longer utilized in the U.S.

▶ *Test-taking Tip: According to guidelines issued from the CDC, TB is a reportable disease.*

**Content Area:** Fundamentals; **Concept:** Infection; Legal; **Integrated Processes:** Nursing Process: Analysis; **Client Needs:** Safe and Effective Care Environment: Management of Care; **Cognitive Level:** Application [Applying]

**538. ANSWER: 1**

1. **Occupational exposure is an urgent medical concern, and medical care should be sought immediately. Prophylactic antiretroviral treatment is started preferably within 1 to 2 hours and lasts for 4 weeks. If results of HIV antibody testing return positive, treatment continues.**
2. HIV antibody testing should be completed now (baseline) and then at 6 weeks, 3 months, and 6 months after exposure.

3. Waiting until the end of the clinical shift may delay starting treatment, thus narrowing the opportunity when prophylaxis against HIV may be effective.
4. The exposure site should be washed well with soap and water. Flushing with water is required for mucous membrane exposure.

▶ *Test-taking Tip: Apply disease prevention principles. The only option that will prevent developing the disease is Option 1.*

**Content Area:** Fundamentals; **Concept:** Infection; Management; **Integrated Processes:** Nursing Process: Implementation; **Client Needs:** Safe and Effective Care Environment: Safety and Infection Control; **Cognitive Level:** Analysis [Analyzing]

**539. MoC ANSWER: 1**

1. **The nurse should hand the HCP a gown and gloves; these should be worn when touching the client with MRSA to prevent its transmission.**
2. The HCP is part of the health care team and should be held accountable to standards that maintain client safety.
3. Notifying the charge nurse and unit manager does not immediately address the breach in the use of contact precautions.
4. Permitting the HCP to examine the client without PPE increases the risk for transmission of MRSA.

▶ *Test-taking Tip: You should use the nursing code of ethics and standards of care to guide decisions.*

**Content Area:** Fundamentals; **Concept:** Safety; Infection; Management; Nursing Roles; **Integrated Processes:** Communication and Documentation; **Client Needs:** Safe and Effective Care Environment: Management of Care; Safe and Effective Care Environment: Safety and Infection Control; **Cognitive Level:** Application [Applying]

## Chapter Fourteen

# Basic Care and Comfort

**540.** The client began wearing hearing aids 5 weeks earlier. Which statement to the nurse demonstrates that the client is successfully adapting to the hearing aids?

1. "I wear the hearing aids only when I go out in public."
2. "I clean my ears daily with a cotton-tipped swab."
3. "I put my hearing aids within reach on the nightstand."
4. "I clean the ear mold with mild soap and water."

**541.** The nurse is inserting a hearing aid in the adult client's ear. Place an X to indicate where the nurse's fingers should be placed to facilitate insertion of the hearing aid.

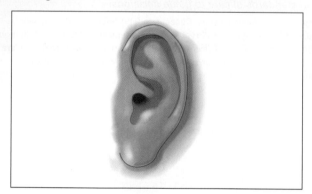

**542.** The hospitalized client with limited mobility is at risk for skin breakdown. Which interventions should the nurse include in the plan of care to maintain the client's skin integrity? **Select all that apply.**

1. Massage vigorously over bony prominences daily.
2. Wear sterile gloves when doing skin inspection.
3. Apply a moisturizing lotion to bony prominences.
4. Teach the client to change position every 2 hours.
5. Apply an overhead trapeze to the client's bed.
6. Apply barrier cream if stool incontinence occurs.

**543.** MoC  The nurse is observing the UAP providing oral hygiene to clients. Which action by the UAP requires follow-up? **Select all that apply.**

1. Replaces the upper denture before the lower one
2. Places the unconscious client in a supine position
3. Inserts a foam swab to pry a lower denture loose
4. Brushes the tongue with a soft-bristled toothbrush
5. Dons exam gloves to perform oral hygiene
6. Uses gauze to move and remove an upper denture

**544.** MoC  The nurse is observing the nursing student caring for the client with a prosthetic eyeball. What action by the student nurse would require intervention?

1. Has the client lie down to remove the eyeball
2. Cleans the prosthetic eye with saline solution
3. Dries the prosthetic eye thoroughly with gauze
4. Teaches to remove and clean the eyeball weekly

**545.** MoC  The nurse is caring for the newly admitted male client who is unconscious. The UAP asks if the client should be shaved. What is the nurse's **best** response?

1. "I need to find out the client's preferences first."
2. "Shave him only after you have bathed him."
3. "Use the electric razor when you shave him."
4. "Avoid shaving him. I need a doctor's order."

**546.** MoC  The nurse is observing the UAP prepare a shower for the client who requires assistance with ambulation and hygiene. Which action(s) by the UAP indicate understanding of the procedure? **Select all that apply.**

1. Sets the water temperature at 100°F to 105°F (37°C to 40°C)
2. Locks the door to provide the client with privacy
3. Uses a chair for the client to sit on in the shower
4. Ensures a nonskid surface is in the shower
5. Helps to wash areas the client cannot reach

**547.** The client is just admitted to a surgical unit following abdominal surgery. Which assessment finding requires the nurse's **immediate** intervention?

1. NG tube to low intermittent suction has small amounts of dark bloody returns.
2. Oxygen saturation level is 92%, and oxygen by nasal cannula is set at 2 liters.
3. The incisional dressing has a 25-cent-piece–sized shadow of new drainage.
4. The Jackson-Pratt (JP) drain is round in shape with 30 mL serosanguinous drainage.

**548.** The nurse is inserting a urinary catheter in the client with urinary retention. During balloon inflation, the client reports pain. What is the nurse's **best** action?

1. Withdraw the sterile water from the balloon and advance the catheter farther.
2. Continue inflating the balloon as this finding is expected during catheter insertion.
3. Remove the catheter and reattempt insertion with a smaller urinary catheter.
4. Reposition the catheter by rotating it slightly and continue to inflate the balloon.

**549.** The client has an indwelling urinary catheter. Which information should the nurse include in the discharge teaching plan? **Select all that apply.**

1. Plan to change the urinary catheter once a week.
2. Clean the perineal area daily with soap and water.
3. Secure the catheter tubing to the thigh with tape.
4. Avoid showering while the catheter is in place.
5. Do hand hygiene before and after catheter care.

**550.** The client voided 300 mL after having an indwelling urinary catheter removed 6 hours ago. A bladder scan immediately after the void showed that the client has a postvoid residual (PVR) volume of 250 mL. What should the nurse conclude from this finding?

1. The finding is expected after catheter removal.
2. The client's bladder function is 50% of normal.
3. The scan should have been done before the void.
4. The client has incomplete bladder emptying.

**551.** **CJ** The client has a sprained right ankle, and the nurse is to apply an elastic bandage. Place an X on the illustration where the nurse should start to wrap and an arrow for the direction that the nurse should continue to wrap.

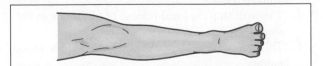

**552.** The client is undergoing a 24-hour urine specimen collection. Twenty hours into the collection period, a single voided urine is accidentally discarded. What is the nurse's **best** action?

1. Resume the urine collection and collect one additional voided specimen.
2. Discard the urine collected and begin a new urine collection immediately.
3. Complete the urine collection and send all urine collected to the laboratory.
4. Dispose of the urine collected and reschedule the test to begin the next morning.

**553.** **PHARM** The client reports pain in the right leg even though it was amputated. Which complementary therapy should the nurse use to control the phantom pain associated with the client's amputation?

1. A small dose of alprazolam at 8-hour intervals in addition to prescribed oxycodone and acetaminophen q6h prn
2. A high-fiber diet and 2000 mL fluid intake in 24 hours while taking hydromorphone at 4- to 6-hour intervals prn
3. Progressive relaxation exercises three times daily in addition to use of a transdermal patch of fentanyl
4. A local anesthetic as a nerve block in addition to prescribed long-acting oxycodone

**554.** The client with a new colostomy asks how to deal with gas coming from the stoma. To respond to the client's concern, the nurse should ask the client to take which action? **Select all that apply.**

1. Describe the dietary intake, including food types.
2. Include cruciferous vegetables in the diet daily.
3. Decrease fluid intake to 1200 mL per 24 hours.
4. Prick the colostomy stoma pouch with a pin.
5. Limit intake of gas-producing carbonated sodas.
6. In the bathroom, open the clamp to release gas.

**555.** The postoperative male client has been unable to urinate into the urinal while lying in bed. Which interventions are appropriate to promote voiding for this client who is to be discharged home within a few hours? **Select all that apply.**

1. Have the client apply an external condom catheter while lying flat in bed.
2. Assist the client to stand at the bedside to attempt to urinate in a urinal.
3. Administer a prescribed analgesic if the client is experiencing pain.
4. Turn on running water so it is heard while the client attempts to void.
5. Ask the client to imagine being at home and voiding in his own bathroom.

**556.** The client was treated for constipation 1 month earlier. On a return clinic visit, which statement would **best** assist the nurse to evaluate that the client is no longer constipated?

1. "I drink 2000 milliliters of fluids daily, including drinking 4 ounces of prune juice."
2. "I have had a soft-formed stool without straining every other day for the past 2 weeks."
3. "I needed to give myself only one disposable enema since my last appointment."
4. "I have a lot of discomfort from hemorrhoids during my daily bowel movements."

**557.** PHARM The client with diarrhea has had four bowel movements in the past 8 hours, measuring 150 mL, 100 mL, 100 mL, and 150 mL. The client is to receive one-to-one replacement with a bolus of IV 0.9% NaCl to be infused over the next 2 hours. How many mL of 0.9% NaCl will the nurse infuse each hour?

_____ mL (Record your answer as a whole number.)

**558.** The client with intermittent abdominal pain recently had a barium enema. The client calls the nurse to report passage of a soft-formed, pale-colored stool. What is the nurse's **best** response?

1. "This is an expected finding after administration of barium."
2. "Describe any abdominal pain you had when passing the stool."
3. "What foods or fluids did you eat after you completed the test?"
4. "You need to increase the amount of water you are drinking."

**559.** The client uses a walker to ambulate with partial weight-bearing after foot surgery. What should the nurse observe when this client is using the walker correctly?

1. Has elbows bent at a 30-degree angle
2. Is bent over the front bar of the walker
3. While walking, lifts the walker 2 inches
4. Has a walker that has four wheels in place

**560.** The nurse learns at shift report that the immobile client has bilateral foot drop. Which finding during the nurse's assessment supports the presence of foot drop?

1. The client's great toe is dorsiflexed, and the other toes are fanned out.
2. The client's feet are unable to be maintained perpendicular to the legs.
3. The client is unable to move the feet into a position of plantar flexion.
4. The client is only able to dorsiflex both feet when asked to bend the feet.

**561.** The client is in skeletal traction with 20 lb of traction applied to a right lower leg fracture. Which intervention should the nurse perform at regular intervals?

1. Perform pin site care.
2. Remove the weights.
3. Reposition the right leg.
4. Do passive ROM to the legs.

**562.** MoC The experienced nurse observes the student nurse caring for the client with the wet plaster cast illustrated. Which conclusion by the experienced nurse is correct?

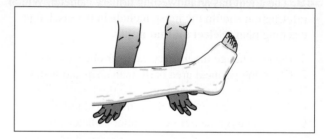

1. The student should not be touching the plaster cast because it is wet.
2. The student should be using a pillow to lift the client's casted extremity.
3. The student is correctly handling a wet plaster cast with the palms.
4. The student should be using fingers and not the palms to handle the cast.

**563.** The nurse applies a warm, moist compress to the site where an IV solution has infiltrated. Which response is correct when the client asks the purpose of the compress?

1. "This will alter tissue sensitivity by producing numbness."
2. "This will decrease the metabolic needs of the involved tissues."
3. "This will stop the local release of histamine in the tissues."
4. "This will increase blood flow and accelerate tissue healing."

**564.** The client requests a kosher meal. Which direction by the nurse to the NA is appropriate?

1. "Avoid eye contact when delivering the meal tray."
2. "Do not remove the wrapping from the plastic utensils."
3. "Have the client sit for the meal facing toward Mecca."
4. "Check that the meal contains both milk and kosher meat."

**565.** The nurse is assessing the female client who is 65 inches tall and has a small body frame. Based on the information in the chart illustrated, what is the client's approximate ideal body weight?

| Rule of 5 for Females | Rule of 6 for Males |
| --- | --- |
| 105 lb for 5 ft of height | 106 lb for 5 ft of height |
| +5 lb for each inch over 5 ft | +6 lb for each inch over 5 ft |
| ±10% for body frame size | ±10% for body frame size |
| Add 10% for large body frame size and subtract 10% for small body frame size. | |

_____ lb (Record your answer as a whole number.)

**566.** The client residing in a nursing home has bilateral weak handgrips and visual and hearing deficits. Which interventions should the nurse implement when the client is eating a meal? **Select all that apply.**

1. Ask the client's permission to open containers and cut up meats on the food tray.
2. Obtain special easy-to-hold, built-up silverware for the client to use when eating.
3. Observe the client, but avoid providing assistance even if the client is frustrated.
4. Help feed the client if the client is eating too slowly so food does not get too cold.
5. Ensure that the client wears eyeglasses and hearing aids before starting to eat.

**567.** MoC The dietitian prescribes a 24-hour calorie count for the malnourished hospitalized client. Which action should be taken by the nurse?

1. Ask the client to recall at the end of the day the food and beverages consumed.
2. Inform the client how to count the calories in the food and beverages consumed.
3. Inform the client that a record will be maintained of food and beverages consumed.
4. Ask the client to identify the food groups and foods that are being consumed in each.

**568.** The hospitalized client is able to stand to use an electronic digital scale for obtaining the client's prescribed daily weight. Which nursing interventions **best** ensure that the client's daily weight is accurate? **Select all that apply.**

1. Ask the client to wear supportive shoes before stepping on the scale.
2. Ensure that the scale is calibrated and "zeroed" before a weight is obtained.
3. Weigh the client by moving the sliding indicator until the scale balances.
4. Weigh the client at different times of the day and then average the weights.
5. Take the weight as soon as the client wakens in the morning and after voiding.

**569.** MoC The nurse should inform the NA to not take a rectal temperature on which unresponsive client?

1. The adult who underwent ileostomy surgery because of a perforated bowel
2. The adult who has a productive cough and is receiving oxygen by nasal cannula
3. The adult who develops thrombocytopenia after receiving chemotherapy treatments
4. The adult who has hypothermia after being outside in a below-zero temperature

**570.** The nurse teaches the client who needs nasotracheal suctioning (NT) and performs hand hygiene. Order the remaining steps to perform NT suctioning correctly.

1. Prepare suction supplies and equipment, and pour sterile saline into a sterile container.
2. Place finger over suction control port; suction intermittently while withdrawing the catheter.
3. Put on sterile gloves.
4. Lubricate the catheter with sterile saline, insert into naris, and advance into pharynx.
5. As the client inhales, advance it into the trachea.
6. Pick up suction catheter with the dominant hand and attach it to connection tubing; avoid contamination of the glove on the dominant hand.
7. Place tip into sterile saline container while applying suction to clear secretions from the tubing.

Answer: _____

**571.** The 11-month-old with a tracheostomy is receiving oxygen at 30%. What should the nurse do when the infant has a decline in oxygen saturation from 96% to 87% and appears anxious and restless?

1. Obtain arterial blood gases (ABGs).
2. Increase oxygen rate from 30% to 50%.
3. Suction the tracheostomy tube.
4. Medicate for anxiety and pain.

**572.** MoC The NA tells the nurse that the unit's small-adult BP cuff cannot be found and that the client's arm is too small to use a regular adult-sized cuff. Which direction should the nurse give to the NA?

1. Document the other vital signs and note that the proper-fitting BP cuff is not available.
2. Go to another nursing unit to obtain their small-adult BP cuff, and take the client's BP.
3. Use the regular-sized BP cuff and add 10 to the diastolic and systolic BP readings.
4. If the cuff closes around the arm, take the client's BP using the regular adult cuff.

**573.** Before the client's initial ambulation, the nurse obtains the client's BP with an automatic BP machine. What should the nurse do **first** when obtaining a BP reading of 86/56 and heart rate of 64?

1. Assess the client for dizziness and feel the temperature of extremities.
2. Obtain a manual BP cuff and machine and retake the client's BP.
3. Elevate the head of the client's bed and assist the client out of bed.
4. Review the medical record and determine the client's normal BP range.

**574.** The nurse is taking the adult client's temperature. What should the nurse do to correctly obtain the temperature with a tympanic thermometer?

1. Ensure that the probe tip seals the ear canal.
2. Remove earwax with a cotton-tipped applicator.
3. Pull the pinna downward to insert the probe tip.
4. Ask whether the client has a tympanostomy tube.

**575.** The nurse is caring for the client with a stage III pressure ulcer to the right heel. Which actions should the nurse plan? **Select all that apply.**

1. Give foods high in vitamin C such as orange juice.
2. Provide analgesics before dressing changes.
3. Check the leg's pedal pulses and capillary refill.
4. Use hydrogen peroxide for cleaning the ulcer.
5. Turn and reposition the client every 1 to 2 hours.
6. Elevate the leg on pillows, with the heel off the pillow.

**576.** The nurse is evaluating the client's ability to perform active ROM. Which illustration demonstrates the client's ability to correctly perform eversion?

1.
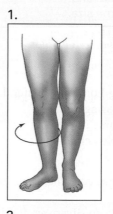

2.
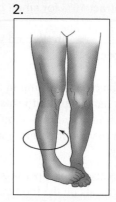

3.
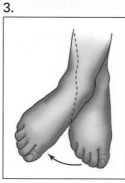

4.
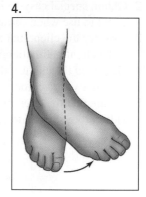

**577.** MoC The experienced nurse and the new nurse are preparing to provide phototherapy to the 4-day-old infant with hyperbilirubinemia. Which information should the experienced nurse include when instructing the new nurse about providing phototherapy for the infant?

1. Keep the infant fully clothed to prevent chilling and hypothermia.
2. Cover the infant's eyes with eye shields to prevent retinal damage.
3. Limit the number of feedings to reduce the number of soiled diapers.
4. Discontinue the phototherapy if the infant develops a mild skin rash.

**578.** The nurse is using a hypothermia blanket for the febrile client. Which findings indicate that the client is now hypothermic? **Select all that apply.**

1. Increased urine output
2. Increased drowsiness
3. Decreased HR
4. Decreased BP
5. Increased core body temperature

# Answers and Rationales

## 540. ANSWER: 4

1. Hearing aids should be worn daily to adjust to their use. Noisy public situations are sometimes difficult for persons with hearing aids.
2. Cotton-tipped swabs should not be inserted into the ear canal due to possible injury and infection.
3. Hearing aids are expensive and delicate, and they should be stored in a protective container in a dry, safe place.
4. **The ear mold can be cleansed with mild soap and water to remove wax build-up.**

▶ *Test-taking Tip: The key phrase in the stem is "successfully adapting to the hearing aids."*

Content Area: Fundamentals; Concept: Self; Sensory Perception; Integrated Processes: Nursing Process: Evaluation; Client Needs: Physiological Integrity: Basic Care and Comfort; Psychosocial Integrity; Cognitive Level: Evaluation [Evaluating]

## 541. ANSWER:

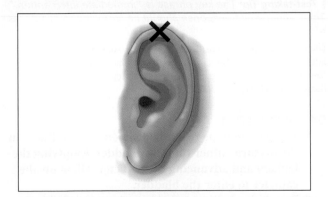

**Placing the fingers on the helix to pull the ear up and back straightens the ear canal.**

▶ *Test-taking Tip: Placement of the nurse's fingers to facilitate insertion of a hearing aid is the same technique used to assess the adult ear with an otoscope.*

Content Area: Fundamentals; Concept: Sensory Perception; Integrated Processes: Nursing Process: Implementation; Client Needs: Physiological Integrity: Basic Care and Comfort; Psychosocial Integrity; Cognitive Level: Application [Applying]

## 542. ANSWER: 3, 4, 5, 6

1. Bony prominences should not be vigorously massaged because this may lead to tissue trauma.
2. Wearing sterile gloves is not necessary when inspecting the client's skin; if skin breakdown is present, examination gloves should be worn.
3. **Combating dry skin with moisturizing lotions helps prevent dryness and maintains the skin's natural integrity.**
4. **A change in position every 2 hours alters the area of the body bearing weight and improves overall circulation to tissues.**
5. **Use of an overhead trapeze allows the client to help lift some of the weight, decreasing friction and shear with lifts.**
6. **A barrier cream to the buttocks and rectal area will protect the skin from coming in contact with incontinent stool.**

▶ *Test-taking Tip: The focus of the question involves nursing interventions that maintain skin integrity. Eliminate harmful or unrelated interventions.*

Content Area: Fundamentals; Concept: Skin Integrity; Integrated Processes: Nursing Process: Implementation; Client Needs: Physiological Integrity: Basic Care and Comfort; Cognitive Level: Synthesis [Creating]

## 543. MoC ANSWER: 2, 3

1. Remove and replace the upper denture first for ease of insertion.
2. **The unconscious client should be placed in a side-lying position with the head turned to the side. Performing oral care in a supine position on the unconscious client can result in aspiration.**

3. **Removing the denture plates with a foam swab to pry the plate loose could injure the client.**

4. A soft-bristled toothbrush removes debris from the tongue, which can act as a reservoir for microorganisms.

5. Oral care is a clean procedure. Donning gloves prior to oral hygiene adheres to standard precautions.

6. Using gauze to grasp the upper plate will prevent it from slipping. Moving it breaks the suction that holds the plate on the roof of the client's mouth.

▶ *Test-taking Tip:* The key phrase is "immediate follow-up." You should be selecting actions that are incorrectly performed by the UAP.

**Content Area:** Fundamentals; **Concept:** Critical Thinking; Management; **Integrated Processes:** Communication and Documentation; **Client Needs:** Physiological Integrity: Basic Care and Comfort; Safe and Effective Care Environment: Management of Care; **Cognitive Level:** Application [Applying]

---

### 544. MoC ANSWER: 3

1. Positioning the client lying down aids with removal of the prosthetic eye; if the eye is accidentally dropped, it will fall onto the bed instead of the floor.

2. NS is an appropriate cleansing agent.

3. **The prosthetic eye should be moist to facilitate insertion. Drying the prosthetic thoroughly with gauze could result in trauma to the eye socket.**

4. The prosthetic eye needs to be removed periodically for cleansing. It is recommended this be done every 1 to 3 weeks.

▶ *Test-taking Tip:* Look at the key words "would require intervention," which indicates one option is unsafe, whereas the other three options are appropriate.

**Content Area:** Fundamentals; **Concept:** Management; **Integrated Processes:** Nursing Process: Evaluation; **Client Needs:** Physiological Integrity: Basic Care and Comfort; Safe and Effective Care Environment: Management of Care; **Cognitive Level:** Evaluation [Evaluating]

---

### 545. MoC ANSWER: 1

1. **Removal of facial hair varies based on personal and cultural preferences. The nurse needs to assess the client's preferences before proceeding. If the client is unable to share his preferences, the family or significant other is consulted.**

2. The nurse should not assert personal preferences with client grooming.

3. An electric shaver is a safe alternative to a razor, but the client's preferences are not known.

4. Shaving the client does not require a doctor's order.

▶ *Test-taking Tip:* You should note that one option is client-centered. The remaining options are nurse-centered.

**Content Area:** Fundamentals; **Concept:** Management; **Integrated Processes:** Nursing Process: Assessment; **Client Needs:** Physiological Integrity: Basic Care and Comfort; Safe and Effective Care Environment: Management of Care; **Cognitive Level:** Application [Applying]

---

### 546. MoC ANSWER: 3, 4, 5

1. Water temperature should range from 110°F to 115°F (43°C to 46°C); the water temperature is too cool.

2. The client who requires assistance should not be left unattended behind a locked door. The UAP will not be able to reach the client.

3. **This client requires assistance with ambulation and would be at risk for falling if attempting to shower without a shower chair.**

4. **A nonskid surface promotes safety in a wet environment where slips and falls may occur.**

5. **Assisting the client with hygiene in areas that the client cannot reach allows for active participation according to the client's ability.**

▶ *Test-taking Tip:* Use the process of elimination to narrow the options that promote client safety.

**Content Area:** Fundamentals; **Concept:** Management; **Integrated Processes:** Nursing Process: Evaluation; **Client Needs:** Safe and Effective Care Environment: Safety and Infection Control; Safe and Effective Care Environment: Management of Care; **Cognitive Level:** Evaluation [Evaluating]

---

### 547. ANSWER: 4

1. An NG tube to low intermittent suction with small amounts of dark bloody returns would be normal immediately after surgery if there were any trauma associated with insertion of tube; thus no intervention would be required.

2. The oxygen saturation of 92% is normal. The 2 liters of oxygen by nasal cannula is maintaining this level. No intervention is required.

3. The nurse should monitor the dressing for additional drainage, but no intervention is required.

4. **A round JP drain requires immediate intervention; the drain needs to be emptied and compressed to create suction and collect fluid. Suction is lost when there is too much drainage or there is a leak in the system.**

▶ *Test-taking Tip:* The key phrase is "immediate intervention." Think about which response should be corrected to avoid loss of life or limb.

**Content Area:** Fundamentals; **Concept:** Critical Thinking; Perioperative; **Integrated Processes:** Nursing Process: Assessment; **Client Needs:** Physiological Integrity: Physiological Adaptation; **Cognitive Level:** Application [Applying]

---

### 548. ANSWER: 1

1. **The pain may be from the balloon being inflated in the urethra rather than the bladder. Emptying the balloon and advancing the catheter will allow the catheter to enter the bladder.**

2. Pain during balloon inflation is abnormal. Continuing to inflate the balloon could damage the urethra.

3. The catheter should be removed if an attempt to advance the catheter fails. The size of the catheter does influence pain experienced during balloon inflation when improperly located.

4. Repositioning a catheter with a partially inflated balloon could damage the urethra and cause more pain for the client.

▶ *Test-taking Tip: Note the words "best action." Three options are similar with keeping the balloon partially inflated, and the other is different.*

Content Area: Fundamentals; Concept: Urinary Elimination; Safety; Integrated Processes: Nursing Process: Implementation; Client Needs: Physiological Integrity: Reduction of Risk Potential; Cognitive Level: Analysis [Analyzing]

## 549. ANSWER: 2, 3, 5

1. For clients with long-term indwelling urinary catheters, monthly catheter changes are recommended unless there is a greater risk for catheter blockage.
2. **Soap and water is an appropriate perineal cleansing agent; routine use of antimicrobial cleansers is not recommended.**
3. **Securing the catheter to the thigh anchors the catheter and minimizes trauma to the urethra and bladder neck.**
4. An indwelling catheter does not alter the client's method of meeting hygiene needs. The client may shower if the client's condition permits.
5. **Performing hand hygiene prior to and after catheter care reduces the risk of transmission of microorganisms that could cause UTI.**

▶ *Test-taking Tip: Identify options that will have a positive effect on the client. Also, eliminate options that increase the client's risk for infection.*

Content Area: Fundamentals; Concept: Nursing Roles; Integrated Processes: Nursing Processs: Planning; Teaching/Learning; Client Needs: Physiological Integrity: Basic Care and Comfort; Health Promotion and Maintenance; Cognitive Level: Application [Applying]

## 550. ANSWER: 4

1. This is not an expected finding. If the bladder is functioning normally, PVR volume should be less than 50 mL.
2. It is not possible to estimate the percent of bladder functioning from this finding.
3. PVR volume should be measured within 20 minutes after voiding. A bladder scan before voiding is not necessary.
4. **If the bladder scan is completed within 20 minutes of voiding, the PVR volume should be less than 50 mL. The 250 mL indicates that the client has incomplete bladder emptying.**

▶ *Test-taking Tip: The PVR volume should be less than 50 mL when measured by a bladder scan within 20 minutes of voiding.*

Content Area: Fundamentals; Concept: Critical Thinking; Urinary Elimination; Integrated Processes: Nursing Process: Analysis; Client Needs: Physiological Integrity: Physiological Adaptation; Cognitive Level: Analysis [Analyzing]

## 551. CJ ANSWER:

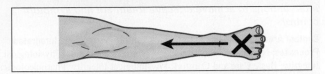

**To wrap a sprained ankle, the elastic bandage should be placed first on the top of the foot (noted with the X), wrapped under the ball of the foot, repeated again, then moved upward around the ankle, and then proceed around and up the leg. The direction of the arrow is upward. This direction promotes the flow of circulation to the heart.**

▶ *Test-taking Tip: This is an enhanced hot spot item. You need to insert both an X and an arrow.*

Content Area: Fundamentals; Concept: Perfusion; Integrated Processes: Nursing Process: Implementation; Client Needs: Physiological Integrity: Basic Care and Comfort; Cognitive Level: Application [Applying]

## 552. ANSWER: 2

1. Resuming the collection and adding one additional voided specimen will result in test inaccuracies.
2. **The urine collected must be discarded and restarted. When starting a 24-hour urine collection, the first void is discarded, and all urine is collected for the next 24 hours.**
3. The specimen will be 4 hours short of 24 hours and could result in inaccurate test results.
4. There is no need to reschedule the test for the morning. The start time for a 24-hour urine does not affect test results. The first void is discarded. The accidentally discarded void is the first void.

▶ *Test-taking Tip: For a 24-hour urine collection, the time that the test starts is when the first void is discarded.*

Content Area: Fundamentals; Concept: Critical Thinking; Urinary Elimination; Integrated Processes: Nursing Process: Implementation; Client Needs: Physiological Integrity: Reduction of Risk Potential; Cognitive Level: Application [Applying]

## 553. PHARM ANSWER: 3

1. Combining an antianxiety medication such as alprazolam (Xanax) with an analgesic such as oxycodone and acetaminophen (Percocet) is a conventional medicinal intervention.
2. Dietary interventions help control constipation associated with opioids such as hydromorphone (Dilaudid) and are not a complementary therapy to control phantom limb pain.
3. **Progressive relaxation therapy, used along with prescribed analgesic medication such as fentanyl (Duragesic) to control phantom pain, is an example of complementary therapy.**
4. A nerve block with an analgesic such as oxycodone (OxyContin) is using conventional medicinal practice.

▶ **Test-taking Tip:** *Complementary interventions are holistic therapies used in addition to conventional medicinal interventions to achieve effective treatment and symptom control.*

**Content Area:** Fundamentals; **Concept:** Comfort; Medication; **Integrated Processes:** Nursing Process: Implementation; **Client Needs:** Physiological Integrity: Basic Care and Comfort; Physiological Integrity: Pharmacological and Parenteral Therapies; **Cognitive Level:** Application [Applying]

### 554. ANSWER: 1, 5, 6

1. **The nurse can assess for foods and beverages known to produce gas if the usual dietary intake is described by the client.**
2. Cruciferous vegetables, which include vegetables of the cabbage family, are known to cause gas formation.
3. The client needs at least 2000 mL of fluid daily to maintain proper function of the colostomy.
4. Pricking the colostomy pouch with a pin leads to constant gas release and an unpleasant odor.
5. **Limiting carbonated beverages reduces gas formation in the intestinal tract.**
6. **Gas in the pouch should be released by opening the clamp in a restroom environment.**

▶ **Test-taking Tip:** *Evaluate each option to determine if it has a positive or negative effect on gas from the stoma.*

**Content Area:** Fundamentals; **Concept:** Bowel Elimination; Nutrition; **Integrated Processes:** Nursing Process: Implementation; **Client Needs:** Physiological Integrity: Basic Care and Comfort; **Cognitive Level:** Analysis [Analyzing]

### 555. ANSWER: 2, 3, 4, 5

1. Use of an external catheter will not assist the client to void; it may be used for incontinence.
2. **The nurse should try to assist the client to void by assisting him to the normal position of standing.**
3. **Pain may be interfering with the ability to urinate and should be treated.**
4. **Using the sound of running water stimulates the voiding reflex.**
5. **Guided imagery is a relaxation technique that may help the client to void.**

▶ **Test-taking Tip:** *One option is different from the others. Often the option that is different can be eliminated as the answer.*

**Content Area:** Fundamentals; **Concept:** Urinary Elimination; **Integrated Processes:** Nursing Process: Implementation; **Client Needs:** Physiological Integrity: Basic Care and Comfort; **Cognitive Level:** Application [Applying]

### 556. ANSWER: 2

1. The fluid intake, which includes prune juice, shows the client is taking action to prevent constipation, but it does not indicate that the client is not constipated.
2. **Constipation is having fewer than three bowel movements per week. The client is no longer constipated when having a soft-formed stool without straining every other day.**

3. A disposable enema is used to stimulate bowel function. Using only one does not indicate that the client is no longer constipated.
4. Although the client is having a daily stool, there is insufficient information in this statement to evaluate what the client used to stimulate daily bowel movements or the consistency of the stool.

▶ **Test-taking Tip:** *The key word is "best," indicating that there may be more than one correct answer, but one option is better than the other. Choose the option that is most descriptive of the stools.*

**Content Area:** Fundamentals; **Concept:** Bowel Elimination; **Integrated Processes:** Nursing Process: Evaluation; **Client Needs:** Physiological Integrity: Basic Care and Comfort; **Cognitive Level:** Evaluation [Evaluating]

### 557. PHARM ANSWER: 250

**The total fluid loss from the client's diarrhea is 500 mL (150 + 100 + 100 + 150). One-to-one replacement equals 500 mL of NaCl to be infused. The amount to be delivered over 2 hours is 500 mL; the amount for each hour is 500 ÷ 2 = 250 mL.**

▶ **Test-taking Tip:** *A "one-to-one replacement" means that the replacement volume should equal the volume of fluid lost. Calculate the total fluid loss from the diarrhea to calculate the replacement of the same volume of intravenous fluids.*

**Content Area:** Fundamentals; **Concept:** Fluid and Electrolyte Balance; Medication; **Integrated Processes:** Nursing Process: Analysis; **Client Needs:** Physiological Integrity: Basic Care and Comfort; Physiological Integrity: Pharmacological and Parenteral Therapies; **Cognitive Level:** Analysis [Analyzing]

### 558. ANSWER: 1

1. **Barium administered in the GI tract results in pale or white-colored stools due to residual barium being evacuated from the bowel.**
2. Passage of stool may or may not result in additional abdominal pain; however, abdominal pain does not result in pale-colored stools.
3. Dietary intake after barium enema does not result in a pale stool color.
4. Water is important to drink after a barium enema, but there is no indication that the client requires additional water. If the stool had been firm or difficult to pass, additional water would have been beneficial.

▶ **Test-taking Tip:** *You will need to know what is normal to expect after specific diagnostic tests.*

**Content Area:** Fundamentals; **Concept:** Bowel Elimination; **Integrated Processes:** Communication and Documentation; **Client Needs:** Physiological Integrity: Reduction of Risk Potential; **Cognitive Level:** Analysis [Analyzing]

### 559. ANSWER: 1

1. **When a walker is at the proper height, the client's elbows will be bent at a 30-degree angle.**
2. The client should stand erect and not bent over while using the walker.

3. The client cannot be ambulating with partial weight-bearing if the client lifts the walker off the floor.
4. The client cannot be ambulating with partial weight-bearing if using a walker with four wheels.

▶ **Test-taking Tip:** *The topic of the question is the correct use of a walker with partial weight-bearing. Use the process of elimination, eliminating Option 2 because the client should be erect, and Options 3 and 4 because these would require full weight-bearing.*

**Content Area:** Fundamentals; **Concept:** Mobility; **Integrated Processes:** Nursing Process: Evaluation; **Client Needs:** Physiological Integrity: Basic Care and Comfort; **Cognitive Level:** Evaluation [Evaluating]

## 560. ANSWER: 2

1. A positive Babinski's sign occurs when the great toe dorsiflexes and the toes fan out in response to stroking the lateral surface of the foot.
2. **The client with foot drop is unable to hold the feet up in dorsiflexion or in a perpendicular position to the leg.**
3. With foot drop, the feet stay in plantar flexion.
4. The client with bilateral foot drop is unable to dorsiflex the feet.

▶ **Test-taking Tip:** *The topic of the question is the definition of foot drop. Define foot drop in terms of dorsal or plantar flexion.*

**Content Area:** Fundamentals; **Concept:** Mobility; Assessment; **Integrated Processes:** Nursing Process: Assessment; **Client Needs:** Physiological Integrity: Basic Care and Comfort; **Cognitive Level:** Analysis [Analyzing]

## 561. ANSWER: 1

1. **Pin site care should be routinely performed per agency policy to reduce the risk of infection.**
2. With skeletal traction, the weights should never be removed except for emergencies.
3. The leg in traction needs to stay in proper alignment, so it would not be repositioned.
4. The leg in traction needs to stay in proper alignment, so ROM would not be performed on that leg.

▶ **Test-taking Tip:** *Remember that with skeletal traction a pin is placed through the bone and is used for applying traction to pull the bones into alignment. With this knowledge, only Option 1 is the plausible option.*

**Content Area:** Fundamentals; **Concept:** Mobility; **Integrated Processes:** Nursing Process: Implementation; **Client Needs:** Physiological Integrity: Reduction of Risk Potential; **Cognitive Level:** Application [Applying]

## 562. MoC ANSWER: 3

1. A plaster cast takes hours to dry and should be repositioned to allow drying of the underside of the cast and to prevent indentations.
2. Handling a wet plaster cast only with a pillow will not allow inspection of the underside of the cast.

3. **The student nurse is observed safely handling the wet plaster cast with the palms of the hands to prevent indentations from the fingers. This technique prevents pressure areas from developing on the skin underneath the cast.**
4. Using the fingers will cause indentations in the cast that will cause pressure areas.

▶ **Test-taking Tip:** *Study the illustration. Compare the conclusion in each option with the illustration. Use the process of elimination to rule out incorrect options.*

**Content Area:** Fundamentals; **Concept:** Safety; Mobility; Management; **Integrated Processes:** Nursing Process: Evaluation; **Client Needs:** Physiological Integrity: Reduction of Risk Potential; Safe and Effective Care Environment: Management of Care; **Cognitive Level:** Evaluation [Evaluating]

## 563. ANSWER: 4

1. Application of cold, not hot, alters the sensitivity of nerves in the area and causes numbness.
2. Heat causes an increase, not a decrease, in tissue metabolism.
3. Cold, not hot, decreases the inflammatory response by reducing the release of histamine from inflamed tissues.
4. **Application of the warm, moist compress dilates the blood vessels, thus increasing local blood flow and capillary permeability. This accelerates the inflammatory response and promotes healing to the involved tissues.**

▶ **Test-taking Tip:** *The topic of the question is the effect of heat on an area of sustained inflammation. Recall the effects of heat on tissues. Evaluate each option to determine whether it accurately describes the effect of heat.*

**Content Area:** Fundamentals; **Concept:** Perfusion; Comfort; **Integrated Processes:** Nursing Process: Analysis; Caring; **Client Needs:** Physiological Integrity: Basic Care and Comfort; **Cognitive Level:** Knowledge [Remembering]

## 564. ANSWER: 2

1. Avoiding eye contact is not associated with a kosher meal. There is no information suggesting that eye contact should be avoided.
2. **The NA should not unwrap the utensils. The client should do the unwrapping to be sure that the utensils have not been tainted by nonkosher items.**
3. There is no need for the client who requests a kosher meal to face toward Mecca when eating.
4. A kosher meal would not include both milk and kosher meat; milk or dairy products are kept separate from meat.

▶ **Test-taking Tip:** *Narrow the options to the only two that pertain to items for the meal. Then decide whether the utensils or food are kosher as described in the options.*

**Content Area:** Fundamentals; **Concept:** Management; Nutrition; Diversity; **Integrated Processes:** Caring; Culture and Spirituality; **Client Needs:** Physiological Integrity: Basic Care and Comfort; **Cognitive Level:** Application [Applying]

## 565. ANSWER: 117

**First calculate the client's height in feet and inches. Because 1 foot equals 12 inches, the client's height is 5 feet, 5 inches (65 in/12 in = 5 remainder of 5). Next, apply the formula from the chart: 105 lb for 5 ft height**

**5 lb × 5 = 25 lb; 105 lb + 25 lb = 130 lb Because the client has a small body frame size, calculate 10% of 130 lb.**

**10% = 0.1; 0.1 × 130 lb =13 lb Subtract the 10% due to small body frame size: 130 lb – 13 lb = 117 lb.**

♦ *Test-taking Tip: Focus on the information in the question. Utilize the formula given in the chart. Verify your calculation, especially if it seems like an unusual amount.*

**Content Area:** Fundamentals; **Concept:** Nutrition; **Integrated Processes:** Nursing Process: Analysis; **Client Needs:** Physiological Integrity: Basic Care and Comfort; **Cognitive Level:** Analysis [Analyzing]

## 566. ANSWER: 1, 2, 5

1. **Asking permission allows the nurse to determine whether opening containers and cutting up meat are activities that the client is unable to perform. This promotes client autonomy and independence in decision making.**
2. **With easy-to-hold, built-up silverware, the client can maintain independence with eating.**
3. The nurse should observe the client and assist with specific obstacles to limit client frustration.
4. Feeding the client who is slow at eating will tend to extinguish independent behaviors.
5. **The client will have greater independence with eating if eyeglasses and hearing aids are in place. The client should also have dentures in place if used.**

♦ *Test-taking Tip: Consider each option as to whether it will assist the client to overcome sensory or mobility deficits and promote independence with eating.*

**Content Area:** Fundamentals; **Concept:** Nutrition; Sensory Perception; **Integrated Processes:** Nursing Process: Implementation; **Client Needs:** Physiological Integrity: Basic Care and Comfort; Psychosocial Integrity; **Cognitive Level:** Analysis [Analyzing]

## 567. MoC ANSWER: 3

1. Having the client recall foods may or may not result in an accurate calorie count.
2. When hospitalized, the dietitian (not the client) will determine the number of calories the client consumed in 24 hours.
3. **In a hospital, a calorie count involves the observation and documentation of the amount of foods eaten by the client from meal trays and snacks provided.**
4. Identifying the food groups and foods obtained does not accurately describe a calorie count.

♦ *Test-taking Tip: Options 1, 2, and 4 expect the client to track foods being consumed, but Option 3 is different. Often the option that is different is the answer.*

**Content Area:** Fundamentals; **Concept:** Nutrition; Management; **Integrated Processes:** Nursing Process: Implementation; **Client Needs:** Safe and Effective Care Environment: Management of Care; **Cognitive Level:** Analysis [Analyzing]

## 568. MoC ANSWER: 2, 5

1. The client should not wear shoes because this will add to the weight.
2. **Electronic digital scales should be calibrated and "zeroed" before weighing the client to ensure accuracy.**
3. The nurse moves a slide indicator until the scale balances with a balancing arm scale, not an electronic digital scale.
4. For accuracy, it is best to weigh clients at the same time each day.
5. **For accuracy, the client should be weighed at the same time each day with an empty bladder; a full bladder adds weight.**

♦ *Test-taking Tip: Visualize the process of weighing the client using an electronic digital scale. Evaluate each option and consider if it is correct in describing the process.*

**Content Area:** Fundamentals; **Concept:** Nursing Roles; **Integrated Processes:** Nursing Process: Implementation; **Client Needs:** Physiological Integrity: Basic Care and Comfort; **Cognitive Level:** Analysis [Analyzing]

## 569. MoC ANSWER: 3

1. An ileostomy involves the small bowel and does not affect the rectal area.
2. A rectal temperature is not contraindicated for the client who has a productive cough and is receiving oxygen. The rectal route may be used if the client is unable to keep the thermometer under the tongue due to coughing.
3. **Clients with thrombocytopenia have lower than normal levels of platelets and are at increased risk of bleeding. Measuring the temperature rectally exposes the client to the risk of rectal bleeding.**
4. Monitoring rectal temperature is often used in clients with hypothermia; the temperature may be too low to be measured orally.

♦ *Test-taking Tip: The question calls for a negative answer. Select the option in which taking a temperature rectally would harm the client.*

**Content Area:** Fundamentals; **Concept:** Clotting; Safety; Management; **Integrated Processes:** Nursing Process: Analysis; **Client Needs:** Physiological Integrity: Reduction of Risk Potential; Safe and Effective Care Environment: Management of Care; **Cognitive Level:** Application [Applying]

## 570. ANSWER: 1, 3, 6, 4, 5, 2, 7

1. **Prepare suction supplies and equipment and pour sterile saline into a sterile container. Supplies should be prepared before donning sterile gloves.**
3. **Put on sterile gloves. Sterile gloves are worn when performing NT suctioning to avoid introducing microorganisms.**

6. **Pick up suction catheter with the dominant hand and attach it to connection tubing; avoid contamination of the glove on the dominant hand. The dominant hand is used to insert the catheter into the client's naris, and the glove should remain sterile.**

4. **Lubricate the catheter with the sterile saline, insert into naris, and advance into pharynx. The catheter is lubricated to avoid trauma to the nares and for ease of passage.**

5. **As the client inhales, advance it into the trachea. Advancing the catheter while the client is swallowing will result in misplacement into the esophagus.**

2. **Place finger over suction control port and suction intermittently while withdrawing the catheter. Intermittent suction is used to avoid trauma to tissues.**

7. **Place tip into sterile saline container while applying suction to clear secretions from the tubing. The tubing should be cleared of secretions before advancing the catheter again.**

▶ *Test-taking Tip: Visualize the steps; then identify the first and last options to make ordering easier.*

Content Area: Fundamentals; Concept: Nursing Roles; Oxygenation; Integrated Processes: Nursing Process: Implementation; Client Needs: Physiological Integrity: Physiological Adaptation; Cognitive Level: Synthesis [Creating]

## 571. ANSWER: 3

1. Obtaining ABGs may be helpful if oxygen saturations remain low after suctioning and the infant remains in distress, but clearing the airway should have priority.

2. Increasing the oxygen rate will not be effective if the airway is occluded by secretions.

3. **Suctioning the tracheostomy has priority. A lowering of oxygen saturation and signs of respiratory distress can occur with secretions and a mucus plug.**

4. Medicating for anxiety and pain would not improve oxygen saturations if the airway is not patent due to secretions. Medicating the infant may reduce respiratory drive and cause further distress.

▶ *Test-taking Tip: Use the ABC's. Airway management has priority.*

Content Area: Fundamentals; Concept: Oxygenation; Integrated Processes: Nursing Process: Implementation; Client Needs: Physiological Integrity: Physiological Adaptation; Cognitive Level: Analysis [Analyzing]

## 572. MoC ANSWER: 2

1. The NA should not omit the BP but should obtain the correct-sized cuff.

2. **For an accurate reading, the BP must be taken with the correct-sized BP cuff. When one is not available on the unit, one option is to direct the NA to obtain one from another unit.**

3. Adding numbers to a BP when using an improperly sized cuff will not result in a correct BP measurement.

4. A BP cuff that is too large will result in a lower BP reading.

▶ *Test-taking Tip: Consider that the only acceptable option is one that results in a correct BP measurement.*

Content Area: Fundamentals; Concept: Safety; Management; Integrated Processes: Nursing Process: Implementation; Client Needs: Physiological Integrity: Reduction of Risk Potential; Safe and Effective Care Environment: Management of Care; Cognitive Level: Analysis [Analyzing]

## 573. ANSWER: 1

1. **The nurse should first assess the condition of the client and ascertain if there are physical signs consistent with hypotension. Dizziness is a sign of decreased perfusion to the brain; cool, clammy extremities are a sign of decreased peripheral circulation.**

2. After assessing the client's condition, the nurse should recheck the BP to verify the accuracy of the reading.

3. The nurse should not elevate the head of the client's bed; this action would further lower the BP. The nurse should first assess the client before getting the client out of bed.

4. Determining the client's normal BP range is indicated after assessing the client's condition and verifying the reading.

▶ *Test-taking Tip: The key word is "first." Use the nursing process; assessment is the first step in the process.*

Content Area: Fundamentals; Concept: Perfusion; Safety; Management; Integrated Processes: Nursing Process: Implementation; Client Needs: Physiological Integrity: Reduction of Risk Potential; Cognitive Level: Analysis [Analyzing]

## 574. ANSWER: 1

1. **Failing to seal the ear canal will result in an inaccurate temperature reading.**

2. Earwax does not affect the temperature and results.

3. With an adult, the pinna of the ear should be pulled slightly upward to straighten the ear canal.

4. The presence of tympanostomy tubes does not affect the accuracy of the temperature reading; for comfort, a tympanic temperature should not be taken for a week after placement of the tubes.

▶ *Test-taking Tip: The tympanic thermometer measures the core body temperature by sensing the heat given off from the tympanic membrane (eardrum).*

Content Area: Fundamentals; Concept: Safety; Integrated Processes: Nursing Process: Implementation; Client Needs: Physiological Integrity: Reduction of Risk Potential; Cognitive Level: Comprehension [Understanding]

**575. ANSWER: 1, 2, 3, 5, 6**

1. **Vitamin C promotes wound healing and should be encouraged.**
2. **Premedicating with analgesics promotes client comfort.**
3. **Monitoring pedal pulses and capillary refill of the affected extremity alerts the nurse to further vascular compromise as a result of the wound.**
4. Hydrogen peroxide can be excoriating to the wound and will not promote healing.
5. **Repositioning the client promotes circulation and helps prevent further skin breakdown.**
6. **Elevation reduces edema; keeping the heel off the pillow avoids pressure on the ulcer.**

▸ **Test-taking Tip:** Eliminate any options that would worsen wound healing (Option 4).

**Content Area:** Fundamentals; **Concept:** Skin Integrity; **Integrated Processes:** Nursing Process: Planning; **Client Needs:** Physiological Integrity: Physiological Adaptation; **Cognitive Level:** Application [Applying]

**576. ANSWER: 3**

1. This illustration shows external rotation.
2. This illustration shows internal rotation.
3. **Eversion is turning outward.**
4. This illustration shows inversion, turning inward.

▸ **Test-taking Tip:** Use the memory cue that "inversion" is "in." Thus "eversion" is "out." Eliminate options showing inversion and rotation.

**Content Area:** Fundamentals; **Concept:** Comfort; Mobility; **Integrated Processes:** Nursing Process: Evaluation; **Client Needs:** Physiological Integrity: Basic Care and Comfort; **Cognitive Level:** Comprehension [Understanding]

**577. MoC ANSWER: 2**

1. Phototherapy is designed to convert the bilirubin in the superficial capillaries in the skin. Keeping the baby fully clothed does not allow for maximum skin exposure to achieve bilirubin conversion and excretion.

2. **Covering the baby's eyes with eye shields will protect the baby's eyes from the phototherapy light, which could be damaging to the retinas.**
3. Limiting the number of feedings is incorrect because bilirubin is excreted in the urine and stool, and excretion can be increased with increased feedings.
4. A rash can be caused by capillary dilation and is not harmful to the baby. Discontinuing therapy is not warranted.

▸ **Test-taking Tip:** Use the prefix "photo" from "phototherapy" to narrow the options. Think about exposure to eliminate Option 1. Think about light to select Option 2.

**Content Area:** Fundamentals; Childbearing; **Concept:** Management; Safety; Pregnancy; **Integrated Processes:** Teaching/Learning; **Client Needs:** Safe and Effective Care Environment: Management of Care; **Cognitive Level:** Analysis [Analyzing]

**578. ANSWER: 2, 3, 4**

1. Urine output is decreased in the hypothermic client as a result of decreased renal perfusion.
2. **In hypothermia, a low cardiac output affects the CNS, producing drowsiness.**
3. **In hypothermia, the HR decreases due to the effects on the thermoregulation center in the brain.**
4. **In hypothermia, the BP decreases due to the effects on the thermoregulation center in the brain. A lowering of the BP decreases cardiac workload and cardiac output.**
5. The core body temperature would be decreased, not increased, with hypothermia.

▸ **Test-taking Tip:** When using a hypothermia blanket to reduce temperature, the nurse should monitor the client for signs of decreased cardiac output and decreased CNS functions.

**Content Area:** Fundamentals; **Concept:** Thermo-regulation; **Integrated Processes:** Nursing Process: Analysis; **Client Needs:** Physiological Integrity: Reduction of Risk Potential; **Cognitive Level:** Application [Applying]

## Chapter Fifteen

# Medication Administration

**579.** **PHARM** The nurse is checking newly prescribed medications. Which medications require the nurse to contact the HCP to clarify what has been prescribed? **Select all that apply.**

1. Aspirin 325 mg orally qd
2. MS 4 mg IV q1hr prn
3. Furosemide 40 mg IV now
4. D₅W with 20 mEq KCL IV at 125 mL/hr
5. Heparin 5000 u subcutaneously bid

**580.** **PHARM** The client is prescribed ferrous sulfate 300 mg PO bid. What should the nurse do?

1. Administer ferrous sulfate as prescribed.
2. Contact the HCP to clarify the medication route.
3. Contact the HCP to question twice-daily dosing.
4. Withhold the medication; the dose is too much.

**581.** **MoC** The nurse is reviewing the client's prescribed medications. Which medications should the nurse plan to clarify with the HCP? **Select all that apply.**

1. Digoxin 25 mg IV
2. D₅NS with 20 mEq KCL now
3. Aspirin 325 mg tablet oral every a.m.
4. Lisinopril 5 mg oral bid
5. Hydromorphone 1 mg q1h as needed

**582.** **PHARM** The client is to receive prochlorperazine suppository. Which action by the nurse **best** ensures that the medication is correctly administered?

1. Positions the client on the left side
2. Lubricates the suppository prior to insertion
3. Feels the suppository being pulled away when inserting
4. Notes soft, formed stool 30 minutes after insertion

**583.** **PHARM** The client provides a handwritten medication list that includes bupropion XL 150 mg daily. The client shows the nurse the medication bottle labeled bupropion XL 300 mg tablets. Which questions should the nurse ask the client? **Select all that apply.**

1. "Has your dosage of bupropion increased or decreased recently?"
2. "Did you cut the tablets in half to give yourself the correct dose?"
3. "Are you taking bupropion to stop smoking or to treat depression?"
4. "When was the last time you took medication from this bottle?"
5. "Have you had headaches, tremors, or dry mouth while taking bupropion?"

**584.** **PHARM** Before a child's hospital discharge, the nurse is teaching the parents how to administer the child's oral medication. Which instruction would be **most** appropriate?

1. Administer the medication and then give a small glass of milk.
2. Give the child a flavored ice pop just before giving the medication.
3. Use play to show and tell the child that the medication will taste good.
4. Pour out capsule contents, crush pills, and give these with applesauce.

**585.** **PHARM** The client is to receive esomeprazole 40 mg oral daily. The medication is supplied in 20-mg capsules. To give the correct dose, the nurse should administer how many capsules?

_____ capsules (Record your answer as a whole number.)

**586. PHARM** The nurse is administering oral medications to the client. Prioritize the nurse's actions by placing each step in the correct order.

1. Document on the client's MAR administering the medication.
2. Check the label after preparing the medication.
3. Check the client's name band and another agency-approved identifier.
4. Review the medication prescribed on the medication administration record (MAR).
5. Check the medication label against the MAR.
6. Give the medication with a glass of water.
7. Check the medication at the bedside.

Answer: _____

**587. PHARM** The nurse is evaluating whether the client on multiple oral medications is taking the medications correctly. Which finding should be **most** concerning to the nurse because the absorption rate of medications can be increased?

1. Takes afternoon oral medications with a carbonated soft drink
2. Drinks a glass of milk with the tetracycline antibiotic oral medication
3. Takes morning oral medications with water and consumes 2500 mL of water daily
4. Takes mealtime oral medications with a meal low in fiber and high in fatty foods

**588. MoC PHARM** The nurse observes a nursing student prepare and administer medications. Which action by the nursing student warrants the nurse's intervention?

1. Injects air into a vial before withdrawing 20 mg furosemide from a vial labeled 20 mg/mL
2. Selects a 1-mL syringe and 5/8-inch needle for giving 0.5 mL of heparin subcutaneously
3. Instructs the client to place a medication to be taken buccal under the tongue
4. Pours the prescribed "Robitussin 2 tsp now" to the 10 mL mark on a med cup

**589. PHARM** The client with minimal adipose tissue is to receive insulin subcutaneously. Which approach should the nurse plan to use to give the medication?

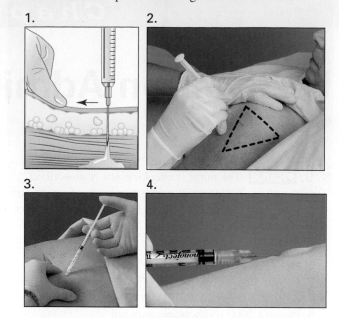

1.  2.

3.  4.

**590. PHARM** The nurse is planning to administer medications through the client's NG tube. Which interventions should the nurse plan after checking the medications, checking client identification, and verifying tube placement? **Select all that apply.**

1. Crush together all medications that are acceptable for crushing.
2. Pour crushed medications into one medication cup, mix with water, and administer.
3. Pour each individual crushed medication into individual medication cups and mix with water.
4. Use a syringe to withdraw one prepared medication from the medication cup and administer.
5. Using a syringe, flush the client's NG tubing with water between each medication.

**591. PHARM** The nurse is to administer promethazine 12.5 mg IM STAT to the client. The medication is supplied in an ampule of 50 mg/mL. How many milliliters should the nurse administer to the client?

_____ mL (Record your answer rounded to hundredths.)

**592.** PHARM The nurse is teaching the client to self-administer a medication dose through an MDI. After having the client sit upright, which instructions should be provided? Prioritize the nurse's instructions by placing each step in the correct order.

1. Press the top of the canister.
2. Shake the canister several times.
3. Close your teeth and lips tightly around the mouthpiece.
4. Exhale slowly through pursed lips.
5. Take a deep breath and exhale until you cannot exhale any more air.
6. Insert the mouthpiece into the mouth over the tongue.
7. Inhale deeply and hold the breath for 10 seconds.

Answer: _____

**593.** PHARM The client who inhales a corticosteroid medication through a metered-dose inhaler states, "I have a foul taste in my mouth after I use the inhaler." Which is the nurse's **best** response?

1. "With time, you will get used to the foul taste."
2. "Be sure that you shake the canister before using it."
3. "Suck on hard candy before you use the inhaler."
4. "Attach an aerosol spacer before using the inhaler."

**594.** MoC PHARM The student nurse is administering a clonidine transdermal patch to the client with hypertension. Which action requires the observing nurse to intervene?

1. Dons nonsterile gloves before removing the medication from the package.
2. Checks the client's armband for name and medical record number.
3. Applies the patch, rubs it against the skin, and secures it in place.
4. Folds the old patch with the medication on the inside to discard it.

**595.** PHARM MoC The experienced nurse is observing the student nurse provide client care. Which action **most** definitely requires the observing nurse to intervene?

1. Places a medication that requires assessment of the client's heart rate in its own cup
2. Places eye drops prescribed O.D. in the middle of the client's right eye conjunctival sac
3. Flushes an injection port with saline before administering the medication by IV push
4. Opens a sustained-release capsule at the client's request to mix its contents with food

**596.** PHARM The clinic nurse is preparing to administer monovalent HepB (hepatitis B vaccine) IM to a newborn. Which site is **best** for the nurse to select?

1. Deltoid
2. Ventrogluteal
3. Dorsogluteal
4. Vastus lateralis

**597.** MoC The client hospitalized with MS provides a handwritten medication list. Interferon beta-1b 25 mg subcutaneously daily is on the list. Which nursing actions are correct related to the client's medication list? **Select all that apply.**

1. Rewrite the medications on official facility documents as written and file per agency policy.
2. Inquire about vitamins, herbals, and over-the-counter medications that may not be on the list.
3. Verify the dose of interferon beta-1b with the prescribing health care provider.
4. Have pharmacy verify the interferon beta-1b with the pharmacy where it was last filled.
5. Photocopy or scan the handwritten list and insert a copy into the client's medical record.
6. Ask a family member to bring the container with the prescription noted for verification.

**598.** PHARM The nurse plans to administer an IM injection into the left dorsogluteal muscle for the client positioned prone. On the illustration, place an X on the area where the nurse should administer the injection.

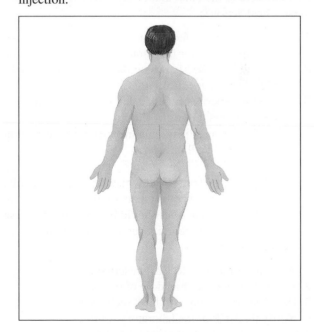

**599.** MoC PHARM An LPN is administering medications to adult clients. Which action requires the RN to intervene?

1. Withdraws 1 mL of purified protein derivative (PPD) from a vial for intradermal injection
2. Holds an insulin pen for 10 seconds on the client's abdomen after administering insulin
3. Measures three finger-breadths below the acromion process for an intramuscular injection
4. Injects 5000 units heparin subcutaneously in the abdomen without first aspirating for blood

**600.** PHARM The client is to receive hydroxyzine 25 mg IM. Which statements should the nurse make before injecting the medication? **Select all that apply.**

1. "You will feel minimal pain as I administer the medication."
2. "Expect to experience relief from nausea within about 10 minutes."
3. "You will feel me pull the skin to the side at the site before I give the medication."
4. "Tense your muscle as I make the injection to avoid focusing on the injection itself."
5. "I will use the deltoid muscle; use of the arm muscles will increase absorption."
6. "You will feel a cold sensation as I cleanse your skin with the alcohol swab."

**601.** MoC PHARM The experienced nurse instructs the new nurse to give an IM injection into the dorsogluteal muscle of the older adult client. Which is the new nurse's **best** action?

1. Position the client onto his or her abdomen and identify the landmarks for injection.
2. Administer the injection using the Z-track method to avoid leakage of medication.
3. Inform the experienced nurse that the ventrogluteal muscle is the preferred IM site.
4. Select a 1-inch needle for administering the medication into the dorsogluteal muscle.

**602.** PHARM MoC Before administering digoxin orally, the nurse determines that the client's serum digoxin level is 2.6 ng/mL. Which actions should be taken by the nurse knowing that the therapeutic range is 0.5 to 2.0 ng/mL? **Select all that apply.**

1. Administer the oral dose as prescribed.
2. Withhold the prescribed dose of digoxin.
3. Have the client's digoxin level rechecked.
4. Notify the HCP of the laboratory results.
5. Call pharmacy to discontinue the digoxin.

**603.** PHARM The nurse, working the evening shift, is planning to administer insulin subcutaneously to a child. Which statement made by the nurse to the mother would be **inappropriate?**

1. "It is okay for your child to say 'ouch,' cry, or even scream when receiving an injection."
2. "I can give the injection while your child is sleeping; then the injection won't be noticed."
3. "I will apply a topical analgesic 1 hour before administering the injection to reduce pain."
4. "The child will need to be lying, but after the injection you can hold and comfort your child."

**604.** PHARM The client has $D_5W/20$ mEq KCL infusing at 75 mL/hr. An antibiotic newly prescribed for the client is to be administered by an IVPB infusion. Which actions should be taken by the nurse? **Select all that apply.**

1. Verify compatibilities between the IV infusion and antibiotic.
2. Check for client allergies to the newly prescribed antibiotic.
3. Initiate a peripherally inserted central catheter for the antibiotic.
4. Ask the HCP if the IV solution and IVPB can be infused together.
5. Determine the infusion rate for administering the antibiotic.

**605.** MoC PHARM The experienced nurse is supervising the new nurse caring for a hospitalized child. Which action indicates that the new nurse needs additional orientation regarding IV therapy for children?

1. Determines that the current solution has been infusing for 24 hours and should be changed
2. Selects a 1000-mL bag of the prescribed IV solution and checks it against the child's chart
3. Prepares new tubing and the prescribed IV solution 1 hour before it is due to be changed
4. Removes the cover from the tubing spike, spikes the bag, and squeezes the drip chamber

**606.** PHARM The client is to receive cefazolin 500 mg in 50 mL of NS IVPB. The medication is to be infused over 20 minutes. The nurse should set the infusion pump to deliver how many milliliters per hour?

_____ mL/hr (Record your answer as a whole number.)

**607.** MoC PHARM The nurse notes that the client has 0.9% NaCl infusing intravenously. On the previous day, the HCP prescribed a change in IV solution to 0.9% NaCl with 10 mEq KCL. Which action should the nurse initiate **first?**

1. Notify the client's health care provider (HCP).
2. Complete an agency variance/incident report.
3. Check the client's serum potassium level.
4. Replace 0.9% NaCl with the correct solution.

**608.** PHARM The client has a low serum potassium level. What should the nurse consider when preparing to administer potassium replacement intravenously?

1. The potassium concentration should not exceed 20 mEq/L.
2. Ice or warm packs may be needed to reduce vein irritation.
3. The potassium should be administered by the IV push route.
4. The potassium should be added to the IV solution that is infusing.

**609.** PHARM The nurse plans to administer an antibiotic IVPB to the client who is on a fluid restriction and strict I&O. On the illustration, which port on the 0.9% NaCl IV line would be **best** for the nurse to add a secondary line for the antibiotic?

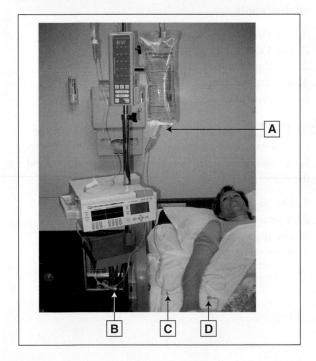

1. A
2. B
3. C
4. D

**610.** MoC PHARM The nurse is preparing to administer cefotaxime. Which action is **most** appropriate when the nurse notes that the client has a cephalosporin allergy and allergic to ceftriaxone?

1. Give the cefotaxime as prescribed by the HCP.
2. Call pharmacy to verify that cefotaxime is a cephalosporin.
3. Ask the client whether cefotaxime had been received in the past.
4. Verify that the HCP is aware that the client has an allergy to cephalosporins.

**611.** MoC PHARM The nurse receives new orders for multiple clients. Which order should be the nurse's **priority?**

1. Nitroglycerin 0.4 mg sublingually (SL) STAT for the client experiencing chest pain
2. Morphine sulfate 4 mg intravenously (IV) now for the client experiencing incisional pain
3. Lorazepam 2 mg IV now for the client experiencing restlessness and picking at tubing
4. One unit packed red blood cells STAT for the client with hemoglobin of 9.5 g

**612.** PHARM The client's assessment findings at 0800 hours include BP 180/88 mm Hg, HR 96 bpm, RR 24 breaths per minute, and T 102.6°F (39.2°C). The client's last bowel movement was 6 days ago. The client prefers to take medications one at a time due to difficulty swallowing. The client is lying flat in bed. In which order should the nurse administer the medications?

1. Timolol 2 gtt right eye
2. Labetalol 20 mg IV push for systolic BP > 160 mm Hg
3. Ramipril 2.5 mg oral daily
4. Docusate sodium rectal suppository this a.m.
5. Cefazolin sodium 1 g IV syringe pump (IVSP)

Answer: _____

**613.** MoC PHARM The nurse notes that a hospital coworker omits treatments for clients, has mood swings, makes frequent requests for help with assignments, and has numerous requests to witness the waste of controlled substances. Which nursing action is **most** appropriate?

1. Report the findings to the nurse's immediate supervisor.
2. Tell the coworker that drug abuse is suspected and offer support.
3. Notify the police, who will investigate because drug abuse is a legal offense.
4. Complete an incident report, noting the times the coworker wasted controlled substances.

**614.** PHARM The client is to receive oxycodone 5 mg with acetaminophen 325 mg, two tablets orally for pain relief. Which actions by the nurse should be corrected by an observing nurse? **Select all that apply.**

1. Obtains apple juice for the client to drink with the medication
2. Goes to the med box in the client's room to obtain the medication
3. Identifies the client by name, birth date, and medical record number
4. Informs the client to expect some pain relief within 10 to 15 minutes
5. Tells the client to place the tablets under the tongue for faster pain relief

**615.** MoC PHARM The client's son asks the hospice nurse to administer larger doses of pain medication. Despite having pain, the client, who is devoutly religious, adamantly refuses increased doses. The client states, "I believe that accepting pain is God's will for me." By withholding larger analgesic doses, the nurse **best** demonstrates ethical practice guided by which principle?

1. Nonmaleficence
2. Autonomy
3. Beneficence
4. Veracity

**616.** MoC The client experiences nausea after an oral dose of cephalexin, and interventions for nausea are unsuccessful. When the nurse attempts to administer the next dose of cephalexin, the client adamantly refuses to take it. Which nursing intervention is **best?**

1. Administer the cephalexin dose 1 hour after repeating the dose of antiemetic.
2. Have the client suck on ice chips for several minutes before taking cephalexin.
3. Crush the cephalexin tablet and mix it with applesauce for administration.
4. Report the information to the client's HCP and request a different medication.

**617.** PHARM The nurse is administering metoclopramide 10 mg IV to the client with decreased peristalsis. Which action would result in a medication error?

1. Gives metoclopramide intravenously over 1 minute
2. Administers the metoclopramide 30 minutes after meals
3. Notes a Y-site incompatibility of metoclopramide and furosemide
4. Holds the infusing $D_5W$ and injects metoclopramide at the most distal port

**618.** PHARM The client with cellular dehydration is to receive an IV solution that will rehydrate cells. Which solution, if prescribed by the HCP, should the nurse plan to administer?

1. Lactated Ringer's
2. 0.9% sodium chloride
3. 0.45% sodium chloride
4. $D_5W$ 0.9% sodium chloride

**619.** PHARM The client with a central venous access device suddenly develops dyspnea, chest pain, tachycardia, and hypotension after the nurse attaches new injection caps during a central line dressing change. Which action should be taken by the nurse **first?**

1. Apply oxygen via a facemask at 4 liters per minute.
2. Turn the client onto the left side with the head lowered.
3. Call for another nurse to notify the HCP.
4. Cleanse the injection caps and flush the catheter with saline.

**620.** PHARM The client has a vesicant solution infusing intravenously in a large peripheral vein. Which assessment findings should prompt the nurse to explore whether extravasation has occurred? **Select all that apply.**

1. The IV solution bag is empty.
2. The IV pump is malfunctioning.
3. Swelling noted at the IV insertion site.
4. Blisters noted at the IV insertion site.
5. The client is having chest pain.

**621.** PHARM The nurse is assessing the veins of the client's hand and arm prior to inserting an IV catheter for a transfusion of RBCs. Which vein would be **best** for the nurse to select?

1. The basic vein that has a bifurcation
2. A vein on the client's nondominant hand
3. The distal cephalic vein above the wrist
4. A dorsal metacarpal vein that is straight

**622.** **PHARM** The nurse is preparing to administer a transfusion of RBCs to the client with blood type AB negative. The blood bank does not have any units of AB negative PRBCs so provides a unit of O negative RBCs. What should the nurse do?

1. Return the unit to the blood bank because it is incompatible.
2. Continue to prepare to administer the unit; it is compatible.
3. Verify with the HCP that the client can receive O negative RBCs.
4. Obtain the client's consent before administering the O negative RBCs.

**623.** **PHARM** The nurse is to administer chlordiazepoxide HCL 25 mg intramuscularly (IM) to the client. The medication package contains 100 mg of sterile, powdered chlordiazepoxide HCL that must be reconstituted with 2 mL of diluent. After reconstitution, how many mL of medication should the nurse withdraw into the syringe illustrated to administer the correct dose?

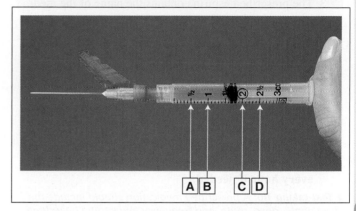

1. A
2. B
3. C
4. D

## *Answers and Rationales*

**579.** **PHARM** **ANSWER: 1, 2, 5**
1. **The nurse should clarify aspirin with the HCP because the abbreviation "qd" is disallowed by The Joint Commission. The "qd" can be mistaken for every other day rather than daily.**
2. **The nurse should clarify "MS" with the HCP. The use of MS is disallowed by The Joint Commission because it can be mistaken for magnesium sulfate rather than morphine sulfate.**
3. Furosemide (Lasix) has the essential components of a medication order—medication name, dose, frequency, and route—and uses acceptable abbreviations.
4. $D_5W$ with 20 mEq KCL has the essential components of a medication order—medication name, dose, frequency, and route—and uses acceptable abbreviations.
5. **The nurse should clarify heparin with the HCP because the abbreviation "u" is disallowed by the Joint Commission. The "u" can be mistaken for "0" (zero), the number "4" (four), or "cc."**

▶ *Test-taking Tip: Read each order carefully to identify the disallowed abbreviations according to The Joint Commission "Do Not Use" list of abbreviations. Eliminate options that use acceptable abbreviations and have the essential components for prescribed medications.*

Content Area: Fundamentals; Concept: Medication; Integrated Processes: Nursing Process: Analysis; Client Needs: Physiological Integrity: Pharmacological and Parenteral Therapies; Cognitive Level: Analysis [Analyzing]

**580.** **PHARM** **ANSWER: 1**
1. **The nurse should administer ferrous sulfate (Feosol) as prescribed. All essential information is included using approved abbreviations.**
2. The abbreviation "PO" is an acceptable abbreviation for the oral route and does not need to be clarified.
3. The abbreviation "bid" is acceptable for twice-daily administration and at this dose.
4. The dose of ferrous sulfate is within the acceptable range and should not be withheld.

▶ *Test-taking Tip: Determine if essential information is included for administering a prescribed medication and whether the information includes The Joint Commission "Do Not Use" list of abbreviations.*

Content Area: Fundamentals; Concept: Medication; Integrated Processes: Nursing Process: Implementation; Client Needs: Physiological Integrity: Pharmacological and Parenteral Therapies; Cognitive Level: Analysis [Analyzing]

**581.** **MoC** **ANSWER: 1, 2, 5**

1. **Digoxin (Lanoxin) is missing the frequency and should be clarified with the HCP; the dosage also is too large and will result in a medication error.**
2. **The IV solution is missing the rate and should be clarified with the HCP.**
3. The prescribed aspirin contains the name of the medication, the dose, the route, and the frequency and is correct.
4. The prescribed lisinopril (Zestril) contains the name of the medication, the dose, the route, and the frequency and is correct. The abbreviation bid means twice daily and is an accepted abbreviation.
5. **The prescribed hydromorphone (Dilaudid) is missing the route. The abbreviation q1h is an acceptable medication-related abbreviation indicating that hydromorphone may be administered every hour if needed.**

♦ *Test-taking Tip:* A prescribed medication should include the drug name, dose, route, and frequency and should be written using approved medication-related abbreviations. Prescriptions using abbreviations on The Joint Commission "Do Not Use" list of abbreviations need to be clarified with the HCP.

**Content Area:** Fundamentals; **Concept:** Safety; Medication; **Integrated Processes:** Nursing Process: Planning; **Client Needs:** Safe and Effective Care Environment: Management of Care; **Cognitive Level:** Evaluation [Evaluating]

**582.** **PHARM** **ANSWER: 3**

1. Although the client should be positioned on the left side, this does not indicate whether the medication is in the correct position.
2. Lubrication makes passage easier but does not ensure the correct placement against the rectal wall and past the sphincter.
3. **Rectal suppositories should be inserted past the internal anal sphincter and against the rectal wall. Stimulation of the bowel, once past the internal anal sphincter, will draw the medication inward. Stool in the bowel could cause incorrect placement of the suppository.**
4. Prochlorperazine (Compazine) is an antiemetic medication. It does not produce bowel peristalsis nd elimination. Digital stimulation may cause passage of stool that is in the bowel, but this does not ensure correct administration.

♦ *Test-taking Tip:* The key word is "best," suggesting that more than one option could be correct, but one is better than the other.

**Content Area:** Fundamentals; **Concept:** Medication; **Integrated Processes:** Nursing Process: Implementation; **Client Needs:** Physiological Integrity: Pharmacological and Parenteral Therapies; **Cognitive Level:** Application [Applying]

**583.** **PHARM** **ANSWER: 1, 3, 4, 5**

1. **The handwritten medication list is half the strength of the tablets in the bottle. Either the dose was increased and this is the correct bottle, or the dose was decreased and the handwritten medication list is correct and this is the wrong bottle.**
2. Bupropion is sustained release; tablets should not be halved for safe administration. This is the wrong question to ask.
3. **Bupropion (Wellbutrin) is commonly used for smoking cessation or treating depression. It can also be used for treating ADHD in adults or to increase sexual desire in women.**
4. **The last time a dose was taken from the bottle will help determine the amount the client is taking and to verify if it is the correct amount.**
5. **Major side effects of bupropion include headaches, tremors, and dry mouth. If the client is taking a higher dose than prescribed, the client could be experiencing side effects.**

♦ *Test-taking Tip:* Carefully read the client's medication list and compare it against the bottle to answer the question. Recall that XL means sustained release.

**Content Area:** Fundamentals; **Concept:** Medication; Assessment; **Integrated Processes:** Communication and Documentation; **Client Needs:** Physiological Integrity: Pharmacological and Parenteral Therapies; Physiological Integrity: Reduction of Risk Potential; **Cognitive Level:** Analysis [Analyzing]

**584.** **PHARM** **ANSWER: 2**

1. Essential foods, such as milk, should not be given with medications. The child may later associate the food with the medicine and refuse the food. Some medications should not be taken with milk.
2. **The cold from the ice pop will help numb the taste buds and weaken the medication's taste.**
3. Providing potentially false information about the taste may affect the child's trust. If the child is old enough, warn the child that the medication is objectionable, but then praise the child after the medication is swallowed.
4. Some capsules are extended release and should not be opened.

♦ *Test-taking Tip:* Note the key words "most appropriate." Recall that cold has a numbing effect.

**Content Area:** Fundamentals; **Concept:** Nursing Roles; Medication; **Integrated Processes:** Teaching/Learning; **Client Needs:** Physiological Integrity: Pharmacological and Parenteral Therapies; Physiological Integrity: Basic Care and Comfort; **Cognitive Level:** Analysis [Analyzing]

**585.** **PHARM** **ANSWER: 2**

**Use a proportion formula, multiply the extremes (outside values) by the means (inside values), and solve for X.**

**20 mg : 1 capsule :: 40 mg : X capsules; 20X = 40; X = 40 ÷ 20; X = 2 capsules**

▸ *Test-taking Tip: Use a formula to calculate the correct dose of esomeprazole (Nexium) and verify the answer if it seems unusually large.*

**Content Area:** Fundamentals; **Concept:** Medication; **Integrated Processes:** Nursing Process: Planning; **Client Needs:** Physiological Integrity: Pharmacological and Parenteral Therapies; **Cognitive Level:** Application [Applying]

**586.** PHARM **ANSWER: 4, 5, 2, 3, 7, 6, 1**

4. **Review the medication prescribed on the MAR.**
5. **Check the medication label against the MAR.**
2. **Check the label after preparing the medication.**
3. **Check the client's name band and another agency-approved identifier.**
7. **Check the medication at the bedside.**
6. **Give the medication with a glass of water.**
1. **Document on the client's MAR administering the medication. The medication should be reviewed three times before administering it to the client: when obtaining the medication, after preparing the medication, and at the bedside after the client's name band has been checked. This sequence is necessary so that the right client receives the right medication and dose at the right time.**

▸ *Test-taking Tip: Use visualization to focus on the information in the question and then visualize the steps of the procedure. A medication should be checked three times before it is administered to the client.*

**Content Area:** Fundamentals; **Concept:** Medication; **Integrated Processes:** Nursing Process: Implementation; **Client Needs:** Physiological Integrity: Pharmacological and Parenteral Therapies; **Cognitive Level:** Synthesis [Creating]

**587.** PHARM **ANSWER: 1**

1. **Carbonated beverages can cause oral medications to dissolve faster, be neutralized, or change the absorption rate in the stomach.**
2. When dairy products are taken with an antibiotic, such as tetracycline, there is decreased drug absorption in the stomach.
3. Medications should be taken with a full glass of water.
4. Foods low in fiber and high in fat will delay stomach emptying and medication absorption by up to 2 hours.

▸ *Test-taking Tip: Focus on key words "absorption rate ... increased." Although options 2 and 4 are concerning, these decrease rather than increase the medication absorption rate and should be deleted.*

**Content Area:** Fundamentals; **Concept:** Medication; **Integrated Processes:** Nursing Process: Analysis; **Client Needs:** Physiological Integrity: Pharmacological and Parenteral Therapies; Physiological Integrity: Reduction of Risk Potential; **Cognitive Level:** Analysis [Analyzing]

**588.** MoC PHARM **ANSWER: 3**

1. Air should be injected into a vial before withdrawing the furosemide (Lasix).
2. A needle size of ½ to ⅝ inch in length should be used for adult subcutaneous injections.
3. **Buccal medications should be held in the cheek rather than under the tongue. The rate of absorption may be affected.**
4. A teaspoon is equivalent to 5 mL; thus 2 teaspoons is 10 mL.

▸ *Test-taking Tip: This is a false-response item. Look for the student nurse's incorrect action. Use the process of elimination to eliminate the correct actions: Options 1, 2, and 4.*

**Content Area:** Fundamentals; **Concept:** Medication; Management; Nursing Roles; **Integrated Processes:** Nursing Process: Evaluation; **Client Needs:** Safe and Effective Care Environment: Management of Care; Physiological Integrity: Pharmacological and Parenteral Therapies; **Cognitive Level:** Evaluation [Evaluating]

**589.** PHARM **ANSWER: 3**

1. An IM and not a subcutaneous injection is given by the Z-track method.
2. The triangle identifies the site for giving an IM and not a subcutaneous injection.
3. **A subcutaneous injection can be given in the abdomen. Pulling the skin to pinch a large skinfold between the thumb and fingers lifts the subcutaneous layer off the muscle. A 90-degree angle is used for someone who has a lot of subcutaneous tissue. A 45-degree angle is used if the person has a small amount of subcutaneous tissue.**
4. A 15-degree needle angle is used for an intradermal and not a subcutaneous injection.

▸ *Test-taking Tip: A subcutaneous injection deposits the medication into the tissue layer below the skin and above the muscle layer.*

**Content Area:** Fundamentals; **Concept:** Medication; Metabolism; **Integrated Processes:** Nursing Process: Planning; **Client Needs:** Safe and Effective Care Environment: Safety and Infection Control; Physiological Integrity: Pharmacological and Parenteral Therapies; **Cognitive Level:** Application [Applying]

**590.** PHARM **ANSWER: 3, 4, 5**

1. Medications should not be combined for crushing to prevent compatibility issues, tube occlusions, and altering the effects of the medications. Medications should be given one at a time and the tube flushed between medications.
2. Pouring crushed medications into one medication cup combines the medications.
3. **Medications to be administered through the NG tube should be crushed, mixed with water, and given separately. This prevents altering the effects of the medications, compatibility issues, and tube occlusions.**

4. **A syringe with the appropriate-sized tip that fits into the NG tube should be used for withdrawing the medication from the med cup and for administration.**

5. **The NG tube should be flushed with water between each medication to prevent occlusion of the NG tube.**

▶ *Test-taking Tip: Visualize the sequence to administer medications through an NG tube. Remember to administer medications separately.*

Content Area: Fundamentals; Concept: Medication; Integrated Processes: Nursing Process: Planning; Client Needs: Physiological Integrity: Pharmacological and Parenteral Therapies; Cognitive Level: Application [Applying]

**591. PHARM ANSWER: 0.25**

Use a proportion formula:

50 mg : 1 mL :: 12.5 mg : $X$ mL

Multiple the extremes (outside values) and then the means (inside values) and solve for $X$.

$50X = 12.5$ mg; $X = 12.5 \div 50 = 0.25$

**Medication dosing less than 1 is always expressed with a 0 preceding the decimal.**

▶ *Test-taking Tip: Think about the dose of promethazine (Phenergan); 12.5 mg is less than 50 mg, so the answer obtained should be less than 1 mL. In medication dosing, the number is never rounded to the nearest whole number.*

Content Area: Fundamentals; Concept: Medication; Integrated Processes: Nursing Process: Implementation; Client Needs: Physiological Integrity: Pharmacological and Parenteral Therapies; Cognitive Level: Application [Applying]

**592. PHARM ANSWER: 2, 6, 3, 5, 1, 7, 4**

2. **Shake the canister several times. This will ensure mixing of the contents.**

6. **Insert the mouthpiece into the mouth over the tongue.**

3. **Close your teeth and lips tightly around the mouthpiece. This ensures that the medication will be delivered.**

5. **Take a deep breath and exhale until you cannot exhale any more air.**

1. **Press the top of the canister.**

7. **Inhale deeply and hold the breath for 10 seconds.**

4. **Exhale slowly through pursed lips.**

▶ *Test-taking Tip: Use visualization to focus on the data in the question and then visualize the remaining steps of the procedure. Prioritizing is placing items in the correct sequence.*

Content Area: Fundamentals; Concept: Medication; Oxygenation; Integrated Processes: Nursing Process: Analysis; Client Needs: Physiological Integrity: Pharmacological and Parenteral Therapies; Cognitive Level: Synthesis [Creating]

**593. PHARM ANSWER: 4**

1. Stating that the client will get used to the taste does not acknowledge the client's concern and is not helpful. The foul taste is from large particles of medication on the client's tongue.

2. Shaking the canister does not change the taste of the medication; it ensures that the medication is dispersed within the canister.

3. Sucking on hard candy may alter the taste and make it worse; it is not the best response.

4. **Using a spacer delivers the medication in smaller particles; fewer particles fall onto the tongue. The spacer promotes deeper delivery of the medication into the lungs.**

▶ *Test-taking Tip: The focus of the question is the client's concern about the taste. Eliminate options that do not address this concern.*

Content Area: Fundamentals; Concept: Medication; Oxygenation; Sensory Perception; Integrated Processes: Teaching/Learning; Client Needs: Physiological Integrity: Pharmacological and Parenteral Therapies; Health Promotion and Maintenance; Cognitive Level: Application [Applying]

**594. MoC PHARM ANSWER: 3**

1. Nonsterile gloves should be worn to avoid contact with the medication.

2. The client should be identified using two unique identifiers.

3. **The clonidine (Catapres) should not be rubbed into the skin. Patches are designed to allow constant, controlled amounts of medication to be released over 24 hours or more.**

4. Folding the patch with the medication on the inside avoids inadvertent contact with the medication.

▶ *Test-taking Tip: Note the key phrase "requires the observing nurse to intervene." Look for the incorrect action, which is Option 3.*

Content Area: Fundamentals; Concept: Medication; Management; Perfusion; Integrated Processes: Teaching/Learning; Client Needs: Safe and Effective Care Environment: Management of Care; Physiological Integrity: Pharmacological and Parenteral Therapies; Cognitive Level: Analysis [Analyzing]

**595. MoC PHARM ANSWER: 4**

1. A medication that requires special assessments should be separated from other medications in case it needs to be held. It is best not to open the medication until the assessments are complete.

2. The abbreviation O.D. means right eye. Eye drops should be placed in the right eye conjunctival sac, where they are absorbed.

3. Saline (0.9% NaCl) should be used to check the patency of the IV site before administering an IV medication.

4. **A sustained-release medication is meant to be absorbed over 24 hours; the capsule should not be opened and mixed with food.**

▶ *Test-taking Tip: The key word is "intervene." You should select an incorrect action by the student nurse.*

Content Area: Fundamentals; Concept: Medication; Management; Integrated Processes: Nursing Process: Evaluation; Client Needs: Physiological Integrity: Pharmacological and Parenteral Therapies; Safe and Effective Care Environment: Management of Care; Cognitive Level: Evaluation [Evaluating]

**596.** **PHARM** **ANSWER: 4**

1. The deltoid muscle is not well developed in neonates.
2. Although 0.5 mL of medication can be administered into the ventrogluteal muscle of neonates, it is not a recommended site because the muscle is not bulky enough to absorb medications.
3. Dorsogluteal muscles are not well developed in neonates and not bulky enough to absorb medications.
4. **The vastus lateralis muscle on the anterolateral thigh is recommended as the site for IM injections for neonates less than 1 month old. It has a larger muscle mass than other IM injection sites, which is needed for adequate medication absorption. Using this site avoids the risk of sciatic nerve damage.**

♦ *Test-taking Tip: Think about the largest muscle in neonates before selecting an option. The key word is "best."*

**Content Area:** Fundamentals; **Concept:** Medication; Immunity; **Integrated Processes:** Nursing Process: Planning; **Client Needs:** Physiological Integrity: Pharmacological and Parenteral Therapies; Health Promotion and Maintenance; **Cognitive Level:** Knowledge [Remembering]

**597.** **MoC** **ANSWER: 2, 3, 4, 6**

1. Rewriting the medications into the client's medical record without verifying the dose and frequency can result in a medication overdose.
2. **Vitamins, herbals, and OTC medications can affect the action of other medications.**
3. **The usual dose and frequency of interferon beta-1b (Betaseron) is 0.25 mg (8 million IU) every other day, so the dose and frequency should be verified. Medications can be verified by contacting the prescribing physician.**
4. **The nurse can ask pharmacy to contact the pharmacy where the medication was last filled to verify the dose.**
5. Inserting an unaltered copy into the client's medical record without verifying the dose and frequency can result in a medication overdose.
6. **Medications can be verified by asking a family member to bring the container that has the prescribing information noted.**

♦ *Test-taking Tip: Medication reconciliation (verifying medications) is an important safety procedure and is a Joint Commission requirement for health care facilities.*

**Content Area:** Fundamentals; **Concept:** Medication; Immunity; **Integrated Processes:** Nursing Process: Implementation; **Client Needs:** Safe and Effective Care Environment: Management of Care; Physiological Integrity: Reduction of Risk Potential; **Cognitive Level:** Analysis [Analyzing]

**598.** **PHARM** **ANSWER:**

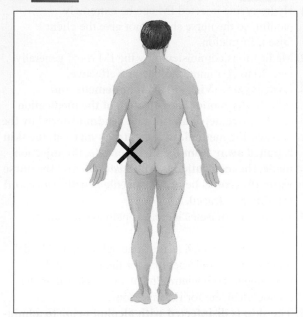

The left dorsogluteal muscle is best located above and outside a line drawn from the left posterior superior iliac spine to the left greater trochanter of the femur. An alternative method is to divide the buttock into four quadrants and make the injection in the upper outer quadrant, about 2 to 3 inches (5–7.6 cm) below the iliac crest. A combination of these methods is often used to identify the correct location and avoid the sciatic nerve.

♦ *Test-taking Tip: Read the stem carefully, noting the term "left dorsogluteal muscle." Apply knowledge of underlying anatomy to answer this question.*

**Content Area:** Fundamentals; **Concept:** Medication; **Integrated Processes:** Nursing Process: Planning; **Client Needs:** Physiological Integrity: Pharmacological and Parenteral Therapies; **Cognitive Level:** Application [Applying]

**599.** **MoC** **PHARM** **ANSWER: 1**

1. **The RN should intervene because 1 mL is too much for an intradermal injection. Only small amounts are administered intradermally, usually no more than 0.1 mL.**
2. Holding an insulin pen at the site for 10 seconds will ensure that the insulin is administered.
3. The deltoid muscle is located three finger-breadths below the acromion process.
4. The nurse should not aspirate for blood when giving heparin subcutaneously.

♦ *Test-taking Tip: The RN should intervene when observing the LPN perform a procedure incorrectly.*

**Content Area:** Fundamentals; **Concept:** Medication; Management; **Integrated Processes:** Nursing Process: Evaluation; **Client Needs:** Safe and Effective Care Environment: Management of Care; Physiological Integrity: Pharmacological and Parenteral Therapies; **Cognitive Level:** Evaluation [Evaluating]

**600.** **PHARM** **ANSWER: 3, 6**

1. Hydroxyzine injected IM can be extremely painful, so the nurse should not give the client false information.
2. Medications administered by the IM route generally take 20 to 30 minutes to become effective.
3. **Hydroxyzine (Vistaril) is an antiemetic and sedative/hypnotic. The injection of the medication can be extremely painful, so it is administered by the Z-track IM method. In the Z-track method, the skin is pulled away from the injection site, the injection made, the medication is administered, and the nurse waits 10 seconds before the needle is withdrawn and the skin is released.**
4. Tensing the muscles increases pain and should be avoided.
5. A large muscle such as the ventrogluteal, not the deltoid muscle, should be used for the injection. Literature suggests the ventrogluteal site is safer than the dorsogluteal site for IM injections.
6. **The skin is disinfected with alcohol prior to administration, which will feel cool when applied.**

♦ **Test-taking Tip:** *The Z-track method is used for giving IM medications.*

**Content Area:** Fundamentals; **Concept:** Medication; **Integrated Processes:** Nursing Process: Implementation; **Client Needs:** Physiological Integrity: Pharmacological and Parenteral Therapies; Physiological Integrity: Reduction of Risk Potential; **Cognitive Level:** Application [Applying]

**601.** **MoC** **PHARM** **ANSWER: 3**

1. Positioning the client prone may help to identify landmarks for an IM injection into the dorsogluteal muscle, but this site is not recommended for older adults due to difficulty in identifying the landmarks and the proximity of the sciatic nerve and superior gluteal artery.
2. All IM injections should be administered by a Z-track method regardless of site. The dorsogluteal muscle should not be used for injection in an older adult.
3. **The new nurse should inform the experienced nurse that the preferred site for an IM injection is the ventrogluteal muscle. It is the safest and least painful site for an IM injection; it is located away from major blood vessels and nerves.**
4. The needle size should be based on the site, the muscle size, and the amount of medication; no information is provided to determine if a 1-inch needle is appropriate.

♦ **Test-taking Tip:** *Even though the nurse is inexperienced, the nurse should speak up if another colleague is not performing procedures according to current nursing practice.*

**Content Area:** Fundamentals; **Concept:** Safety; Medication; **Integrated Processes:** Nursing Process: Evaluation; **Client Needs:** Safe and Effective Care Environment: Management of Care; Physiological Integrity: Pharmacological and Parenteral Therapies; **Cognitive Level:** Evaluation [Evaluating]

**602.** **MoC** **PHARM** **ANSWER: 2, 4**

1. Digoxin should not be administered; the serum digoxin level is higher than the therapeutic range.
2. **Digoxin should be withheld; the serum digoxin level is higher than the therapeutic range.**
3. There is no indication that the digoxin level is inaccurate; a recheck is costly and unnecessary.
4. **The HCP should be informed of the digoxin results; also, the nurse should address that the digoxin was withheld and obtain an order for this.**
5. Only the HCP can discontinue the digoxin order. Once written, the paper or electronic record is received by pharmacy; the nurse does not need to call pharmacy.

♦ **Test-taking Tip:** *The therapeutic range is a range of concentration whereby the medication produces its desired effect. When administering digoxin (Lanoxin), the digoxin level should be within the therapeutic range. Also, consider appropriate communication protocol and the nursing scope of care when determining if an option is correct.*

**Content Area:** Fundamentals; **Concept:** Safety; Medication; Nursing Roles; **Integrated Processes:** Nursing Process: Implementation; **Client Needs:** Safe and Effective Care Environment: Management of Care; Physiological Integrity: Pharmacological and Parenteral Therapies; Physiological Integrity: Reduction of Risk Potential; Psychosocial Integrity; **Cognitive Level:** Application [Applying]

**603.** **PHARM** **ANSWER: 2**

1. Giving approval for the child to vent his or her feelings provides the child with a better sense of control.
2. **Injections should never be administered to a sleeping child because the injection is painful, and the child will wake up and be terrified.**
3. A topical analgesic such as lidocaine/prilocaine (EMLA) cream can reduce the pain with insertion, but pain may still be felt as the medication is injected.
4. The child can be lying flat during the injection.

♦ **Test-taking Tip:** *The key word is "inappropriate."*

**Content Area:** Fundamentals; **Concept:** Medication; Communication; **Integrated Processes:** Communication and Documentation; **Client Needs:** Psychosocial Integrity; Physiological Integrity: Pharmacological and Parenteral Therapies **Cognitive Level:** Analysis [Analyzing]

**604.** **PHARM** **ANSWER: 1, 2, 5**

1. **Although most antibiotics are compatible at the injection site with D₅W/20 mEq KCL, the nurse should check for compatibilities. If incompatible, the nurse must stop the infusion and flush the line before administering the antibiotic.**
2. **Because this is a newly prescribed medication, it is especially important for the nurse to check for allergies.**
3. Antibiotics can be administered in hand and arm veins; initiating a PICC is unnecessary.

4. The nurse would not need to consult with the HCP; if unfamiliar with how to administer an IVPB, the nurse should consult an experienced nurse or consult the agency procedure manual.

5. **The rate for administering antibiotics varies by the type of antibiotic and the amount of solution in the IVPB. The nurse should determine the rate by checking the recommended rate noted on the IVPB and, if not noted, consult a medication book or pharmacy and then calculate the correct rate if necessary.**

▸ *Test-taking Tip: With multiple response options, treat each option as a true/false statement. Remember that if the nurse is unfamiliar with a procedure, the nurse should use unit resources for reviewing the procedure.*

Content Area: Fundamentals; Concept: Safety; Infection; Integrated Processes: Nursing Process: Implementation; Client Needs: Physiological Integrity: Pharmacological and Parenteral Therapies; Cognitive Level: Analysis [Analyzing]

## 605. MoC PHARM ANSWER: 2

1. IV solutions that are open longer than 24 hours are no longer considered sterile.

2. **IV solutions in 250- and 500-mL containers should be selected to guard against circulatory overload. IV solutions are considered medications, and errors in administration can have negative consequences.**

3. Tubing is changed every 72 to 96 hours, depending on agency policy.

4. The procedure for spiking the bag is correct. The bag could either be hung first or after being spiked.

▸ *Test-taking Tip: The key words are "needs additional orientation." Read each option carefully to determine which option has the greatest potential for producing harm.*

Content Area: Fundamentals; Concept: Medication; Management; Safety; Integrated Processes: Nursing Process: Evaluation; Client Needs: Safe and Effective Care Environment: Management of Care; Physiological Integrity: Pharmacological and Parenteral Therapies; Cognitive Level: Evaluation [Evaluating]

## 606. PHARM ANSWER: 150

**50 mL : 20 min :: $X$ mL/h: 60 min/h**
**Multiply the means (inside values) and then the extremes (outside values) to solve for $X$.**
**$20X = 3000$; $X = 3000 \div 20$; $X = 150$ mL/h**
**The nurse should set the infusion pump to deliver cefazolin (Ancef) at 150 mL/h.**

▸ *Test-taking Tip: Use an IV rate formula to calculate the correct rate and verify the answer if it seems unusually large.*

Content Area: Fundamentals; Concept: Medication; Integrated Processes: Nursing Process: Analysis; Client Needs: Physiological Integrity: Pharmacological and Parenteral Therapies; Cognitive Level: Application [Applying]

## 607. MoC PHARM ANSWER: 3

1. The current serum potassium level should be known before notifying the HCP. The HCP may decide to change the amount of potassium based on the client's level.

2. An agency incident report should be completed by the nurse after caring for the client.

3. **Because the order was written the previous day and not implemented, the nurse should first check the client's serum potassium level and then notify the HCP.**

4. The nurse should determine if there are order changes before replacing the solution.

▸ *Test-taking Tip: Note the key word "first." Remember that KCL is potassium chloride. The nurse should have essential information prior to notifying the HCP.*

Content Area: Fundamentals; Concept: Quality Improvement; Legal; Management; Integrated Processes: Nursing Process: Implementation; Client Needs: Safe and Effective Care Environment: Management of Care; Physiological Integrity: Pharmacological and Parenteral Therapies; Physiological Integrity: Reduction of Risk Potential; Cognitive Level: Application [Applying]

## 608. PHARM ANSWER: 2

1. Although the usual replacement dose is 20 mEq/100 mL with administration of 10 to 20 mEq/hour, IV concentrations can safely range from 10 to 40 mEq/L.

2. **Potassium can be irritating to the vein, and the client may experience burning. Strategies to minimize pain and inflammation include applying ice or warm packs.**

3. Potassium is never administered as an IV push; it will cause cardiac dysrhythmias.

4. Adding medication to an already-infusing IV solution is unsafe and can result in a faster or slower rate of administration depending on the volume of solution remaining.

▸ *Test-taking Tip: Note that Options 3 and 4 both address methods of administration. Because both cannot be correct, either one or both are incorrect.*

Content Area: Fundamentals; Concept: Medication; Fluid and Electrolyte Balance; Integrated Processes: Nursing Process: Planning; Client Needs: Physiological Integrity: Pharmacological and Parenteral Therapies; Physiological Integrity: Reduction of Risk Potential; Cognitive Level: Application [Applying]

## 609. PHARM ANSWER: 2

1. Placing the secondary line into the existing IV solution bag will cause mixing of the antibiotic with the IV solution.

2. **The IVPB secondary line should be inserted at the port immediately distal to the back-check valve on the tubing and before the pump (line B). The antibiotic should run through the IV infusion pump to control the rate and ensure that the medication is delivered.**

3. Placing the IVPB secondary line into a port after the infusion pump (line C) would allow an uncontrolled rate for the antibiotic; the IV solution will also be infusing, increasing the volume that the client should receive.

4. Line D is the port closest to the client and after the pump. The rate of administration of the antibiotic would not be controlled by the pump.

▶ **Test-taking Tip:** *Note the key words "strict I&O." The volume delivered is best controlled by delivering the medication through the pump. A port above the pump should be selected.*

**Content Area:** Fundamentals; **Concept:** Medication; Infection; **Integrated Processes:** Nursing Process: Planning; **Client Needs:** Physiological Integrity: Pharmacological and Parenteral Therapies; **Cognitive Level:** Application [Applying]

**610. MoC PHARM ANSWER: 4**

1. Both cefotaxime (Claforan) and ceftriaxone (Rocephin) are third-generation cephalosporins; there could be cross allergies between the medications. If the nurse administers the medication without verifying that the HCP is aware of the allergy to cephalosporins, the nurse would deviate from the standard of care owed to the client.

2. Although the nurse may call pharmacy to verify that the prescribed medication is a cephalosporin and to confirm the risks associated with administering it based on the client's allergy, the most important action is to notify the HCP.

3. The nurse could question the client about receiving the medication previously, but the most important action is for the nurse to verify that the HCP is aware of the allergy.

4. **The nurse should call the HCP to verify that the allergy was known and that the allergy was considered when cefotaxime (Claforan) was prescribed. Even though the medications are different, they are from the same drug classifications.**

▶ **Test-taking Tip:** *Be sure to read drug names carefully. If the nurse fails to identify a known allergy and the client has an adverse reaction when the medication is administered, the nurse will have provided negligent care.*

**Content Area:** Fundamentals; **Concept:** Medication; Immunity; Management; **Integrated Processes:** Nursing Process: Implementation; **Client Needs:** Safe and Effective Care Environment: Management of Care; Physiological Integrity: Pharmacological and Parenteral Therapies; **Cognitive Level:** Analysis [Analyzing]

**611. MoC PHARM ANSWER: 1**

1. **Administering SL nitroglycerin (Nitrostat) has priority. This can be performed more quickly than the other orders and has the greatest potential of changing client outcomes. Nitroglycerin increases coronary blood flow, reducing anginal pain and the potential of MI.**

2. Morphine is a controlled substance requiring the nurse to retrieve it and sign it out from a secure location. Administering IV medications takes longer than SL medications.

3. Lorazepam (Ativan) is a controlled substance requiring the nurse to retrieve it and sign it out from a secure location. Administering IV medications takes longer than SL medications.

4. Obtaining blood from the blood bank will take longer than administering an SL medication.

▶ **Test-taking Tip:** *Use the ABC's and the time it takes to implement each action to establish the priority. Because nitroglycerin affects the circulatory system, this action should be first.*

**Content Area:** Fundamentals; **Concept:** Critical Thinking; Medication; Management; **Integrated Processes:** Nursing Process: Planning; **Client Needs:** Safe and Effective Care Environment: Management of Care; Physiological Integrity: Pharmacological and Parenteral Therapies; **Cognitive Level:** Analysis [Analyzing]

**612. PHARM ANSWER: 2, 5, 1, 3, 4**

2. **Labetalol (Normodyne) 20 mg IV push for systolic BP >160 mm Hg. Labetalol is a beta blocker that will lower the BP. This should be administered first because the client's BP is elevated and the onset of action is 2 to 5 minutes.**

5. **Cefazolin sodium (Ancef) 1 g IVSP should be next. The nurse is working with the IV lines, and the client's temperature is also elevated, suggesting an infection. Cefazolin sodium is a cephalosporin antibiotic.**

1. **Timolol (Timoptic) 2 gtt right eye should be third. The client is lying flat in bed. Timolol is used for treating glaucoma. It is easier to administer into the conjunctival sac if given while lying in bed.**

3. **Ramipril (Altace) 2.5 mg oral daily should be next. It is an ACE inhibitor with an onset of 1 to 2 hours, and the client's BP is already elevated.**

4. **Docusate sodium (Docusate) rectal suppository this a.m. should be last. The client needs to assume a side-lying position for the rectal suppository to be administered. It is used to soften stool and promote defecation. It should be retained as long as possible.**

▶ **Test-taking Tip:** *Use the ABC's to determine the priority action; focus on using aseptic technique, starting with the cleanest areas first.*

**Content Area:** Fundamentals; **Concept:** Critical Thinking; Medication; **Integrated Processes:** Nursing Process: Analysis; **Client Needs:** Physiological Integrity: Pharmacological and Parenteral Therapies; Physiological Integrity: Reduction of Risk Potential; **Cognitive Level:** Synthesis [Creating]

**613.** MoC PHARM **ANSWER: 1**

1. **The findings should be reported to the coworker's supervisor, who should collect additional information and approach the coworker with the concern.**
2. Telling the coworker of suspicions may cause the coworker to hide the problem, if one exists, and could jeopardize client safety.
3. The immediate supervisor, and not the police, should be collecting additional data to either support or refute the nurse's suspicions.
4. The nurse should document suspicions, but completing an incident report is unnecessary because there are no data to support that an incident has occurred.

▶ *Test-taking Tip: Identify the focus of the question from the behaviors described, which suggest suspected drug abuse. Then note the key words "most appropriate." Eliminate Options 2, 3, and 4 because these actions are inappropriate until additional information is collected to eliminate other potential problems.*

**Content Area:** Fundamentals; **Concept:** Quality Improvement; Legal; Management; **Integrated Processes:** Communication and Documentation; **Client Needs:** Safe and Effective Care Environment: Management of Care; Physiological Integrity: Pharmacological and Parenteral Therapies; **Cognitive Level:** Analysis [Analyzing]

**614.** PHARM **ANSWER: 2, 5**

1. Oxycodone with acetaminophen can be taken with apple juice.
2. **Oxycodone with acetaminophen (Percocet) is a Schedule II controlled substance. The Controlled Substances Act requires facilities to keep controlled substances in a locked drawer, box, or automated dispensing machine in a location that is inaccessible to clients.**
3. Two unique client identifiers should be used to administer medications safely, usually the name and medical record number.
4. The time of onset for analgesic effect from oxycodone with acetaminophen is 10 to 15 minutes.
5. **A medication is to be administered by the route it was ordered.**

▶ *Test-taking Tip: Controlled substances are kept in a controlled location; a count is performed at specified times (usually at the end of a shift); thus select Option 2. Oral medications should be swallowed; thus select Option 5.*

**Content Area:** Fundamentals; **Concept:** Medication; Informatics; Management; **Integrated Processes:** Nursing Process: Evaluation; **Client Needs:** Physiological Integrity: Pharmacological and Parenteral Therapies; **Cognitive Level:** Evaluation [Evaluating]

**615.** MoC PHARM **ANSWER: 2**

1. Nonmaleficence is to do no harm. Withholding larger doses should not cause harm.
2. **Autonomy refers to the client's right to make individual choices and to have those choices honored by the nurse.**

3. Beneficence is the promotion of good. The good actions must be weighed against any possible harm.
4. Veracity means truthfulness. No statement was made by the nurse.

▶ *Test-taking Tip: Focus on the definition of the ethical principles in the options. The nurse is adhering to the client's wishes. Persons who are devoutly religious may view pain as the will of God.*

**Content Area:** Fundamentals; **Concept:** Ethics; Medication; Diversity; **Integrated Processes:** Caring; Culture and Spirituality; **Client Needs:** Safe and Effective Care Environment: Management of Care; Physiological Integrity: Pharmacological and Parenteral Therapies; Psychosocial Integrity; **Cognitive Level:** Application [Applying]

**616.** MoC **ANSWER: 4**

1. Giving cephalexin (Keflex) 1 hour after a repeat dose of antiemetic involves administering the medication against the client's wishes.
2. Sucking on ice chips may increase the client's nausea. The stem indicates that the nurse has already tried to manage the client's nausea and that interventions were unsuccessful.
3. Applesauce could increase the client's nausea, and administering cephalexin is against the client's wishes.
4. **In this situation, the client has the right to refuse medications and treatments regardless of the reasons and the consequences.**

▶ *Test-taking Tip: Note that Options 1, 2, and 3 are similar and involve giving the medication. Option 4 is different. Often the option that is different is the answer.*

**Content Area:** Fundamentals; **Concept:** Medication; Ethics; Management; **Integrated Processes:** Nursing Process: Implementation; **Client Needs:** Safe and Effective Care Environment: Management of Care; Psychosocial Integrity; **Cognitive Level:** Application [Applying]

**617.** PHARM **ANSWER: 2**

1. It is safe to administer 10 mg of metoclopramide IV over 1 minute.
2. **Metoclopramide (Reglan) should be administered 30 minutes before (not after) meals to increase GI motility and prevent nausea at mealtime.**
3. The nurse should note any medication incompatibilities and select an IV line with compatible solution, flush the IV line with saline before and after administration, or start another IV access for administering IV medications.
4. Metoclopramide is compatible with $D_5W$, and the most distal port would be the one closest to the client's insertion site.

▶ *Test-taking Tip: Note the key word "error." Look for the action that is incorrect. Use key words in the stem to identify relationships with the options. Note peristalsis in the stem and meals in Option 2.*

**Content Area:** Fundamentals; **Concept:** Medication; Digestion; **Integrated Processes:** Nursing Process: Analysis; **Client Needs:** Physiological Integrity: Pharmacological and Parenteral Therapies; Physiological Integrity: Physiological Adaptation; **Cognitive Level:** Application [Applying]

**618.** **PHARM** **ANSWER: 3**

1. Lactated Ringer's is isotonic. It expands vascular volume and does not enter the cells to treat cellular dehydration.
2. NS (0.9% sodium chloride) is isotonic. It expands vascular volume and does not enter the cells to treat cellular dehydration.
3. **0.45% sodium chloride is hypotonic. It will expand vascular volume and enter cells to rehydrate them and treat cellular dehydration.**
4. $D_5W$ 0.9% sodium chloride is hypertonic. Once dextrose is metabolized, it leaves isotonic 0.9% sodium chloride, which remains in the vascular compartment and does not enter cells.

▶ *Test-taking Tip:* Hypotonic solutions enter cells to treat cellular dehydration.

Content Area: Fundamentals; Concept: Fluid and Electrolyte Balance; Medication; Integrated Processes: Nursing Process: Planning; Client Needs: Physiological Integrity: Pharmacological and Parenteral Therapies; Physiological Integrity: Physiological Adaptation; Cognitive Level: Comprehension [Understanding]

**619.** **PHARM** **ANSWER: 2**

1. Although oxygen should be applied because the client has dyspnea, it should be administered by nasal cannula, not a mask. Applying oxygen is not the first action.
2. **The symptoms suggest air embolism. Turning the client onto the left side with the head lower than the feet will trap the embolism in the right atrium.**
3. Although the HCP should be notified, the first action is to turn the client onto the left side.
4. Air likely entered the vascular system when the injection caps were changed. Injecting saline increases the risk of additional air entering the vascular system. Blood should be aspirated to remove air from the injection caps and central line catheter.

▶ *Test-taking Tip:* An air embolus can occur when inserting the central venous access device or when changing the cap or tubing. During a cap or tubing change, the client should be flat and asked to hold a breath and "bear down" to prevent air from entering the bloodstream.

Content Area: Fundamentals; Concept: Critical Thinking; Safety; Integrated Processes: Nursing Process: Implementation; Client Needs: Physiological Integrity: Pharmacological and Parenteral Therapies; Physiological Integrity: Reduction of Risk Potential; Cognitive Level: Analysis [Analyzing]

**620.** **PHARM** **ANSWER: 3, 4**

1. An empty solution bag indicates the need for a new bag. It is not a sign of extravasation.
2. A malfunctioning IV pump could cause the vesicant to infuse too rapidly and lead to extravasation, but it is not a sign of extravasation.
3. **Swelling surrounding the IV site is a sign of infiltration from fluid leaking into the tissues and not infusing into the vein. A vesicant solution can cause extravasation.**
4. **Blistering at the IV site is a sign of extravasation from leakage of vesicant solution into the tissues.**
5. Chest pain is unrelated to extravasation at a peripheral IV site.

▶ *Test-taking Tip:* Extravasation is leakage of a vesicant IV fluid or medication into tissues near the IV site that can lead to blistering, tissue necrosis, and tissue sloughing.

Content Area: Fundamentals; Concept: Critical Thinking; Inflammation; Integrated Processes: Nursing Process: Assessment; Client Needs: Physiological Integrity: Pharmacological and Parenteral Therapies; Physiological Integrity: Reduction of Risk Potential; Cognitive Level: Application [Applying]

**621.** **PHARM** **ANSWER: 3**

1. It is difficult to advance the catheter in a vein with a bifurcation (point where two veins meet) due to the presence of valves in the veins.
2. A vein in the client's nondominant hand may not be large enough to insert a larger-sized needle for a blood transfusion. Too small a catheter may destroy RBCs being infused.
3. **The cephalic vein is a larger vein located on the thumb side of the arm. Selecting the vein above the wrist will allow movement of the wrist and minimize possible displacement of the catheter.**
4. The dorsal metacarpal veins are in the hand. Hand veins may not be large enough to insert a larger-sized needle for a blood transfusion. Too small a catheter may destroy RBCs being infused.

▶ *Test-taking Tip:* You should note that two options are the same but use different terminology. Eliminating Options 2 and 4 narrows your choices.

Content Area: Fundamentals; Concept: Nursing Roles; Assessment; Medication; Integrated Processes: Nursing Process: Assessment; Client Needs: Physiological Integrity: Pharmacological and Parenteral Therapies; Cognitive Level: Application [Applying]

**622.** **PHARM** **ANSWER: 2**

1. The nurse should not return the blood to the blood bank. The client with AB negative blood type can receive type O negative RBCs. Type O negative has no antigens on the RBC to react with the A and B antigens on the type AB negative RBC.
2. **The nurse should continue to prepare the blood because it is compatible. A person with type AB blood has A and B antigens on the RBC, but type O has none.**
3. It is unnecessary to verify compatible RBCs with the HCP; this will delay administering the transfusion.

4. The client's consent for blood administration should have been received before obtaining the blood. Blood must be started within 30 minutes of obtaining it from the blood bank.

▶ **Test-taking Tip:** *Remember that a person with blood type O negative has no antigens on the RBC and is the universal donor of RBCs.*

**Content Area:** Fundamentals; **Concept:** Safety; Medication; **Integrated Processes:** Nursing Process: Analysis; **Client Needs:** Physiological Integrity: Pharmacological and Parenteral Therapies; **Cognitive Level:** Analysis [Analyzing]

**623.** PHARM **ANSWER: 1**
The line is pointing to the ½ mL or 0.5 mL mark on the syringe. Use a proportion formula to calculate the correct dose.
100 mg : 2 mL :: 25 mg : $X$ mL
Multiply the extremes and then the means.
$100X = 50$; $X = 50 \div 100$ or 0.5 mL

▶ **Test-taking Tip:** *Carefully read what the question is asking. Be sure that you choose the option that corresponds to the syringe and not the amount of chlordiazepoxide HCL (Librium) you calculated.*

**Content Area:** Fundamentals; **Concept:** Medication; **Integrated Processes:** Nursing Process: Implementation; **Client Needs:** Physiological Integrity: Pharmacological and Parenteral Therapies; **Cognitive Level:** Application [Applying]

## Chapter Sixteen

# Perioperative Care

**624.** The nurse is performing presurgical assessment of multiple clients. The nurse determines that which client has the greatest risk for developing an infection postoperatively?

1. The client with new-onset neutropenia of unknown etiology
2. The client with thrombocytopenia secondary to taking aspirin
3. The child newly diagnosed with type 1 diabetes mellitus (DM)
4. The client who needs assistance with ambulation due to arthritis

**625.** MoC The client being admitted for same-day surgery has inspiratory crackles and bilateral wheezes, and reports shortness of breath for several days. Which intervention should the nurse implement **first?**

1. Notify the surgeon of the findings.
2. Document the assessment findings.
3. Apply 4 liters oxygen by nasal cannula.
4. Instruct on using an incentive spirometer (IS).

**626.** PHARM MoC All of the following must be completed for the client being prepared for surgery. Which intervention should the nurse plan to do **first?**

1. Complete the preoperative checklist.
2. Assess the client's preoperative vital signs.
3. Send the client to radiology for a chest x-ray.
4. Give 10 mEq KCL IV for a serum potassium level of 3.0 mEq/L.

**627.** PHARM The nurse is performing a presurgical admission assessment of the client. Which client statement needs the most immediate follow-up?

1. "I feel very hungry; I haven't eaten foods or had any fluids for the past 12 hours."
2. "I donated my own blood in case I need a transfusion; the last donation was 4 days ago."
3. "I took all my meds including warfarin and atenolol with a sip of water this morning."
4. "I brought a copy of my health care directive in case my heart stops during surgery."

**628.** MoC The nurse is to witness the signature of a surgical consent for multiple clients scheduled for surgery the following day. After evaluating the health history of each client, for which client should the nurse plan to obtain a signature from the next of kin?

1. The 75-year-old client who is legally blind
2. The 60-year-old client who does not understand English
3. The 50-year-old client who is forgetful but fully oriented
4. The 16-year-old client who fully understands the surgery

**629.** MoC The nurse receives the written laboratory results of a positive pregnancy test for the client scheduled for an emergency appendectomy. Which intervention should the nurse implement **first?**

1. Call the laboratory to verify the test results.
2. Inform the client of the pregnancy test results.
3. Report the pregnancy test results to the surgeon.
4. Notify the client's primary HCP of the results.

**630.** PHARM During a presurgical admission assessment, the client states, "I've told my surgeon that I am Jehovah's Witness and I won't accept a blood transfusion." Which statement by the nurse would be **most** appropriate?

1. "Tell me more about your fear of receiving a blood transfusion."
2. "Your request not to receive a transfusion would be honored."
3. "Don't worry; there is less blood loss with our newer equipment."
4. "Are you sure you wouldn't want a transfusion if one is needed?"

**631.** MoC The nurse is analyzing serum laboratory results for a 73-year-old female scheduled for surgery in 2 hours. Which result should the nurse inform the surgeon about **immediately?**

1. Hemoglobin 10 g/dL
2. Creatinine 1.0 mg/dL
3. Potassium 4.5 mEq/dL
4. Prothrombin time (PT) 22 seconds

**632.** MoC The nurse is reviewing preoperative orders for the client who is to have surgery on the large intestine the next day. Which written orders should the nurse question? **Select all that apply.**

1. Erythromycin 500 mg bid
2. Nothing by mouth (NPO) after midnight
3. Tap water enemas until hard stool passed
4. Clear liquid diet the day before surgery
5. Start incentive spirometer (IS) today

**633.** MoC PHARM The HCP writes an order to hold all medications the morning of surgery for the client with a history of type 1 DM and hypertension. Which medication(s) placed on hold should the nurse clarify with the HCP?

1. Acetylsalicylic acid (aspirin)
2. Docusate sodium
3. Regular and NPH insulin
4. Lotensin HCT

**634.** MoC The nurse is preparing the client for an operation. The nurse should delegate which tasks to the NA? **Select all that apply.**

1. Taking the client to radiology for a chest x-ray
2. Obtaining the vital signs and pulse oximetry
3. Recording output after emptying the urostomy bag
4. Completing the client's preoperative checklist
5. Helping the client change into a hospital gown

**635.** PHARM The preoperative client has a fear of postoperative pain. Which nursing action would be **best?**

1. Provide diversional activities when the client reports fear of pain.
2. Encourage the client to verbalize concerns regarding the fear of pain.
3. Inform the client of experiences and the likelihood of pain pre- and postoperatively.
4. Explain the medications prescribed for pain control, availability, and treatment goals.

**636.** The nurse observes the preoperative client using a volume IS. Which action demonstrates the client's proper use of the IS?

1. Sits upright, inserts the mouthpiece, and blows until the lungs are emptied of air
2. Sits upright, exhales, seals lips around the mouthpiece, inhales, and holds breath for 5 seconds
3. Sits at the edge of the bed, coughs, inserts the mouthpiece, and blows slowly for 10 seconds
4. Sits at the edge of the bed, exhales deeply, inserts the mouthpiece, and inhales quickly

**637.** The nurse is teaching the client prior to surgery about the device illustrated. The nurse teaches the client that the **primary purpose** of this device is to perform which function?

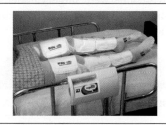

1. Improve the client's circulation prior to surgery
2. Prevent intra- and postoperative deep vein thrombosis (DVT)
3. Assist in keeping the client warm during surgery
4. Promote dehiscence and wound healing postoperatively

**638.** The nurse is caring for the client who received conscious sedation during a surgical procedure. Which assessment is **most** important postoperatively?

1. Bilateral lung sounds
2. Amount of urine output
3. Ability to swallow liquids
4. Rate and depth of breathing

**639.** The client, who is to receive general anesthesia, reports having a dry mouth because food and fluids have been withheld for 8 hours. Which nursing intervention is **most** appropriate?

1. Inform the client that food and fluids have been withheld to prevent vomiting and potential complications.
2. Clarify that fluids should have been withheld for only 4 hours and offer a small sip of water.
3. Explain that a full stomach puts pressure on the diaphragm and will prevent full lung expansion.
4. Tell the client that the general anesthetic will soon make the client sleepy and unaware of the dryness.

**640.** While in the OR holding area, the client who is to receive general anesthesia is noted to have replaced a tongue ring that was previously removed. What should the nurse do **initially?**

1. Document the findings on the client's medical record.
2. Request that the client once again remove the tongue ring.
3. Complete a variance report, noting that the client has reinserted the tongue ring.
4. Notify the surgeon and the anesthesiologist of the reinsertion of the tongue ring.

**641.** The nurse in the PACU obtains the VS illustrated for the client who underwent surgery under general anesthesia. Which should be the nurse's **priority** intervention?

| Client Vital Signs | |
| --- | --- |
| Blood Pressure (mm Hg) | 95/60 |
| Heart Rate (bpm) | 110 |
| Respirations (breaths per min) | 8, shallow |
| Temperature | 96.4°F (35.8°C) |
| SpO$_2$ | 89% on room air |

1. Apply additional warm blankets.
2. Increase the IV infusion rate.
3. Give oxygen by nasal cannula.
4. Assess the surgical incision site.

**642.** The client newly admitted to the PACU is showing signs of airway obstruction, and the nurse intervenes. Which assessment finding should **initially** indicate to the nurse that insertion of an oral airway has been effective?

1. Abdominal breathing pattern
2. Oxygen saturation at 92%
3. Lung sounds clear to auscultation
4. BP within desired range

**643.** MoC PHARM The nurse is preparing to administer the postoperative client's first dose of morphine sulfate through PCA. The nurse should also ensure that which antagonist medication is readily available?

1. Flumazenil
2. Naloxone hydrochloride
3. Digoxin immune fab
4. Protamine sulfate

**644.** The nurse collects the following information on the postoperative client: serum sodium level of 127 mEq/L; weight gain of 3 lb in 24 hours; crackles in lung bases, BP 154/70 mm Hg; 1+ pitting edema at the ankles. If prescribed, which intervention should the nurse implement?

1. 1500 mL fluid restriction
2. 5% NaCl IV at 100 mL/hour
3. Furosemide 80 mg IV now
4. 2000 milligram sodium diet

**645.** The client who had an exploratory laparotomy has a history of chronic back pain and limited ability to ambulate. Which statement by the client indicates that teaching is needed?

1. "I will no longer need to wear my elastic compression stockings once I get home."
2. "I plan to eat foods high in protein, calories, and vitamin C when I get home."
3. "Applying ice to my incision will help to control pain and reduce swelling."
4. "I am almost at my presurgery volume goal on my incentive spirometer."

**646.** Prior to emergency surgery for an appendectomy, the client has an NG tube inserted for gastric decompression. Which assessment finding from the NG returns should the nurse evaluate as normal?

1. Returns coffee-ground in color
2. Returns greenish-yellow in color
3. Has an alkalotic hydrogen level (pH)
4. Measures less than 25 mL in volume

**647.** The client return demonstrates to the nurse proper care and securement of a Jackson-Pratt (JP) drain. Which image shows that the client can properly care for and secure the JP drain?

1.

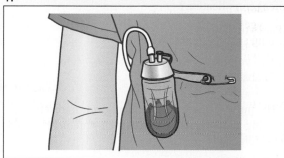

2.

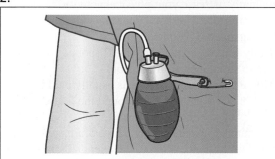

3.

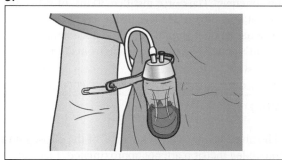

4.

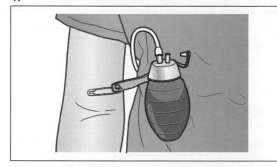

**648.** The nurse is caring for the postoperative client who reports an inability to void for the past 6 hours. What should the nurse do **first**?

1. Notify the HCP.
2. Insert a urinary catheter.
3. Perform a bladder scan.
4. Check the amount of the client's last void.

**649.** The postoperative client who received a spinal anesthetic is experiencing a headache, photophobia, and double vision. What should be the nurse's **initial** intervention?

1. Immediately notify the surgeon.
2. Position the client flat in bed.
3. Limit the client's fluid intake.
4. Administer a steroid medication.

**650.** The progress notes of the postoperative client who has a wound infection state that the client has a shift to the left in the WBC differential count. Which finding by the nurse reviewing the client's laboratory report would support the HCP's documentation?

1. Decreased WBC count
2. Increased band cells
3. Increased eosinophil count
4. Increased C-reactive protein

**651.** PHARM The nurse is caring for the postoperative client. The nurse should determine that which HCP order is specifically written to prevent thrombophlebitis and pulmonary embolism?

1. Dangle client the evening of surgery.
2. Give enoxaparin 40 mg subcutaneously daily.
3. Give hydromorphone 1 to 4 mg IV q4h prn.
4. Have client use IS and cough q2h while awake.

**652.** On the client's second postoperative day, the nurse assesses that the client has diminished breath sounds in both lung bases, is taking shallow breaths, and achieves only 500 mL on an IS. The client smoked cigarettes for the past 30 years. Which is the nurse's **best** interpretation of these findings?

1. The client has atelectasis.
2. The client has pneumonia.
3. The findings are normal for this client.
4. The client's airway is obstructing.

**653.** The nurse is caring for the postsurgical client. Which outcome should indicate to the nurse that the client's coughing and deep breathing (C&DB) are **most** effective?

1. Respirations are 16 per minute and unlabored.
2. Lung sounds are audible and clear on auscultation.
3. Coughs up small amount of clear secretions.
4. Cough effort is strong with productive results.

**654.** The nurse assesses redness, swelling, and warmth at the client's leg incision 48 hours after femoral popliteal bypass surgery. Which is the nurse's **best** interpretation of the findings?

1. The incision is healing normally for the second postoperative day.
2. The incision is showing signs of rejection of the suture materials.
3. The incision is inflamed and may indicate that it is infected.
4. The incision is infected and showing signs of wound dehiscence.

**655.** **MoC** The nurse receives morning report on four postoperative clients. Place the clients in the order that the nurse should plan to attend to the assigned clients.

1. The client who had a thyroidectomy 4 hours ago and reports inability to swallow
2. The client admitted 1 hour ago from PACU has incisional pain at 7 on a 0 to 10 scale
3. The client who had a total abdominal hysterectomy (TAH) yesterday and reports nausea
4. The client who reports a sudden increase in bloody drainage on the surgical bandage

Answer: _____

**656.** **PHARM** When the nurse hands the client a second dose of oxycodone/acetaminophen for incisional pain, the client says, "This medication makes me feel sick." Which statement is the most appropriate **initial** response by the nurse?

1. "I'll call your doctor to see if another medication can be ordered for your pain."
2. "Describe what you feel when you say that the medication makes you feel sick."
3. "The doctor prescribed an antacid. I can give you this along with the medication."
4. "The aspirin in the pain med is hard on your stomach. Eating a cracker may help."

**657.** **MoC** Five days after an exploratory laparotomy, the nurse assesses that the client has a distended abdomen, abdominal pain, absence of flatus, and absent bowel sounds. The nurse notifies the HCP concerned that the client could be experiencing which **typical** complication?

1. Paralytic ileus
2. Silent peritonitis
3. Fluid volume excess
4. Malabsorption syndrome

**658.** The nurse is teaching the client prior to discharge following abdominal surgery. Which statement should the nurse include?

1. "Return to work in about 4 weeks; working helps to gradually increase your physical activity."
2. "The prescribed iron and vitamins will promote wound healing and red blood cell growth."
3. "Daily walking while carrying 10-pound weights will help to strengthen your incision."
4. "Home-care nursing service is usually paid by insurance if you need help around the house."

**659.** The nurse is calculating NG tube drainage for the postoperative client. At 0700, the client's drainage container was marked at 150 mL. At 1500, there was 575 mL in the container. The nurse instilled 30 mL of saline irrigation into the tube four times as prescribed by the surgeon. What amount should the nurse document for the client's actual NG tube drainage from 0700 to 1500 hours?

_____ mL (Record your answer as a whole number.)

**660.** The nurse assesses that two areas of the client's postoperative leg incision are not approximated. Place an X on the two areas in the illustration that correctly describe the nurse's wound assessment.

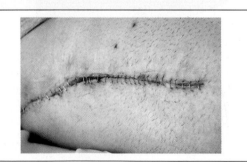

**INSTRUCTIONS:** Use the information provided to answer Questions 661 and 662.

**661.** `PHARM` `CJ` The nurse is interpreting the serum laboratory report illustrated for the postoperative client. Which STAT order should the nurse plan to implement after notifying the HCP of the laboratory results?

| Serum Laboratory Test | Client's Value | Normal Values |
| --- | --- | --- |
| BUN | 40 | 5–25 mg/dL |
| Creatinine | 1.9 | 0.5–1.5 mg/dL |
| Na | 136 | 135–145 mEq/L |
| K | 3.2 | 3.5–5.3 mEq/L |
| Cl | 99 | 95–105 mEq/L |
| $CO_2$ | 16 | 22–30 mEq/L |
| Phosphate | 1.9 | 1.7–2.6 mEq/L |
| Calcium | 9 | 9–11 mg/dL |
| Hgb | 11 | 13.5–17 g/dL |
| Hct | 33% | 40%–54% |

1. Administer 1 unit homologous packed red blood cells (RBCs).
2. Give potassium chloride 10 mEq in 100 mL 0.9% NaCl per IVPB.
3. Hold the ACE inhibitor enalapril due to the potassium level.
4. Give calcium gluconate 10 mEq in 100 mL 0.9% NaCl per IVPB.

**662.** `CJ` `MoC` Based on the information in the client's chart, which two most important lab findings should prompt the nurse to assess the client's renal function? Insert the lab values in the box below.

```


```

**663.** `MoC` The nurse is preparing to discharge the client who had a surgical procedure earlier in the day. The client lives alone. Which information would require the nurse to collaborate with the multidisciplinary team for skilled nursing care at home?

1. Has a dressing on the dominant arm requiring daily changes
2. States uncertainty regarding who will drive the client to appointments
3. Demonstrates ability to empty and compress the Jackson-Pratt drain
4. Able to use nondominant hand to prepare prescribed medications

## Answers and Rationales

**624. ANSWER: 1**
1. **Neutropenia is a reduction in neutrophils, the body's first line of defense in phagocytosis of invading microorganisms. Neutropenia predisposes the client to infection with nonpathogenic organisms that are present in normal body flora as well as opportunistic pathogens.**
2. Thrombocytopenia is a reduction in platelets. Thrombocytopenia predisposes the client to bleeding.
3. The client with DM is more susceptible to infections because there is a defect in the mobilization of inflammatory cells and an impairment of phagocytosis by neutrophils and monocytes. Although at risk, the client with neutropenia has a greater risk.
4. If assistance is provided for activity, there should not be an increased risk.

♦ **Test-taking Tip:** Note the key words "greatest risk." Neutrophils are one type of WBC.

Content Area: Fundamentals; Concept: Infection; Assessment; Integrated Processes: Nursing Process: Assessment; Client Needs: Health Promotion and Maintenance; Physiological Integrity: Reduction of Risk Potential; Cognitive Level: Analysis [Analyzing]

**625.** `MoC` **ANSWER: 1**
1. **The nurse should notify the surgeon of unanticipated changes in the health status of the preoperative client. Surgery may need to be postponed.**
2. The nurse should first notify the surgeon and then document the findings and the notification.
3. There are no objective data supporting the need for oxygen.
4. Although an IS may be prescribed, notifying the surgeon has priority.

▶ *Test-taking Tip:* You should use Maslow's Hierarchy of Needs to prioritize care. Remember a nursing intervention should not be initiated without objective evidence that the intervention is needed.

**Content Area:** Fundamentals; **Concept:** Oxygenation; **Integrated Processes:** Communication and Documentation; **Client Needs:** Safe and Effective Care Environment: Management of Care; **Cognitive Level:** Application [Applying]

### 626. MoC PHARM **ANSWER: 4**

1. Completing the preoperative checklist ensures that all requirements are completed. This would be the third intervention.
2. Although important, assessing the client's preoperative VS does not have priority.
3. The client's chest x-ray must be completed before surgery, but giving the KCL has priority.
4. **Giving KCL has priority. Abnormalities must be corrected before surgery. A low serum potassium level can induce cardiac dysrhythmias and delay surgery.**

▶ *Test-taking Tip:* Use the process of elimination and Maslow's Hierarchy of Needs. Physiological needs have priority over safety needs, unless life-threatening. Replacing serum potassium poses both a physiological and safety need and could be life-threatening.

**Content Area:** Fundamentals; **Concept:** Safety; Medication; **Integrated Processes:** Nursing Process: Planning; **Client Needs:** Safe and Effective Care Environment: Management of Care; Physiological Integrity: Pharmacological and Parenteral Therapies; **Cognitive Level:** Application [Applying]

### 627. PHARM **ANSWER: 3**

1. The exact amount of time the client must be NPO before surgery is controversial. Older adults may have imbalances of fluids, electrolytes, and blood glucose levels from fasting longer. However, there is no indication that this is a concern.
2. Blood can be donated up to 72 hours before the scheduled surgery.
3. **Warfarin (Coumadin) is an anticoagulant. Usually this is stopped a few days before surgery to reduce the risk of bleeding. The nurse should notify the HCP immediately.**
4. Clients should be encouraged to bring a copy of the HCD so others are aware of the client's wishes. The nurse may want to follow up regarding the client's statement "in case my heart stops during surgery," but this is not the most immediate concern.

▶ *Test-taking Tip:* Note the key words "most immediate." Applying knowledge of the anticoagulant effects of warfarin should direct you to Option 3.

**Content Area:** Fundamentals; **Concept:** Safety; Clotting; Medication; **Integrated Processes:** Nursing Process: Implementation; **Client Needs:** Physiological Integrity: Reduction of Risk Potential; Physiological Integrity: Pharmacological and Parenteral Therapies; **Cognitive Level:** Application [Applying]

### 628. MoC **ANSWER: 4**

1. The client who is legally blind may sign his or her signature with an "X" as long as the client understands the nature and reason for surgery, who will perform the surgery, available options, the benefits and risks of surgery, and the consent form that is read to the client. Another person besides the nurse should witness the client's "X" signature.
2. An interpreter should be available to read the consent in the client's native language. The client can then provide written consent in the presence of two witnesses.
3. The client is able to sign a consent form unless determined incompetent. If the client is fully oriented, a signed consent can be obtained from the client.
4. **The legal age for consent is 18 years unless the adolescent has emancipated status granted by a judge.**

▶ *Test-taking Tip:* Note the key words "next of kin." Focus on the ages of the clients and the information provided.

**Content Area:** Fundamentals; **Concept:** Safety; Legal; **Integrated Processes:** Nursing Process: Planning; **Client Needs:** Safe and Effective Care Environment: Management of Care; Psychosocial Integrity; **Cognitive Level:** Application [Applying]

### 629. MoC **ANSWER: 3**

1. Verifying laboratory results is unnecessary. Some hospitals may require repeating critical laboratory tests.
2. Discussing laboratory results with the client is the HCP's responsibility.
3. **The surgeon should be notified because a positive pregnancy test result could influence the choice of anesthetic agents, medications, and surgical approach.**
4. As a courtesy, the primary HCP should be notified. But, it is more important to notify the surgeon.

▶ *Test-taking Tip:* Note the key word "first." Think about the impact that surgery can have on a developing fetus.

**Content Area:** Fundamentals; Childbearing; **Concept:** Safety; Pregnancy; **Integrated Processes:** Nursing Process: Implementation; **Client Needs:** Safe and Effective Care Environment: Management of Care; **Cognitive Level:** Application [Applying]

### 630. PHARM **ANSWER: 2**

1. There is no indication that the client is fearful. The client is refusing blood for religious reasons.
2. **The client's consent is needed prior to administering blood or blood products. Even in a life-threatening situation, the client has the right to refuse blood and blood products for religious reasons.**
3. Telling the client not to worry belittles the client and does not address the client's statement about not receiving a blood transfusion.

4. Asking if the client is sure about not wanting a transfusion is requesting an explanation and questions the client's decision. The client has a right to his or her religious beliefs.

▶ *Test-taking Tip: Use therapeutic communication principles to answer this question. Eliminate nontherapeutic options that misinterpret the client's feelings, belittle the client's feelings, and question the client's decision.*

Content Area: Fundamentals; Concept: Communication; Diversity; Medication; Integrated Processes: Communication and Documentation; Culture and Spirituality; Client Needs: Physiological Integrity: Pharmacological and Parenteral Therapies; Cognitive Level: Application [Applying]

## 631. MoC ANSWER: 4

1. Normal Hgb for a 73-year-old female is 11.7 to 16.1 g/dL. Although a little low at 10 g/dL, this does not warrant the most immediate notification.
2. The creatinine of 1.0 mg/dL is within the normal range of 0.6 to 1.2 mg/dL for a 73-year-old female.
3. The normal potassium of 4.5 mEq/dL is within the normal range of 3.5 to 5.0 mEq/dL.
4. **The nurse should inform the surgeon of a PT time of 22 seconds. Normal PT is 11 to 12.5 seconds. Because it is prolonged, the client is at risk for bleeding.**

▶ *Test-taking Tip: The nurse would be expected to know ranges of these essential laboratory values. Analyze each laboratory value against the normal ranges to determine which value is abnormal.*

Content Area: Fundamentals; Concept: Clotting; Integrated Processes: Nursing Process: Analysis; Client Needs: Physiological Integrity: Reduction of Risk Potential; Safe and Effective Care Environment: Management of Care; Physiological Integrity: Reduction of Risk Potential; Cognitive Level: Analysis [Analyzing]

## 632. MoC ANSWER: 1, 3

1. **Antibiotics such as erythromycin (E Mycin) are administered to sterilize the bowel prior to surgery, but no route is prescribed.**
2. The client should be NPO after midnight to prevent aspiration of gastric contents during surgery.
3. **Tap water enemas would be administered until he returns are clear. Stool present in the colon could predispose the client to peritonitis and infection.**
4. A clear liquid diet the day before surgery minimizes roughage in the bowel.
5. IS use allows for presurgical evaluation of lung capacity.

▶ *Test-taking Tip: Written orders should be complete and appropriate to the client and the client's condition. Option 1 is incomplete, and Option 3 poses a risk to the client.*

Content Area: Fundamentals; Concept: Safety; Management; Nursing Roles; Integrated Processes: Nursing Process: Analysis; Client Needs: Safe and Effective Care Environment: Management of Care; Physiological Integrity: Physiological Adaptation; Cognitive Level: Application [Applying]

## 633. MoC PHARM ANSWER: 3

1. Acetylsalicylic acid (aspirin) has anticoagulant properties and should be discontinued prior to surgery to avoid bleeding complications.
2. Docusate sodium (Colace) is a stool softener. It is appropriate to hold this the morning of surgery.
3. **The diabetic client, who takes insulin, should be given a reduced dose of intermediate- or long-acting insulin based on the client's blood glucose levels. Regular insulin in divided doses or an insulin drip may be initiated on the day of surgery for tight glucose control.**
4. Antihypertensive medications such as Lotensin HCT (Benazepril HCL) are often held prior to surgery to prevent intraoperative hypotension.

▶ *Test-taking Tip: Focus on the medication actions. Remember that stress increases blood glucose levels.*

Content Area: Fundamentals; Concept: Medication; Management; Nursing Roles; Integrated Processes: Nursing Process: Implementation; Client Needs: Safe and Effective Care Environment: Management of Care; Physiological Integrity: Pharmacological and Parenteral Therapies; Cognitive Level: Analysis [Analyzing]

## 634. MoC ANSWER: 1, 2, 3, 5

1. **Transporting the client to radiology is within the NA's scope of practice.**
2. **Obtaining VS and pulse oximetry is within the NA's scope of practice.**
3. **Emptying a urostomy bag and documenting output is within the NA's scope of practice.**
4. The nurse should complete the preoperative checklist. Assessment, analysis, teaching, and evaluation are responsibilities only within the RN scope of practice.
5. **Helping the client change into a hospital gown is within the NA's scope of practice.**

▶ *Test-taking Tip: The nurse should never delegate tasks that require assessments, analysis, teaching, or evaluation. The nurse should consider the knowledge and skills of the person receiving the delegation.*

Content Area: Fundamentals; Concept: Collaboration, Regulations; Integrated Processes: Communication and Documentation; Client Needs: Safe and Effective Care Environment: Management of Care; Cognitive Level: Application [Applying]

## 635. PHARM ANSWER: 4

1. Diversional activities are used to enhance the pharmacological effect. Pharmacological management is the mainstay for acute pain.
2. Although allowing the client to verbalize fears is a therapeutic communication technique, allaying the fear is best.
3. Informing the client of experiences may heighten the client's fear. The client needs reassurance that the pain will be controlled.
4. **The client should be reassured that there are medications available to prevent and treat pain.**

▶ *Test-taking Tip: Note the key word "best." Look at the verbs "provide," "encourage," "inform," and "explain." Providing diversional activities does not address the client's verbalization. Eliminate Options 2 and 3 because they are lower-level verbs.*

**Content Area:** Fundamentals; **Concept:** Comfort; Medication; **Integrated Processes:** Nursing Process: Implementation; Caring; **Client Needs:** Physiological Integrity: Pharmacological and Parenteral Therapies; Psychosocial Integrity; **Cognitive Level:** Application [Applying]

## 636. ANSWER: 2

1. The client should inhale, not blow, when using the IS.
2. **Sitting upright promotes lung expansion. With all types of IS's, the client must be able to seal the lips tightly around the mouthpiece and inhale slowly. The client then holds the breath for 3 to 5 seconds for effective lung expansion.**
3. Coughing will help expel secretions and allow for full lung aeration, but the client should inhale, not blow, when using the IS.
4. The client should inhale slowly, not quickly, and hold the breath before exhalation to promote lung expansion.

▶ *Test-taking Tip: Visualize the client using an IS before trying to answer this question. Examine like options first and eliminate one or both of these. Options 1 and 3 include blowing into the IS, whereas Options 2 and 4 include inhaling.*

**Content Area:** Fundamentals; **Concept:** Safety; Oxygenation; **Integrated Processes:** Nursing Process: Evaluation; **Client Needs:** Health Promotion and Maintenance; Physiological Integrity: Reduction of Risk Potential; **Cognitive Level:** Evaluation [Evaluating]

## 637. ANSWER: 2

1. Circulation may be improved with a sequential compression device (SCD), but this is not the primary purpose.
2. **A sequential compression device (SCD) is used to prevent DVT. The device promotes fluid movement by simulating leg muscle contraction. The stocking compartments inflate to 35 to 55 mm Hg, inflating from the ankle, to the calf, and finally the thigh.**
3. SCDs have a cooling and warming option, but keeping the client warm is not the primary purpose.
4. SCDs will have no effect on wound healing.

▶ *Test-taking Tip: Note the key words "primary purpose." First eliminate Option 4 because it is unrelated to the location of the SCD. Recognizing that DVT is a complication following surgery, select Option 2 and eliminate Options 1 and 3.*

**Content Area:** Fundamentals; **Concept:** Safety; Perfusion; Nursing Roles; **Integrated Processes:** Teaching/Learning; **Client Needs:** Health Promotion and Maintenance; Physiological Integrity: Reduction of Risk Potential; **Cognitive Level:** Comprehension [Understanding]

## 638. ANSWER: 4

1. Lung sounds are assessed to determine the adequacy of ventilation of all lung lobes or the presence of fluid or secretions in the airways and lung tissue. Although assessing lung sounds is important postoperatively, assessing the rate and depth of breathing is *most* important with conscious sedation.
2. Although urine output should be at least 30 mL/hr and medications administered can potentially be nephrotoxic, it is more important to assess the rate and depth of respirations with conscious sedation.
3. The client's swallowing ability should be assessed prior to administering liquids; however, it is not the most important assessment with conscious sedation.
4. **The rate and depth of breathing should be assessed to determine the adequacy of air exchange. A respiratory rate of less than 10 breaths per minute indicates drug-induced respiratory depression. The primary concern with conscious sedation is the effect of the medications on the CNS.**

▶ *Test-taking Tip: Note the key words "most important." Use the ABC's to identify the correct option.*

**Content Area:** Fundamentals; **Concept:** Oxygenation; **Integrated Processes:** Nursing Process: Assessment; **Client Needs:** Physiological Integrity: Reduction of Risk Potential; **Cognitive Level:** Application [Applying]

## 639. ANSWER: 1

1. **The client should be NPO for 6 to 8 hours prior to general anesthesia to prevent vomiting and aspiration. The client may take prescribed medications with a sip of water (about 20 mL).**
2. The client should be NPO for 6 to 8 hours, not 4 hours, to reduce the risk of aspiration during surgery.
3. Although a full stomach does put pressure on the diaphragm and may prevent full lung expansion, this is not the primary reason for the NPO status.
4. Telling the client that the anesthesia will soon cause unawareness of the dry mouth disregards the client's concerns.

▶ *Test-taking Tip: Note the key words "most appropriate." Client teaching is most appropriate in the preoperative period.*

**Content Area:** Fundamentals; **Concept:** Nursing Roles; Safety; **Integrated Processes:** Nursing Process: Implementation; **Client Needs:** Physiological Integrity: Reduction of Risk Potential; **Cognitive Level:** Application [Applying]

## 640. ANSWER: 2

1. Documentation regarding finding the tongue ring replaced should occur after the intervention.
2. **Because anesthesia and surgery have not yet started, it is safe to ask the client to remove the tongue ring. If the client refuses, then the surgeon and anesthesiologist should be notified.**

3. A variance report should be completed because the item should have been removed before the client arrived to the holding area. Tongue rings increase the risk of aspiration, burns, and injury during surgery.

4. Notifying the surgeon and the anesthesiologist is not the initial action. If the client removes the tongue ring, the surgeon and anesthesiologist would not need to be notified.

▶ *Test-taking Tip: Note the key word "initial." Use the nursing process. The nurse has already assessed and analyzed information. The next step is implementation.*

Content Area: Fundamentals; Concept: Safety; Perioperative; Integrated Processes: Nursing Process: Implementation; Client Needs: Physiological Integrity: Reduction of Risk Potential; Cognitive Level: Application [Applying]

## 641. ANSWER: 3

1. Although the client is hypothermic, applying additional warm blankets is not the priority.

2. Although the client is tachycardic with a low-normal BP, oxygenation is the priority.

3. **Oxygen is indicated because the client has low oxygen saturation and is hypoventilating; hypoventilation is a common effect of general anesthesia.**

4. Although the nurse should assess the surgical site, this is not the priority.

▶ *Test-taking Tip: You should address the ABC's before addressing other problems. Option 4 can be eliminated because this is an assessment and not an intervention.*

Content Area: Fundamentals; Concept: Oxygenation; Integrated Processes: Nursing Process: Implementation; Client Needs: Physiological Integrity: Reduction of Risk Potential; Cognitive Level: Analysis [Analyzing]

## 642. ANSWER: 2

1. An abdominal breathing pattern is an indication of muscle weakness and is a poor sign in the postoperative client.

2. **The purpose of an oral airway is to prevent the tongue from blocking the airway. Oxygen saturation of 92% is within the normal range.**

3. If the cause of the airway obstruction were secretions, the intervention would be suctioning, and the evaluation of the effectiveness would be clear lung sounds.

4. Although VS may vary with airway obstruction, it is not a measure for determining the effectiveness of the oral airway in relieving the obstruction.

▶ *Test-taking Tip: Be clear about what the question is asking. Only one option indicates an effective breathing pattern.*

Content Area: Fundamentals; Concept: Oxygenation; Integrated Processes: Nursing Process: Evaluation; Client Needs: Physiological Integrity: Reduction of Risk Potential; Cognitive Level: Evaluation [Evaluating]

## 643. PHARM ANSWER: 2

1. Flumazenil (Romazicon) antagonizes the effects of benzodiazepines on the CNS. It does not reverse the effect of opioids.

2. **Naloxone hydrochloride (Narcan) is an antagonist for opioids and is used for reversing the respiratory-depressive effects of opioid analgesics.**

3. Digoxin immune fab (Digibind) is an antagonist for digoxin and digitoxin, thereby preventing the drug binding at receptor sites.

4. Protamine sulfate is an antidote for heparin. Because it is strongly basic and heparin is acidic, it neutralizes the effect of both drugs.

▶ *Test-taking Tip: Focus on the key word "antagonistic." Look for the drug that reverses the effects of morphine sulfate.*

Content Area: Fundamentals; Concept: Medication; Integrated Processes: Nursing Process: Implementation; Client Needs: Safe and Effective Care Environment: Safety and Infection Control; Physiological Integrity: Pharmacological and Parenteral Therapies; Cognitive Level: Knowledge [Remembering]

## 644. ANSWER: 1

1. **The client is experiencing hyponatremia (serum sodium level less than 135 milliequivalents [mEq/L]), likely from fluid volume excess. When hyponatremia is caused by hypervolemia, treatment is fluid restriction.**

2. Hypertonic solutions are prescribed when there is hypernatremia with fluid volume deficit. The usual rate is 3 milliliters per kilogram per hour (mL/kg/hr).

3. Osmotic diuretics, rather than loop diuretics such as furosemide (Lasix), are prescribed. Water, potassium, and sodium loss occur with loop diuretics.

4. A low-sodium diet would not raise the serum sodium level, which is low.

▶ *Test-taking Tip: Note that the serum sodium level is low and that the client has signs of hypervolemia. Remember that hemodilution can cause hyponatremia. Normal serum sodium is 135 to 145 mEq/L.*

Content Area: Fundamentals; Concept: Fluid and Electrolyte Balance; Integrated Processes: Nursing Process: Analysis; Client Needs: Physiological Integrity: Physiological Adaptation; Cognitive Level: Analysis [Analyzing]

## 645. ANSWER: 1

1. **Due to the client's limited ability to ambulate, the client should continue to wear the antiembolic stockings at home to prevent DVT. The stockings should be removed one to two times daily for skin care and inspection.**

2. A diet high in protein, calories, and vitamin C will promote wound healing.

3. A nonpharmacological method to reduce postoperative pain and promote comfort includes ice application.

4. Specific volume goals are usually set based on the client's ability and the type of IS. Achievement of the volume goal is an expected postoperative outcome that should be met prior to discharge.

▶ *Test-taking Tip: Focus on the key words "limited ability to ambulate." Antiembolic stockings will promote venous return.*

**Content Area:** Fundamentals; **Concept:** Nursing Roles; Clotting; **Integrated Processes:** Teaching/Learning; **Client Needs:** Health Promotion and Maintenance; Physiological Integrity: Reduction of Risk Potential; **Cognitive Level:** Application [Applying]

## 646. ANSWER: 2

1. NG drainage with a "coffee-ground" appearance indicates old bleeding.
2. **Normal NG drainage fluid is greenish-yellow in color.**
3. The pH of gastric secretions would be acidic, not alkalotic.
4. Large amounts of output would be expected because it is unlikely that the client's stomach was empty when inserted in an emergency.

▶ *Test-taking Tip: Rule out options by focusing on the purpose of the NG tube in this situation.*

**Content Area:** Fundamentals; **Concept:** Nursing Roles; **Integrated Processes:** Nursing Process: Evaluation; **Client Needs:** Physiological Integrity: Reduction of Risk Potential; **Cognitive Level:** Evaluation [Evaluating]

## 647. ANSWER: 1

1. **Illustration 1 demonstrates proper care of the JP drain. It is compressed to provide suction, the cap is secure, and the drain is secured to the client's clothing to prevent traction on the skin.**
2. In Illustration 2, the JP drain is capped and secured but is not compressed; the drain will not provide suction.
3. In Illustration 3, the JP drain is capped and compressed but is not secured to the client's clothing; the drain could become entangled and dislodge.
4. In Illustration 4, the JP drain is not capped, compressed, or secured; this increases the risk for infection.

▶ *Test-taking Tip: Remember that the wound drainage systems need to be compressed to allow for negative pressure. Maintain aseptic technique when handling the cap to empty the drain, and secure the drain so that it does not pull on the client's skin.*

**Content Area:** Fundamentals; **Concept:** Safety; **Integrated Processes:** Nursing Process: Evaluation; **Client Needs:** Safe and Effective Care Environment: Safety and Infection Control; **Cognitive Level:** Evaluation [Evaluating]

## 648. ANSWER: 3

1. If intermittent urinary catheterization has not been prescribed, the HCP will want to know the urine volume result from the bladder scan.
2. A urinary catheter should be inserted only if the client has a full bladder and other measures to initiate voiding have been unsuccessful.

3. **A bladder scan will inform the nurse about the urine volume in the bladder and whether intermittent urinary catheterization is indicated.**
4. Reviewing the chart for the amount of the last void may assist in determining if there is a problem, but knowing the amount currently in the bladder is more important.

▶ *Test-taking Tip: Use the steps in the nursing process to identify the answer. Assessment should be completed before interventions are implemented.*

**Content Area:** Fundamentals; **Concept:** Urinary Elimination; **Integrated Processes:** Nursing Process: Assessment; **Client Needs:** Physiological Integrity: Basic Care and Comfort; **Cognitive Level:** Application [Applying]

## 649. ANSWER: 2

1. The surgeon as well as the anesthesiologist should be notified of the client's symptoms, especially if the headache persists despite interventions or there is noticeable leakage of CSF, but this is not the initial intervention.
2. **The client is experiencing a postdural puncture headache caused by leakage of CSF from the needle insertion into the dura for the spinal anesthetic. Placing the client in the flat position minimizes the leakage of CSF.**
3. Fluids should be increased to hydrate the client and replace fluids lost from the CSF leakage, but first the anesthesiologist and surgeon should be notified.
4. If the headache persists, steroids may be prescribed to decrease inflammation, but this is not an initial intervention.

▶ *Test-taking Tip: Note the key word "initial." Positioning the client flat in bed can be accomplished quickly to reduce the client's headache.*

**Content Area:** Fundamentals; **Concept:** Nursing Roles; Perioperative; **Integrated Processes:** Nursing Process: Implementation; **Client Needs:** Physiological Integrity: Physiological Adaptation; **Cognitive Level:** Application [Applying]

## 650. ANSWER: 2

1. The total WBC count should be elevated, not decreased. However, this does not describe the left shift.
2. **An early indication of infection is an increase in the band cells, which are immature neutrophils in the WBC differential count. The increase is termed a *shift to the left*.**
3. Although eosinophils are a component of the WBC differential count, they are associated with an allergic reaction and not an infection.
4. An increased C-reactive protein indicates nonspecific inflammation and is not part of the WBC differential count.

▶ *Test-taking Tip: Associate key words "WBC differential" with words in the options. Decreased Hgb and increased C-reactive protein do not pertain to the WBC count.*

Content Area: Fundamentals; **Concept:** Infection; **Integrated Processes:** Nursing Process: Analysis; **Client Needs:** Physiological Integrity: Reduction of Risk Potential; **Cognitive Level:** Analysis [Analyzing]

## 651. PHARM **ANSWER: 2**

1. Early postoperative ambulation instead of dangling is a major technique for preventing thrombophlebitis.
2. **Enoxaparin (Lovenox), an anticoagulant that potentiates the inhibitory effect of antithrombin on factor Xa and thrombin, is given to prevent postoperative thrombophlebitis and pulmonary embolism.**
3. Hydromorphone (Dilaudid) is a narcotic analgesic for pain control.
4. IS use and coughing promote lung expansion and removal of secretions. These help to prevent atelectasis and pneumonia.

▶ **Test-taking Tip:** *An anticoagulant is often administered after surgery to prevent thrombophlebitis and pulmonary embolism.*

Content Area: Fundamentals; **Concept:** Clotting; Medication; **Integrated Processes:** Nursing Process: Analysis; **Client Needs:** Physiological Integrity: Pharmacological and Parenteral Therapies; Physiological Integrity: Reduction of Risk Potential; **Cognitive Level:** Analysis [Analyzing]

## 652. ANSWER: 1

1. **Atelectasis is a common finding in smokers after surgery due to the accumulation of secretions. It is caused from collapsed alveoli or mucus that prevents some alveoli from opening. It manifests with diminished breath sounds, diminished vital capacity, and decreased oxygen saturation.**
2. There is no indication, such as elevated temperature or increased WBCs, that the client has an infection.
3. The findings are abnormal for the second postoperative day.
4. The diminished lung bases suggest alveoli are not expanding. The problem is not occurring at the trachea or bronchus, indicating a possible airway obstruction.

▶ **Test-taking Tip:** *The client is 2 days postsurgery. You need to think about the most common respiratory problem in the postsurgical client.*

Content Area: Fundamentals; **Concept:** Oxygenation; Nursing Roles; **Integrated Processes:** Nursing Process: Analysis; **Client Needs:** Physiological Integrity: Physiological Adaptation; **Cognitive Level:** Analysis [Analyzing]

## 653. ANSWER: 2

1. Secretions could still be present in the lungs with normal respirations and unlabored breathing.
2. **The purpose of postoperative C&DB is to expel secretions, keep the lungs clear, allow full aeration, and prevent atelectasis and pneumonia. Auscultating for clear and audible lung sounds is a definitive means for evaluating the effectiveness of C&DB.**

3. Coughing up clear secretions indicates that mucus may still be present in the lungs.
4. A productive cough indicates that secretions are still present in the lungs.

▶ **Test-taking Tip:** *Often the option that is different from the other options is the answer. Only Option 2 includes an assessment other than observation.*

Content Area: Fundamentals; **Concept:** Nursing Roles; Oxygenation; **Integrated Processes:** Nursing Process: Evaluation; **Client Needs:** Physiological Integrity: Reduction of Risk Potential; **Cognitive Level:** Evaluation [Evaluating]

## 654. ANSWER: 3

1. These are not normal findings. Slight crusting, a pink color to the incision line, and slight swelling under the sutures or staples are normal for the second postoperative day due to inflammation from the procedure.
2. Although these findings could indicate rejection of the sutures, rejection occurs less frequently than a wound infection.
3. **Redness, swelling, and warmth are signs of inflammation and could indicate the presence of an infection. Other signs of an infection include excessive pain or tenderness on palpation and purulent or odorous drainage.**
4. Bloody or serosanguineous drainage would be present if the wound were dehiscing.

▶ **Test-taking Tip:** *Narrow the options by eliminating the extreme interpretations.*

Content Area: Fundamentals; **Concept:** Inflammation; Nursing Roles; **Integrated Processes:** Nursing Process: Analysis; **Client Needs:** Physiological Integrity: Reduction of Risk Potential; **Cognitive Level:** Analysis [Analyzing]

## 655. MoC **ANSWER: 1, 4, 2, 3**

1. **The client who had a thyroidectomy 4 hours ago and reports inability to swallow. This client should be assessed first because the client's airway is in imminent danger of compromise.**
4. **The client who reports a sudden increase in bloody drainage on the surgical bandage. The sudden increase in bloody drainage could indicate hemorrhage.**
2. **The client admitted 1 hour ago from PACU has incisional pain at 7 on a 0 to 10 scale. Although pain should be managed, the other two clients are priority.**
3. **The client who had a TAH yesterday and reports nausea. This client is relatively stable but needs medication for nausea.**

▶ **Test-taking Tip:** *Use the ABC's to establish priority. Airway issues take precedence; hemorrhage (circulation) is the next priority. Acute pain in the client who has just had surgery is more urgent than nausea in the stable client.*

Content Area: Fundamentals; **Concept:** Critical Thinking; Management; **Integrated Processes:** Nursing Process: Planning; **Client Needs:** Safe and Effective Care Environment: Management of Care; **Cognitive Level:** Synthesis [Creating]

**656.** PHARM **ANSWER: 2**

1. Without first questioning the client, the nurse has insufficient information to give to the HCP about the client's reaction. Simply offering a different medication avoids the client's feelings.

2. **The nurse is using the therapeutic communication technique, known as clarifying, to determine the effects of the medication on the client. This focuses on the client's feelings.**

3. Offering an antacid assumes that the client has a GI reaction.

4. Oxycodone/acetaminophen (Percocet) does not contain aspirin. Offering a cracker assumes the client has a GI reaction.

▶ *Test-taking Tip: Use therapeutic communication techniques and focus on the client's concern to collect additional information. Only one option focuses on the client.*

**Content Area:** Fundamentals; **Concept:** Medication; Communication; **Integrated Processes:** Communication and Documentation; Caring; **Client Needs:** Psychosocial Integrity; Physiological Integrity: Pharmacological and Parenteral Therapies; **Cognitive Level:** Application [Applying]

**657.** MoC **ANSWER: 1**

1. **Paralytic ileus (paralysis of the intestinal muscles) is a typical complication of abdominal surgery. Manifestations include distended abdomen, abdominal pain, absence of flatus, diminished or absent bowel sounds, and sometimes nausea and vomiting.**

2. The client would not have any signs or symptoms with silent peritonitis.

3. The distended abdomen could indicate that fluid may have shifted into the abdomen. However, fluid volume deficit would then occur and not excess.

4. There is an interference with absorption of nutrients in malabsorption syndrome. Typical manifestations include weight loss, bloating and flatus, edema, bone pain, anemia, easy bruising, and decreased libido.

▶ *Test-taking Tip: Note the key words "typical complication" and eliminate options that occur over a longer period of time.*

**Content Area:** Fundamentals; **Concept:** Collaboration; Management; Perioperative; **Integrated Processes:** Nursing Process: Analysis; **Client Needs:** Safe and Effective Care Environment: Management of Care; **Cognitive Level:** Analysis [Analyzing]

**658. ANSWER: 2**

1. Surgery stresses the body, and time and rest are needed for healing. The client should return to work only after consulting with the surgeon. If work involves a moderate amount of physical labor, up to 6 weeks or more time off may be needed for recovery.

2. **In addition to vitamins and iron, supplemental vitamin C and a diet high in protein and calories will promote wound healing.**

3. Daily walking should be encouraged, but carrying 10-lb weights or lifting heavy objects stresses the incision. Although the wound may appear to be healed in 2 to 3 weeks, it takes up to 2 years for complete wound healing and strengthening of the scar.

4. A referral is made to a home-care agency if skilled nursing care is needed such as complex dressing changes. Nursing service does not include household help.

▶ *Test-taking Tip: Narrow the options by eliminating options with extremes, Options 1 and 3. Then note the key words "nursing" and "help around the house" in Option 4 to eliminate this option.*

**Content Area:** Fundamentals; **Concept:** Nursing Roles; Perioperative; **Integrated Processes:** Teaching/Learning; **Client Needs:** Physiological Integrity: Physiological Adaptation; **Cognitive Level:** Analysis [Analyzing]

**659. ANSWER: 305**

**575 mL – 150 mL = 425 mL of drainage in the container**

**30 mL × 4 = 120 mL of irrigation solution**

**425 mL – 120 mL = 305 mL of actual drainage**

▶ *Test-taking Tip: Be sure to subtract the before shift amount of 150 mL and the amount of irrigation solution used to obtain the correct amount of output from 0700 to 1500 hours.*

**Content Area:** Fundamentals; **Concept:** Nursing Roles; **Integrated Processes:** Nursing Process: Implementation; **Client Needs:** Safe and Effective Care Environment: Safety and Infection Control; **Cognitive Level:** Analysis [Analyzing]

**660. ANSWER:**

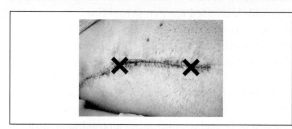

**A nonapproximated incision is one in which wound edges are not closed. The wound will close by secondary intention healing.**

▶ *Test-taking Tip: Read the stem carefully, noting the words "not approximated." Eliminate puncture sites.*

**Content Area:** Fundamentals; **Concept:** Assessment; Perioperative; **Integrated Processes:** Nursing Process: Assessment; **Client Needs:** Physiological Integrity: Reduction of Risk Potential; **Cognitive Level:** Application [Applying]

**661.** PHARM CJ **ANSWER: 2**

1. Unless the client is showing symptoms of inadequate tissue perfusion, blood would not be replaced with a Hgb level of 11.0.

2. **The nurse should plan to administer potassium. A low serum potassium (K) level can cause cardiac dysrhythmias. Potassium is lost through NG suctioning and tissue destruction. The potassium needs to be replaced immediately.**

3. The nurse should be alert for the development of hyperkalemia, not hypokalemia, with ACE inhibitors such as enalapril (Vasotec), especially if the client has DM, impaired kidney function, or CHF.

4. Calcium gluconate is given in acute hypocalcemia to replace calcium, or when the serum potassium level is elevated to raise the threshold for cardiac muscle excitation and prevent life-threatening dysrhythmias. Neither situation is present.

▶ **Test-taking Tip:** *Use the ABC's to determine the priority intervention. Both the serum K level and the Hgb/Hct affect oxygenation and circulation. However, the low serum K level is more critical than the low Hgb/Hct level because the serum K level affects cardiac muscle function.*

**Content Area:** Fundamentals; **Concept:** Fluid and Electrolyte Balance; Medication; **Integrated Processes:** Nursing Process: Analysis; **Client Needs:** Physiological Integrity: Pharmacological and Parenteral Therapies; Physiological Integrity: Physiological Adaptation; **Cognitive Level:** Analysis [Analyzing]

**662.** CJ MoC **ANSWER:**

---
**BUN and creatinine**
---

**An elevated BUN and serum creatinine may indicate either impaired renal function or dehydration.**

▶ **Test-taking Tip:** *Narrow the options to only those with abnormal values.*

**Content Area:** Fundamentals; **Concept:** Assessment; Perioperative; **Integrated Processes:** Nursing Process: Planning; **Client Needs:** Safe and Effective Care Environment: Management of Care; **Cognitive Level:** Application [Applying]

**663.** MoC **ANSWER: 1**

1. **Because the client lives alone and needs to use the nondominant hand for dressing changes, the nurse should collaborate with a social worker or case manager to arrange for home health services for skilled nursing care to assist with daily dressing changes.**

2. Collaboration with the multidisciplinary team is necessary if the client needs transportation assistance, but skilled nursing care does not provide this service.

3. Collaboration with the multidisciplinary team is unnecessary if the client is able to demonstrate necessary self-care measures.

4. Collaboration with the multidisciplinary team is unnecessary if the client is able to manage self-administration of home medications.

▶ **Test-taking Tip:** *The nurse should evaluate the client's ability to perform self-care prior to discharge. If unable to perform self-care measures and support systems are unavailable such as significant others, then the nurse should collaborate with interdisciplinary team members, such as a case manager or social worker, to obtain the needed services. Although the client needs both skilled nursing care and transportation, select the option that pertains to the role of the nurse.*

**Content Area:** Fundamentals; **Concept:** Collaboration; Management; **Integrated Processes:** Nursing Process: Planning; **Client Needs:** Safe and Effective Care Environment: Management of Care; **Cognitive Level:** Application [Applying]

## Chapter Seventeen

# Disaster Preparedness and Basic Life Support

**664.** The nurse has been asked to review an agency's emergency response plan as a member of the Emergency Operations Committee. Which components should the nurse identify for inclusion in the agency's emergency plan? **Select all that apply.**

1. The emergency response number of 911
2. A plan for internal and external communication
3. Documentation of available external resources
4. The agency plan for performing practice drills
5. List of expendable resources that may be needed
6. Methods to be used for educating agency personnel

**665.** MoC The hospital is overloaded with victims from a tornado that leveled a nearby community of 75,000 people, and the hospital is short-staffed. Which actions might be necessary in this situation? **Select all that apply.**

1. Nurses performing duties outside of their expertise
2. Family providing nonskilled care to their children
3. Giving care to persons with extensive injuries and little chance of survival first
4. Setting up a hospital ward in a community shelter
5. Asking if anyone can interpret for clients who only speak a foreign language

**666.** MoC Five families of clients injured in an apartment fire come to the ED to ask about the status of their family members. Which is the nurse's **best** action?

1. Take the families to the triage area so they can be with their loved ones.
2. Ask the families to wait in the waiting area until information is available.
3. Have families taken to a designated room that is staffed by a social worker or clergy.
4. Direct families to a lounge where a receptionist will keep families informed.

**667.** MoC The hospital's disaster response plan is initiated to prepare for receiving victims from a bridge collapse. To increase bed capacity, which clients on a maternal-infant unit should the nurse identify as appropriate for discharge? **Select all that apply.**

1. The 1-day-old healthy full-term infant with a strong suck; mother is healthy
2. The 2-day-old infant with a total serum bilirubin of 16 mg/dL; mother is healthy
3. The multipara woman who delivered 20 hours ago and has an intact perineum
4. The woman who had a cesarean section; just put on IV antibiotics for an infection
5. The infant born 28 hours ago who was at 34 weeks of gestation; mother is fatigued

**668.** The community nurse is teaching disaster preparedness to community members. Which statement is **most** appropriate?

1. "Yearly, discard and replace the disaster kit's supply of bottled water."
2. "Keep on hand a 3-day supply of water, 1 gallon per person per day."
3. "Animals will be able to fend for themselves for a few days in a disaster."
4. "Include a 1-day supply of food for each person in the disaster kit."

**669.** Clients who were exposed to a white phosphorus chemical spill are arriving to the ED. Which intervention should the nurse plan to do **first**?

1. Triage clients before transport to designated areas.
2. Put on personal protective equipment (PPE).
3. Flush the clients' skin and clothing with water.
4. Brush the chemical off of the clients' skin.

**670.** An explosion occurred at a nearby factory. The ED charge nurse receives a call from EMS personnel that 35 clients will arrive by ambulance within 10 minutes. These clients were triaged at the scene as red and yellow according to the NATO mass casualty categories; others will be arriving, and the unit is short-staffed. Which action should the nurse initiate **first?**

1. Activate the hospital's emergency response plan.
2. Contact the ED's director of nursing.
3. Notify other nurses of the need for extra help.
4. See if 15 clients could be rerouted to another facility.

**671.** A passenger train derailed with more than 500 casualties. The nurse is receiving clients who were triaged according to the NATO triage system. Place the clients in the order in which they should be further assessed and treated.

1. Client with an upper arm fracture and minor burn tagged as green
2. Client who has wounds involving multiple anatomical sites tagged as black
3. Client who has an incomplete leg amputation tagged as red
4. Client who has an eye injury, broken jaw, and facial wounds tagged as yellow

Answer: _____

**672.** PHARM The ED charge nurse is informed that an unknown number of clients were exposed to a nerve agent. Which medication should the nurse plan to have available in sufficient quantities to treat the clients?

1. Atropine sulfate
2. Labetalol
3. Dopamine
4. Phentolamine

**673.** MoC PHARM Clients from an alleged inhalation anthrax exposure are being admitted to an ED. Which actions should the nurse plan in treating the clients? **Select all that apply.**

1. Don level D personal protective equipment (PPE).
2. Prepare to administer ciprofloxacin orally.
3. Prepare to give postexposure prophylaxis (PEP).
4. Assess for dyspnea, fever, cough, or chest pain.
5. Prepare clients to receive an abdominal x-ray.

**674.** MoC The triage nurse in an ED is caring for clients injured in a mass casualty disaster. Which client should the nurse establish as the **priority** client?

1. Unresponsive client with a penetrating head injury
2. Partially responsive client with a sucking chest wound
3. Client with a maxilla fracture and facial wounds without airway compromise
4. Client with third-degree burns over 65% of the body surface area

**675.** An emergency trauma center receives a call to expect to receive the infant illustrated. Which precautions should the nurse plan when preparing for the infant's care? **Select all that apply.**

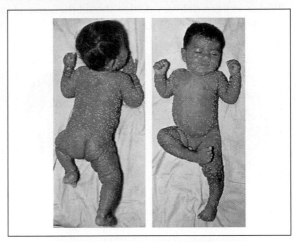

1. Placing the infant in a negative-air-pressure isolation room
2. Wearing a surgical mask when in contact with the infant's lesions
3. Wearing an N95 (HEPA) particulate mask when in contact with the infant
4. Wearing gloves and a gown when entering the room to assess the infant
5. Notifying the Centers for Disease Control of possible bioterrorism
6. Decontaminating the infant because of suspected smallpox exposure

**676.** MoC The nurse is triaging four clients who enter the ED at the same time. Which client should be assigned as the **highest** priority?

1. The 16-year-old with a severe sunburn injury that is blistering
2. The 55-year-old client experiencing dyspnea, diaphoresis, and chest pain
3. The 40-year-old client with a leg laceration that appears to need stitches
4. The 19-year-old who has headaches, diplopia, and fever of 102.8°F (39.3°C)

**677.** MoC The school nurse is planning an intervention program for children who lost their homes due to a tornado and are now residing in temporary housing. Which group should be the nurse's **initial** focus?

1. Older age female children of higher socioeconomic status
2. Older age male children of higher socioeconomic status
3. Younger age female children of lower socioeconomic status
4. Younger age male children of lower socioeconomic status

**678.** The client is in respiratory distress following exposure to an unknown substance, and requires oxygen. Which oxygen delivery device should the nurse plan to select to deliver an $F_{IO_2}$ of 100%?

1.

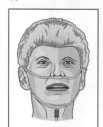

2.

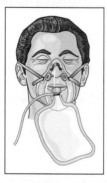

3.

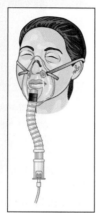

4.

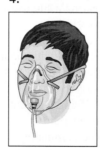

**679.** Members of a resuscitation team arrive at the client's bedside with a defibrillator. The nurse and an NA are performing CPR. What should the nurse do **next**?

1. Stop CPR while the resuscitation team applies the conduction pads and analyzes the rhythm.
2. Complete a full minute of CPR, then apply the conduction pads and analyze the rhythm.
3. Continue with CPR while the conduction pads are being applied and the rhythm analyzed.
4. Continue with CPR until the resuscitation team is ready to analyze the rhythm.

**680.** The nurse applies AED pads to the client's chest, and a shock is advised. What should the nurse do **next**?

1. Push the AED button to deliver a shock.
2. Clear everyone from touching the client.
3. Place the client into the shock position.
4. Nothing; the AED will deliver a shock.

**681.** When placing defibrillator pads on the client, the nurse observes that the client possibly has an implanted pacemaker on the left upper chest. Which statement demonstrates that the nurse knows where to correctly place the defibrillator pad?

1. "One of the defibrillator pads should be placed directly over the pacemaker."
2. "The defibrillator pads should be placed at least 8 cm away from the pacemaker."
3. "The pads should not be used because defibrillation may damage the pacemaker."
4. "One defibrillator pad should be placed on the upper back, the other a little lower."

**682.** While jogging, the nurse finds an adult lying on the ground. The nurse determines that the client is unresponsive. What should the nurse do **next**?

1. Dial 911 to activate emergency medical services.
2. Check whether the carotid pulse is present.
3. Open the airway by the head-tilt, chin-lift method.
4. Do chest compressions at a rate of 100 per minute.

**683.** PHARM The nurse is to administer epinephrine 1 mg to the client during a cardiac arrest. Epinephrine injection 1:10,000 is supplied in a syringe for administration. The 10-mL syringe states 0.1 mg/mL. How many milliliters should the nurse administer?

_____ mL (Record your answer as a whole number.)

**684.** MoC During resuscitation efforts of a trauma victim, the spouse tells the nurse that her husband has terminal cancer, has completed an advance HCD, and does not want CPR. What should be the nurse's **next** action?

1. Contact medical records to see if the client's HCD is on file.
2. In honor of the client's wishes, stop the resuscitation team's actions.
3. Document the spouse's statement in the client's medical record.
4. Inform the HCP in charge of the resuscitation team.

**685.** The client's spouse is allowed to be present during resuscitation efforts. Which statement made by the nurse is **most** appropriate?

1. "Hold your loved one's hand; sometimes a recovering person will remember that touch."
2. "I will show you where you can stand near your husband; another staff will be with you."
3. "The resuscitation team needs to work quickly, so stay out of the way and do not interfere."
4. "If resuscitation fails, the HCP will ask you if you want resuscitation efforts terminated."

**686.** Two nurses are performing CPR on an adult. The nurse performing chest compressions is on the right side of the client, and the nurse performing rescue breathing is on the left. The nurse performing rescue breathing checks the client's pulse to determine if the nurse's compressions are perfusing. Place an X at the location where the nurse should check the client's pulse.

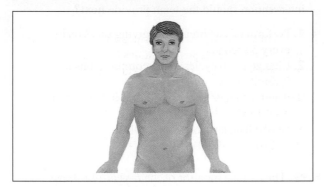

**687.** The nurse is teaching rescue breathing to the son of an adult client. Which statement indicates the son understands how to perform rescue breathing?

1. "I should provide one breath every 5 to 6 seconds."
2. "I should provide one breath every 3 seconds."
3. "I should provide at least 20 breaths per minute."
4. "I should provide a breath every few minutes."

**688.** MoC The nurse finds an unresponsive, pulseless client lying in a puddle of water in a shower. The resuscitation team would like to attach the AED to the client immediately. What intervention should the nurse implement **first**?

1. Assist with defibrillator pad placement quickly to facilitate early defibrillation.
2. Assist the team to move the client from the puddle of water before defibrillation.
3. Dry the chest off and place the defibrillator pads on the client's anterior chest.
4. Ensure that the team is performing adequate compressions during defibrillation.

**689.** The nurse finds an unresponsive adult client. What should the nurse do? **Select all that apply.**

1. Assess the client's pulse for at least 15 seconds.
2. Quickly activate emergency medical services.
3. Provide 100 chest compressions over a minute.
4. Auscultate the client's heart and lung sounds.
5. Use the fist to quickly hit the client's chest.

**690.** The nurse is providing postresuscitation care to the client. The client's HR is 80 bpm, and the RR is 14 breaths per minute and regular. Which action should the nurse perform **next**?

1. Resume with bag-valve-mask ventilations at a rate of one breath every 6 seconds.
2. Continue the chest compressions at a depth of 2 inches and rate of 100 per minute.
3. Monitor the client closely until advanced life support personnel arrive at the scene.
4. Press the "analyze" button on the AED to decide if defibrillation is needed at this time.

**691.** The nurse is performing abdominal thrusts on a conscious, choking client. Place the nurse's actions in the sequence in which they should be performed.

1. Place both arms around the person's waist.
2. Place the thumb side of the fist against the person's abdomen above the navel and below the xiphoid process.
3. Press upward with firm, quick thrusts 6 to 10 times until the obstruction is cleared.
4. Stand behind the person who is choking.
5. Grasp the fist with the other hand.

Answer: _____

**692.** The nurse enters the client's room and notes the client in the position illustrated. Which action should be taken by the nurse?

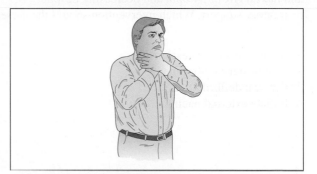

1. Immediately yell for help.
2. Ask the client if he is okay.
3. Ask the client if he is choking.
4. Call for the acute response team.

**693.** The adult client reports to the nurse that he feels like he is choking. The client is coughing loudly, and his skin is acyanotic. What should the nurse do **next**?

1. Monitor the client closely for any deterioration.
2. Implement immediate use of the Heimlich maneuver.
3. Assist the client to the floor and begin rescue breathing.
4. Perform chest thrusts over the lower half of the sternum.

**694.** The nurse sees the coworker assisting the pregnant client who appears to be choking. The coworker's fist and hand placement is appropriate. Which location **best** describes the coworker's hand placement?

1. At the level of the sternum
2. At the level of the umbilicus
3. Between the umbilicus and the sternum
4. At the level of the sternal notch

**695.** During transport for an emergency surgery, the client experiences a cardiac arrest and dies. The client's family witnesses the arrest and is present when the client is pronounced dead. Which action by the nurse **best** demonstrates compassionate care?

1. Explaining the actions of the code team in trying to save the life of their loved one
2. Accompanying the family to a waiting room where they can contact other relatives
3. Closing doors to allow the family to be alone with their loved one to say good-bye
4. Asking questions to determine if there was some underlying cause for the arrest

**696.** The nurse is caring for the 4-year-old with respiratory distress. The child has pale, cool skin; is hypotensive; and has an HR of 54 bpm and decreasing despite respiratory support. Which intervention should the nurse implement?

1. Begin chest compressions.
2. Administer IV atropine.
3. Perform defibrillation.
4. Initiate external pacing.

**697.** The resuscitation team has been performing CPR on the child for 15 minutes. The mother, who is present, asks when CPR would be stopped. What is the **most** appropriate response by the nurse?

1. "The physician will consider the amount of time passed before CPR is started and multiple factors before making a decision to stop CPR."
2. "Every effort will be made to save your child. Sometimes CPR is performed for a long time, and a child is revived."
3. "The physician will likely ask you about your feelings before making the decision to terminate CPR."
4. "You seem concerned. Are you worried that CPR will be stopped too soon or that it will be performed too long?'

**698.** The nurse is performing CPR on the 5-year-old in asystolic cardiac arrest. A second rescuer arrives. The client remains pulseless and apneic. What intervention should the team provide **next?**

1. Perform rescue breathing, giving one breath every 5 seconds.
2. Change to 10 cycles of 15 compressions to 2 ventilations.
3. Continue chest compressions at a depth of at least 1 inch.
4. Defibrillate as soon as possible at 1 joule per kilogram.

**699.** The cardiac monitor of the 6-year-old shows ventricular fibrillation. Which interventions should the two responding nurses implement? **Select all that apply.**

1. Auscultate the child's apical pulse for 10 seconds.
2. Activate the facility emergency response system.
3. Provide at least 100 chest compressions per minute.
4. Prepare to cardiovert the child as soon as possible.
5. Prepare to defibrillate the child as soon as possible.

**700.** The nurse is performing CPR on a neonate. Which action indicates that the nurse needs further instruction on performing CPR on a neonate?

1. Compresses the chest with two thumbs while the fingers encircle the chest.
2. Delivers chest compressions on the lower third of the neonate's sternum.
3. Completes a total of 100 compressions and 30 breaths over each minute.
4. Raises the thumbs an inch from the chest between chest compressions.

**701.** Resuscitation efforts have been provided for 2 minutes for the 4-month-old in cardiac arrest, and CPR is now paused. The cardiac monitor shows sinus tachycardia. What action should the nurse take **next**?

1. Check the brachial pulse.
2. Ready the defibrillator.
3. Check for breathing.
4. Prepare for transport.

**702.** The nurse is attempting to relieve a foreign body airway obstruction from an infant. The infant suddenly becomes unresponsive. Which action should the nurse perform **next**?

1. Begin delivering back blows.
2. Go and locate an AED.
3. Begin chest compressions.
4. Deliver rescue breathing.

## Answers and Rationales

**664. ANSWER: 2, 3, 4, 5, 6**

1. An activation response defines where, how, and when the response is initiated. Calling 911 would not be an appropriate activation.
2. **Communication to and from the prehospital arena and to all parties involved is needed for a rapid and orderly response to a disaster.**
3. **Local, state, and federal resources should be identified as well as how to activate these resources.**
4. **Practice drills with community participation allow for troubleshooting problems before an event happens and give persons an opportunity to practice their roles.**
5. **Expendable resources such as food, water, and supplies must be available and sources for these identified.**
6. **Educating personnel allows for improved readiness and additional input for refining the process.**

▶ *Test-taking Tip: Read each option carefully to determine if the option is a necessary component for a health care facility to respond to a disaster.*

Content Area: Management of Care; **Concept:** Safety; Trauma; **Integrated Processes:** Communication and Documentation; **Client Needs:** Safe and Effective Care Environment: Safety and Infection Control; Physiological Integrity: Basic Care and Comfort; **Cognitive Level:** Application [Applying]

**665. MoC ANSWER: 1, 2, 4, 5**

1. **Due to staff shortages, nurses may be asked to take on responsibilities normally held by HCPs or advanced practice nurses.**
2. **When insufficient health care personnel are available, family members may take on nonskilled responsibilities.**
3. Victims with extensive injuries and unlikely to survive should be triaged and treated last. Nursing care in a disaster focuses on essential care from the perspective of what is best for all persons.
4. **In a disaster, care may need to be provided outside of the hospital setting.**

5. **Although client confidentially is important, a medical emergency may require the services of laypersons to interpret for non–English-speaking clients.**

▶ *Test-taking Tip: In a disaster, atypical roles occur for health care personnel, victims, and families. Consider whether each option contributes to providing essential care from the perspective of what is best for all persons given the circumstances.*

Content Area: Management of Care; **Concept:** Critical Thinking; Management; Legal; Trauma; **Integrated Processes:** Nursing Process: Implementation; Culture and Spirituality; **Client Needs:** Safe and Effective Care Environment: Management of Care; Safe and Effective Care Environment: Safety and Infection Control; **Cognitive Level:** Application [Applying]

**666. MoC ANSWER: 3**

1. To protect the privacy of other clients and to prevent congestion or interference with treatment measures, families should not be in the triage or treatment areas.
2. Support systems would be unavailable in a waiting area or in a lounge.
3. **Families should be in a designated area where social workers, counselors, therapists, or clergy members are available for support. Family should be provided with information and updates as soon as possible.**
4. Family members may be feeling intense anxiety, shock, or grief. A receptionist would not have the expertise to handle these emotions.

▶ *Test-taking Tip: Think about the support families will need in coping with disaster-related injuries or death, and select the option that would provide the families with the most support.*

Content Area: Management of Care; **Concept:** Family; Management; Trauma; **Integrated Processes:** Nursing Process: Implementation; **Client Needs:** Safe and Effective Care Environment: Management of Care; Psychosocial Integrity; **Cognitive Level:** Application [Applying]

**667. MoC ANSWER: 1, 2, 3**

1. **The 1-day-old healthy infant and the infant's mother can be discharged because they are both healthy.**

2. **Although the 2-day-old infant has an elevated serum bilirubin, a home phototherapy blanket can be prescribed. Phototherapy is prescribed when the total serum bilirubin level rises to 15 mg/dL at 25 to 28 hours of age.**
3. **The multipara woman is stable; a mother can be discharged even if the infant needs to remain hospitalized.**
4. The woman on antibiotics should remain hospitalized because the antibiotic's effectiveness is unknown.
5. An infant born before 34 weeks of gestation is preterm. Preterm infants can have respiratory or other health problems and should remain hospitalized.

▶ *Test-taking Tip: The key words are "appropriate for discharge," which means that the mothers and infants are stable and likely to remain stable. Consider the age of infants and the health status of the mothers and infants.*

Content Area: Management of Care; Concept: Critical Thinking; Management; Trauma; Integrated Processes: Nursing Process: Analysis; Client Needs: Safe and Effective Care Environment: Management of Care; Psychosocial Integrity; Cognitive Level: Analysis [Analyzing]

### 668. ANSWER: 2
1. Bottled water that is stored for use in an emergency should be replaced before it expires or, if self-prepared, every 6 months.
2. **The amount of water to keep on hand is calculated according to family size (1 gallon per person per day) for a 3-day supply of water.**
3. A disaster kit should contain water, food, and other necessary items for household pets.
4. The disaster kit should contain a 3-day (not 1-day) supply of food that will not spoil.

▶ *Test-taking Tip: You should take note of the time periods when answering this question. Think about how long it may be before help would arrive in a disaster.*

Content Area: Management of Care; Concept: Safety; Nursing Roles; Management; Trauma; Integrated Processes: Teaching/Learning; Client Needs: Safe and Effective Care Environment: Safety and Infection Control; Health Promotion and Maintenance; Cognitive Level: Analysis [Analyzing]

### 669. ANSWER: 2
1. The clients need to be decontaminated before being triaged and separated to maintain safety of the hospital environment.
2. **The nurse should first don PPE because white phosphorus can burn the skin.**
3. Because of the potential for an explosion or for deepening the burn, all evidence of white phosphorus should be brushed off of the clients' skin before any flushing occurs.
4. All evidence of white phosphorus should be brushed off of the clients' skin to prevent an explosion or deepening of the burn, but first the nurse should don PPE.

▶ *Test-taking Tip: Safety has priority. In this situation, personal safety is first, followed by the safety of the hospital environment and clients.*

Content Area: Management of Care; Concept: Safety; Management; Trauma; Integrated Processes: Nursing Process: Planning; Client Needs: Safe and Effective Care Environment: Safety and Infection Control; Cognitive Level: Application [Applying]

### 670. ANSWER: 1
1. **Every health care facility is required by The Joint Commission to have a plan in place for emergency preparedness. The activation response defines where, how, and when the response should be initiated.**
2. The nursing director would be notified as part of the emergency response plan.
3. The nurse receiving the call should be getting ready to receive the victims and would not call for extra staff. The agency's emergency response plan would identify the person who would make calls to obtain additional staff.
4. The agency's emergency response plan would identify the person who would make decisions about rerouting clients. The nurse should be getting ready to receive the victims.

▶ *Test-taking Tip: Consider that emergency response plans are broad and that contacting the director, requesting extra help, and rerouting clients are included in the emergency response plan. Thus eliminate Options 2, 3, and 4.*

Content Area: Management of Care; Concept: Safety; Management; Trauma; Integrated Processes: Nursing Process: Implementation; Client Needs: Safe and Effective Care Environment: Safety and Infection Control; Cognitive Level: Application [Applying]

### 671. ANSWER: 3, 4, 1, 2
3. **Client who has an incomplete leg amputation tagged as red. Red is priority according to the NATO triage system.**
4. **Client who has an eye injury, broken jaw, and facial wounds tagged as yellow. Yellow follows red in priority according to the NATO triage system.**
1. **Client with an upper arm fracture and minor burn tagged as green. Green is after red and yellow in priority according to the NATO triage system.**
2. **Client who has wounds involving multiple anatomical sites tagged as black. The client tagged black according to the NATO triage system has the least chance of survival.**

▶ *Test-taking Tip: The priority order according to the NATO triage system is red, yellow, green, and then black. Focus on the colors the clients are tagged and not the injuries. In a disaster with numerous casualties, clients with little chance of survival are tagged black.*

Content Area: Management of Care; Concept: Critical Thinking; Safety; Management; Trauma; Integrated Processes: Nursing Process: Assessment; Client Needs: Physiological Integrity: Physiological Adaptation; Cognitive Level: Synthesis [Creating]

**672. PHARM ANSWER: 1**

1. **Atropine sulfate increases the HR and dries secretions, symptoms caused by the nerve agent.**
2. Labetalol (Trandate) is a beta-adrenergic blocking agent that will decrease the HR.
3. Dopamine (Intropin) is a vasopressor used to treat cardiac output and increase the BP.
4. Phentolamine (Regitine) is an alpha-adrenergic receptor blocker that will produce hypotension. It is given subcutaneously to treat dopamine extravasation.

♦ *Test-taking Tip: Narrow the options by eliminating medications that will lower the HR or BP.*

Content Area: Management of Care; Concept: Medication; Integrated Processes: Nursing Process: Planning; Client Needs: Physiological Integrity: Pharmacological and Parenteral Therapies; Cognitive Level: Knowledge [Remembering]

**673. MoC PHARM ANSWER: 2, 3, 4**

1. Level D is basically the work uniform and is typically used to care for someone infected with anthrax. However, level A PPE is worn in suspected inhalation anthrax exposure because maximum respiratory, skin, eye, and mucous membrane protection is required.
2. **Ciprofloxacin (Cipro) is the treatment of choice for inhalation anthrax exposure. Antibiotics prevent systemic involvement.**
3. **PEP includes the administration of doxycycline or any quinolone (e.g., ciprofloxacin, levofloxacin) antibiotics to prevent inhalational anthrax. PEP should be continued for 60 days.**
4. **Signs of inhalation anthrax are more severe than skin contact or ingestion. Initial signs include dyspnea, fever, cough, chest pain, weakness, and syncope. Within 1 to 3 days, severe respiratory distress, hypotension, and shock can ensue.**
5. With inhalation anthrax exposure a CXR, not an abdominal x-ray, would be prescribed. It can reveal widened mediastinum or hemorrhagic mediastinitis that occurs with anthrax exposure.

♦ *Test-taking Tip: The key word is "inhalation." Select options that relate to oxygenation and the pulmonary system.*

Content Area: Management of Care; Concept: Nursing Roles; Management; Integrated Processes: Nursing Process: Planning; Client Needs: Safe and Effective Care Environment: Management of Care; Physiological Integrity: Pharmacological and Parenteral Therapies; Cognitive Level: Analysis [Analyzing]

**674. MoC ANSWER: 2**

1. The unresponsive client with a penetrating head injury has a limited potential for survival, even with definitive care, and would be categorized as a priority 4 level (black).

2. **A sucking chest wound is a life-threatening but survivable emergency. The client would be triaged as priority 1 (red) according to the NATO triage system.**
3. The client with the facial wounds would be classified as priority 2 (yellow) because injuries are significant and require medical care but can wait hours without threat to life.
4. The severely burned client has a limited potential for survival, even with definitive care, and would be categorized as a priority 4 level (black).

♦ *Test-taking Tip: Use the NATO triage system for mass casualty disasters and the ABC's. Clients with minimal chance of survival would be the last priority.*

Content Area: Management of Care; Concept: Critical Thinking; Safety; Management; Trauma; Integrated Processes: Nursing Process: Analysis; Client Needs: Safe and Effective Care Environment: Management of Care; Cognitive Level: Application [Applying]

**675. ANSWER: 1, 3, 4**

1. **The lesions are characteristic of smallpox, which is highly contagious. Smallpox is airborne and transmitted by both large and small respiratory droplets and by contact with skin lesions or secretions. Airborne, contact, and standard precautions should be used. A negative-air-pressure isolation room is necessary to prevent transmission of smallpox to others.**
2. An N95 particulate mask, not a surgical mask, is required to prevent airborne and droplet transmission of smallpox.
3. **Respiratory protection with an N95 particulate mask is needed to protect against airborne droplet nuclei smaller than 5 microns.**
4. **Smallpox is transmitted by contact with skin lesions or secretions. Contact precautions include wearing a gown and gloves when in contact with the infant or environmental surfaces that could be contaminated.**
5. Although the CDC should be notified by the agency, there is no indication that this is an act of bioterrorism. The nurse caring for the infant would not notify the CDC. In most agencies, a nursing supervisor or other designated person would be notifying the CDC.
6. Environmental surfaces should be decontaminated utilizing low- to intermediate-level chemical germicides or EPA-registered detergent disinfectants. The infant is not decontaminated.

♦ *Test-taking Tip: Even if you are unable to recognize this as smallpox, anyone with a rash lesion should be placed in airborne, contact, and standard precautions until a diagnosis is confirmed.*

Content Area: Management of Care; Concept: Infection; Safety; Integrated Processes: Nursing Process: Planning; Client Needs: Safe and Effective Care Environment: Safety and Infection Control; Cognitive Level: Analysis [Analyzing]

**676. MoC ANSWER: 2**

1. The client with a blistering sunburn is a level 3 priority according to the five-level Emergency Severity Index (ESI).
2. **Among the clients identified, the client with chest pain has priority. According to the five-level ESI, clients with chest pain, multiple trauma (unless responsive), child with fever and lethargy, and disruptive psychiatric clients are classified as threatened and are level 2 priority.**
3. The client with a leg laceration is a level 3 priority according to the ESI.
4. The client with neurological symptoms is a level 3 priority according to the ESI.

▸ *Test-taking Tip: Use the ABC's to determine priority. Select the client with a threat to breathing and circulation. The ESI has five levels of priority. Level 1 priorities include clients with cardiac arrest, intubated, trauma, severe overdose, or SIDS.*

**Content Area:** Management of Care; **Concept:** Critical Thinking; Management; **Integrated Processes:** Nursing Process: Implementation; **Client Needs:** Safe and Effective Care Environment: Management of Care; **Cognitive Level:** Application [Applying]

**677. MoC ANSWER: 3**

1. Older age female children of higher socioeconomic status are not the highest risk group for mental health distress after a natural disaster.
2. Older age male children of higher socioeconomic status are not the highest risk group for mental health distress after a natural disaster.
3. **Clients who are female, younger age, and lower socioeconomic status are more likely to experience symptoms of mental health distress after a natural disaster, and they should be the nurse's initial focus for an intervention program.**
4. Younger age male children of lower socioeconomic status are not the highest risk group for mental health distress after a natural disaster.

▸ *Test-taking Tip: The key word is "initial." Focus on the most vulnerable age group in which the threat to safety and security is most likely to cause mental health distress.*

**Content Area:** Management of Care; **Concept:** Stress; Nursing Roles; Management; **Integrated Processes:** Nursing Process: Planning; **Client Needs:** Safe and Effective Care Environment: Management of Care; Psychosocial Integrity; **Cognitive Level:** Application [Applying]

**678. ANSWER: 3**

1. A nasal cannula will only deliver an $FiO_2$ of 44% with oxygen flow rates at 6 L.
2. The venturi mask will only deliver an $FiO_2$ of 24% to 50%.
3. **The nonrebreather mask can deliver an $FiO_2$ of 100% with oxygen flow rates at 15 L. The oxygen reservoir bag contains only oxygen, and a valve keeps exhaled air from entering the reservoir bag. The bag must be inflated during oxygen delivery.**
4. The simple mask delivers $FiO_2$ of 40% to 60% at an oxygen flow rate of 5 to 10 L.

▸ *Test-taking Tip: Examine each illustration to determine which would best trap oxygen to provide higher levels for inspiration.*

**Content Area:** Fundamentals; **Concept:** Safety; Oxygenation; **Integrated Processes:** Nursing Process: Planning; **Client Needs:** Safe and Effective Care Environment: Safety and Infection Control; Physiological Integrity: Physiological Adaptation; **Cognitive Level:** Application [Applying]

**679. ANSWER: 4**

1. CPR should continue, not be stopped; defibrillator pads are placed on the chest, or one on the chest and one on the back.
2. Continuing with CPR for a full minute can delay defibrillation. Every minute that defibrillation is delayed worsens the prognosis.
3. The rhythm cannot be accurately analyzed while CPR is being performed.
4. **CPR should continue until the resuscitation team applies the conduction pads and the team is ready to analyze the rhythm. The client should not be touched while the rhythm is being analyzed.**

▸ *Test-taking Tip: Visualize each option before making a selection.*

**Content Area:** Fundamentals; **Concept:** Safety; **Integrated Processes:** Nursing Process: Implementation; **Client Needs:** Physiological Integrity: Physiological Adaptation; **Cognitive Level:** Application [Applying]

**680. ANSWER: 2**

1. The nurse must push the button to deliver a shock but only after verifying that no one is touching the client.
2. **To deliver a shock, the nurse must first be sure that everyone is clear of the client.**
3. A shock position (modified Trendelenburg) is not used for defibrillation.
4. The AED does not automatically deliver a shock.

▸ *Test-taking Tip: Visualize the steps of using an AED.*

**Content Area:** Fundamentals; **Concept:** Safety; **Integrated Processes:** Nursing Process: Assessment; **Client Needs:** Physiological Integrity: Physiological Adaptation; **Cognitive Level:** Application [Applying]

**681. ANSWER: 2**

1. The defibrillator pads should not be placed over any implanted device such as an internal pacemaker or defibrillator if possible to prevent damage to the implanted device.
2. **It is recommended that the defibrillator pads be placed at least 8 cm away from any implanted device when possible to prevent damage to the implanted device.**
3. The pads can be used on clients with implanted pacemakers, but these cannot be directly over the implanted device site.

4. Placing both defibrillator pads on the back will prevent the correct flow of current to shock the client effectively. The pads may be placed one anterior and one posterior.

▶ *Test-taking Tip: Defibrillator pads should not be placed directly over implanted devices. You should be able to narrow the options based on this information.*

Content Area: Fundamentals; Concept: Safety; Nursing Roles; Integrated Processes: Nursing Process: Evaluation; Client Needs: Safe and Effective Care Environment: Safety and Infection Control; Cognitive Level: Evaluation [Evaluating]

## 682. ANSWER: 2

1. Activating the emergency response system is crucial to this client's care, but according to the adult chain of survival, activation comes second after recognition.
2. **Part of recognition of cardiac arrest is to establish if the client is unresponsive and to determine whether or not a pulse is present. Because the given scenario only describes ascertaining unresponsiveness, it would be most appropriate to check for a pulse next.**
3. The nurse should not attempt to open the airway without first assessing the respiratory status.
4. Until recognition is complete, it would be inappropriate for the nurse to begin chest compressions.

▶ *Test-taking Tip: Review each of the links in the adult chain of survival. Within each link are important details for caring for the client in cardiac arrest in the appropriate sequence.*

Content Area: Fundamentals; Concept: Safety; Perfusion; Integrated Processes: Nursing Process: Assessment; Client Needs: Physiological Integrity: Physiological Adaptation; Cognitive Level: Application [Applying]

## 683. PHARM ANSWER: 10

**Use a proportion formula and multiply the outside values, then the inside values and solve for $X$:**
**0.1 mg : 1 mL :: 1 mg : $X$ mL; 0.1$X$ = 1; $X$ = 1 ÷ 0.1; $X$ = 10.**
**Using a desired over have formula:**

$$\frac{X \text{ mL}}{1 \text{ mg}} = \frac{1 \text{ mL}}{0.1 \text{ mg}}$$

**Cross-multiply to obtain 0.1$X$ = 1; $X$ = 1 ÷ 0.1; $X$ = 10.**

▶ *Test-taking Tip: Do not be confused with the 1:10,000. This is the percent concentration of epinephrine, which means that there is 0.1% epinephrine in the solution. Epinephrine is supplied in 1:1000 and 1:10,000 concentrations. The label has already converted the percent concentration by providing 0.1 mg/mL, and this is the drug amount and volume you should use in your calculation.*

Content Area: Fundamentals; Concept: Perfusion; Medication; Integrated Processes: Nursing Process: Implementation; Client Needs: Physiological Integrity: Pharmacological and Parenteral Therapies; Cognitive Level: Analysis [Analyzing]

## 684. MoC ANSWER: 4

1. Depending on the situation and status of the client, the HCP may want to review the HCD, but this is not the next action because it delays a decision.
2. Even if the client requests no CPR, an HCP's order is required to carry out the request.
3. The spouse's statements should be documented, but this is not the next action.
4. **The HCP must inform the team whether to withhold or terminate CPR even if it is specified in the client's HCD.**

▶ *Test-taking Tip: Note the key phrase "next action." Prioritization is required.*

Content Area: Management of Care; Concept: Collaboration; Management; Integrated Processes: Nursing Process: Implementation; Client Needs: Safe and Effective Care Environment: Management of Care; Psychosocial Integrity; Cognitive Level: Application [Applying]

## 685. ANSWER: 2

1. Touching the client is unsafe. If a shock is delivered and another person is touching the client or bed, that person will also receive a shock.
2. **Family members allowed to be present during resuscitation should have a support person with them who is able to answer their questions and explain expected outcomes of treatment and procedures.**
3. Telling the wife to stay out of the way and not interfere is insensitive.
4. Although the HCP may ask the wife regarding terminating resuscitation should efforts fail, it is insensitive to present a preconceived idea of failure.

▶ *Test-taking Tip: Consider the need of family members for support during resuscitation efforts.*

Content Area: Fundamentals; Concept: Family; Management; Integrated Processes: Communication and Documentation; Caring; Client Needs: Physiological Integrity: Physiological Adaptation; Psychosocial Integrity; Cognitive Level: Analysis [Analyzing]

## 686. ANSWER:

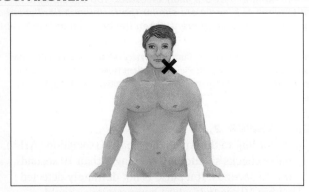

**The person performing rescue breathing is on the left; thus the client's left carotid pulse should be checked.**

▶ *Test-taking Tip: Read the scenario carefully to determine where each nurse is located in relation to the client.*

Content Area: Fundamentals; **Concept:** Perfusion; **Integrated Processes:** Nursing Process: Implementation; **Client Needs:** Physiological Integrity: Physiological Adaptation; **Cognitive Level:** Application [Applying]

### 687. ANSWER: 1

1. **Rescue breaths for adult clients should be administered at a rate of 1 breath every 5 to 6 seconds to provide optimal ventilation.**
2. Administering a breath every 3 seconds provides a rate of 20 breaths per minute. This is faster than recommended by the American Heart Association (AHA) for rescue breathing.
3. A rate of 20 breaths per minute is faster than recommended by the AHA for rescue breathing.
4. A rate of 1 breath every few minutes would be far too slow to provide adequate ventilation.

▶ **Test-taking Tip:** If you do not know the answer, look at all the options and note that two of the options are equivalent (1 breath every 3 seconds and 20 breaths per minute). These options can be eliminated.

Content Area: Fundamentals; **Concept:** Oxygenation; **Integrated Processes:** Teaching/Learning; **Client Needs:** Physiological Integrity: Reduction of Risk Potential; **Cognitive Level:** Comprehension [Understanding]

### 688. MoC ANSWER: 2

1. The defibrillator pads should be placed quickly; however, if the client is in a puddle of water, rescuers may be injured if a shock is delivered.
2. **For the safety of the rescuers, it is recommended that the client be moved from the puddle of water before defibrillation.**
3. The client's chest will need to be dry for the defibrillator pads to stick, but the priority is to move the client from the puddle first.
4. No one should ever be touching the client when the defibrillator's shock is being delivered.

▶ **Test-taking Tip:** Safety of the client or health care team supersedes other interventions. If options put the client or team in danger, they are likely incorrect. You should note that Options 1, 3, and 4 are similar (performing defibrillation), whereas Option 2 is different. Often the option that is different is the answer.

Content Area: Fundamentals; **Concept:** Safety; Collaboration; **Integrated Processes:** Nursing Process: Planning; **Client Needs:** Safe and Effective Care Environment: Management of Care; **Cognitive Level:** Application [Applying]

### 689. ANSWER: 2, 3

1. According to the American Heart Association (AHA), pulse checks should take no longer than 10 seconds, not 15 seconds. If a pulse is not definitely detected within 10 seconds, chest compressions should begin.
2. **Early activation of EMS by calling 911 will provide additional help and activate advanced care.**

3. **Providing chest compressions of at least 100 per minute is an appropriate goal for the client in cardiopulmonary arrest to optimize circulation.**
4. Auscultation of heart and lung sounds is not a recommended action for the client in cardiopulmonary arrest because it will delay CPR.
5. Performing a chest blow may be indicated in a witnessed arrest when an AED is unavailable; this arrest was not witnessed.

▶ **Test-taking Tip:** You should eliminate options that would delay starting CPR.

Content Area: Fundamentals; **Concept:** Safety; Oxygenation; Perfusion; **Integrated Processes:** Nursing Process: Implementation; **Client Needs:** Physiological Integrity: Physiological Adaptation; **Cognitive Level:** Analysis [Analyzing]

### 690. ANSWER: 3

1. Bag-valve-mask ventilation is needed when the client's respirations are inadequate. A respiratory rate of 14 is normal.
2. Chest compressions are needed when the client's HR is insufficient. The client's HR is normal at 80 bpm.
3. **Advanced life support personnel are needed to provide care for any client who was just resuscitated following cardiac arrest because the client may arrest again. When the client's HR and respiratory effort are adequate, the nurse should frequently monitor these until the advanced life support team arrives.**
4. There is no need to reanalyze the client's heart rhythm; the client has a normal heart rate and respiratory rate.

▶ **Test-taking Tip:** Even after experiencing cardiac arrest, the client with adequate HR and respirations should be monitored until more skilled help arrives.

Content Area: Fundamentals; **Concept:** Nursing Roles; **Integrated Processes:** Nursing Process: Evaluation; **Client Needs:** Physiological Integrity: Physiological Adaptation; **Cognitive Level:** Evaluation [Evaluating]

### 691. ANSWER: 4, 1, 2, 5, 3

4. **Stand behind the person who is choking.**
1. **Place both arms around the person's waist.**
2. **Place the thumb side of the fist against the person's abdomen above the navel and below the xiphoid process.**
5. **Grasp the fist with other hand.**
3. **Press upward with firm, quick thrusts 6 to 10 times until the obstruction is cleared.**

▶ **Test-taking Tip:** Read all the steps before placing these in the correct sequence. Often identifying the first and last step will help to sequence the other steps correctly.

Content Area: Fundamentals; **Concept:** Oxygenation; **Integrated Processes:** Nursing Process: Implementation; **Client Needs:** Physiological Integrity: Physiological Adaptation; **Cognitive Level:** Synthesis [Creating]

**692. ANSWER: 3**

1. The nurse should first determine if the client is choking before calling for help.
2. Asking the client if he is okay will elicit a yes or no response if the client were choking, but then the nurse would still need to determine the client's problem.
3. **Hands crossed at the neck is the universal sign for choking. The nurse's first action is to ask the client if he is choking and, if so, to perform the Heimlich maneuver.**
4. The client is still responsive; there may not be a need for the ART if the object can be expelled by the Heimlich maneuver.

▶ *Test-taking Tip: Hands crossed at the neck is the universal sign for choking.*

Content Area: Fundamentals; **Concept:** Oxygenation; **Integrated Processes:** Nursing Process: Analysis; **Client Needs:** Physiological Integrity: Physiological Adaptation; **Cognitive Level:** Application [Applying]

**693. ANSWER: 1**

1. **If the client can verbally communicate to the nurse and cough loudly, and if the skin is not cyanotic, then the airway is not occluded. This client should be closely observed by the nurse for signs of deterioration, but no other intervention is required at this time.**
2. The Heimlich maneuver is used for the client whose airway is obstructed by a foreign object.
3. Rescue breathing is applicable only for the client with a pulse who is not breathing.
4. Chest thrusts over the lower half of the sternum are appropriate for clients who are unresponsive, obese, or gravid.

▶ *Test-taking Tip: Remember that the victim who can cough or speak does not have a complete airway obstruction.*

Content Area: Fundamentals; **Concept:** Oxygenation; **Integrated Processes:** Nursing Process: Analysis; **Client Needs:** Physiological Integrity: Physiological Adaptation; **Cognitive Level:** Application [Applying]

**694. ANSWER: 1**

1. **The woman who is in later stages of pregnancy may require adjustment of hand placement for Heimlich maneuver, with the rescuer's fist and hand placed over the sternum for chest thrusts.**
2. Chest thrusts for choking are not performed at the level of the umbilicus because it could damage the fetus.
3. The usual site for chest thrusts for the choking client is between the umbilicus and the xiphoid; however, this client has a gravid abdomen. The rescuer's fist and hand should be displaced upward over the sternum.
4. The sternal notch is not a recommended site for chest thrusts because it can be damaged.

▶ *Test-taking Tip: Use clues in the question to help find the answer. In this question, you are told that the rescuer's hand placement is correct. You should be selecting the correct placement for the gravid client.*

Content Area: Fundamentals; **Concept:** Oxygenation; Safety; **Integrated Processes:** Nursing Process: Evaluation; **Client Needs:** Physiological Integrity: Physiological Adaptation; **Cognitive Level:** Evaluation [Evaluating]

**695. ANSWER: 3**

1. Explaining the actions of the code team depersonalizes the client and puts the focus on the code team's actions.
2. Accompanying the family to a waiting room demonstrates respect for the family but is not the *best* response.
3. **Allowing family time alone with the deceased demonstrates compassionate care by treating the client with respect and dignity and recognizing that the client is part of a family unit.**
4. Asking questions to determine an underlying cause may induce family guilt about possibly missing the client's symptoms or information in the client's history.

▶ *Test-taking Tip: Focus on the meaning of compassionate care, which is humanizing the client and showing respect and dignity.*

Content Area: Fundamentals; **Concept:** Stress; Grief and Loss; **Integrated Processes:** Nursing Process: Evaluation; Caring; **Client Needs:** Psychosocial Integrity; **Cognitive Level:** Application [Applying]

**696. ANSWER: 1**

1. **For pediatric clients with bradycardia and signs of inadequate perfusion despite appropriate ventilatory support, chest compressions should be started immediately.**
2. Atropine will increase the HR but not necessarily the child's cardiac output. With signs of inadequate perfusion, the child needs more cardiac output in the form of chest compressions.
3. Defibrillation is inappropriate at this time. Defibrillation is suitable only for pulseless ventricular dysrhythmias, such as ventricular fibrillation and pulseless ventricular tachycardia.
4. External pacing is not indicated at this time. The treatment of choice for the pediatric client who is being properly ventilated yet has bradycardia and signs of inadequate perfusion is chest compressions.

▶ *Test-taking Tip: Pediatric basic life support care varies from adult basic life support. Chest compressions are started in the pediatric client when bradycardia and signs of inadequate perfusion are evident. In an adult, chest compressions are performed only in the absence of an HR.*

Content Area: Fundamentals; **Concept:** Nursing Roles; **Integrated Processes:** Nursing Process: Implementation; **Client Needs:** Physiological Integrity: Physiological Adaptation; **Cognitive Level:** Application [Applying]

**697. ANSWER: 1**

1. **The decision to terminate resuscitative efforts rests with the resuscitation team physician and is based on many factors, such as the amount of time passed before starting CPR and defibrillation, comorbid disease, prearrest state, and initial arrest rhythm. This response directly answers the mother's question.**
2. Although the nurse is attempting to be reassuring, telling the mother that CPR is sometimes performed for a long time does not answer the mother's question.
3. The physician may ask the parents' feelings about terminating CPR, but depending on the parents' emotional reaction to the situation, this may not happen.
4. Using a therapeutic communication technique of reflection does not answer the mother's question.

♦ *Test-taking Tip: Determine the option that best answers the mother's question.*

Content Area: Fundamentals; Concept: Communication; Nursing Roles; Integrated Processes: Communication and Documentation; Client Needs: Physiological Integrity: Physiological Adaptation; Psychosocial Integrity; Cognitive Level: Application [Applying]

**698. ANSWER: 2**

1. Although the correct rate of rescue breathing for the pediatric client is one breath every 3 to 5 seconds, rescue breathing is not an appropriate intervention for the client in cardiac arrest.
2. **Once a second rescuer arrives to the scene of a pediatric cardiac arrest, the compression/ventilation ratio changes from 30 compressions and 2 ventilations to 15 compressions and 2 ventilations.**
3. Chest compressions for the pediatric client over 1 year of age should be delivered at a depth of 2 inches, not 1 inch. Proper depth is important for providing suitable cardiac output.
4. Defibrillation is not indicated in asystole, only ventricular fibrillation and pulseless ventricular tachycardia. For the pediatric client, 2 joules per kilogram is given for the initial shock and 4 joules per kilogram for subsequent shocks.

♦ *Test-taking Tip: The ventilation/compression ratios for both the child and infant vary from that for the adult and are based on whether there is a lone rescuer or multiple rescuers. With the arrival of the second rescuer in the scenario, you should be alert to the key word "change" in Option 2.*

Content Area: Fundamentals; Concept: Perfusion; Integrated Processes: Nursing Process: Implementation; Client Needs: Physiological Integrity: Physiological Adaptation; Cognitive Level: Application [Applying]

**699. ANSWER: 2, 3, 5**

1. A pulse check should not take longer than 10 seconds. The carotid artery is the recommended pulse check site for the adult or child, not the apical pulse.
2. **Activating the emergency response system early is recommended to gain access to additional help and to activate advanced care.**
3. **It is recommended that at least 100 chest compressions be provided per minute for the child in cardiopulmonary arrest.**
4. Cardioversion is not recommended for ventricular fibrillation because there is no QRS complex for synchronization.
5. **The child is in ventricular fibrillation; early defibrillation is indicated.**

♦ *Test-taking Tip: You should consider that ventricular fibrillation is a pulseless cardiac dysrhythmia as you review each option.*

Content Area: Fundamentals; Concept: Perfusion; Collaboration; Integrated Processes: Nursing Process: Implementation; Client Needs: Physiological Integrity: Physiological Adaptation; Cognitive Level: Application [Applying]

**700. ANSWER: 4**

1. Compressions can be performed with two thumbs or with two fingers while a second hand supports the neonate's back.
2. Compressions are performed on the lower third of the sternum to a depth of approximately one-third of the anterior-posterior diameter of the chest, or about 1½ inches.
3. The compressions rate is 100 compressions and 30 breaths per minute to achieve approximately 130 events per minute.
4. **The thumbs should remain on the chest between chest compressions to maintain the correct position.**

♦ *Test-taking Tip: The phrase "needs further instruction" indicates this is a false-response item. Select the action that is incorrect. The 2010 American Heart Association Guidelines for CPR recommends 100 compressions per minute for adults, children, and infants.*

Content Area: Fundamentals; Childbearing; Concept: Critical Thinking; Perfusion; Integrated Processes: Nursing Process: Evaluation; Client Needs: Physiological Integrity: Physiological Adaptation; Cognitive Level: Evaluation [Evaluating]

**701. ANSWER: 1**

1. **Pauses between 2-minute rounds of CPR should be limited to less than 10 seconds. During this time, the team should perform a pulse check and rhythm check. This will direct the team on how best to proceed with resuscitative care.**

2. Defibrillation is not indicated for sinus tachycardia. It is only necessary when the client is experiencing ventricular fibrillation or pulseless ventricular tachycardia.

3. The pulse should be checked before observing for spontaneous breathing. The monitor could be displaying a rhythm in the absence of a pulse.

4. The presence of a rhythm on the cardiac monitor does not necessarily indicate that a pulse has returned and that the infant is stable enough for transport to a higher level of care.

▸ **Test-taking Tip:** *Remember the sequence CAB for circulation, airway, and breathing. Knowing this should direct you to the only option that pertains to circulation.*

**Content Area:** Fundamentals; **Concept:** Perfusion; **Integrated Processes:** Nursing Process: Assessment; **Client Needs:** Physiological Integrity: Physiological Adaptation; **Cognitive Level:** Application [Applying]

## 702. ANSWER: 3

1. Back blows in the infant client with a foreign body airway obstruction are used only while the infant remains responsive.

2. Leaving the infant to retrieve an AED could cause the infant harm.

3. **Initiation of chest compressions and CPR is recommended for all clients with foreign body airway obstruction who become unresponsive.**

4. Rescue breaths will not be effective in cases where the airway is occluded by a foreign body.

▸ **Test-taking Tip:** *Remember that all clients with foreign body airway obstruction who become unresponsive should be treated with CPR.*

**Content Area:** Fundamentals; **Concept:** Oxygenation; Perfusion; **Integrated Processes:** Nursing Process: Implementation; **Client Needs:** Physiological Integrity: Physiological Adaptation; **Cognitive Level:** Application [Applying]

# Prenatal and Antepartum Management

**703.** The nurse is counseling the client who is trying to become pregnant. To promote fetal health when the client is unaware of a pregnancy, which nutrient should the nurse stress to include in daily food intake?

1. Potassium
2. Calcium
3. Folic acid
4. Sodium

**704.** **PHARM** The nurse is reviewing the medication history of the client during preconception counseling. The client reports taking isotretinoin for acne. Which is the nurse's **best** response?

1. "Stop taking isotretinoin now! It can cause serious birth defects if you become pregnant."
2. "You need to be on some type of birth control right now. Getting pregnant is not an option."
3. "Talk with your HCP about changing isotretinoin before you consider becoming pregnant."
4. "Once you are off of isotretinoin for treating acne, you can then safely become pregnant."

**705.** The nurse is counseling the client who has SLE. The client tells the nurse that she plans to become pregnant in the next year. Which response by the nurse is correct?

1. "It is best to plan for your pregnancy when you have been in remission for 6 months."
2. "Having systemic lupus erythematosus will not impact your pregnancy in any way."
3. "Your chances of having an infant with congenital malformations are increased with SLE."
4. "You will need to be scheduled for a cesarean delivery to prevent disease transmission."

**706.** The 22-year-old client tells the clinic nurse that her last menstrual period was 3 months ago, which began on November 21. She has a positive urine pregnancy test. Using Naegele's rule, which date should the nurse calculate to be the client's estimated date of confinement (EDC)?

1. August 28
2. January 28
3. August 15
4. January 15

**707.** The client is pregnant and receiving diet counseling. Which response by the nurse is most helpful when the client states she does not consume any dairy products due to her cultural heritage?

1. "Tell me how you perceive dairy products in your culture."
2. "Try having a glass of soy milk at each meal and at bedtime."
3. "Tell me about your intake of fortified tofu and leafy green vegetables."
4. "Rice milk fortified with calcium and nettle tea are good calcium choices."

**708.** The client tells the nurse, "Most days, I am so happy I am pregnant, but other days, I am not sure that I am ready to have a baby." Which is the most accurate response from the nurse?

1. "This is such a happy time in your life. You need to be optimistic to feel happy."
2. "How does your spouse feel about the pregnancy? I hope he is happy about the baby."
3. "Feeling differently from day to day is normal. How do you feel today?"
4. "Why do you feel this way? Is there something I can do to make it better for you?"

**709.** The nurse is teaching the pregnant client during her first trimester. The nurse identifies that which decision is most important for her to make **first?**

1. Bottle versus breastfeeding
2. Labor and delivery location
3. Pain management during labor
4. Method for delivery of the baby

**710.** The pregnant client is experiencing low back pain. After determining that the client is not in labor, the nurse instructs the client to perform which exercises to increase comfort and decrease the incidence of the low back pain? **Select all that apply.**

1. Kegel exercises
2. Pelvic tilt exercises
3. Leg raises
4. Back stretch
5. Stepping

**711.** The nurse's assessment findings of the pregnant client include darkening of areola and nipple, presence of Goodell's sign, leukorrhea, HR 124 bpm, dysuria, and heartburn. Of these findings, how many require further evaluation?

_____ findings (Record your answer as a whole number.)

**712.** **MoC** The pregnant client and her significant other are attending childbirth classes. The client asks for guidance on preparing her school-aged child for the new baby's birth. Which strategies might the nurse suggest that the client use with her child? **Select all that apply.**

1. Read books about bringing home a new baby.
2. Think of unique names for the new baby.
3. Help pack a bag for bringing the new baby home.
4. Explain how pregnancy occurred, if asked.
5. Help the child buy presents for the new baby.

**713.** The nurse is counseling the client who is pregnant. The nurse should teach that which assessment finding requires follow-up with the HCP?

1. Dependent edema
2. Edema in the hands
3. Generalized edema
4. Edema occurring every evening

**714.** The client expresses concerns related to nausea in the first trimester of pregnancy. Which recommendation should the nurse make?

1. Eat crackers while still in bed in the morning.
2. Lie down and rest whenever nausea occurs.
3. Eat more frequently throughout the day.
4. Avoid food items containing ginger.

**715.** The nurse is providing nutrition counseling to the client during her first prenatal clinical visit. Which statement, if made by the client, indicates that the client has an understanding of some of the nutritional requirements during pregnancy?

1. "I can eat cheese as an alternative to milk, as I don't care for milk."
2. "I should be eating more at each meal because I'm eating for two."
3. "I will need to limit my calories because I am already overweight."
4. "I should limit myself to eating only three healthy meals per day."

**716.** The nurse is providing nutrition counseling to a primigravida who is 10 weeks pregnant. Which meal choice stated by the client indicates she needs additional information?

1. Black beans, wild rice, collard greens
2. Dry cereal, milk, dried cranberries
3. Tuna, broccoli, baked potato
4. Beef strips, lentils, red peppers

**717.** The nurse evaluates the pregnant client with sickle cell disease during her second trimester. The nurse should identify which manifestation as being related to sickle cell disease and not the pregnancy?

1. Hand and lower extremities edema
2. Elevated serum blood glucose level
3. Decreased oxygen saturation level
4. Elevated BP

**718.** The nurse is assessing the client who is 34 weeks' gestation. Place an X where the nurse should place the Doppler **first** to assess the FHR when the fetus is thought to be left occiput anterior (LOA).

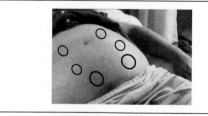

**719.** The client who is 32 weeks pregnant asks how the nurse will monitor the baby's growth and determine if the baby is "really okay." Which assessments should the nurse identify for evaluating the fetus for adequate growth and viability? **Select all that apply.**

1. Auscultate maternal heart tones.
2. Measure the height of the fundus.
3. Measure the client's abdominal girth.
4. Complete a third-trimester ultrasound.
5. Auscultate the fetal heart tones (FHT).

**720.** The client tells the nurse that she is using cocoa butter on her abdomen to prevent stretch marks. Which is the most accurate response from the nurse?

1. "That is wonderful. If you continue to use cocoa butter daily, you should have no stretch marks after delivery."
2. "The cocoa butter will not prevent stretch marks completely, but it will help to reduce their number."
3. "The cocoa butter will not prevent stretch marks but will decrease the appearance of the linea nigra."
4. "Cocoa butter does not prevent stretch marks, but it soothes itching that occurs as your abdomen enlarges."

**721.** The nurse is caring for the 24-year-old client whose pregnancy history is as follows: elective termination age 18 years, spontaneous abortion age 21 years, term vaginal delivery at 22 years old, and currently pregnant again. Which documentation by the nurse of the client's gravidity and parity is correct?

1. G4P1
2. G4P2
3. G3P1
4. G2P1

**722.** The nurse is caring for the pregnant client at 20 weeks' gestation. At what level should the clinic nurse expect to palpate the client's uterine height?

1. Two finger-breadths above the symphysis pubis
2. Halfway between the symphysis pubis and the umbilicus
3. At the level of the umbilicus
4. Two finger-breadths above the umbilicus

**723.** The nurse assesses the fundal height for multiple pregnant clients. For which client should the nurse conclude that a fundal height measurement is most accurate?

1. The pregnant client with uterine fibroids
2. The pregnant client who is obese
3. The pregnant client with polyhydramnios
4. The pregnant client having fetal movement

**724.** The nurse is conducting a physical assessment of the pregnant client. Which physiological cervical changes associated with pregnancy should the nurse expect to find? **Select all that apply.**

1. Formation of mucus plug
2. Chadwick's sign
3. Presence of colostrum
4. Goodell's sign
5. Cullen's sign

**725.** The nurse is assessing pregnant clients. During which time frames should the nurse expect clients to report frequent urination throughout the night? **Select all that apply.**

1. Before the first missed menstrual period
2. During the first trimester
3. During the second trimester
4. During the third trimester
5. One week following delivery

**726.** The pregnant client asks the nurse, who is teaching a prepared childbirth class, when she should expect to feel fetal movement. The nurse responds that fetal movement usually can **first** be felt during which time frame?

1. 8 to 12 weeks of pregnancy
2. 12 to 16 weeks of pregnancy
3. 18 to 20 weeks of pregnancy
4. 22 to 26 weeks of pregnancy

**727.** The nurse is caring for the pregnant client at the initial prenatal visit. Which universal screenings should the nurse complete? **Select all that apply.**

1. Taking the client's BP
2. Doing a urine dipstick test for protein
3. Doing a urine dipstick test for glucose
4. Asking questions about domestic violence
5. Asking questions about use of tobacco

**728.** While assessing the prenatal client, the nurse found a number of concerning problems. Place the concerning problems in the sequence that they should be addressed by the nurse.

1. Currently bleeding and cramping
2. Previous varicella infection
3. Currently using tobacco
4. Has intense pelvic pain

Answer: _____

**729.** The nurse is reviewing the laboratory report from the first prenatal visit of the pregnant client. Which laboratory result should the nurse most definitely discuss with the HCP?

1. Hemoglobin 11 g/dL; hematocrit 33%
2. White blood cell (WBC) count: 7000/mm$^3$
3. Pap smear: human papilloma virus changes
4. Urine pH: 7.4; specific gravity 1.015

**730.** The nurse is taking the health history of the 40-year-old pregnant client. Which identified medical conditions increase the client's risk for complications during her pregnancy? **Select all that apply.**

1. Diabetes mellitus type 2
2. Previous full-term pregnancy
3. Controlled chronic hypertension
4. New onset of iron-deficiency anemia
5. Hemorrhage with a previous pregnancy

**731.** Multiple women are being seen in a clinic for various conditions. From which clients should the nurse prepare to obtain a group beta streptococcus (GBS) culture? **Select all that apply.**

1. The client who is having symptoms of preterm labor
2. The women who had a neonatal death 1 year ago
3. All pregnant women coming to the clinic for care
4. The women who had a spontaneous abortion 1 week ago
5. The women who had an abortion for an unwanted pregnancy

**732.** MoC The experienced nurse is observing the new nurse determine the fetal position of the pregnant client using Leopold maneuver. The experienced nurse determines that the new nurse correctly identifies the first Leopold maneuver when placing the hands in which position illustrated **first?**

1.

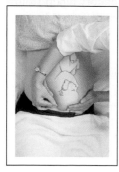

2.

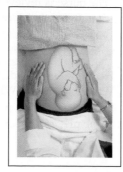

3.

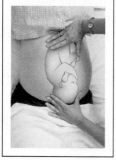

4.

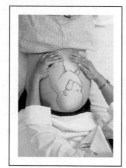

**733.** The pregnant client has an abnormal 1-hour glucose screen and completes a 3-hour, 100-g oral glucose tolerance test (OGTT). Which test results should the nurse interpret as being abnormal?

1. Fasting blood glucose = 104 mg/dL
2. 1 hour = 179 mg/dL
3. 2 hour = 146 mg/dL
4. 3 hour = 129 mg/dL

**734.** The nurse is reviewing the laboratory test results of the pregnant client. Which laboratory test findings would require further follow-up from the nurse?

| Laboratory Test | Result |
| --- | --- |
| Hgb | 10.6 g/dL |
| Indirect Coombs' test | Negative |
| 50-g 1-hour glucose test | 137 |
| Glucosuria | Negative |
| Proteinuria | Trace |
| Group beta streptococcus (GBS) | Negative |

1. Hemoglobin
2. 50-g, 1-hour glucose test
3. Glucosuria
4. Proteinuria

**735.** The nurse assesses the 34-week pregnant client (G2P1). Place the assessment findings in the sequence that they should be addressed by the nurse from the most significant to the least significant.

1. Pedal edema at +3
2. BP 144/94 mm Hg
3. Positive group beta streptococcus vaginal culture
4. Fundal height increase of 4.5 cm in 1 week

Answer: _____

**736.** The pregnant client tells the nurse that she thinks she is carrying twins. In reviewing the client's history and medical records, the nurse should determine that which factors are associated with a multiple gestation? **Select all that apply.**

1. Elevated serum alpha-fetoprotein
2. Use of reproductive technology
3. Maternal age greater than 40
4. History of twins in the family
5. Elevated hemoglobin levels

**737.** The 22-year-old client, who is experiencing vaginal bleeding in the first trimester of pregnancy, fears that she has lost her baby at 8 weeks. Which definitive test result should indicate to the nurse that the client's fetus has been lost?

1. Falling beta human chorionic gonadotropin (BHCG) measurement
2. Low progesterone measurement
3. Ultrasound showing a lack of fetal cardiac activity
4. Ultrasound determining crown–rump length

**738.** The pregnant client (G1P0) in the first trimester tells the nurse that she is anxious about losing her baby, prenatal care, and her labor and birth. Which teaching need should the nurse identify as **priority**?

1. Sexual relations with her spouse
2. Fetal growth and development
3. Options for labor and delivery
4. Preparing needed items for the baby

**739.** The nurse is teaching the client who is wishing to travel by airplane during the first 36 weeks of her pregnancy. Which is the **primary** risk of air travel for this client that the nurse should address?

1. Risk of preterm labor
2. Deep vein thrombosis
3. Spontaneous abortion
4. Nausea and vomiting

**740.** The first-trimester pregnant client asks the nurse if the activities in which she participates are safe in the first trimester. Which activity should the nurse verify as a **safe** activity during the client's first trimester?

1. Hair coloring
2. Hot tub use
3. Pesticide use
4. Sexual activity

**741.** The nurse is counseling the pregnant client who has painful hemorrhoids. Which **initial** recommendation should be made by the nurse?

1. Apply steroid-based creams.
2. Modify the diet to include more fiber.
3. Treat these surgically before delivery.
4. Increase intake of foods with flavonoids.

**742.** The client presents with vaginal bleeding at 7 weeks. Which action should be taken by the nurse **first?**

1. Take the client's vital signs.
2. Prepare examination equipment.
3. Give 2 liters oxygen per nasal cannula.
4. Assess the client's response to the situation.

**743.** The client who is actively bleeding after a spontaneous abortion asks the nurse why she lost the baby. The nurse responds that the majority of first-trimester losses are related to which problem?

1. Cervical incompetence
2. Chronic maternal disease
3. Poor implantation
4. Chromosomal abnormalities

**744.** The pregnant client presents with vaginal bleeding and increasing cramping. Her exam reveals that the cervical os is open. Which term should the nurse expect to see in the client's chart notation to most accurately describe the client's condition?

1. Ectopic pregnancy
2. Complete abortion
3. Imminent abortion
4. Incomplete abortion

**745.** The HCP prescribes interventions for the client with decreased fetal movement at 35 weeks' gestation. Place the prescribed interventions in the sequence that they should be performed by the nurse.

1. Prepare for a nonstress test.
2. Prepare for a biophysical profile.
3. Palpate for fetal movement.
4. Apply and explain the external fetal monitor.

Answer: _____

**746.** The pregnant client tells the nurse that she smokes two packs per day (PPD) of cigarettes, has smoked in other pregnancies, and has never had any problems. What is the nurse's **best** response?

1. "I'm glad that your other pregnancies went well. Smoking can cause both maternal and fetal problems, and it is best if you could quit smoking."
2. "You need to stop smoking for the baby's sake. You could have a spontaneous abortion with this pregnancy if you continue to smoke."
3. "Smoking can lead to having a large baby, which can make delivery difficult. You may even need a cesarean section."
4. "Smoking less would eliminate the risk for your baby, and you would feel healthier during your pregnancy."

**747.** The 28-year-old pregnant client (G3P2) has just been diagnosed with gestational diabetes at 30 weeks. The client asks what types of complications may occur with this diagnosis. Which complications should the nurse identify as being associated with gestational diabetes? **Select all that apply.**

1. Seizures
2. Large-for-gestational-age infant
3. Low-birth-weight infant
4. Congenital anomalies
5. Preterm labor

**748.** **PHARM** The client is diagnosed with pregnancy-related diabetes at 28 weeks' gestation. In teaching the client, the nurse should include what information for managing her blood glucose? **Select all that apply.**

1. Having glycosylated hemoglobin $A_{1c}$ lab tests
2. Performing home blood glucose monitoring
3. Developing a weight management plan
4. Engaging in appropriate daily exercise
5. Taking oral diabetic agents in the a.m.

**749.** The nurse informs the pregnant client that her test results indicate that she has iron-deficiency anemia. Based on this diagnosis, the nurse should monitor the client for which problems? **Select all that apply.**

1. Susceptibility to infection
2. Easily fatigued
3. Increased risk for preeclampsia
4. Increased risk of diabetes
5. Congenital defects

**750.** The nurse is caring for the client admitted to the antepartum unit at 32 weeks' gestation with possible preterm labor. The nurse is performing a fetal fibronectin (fFN) test. Which event, if it occurred, would require the nurse to recollect the specimen?

1. The specimen is collected before a vaginal examination.
2. A lubricant was used to facilitate insertion of the swab.
3. The client reports that she has not had intercourse for 3 days.
4. The specimen is collected before other specimens are collected.

**751.** The client admitted in preterm labor is told that an amniocentesis needs to be performed. The client asks the nurse why this is necessary when the HCP has been performing ultrasounds throughout the pregnancy. Which is an appropriate response by the nurse?

1. "Your baby is older now, and an amniocentesis provides us with more information on how your baby is doing."
2. "An amniocentesis could not be performed before 32 weeks, so you will be having this test from now until delivery."
3. "Your doctor wants to make sure that there are no problems with the baby that an ultrasound might not be able to identify."
4. "With your preterm labor your doctor needs to know your baby's lung maturity; this is best identified by amniocentesis."

**752.** The pregnant client presents to the ED with a large amount of painless, bright red bleeding. She looks to be about 30 to 34 weeks pregnant based on her uterine size. She speaks limited English and is unable to communicate with the staff. Which actions should be taken by the nurse? **Select all that apply.**

1. Call for an interpreter for this client.
2. Establish an intravenous access.
3. Auscultate for FHT.
4. Place the client into a lithotomy position.
5. Perform a digital pelvic examination.

**753.** The nurse assesses the client in her third trimester with suspected placenta previa. Which finding should the nurse associate with placenta previa?

1. Cervix is 100% effaced
2. Painless vaginal bleeding
3. The fetal lie is transverse
4. Absence of fetal movement

**754.** The client at 32 weeks' gestation presents to the ED with a severe headache. Her BP is 184/104 mm Hg. Based on the assessment and the serum laboratory report results, which **most** severe complication warrants the nurse's further assessment?

| Serum Laboratory Test | Client Results |
| --- | --- |
| Serum bilirubin | 2.1 mg/dL |
| LDH | 782 units/L |
| AST (SGOT) | 84 units/L |
| ALT (SGPT) | 51 units/L |
| Plt | 99,000/mm³ |
| Hgb | 12.1 g/dL |
| Hct | 36.3% |

1. Renal failure
2. Liver failure
3. Preeclampsia
4. HELLP syndrome

**755.** The 29-weeks-pregnant client presents to triage with decreased fetal movement. Her initial BP is 140/90 mm Hg. She states she "doesn't feel well" and her vision is "blurry." Additional assessment findings include normal reflexes, +2 proteinuria, trace pedal edema, and puffy face and hands. What is the **most** important information that the nurse should obtain from the client's prenatal record?

1. Depressed liver enzymes
2. BP at her first prenatal visit
3. Urine dipstick from last visit
4. The pattern of weight gain

**756.** The client at 31 weeks' gestation is diagnosed with mild preeclampsia and placed on home management. What information should the nurse include when educating the client? **Select all that apply.**

1. "Plan for hospitalization when nearing 36 weeks' gestation."
2. "Weigh daily and inform the HCP of a sudden increase in weight."
3. "Home care will be consulted to take your BP daily."
4. "Perform stretching and range-of-motion exercises twice daily."
5. "Rest as much as possible, especially in the lateral recumbent position."

**757.** The nurse is caring for the client with mild preeclampsia. The nurse should monitor for which complications associated with mild preeclampsia? **Select all that apply.**

1. Placental abruption
2. Hyperbilirubinemia
3. Nonreassuring fetal status
4. Severe preeclampsia
5. Gestational diabetes

**758.** MoC PHARM The nurse is caring for the client who is Rh negative at 13 weeks' gestation. The client is having cramping and has moderate vaginal bleeding. Which HCP order should the nurse question?

1. Administer Rho(D) immune globulin (RhoGAM).
2. Obtain a beta human chorionic gonadotropin level (BHCG).
3. Schedule for an immediate ultrasound.
4. Place on continuous external fetal monitoring.

**759.** The nurse is caring for the client with a grade 3 placental abruption. Prioritize how the nurse should implement the prescribed interventions.

1. Obtain serum blood draw for clotting disorders.
2. Administer 1 unit whole blood.
3. Start oxygen at 2 to 4 liters per nasal cannula.
4. Administer lactated Ringer's at 200 mL/hr.
5. Prepare for cesarean delivery if fetal distress.
6. Do continuous external fetal monitoring.

Answer: _____

**760.** The client diagnosed with velamentous cord insertion asks, "What symptom will I experience first if one of the vessels tears?" Which symptom should the nurse address?

1. Vaginal bleeding
2. Abdominal cramping
3. Uterine contractions
4. Placental abruption

**INSTRUCTIONS:** Use the information provided to answer Question 761.

**761.** `CJ` `PHARM` The nurse is reviewing the medical record of the client.

| | |
|---|---|
| **Client** | 46-year-old female |
| **Allergies** | Macrodantin |
| **Medical History** | Hypothyroidism, depression, hyperlipidemia, DM type 2 |
| **Presenting Symptoms** | Dysuria, urinary urgency and frequency, a sensation of bladder fullness and lower abdominal discomfort, suprapubic tenderness<br>States recent 10-lb weight gain; last menstrual period unknown. Started menstruation age 13 years. |
| **Laboratory Test Results** | **Complete blood count:** hemoglobin 15.6 g/dL (166 g/L), platelets 480 × 10³/microL (480,000/mm³), WBC 11.1 × 10³/microL (11,100/mm³)<br>**Serum chemistry:** sodium 140 mEq/L (140 mmol/L), potassium 4.6 mEq/L (4.6 mmol/L), creatinine 1.0 mg/dL, BUN 20 mg/dL, glucose 90 mg/dL<br>**Urinalysis:** Color red, specific gravity 1.026, glucose neg, ketones trace, nitrates positive, leukocytes mod, WBC 12/mL, bacteria few<br>**Urine culture:** >100,000 cfu/mL *Escherichia coli*<br>**Pregnancy test:** Positive<br>**TSH:** 7.00 UIU/mL (range = 0.47–5.00 UIU/mL)<br>**Free T4:** 0.2 ng/dL (range = 0.7–2.0 ng/dL) |
| **Current Vital Signs** | BP 138/80; pulse 82; respirations 20; oral temperature 101°F (38.3°C) |
| **Medications** | Atorvastatin Lipitor 20 mg oral daily<br>Insulin aspart: 10 units subcut at breakfast and 10 units at evening meal<br>Levothyroxine 75 mcg oral daily in am<br>Multivitamin 1 tablet oral daily<br>Nitrofurantoin 100 mg oral twice daily for 7 days<br>Sertraline 50 mg oral daily |

Which three medications should the nurse bring to the attention of the HCP? Complete the following statements by choosing the number for the medication from the left column that should be clarified with the HCP and the letter for the correct reason to clarify the medication with the HCP from the right column. Place the number and letter of the correct answer in the blank lines that follow.

| The Medications Brought to the HCP Attention Should Be: | Because: |
|---|---|
| 1. atorvastatin<br>2. insulin aspart<br>3. levothyroxine<br>4. multivitamin<br>5. nitrofurantoin<br>6. sertraline | A. The serum creatinine and BUN are elevated.<br>B. The client has an allergy to Macrodantin.<br>C. The client has hypoglycemia.<br>D. The client has thrombocytopenia.<br>E. The dose is too low.<br>F. The medication is contraindicated in pregnancy. |

Answer:

Medication number _____ Reason letter _____

Medication number _____ Reason letter _____

Medication number _____ Reason letter _____

## Answers and Rationales

**703. ANSWER: 3**

1. Potassium is important in preventing leg cramps during pregnancy, but this is usually not an issue during the first 4 weeks of gestation.
2. Calcium is important for fetal development of bones, teeth, heart, nerves, and muscles, but the fetus will take calcium from the mother. Calcium is more important to maternal health than fetal development.
3. **The nurse should educate the client about the need for adequate folic acid intake. Folic acid is important in preventing neural tube defects, especially during the first 4 weeks of fetal development.**
4. Sodium is important for maintaining optimal electrolyte balance but is typically ingested in more than adequate amounts in a typical diet.

▸ *Test-taking Tip: The key words are "unaware of a pregnancy." Think about the nutrient most important during the early stages of fetal development.*

Content Area: Childbearing; Concept: Promoting Health; Nutrition; Integrated Processes: Nursing Process: Implementation; Client Needs: Health Promotion and Maintenance; Cognitive Level: Knowledge [Remembering]

**704. PHARM ANSWER: 3**

1. Responding to the client emphatically can create anxiety and fear.
2. Telling the client that getting pregnant is not an option is a paternal response and does not facilitate open communication.
3. **The best response is to have the client consult her HCP so another medication can be prescribed. This response indicates that isotretinoin (Accutane) is not safe but that alternative medications can be prescribed.**
4. Clients must wait 1 month after cessation of isotretinoin before becoming pregnant.

▸ *Test-taking Tip: Not only is it important for you to know the FDA classifications of medications used during pregnancy, but the information must also be provided to the client in a way that is therapeutic.*

Content Area: Childbearing; Concept: Female Reproduction; Medication; Integrated Processes: Communication and Documentation; Client Needs: Physiological Integrity: Pharmacological and Parenteral Therapies; Cognitive Level: Analysis [Analyzing]

**705. ANSWER: 1**

1. **Planning for pregnancy with SLE when in remission for 6 months is correct. Pregnancy planned during periods of inactive or stable disease often results in giving birth to a healthy full-term baby without increased risks of pregnancy complications.**

2. Exacerbations of SLE can occur during pregnancy and impact pregnancy outcomes.
3. There is no risk of congenital malformations associated with maternal SLE. However, the risk for spontaneous abortion, preterm labor and birth, and neonatal death is increased.
4. SLE is not a transmissible disease, and there is no reason for a cesarean delivery.

▸ *Test-taking Tip: SLE is an autoimmune disease characterized by remissions and exacerbations.*

Content Area: Childbearing; Concept: Pregnancy; Immunity; Integrated Processes: Teaching/Learning; Client Needs: Health Promotion and Maintenance; Physiological Integrity: Reduction of Risk Potential; Cognitive Level: Application [Applying]

**706. ANSWER: 1**

1. **Naegele's rule is a common method to determine the EDC. To calculate the EDC, subtract 3 months and add 7 days. This makes the EDC August 28.**
2. An EDC of January 28 was calculated by adding 2 months and 7 days.
3. An EDC of August 15 was calculated by subtracting 3 months and 6 days.
4. An EDC of January 15 was calculated by adding 2 months and subtracting 6 days.

▸ *Test-taking Tip: Using Naegele's rule to calculate EDC, you should subtract 3 months and add 7 days to the date when the last menstrual cycle began.*

Content Area: Childbearing; Concept: Pregnancy; Assessment; Integrated Processes: Nursing Process: Assessment; Client Needs: Health Promotion and Maintenance; Cognitive Level: Analysis [Analyzing]

**707. ANSWER: 3**

1. Although asking about the client's perception of dairy products shows cultural sensitivity, the client has already stated she does not consume these. This statement is not the most helpful regarding helping the client to increase calcium intake in her diet.
2. The nurse is making a recommendation without further assessing the client's dietary preferences. Soy milk should be calcium fortified; yet, according to research the calcium content can be as much as 85% less than the amount indicated on the product label.
3. **Assessing the client's intake of calcium-rich foods is the best response.**
4. Both rice milk fortified with calcium and nettle tea are sources of calcium; however, the nurse is making an assumption that the client consumes these beverages.

▸ *Test-taking Tip: The focus of the question is about increasing calcium in the diet. Use the nursing process step of assessment to narrow options.*

Content Area: Childbearing; Concept: Pregnancy; Nutrition; Diversity; Integrated Processes: Nursing Process: Assessment; Culture and Spirituality; Client Needs: Physiological Integrity: Basic Care and Comfort; Cognitive Level: Analysis [Analyzing]

### 708. ANSWER: 3

1. Not all clients consider pregnancy a happy time in their lives, and the nurse should never tell the client how to feel.
2. The nurse should not divert the client's concerns away from self by bringing up the father's adaptation to the pregnancy, even though paternal adaptation is related to maternal adaptation.
3. **It is most therapeutic to acknowledge the client's feelings and probe for more information on her thoughts and feelings about the pregnancy.**
4. The client may not be able to identify why she has the feelings she is experiencing or how the nurse can make her feel better. This response does not provide an avenue for further exploration of the client's concerns.

♦ *Test-taking Tip: Identifying the statements that offer caring and an openness to more communication will lead to the correct option.*

Content Area: Childbearing; Concept: Communication; Integrated Processes: Caring; Client Needs: Psychosocial Integrity; Cognitive Level: Analysis [Analyzing]

### 709. ANSWER: 2

1. The decision on feeding the newborn can be made up to the time of the first feeding.
2. **A decision regarding labor and delivery location has priority for the client to properly plan for a home birth versus a hospital birth, HCP availability at the location, and type of labor and delivery settings available at the location.**
3. The decision on pain management can be made early but can be changed up through the early stages of labor.
4. The decision of delivery method should be made early but cannot be determined until the decision is made on labor and delivery location.

♦ *Test-taking Tip: The key words are "most important." Think about which decision should be made the earliest.*

Content Area: Childbearing; Concept: Pregnancy; Integrated Processes: Nursing Process: Evaluation; Client Needs: Health Promotion and Maintenance; Cognitive Level: Evaluation [Evaluating]

### 710. ANSWER: 2, 3, 4

1. Kegel exercises strengthen the pubococcygeal muscle, decreasing urinary leakage, but do not relieve back pain.
2. **Pelvic tilt exercises strengthen and stretch the abdominal and back muscles to relieve pain.**
3. **Leg raises strengthen and stretch leg and abdominal muscles to relieve pain.**

4. **Back stretch relieves pain from the back muscles caused by lordosis.**
5. Stepping provides aerobic exercise, which is good for circulation but is not recommended to decrease low back pain.

♦ *Test-taking Tip: Identify first how the exercises work in the body, then what effects they would have on relieving back pain, if any. Focus on those exercises that strengthen abdominal and back muscles.*

Content Area: Childbearing; Concept: Pregnancy; Comfort; Nursing Roles; Integrated Processes: Teaching/Learning; Client Needs: Health Promotion and Maintenance; Cognitive Level: Application [Applying]

### 711. ANSWER: 3

**There are three abnormal findings that require further evaluation. Leukorrhea needs to be distinguished from a vaginal infection, such as *Candida albicans* or a sexually transmitted infection. Heart rate can increase by 10 to 15 bpm during pregnancy, but an increase to 124 bpm is too high. Dysuria may be a sign of a UTI.**

♦ *Test-taking Tip: Darkening of the areola and nipple, Goodell's sign, and heartburn are common physiological changes and discomforts during pregnancy.*

Content Area: Childbearing; Concept: Pregnancy; Integrated Processes: Nursing Process: Analysis; Client Needs: Health Promotion and Maintenance; Cognitive Level: Analysis [Analyzing]

### 712. MoC ANSWER: 1, 2, 3, 5

1. **Engaging the child in activities such as reading books about bringing the new baby home helps the child to feel a part of the experience.**
2. **Engaging the child in activities such as naming the new baby helps the child to feel a part of the experience.**
3. **Engaging the child in activities such as packing a bag for the new baby's coming home helps the child to feel a part of the experience.**
4. Children younger than adolescents do not fully understand conception and pregnancy due to preoperational and concrete operational thinking. They are not usually asking for an explanation of sex during this time.
5. **Engaging the child in activities such as buying presents for the new baby helps the child to feel a part of the experience.**

♦ *Test-taking Tip: The developmental level and need to know information should be considered when selecting appropriate strategies for preparing a sibling at home.*

Content Area: Childbearing; Concept: Pregnancy; Integrated Processes: Teaching/Learning; Nursing Process: Planning; Client Needs: Safe and Effective Care Environment: Management of Care; Cognitive Level: Application [Applying]

### 713. ANSWER: 3

1. Dependent edema is typical during pregnancy, resulting from relaxation of the blood vessels in the legs and decreased venous return.

2. Edema in the hands is typical during pregnancy, particularly when a high-sodium diet is consumed.
3. **The nurse needs to teach the client that generalized edema is a sign of preeclampsia and requires follow-up by an HCP for further evaluation.**
4. Edema that occurs every evening is a normal finding associated with decreased venous return and pelvic congestion from daily activity.

▶ *Test-taking Tip: Often the most global option is the answer.*

Content Area: Childbearing; Concept: Pregnancy; Nursing Roles; Integrated Processes: Teaching/Learning; Client Needs: Physiological Integrity: Reduction of Risk Potential; Cognitive Level: Application [Applying]

**714. ANSWER: 1**

1. **The nurse should instruct the client to eat dry crackers before rising from bed. This typically relieves some of the nausea.**
2. Lying down when the nausea occurs may increase heartburn and reflux, thereby increasing nausea.
3. Eating frequently may increase heartburn and reflux, thereby increasing nausea.
4. Food items with ginger may help to alleviate nausea and are recommended (rather than avoided), including ginger tea.

▶ *Test-taking Tip: Use process of elimination to eliminate options that will increase nausea.*

Content Area: Childbearing; Concept: Pregnancy; Integrated Processes: Teaching/Learning; Client Needs: Physiological Integrity: Basic Care and Comfort; Cognitive Level: Application [Applying]

**715. ANSWER: 1**

1. **Cheese is a milk product and is an alternative to milk. This statement indicates understanding of nutritional requirements regarding milk and milk products.**
2. Caloric intake needs to increase by 300 kcal per day during pregnancy to meet increased metabolic needs. However, "I'm eating for two" is a common misconception and leads to caloric intake greater than necessary.
3. Caloric intake needs to increase by 300 kcal per day and should not be limited during pregnancy.
4. Nutritional snacks throughout the day can provide for steady blood glucose levels and decrease the nausea associated with pregnancy. A limit of only three meals per day may not provide the client with enough calories to meet increased metabolic needs or may cause the client to eat more at each meal and increase nausea and bloating.

▶ *Test-taking Tip: Options with absolute words are often incorrect and should be eliminated. The nurse should provide alternate sources of nutrients when a food item is not preferred by the client.*

Content Area: Childbearing; Concept: Pregnancy; Nursing Roles; Integrated Processes: Nursing Process: Evaluation; Client Needs: Health Promotion and Maintenance; Cognitive Level: Evaluation [Evaluating]

**716. ANSWER: 3**

1. Black beans provide a good source of calcium, iron, and protein. Black beans, wild rice, and collard greens provide fiber. Collard greens provide a good source of calcium and folic acid.
2. Dry cereal provides a good source of vitamin D, milk provides a good source of calcium, and dried cranberries provide a good source of calcium and iron.
3. **Tuna contains mercury and should be limited in pregnancy due to risk of mercury poisoning. The nurse should provide this additional information.**
4. Beef provides a good source of protein and iron, lentils provide a good source of iron, and red peppers provide a good source of vitamin C.

▶ *Test-taking Tip: The key words are "additional information." Identify the food that if used in excess in pregnancy can result in poisoning.*

Content Area: Childbearing; Concept: Pregnancy; Nutrition; Promoting Health; Integrated Processes: Nursing Process: Evaluation; Client Needs: Health Promotion and Maintenance; Cognitive Level: Evaluation [Evaluating]

**717. ANSWER: 3**

1. Edema is a normal finding related to pregnancy. A decrease in osmotic pressure causes a shift of body fluids into interstitial spaces, leading to edema.
2. Elevated serum blood glucose levels after a meal help ensure that there is a sustained supply of glucose available for the fetus. Sustained elevation may be associated with pregnancy-related diabetes, not sickle cell disease.
3. **Decreased oxygen saturation level is a clinical manifestation of sickle cell disease. Dehydration and anemia during pregnancy can result in vaso-occlusive crisis, which causes damage to RBCs and decreased oxygenation. The decrease in oxygenation manifests in decreased oxygen saturation levels.**
4. Elevated BP is associated with essential hypertension or preeclampsia.

▶ *Test-taking Tip: Identify the clinical manifestations that can be related to pregnancy first. Then, by process of elimination, you should be able to identify the answer.*

Content Area: Childbearing; Concept: Hematologic Regulation; Pregnancy; Integrated Processes: Nursing Process: Analysis; Client Needs: Physiological Integrity: Physiological Adaptation; Cognitive Level: Application [Applying]

## 718. ANSWER:

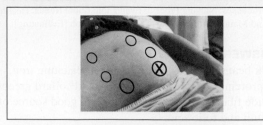

**FHT are best heard in the lower left quadrant of the client's abdomen when the fetus is LOA.**

▶ *Test-taking Tip: The FHT varies according to the fetal position. The FHR is heard most clearly directly over the fetal upper back. Think about where the fetal back is located when positioned LOA.*

Content Area: Childbearing; Concept: Pregnancy; Assessment; Integrated Processes: Nursing Process: Assessment; Client Needs: Health Promotion and Maintenance; Cognitive Level: Application [Applying]

## 719. ANSWER: 2, 5

1. The presence of fetal (not maternal) heart tones is a standard to assess fetal growth and viability.
2. **Adequate fetal growth is evaluated by measuring the fundal height.**
3. The abdominal circumference does not provide information about fetal growth. The increase in abdominal girth could be due to weight gain or fluid retention, not just growth of the baby.
4. Third-trimester ultrasound is neither routine nor advised for routine prenatal care because of the added cost and potential risk to the fetus.
5. **Auscultating the FHT assesses fetal viability.**

▶ *Test-taking Tip: The client is in her third trimester. Select only options that pertain to the fetus.*

Content Area: Childbearing; Concept: Pregnancy; Assessment; Integrated Processes: Nursing Process: Assessment; Client Needs: Health Promotion and Maintenance; Cognitive Level: Analysis [Analyzing]

## 720. ANSWER: 4

1. Cocoa butter does not prevent striae gravidarum.
2. Cocoa butter does not decrease the incidence of striae gravidarum.
3. Cocoa butter does not prevent the appearance of linea nigra.
4. **Cocoa butter is an emollient and provides moisture to the skin, thereby decreasing the itching associated with stretching of the skin as the abdomen enlarges.**

▶ *Test-taking Tip: Nothing can "prevent" striae gravidarum.*

Content Area: Childbearing; Concept: Pregnancy; Comfort; Nursing Roles; Integrated Processes: Teaching/Learning; Client Needs: Physiological Integrity: Basic Care and Comfort; Cognitive Level: Application [Applying]

## 721. ANSWER: 1

1. **The client has been pregnant four times in all (gravidity). This client has delivered once (parity) and is currently pregnant, so the parity is 1.**
2. Although the client has been pregnant four times in all (gravidity), she would have had to deliver two fetuses over 20 weeks old, regardless of whether either fetus survived.
3. The client has been pregnant four times in all, not three (gravidity). Parity of 1 is correct.
4. The client has been pregnant four times in all, not two times (gravidity). Parity of 1 is correct.

▶ *Test-taking Tip: Each time the client is pregnant counts as a pregnancy regardless of the outcome (gravidity). Parity is counted once the client delivers a fetus over 20 weeks old, regardless of whether the fetus survived.*

Content Area: Childbearing; Concept: Pregnancy; Integrated Processes: Communication and Documentation; Client Needs: Health Promotion and Maintenance; Cognitive Level: Analysis [Analyzing]

## 722. ANSWER: 3

1. The uterine height is too low for 20 weeks' gestation. At 13 weeks, the uterus would be approximately two finger-breadths above the symphysis pubis.
2. The uterine height is too low for 20 weeks' gestation. At 16 weeks, the uterus would be approximately halfway between the umbilicus and symphysis pubis.
3. **At 20 gestational weeks, the uterus should be at the level of the umbilicus.**
4. The uterine height is too high for 20 weeks' gestation. At 22 weeks, the uterus would be two finger-breadths above the umbilicus.

▶ *Test-taking Tip: Consider that the client is approximately at the halfway point in her pregnancy.*

Content Area: Childbearing; Concept: Pregnancy; Integrated Processes: Nursing Process: Assessment; Client Needs: Health Promotion and Maintenance; Cognitive Level: Application [Applying]

## 723. ANSWER: 4

1. Fibroids can increase fundal height and give a false measurement.
2. Obesity can increase fundal height and give a false measurement.
3. Polyhydramnios can increase fundal height and give a false measurement.
4. **Excessive fetal movement may make it difficult to measure the client's fundal height; however, it should not cause an inaccuracy in the measurement.**

▶ *Test-taking Tip: Consider what factors would increase the fundal height measurement and eliminate these options.*

Content Area: Childbearing; Concept: Pregnancy; Assessment; Integrated Processes: Nursing Process: Analysis; Client Needs: Physiological Integrity: Physiological Adaptation; Cognitive Level: Application [Applying]

**724. ANSWER: 1, 2, 4**

1. **Cervical changes associated with pregnancy include the formation of the mucus plug. Endocervical glands secrete a thick, tenacious mucus, which accumulates and thickens to form the mucus plug that seals the endocervical canal and prevents the ascent of bacteria or other substances into the uterus. This plug is expelled when cervical dilatation begins.**
2. **Cervical changes associated with pregnancy include a bluish-purple discoloration of the cervix (Chadwick's sign) from increased vascularization.**
3. Colostrum does occur with pregnancy but is a physiological change associated with the breasts and not with a cervical change.
4. **Cervical changes associated with pregnancy include the softening of the cervix (Goodell's sign) from increased vascularization and hypertrophy and engorgement of the vessels below the growing uterus.**
5. Cullen's sign is a bluish discoloration of the periumbilical skin caused by intraperitoneal hemorrhage. It can occur with a ruptured ectopic pregnancy or acute pancreatitis.

▶ *Test-taking Tip: The key words are "cervical changes." Use the process of elimination to eliminate a breast change or a sign of an ectopic pregnancy. "Expect to find" implies that it is a normal pregnancy.*

**Content Area:** Childbearing; **Concept:** Pregnancy: Assessment; **Integrated Processes:** Nursing Process: Assessment; **Client Needs:** Health Promotion and Maintenance; **Cognitive Level:** Analysis [Analyzing]

**725. ANSWER: 2, 4**

1. Women do not typically experience urinary changes before the first missed menstrual period.
2. **Urinary frequency is most likely to occur in the first and third trimesters. First-trimester urinary frequency occurs as the uterus enlarges in the pelvis and begins to put pressure on the bladder.**
3. During the second trimester, the uterus moves into the abdominal cavity, putting less pressure on the bladder.
4. **In the third trimester, urinary frequency returns due to the increased size of the fetus and uterus placing pressure on the bladder.**
5. Nocturnal frequency occurring a week after delivery may be a sign of a UTI.

▶ *Test-taking Tip: Consider how pressure is placed on the bladder during the time frames as you review the options.*

**Content Area:** Childbearing; **Concept:** Urinary Elimination; Pregnancy; **Integrated Processes:** Nursing Process: Assessment; **Client Needs:** Physiological Integrity: Physiological Adaptation; **Cognitive Level:** Application [Applying]

**726. ANSWER: 3**

1. Eight to 12 weeks of pregnancy is too early to expect the first fetal movement to be felt.
2. Twelve to 16 weeks of pregnancy is too early to expect the first fetal movement to be felt.
3. **Subtle fetal movement (quickening) can be felt as early as 18 to 20 weeks of gestation, and it gradually increases in intensity.**
4. Twenty-two to 26 weeks of pregnancy is later than expected to feel the first fetal movement.

▶ *Test-taking Tip: The key phrase is "usually ... first felt." Think about each option and the growth of the fetus during each week.*

**Content Area:** Childbearing; **Concept:** Pregnancy; Nursing Roles; **Integrated Processes:** Nursing Process: Assessment; **Client Needs:** Physiological Integrity: Physiological Adaptation; **Cognitive Level:** Comprehension [Understanding]

**727. ANSWER: 1, 4, 5**

1. **BP screening should be performed at the initial prenatal visit to establish a baseline and to evaluate for actual or potential problems.**
2. The use of routine urine dip assessments is unreliable in detecting proteinuria and is not always considered accurate. A urine sample should be collected and a UA completed to check for a UTI.
3. The urine dipstick test is of insufficient sensitivity to be used as a screening tool for glycosuria and is not always considered accurate. A urine sample should be collected and a UA completed to check for the presence of glucose.
4. **Domestic violence screening should be performed at the initial prenatal visit to determine fetal and maternal risk for harm.**
5. **Screening for tobacco use should be performed at the initial prenatal visit to determine fetal and maternal risk. Smoking is associated with an increased risk for spontaneous abortion, preterm labor, and low birth weight.**

▶ *Test-taking Tip: Urine dipstick tests are of insufficient sensitivity to be used as a screening tool in an asymptomatic population.*

**Content Area:** Childbearing; **Concept:** Pregnancy; Promoting Health; **Integrated Processes:** Nursing Process: Implementation; **Client Needs:** Health Promotion and Maintenance; **Cognitive Level:** Application [Applying]

**728. ANSWER: 4, 1, 3, 2**

4. **Has intense pelvic pain is most concerning and should be addressed first by the nurse. It could be a symptom of a serious medical condition, such as a miscarriage, ectopic pregnancy, or appendicitis. This symptom represents a possible pathology that could warrant immediate surgical intervention.**

1. Currently bleeding and cramping should be addressed next. It could be associated with the pelvic pain and could be a symptom of a serious medical condition, such as a miscarriage or ectopic pregnancy.

3. Currently using tobacco can put the client at risk for multiple adverse outcomes and should be addressed, although it is not an immediately concerning factor.

2. Previous varicella infection is important to document but poses no risk to the client or the fetus, so it is the least important to address.

▸ *Test-taking Tip: Consider the possible etiology for each abnormal finding. Prioritize the most serious as first (intense pelvic pain) and proceed to rank the remaining concerning problems.*

Content Area: Childbearing; Concept: Safety; Assessment; Integrated Processes: Nursing Process: Assessment; Client Needs: Physiological Integrity: Physiological Adaptation; Cognitive Level: Synthesis [Creating]

## 729. ANSWER: 3

1. A normal Hgb is 12 to 15 g/dL; nutritional counseling should be initiated when the Hgb is less than 12 g/dL. An Hct of 33% is also low (normal Hct value = 38% to 47%; this decreases by 4% to 7% in pregnancy), but increasing the Hgb with iron-rich foods should also raise the Hct.

2. A WBC count of 7000/mm$^3$ is within the normal range of 5000 to 12,000/mm$^3$.

3. **A Pap smear with HPV changes reflects an abnormal result. HPV changes are a risk factor for cervical cancer. The nurse should discuss the result with the HCP because it requires further assessment and follow-up.**

4. A urine pH of 7.4 is within the normal range of 4.6 to 8.0; the specific gravity is within the normal range of 1.010 to 1.025.

▸ *Test-taking Tip: The key phrase is "most definitely," indicating that more than one option has abnormal values, but one is more important than the other to address with the HCP.*

Content Area: Childbearing; Concept: Assessment; Pregnancy; Integrated Processes: Nursing Process: Evaluation; Client Needs: Physiological Integrity: Reduction of Risk Potential; Cognitive Level: Evaluation [Evaluating]

## 730. ANSWER: 1, 3, 4, 5

1. **DM is a risk factor for complications such as preeclampsia, eclampsia, dystocia, fetal macrosomia, recurrent monilial vaginitis and UTIs, ketoacidosis, congenital abnormalities, and others.**

2. Having a previous full-term pregnancy is not a risk factor for a current pregnancy.

3. **Controlled chronic hypertension may become uncontrolled during pregnancy due to water retention and other factors related to pregnancy. It is a risk factor for complications such as preeclampsia, placental abruption, and fetal hypoxia.**

4. **Iron-deficiency anemia is associated with an increased incidence of preterm birth, low-birth-weight infants, and maternal and infant mortality.**

5. **Previous pregnancy complications are a risk factor for complications.**

▸ *Test-taking Tip: Focus on the topic, risk factors for complications. Select options that are medical problems.*

Content Area: Childbearing; Concept: Pregnancy; Integrated Processes: Nursing Process: Evaluation; Client Needs: Physiological Integrity: Reduction of Risk Potential; Cognitive Level: Evaluation [Evaluating]

## 731. ANSWER: 1, 3

1. **The client in preterm labor should be screened for GBS infection. Between 10% and 30% of all women are colonized for GBS.**

2. There is no indication that the client with a previous neonatal death is pregnant.

3. **All pregnant women, regardless of risk status, should be screened for GBS infection. Between 10% and 30% of all women are colonized for GBS.**

4. The client would not be screened for GBS solely because of a history of spontaneous abortion.

5. The client would not be screened for GBS solely because of an elective abortion.

▸ *Test-taking Tip: You should eliminate options that do not indicate whether the women are pregnant. All pregnant women should be screened for GBS.*

Content Area: Childbearing; Concept: Infection; Pregnancy; Integrated Processes: Nursing Process: Planning; Client Needs: Health Promotion and Maintenance; Cognitive Level: Analysis [Analyzing]

## 732. MoC ANSWER: 2

1. This illustration shows the fourth Leopold maneuver. The nurse's fingertips are used to determine the location of the cephalic prominence.

2. **This illustration shows that the new nurse identifies the first step of Leopold's maneuver. The nurse palpates the fundus to determine which fetal body part (e.g., head or buttocks) occupies the uterine fundus.**

3. This illustration shows the third Leopold maneuver ("Pawlik maneuver"). During this maneuver the fetal part in the fundal region is compared with the part in the lower uterine segment. It is completed primarily to confirm that the fetus is in a cephalic (head) presentation.

4. This illustration shows the second Leopold maneuver. The second maneuver determines the location of the fetal back or spine.

▸ *Test-taking Tip: Consider that Leopold maneuver palpation begins at the top of the fundus.*

Content Area: Childbearing; Concept: Pregnancy; Integrated Processes: Nursing Process: Evaluation; Client Needs: Safe and Effective Care Environment: Management of Care; Cognitive Level: Evaluation [Evaluating]

**733. ANSWER: 1**

1. **The fasting blood glucose of 104 mg/dL is abnormal for the OGTT; normal is 95 mg/dL or lower.**
2. A 1-hour OGTT value of 179 mg/dL is normal; normal is 180 mg/dL or lower.
3. The 2-hour OGTT value of 146 mg/dL is normal; an abnormal value is 155 mg/dL or higher.
4. The 3-hour OGTT value of 129 mg/dL is normal; an abnormal value is 140 mg/dL or higher.

▶ *Test-taking Tip: Normal expected values for a glucose tolerance test include fasting blood sugar = 95 mg/dL, 1 hr = 180 mg/dL, 2 hr = 155 mg/dL, and 3 hr = 140 mg/dL.*

Content Area: Childbearing; Concept: Metabolism; Integrated Processes: Nursing Process: Assessment; Client Needs: Physiological Integrity: Physiological Adaptation; Cognitive Level: Knowledge [Remembering]

**734. ANSWER: 1**

1. **The normal Hgb level should be 12 to 16 g/dL in the pregnant client. The nurse should encourage iron-rich foods.**
2. The 50-g 1-hour glucose test should be less than 140. Values over 140 warrant a 3-hour glucose screen to determine if the client has gestational diabetes.
3. The presence of glucose in the urine (glucosuria) is negative, which is a normal finding.
4. Proteinuria in trace amounts is common in pregnant women, although higher protein concentrations should be evaluated.

▶ *Test-taking Tip: Evaluate each lab result and identify normal pregnancy levels. Evaluate which lab result is abnormal and select the appropriate levels.*

Content Area: Childbearing; Concept: Pregnancy; Integrated Processes: Nursing Process: Planning; Client Needs: Physiological Integrity: Reduction of Risk Potential; Cognitive Level: Analysis [Analyzing]

**735. ANSWER: 2, 4, 1, 3**

2. **BP 144/94 mm Hg warrants immediate evaluation. It could indicate preeclampsia, a condition that can progress to serious complications.**
4. **Fundal height increase of 4.5 cm in 1 week is abnormal and requires further follow-up. Normal fundal height increase is 1 to 2 cm per week. An increase in fundal size can be related to gestational diabetes, large-for-gestational-age fetus, fetal anomalies, or polyhydramnios.**
1. **Pedal edema at +3 may be a normal physiological process if it is an isolated finding. Pedal edema warrants further assessment because it can be a symptom of preeclampsia.**
3. **Positive group beta streptococcus vaginal culture warrants antibiotic treatment in labor but does not warrant intervention during the pregnancy.**

▶ *Test-taking Tip: Consider the possible etiology for each listed abnormal finding. Prioritize the most serious as first (elevated BP) and proceed to rank the other abnormalities by the seriousness of each condition.*

Content Area: Childbearing; Concept: Pregnancy; Assessment; Integrated Processes: Nursing Process: Assessment; Client Needs: Physiological Integrity: Physiological Adaptation; Cognitive Level: Synthesis [Creating]

**736. ANSWER: 1, 2, 4**

1. **An elevated serum alpha-fetoprotein level (an oncofetal protein normally produced by the fetal liver and yolk sac) is associated with a multiple gestation.**
2. **The use of reproductive technology such as artificial insemination or fertility drugs is associated with a multiple gestation.**
3. Maternal age greater than 40 is not associated with multiple gestation.
4. **History of twins in the family is associated with a multiple gestation.**
5. An elevated Hgb is not associated with multiple gestation.

▶ *Test-taking Tip: Consider which options might lead to or be caused by a multiple gestation.*

Content Area: Childbearing; Concept: Pregnancy; Integrated Processes: Nursing Process: Assessment; Client Needs: Physiological Integrity: Physiological Adaptation; Cognitive Level: Application [Applying]

**737. ANSWER: 3**

1. Falling BHCG levels do not conclusively diagnose fetal demise.
2. Low progesterone levels do not conclusively diagnose fetal demise.
3. **Ultrasound is used to determine if the fetus has died. The lack of fetal heart activity in a pregnancy over 6 weeks determines a fetal loss.**
4. Crown–rump length determines only the fetal gestational age.

▶ *Test-taking Tip: Identify closely associated words in the stem and the options to select the answer.*

Content Area: Childbearing; Concept: Pregnancy; Integrated Processes: Nursing Process: Analysis; Client Needs: Physiological Integrity: Reduction of Risk Potential; Cognitive Level: Analysis [Analyzing]

**738. ANSWER: 2**

1. There is no indication that sexual relations are a concern for the client. Sexual relations, including intercourse, are safe during the first trimester.
2. **Information about fetal growth and development is priority and important to address during the first trimester, especially when the client expresses concerns about losing her baby.**
3. Labor and delivery options for the baby are priorities in the third trimester.
4. The completion of preparations for the baby is a priority in the third trimester.

▶ **Test-taking Tip:** *The priorities for teaching should focus on the learning needs of each trimester and the concerns of the client.*

**Content Area:** Childbearing; **Concept:** Pregnancy; Nursing Roles; **Integrated Processes:** Teaching/Learning; Caring; **Client Needs:** Health Promotion and Maintenance; **Cognitive Level:** Application [Applying]

## 739. ANSWER: 2

1. Preterm labor is not associated with air travel.
2. **The primary risk with air travel during pregnancy is DVT. Pregnancy increases the risk of blood coagulation, and prolonged sitting produces venous stasis.**
3. The threat of spontaneous abortion diminishes during the second trimester. Spontaneous abortion is not associated with air travel.
4. Although nausea and vomiting can occur, they are not dangerous.

▶ **Test-taking Tip:** *When reviewing options, consider the vascular changes occurring with pregnancy and the prolonged sitting associated with air travel.*

**Content Area:** Childbearing; **Concept:** Pregnancy; Nursing Roles; **Integrated Processes:** Nursing Process: Planning; **Client Needs:** Safe and Effective Care Environment: Safety and Infection Control; **Cognitive Level:** Application [Applying]

## 740. ANSWER: 4

1. Hair coloring should be avoided in the first trimester because the chemicals can be absorbed and pose a risk to the developing fetus.
2. Hot tub use should be avoided because it increases the client's body temperature. Maternal hyperthermia during the first trimester raises concerns about possible spontaneous abortion, CNS defects, and failure of neural tube closure.
3. Exposure to pesticides during pregnancy increases the risk for preterm birth, intrauterine growth restriction, childhood developmental delays, and infertility later in adulthood.
4. **Sexual activity is not contraindicated in pregnancy unless a specific risk factor is identified.**

▶ **Test-taking Tip:** *Chemicals are associated with two options and should be eliminated.*

**Content Area:** Childbearing; **Concept:** Safety; Pregnancy; **Integrated Processes:** Nursing Process: Implementation; **Client Needs:** Safe and Effective Care Environment: Safety and Infection Control; **Cognitive Level:** Application [Applying]

## 741. ANSWER: 2

1. Steroid-based creams are frequently used for hemorrhoids, although evidence does not support their effectiveness.
2. **An initial recommendation should be a high-fiber diet because high-fiber foods increase intestinal bulk and make passage of stool easier.**
3. Surgical intervention to remove hemorrhoids is not recommended in pregnancy because hemorrhoids frequently resolve after pregnancy.

4. Flavonoids aid in symptom relief, although they are not recommended as the first line of treatment.

▶ **Test-taking Tip:** *Determine the interventions that are least invasive as an initial recommendation (Options 2 and 4). Of these options, determine which option aids in elimination to prevent straining and which option provides symptom relief. Select the option that aids in elimination.*

**Content Area:** Childbearing; **Concept:** Bowel Elimination; Pregnancy; **Integrated Processes:** Nursing Process: Implementation; **Client Needs:** Physiological Integrity: Physiological Adaptation; **Cognitive Level:** Analysis [Analyzing]

## 742. ANSWER: 1

1. **Assessing the client's VS should be completed first. Bleeding can cause hypotension.**
2. Although preparing examination equipment is important, the nurse should first focus on the client.
3. Having oxygen available is important, but there is no indication that the client needs oxygen at this time.
4. Assessing the client's response is important, but assessment of physiological problems should occur first.

▶ **Test-taking Tip:** *Use the nursing process. Assessment should be first. Then use Maslow's Hierarchy of Needs to narrow the options further; physiological needs have priority over psychosocial needs.*

**Content Area:** Childbearing; **Concept:** Pregnancy; Perfusion; **Integrated Processes:** Nursing Process: Assessment; **Client Needs:** Physiological Integrity: Physiological Adaptation; **Cognitive Level:** Application [Applying]

## 743. ANSWER: 4

1. Cervical incompetence can result in spontaneous abortion but does not account for the majority.
2. Chronic maternal disease can result in spontaneous abortion but does not account for the majority.
3. Poor implantation can result in spontaneous abortion but does not account for the majority.
4. **Chromosomal abnormalities account for the majority of first-trimester spontaneous abortions.**

▶ **Test-taking Tip:** *The key word is "majority."*

**Content Area:** Childbearing; **Concept:** Pregnancy; **Integrated Processes:** Teaching/Learning; **Client Needs:** Physiological Integrity: Physiological Adaptation; **Cognitive Level:** Application [Applying]

## 744. ANSWER: 3

1. In ectopic pregnancy, the pregnancy is outside of the uterus, and intervention is indicated to resolve the pregnancy.
2. A complete abortion indicates that the contents of the pregnancy have been passed.
3. **In imminent abortion, the client's bleeding and cramping increase and the cervix is open, which indicates that abortion is imminent or inevitable.**

4. In an incomplete abortion, a portion of the pregnancy has been expelled, and a portion remains in the uterus.

▸ *Test-taking Tip: Narrow the options to abortion and then focus on the client's symptoms to identify the answer.*

Content Area: Childbearing; Concept: Pregnancy; Management; Integrated Processes: Communication and Documentation; Client Needs: Physiological Integrity: Physiological Adaptation; Cognitive Level: Comprehension [Understanding]

### 745. ANSWER: 3, 4, 1, 2

3. **Palpate for fetal movement should be performed first. Assessment should be first to verify fetal movement.**
4. **Apply and explain the external fetal monitor should be next. The fetus should be monitored for heart rate changes.**
1. **Prepare for an NST. The NST is performed to determine fetal well-being.**
2. **Prepare for a biophysical profile (BPP). The BPP is an assessment of five fetal biophysical variables: FHR acceleration, fetal breathing, fetal movements, fetal tone, and amniotic fluid volume. The first criterion is assessed with the NST. The other variables are assessed by ultrasound scanning.**

▸ *Test-taking Tip: Consider which testing is most in-depth and which testing is used for initial screening. Use this information to prioritize nursing care.*

Content Area: Childbearing; Concept: Pregnancy; Management; Integrated Processes: Nursing Process: Planning; Client Needs: Physiological Integrity: Physiological Adaptation; Cognitive Level: Synthesis [Creating]

### 746. ANSWER: 1

1. **The nurse is acknowledging that the client did not experience problems with her other pregnancies but is also informing the client that smoking can cause maternal and fetal problems during pregnancy.**
2. Telling the client to stop smoking for the baby's sake is confrontational, making the client less likely to listen to the nurse's teaching. Although spontaneous abortion is associated with tobacco use during pregnancy, the nurse is using a scare tactic rather than therapeutic communication.
3. Smoking can lead to a fetus that is small for gestational age, not a large baby.
4. Decreasing her smoking intake should be suggested; however, it does not eliminate the risk to the baby completely.

▸ *Test-taking Tip: First eliminate Option 3 because it contains incorrect information. Then eliminate Options 2 and 4 because these statements do not use therapeutic communication techniques.*

Content Area: Childbearing; Concept: Communication; Pregnancy; Integrated Processes: Teaching/Learning; Caring; Client Needs: Health Promotion and Maintenance; Psychosocial Integrity; Cognitive Level: Analysis [Analyzing]

### 747. ANSWER: 2, 4

1. Seizures do not occur as a result of diabetes but can be associated with preeclampsia, another pregnancy complication.
2. **Infants of diabetic mothers can be large as a result of excess glucose to the fetus.**
3. Infants of diabetic mothers are usually large for gestational age and do not have a low birth weight.
4. **Congenital anomalies are more common in diabetic pregnancies.**
5. Preterm labor is not typically associated with maternal diabetes.

▸ *Test-taking Tip: Note that Options 2 and 3 are opposites. Only one can be correct.*

Content Area: Childbearing; Concept: Metabolism; Pregnancy; Integrated Processes: Nursing Process: Analysis; Client Needs: Physiological Integrity: Physiological Adaptation; Cognitive Level: Application [Applying]

### 748. PHARM ANSWER: 1, 2, 3, 4

1. **Hgb $A_{1c}$ will be drawn and monitored throughout the pregnancy, with a goal of reaching a level of less than 7%.**
2. **Home blood glucose monitoring will help the client identify when her blood glucose is outside normal parameters.**
3. **Excessive weight gain worsens control of glucose levels.**
4. **Exercise adapted for the pregnant body is important to glucose control.**
5. Oral diabetic agents are contraindicated in pregnant clients.

▸ *Test-taking Tip: For the NCLEX-RN® exam, multiple-response items will have at least one option that is not the answer.*

Content Area: Childbearing; Concept: Metabolism; Pregnancy; Nursing Roles; Integrated Processes: Teaching/Learning; Client Needs: Physiological Integrity: Pharmacological and Parenteral Therapies; Physiological Integrity: Physiological Adaptation; Cognitive Level: Application [Applying]

### 749. ANSWER: 1, 2, 3

1. **Iron-deficiency anemia is associated with susceptibility to infection because oxygen is not transported effectively.**
2. **Iron-deficiency anemia is associated with fatigue because oxygen is not transported effectively.**
3. **Iron-deficiency anemia is associated with risk of preeclampsia because oxygen is not transported effectively.**
4. Iron-deficiency anemia is not associated with an increased risk of diabetes.
5. Iron-deficiency anemia is not associated with an increased risk of congenital defects.

▸ *Test-taking Tip: Consider which conditions could be caused from a reduction in the Hgb and Hct levels that occur with iron-deficiency anemia.*

Content Area: Childbearing; Concept: Nutrition; Hematologic Regulation; Pregnancy; Integrated Processes: Nursing Process: Assessment; Client Needs: Physiological Integrity: Reduction of Risk Potential; Cognitive Level: Analysis [Analyzing]

## 750. ANSWER: 2

1. The specimen needs to be collected before a vaginal examination to ensure that the fluids are not contaminated.
2. **When collecting a fetal fibronectin test swab, the nurse must not use lubricant, as it will interfere with the collection of the specimen and contaminate the specimen. If this occurs, the test will need to be repeated.**
3. The client must not have had sexual intercourse within 24 hours of the specimen collection, as semen will contaminate the specimen.
4. The specimen must be collected before other specimens are collected to maintain the integrity of the specimen.

♦ *Test-taking Tip: In making your selection, you should consider whether or not each option contaminates the specimen.*

Content Area: Childbearing; Concept: Pregnancy; Integrated Processes: Nursing Process: Evaluation; Client Needs: Physiological Integrity: Reduction of Risk Potential; Cognitive Level: Evaluation [Evaluating]

## 751. ANSWER: 4

1. Although an amniocentesis can provide fetal information that an ultrasound cannot, the rationale for the amniocentesis is to determine lung maturity. Stating additional information is too broad.
2. An amniocentesis can be performed as early as 12 weeks' gestation, not after 32 weeks.
3. The amniocentesis is not being performed to identify fetal anomalies.
4. **The amniocentesis is being performed to determine fetal lung maturity. Once fetal lung maturity is determined, appropriate care can be planned, including administration of betamethasone, administration of tocolytics, or delivery of the baby.**

♦ *Test-taking Tip: Determine the rationale for the amniocentesis being performed for this client, who is in preterm labor.*

Content Area: Childbearing; Concept: Pregnancy; Nursing Roles; Integrated Processes: Teaching/Learning; Caring; Client Needs: Physiological Integrity: Reduction of Risk Potential; Cognitive Level: Application [Applying]

## 752. ANSWER: 1, 2, 3

1. **The nurse should call for an interpreter so that the client is able to communicate.**
2. **An IV access should be performed by the nurse to administer any needed medications.**
3. **Auscultating FHT will provide information about fetal well-being.**

4. Positioning the client in a lithotomy position can cause abdominal pain, and there is no indication that birth is imminent.
5. The pregnant client who presents in later pregnancy should never have a digital pelvic examination because this could cause additional bleeding, especially if she has placenta previa.

♦ *Test-taking Tip: The nurse should not be performing invasive procedures on the client who is bleeding in late pregnancy.*

Content Area: Childbearing; Concept: Pregnancy; Diversity; Integrated Processes: Nursing Process: Implementation; Culture and Spirituality; Client Needs: Psychosocial Integrity; Physiological Integrity: Physiological Adaptation; Cognitive Level: Analysis [Analyzing]

## 753. ANSWER: 2

1. The nurse should not perform a vaginal examination to determine effacement on the client with suspected placenta previa.
2. **In placenta previa, the abnormal location of the placenta causes painless, bright red vaginal bleeding as the lower uterine segment stretches and thins.**
3. The lie of the fetus is not associated with placenta previa.
4. An absence of fetal movement is always cause for concern but is not a primary symptom of placenta previa.

♦ *Test-taking Tip: In placenta previa, implantation of the placenta is in the lower uterine segment, near or over the internal cervical os. The nurse should not perform a vaginal examination on the client with suspected placenta previa.*

Content Area: Childbearing; Concept: Assessment; Pregnancy; Integrated Processes: Nursing Process: Evaluation; Client Needs: Physiological Integrity: Physiological Adaptation; Cognitive Level: Evaluation [Evaluating]

## 754. ANSWER: 4

1. The laboratory results do not show the serum creatinine level, so no inferences can be made about renal failure.
2. Although liver enzymes are elevated, HELLP syndrome is a more severe complication associated with pregnancy.
3. Preeclampsia commonly coexists with HELLP syndrome; however, these laboratory findings show worsening symptoms that are associated with HELLP syndrome.
4. **It is most important for the nurse to further assess for HELLP syndrome, a variation of pregnancy-induced hypertension characterized by hemolysis (elevated bilirubin), elevated liver enzymes, and low platelets.**

♦ *Test-taking Tip: Of the options, consider the most severe complication, which may be an umbrella for other options.*

Content Area: Childbearing; Concept: Pregnancy; Perfusion; Integrated Processes: Nursing Process: Assessment; Client Needs: Physiological Integrity: Physiological Adaptation; Cognitive Level: Analysis [Analyzing]

**755. ANSWER: 2**

1. Generalized vasospasm in preeclampsia would result in reduced blood flow to the liver and elevated, not depressed, liver enzymes.
2. **The pregnant client with a BP that is greater than 140/90 mm Hg with the presence of proteinuria may have preeclampsia. New-onset hypertension is associated with preeclampsia.**
3. The urine dip from the last visit should be reviewed but is not the most important to review because the significant information is the client's elevated BP.
4. The weight gain pattern should be reviewed but is not the most important to review because the significant information is the client's elevated BP.

▶ *Test-taking Tip: Identify two parameters that are stated in both the stem and the options. Narrow these two options to the most significant information that can result in complications.*

Content Area: Childbearing; Concept: Pregnancy; Assessment; Management; Integrated Processes: Nursing Process: Assessment; Client Needs: Physiological Integrity: Reduction of Risk Potential; Cognitive Level: Analysis [Analyzing]

**756. ANSWER: 2, 4, 5**

1. A diagnosis of mild preeclampsia does not require hospitalization during the antepartum period unless home management fails to reduce the client's BP or other complications occur.
2. **A sudden weight gain could indicate that the mild preeclampsia is uncontrolled and the client is retaining fluid. The HCP should be consulted.**
3. BP monitoring every 4 to 6 hours is recommended for the client with mild preeclampsia, but the BP can be taken by the client and does not require a consult with home care.
4. **Stretching and ROM exercises can help prevent thrombophlebitis and venous stasis.**
5. **The lateral recumbent position improves uteroplacental blood flow, reduces maternal BP, and promotes diuresis.**

▶ *Test-taking Tip: As you review the options, consider whether the client could monitor her own BP daily.*

Content Area: Childbearing; Concept: Pregnancy; Management; Integrated Processes: Teaching/Learning; Client Needs: Health Promotion and Maintenance; Physiological Integrity: Reduction of Risk Potential; Cognitive Level: Application [Applying]

**757. ANSWER: 1, 2, 3, 4**

1. **Placental abruption can occur as a complication of preeclampsia due to hypoperfusion of the placenta and endothelial injury.**
2. **Hyperbilirubinemia can occur as a complication of preeclampsia due to hypoperfusion to the liver.**
3. **Nonreassuring fetal status can occur as a complication of preeclampsia due to hypoperfusion to the placenta.**
4. **Severe preeclampsia can occur as a complication of preeclampsia if the BP remains uncontrolled.**
5. Gestational diabetes is not associated with preeclampsia.

▶ *Test-taking Tip: The underlying mechanisms involved with preeclampsia are vasospasm, hypertension, and hypoperfusion of the brain, liver, kidneys, placenta, and lungs. Endothelial injury occurs, leading to platelet adherence, fibrin deposits, and the presence of schistocytes (fragment of an erythrocyte). Knowing this, you should be able to select the correct options.*

Content Area: Childbearing; Concept: Pregnancy; Integrated Processes: Nursing Process: Implementation; Client Needs: Physiological Integrity: Physiological Adaptation; Cognitive Level: Analysis [Analyzing]

**758. MoC PHARM ANSWER: 2**

1. RhoGAM is indicated for any pregnant client with bleeding who is Rh negative.
2. **Obtaining the BHCG level is not indicated at 13 weeks' gestation. BHCG levels are followed in early pregnancy before a fetal heartbeat can be confirmed.**
3. An ultrasound can identify the cause of bleeding and confirm fetal viability.
4. Continuous external fetal monitoring can be used to confirm a fetal heartbeat, fetal viability, and fetal risk.

▶ *Test-taking Tip: Questioning an HCP indicates that an option would be incorrect for the client at 13 weeks' gestation with these symptoms.*

Content Area: Childbearing; Concept: Pregnancy; Management; Safety; Integrated Processes: Nursing Process: Assessment; Client Needs: Safe and Effective Care Environment: Management of Care; Physiological Integrity: Pharmacological and Parenteral Therapies; Cognitive Level: Analysis [Analyzing]

**759. ANSWER: 3, 4, 6, 1, 2, 5**

3. **Start oxygen at 2 to 4 liters per nasal cannula is priority to maximize fetal oxygenation.**
4. **Administer lactated Ringer's at 200 mL/hr to treat hypovolemia, increase blood flow, and maximize oxygenation.**
6. **Continuous external fetal monitoring should be performed to identify fetal distress early.**
1. **Obtain serum blood draw for clotting disorders, specifically DIC.**
2. **Administer 1 unit whole blood is next and will depend on the amount of blood loss.**
5. **Prepare for cesarean delivery if fetal distress would be last because it would depend on the client and fetal status.**

▶ *Test-taking Tip: Note the option that has the most immediate impact on maternal and fetal well-being and can be accomplished the fastest. Prioritize this as the first action for the nurse. Consider that oxygenation is the most critical aspect to promote oxygenation.*

Content Area: Childbearing; Concept: Pregnancy; Medication; Integrated Processes: Nursing Process: Planning; Client Needs: Physiological Integrity: Physiological Adaptation; Cognitive Level: Synthesis [Creating]

**760. ANSWER: 1**

1. **In a velamentous cord insertion, vessels of the cord divide some distance from the placenta in the placental membrane. Thus the most likely first symptom would be vaginal bleeding.**

2. Abdominal cramping is unlikely to occur; velamentous cord insertion is not related to uterine activity.

3. Contractions are unlikely to occur; velamentous cord insertion is not related to uterine activity.

4. An abruption, when the placenta comes off the uterine wall, results in severe abdominal pain.

▶ *Test-taking Tip:* Associate key information in the stem, "vessels ... tear," to one of the options.

Content Area: Childbearing; Concept: Pregnancy; Nursing Roles; Integrated Processes: Teaching/Learning; Client Needs: Physiological Integrity: Physiological Adaptation; Cognitive Level: Application [Applying]

**761.** CJ PHARM **ANSWER: 1F, 3E, 5B**

1. **Atorvastatin (Lipitor), a HMG-CoA reductase inhibitor used to lower cholesterol levels, is contraindicated in pregnancy.**

2. Insulin aspart (NovoLog) is used to control hyperglycemia with type 1 or type 2 DM. It is safe to use in pregnancy. The client's blood glucose level of 90 mg/dL is within the normal range of 70 to 100 mg/dL (3.9 and 5.5 mmol/L).

3. **Levothyroxine (Synthroid) is a thyroid hormone supplement used to treat hypothyroidism. The elevated TSH and low free T4 values indicate that the dose is too low and should be increased.**

4. A multivitamin is safe to use in pregnancy. There are no reasons among the options to bring it to the attention of the HCP.

5. **Nitrofurantoin (Macrodantin), an antibiotic, is used in the treatment of a UTI. Although it can be used during pregnancy, the client is allergic to Macrodantin.**

6. Sertraline (Zoloft) is an SSRI antidepressant. There are no reasons among the options to bring it to the attention of the HCP.

▶ *Test-taking Tip:* This is a new item type that is being trialed on the NCLEX-RN®. The medications and reasons will have drop-down menus for selecting these. With large amounts of information in the chart, it is best to read the question and the options first. Then go to the information in the chart.

Content Area: Childbearing; Concept: Pregnancy; Medications; Nursing Roles; Integrated Processes: Nursing Process: Analysis; Client Needs: Physiological Integrity: Pharmacological and Parenteral Therapies; Cognitive Level: Analysis [Analyzing]

## Chapter Nineteen

# Intrapartum Management

**762.** **MoC** The pregnant client arrives at the triage unit. The nurse assesses that she is at 4/50/–1 and that the fetal HR is 148. What **priority** information should the nurse collect before proceeding?

1. Time and amount of last meal
2. Number of weeks' gestation
3. Who is attending the delivery
4. History of previous illnesses

**763.** The nurse, admitting a 40-week primigravida to the labor unit, just documented the results of a recent vaginal exam: 3/100/–2, RSP. How should the oncoming shift nurse interpret this documentation?

1. The fetus is approximately 2 cm below maternal ischial spines.
2. The cervix is totally dilated and effaced, with fetal engagement.
3. The fetus is breech and posterior to the client's pelvis.
4. The fetal lie is transverse, and the fetal attitude is flexion.

**764.** **PHARM** The nurse is caring for the low-risk client during the first stage of labor. When should the nurse assess the fetal heart rate (FHR) pattern? **Select all that apply.**

1. Before administering medications
2. At least every 15 minutes
3. After vaginal examinations
4. During a hard contraction
5. When giving oxytocin

**765.** **MoC** **PHARM** The laboring client just had a convulsion after being given regional anesthesia. Which interventions should the nurse implement? **Select all that apply.**

1. Establish an airway.
2. Position on her right side.
3. Provide 100% oxygen.
4. Administer diazepam.
5. Page the anesthesiologist STAT.

**766.** After performing Leopold's maneuvers and determining that the fetus is in the RSA position, the nurse plans to assess the FHR. Place an X on the area of the client's abdomen where the nurse would **best** be able to listen to and count the FHR.

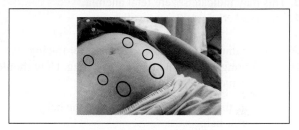

**767.** The laboring client in the first stage of labor is talking and laughing with her husband. The nurse should conclude that the client is probably in what phase?

1. Transition
2. Active
3. Active pushing
4. Latent

**768.** **PHARM** The nurse administers butorphanol tartrate to the client in active labor. What is the nurse's **most** important action to help prevent side effects from the medication?

1. Assess the client's bladder for distention.
2. Place the client on seizure precautions.
3. Assess the client's body for itchy rash.
4. Evaluate the client's vital signs and pulse oximetry.

**769.** The nurse admits the client at 34 weeks' gestation for preterm labor as a result of a battledore placenta. The nurse should plan to monitor for which most common complication associated with battledore placenta?

1. Late abortion
2. Fetal demise
3. Postpartum hemorrhage
4. Preterm labor with bleeding

**770.** The laboring client is at 5/100/0, ROA, and having difficulty coping with her contractions. She does not want epidural analgesia or medications. How can the nurse **best** assist the client and her partner?

1. Apply counterpressure to sacral area with a firm object.
2. Implement effleurage (light massage) of the abdomen.
3. Provide a quiet, calm, and relaxed labor environment.
4. Reemphasize modified-paced breathing techniques.

**771.** The labor nurse observes a sinusoidal FHR pattern on the monitor. How should the nurse interpret this?

1. The fetus may be in a sleep state.
2. Congenital anomalies are possible.
3. This may indicate severe fetal anemia.
4. This predicts normal fetal well-being.

**772.** The continuous electronic FHR monitor tracing on the laboring client is no longer recording. How should the nurse immediately respond?

1. Conclude that there is a problem with the baby and call for help.
2. Check that there is adequate gel under the transducer and reposition.
3. Give the client oxygen via facemask at 8 to 10 liters per minute.
4. Auscultate FHR by fetoscope and assess maternal vital signs.

**773.** The nurse is caring for the client in labor. Which assessment finding would help the nurse determine whether the client is in the third stage of labor?

1. Lengthening of fetal cord
2. Increased bloody show
3. A strong urge to push
4. More frequent contractions

**774.** The client in labor tells the nurse that it feels like her membranes just ruptured. Which assessment finding of the amniotic fluid would indicate that it is normal?

1. Cloudy in color
2. Has a strong odor
3. Meconium stained
4. Has a pH of 7.1

**775.** **MoC** The laboring multigravida client's last vaginal examination was 8/90/+1. The client now states feeling rectal pressure. Which action should the nurse perform **first**?

1. Encourage the client to push.
2. Notify the obstetrician or midwife.
3. Help the client to the bathroom.
4. Complete another vaginal exam.

**776.** **MoC** The laboring client's amniotic membranes have just ruptured. Which nursing action should be **priority**?

1. Monitor maternal temperature.
2. Inspect characteristics of the fluid.
3. Perform a sterile vaginal examination.
4. Assess the FHR pattern.

**777.** **MoC** The client in labor received an epidural anesthesia 20 minutes ago. The nurse assesses that the client's BP is 98/62 mm Hg and that the client is lying supine. What should the nurse do **next**?

1. Increase the lactated Ringer's infusion rate.
2. Elevate the client's legs for 2 to 3 minutes.
3. Place the bed in 10- to 20-degree Trendelenburg.
4. Position the client in a left side-lying position.

**778.** The nurse explained the process of cervical efface-ment to the client in early labor. Which statement indicates that she understands the information?

1. "The cervix will widen from less than 1 cm to about 10 cm."
2. "The cervix will pull or draw up and become paper-thin."
3. "The cervical changes will cause my membranes to rupture."
4. "The cervical changes will help my baby to change position."

**779.** **MoC** The nurse observes on the monitor tracing of the client in the transition phase of labor that the baseline FHR is 160 and that there is moderate variability with V-shaped decelerations unrelated to contractions. What should the nurse do **first?**

1. Prepare for delivery.
2. Notify the obstetrician.
3. Apply oxygen nasally.
4. Reposition the client.

**780.** The nurse is caring for the pregnant client. Which assessment findings help the nurse determine that she may be in true labor? **Select all that apply.**

1. Progressive cervical dilation and effacement
2. Walking usually increases contraction intensity
3. Warm tub baths and rest lessen contractions
4. Discomfort is usually in the client's abdomen
5. Contractions increase in duration and intensity

**781.** The nurse is unable to determine the fetal position for the laboring client who is morbidly obese. What should the nurse plan do to obtain the **most** accurate method of determining fetal position in this client?

1. Inspect the client's abdomen.
2. Palpate the client's abdomen.
3. Perform a vaginal examination.
4. Perform transabdominal ultrasound.

**782.** The nurse is caring for multiple clients. The nurse determines that which client would be a candidate for intermittent fetal monitoring during labor?

1. The client with a previous cesarean birth
2. The primigravida client at 41 weeks
3. The client with preeclampsia
4. The client with gestational diabetes

**783.** The laboring client is experiencing dyspnea, diaphoresis, tachycardia, and hypotension while lying on her back. Which intervention should the nurse implement **immediately?**

1. Turn the client onto her left side.
2. Turn the client onto her right side.
3. Notify the attending obstetrician.
4. Apply oxygen by nasal cannula.

**784.** MoC PHARM The nurse notifies the HCP after feeling a pulsating mass during the vaginal examination of a newly admitted full-term pregnant client. Which HCP order should the nurse question?

1. Prepare for possible cesarean section.
2. Place the client in a knee-chest position.
3. Initiate a low-dose oxytocin IV infusion.
4. Give terbutaline 0.25 mg subcutaneously.

**785.** The primigravida client has been pushing for 2 hours when the infant's head emerges. The infant fails to deliver, and the obstetrician states that the turtle sign has occurred. Which should be the nurse's interpretation of this information?

1. There is cephalopelvic disproportion.
2. The infant has a shoulder dystocia.
3. The infant's position is occiput posterior.
4. The infant's umbilical cord is prolapsed.

**786.** The nurse is caring for the client who has been in the second stage of labor for the last 12 hours. The nurse should monitor for which cardiovascular change that occurs during this stage of labor?

1. An increase in maternal HR
2. A decrease in the cardiac output
3. An increase in the WBC count
4. A decrease in intravascular volume

**787.** The pregnant client presents with regular contractions that she describes as "strong." Her cervical exam indicates that she is dilated to 3 cm. Which conclusion should the nurse make based on this information?

1. The client is experiencing early labor.
2. The client is experiencing false labor.
3. The client has experienced cervical ripening.
4. The client has experienced lightening.

**788.** MoC The nurse is reviewing laboratory results of the client in labor prior to her receiving epidural anesthesia. Which result is **most** important to report to the HCP prior to the initiation of the epidural?

1. White blood cells: 24,000/mm$^3$
2. Glucose: 78 grams/dL
3. Hemoglobin: 10.2 g/dL
4. Platelets: 100,000/mm$^3$

**789.** MoC The nurse's laboring client presents with ruptured membranes, frequent contractions, and bloody show. She reports a greenish discharge for 2 days. Place the nurse's actions in the order that they should be completed.

1. Perform a sterile vaginal exam.
2. Assess the client thoroughly.
3. Obtain fetal heart tones.
4. Notify the HCP.

Answer: _____

**790.** The nurse is caring for two maternity clients who are in labor. The nurse determines that head entrapment is most likely to occur with which delivery presentation? Place an X on the correct illustration.

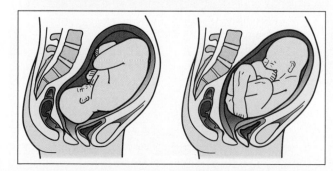

**791.** The nurse is assessing the client who is in the active stage of labor. Which is the **most** crucial information that the nurse should assess related to the client's ethnicity and stage of labor?

1. Choice of pain control measures
2. Desire for hot or cold fluids
3. Persons to be in the room during labor and birth
4. Desire for circumcision if a male infant is born

**792.** PHARM The laboring client is experiencing problems, and the nurse is concerned about possible side effects from the epidural anesthetic just administered. Which problems should the nurse attribute to the epidural anesthetic? **Select all that apply.**

1. Has breakthrough sharp pain
2. Blood pressure is increased
3. Has a pounding headache
4. Unable to feel a full bladder
5. Has an elevated temperature

**793.** The client in labor is requesting water therapy (hydrotherapy) to help provide pain relief and relaxation. Her recent vaginal exam was 2/50/−2. How should the nurse respond to the client's request?

1. "Usually we initiate hydrotherapy during active labor."
2. "You will not need to change positions quite as much."
3. "We will not be able to monitor FHR as easily."
4. "You can use hydrotherapy for up to 60 minutes at a time."

**794.** MoC A new nurse observes the FHR pattern illustrated. Which documentation should the experienced nurse evaluate as correct regarding electronic fetal monitoring (EFM)?

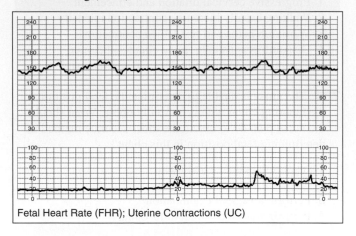

Fetal Heart Rate (FHR); Uterine Contractions (UC)

1. EFM shows FHR accelerations with uterine contractions.
2. EFM shows normal FHR baseline; no change in response to contractions.
3. EFM shows FHR early decelerations in response to uterine contractions.
4. EFM shows FHR late decelerations in response to uterine contractions.

**795.** The nurse's laboring client is being electronically monitored during her labor. The baseline FHR throughout the labor has been in the 130s. In the last 2 hours, the baseline has decreased to the 100s. How should the nurse document this FHR?

1. Tachycardia
2. Bradycardia
3. Late deceleration
4. Within normal limits

**796.** **MoC** The nurse is caring for the pregnant client whose FHR tracing reveals a reduction in variability over the last 40 minutes. The client has had occasional decelerations after the onset of a contraction that did not resolve until the contraction was over. The client suddenly has a prolonged deceleration that does not resolve, and the nurse immediately intervenes by calling for assistance. Place the nurse's interventions in the sequence that they should occur.

1. Administer oxygen via facemask.
2. Have the HCP paged if the prolonged decelerations have not resolved.
3. Place an indwelling urinary catheter in anticipation of emergency cesarean birth if the HR remains low.
4. Increase the rate of the intravenous (IV) fluids.
5. Assist the client into a different position.
6. Prepare for a vaginal examination and fetal scalp stimulation.

Answer: _____

**797.** The nurse is caring for the client who is being evaluated for a suspected malpresentation. The fetus's long axis is lying across the maternal abdomen, and the contour of the abdomen is elongated. Which should be the nurse's documentation of the lie of the fetus?

1. Vertex
2. Breech
3. Transverse
4. Brow

**798.** The full-term pregnant client presents with bright red vaginal bleeding and intense abdominal pain. Her BP is 150/96 mm Hg, and her pulse is 109 bpm. The nurse should immediately implement interventions for which possible complication?

1. Placenta previa
2. Placental abruption
3. Bloody show
4. Succenturiate placenta

**799.** The nurse is evaluating the client in triage for possible labor. The client's contractions are every 3 to 4 minutes, 60 to 70 seconds in duration, and moderate by palpation. Her cervical exam in the office was Illustration 1. Her current exam is Illustration 2. What conclusions should the nurse draw from Illustration 2?

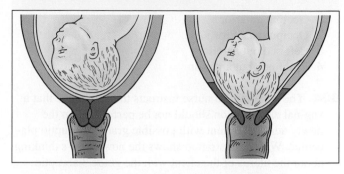

1. The client is not dilated or effaced.
2. The client is completely dilated but not effaced.
3. The client has minimally dilated but completely effaced.
4. The client is not dilated but completely effaced.

**800.** **PHARM** The laboring client is requesting IV pain medication instead of epidural anesthesia. The nurse determines that which factor would most definitely contraindicate the administration of nalbuphine hydrochloride?

1. Completely dilated and 100% effaced
2. FHR of 120 beats per minute
3. Reassuring FHR variability and accelerations
4. Variable decelerations with reassuring FHR

**801.** The client on the labor unit has been experiencing frequent, painful contractions for the last 6 hours. The contractions are of poor quality, and there has been no cervical change. Which interventions should the nurse implement? **Select all that apply.**

1. Maintain bedrest.
2. Administer a sedative.
3. Administer an analgesic.
4. Prepare for cesarean delivery.
5. Prepare to start oxytocin.

**802.** **MoC** The nurse reviews information and assesses the laboring client at 42 weeks' gestation before an HCP induces labor. Which findings should be reported to the HCP because they are contraindications to labor induction? **Select all that apply.**

1. Umbilical cord prolapse
2. Transverse fetal lie
3. Cervical dilation not progressing
4. Premature rupture of membranes
5. Previous cesarean incision

**803.** MoC The client in active labor has moderate to strong contractions occurring every 2 minutes and lasting 60 to 70 seconds. The client states extreme pain in the small of her back. Her abdomen reveals a small depression under the umbilicus. Which fetal position should the nurse document?

1. Occiput anterior
2. Occiput posterior
3. Left occiput anterior
4. Right occiput anterior

**804.** The experienced nurse instructs the new nurse that a vaginal examination should not be performed on the newly admitted client with possible grade 3 abruptio placentae. Which illustration shows the new nurse's thinking about the uterus of the client with the grade 3 abruptio placentae?

**1.**

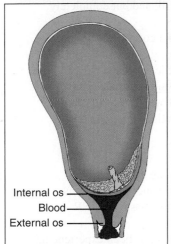

Internal os
Blood
External os

**2.**

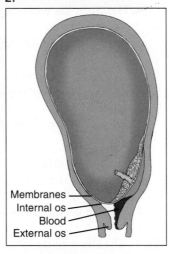

Membranes
Internal os
Blood
External os

**3.**

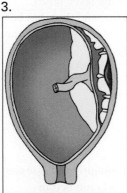

**4.**

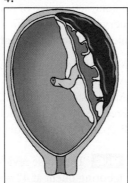

**805.** The nurse is about to auscultate the FHR on the client in triage. What information should be determined **first** to find the correct placement for auscultation?

1. Position of the fetus
2. Position of the placenta
3. Presence of contractions
4. Where to apply the ultrasonic gel

**806.** MoC The pregnant client has been pushing for 2.5 hours. After some difficulty, the large fetal head emerges. The HCP attempts to deliver the shoulders without success. Place the nurse's actions in caring for this client in the correct sequence.

1. Apply suprapubic pressure per direction of the HCP.
2. Place the client in exaggerated lithotomy position.
3. Catheterize the client's bladder.
4. Call for the neonatal resuscitation team to be present.
5. Prepare for an emergency cesarean birth.

Answer: _____

**807.** The laboring client suddenly experiences a dramatic drop in the FHR from the 150s to the 110s. A vaginal exam reveals the presence of the fetal cord protruding through the cervix. What should the nurse do **first**?

1. Put continuous pressure on the presenting part to keep it off the cord.
2. Place the bed in Trendelenburg position.
3. Insert a urinary catheter and instill saline.
4. Continue to monitor the FHR.

**808.** MoC PHARM The nurse is caring for the 30-weeks-pregnant client who is having contractions every 1.5 to 2 minutes with spontaneous rupture of membranes 2 hours ago. Her cervix is 8 cm dilated and 100% effaced. Delivery is imminent. What intervention is **most** important now?

1. Administer a tocolytic agent.
2. Provide teaching on premature infant care.
3. Notify neonatology of the impending birth.
4. Prepare for a cesarean section birth.

**809.** The nurse is evaluating the 39-weeks-pregnant client who reports greenish, foul-smelling vaginal discharge. Her temperature is 101.6°F (38.7°C), and the FHR is 120 with minimal variability and no accelerations. The client's group beta streptococcus (GBS) culture is positive. Which interventions should the nurse plan to implement? **Select all that apply.**

1. Prepare for cesarean birth due to chorioamnionitis.
2. Start oxytocin for labor induction.
3. Start antibiotics as directed for the GBS infection.
4. Prepare the client for epidural anesthesia.
5. Notify the neonatologist of the client's status.
6. Administer a cervical ripening agent.

**810.** At 1 minute after birth, a neonate is pink, except for blue extremities. The neonate is crying, gagging, and grimacing when the bulb syringe is used and has some flexion of extremities and an HR of 97. Based on the Apgar score, what should the nurse do **next**?

1. Notify the HCP.
2. Recheck the Apgar at 5 minutes after birth.
3. Initiate resuscitation measures immediately.
4. Swaddle and hand to mother for breastfeeding.

**811.** A 5-minute-old newborn in a delivery room has a good cry, HR 88, well flexed, good reflex irritability, and blue extremities with a completely pink body. What Apgar score would the nurse document for this newborn?

_____ Apgar score (Record your answer as a whole number.)

## Answers and Rationales

**762. ANSWER: 2**

1. The time and amount of last meal is important to know, but number of weeks' gestation is more important. This client is dilated at 4 cm and in active labor.
2. **Knowing the weeks of gestation is most important because if she is in premature labor, she may need to be given tocolytics to stop the process and to ensure adequate fetal lung maturity. If she is full term, the labor process could continue.**
3. Who will attend the delivery should be identified during admission to the labor unit, but it is not the most important when being evaluated in triage.
4. History of previous illnesses should be collected during admission to the labor unit, but it is not the most important when being evaluated in triage.

▶ *Test-taking Tip: The key word is "priority." All options include information that the nurse should collect as part of an initial assessment of the client in possible labor, but you need to think about what information is missing from the scenario that determines whether or not to allow labor to continue.*

**Content Area:** Childbearing; **Concept:** Pregnancy; Assessment; **Integrated Processes:** Nursing Process: Assessment; **Client Needs:** Safe and Effective Care Environment: Management of Care; **Cognitive Level:** Nursing Process: Analysis

**763. ANSWER: 3**

1. At –2, the fetus is 2 cm above, not below, the maternal ischial spines. Two centimeters below the ischial spines would be recorded as +2.
2. The cervix is 3 cm, not totally dilated. Total dilation would be documented as 10 for the first number. Also, the cervix is 100% effaced, which is total effacement (shortening and thinning out).
3. **The nurse should interpret 3/100/–2, RSP as the cervix is 3 cm dilated, 100% effaced, and the fetus is 2 cm above the maternal ischial spines. RSP means that the fetus is to the right of the mother's pelvis (R), with the sacrum as the specific presenting part (S), which is a breech position. This fetus is also posterior (P).**

4. Fetal lie (relationship of long axis or spine of fetus to long axis of mother) is longitudinal, not transverse. The documentation does not specify if the fetal attitude is flexion.

▶ *Test-taking Tip: To interpret the documentation of 3/100/–2, RSP, remember the first number represents cervical dilation in centimeters, the second number represents cervical effacement, and the third number represents cm above (–), at (0), or below (+) the maternal ischial spines. The final abbreviations represent fetal position. Fetal position is the relationship of a reference point on the presenting part to the four quadrants of the mother's pelvis and is designated by three letters. The first letter is the location of the presenting part to either the right or left of the mother's pelvis (R or L). The middle letter refers to the specific presenting part of the fetus (O for occiput, S for sacrum, M for mentum or chin, and Sc for scapula or shoulder). The third letter is the location of the presenting part in relation to the anterior (A), posterior (P), or transverse (T) portion of the maternal pelvis.*

**Content Area:** Childbearing; **Concept:** Pregnancy; Communication; **Integrated Processes:** Nursing Process: Analysis; **Client Needs:** Physiological Integrity: Reduction of Risk Potential; **Cognitive Level:** Application [Applying]

**764.** PHARM **ANSWERS: 1, 3**

1. **The FHR may be affected by medications given to the mother. Therefore a baseline FHR should be determined before giving any medication to the laboring client and then assessed again after giving the medication.**
2. The FHR should be assessed every 30 minutes (not 15 minutes) during the first stage of labor if the client is categorized as low risk. The FHR should be assessed every 15 minutes during the second stage of labor.
3. **The FHR should be assessed after each vaginal examination because the fetus could change positions, or be stressed by the intrusion of the examiner's fingers, or intact membranes could have ruptured.**
4. Although the FHR could be listened to during a contraction, it may be difficult due to muffling of the sounds and maternal movement. It is most important to listen before and after the contraction to more accurately detect FHR decelerations.

5. If the client is classified as low risk, she should not be receiving oxytocin (Pitocin) for labor augmentation or induction.

▶ *Test-taking Tip: Focus on the client as you review the options; she is a low-risk laboring client during the first stage of labor. Low-risk status for the laboring client means that she has no pregnancy risk factors, no meconium-stained fluid, and normal labor patterns, and labor is without augmentation or induction. Use this information to narrow the options.*

**Content Area:** Childbearing; **Concept:** Pregnancy; Assessment; **Integrated Processes:** Nursing Process: Assessment; **Client Needs:** Physiological Integrity: Pharmacological and Parenteral Therapies; Physiological Integrity: Reduction of Risk Potential; **Cognitive Level:** Analysis [Analyzing]

**765. MoC PHARM ANSWER: 1, 3, 4, 5**

1. **The client experiencing a convulsion related to anesthesia should first have an airway established.**
2. The client's head should be turned to the side if vomiting occurs, but the client typically remains in a left lateral tilt position so an airway can be maintained. Positioning on the right side can cause aortocaval compression.
3. **The client experiencing a convulsion related to anesthesia should receive 100% oxygen so that the mother and fetus remain oxygenated.**
4. **Small doses of diazepam (Valium) or thiopental (Pentothal) can be administered to stop the convulsions.**
5. **The anesthesiologist should be STAT paged to provide assistance; the convulsion was initiated by the regional anesthetic.**

▶ *Test-taking Tip: You should use the ABC's to establish the most important interventions. Eliminate any option that can increase risk to the fetus.*

**Content Area:** Childbearing; **Concept:** Safety; Pregnancy; Management; **Integrated Processes:** Nursing Process: Implementation; **Client Needs:** Safe and Effective Care Environment: Management of Care; Physiological Integrity: Physiological Adaptation; Physiological Integrity: Pharmacological and Parenteral Therapies; **Cognitive Level:** Analysis [Analyzing]

**766. ANSWER:**

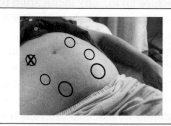

**The right upper quadrant of the client's abdomen is the best area to listen to and count the FHR when the fetus is in the RSA (right sacrum anterior) position. When the fetus is in RSA position, the fetal back faces the client's right side. The fetal presentation is breech, and the fetal head is in the upper segment of the client's abdomen. The FHR is heard most clearly through the fetal back. This is designated as the area of maximal intensity or loudness, providing clarity of fetal heart sounds.**

▶ *Test-taking Tip: First interpret the abbreviation RSA. The first letter is the right (R) or left (L) side of the maternal pelvis. The second letter is the landmark of the presenting part: occiput (O), mentum (M), sacrum (S), or acromion process (A). The third letter is anterior (A), posterior (P), or transverse (T), depending on whether the landmark is in the front, back, or side of the maternal pelvis. The FHR is heard most clearly through the fetal back.*

**Content Area:** Childbearing; **Concept:** Pregnancy; **Integrated Processes:** Nursing Process: Planning; **Client Needs:** Physiological Integrity: Reduction of Risk Potential; **Cognitive Level:** Application [Applying]

**767. ANSWER: 4**

1. During the transition phase (8 to 10 cm), the client is usually more restless, irritable, and more likely to lose control.
2. During the active phase (4 to 7 cm), the client may become more anxious and fatigued and needs to concentrate on breathing techniques to cope with the increasingly stronger contractions.
3. The client who is actively pushing is focusing on how effective she is in the descent of the fetus and concentrating on how she is coping with contractions. She is usually not expressing happiness or laughter, and is not talkative.
4. **During the latent phase (1 to 3 cm), the client is usually happy and talkative.**

▶ *Test-taking Tip: The latent, active, and transition phases are components of the first stage of labor. Uterine contractions become stronger and closer together throughout the first stage, with characteristic responses of the client.*

**Content Area:** Childbearing; **Concept:** Pregnancy; Assessment; **Integrated Processes:** Nursing Process: Analysis; **Client Needs:** Physiological Integrity: Physiological Adaptation; **Cognitive Level:** Comprehension [Understanding]

**768. PHARM ANSWER: 4**

1. Although bladder distention is a possible side effect of butorphanol tartrate, it is not common and is not the most important assessment.
2. Seizures are not a potential side effect of butorphanol tartrate.
3. An itchy rash is not a potential side effect of butorphanol tartrate.
4. **Evaluating maternal VS and pulse oximetry would determine changes in respiratory and cardiac status. Respiratory depression in both the mother and fetus can occur with butorphanol tartrate (Stadol).**

▶ *Test-taking Tip: Butorphanol tartrate (Stadol) is an opioid agonist-antagonist analgesic frequently used for laboring women. Use the ABC's to determine the priority assessment.*

Content Area: Childbearing; Concept: Medication; Pregnancy; Integrated Processes: Nursing Process: Evaluation; Client Needs: Physiological Integrity: Pharmacological and Parenteral Therapies; Cognitive Level: Evaluation [Evaluating]

## 769. ANSWER: 4

1. Late abortions occur most commonly with circumvallate placenta where the fetal side of the placenta is covered to some extent with chorion.
2. Fetal demise occurs most commonly with circumvallate placenta where the fetal side of the placenta is covered to some extent with chorion.
3. Postpartum hemorrhage occurs more commonly in a succenturiate placenta where one or more accessory lobes are connected to the main placenta by blood vessels.
4. **A battledore placenta occurs when the umbilical cord is inserted at or near the placenta margin. It most commonly results in preterm labor and bleeding.**

▸ *Test-taking Tip: Battledore placenta is an umbilical cord abnormality where the umbilical cord is located near the placenta margin and bleeding can occur. Consider the gestation of the client to narrow the options.*

Content Area: Childbearing; Concept: Pregnancy; Integrated Processes: Nursing Process: Planning; Client Needs: Physiological Integrity: Physiological Adaptation; Cognitive Level: Analysis [Analyzing]

## 770. ANSWER: 4

1. Counterpressure can be helpful to cope with internal pressure sensations and pain in the lower back when the fetus is in posterior position. The fetus is ROA or right occiput anterior position.
2. Effleurage can distract from contraction pain during the latent phase of the first stage of labor. This client is in active labor, and as labor progresses, hyperesthesia occurs, increasing the likelihood that effleurage will be uncomfortable and less effective.
3. Providing a quiet, calm, and relaxed labor environment should be part of the nursing responsibilities to help the client cope with contractions, but doing something more is best.
4. **Breathing techniques provide distraction, reduce pain perception, and help the client maintain control during labor. The modified-paced breathing technique is usually more effective during active labor (4 to 7 cm). The client is at 5 cm. The modified-paced technique is performed at about twice the normal breathing rate and requires that the client remain alert and concentrate fully on her breathing.**

▸ *Test-taking Tip: The client is at 5 cm, in active labor, and has a fetus in ROA or right occiput anterior position. Narrow the options to a technique that can be used during active labor with a fetus positioned ROA.*

Content Area: Childbearing; Concept: Pregnancy; Comfort; Integrated Processes: Nursing Process: Implementation; Client Needs: Physiological Integrity: Basic Care and Comfort; Psychosocial Integrity; Cognitive Level: Application [Applying]

## 771. ANSWER: 3

1. An FHR pattern having minimal variability (not a sinusoidal pattern) might indicate that the fetus is in a sleep state.
2. Absent or minimal variability, not a sinusoidal FHR pattern, could indicate possible congenital anomalies.
3. **A sinusoidal pattern, which is regular, smooth, undulating, and uncommon, classically occurs with severe fetal anemia as a result of abnormal perinatal conditions.**
4. Moderate variability of the FHR (not a sinusoidal pattern) reflects normal fetal well-being.

▸ *Test-taking Tip: Options 1 and 4 are normal, whereas Options 2 and 3 are abnormal. A sinusoidal pattern is regular, smooth, and undulating and is uncommon. Use this information to eliminate Options 1 and 4. Of the two remaining options, you should select the option that identifies a real problem.*

Content Area: Childbearing; Concept: Pregnancy; Integrated Processes: Nursing Process: Analysis; Client Needs: Physiological Integrity: Reduction of Risk Potential; Cognitive Level: Application [Applying]

## 772. ANSWER: 2

1. Assessing for adequate gel under the transducer and repositioning should be done before assuming there is a problem with the baby's HR.
2. **When the FHR monitor tracing is no longer recording, the nurse should first check for adequate gel under the transducer. There needs to be adequate gel under the transducer for good conduction, and adding gel frequently corrects the problem.**
3. There is no indication to give oxygen to the client.
4. Auscultating FHR by fetoscope and assessing maternal VS could be completed, but not until the transducer has been checked.

▸ *Test-taking Tip: This question emphasizes that common-sense independent actions can be implemented by the nurse before making an assumption.*

Content Area: Childbearing; Concept: Pregnancy; Communication; Integrated Processes: Nursing Process: Analysis; Client Needs: Safe and Effective Care Environment: Safety and Infection Control; Cognitive Level: Application [Applying]

## 773. ANSWER: 1

1. **The third stage of labor lasts from the birth of the baby until the placenta is expelled. Lengthening of the fetal cord is one of several signs indicating placental separation.**
2. Bloody show is pink and mucoid in nature and occurs during the first and second stages of labor. During the third stage, there may be increased vaginal bleeding that is bright or dark red.

3. A strong urge to push may occur during the first and second stages of labor.

4. More frequent contractions occur during the first and second stages of labor.

▶ *Test-taking Tip:* *The third stage of labor lasts from the birth of the baby until the placenta is expelled. Only one option pertains to the fetus.*

**Content Area:** Childbearing; **Concept:** Pregnancy; Assessment; **Integrated Processes:** Nursing Process: Assessment; **Client Needs:** Health Promotion and Maintenance; **Cognitive Level:** Application [Applying]

### 774. ANSWER: 4

1. Normal amniotic fluid should be clear. Cloudiness could indicate the presence of meconium or an intrauterine infection.

2. Amniotic fluid should have no odor. Any odor may indicate the presence of infection.

3. Amniotic fluid should be clear. Meconium stained could indicate fetal distress.

4. **The pH of amniotic fluid is usually between 6.5 and 7.5, which is more alkaline than urine or purulent material.**

▶ *Test-taking Tip:* *If uncertain, carefully think through Options 1, 2, and 3 to determine if these would be normal findings with any fluid.*

**Content Area:** Childbearing; **Concept:** Pregnancy; **Integrated Processes:** Nursing Process: Evaluation; **Client Needs:** Physiological Integrity: Reduction of Risk Potential; **Cognitive Level:** Evaluation [Evaluating]

### 775. MoC ANSWER: 4

1. The client needs to be fully dilated (10 cm, not 8 cm) and fully effaced (100%, not 90%) before being encouraged to push. Pushing too early may cause cervical edema and lacerations and may slow the labor process.

2. Rectal pressure may indicate that the client has progressed since the last vaginal exam. Another vaginal exam should be performed before contacting the obstetrician or midwife.

3. During labor, rectal pressure is usually not due to the need for a bowel movement because intestinal motility decreases.

4. **The nurse should first evaluate labor progress by performing another vaginal exam. Previously the client was almost fully effaced (90%), and fetal station was 1 cm below the ischial spines (+1). Rectal pressure is often due to pressure exerted during descent of the fetal presenting part.**

▶ *Test-taking Tip:* *Notice that all options are interventions except for Option 4, which is an assessment. Remember to assess the client before intervening.*

**Content Area:** Childbearing; **Concept:** Pregnancy; Management; **Integrated Processes:** Nursing Process: Implementation; **Client Needs:** Safe and Effective Care Environment: Management of Care; **Cognitive Level:** Application [Applying]

### 776. MoC ANSWER: 4

1. The maternal temperature should be monitored during labor and at least every 2 hours after the membranes rupture to assess for possible infection. However, this is not the priority nursing action.

2. Characteristics of the fluid (color, odor, and estimated amount) should be assessed and documented after rupture, but this is not the priority at this time.

3. A vaginal exam that assesses the progress of labor does need to be performed right after membrane rupture, but it is not the priority.

4. **The priority nursing action is to assess the FHR pattern for several minutes immediately after membrane rupture to determine fetal well-being. The umbilical cord may prolapse as a result of the rupture, causing life-threatening changes in the FHR.**

▶ *Test-taking Tip:* *Three options pertain to the client and one to the fetus. Often the option that is different is the answer.*

**Content Area:** Childbearing; **Concept:** Pregnancy; Management; **Integrated Processes:** Nursing Process: Assessment; **Client Needs:** Safe and Effective Care Environment: Management of Care; **Cognitive Level:** Application [Applying]

### 777. MoC ANSWER: 4

1. Increasing the infusion rate may be implemented if repositioning the client does not correct the hypotension.

2. Elevating the client's legs for 2 to 3 minutes is done with severe or prolonged hypertension to increase blood return from the extremities. It may be implemented after repositioning to left side, increasing the IV rate, and placing in Trendelenburg position.

3. Placing in 10- to 20-degree Trendelenburg position is usually implemented if the BP does not increase within 1 to 2 minutes after repositioning to left side and increasing the IV flow rate.

4. **The first action is to place the client in a left side-lying position. This displaces the uterus and alleviates aortocaval compression.**

▶ *Test-taking Tip:* *The key in the stem is that the client is lying supine and has hypotension. Think about aortocaval compression and what action will alleviate this.*

**Content Area:** Childbearing; **Concept:** Pregnancy; Management; **Integrated Processes:** Nursing Process: Implementation; **Client Needs:** Safe and Effective Care Environment: Management of Care; **Cognitive Level:** Application [Applying]

### 778. ANSWER: 2

1. Widening of the cervix describes cervical dilation, not effacement.

2. **In cervical effacement, the cervix progressively changes from a thick and long structure to paper thin. This statement indicates that the client understands the information.**

3. Cervical changes will not cause membranes to rupture. The power of contractions causes cervical changes (effacement and dilation) and, possibly, membrane rupture.

4. Cervical changes will not help the fetus to change position. Fetal descent is thought to occur from the pressure of contractions, especially from the fundus, and from the pressure of the amniotic fluid. Fetal position changes also occur from the fetal head and body adjusting to the maternal pelvis as they descend.

▶ *Test-taking Tip: Narrow the options to the process (Options 1 and 2) and eliminate Options 3 and 4, which address incorrect information about the cervical changes.*

**Content Area:** Childbearing; **Concept:** Pregnancy; Nursing Roles; **Integrated Processes:** Teaching/Learning; Nursing Process: Evaluation; **Client Needs:** Health Promotion and Maintenance; **Cognitive Level:** Evaluation [Evaluating]

## 779. MoC ANSWER: 4

1. The fetus has a normal baseline HR and good variability. There is no indication that immediate delivery is necessary. Other measures could correct the V-shaped (variable) decelerations.

2. Other nursing measures are used to correct the V-shaped (variable) decelerations prior to contacting the obstetrician (or midwife).

3. Repositioning the client should be implemented prior to giving her oxygen.

4. **Repositioning the client to her side or to knee-chest should be done first to take the pressure off the umbilical cord. Variable decelerations usually result from cord compression and stretching during fetal descent.**

▶ *Test-taking Tip: The baseline and variability are WNL, but the V-shaped deceleration unrelated to contractions is abnormal. This is a typical variable pattern that can occur during the transition phase of the first stage of labor, caused by umbilical cord compression. Knowing this, think about the action that will relieve the cord compression.*

**Content Area:** Childbearing; **Concept:** Pregnancy; Management; **Integrated Processes:** Nursing Process: Implementation; **Client Needs:** Safe and Effective Care Environment: Management of Care; Physiological Integrity: Reduction of Risk Potential; **Cognitive Level:** Application [Applying]

## 780. ANSWERS: 1, 2, 5

1. **Progressive cervical dilation and effacement indicate true labor. In false labor, the contractions may occur for several hours, but there is no cervical change.**

2. **In true labor, walking usually increases the intensity of contractions. In false labor, walking usually has little or no effect on contractions and may sometimes decrease the frequency, intensity, and duration of contractions.**

3. Warm tub baths and rest lessen contractions during false labor. In true labor, contractions do not decrease with warm tub baths or rest.

4. Discomfort is usually in the client's abdomen during false labor. Discomfort begins in the back and radiates around to the abdomen during true labor.

5. **Contractions increase in duration and intensity during true labor, while there is usually no change in contractions during false labor.**

▶ *Test-taking Tip: Look in the options for key words such as "increase" or "progressive" that would be indicators of true labor. The words "lessen" and "discomfort" should cue you that these may indicate false labor.*

**Content Area:** Childbearing; **Concept:** Pregnancy; **Integrated Processes:** Nursing Process: Evaluation; **Client Needs:** Health Promotion and Maintenance; **Cognitive Level:** Evaluation [Evaluating]

## 781. ANSWER: 4

1. Inspection of the abdomen can be used to determine fetal position, but because the client is obese, this is not the most accurate method.

2. Palpation of the abdomen can be used to determine fetal position, but because the client is obese, this is not the most accurate method.

3. Vaginal examination can be used to determine fetal position, but because the client is obese, this is not the most accurate method.

4. **Real-time transabdominal ultrasound (US) is the most accurate assessment measure to determine the fetal position and is frequently available in the birthing setting. US images may be used to assess fetal lie, presentation, and position in the morbidly obese client.**

▶ *Test-taking Tip: Determine the accuracy and ease of use of each assessment method to determine the best option. Note that three options are similar, using only the hands, and one option is different. Often the option that is different is the answer.*

**Content Area:** Childbearing; **Concept:** Assessment; Pregnancy; **Integrated Processes:** Nursing Process: Planning; **Client Needs:** Health Promotion and Maintenance; **Cognitive Level:** Application [Applying]

## 782. ANSWER: 2

1. Women with a previous cesarean birth are at an increased risk for uterine rupture.

2. **The client who is overdue by 7 days but has a reassuring FHR pattern is able to have intermittent fetal monitoring.**

3. Women with preeclampsia are at an increased risk for placental insufficiency and need continuous monitoring during labor.

4. Women with gestational diabetes are at an increased risk for placental insufficiency and need continuous monitoring during labor.

▶ *Test-taking Tip: The key word is "intermittent." Eliminate options that include a risk factor that would require continuous fetal monitoring. One option is different from the other options. Often the option that is different is the answer.*

Content Area: Childbearing; Concept: Pregnancy; Integrated Processes: Nursing Process: Analysis; Client Needs: Safe and Effective Care Environment: Safety and Infection Control; Cognitive Level: Application [Applying]

## 783. ANSWER: 1

1. **When the laboring client lies flat on her back, the gravid uterus completely occludes the inferior vena cava and laterally displaces the subrenal aorta. This aortocaval compression reduces maternal cardiac output, producing dyspnea, diaphoresis, tachycardia, and hypotension. Other symptoms include air hunger, nausea, and weakness. A left side-lying position decreases aortocaval compression.**

2. Lying on the right side increases aortocaval compression.

3. Notifying the obstetrician is not the first intervention. The obstetrician would be notified if symptoms are not relieved by a left side-lying position.

4. Applying oxygen may be needed, but first the client should be placed left side-lying.

▶ *Test-taking Tip: Think of the maternal structures on the right side that would result in decreased cardiac output when compressed by the gravid uterus.*

Content Area: Childbearing; Concept: Pregnancy; Integrated Processes: Nursing Process: Implementation; Client Needs: Physiological Integrity: Physiological Adaptation; Cognitive Level: Application [Applying]

## 784. MoC PHARM ANSWER: 3

1. The pulsating mass indicates umbilical cord prolapse, which is a medical emergency. If vaginal birth is not imminent, a cesarean section is preferred to prevent hypoxic acidosis.

2. Placing the client in a knee-chest position relieves pressure on the umbilical cord.

3. **The nurse should question the administration of oxytocin (Pitocin). Oxytocin is used for stimulating contraction of the uterus. Uterine contractions can cause further umbilical cord compression.**

4. Terbutaline (Brethine) is a tocolytic agent used to reduce contractions.

▶ *Test-taking Tip: You need to consider that oxytocin and terbutaline have two different, opposing actions.*

Content Area: Childbearing; Concept: Assessment; Medication; Management; Integrated Processes: Nursing Process: Implementation; Client Needs: Safe and Effective Care Environment: Management of Care; Physiological Integrity: Pharmacological and Parenteral Therapies; Cognitive Level: Analysis [Analyzing]

## 785. ANSWER: 2

1. Cephalopelvic disproportion occurs when the head is too large to fit through the client's pelvis. Fetal descent ceases, and infant's head would not emerge.

2. The "turtle sign" occurs when the infant's head suddenly retracts back against the mother's perineum after emerging from the vagina, resembling a turtle pulling its head back into its shell. This head retraction is caused by the infant's anterior shoulder being caught on the back of the maternal pubic bone (shoulder dystocia), preventing delivery of the remainder of the infant.

3. Persistent occiput posterior results in prolonged pushing; however, once the head is born, the remainder of the birth occurs without difficulty.

4. A cord prolapse occurs when the umbilical cord enters the cervix before the fetal presenting part and is considered a medical emergency.

▶ *Test-taking Tip: Note in the stem that the baby's head emerges. Think about the head of the turtle retracting back with the "turtle sign." This occurs because the infant is caught. Of the options, think about the part that could be caught on the mother's body.*

Content Area: Childbearing; Concept: Pregnancy; Integrated Processes: Nursing Process: Analysis; Client Needs: Physiological Integrity: Physiological Adaptation; Cognitive Level: Comprehension [Understanding]

## 786. ANSWER: 1

1. **Maternal HR is normally increased due to pain resulting from increased catecholamine secretion, fear, anxiety, and increased blood volume.**

2. When the laboring client holds her breath and pushes against a closed glottis, intrathoracic pressure rises. Blood in the lungs is forced into the left atrium, leading to a transient increase (not decrease) in cardiac output.

3. Although the WBCs increase to 25,000/mm$^3$ to 30,000/mm$^3$ during labor and early postpartum as a physiological response to stress, this is not a cardiovascular change.

4. During the second stage of labor, the maternal intravascular volume is increased (not decreased) by 300 to 500 mL of blood from the contracting uterus.

▶ *Test-taking Tip: The key word is "cardiovascular"; thus eliminate Option 3. Of the remaining options, consider that two options are a decrease and one is an increase. Often the option that is different is the answer.*

Content Area: Childbearing; Concept: Perfusion; Pregnancy; Integrated Processes: Nursing Process: Assessment; Client Needs: Physiological Integrity: Physiological Adaptation; Cognitive Level: Application [Applying]

## 787. ANSWER: 1

1. **Early labor is a pattern of labor that occurs when contractions become regular and the cervix dilates to 3 cm.**

2. False labor occurs when Braxton-Hicks contractions are strong enough for the client to believe she is in actual labor. The contractions are infrequent or do not have a definite pattern. This client's contractions are regular and strong.
3. Cervical ripening (softening, effacement, and increased distensibility) begins about 4 weeks before birth. There is no information in the stem about cervical ripening.
4. Lightening is settling or lowering of the fetus into the pelvis. Lightening can occur a few weeks or a few hours before labor. There is no information in the stem about lightening.

▶ *Test-taking Tip: If there is no information in the stem pertaining to an option, then the option should be eliminated (Options 3 and 4). You should consider that the contractions are regular but that dilation is only at 3 cm when choosing between Options 1 and 2.*

Content Area: Childbearing; **Concept:** Pregnancy; **Integrated Processes:** Nursing Process: Analysis; **Client Needs:** Physiological Integrity: Physiological Adaptation; **Cognitive Level:** Application [Applying]

### 788. MoC ANSWER: 4

1. The WBC count in labor is normally increased due to the stress of labor and can be as high as 25,000/mm³ to 30,000/mm³.
2. The glucose level normally falls during labor because of an expenditure of energy in labor.
3. Anemia or a reduction in the Hgb and Hct is common in pregnancy. Hgb levels less than 10 g/dL are considered abnormal in pregnancy.
4. **The nurse should report the low platelet count of 100,000/mm³ (normal is 150,000 to 450,000/mm³). A low count can contribute to bleeding and affect the use of epidural anesthesia.**

▶ *Test-taking Tip: Although a number of the laboratory values are abnormal, only one places the client at a high risk for bleeding and can affect the use of epidural anesthesia. Focus on selecting the laboratory value result that affects bleeding.*

Content Area: Childbearing; **Concept:** Pregnancy; Management; **Integrated Processes:** Nursing Process: Analysis; **Client Needs:** Safe and Effective Care Environment: Management of Care; Physiological Integrity: Reduction of Risk Potential; **Cognitive Level:** Application [Applying]

### 789. MoC ANSWER: 3, 1, 2, 4

3. **Obtain FHT should be first. The client has ruptured membranes with greenish fluid, and the fetus could be experiencing nonreassuring fetal status.**
1. **Perform a sterile vaginal exam to determine labor progression.**
2. **Assess the client thoroughly. This needs to be completed prior to notifying the HCP with the information.**

4. **Notify the HCP is the last of the options. Assessment findings would need to be reported to the HCP. The client should then be moved into an inpatient room.**

▶ *Test-taking Tip: Use the nursing process. You will want to have completed your assessment prior to notifying the HCP.*

Content Area: Childbearing; **Concept:** Critical Thinking; Pregnancy; Management; **Integrated Processes:** Nursing Process: Planning; **Client Needs:** Safe and Effective Care Environment: Management of Care; **Cognitive Level:** Synthesis [Creating]

### 790. ANSWER:

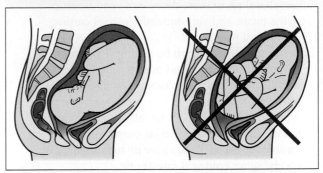

**A breech delivery is most likely to be associated with head entrapment because the head is the largest part of the fetal body, and it is delivered last in a breech delivery.**

▶ *Test-taking Tip: View each delivery mentally and predict which image is most likely to result in head entrapment.*

Content Area: Childbearing; **Concept:** Pregnancy; **Integrated Processes:** Nursing Process: Planning; **Client Needs:** Physiological Integrity: Reduction of Risk Potential; **Cognitive Level:** Application [Applying]

### 791. ANSWER: 1

1. **Because cultural variations exist in pain control measures used and pain tolerance, the most crucial assessment in the active stage of labor is the client's choice of pain control measures.**
2. A desire for hot or cold fluids is an important aspect that should be determined during the early stage of labor.
3. Determination of support persons is an important aspect that should be made during the early stage of labor.
4. The desire for circumcision is an important consideration, but it is not the primary need during the active stage of labor.

▶ *Test-taking Tip: Although all of the options have cultural implications that require the nurse to have an understanding of cultural diversity and needs, only one would be most crucial during the "active stage of labor."*

Content Area: Childbearing; **Concept:** Diversity; Pregnancy; Assessment; **Integrated Processes:** Nursing Process: Assessment; Culture and Spirituality; **Client Needs:** Psychosocial Integrity; **Cognitive Level:** Application [Applying]

**792.** PHARM **ANSWER: 1, 3, 4, 5**

1. **Breakthrough pain can occur when the continuous infusion rate of the anesthetic agent is below the recommended rate for a therapeutic dose. Breakthrough pain can also occur when the client has a full bladder or when the cervix is completely dilated.**

2. Hypertension is a contraindication for epidural anesthesia. A major side effect of epidural anesthesia is hypotension (not hypertension) caused by a spinal blockade, which lowers peripheral resistance, decreases venous return to the heart, and subsequently lessens cardiac output and lowers BP.

3. **A spinal headache can be a complication of epidural anesthesia and occurs when the dura is accidently punctured during epidural placement.**

4. **A sensory level of $T_{10}$ is usually maintained during epidural anesthesia; most women are unable to feel a full bladder or to void after receiving an epidural anesthetic.**

5. **Maternal temperature may be elevated to 100. 1°F (37.8°C) or higher with an epidural. Sympathetic blockade may decrease sweat production and diminish heat loss.**

▶ *Test-taking Tip: Only one option should be eliminated because it is opposite of the expected side effects with epidural anesthesia.*

**Content Area:** Childbearing; **Concept:** Medication; Pregnancy; **Integrated Processes:** Nursing Process: Analysis; **Client Needs:** Physiological Integrity: Pharmacological and Parenteral Therapies; **Cognitive Level:** Analysis [Analyzing]

**793. ANSWER: 1**

1. **Hydrotherapy is usually initiated when the client is in active labor, at approximately 4 or 5 cm. This timing will help reduce the risk of prolonged labor and provide a welcome change when the contractions are becoming stronger and closer together.**

2. Changing position takes less effort while immersed in water, so women are encouraged to change positions more frequently to help facilitate the process of labor.

3. FHR monitoring can be done just as easily during hydrotherapy, using a wireless external monitor, Doppler, or fetoscope. Internal electrodes can be placed during most types of hydrotherapy but is contraindicated during jet hydrotherapy.

4. There is no time limit for laboring women to use hydrotherapy; they may stay as long as desired, unless complications develop during the labor process.

▶ *Test-taking Tip: Note that Options 2, 3, and 4 are similar with negative phrasing. The only option that is positive is Option 1.*

**Content Area:** Childbearing; **Concept:** Nursing Roles; Pregnancy; Comfort; **Integrated Processes:** Teaching/Learning; Caring; **Client Needs:** Physiological Integrity: Basic Care and Comfort; Psychosocial Integrity; **Cognitive Level:** Application [Applying]

**794.** MoC **ANSWER: 1**

1. **The illustration shows FHR accelerations in the top graph and uterine contractions in the bottom graph. Acceleration is an increase in the FHR of 15 bpm above the FHR baseline that lasts for at least 15 to 30 seconds.**

2. Option 2 is incorrect because the FHR increases in response to uterine contractions.

3. With FHR early decelerations, there would be a decrease in FHR below the baseline FHR in response to uterine contractions.

4. With FHR late decelerations, there is a decrease in the FHR beginning at or after the peak of the uterine contraction and returning to baseline only after the contraction has ended.

▶ *Test-taking Tip: The term acceleration refers to an increase in FHR and decelerations to a decrease in FHR. Use this information to eliminate options.*

**Content Area:** Childbearing; **Concept:** Assessment; Management; Pregnancy; **Integrated Processes:** Nursing Process: Evaluation; **Client Needs:** Safe and Effective Care Environment: Management of Care; Safe and Effective Care Environment: Safety and Infection Control; **Cognitive Level:** Evaluation [Evaluating]

**795. ANSWER: 2**

1. Tachycardia occurs when the baseline is greater than 160 bpm.

2. **An FHR baseline less than 110 is classified as bradycardia.**

3. A prolonged deceleration is defined as a change from the baseline FHR that occurs for 2 to 10 minutes before returning to baseline. A late deceleration is a gradual decrease and return of the FHR to baseline, associated with a uterine contraction.

4. A decrease to the 100s is not within the normal range. The normal FHR is 120 to 160 bpm.

▶ *Test-taking Tip: The normal FHR is 120 to 160 bpm.*

**Content Area:** Childbearing; **Concept:** Pregnancy; Communication; **Integrated Processes:** Communication and Documentation; **Client Needs:** Safe and Effective Care Environment: Safety and Infection Control; **Cognitive Level:** Application [Applying]

**796.** MoC **ANSWER: 5, 1, 4, 2, 6, 3**

5. **Assist the client into a different position should be first. Repositioning is an attempt to increase the FHR in case of cord obstruction.**

1. **Administer oxygen via facemask is next to increase oxygenation to the fetus.**

4. **Increase the rate of the IV fluids next to treat possible hypotension, the most common cause of fetal bradycardia.**

2. **Have the HCP paged if the prolonged decelerations have not resolved. The immediate focus should be on attempting to relieve the prolonged decelerations.**

6. **Prepare for a vaginal examination and fetal scalp stimulation. This is performed to rule out cord prolapse and to provide stimulation to the fetal head.**

3. Place an indwelling urinary catheter in anticipation of emergency cesarean birth if the HR remains low.

▶ *Test-taking Tip:* Use the ABC's to establish that the initial actions are promoting oxygenation to the fetus and then to the client.

Content Area: Childbearing; Concept: Critical Thinking; Pregnancy; Management; Integrated Processes: Nursing Process: Planning; Client Needs: Safe and Effective Care Environment: Management of Care; Cognitive Level: Synthesis [Creating]

## 797. ANSWER: 3

1. Vertex presentations result in the lie's being vertical.
2. Breech presentations result in the lie's being vertical.
3. **A transverse lie occurs in 1 in 300 births and is marked by the fetus's lying in a side-lying position across the abdomen.**
4. A brow presentation is also a vertical lie.

▶ *Test-taking Tip:* The key phrase is "lying across the maternal abdomen." Recall that transverse is a side-lying position. This should direct you to Option 3.

Content Area: Childbearing; Concept: Pregnancy; Integrated Processes: Communication and Documentation; Client Needs: Physiological Integrity: Physiological Adaptation; Cognitive Level: Application [Applying]

## 798. ANSWER: 2

1. Placenta previa is marked by painless vaginal bleeding.
2. **The nurse should immediately implement interventions for placental abruption. This occurs when the placenta separates from the uterine wall before the birth of the fetus. It is commonly associated with preeclampsia.**
3. Bloody show is a normal physiological sign associated with normal labor progression and is marked by bloody, mucus-like consistency.
4. Succenturiate placenta is the presence of one or more accessory lobes that develop on the placenta with vascular connections of fetal origin.

▶ *Test-taking Tip:* You should narrow the options by eliminating the one normal sign. Of the other three options, you should focus on the client's BP and bleeding.

Content Area: Childbearing; Concept: Pregnancy; Integrated Processes: Nursing Process: Analysis; Client Needs: Physiological Integrity: Physiological Adaptation; Cognitive Level: Application [Applying]

## 799. ANSWER: 3

1. Illustration 1 (not Illustration 2) shows that the client is neither effaced nor dilated.
2. The cervical opening is minimally dilated, not completely dilated, and completely effaced.
3. **In Illustration 2, the client is completely effaced and has some dilation.**
4. Illustration 2 shows some dilation.

▶ *Test-taking Tip:* Effacement refers to a thinning of the cervix, whereas dilation refers to the opening of the cervix. Be sure to focus on Illustration 2 when reading the options.

Content Area: Childbearing; Concept: Pregnancy; Integrated Processes: Nursing Process: Analysis; Client Needs: Physiological Integrity: Physiological Adaptation; Cognitive Level: Application [Applying]

## 800. PHARM ANSWER: 1

1. **Systemic medications, such as nalbuphine hydrochloride (Nubain), should not be administered when advanced dilation is present (transition stage of labor) because its use can lead to respiratory depression if given too close to the time of delivery.**
2. An FHR of 120 bpm is within normal parameters of 120 to 160 bpm.
3. Reassuring FHR variability and accelerations are interpreted as adequate placental oxygenation and do not contraindicate administration of nalbuphine hydrochloride.
4. If mild variable decelerations are present but the FHR pattern remains reassuring, nalbuphine hydrochloride can still be administered.

▶ *Test-taking Tip:* Nalbuphine hydrochloride (Nubain) should not be administered during the transition stage of labor. You should identify which option best describes the transition stage.

Content Area: Childbearing; Concept: Medication; Pregnancy; Integrated Processes: Nursing Process: Evaluation; Client Needs: Physiological Integrity: Pharmacological and Parenteral Therapies; Cognitive Level: Evaluation [Evaluating]

## 801. ANSWER: 1, 2, 3, 5

1. **This client is experiencing a hypertonic labor pattern in which her contractions are frequent and painful, but no cervical change has occurred. This client should be encouraged to rest often.**
2. **A sedative should be given to assist the client to rest.**
3. **Because the contractions are painful, an analgesic should be administered to help the client relax and cope more effectively.**
4. A cesarean birth is not a treatment for a hypertonic labor pattern unless a nonreassuring FHR pattern is present.
5. **If the hypertonic labor pattern continues, augmentation should be initiated with either an oxytocin infusion or amniotomy.**

▶ **Test-taking Tip:** *This client is experiencing a hypertonic labor pattern in which her contractions are frequent and painful, but no cervical change has occurred. You should focus on selecting options that will help the client feel more comfortable or enhance labor progression.*

**Content Area:** Childbearing; **Concept:** Pregnancy; **Integrated Processes:** Nursing Process: Implementation; **Client Needs:** Physiological Integrity: Reduction of Risk Potential; **Cognitive Level:** Analysis [Analyzing]

### 802. MoC ANSWER: 1, 2, 5

1. **Inducing labor with an umbilical cord prolapse can cause fetal trauma and is contraindicated. This should be reported to the HCP.**
2. **Inducing labor with a transverse fetal lie can produce trauma to the fetus and mother and is contraindicated. This should be reported to the HCP.**
3. Lack of progressive cervical dilation is an indication for labor induction, not a contraindication.
4. Premature rupture of the membranes is an indication for labor induction, not a contraindication.
5. **Women with a previous cesarean incision should not be stimulated because it is a contraindication for a vaginal birth and warrants an immediate repeat cesarean birth. This should be reported to the HCP.**

▶ **Test-taking Tip:** *Options that could cause fetal or maternal trauma would be contraindications for inducing labor.*

**Content Area:** Childbearing; **Concept:** Pregnancy; Management; **Integrated Processes:** Nursing Process: Analysis; **Client Needs:** Safe and Effective Care Environment: Management of Care; **Cognitive Level:** Application [Applying]

### 803. MoC ANSWER: 2

1. When a fetus presents anterior, it is uncommon for the mother's chief symptom to be back pain, and the uterus should appear smooth.
2. **An occiput posterior position is characterized by intense back pain (back labor). A depression under the umbilicus occurs as a result of the posterior shoulder.**
3. When a fetus presents anterior, it is uncommon for the mother's chief symptom to be back pain, and the uterus should appear smooth.
4. When a fetus presents anterior, it is uncommon for the mother's chief symptom to be back pain, and the uterus should appear smooth.

▶ **Test-taking Tip:** *Remember when the fetal back (occiput posterior) is against the mother's spine, back pain is the chief symptom. All options except 2 include the word anterior. Thus eliminate Options 1, 3, and 4.*

**Content Area:** Childbearing; **Concept:** Pregnancy; Communication; **Integrated Processes:** Communication and Documentation; **Client Needs:** Safe and Effective Care Environment: Management of Care; **Cognitive Level:** Application [Applying]

### 804. ANSWER: 4

1. Illustration 1 shows complete placenta previa and not abruptio placentae.
2. Illustration 2 shows partial placenta previa and not abruptio placentae.
3. Illustration 3 shows mild grade 1 abruptio placentae. Less than 15% of the placenta separates with concealed hemorrhage.
4. **Illustration 4 shows severe grade 3 abruptio placentae. More than 50% of the placenta separates with concealed hemorrhage.**

▶ **Test-taking Tip:** *Think about the risk to the mother and neonate.*

**Content Area:** Childbearing; **Concept:** Pregnancy; **Integrated Processes:** Nursing Process: Analysis; **Client Needs:** Safe and Effective Care Environment: Safety and Infection Control; **Cognitive Level:** Knowledge [Remembering]

### 805. ANSWER: 1

1. **The nurse should first perform Leopold's maneuvers to determine the fetal position. This will enable proper placement of the Doppler device over the location of the FHR.**
2. The position of the placenta can provide important information. However, if the Doppler device is placed over the placenta, the nurse will hear a swishing sound and not the FHR.
3. The FHR is still assessed regardless of the presence of contractions. The nurse who has difficulty obtaining an FHR because of a contraction can listen again once the contraction has concluded.
4. Ultrasonic gel is used with any ultrasound device and allows for the conduction of sound and continuous contact of the device with the maternal abdomen. To apply the gel to the correct location, the position of the fetus must be known.

▶ **Test-taking Tip:** *The key word in both the stem and options is "fetal." Carefully read the question to determine what is being asked.*

**Content Area:** Childbearing; **Concept:** Pregnancy; **Integrated Processes:** Nursing Process: Planning; **Client Needs:** Health Promotion and Maintenance; **Cognitive Level:** Application [Applying]

### 806. MoC ANSWER: 4, 2, 1, 3, 5

4. **Call for the neonatal resuscitation team to be present because of fetal distress.**
2. **Place the client in exaggerated lithotomy position so the McRoberts' maneuver can be performed (flexing her thighs sharply on her abdomen may widen the pelvic outlet and let the anterior shoulder be delivered).**
1. **Apply suprapubic pressure per direction of the HCP. This is completed in an effort to dislodge the shoulder from under the pubic bone.**
3. **Catheterize the client's bladder. This will empty the bladder to make more room for the fetal head.**

5. **Prepare for an emergency cesarean birth. This will be performed if all efforts for a vaginal birth fail.**

▶ *Test-taking Tip: The client is experiencing shoulder dystocia. Calling for help has priority. Identifying the last action may help in ordering the remainder of the actions.*

Content Area: Childbearing; Concept: Safety; Pregnancy; Management; Integrated Processes: Nursing Process: Implementation; Client Needs: Safe and Effective Care Environment: Management of Care; Cognitive Level: Synthesis [Creating]

## 807. ANSWER: 1

1. **The nurse should first exert continuous pressure on the presenting part to prevent further cord compression. This is continued until birth, which is usually by cesarean section.**
2. The bed should be placed in Trendelenburg position to further prevent pressure on the cord, but only after pressure is placed on the presenting part.
3. A catheter may be inserted and 500 mL of warmed saline instilled to help float the head and prevent further compression, but only after pressure is placed on the presenting part.
4. The fetus is continually monitored throughout until birth.

▶ *Test-taking Tip: Use the ABC's to determine priority and eliminate options. One option is an assessment; the stem calls for an intervention.*

Content Area: Childbearing; Concept: Perfusion; Pregnancy; Integrated Processes: Nursing Process: Implementation; Client Needs: Safe and Effective Care Environment: Safety and Infection Control; Cognitive Level: Application [Applying]

## 808. MoC PHARM ANSWER: 3

1. Tocolytic agents, such as nifedipine (Procardia), can be used for short-term intervention to slow down contractions and delay birth, but it is too late to administer a tocolytic agent.
2. Teaching is important but is not appropriate at this time.
3. **The most important intervention is to notify the neonatal team of the delivery because the team members will be needed for respiratory support and possible resuscitation.**
4. A cesarean birth is indicated if there are other obstetrical needs.

▶ *Test-taking Tip: Focus on the gestational age and the most important needs at this time. Associate "delivery is imminent" with "impending birth" and select Option 3.*

Content Area: Childbearing; Concept: Pregnancy; Management; Integrated Processes: Nursing Process: Implementation; Client Needs: Safe and Effective Care Environment: Management of Care; Physiological Integrity: Pharmacological and Parenteral Therapies; Cognitive Level: Application [Applying]

## 809. ANSWER: 1, 3, 4, 5

1. **Because this client is not in labor and chorioamnionitis is possible, a cesarean birth is indicated.**
2. Starting oxytocin (Pitocin) would prolong the time to delivery.
3. **The client should be given antibiotics as prescribed to treat the infection.**
4. **Because epidural anesthesia offers the least risk to the fetus, preparation for epidural anesthesia should begin.**
5. **The pediatrician or neonatologist should be notified and available for the impending delivery.**
6. Administering a cervical ripening agent would prolong the time to delivery.

▶ *Test-taking Tip: Chorioamnionitis is an intra-amniotic infection resulting from bacterial invasion and inflammation of the membranes before birth. This client needs to deliver as soon as possible. Identify which interventions would result in the quickest and safest delivery method.*

Content Area: Childbearing; Concept: Infection; Pregnancy; Integrated Processes: Nursing Process: Planning; Client Needs: Physiological Integrity: Reduction of Risk Potential; Cognitive Level: Synthesis [Creating]

## 810. ANSWER: 2

1. Notifying the HCP is not necessary at this time. The 1-minute Apgar score is 6, very close to the 7 to 10 normal limits. This newborn has a good cry, indicating good transition to the extrauterine environment thus far.
2. **Rechecking the Apgar score at 5 minutes after birth will determine if the newborn is continuing to make a good transition to the extrauterine environment.**
3. Initiating resuscitation measures immediately is not necessary. This would be done if the newborn were not crying and demonstrated a blue or pale body.
4. Swaddling and giving the newborn to the mother for breastfeeding are important but should occur after the 5-minute Apgar, if the score is WNL. Keeping this newborn in the radiant warmer, rather than giving him or her to the mother, will help prevent hypothermia and promote better transition to extrauterine life.

▶ *Test-taking Tip: You need to first calculate the Apgar score and then decide the appropriate action based on knowing the score. This newborn's 1-minute Apgar score is 6: 1 out of 2 because the HR is below 100, 1 of out 2 for grimace, 1 out of 2 for a pink body with blue extremities, 2 points for crying, and 1 point for some flexion of extremities. A score of 7 to 10 is WNL, and 6 is close. The good cry indicates good transition to extrauterine life. Using this information should assist you in identifying the answer.*

**Content Area:** Childbearing; **Concept:** Pregnancy; **Integrated Processes:** Nursing Process: Implementation; **Client Needs:** Health Promotion and Maintenance; **Cognitive Level:** Analysis [Analyzing]

### 811. ANSWER: 8

**The newborn would receive 1 point because the HR is below 100 bpm, 2 points for a good cry (respiratory effort), 2 points for being well flexed (muscle tone), 2 points for good reflex irritability (reflex response), and 1 point for a pink body with blue extremities (color).**

▶ **Test-taking Tip:** The 10-point Apgar scoring system includes five signs: 2 points for a HR greater than 100 beats/minute, 2 points for respiration good with crying, 2 points for muscle tone of active movement of extremities, 2 points for reflex response of vigorous cry, coughs, sneezes, and pulls away when touched, and 2 points for skin color of pink body and extremities. The score for each sign is reduced to 1 or 0 if not within the parameter for that sign.

**Content Area:** Childbearing; **Concept:** Development; Pregnancy; Communication; **Integrated Processes:** Communication and Documentation; **Client Needs:** Physiological Integrity: Physiological Adaptation; **Cognitive Level:** Application [Applying]

## Chapter Twenty

# Postpartum Management

**812.** The delivery nurse is reporting to the postpartum nurse about the client who just delivered her first baby, a term newborn. Which number should the delivery nurse report for the client's parity?

_____ Parity (Record your answer as a whole number.)

**813.** Immediately after delivery of the client's placenta, the nurse palpates the client's uterine fundus. The fundus is firm and located halfway between the umbilicus and symphysis pubis. Which action should the nurse take based on the assessment findings?

1. Immediately begin to massage the uterus.
2. Document the findings of the fundus.
3. Assess the client for bladder distention.
4. Monitor for increased vaginal bleeding.

**814.** MoC The client, who delivered a 4200-g baby 4 hours ago, continues to have bright red, heavy vaginal bleeding. The nurse assesses the client's fundus and finds it to be firm and midway between the symphysis pubis and umbilicus. What should the nurse do **next?**

1. Continue to monitor the client's bleeding and weigh the peri-pads.
2. Call the client's HCP and request an additional visual examination.
3. Prepare to give oxytocin to stimulate uterine muscle contraction.
4. Document the findings as normal with no interventions needed at that time.

**815.** When looking in the mirror at her abdomen, the postpartum client says to the nurse, "My stomach still looks like I'm pregnant!" The nurse explains that the abdominal muscles, which separate during pregnancy, will undergo which change?

1. Regain tone within the first week after birth
2. Regain prepregnancy tone with exercise
3. Remain separated, giving the abdomen a slight bulge
4. Regain tone as the weight gained during pregnancy is lost

**816.** The clinic nurse reviews the laboratory results illustrated from the postpartum client who is 3 days postdelivery. What should the nurse do in response to these results?

| Laboratory Value | Result |
|---|---|
| Hct | 35% |
| Hgb | 11 g/dL |
| WBCs | 20,000/mm³ |

1. Document the laboratory report findings.
2. Assess the client for increased lochia.
3. Assess the client's temperature orally.
4. Notify the HCP immediately.

**817.** The Caucasian postpartum client asks the nurse if the stretch marks (striae gravidarum) on her abdomen will ever go away. Which response by the nurse is **most** accurate?

1. "Your stretch marks should totally disappear over the next month."
2. "Your stretch marks will always appear raised and reddened."
3. "Your stretch marks will lighten in color with good skin hydration."
4. "Your stretch marks will fade to pale white over the next 3 to 6 months."

**818.** Twenty-four hours post-vaginal delivery, the postpartum client tells the nurse that she is concerned because she has not had a bowel movement (BM) since before delivery. Which action should be taken by the nurse?

1. Document the data in the client's medical record.
2. Notify the HCP immediately.
3. Administer a laxative that was prescribed prn.
4. Assess the client's abdomen and bowel sounds.

**819.** MoC The RN and the student nurse are caring for the postpartum client who is 16 hours postdelivery. The RN evaluates that the student needs more education about uterine assessment when the student is observed doing which activity?

1. Elevating the client's head 30 degrees before doing the assessment
2. Supporting the lower uterine segment during the assessment
3. Gently palpating the uterine fundus for firmness and location
4. Observing the abdomen before beginning palpation

**820.** The nurse is assessing the postpartum client, who is 5 hours postdelivery. Initially, the nurse is unable to palpate the client's uterine fundus. Prioritize the nurse's actions to locate the client's fundus by placing each step in the correct sequence.

1. Place the side of one hand just above the client's symphysis pubis.
2. Press deeply into the abdomen.
3. Place the other hand at the level of the umbilicus.
4. Massage the abdomen in a circular motion.
5. Position the client in the supine position.
6. If the fundus is not felt, move the upper hand lower on the abdomen and repeat the massage.

Answer: _____

**821.** PHARM The client delivered a healthy newborn 4 hours ago after being induced with oxytocin. While being assisted to the bathroom to void for the first time after delivery, the client tells the nurse that she doesn't feel a need to urinate. Which explanation should the nurse provide when the client expresses surprise after voiding 900 mL of urine?

1. "A decreased sensation of bladder filling is normal after childbirth."
2. "The oxytocin you received in labor makes it difficult to feel voiding."
3. "You probably didn't empty completely. I will need to scan your bladder."
4. "Your bladder capacity is large; you likely won't void again for 6 to 8 hours."

**822.** PHARM The nurse is preparing to administer 2 mg hydromorphone hydrochloride to the client who is 28 hours post–cesarean section. The medication available is in a concentration of 4 mg/mL. How many milliliters should the nurse administer?

_____ mL (Record your answer in tenths.)

**823.** MoC Before hospitalization, an adolescent client had decided to give up her newborn for adoption. The client had an uncomplicated vaginal delivery and is still committed to her decision. Which intervention should the nurse exclude?

1. Offer the client a transfer to a different unit within the hospital.
2. Talk to the client about having possible feelings of ambivalence.
3. Initiate a case management or social work consult for the client.
4. Notify her family to ensure that support is available upon her discharge.

**824.** MoC PHARM The client, who had preeclampsia and delivered vaginally 4 hours ago, is still receiving magnesium sulfate IV. When assessing the client's deep tendon reflexes (DTRs), the nurse finds that they are both weak, at 1+, whereas previously they were 2+ and 3+. What should be the nurse's plan? **Select all that apply.**

1. Notify the client's HCP about the reduced DTRs.
2. Prepare to increase the magnesium sulfate dose.
3. Prepare to administer calcium gluconate IV.
4. Assess the level of consciousness and vital signs.
5. Ask the HCP about drawing a serum calcium level.

**825.** The postpartum client delivered a full-term infant 2 days previously. The client states to the nurse, "My breasts seem to be growing, and my bra no longer fits." Which statement should be the basis for the nurse's response to the client's concern?

1. Rapid enlargement of breasts usually is a symptom of infection.
2. Increasing breast tissue may be a sign of postpartum fluid retention.
3. Thrombi may form in veins of the breast and cause increased breast size.
4. Breast tissue increases in the early postpartum period as milk forms.

**826.** While assessing the postpartum client who is 10 hours post–vaginal delivery, the nurse notes a perineal pad that is totally saturated. To determine the significance of this finding, which question should the nurse ask the client **first?**

1. "How often are you having uterine cramping?"
2. "When was the last time you changed your pad?"
3. "Do you have any bladder urgency or frequency?"
4. "Did you pass clots that required a pad change?"

**827.** **MoC** Two hours after the client's vaginal delivery, she reports feeling "several large, warm gushes of fluid" from her vagina. The nurse assesses the client's perineum and finds a large pool of blood on the client's bed. Which nursing action is **priority?**

1. Encourage the client to ambulate to the bathroom to empty her bladder.
2. Place two hands on the uterine fundus and prepare to vigorously massage the uterus.
3. Reassure the client that heavy bleeding is expected in the first few hours postpartum.
4. Support the lower uterine segment with one hand and assess the fundus with the other.

**828.** The oncoming shift nurse assesses the fundus of the postpartum client 6 hours after a vaginal birth and finds that it is firm. When the nurse then assists the client out of bed for the first time, blood begins to run down the client's leg. Which action by the nurse in response to the client's bleeding is correct?

1. Explain that extra bleeding can occur with initial standing.
2. Immediately assist the client back into bed.
3. Push the emergency call light in the room.
4. Call the HCP to report this increased bleeding.

**829.** **MoC** An LPN asks an RN to assist in locating the fundus of the client who is 8 hours post–vaginal delivery. Place an X at the location on the client's abdomen where the RN should direct the LPN to begin to palpate the fundus.

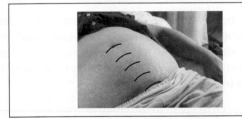

**830.** The nurse is caring for the client who just gave birth. Which observation should lead the nurse to be concerned about the client's attachment to her male infant?

1. Asking the caregiver about how to change his diaper
2. Comparing her newborn's nose to her brother's nose
3. Calling the baby "Kelly," which was the name selected
4. Repeatedly telling her husband that she wanted a girl

**831.** The nurse is caring for the postpartum family. The nurse determines that paternal engrossment is occurring when which observation is made of the newborn's father?

1. Talks to his newborn from across the room
2. Shows similarities between his and the baby's ears
3. Expresses feeling frustrated when the infant cries
4. Seems to be hesitant to touch his newborn

**832.** The nurse is caring for the postpartum primiparous client who is 13 hours post–vaginal delivery. The nurse observes that the client is passive and hesitant about making decisions about her own and her newborn's care. In response to this observation, which interventions should be implemented by the nurse? **Select all that apply.**

1. Question her closely about the presence of pain.
2. Ask if she would like to talk about her birth experience.
3. Encourage her to nap when her infant is napping.
4. Encourage attendance in teaching sessions about infant care.
5. Suggest that she begin to write her birth announcements.

**833.** The client has a vaginal delivery of a full-term newborn. Immediately after delivery, the nurse assesses that the client's perineum and labia are edematous, but she does not have an episiotomy or a perineal laceration. Which intervention should the nurse implement?

1. Give her an ice pack to apply to the perineum.
2. Teach her to relax her buttocks before sitting.
3. Apply warm packs to the affected areas.
4. Provide a plastic donut cushion for sitting.

**834.** The nurse observes the postpartum multiparous client rubbing her abdomen. When asked if she is having pain, the client says, "It feels like menstrual cramps." Which intervention should the nurse implement?

1. Offer a warm blanket for her to place on her abdomen.
2. Encourage her to lie on her stomach until the cramps stop.
3. Instruct the client to avoid ambulation while having pain.
4. Check her lochia flow; pain sometimes precedes hemorrhage.

**835.** The postpartum client tells the nurse that she has pain when she breastfeeds. The nurse identifies that the infant has poor latch during breastfeeding. Which breast appearance shows that the client is experiencing symptoms associated with poor latch?

1.
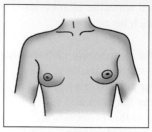

Illustration by Linda Ostwald-Boelke.

2.
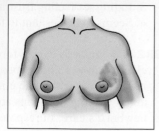

Illustration by Linda Ostwald-Boelke.

3.
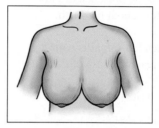

Illustration by Linda Ostwald-Boelke.

4.
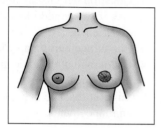

Illustration by Linda Ostwald-Boelke.

**836.** Two hours after delivery, the mother tells the nurse that she will be bottle feeding. She asks what she can do to prevent the terrible pain experienced when her milk came in with her last baby. Which response by the nurse is **most** appropriate?

1. "Once you have recovered from the birth, I will help you bind your breasts."
2. "Engorgement is familial. If you had it with your last baby, it is inevitable."
3. "I can help you put on a supportive bra; wear one constantly for 1 to 2 weeks."
4. "Engorgement occurs right after birth; if you don't have it yet, it won't occur."

**837.** The client, who had a vaginal delivery 18 hours ago, asks the nurse how she should take care of her perineal laceration. Which statements by the nurse are appropriate? **Select all that apply.**

1. "You should change your peri-pad at least twice each day."
2. "Once home, use a warm sitz bath to sooth your perineum."
3. "Keep your perineum warm and dry until stitches are removed."
4. "Use your peri-bottle to apply water to the perineum after each void."
5. "Wash your perineum with mild soap at least once each 24 hours."
6. "Check your perineum for foul odor or increased redness, heat, or pain."

**838.** The postpartum client, who is 24 hours post–cesarean section, tells the nurse that she has much less lochial discharge after this birth than with her vaginal birth 2 years ago. The client asks if this is normal after a cesarean birth. Which statement should be the basis for the nurse's response?

1. A decrease in her lochia is not expected; further assessment is needed.
2. Women usually have increased lochial discharge after cesarean births.
3. Women normally have less lochial discharge after a cesarean birth.
4. The lochia amount depends on whether surgery was emergent or planned.

**839.** The client, who is 12 days postpartum, telephones the clinic and tells the nurse that she is concerned that she may have an infection because her vaginal discharge has been creamy white for 2 days now. Which response by the nurse is correct?

1. "You need to come to the clinic as soon as possible."
2. "You'll need an antibiotic; which pharmacy do you use?"
3. "Take your temperature and let me know if it is elevated."
4. "A creamy, white discharge 10 days postpartum is normal."

**840.** MoC The nurse receives report for four postpartum clients. In which order should the nurse assess the clients? Prioritize the clients in order from first to last.

1. The client who had a normal, spontaneous vaginal delivery 30 minutes ago
2. The client who had a cesarean section 48 hours ago and is bottle feeding her newborn infant
3. The client who had a vaginal delivery 32 hours ago and is having difficulty breastfeeding
4. The client who delivered her newborn via scheduled C-section 8 hours ago and has a PCA pump with morphine for pain control

Answer: _____

**841.** MoC The nurse is caring for four postpartum clients. Which client should be the nurse's **priority** for monitoring for uterine atony?

1. The client who is 2 hours post–cesarean birth for a breech baby
2. The client who delivered a macrosomic baby after a 12-hour labor
3. The client who has a firm fundus after a vaginal delivery 4 hours ago
4. The client receiving oxytocin intravenously for past 2 hours

**842.** The postpartum client, who is 24 hours post–vaginal birth and breastfeeding, asks the nurse when she can begin exercising to regain her prepregnancy body shape. Which response by the nurse is correct?

1. "Simple abdominal and pelvic exercises can begin right now."
2. "You will need to wait until after your 6-week postpartum checkup."
3. "Once your lochia has stopped, you can begin exercising."
4. "You should not exercise while you are breastfeeding."

**843.** In the process of preparing the client for discharge after a cesarean section, the nurse addresses all of the following areas during discharge education. Which should be the **priority** advice for the client?

1. How to manage her incision
2. Planning for assistance at home
3. Infant care procedures
4. Increased need for rest

**844.** The nurse asks the 12-hour postpartum client, who is breastfeeding her baby now, why she has not yet received a dinner tray. The client states that her mother is bringing curry and that she won't be eating the hospital food tonight. Which response by the nurse is **best?**

1. "Please let me know if you change your mind. I can order food for you later."
2. "Because you are breastfeeding, you should avoid eating highly spiced food."
3. "I will ask the dietitian to meet with you so you can discuss your nutritional needs."
4. "You should not be eating highly spiced food 12 hours after delivery."

**845.** The nurse is evaluating a breastfeeding session. The nurse determines that the infant has appropriately latched on to the mother's breast when which observations are made? **Select all that apply.**

1. The mother reports a firm tugging feeling on her nipple.
2. A smacking sound is heard each time the baby sucks.
3. The infant's mouth covers only the mother's nipple.
4. The baby's nose, mouth, and chin are touching the breast.
5. The infant's cheeks are rounded when sucking.
6. The infant's swallowing can be heard after sucking.

**846.** The primiparous client, who is bottle feeding her infant, asks the nurse when she can expect to start having her menstrual cycle again. Which response by the nurse is **most** accurate?

1. "Most women who bottle feed can expect their period within 6 to 10 weeks after birth."
2. "Your period should return a few days after your lochial discharge stops."
3. "Your lochia will change from pink to white; when white, your period should return."
4. "Bottle feeding delays the return of a normal menstrual cycle until 6 months postbirth."

**847.** Twenty-four hours after the birth of her first child, the 25-year-old single client tells the nurse that she has several different male sex partners and asks the nurse to recommend an appropriate birth control method for her. Considering her lifestyle, which method of birth control should the nurse suggest?

1. An intrauterine device (IUD)
2. Depot-medroxyprogesterone acetate injections
3. A female condom with nonoxynol-9
4. A diaphragm

**848.** **PHARM** After delivering the full-term infant, the breastfeeding mother asks the nurse if there is any contraceptive method that she should avoid while she is breastfeeding. Which contraceptive should the nurse advise the client to avoid?

1. A diaphragm
2. An intrauterine device (IUD)
3. The combined oral contraceptive (COC) pill
4. The progesterone-only mini pill

**849.** While assessing the breastfeeding mother 24 hours postdelivery, the nurse notes that the client's breasts are hard and painful. Which interventions should be implemented by the nurse? **Select all that apply.**

1. Tell her to feed a small amount from both breasts at each feeding.
2. Apply ice packs to the breasts at intervals between feedings.
3. Give supplemental formula at least once in a 24-hour period.
4. Administer an anti-inflammatory medication prescribed prn.
5. Apply warm, moist packs to the breasts between feedings.
6. Pump the breasts as needed to ensure complete emptying.

**850.** The nurse is teaching the client, who is breastfeeding, about returning to sexual activity after vaginal delivery. Which statement should the nurse include?

1. "Orgasm may decrease the amount of breast milk you produce."
2. "You may need to use lubrication when resuming sexual intercourse."
3. "You should not have sexual intercourse until two months postpartum."
4. "Your HCP will let you know when you can resume sexual activity."

**851.** **PHARM** The postpartum client's blood type is A negative, and her newborn infant's blood type is AB negative. The client received RhoGAM in her second trimester and another dose in her third trimester, after a minor car accident. The client is preparing for discharge and asks the nurse when she will receive her RhoGAM injection. The nurse correctly responds with which statement?

1. "You already received two doses of RhoGAM and do not need an additional dose."
2. "I will give your last dose of RhoGAM today, before you are discharged to home."
3. "You and your baby have negative blood types; a dose of RhoGAM is not needed."
4. "RhoGAM would have been already given while you were in the delivery room."

**852.** The client with mastitis asks the nurse if she should stop breastfeeding because she has developed a breast infection. Which response by the nurse is **best**?

1. "Continuing to breastfeed will decrease the duration of your symptoms."
2. "Breastfeeding should only be continued if your symptoms decrease."
3. "Stop feeding for 24 hours until antibiotic therapy begins to take effect."
4. "It is best to stop breastfeeding because the infant may become infected."

**853.** The postpartum client is being admitted for mastitis. The nurse should prepare the client for which interventions? **Select all that apply.**

1. Walking at least four times in 24 hours
2. Receiving a prescribed oral antibiotic
3. Applying warm packs to the breasts
4. Getting a prescribed anti-inflammatory drug
5. Limiting oral fluid intake to 1000 mL per day
6. Emptying the milk from her breasts frequently

**854.** The nurse educates the breastfeeding client diagnosed with mastitis. The nurse evaluates that the client has an adequate understanding of how to prevent mastitis in the future when the client makes which statements? **Select all that apply.**

1. "Incorrect latch of my baby can lead to mastitis."
2. "I should perform hand hygiene before I breastfeed."
3. "I should rinse my baby's mouth before I let her latch."
4. "A tight underwire bra has support that prevents mastitis."
5. "I should allow my nipples to air-dry after breastfeeding."

**855.** The client delivered vaginally six hours ago, and is upset about bleeding too much. She shows the nurse the peri-pad that was just removed. What should the nurse do **first**?

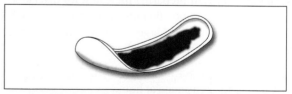

Illustration by Linda Ostwald-Boelke.

1. Ask her how long she has been wearing this pad.
2. Notify the HCP of this increased amount of lochia.
3. Prepare to give oxytocin to decrease bleeding.
4. Document the finding; this amount is normal

**856.** The client, who is 20 days postpartum, telephones the perinatal clinic to tell the nurse that she is having heavy, bright red bleeding since hospital discharge 18 days ago. Which instruction to the client is correct?

1. "You need to come to the clinic immediately."
2. "Limit physical activity until the bleeding stops."
3. "There is no need for concern; this is expected."
4. "Call next week if the bleeding has not stopped."

**857.** The postpartum client suffered a fourth-degree perineal laceration during her vaginal birth. Which interventions should the nurse add to the client's plan of care? **Select all that apply.**

1. Limit ambulation to bathroom privileges only.
2. Decrease fluid intake to 1000 mL every 24 hours.
3. Instruct the client on a high-fiber diet.
4. Monitor the uterus for firmness every 2 hours.
5. Give prn prescribed stool softeners in the a.m. and at h.s.

**858.** The client, who had a forceps-assisted vaginal birth 4 hours ago, tells the nurse that she is having continuing perineal pain rated at 7 out of 10 and rectal pressure. An oral analgesic was given and ice applied to the perineum earlier. What should the nurse do now?

1. Call the HCP to report the pain.
2. Closely reinspect the perineum.
3. Help her out of bed to ambulate.
4. Administer a stool softener.

**859.** **MoC** The nurse is caring for the client who is 28 hours postpartum. Which assessment findings should prompt the nurse to notify the HCP of possible puerperal infection? **Select all that apply.**

1. Oral temperature of 102.2°F (39°C)
2. Telangiectasis on the neck and chest
3. Mild abdominal tenderness with palpation
4. Lochial discharge that is foul smelling
5. White blood cell count of 16,500 cells/mm³

**860.** The postpartum client is being discharged to home with a streptococcal puerperal infection. The client is taking antibiotics but asks the nurse what precautions she should take at home to prevent spreading the infection to her husband, newborn, and toddler. Which is the **best** response by the nurse?

1. "No precautions are necessary because you are taking antibiotics."
2. "You should always wear a mask when caring for your newborn and toddler."
3. "Wash your hands before caring for your children and after toileting and perineal care."
4. "Your husband should provide all cares for both children until your infection is gone."

**861.** **MoC** The student nurse reports to an experienced nurse finding a warm, red, tender area on the left calf of the client who is 48 hours post–vaginal delivery. The nurse assesses the client and explains that postpartum clients are at increased risk for thrombophlebitis due to which factors? **Select all that apply.**

1. The fibrinogen levels in the blood of postpartum clients are elevated.
2. Fluids normally shift from the interstitial to the intravascular space.
3. Postpartum hormonal shifts irritate vascular basement membranes.
4. Pressure is placed on the legs when elevated in stirrups during delivery.
5. Dilation of veins in the lower extremities occurs during pregnancy.
6. Compression of the common iliac vein occurs during pregnancy.

**862.** The postpartum client delivered a healthy newborn 36 hours previously. The nurse finds the client crying and asks what is wrong. The client replies, "Nothing, really. I'm not in pain or anything, but I just seem to cry a lot for no reason." What should be the nurse's **first** intervention?

1. Call the client's support person to come and sit with her.
2. Remind her that she has a healthy baby and that she shouldn't be crying.
3. Contact the HCP to have the counselor come see the client.
4. Ask the client to discuss her birth experience.

**863.** The husband of the postpartum client diagnosed with moderate postpartum depression (PPD) asks the nurse about the treatments his wife will require. The nurse's response should be based on knowing that which treatments are included in the **initial** collaborative plan of care? **Select all that apply.**

1. Antidepressant medication
2. Individual or group psychotherapy
3. Removal of the infant from the home
4. Sedative-hypnotic agents
5. Electroconvulsive therapy (ECT)

**864.** The client is diagnosed with moderate postpartum depression (PPD) after vaginal delivery of a 10-lb baby. One week following the delivery, the nurse completes a home visit. Which finding is the **priority?**

1. Lochia has a foul-smelling odor.
2. Small but tender hemorrhoids.
3. Yells at her baby to stop crying.
4. Client cries throughout the visit.

**865.** The client, whose parity is 1, had a vaginal delivery 6 days ago and arrived home yesterday after treatment for endometritis. The home health nurse visits the client and plans teaching after seeing which **most** concerning item in the client's bathroom?

1. A box of tampons on the floor outside of the shower stall.
2. Loofa bath sponge sitting on the seat of the shower stall.
3. Damp towel bunched on the towel bar and near the floor.
4. Can of bathroom cleaner on the floor of the shower stall.

**866.** The home care nurse is visiting the mother and her 6-day-old son. The nurse observes that the infant is sleeping in a crib on his back and has a blanket draped over his body. The mother had been sleeping in a nearby room. Which statements are appropriate for the nurse to make in response to this situation? **Select all that apply.**

1. "I'm glad to see that you are sleeping while your baby sleeps."
2. "Having your baby sleep on his back reduces the risk of SIDS."
3. "It is best for you to sleep in the same room as your newborn."
4. "Position your baby on his tummy and side when he is awake."
5. "When using a blanket, always tuck its sides under the mattress."

# Answers and Rationales

## 812. ANSWER: 1

**The client has given birth to her first child; her parity is 1.**

▶ *Test-taking Tip: Parity refers to the number of births after 20 weeks' gestation.*

**Content Area:** Childbearing; **Concept:** Pregnancy; Communication; Integrated Processes: Communication and Documentation; **Client Needs:** Health Promotion and Maintenance; **Cognitive Level:** Application [Applying]

## 813. ANSWER: 2

1. Uterine massage is indicated only if the uterus does not feel firm and contracted.
2. **Immediately after birth, the uterus should contract, and the fundus should be located one-half to two-thirds of the way between the symphysis pubis and umbilicus. Thus the only action required is to document the assessment finding.**
3. There is no indication that the bladder is full. A full bladder will cause uterine displacement to either side of the abdomen.
4. The uterus is firm; there is no reason to infer that increased vaginal bleeding would occur.

▶ *Test-taking Tip: The assessment findings of the fundus are normal.*

**Content Area:** Childbearing; **Concept:** Pregnancy; Integrated Processes: Communication and Documentation; **Client Needs:** Physiological Integrity Reduction of Risk Potential; **Cognitive Level:** Application [Applying]

## 814. MoC ANSWER: 2

1. Although the nurse would definitely need to continue to monitor the amount and quality of bleeding, additional intervention is also needed.

2. **The nurse should consider the possibility of a vaginal wall or cervical laceration, which could produce heavy, bright red bleeding. The HCP should be notified and asked to perform a visual exam of the vagina to assess for possible lacerations in need of repair.**
3. Preparing to administer oxytocin (Pitocin) would be appropriate if the source of bleeding was suspected to be uterine atony, but the uterus is firm and in the expected location.
4. Documenting the findings without further intervention would lead to a failure to identify the source of increased bleeding resulting in possible client injury. Further assessments and interventions are needed.

▶ *Test-taking Tip: Choose the option that indicates the action that should be taken **next**. Rule out Options 1 and 4 because additional intervention is needed. Then rule out Option 3 because the client's uterus is already firm and in the correct location, leaving Option 2 as the only choice.*

**Content Area:** Childbearing; **Concept:** Critical Thinking; Pregnancy; Management; Integrated Processes: Nursing Process: Implementation; **Client Needs:** Safe and Effective Care Environment: Management of Care; **Cognitive Level:** Analysis [Analyzing]

## 815. ANSWER: 2

1. For most women, it takes about 6 weeks (not 1 week) to regain abdominal wall muscle tone to the prepregnancy state, and usually only with exercise.
2. **The "still-pregnant" appearance is caused by relaxation of the abdominal wall muscles. With exercise, most women can regain prepregnancy abdominal muscle tone within about 6 weeks.**

3. If the client delivers a very large infant, the abdominal muscles may separate, but the separation will become less apparent over time.

4. Weight loss alone will not strengthen the abdominal muscles.

▶ *Test-taking Tip: Only one option indicates that the client's actions will affect the muscle tone.*

**Content Area:** Childbearing; **Concept:** Pregnancy; Nursing Roles; Integrated Processes: Teaching/Learning; **Client Needs:** Health Promotion and Maintenance; **Cognitive Level:** Application [Applying]

**816. ANSWER: 1**

1. **The only action required is to document the findings; all values are within expected parameters. Nonpathological leukocytosis often occurs during labor and in the immediate postpartum period because labor produces a mild pro-inflammatory state. WBCs should return to normal by the end of the first postpartum week. Hct and Hgb will begin to decrease on postpartum day 3 or 4 from hemodilution.**

2. Assessing the client's lochia is unnecessary with these results.

3. Assessing the client's temperature is unnecessary with these results.

4. Notifying the HCP is unnecessary with these results.

▶ *Test-taking Tip: The client is 5 days postdelivery. WBCs are usually still elevated in the first week postpartum, and hemodilution occurs also near the end of the first postpartum week. Use this information to narrow the options.*

**Content Area:** Childbearing; **Concept:** Pregnancy; Nursing Roles; Integrated Processes: Communication and Documentation; **Client Needs:** Physiological Integrity: Reduction of Risk Potential; **Cognitive Level:** Analysis [Analyzing]

**817. ANSWER: 4**

1. Stretch marks will fade but will not totally disappear.

2. Stretch marks will fade and will not always appear reddened.

3. There is no evidence that keeping the skin hydrated will lighten the appearance of the stretch marks.

4. **In Caucasian women, stretch marks will fade to a pale white over 3 to 6 months.**

▶ *Test-taking Tip: Options 1 and 2 reflect opposite ends of the spectrum of possible changes in striae gravidarum. Eliminate both of these options as too extreme. Of the remaining options, consider which option contains a time element.*

**Content Area:** Childbearing; **Concept:** Nursing Roles; Diversity; Pregnancy; Integrated Processes: Teaching/Learning; Culture and Spirituality; **Client Needs:** Physiological Integrity: Basic Care and Comfort; **Cognitive Level:** Application [Applying]

**818. ANSWER: 1**

1. **A spontaneous BM may not occur for 2 to 3 days after childbirth due to decreased muscle tone in the intestines during labor and the immediate postpartum period, possible prelabor diarrhea, and decreased food intake and dehydration during labor. Thus documentation of the lack of a BM is the only action required.**

2. There is no need to notify the HCP for a normal finding.

3. A laxative is unnecessary because a BM is not expected for 2 to 3 days postdelivery.

4. Bowel sounds are not altered by a vaginal delivery, even though the passage of stool through the intestines is slowed.

▶ *Test-taking Tip: Immediate notification of the HCP implies that a health-threatening problem is occurring. Lack of a bowel movement would not meet this criterion.*

**Content Area:** Childbearing; **Concept:** Bowel Elimination; Pregnancy; Integrated Processes: Nursing Process: Analysis; **Client Needs:** Physiological Integrity: Basic Care and Comfort; **Cognitive Level:** Application [Applying]

**819. MoC ANSWER: 1**

1. **For uterine assessment, the client should be positioned in a supine position so the height of the uterus is not influenced by an elevated position.**

2. When beginning the assessment, one hand should be placed at the base of the uterus just above the symphysis pubis to support the lower uterine segment. This prevents the inadvertent inversion of the uterus during palpation.

3. Once the lower hand is in place, the fundus of the uterus can be gently palpated.

4. The abdomen should be observed prior to palpation for contour to detect distention and for the appearance of striae or a diastasis.

▶ *Test-taking Tip: The statement "needs more education" is a false-response item. Select the incorrect statement.*

**Content Area:** Childbearing; **Concept:** Assessment; Management; Pregnancy; Integrated Processes: Nursing Process: Evaluation; **Client Needs:** Safe and Effective Care Environment: Management of Care; **Cognitive Level:** Evaluation [Evaluating]

**820. ANSWER: 5, 1, 3, 2, 4, 6**

5. **Position the client supine so the height of the uterus is not influenced by an elevated position.**

1. **Place the side of one hand just above the client's symphysis pubis. This supports the lower uterine segment and prevents the inadvertent inversion of the uterus during palpation.**

3. **Place the other hand at the level of the umbilicus. This is the expected location of the uterine fundus on the day of delivery.**

2. **Press deeply into the abdomen to allow the massage to reach the fundus.**

4. **Massage the abdomen in a circular motion. This massage should stimulate the uterus to contract and allow location of the fundus to be determined.**

6. **If the fundus is not felt, move the upper hand lower on the abdomen and repeat the massage. Involution could potentially be occurring more rapidly than expected if the client is breastfeeding and/or had an uncomplicated labor and birth.**

▶ *Test-taking Tip:* The uterine muscle will respond to massage by contracting, but correct positioning and hand placement before massage are important to prevent inversion of the uterus.

**Content Area:** Childbearing; **Concept:** Assessment; Pregnancy; Integrated Processes: Nursing Process: Assessment; **Client Needs:** Health Promotion and Maintenance; **Cognitive Level:** Synthesis [Creating]

## 821. PHARM ANSWER: 1

1. **The nurse should explain about the decreased sensation of bladder filling after childbirth. It is not uncommon for the postpartum client to have increased bladder capacity, decreased sensitivity to fluid pressure, and a decreased sensation of bladder filling.**

2. Oxytocin (Pitocin) is not expected to cause a change in bladder sensation, but it does have an antidiuretic effect.

3. There is no indication that the client didn't completely empty; a volume of 900 mL is a large amount.

4. The postpartum client is at risk for bladder overdistention and should be encouraged to void every 2 to 4 hours.

▶ *Test-taking Tip:* You will need to know the normal findings after childbirth.

**Content Area:** Childbearing; **Concept:** Pregnancy; Nursing Roles; Integrated Processes: Teaching/Learning; **Client Needs:** Physiological Integrity: Basic Care and Comfort; Physiological Integrity: Pharmacological and Parenteral Therapies; **Cognitive Level:** Analysis [Analyzing]

## 822. PHARM ANSWER: 0.5

4 mg : 1 mL :: 2 mg : $X$ mL; $4X = 2$; $2 \div 4 = 0.5$ mL

**The nurse should administer 0.5 mL hydromorphone hydrochloride (Dilaudid).**

▶ *Test-taking Tip:* Amounts less than 1 should have a zero before the decimal point.

**Content Area:** Childbearing; **Concept:** Medication; Pregnancy; Integrated Processes: Nursing Process: Implementation; **Client Needs:** Physiological Integrity: Pharmacological and Parenteral Therapies; **Cognitive Level:** Application [Applying]

## 823. MoC ANSWER: 4

1. Offering to transfer the client is appropriate and would not be excluded. The postpartum unit may be filled with sounds and sights that may distress the client.

2. It would be appropriate for the nurse to discuss possible ambivalence with the client, as she may have increased feelings of attachment, love, and grief after delivery. Having those feelings does not necessarily mean that the client has made the wrong decision.

3. Initiating a case management or social work consult is appropriate and would not be excluded. The client may not have support systems available because she may not have disclosed her pregnancy to others.

4. **The adolescent may not have disclosed the pregnancy to family. Although it would be appropriate for the nurse to explore the client's support system with the client, the nurse should not contact the client's family.**

▶ *Test-taking Tip:* Remember the importance of providing privacy and confidentiality for clients.

**Content Area:** Childbearing; **Concept:** Pregnancy; Integrated Processes: Nursing Process: Evaluation; Caring; **Client Needs:** Safe and Effective Care Environment: Management of Care; **Cognitive Level:** Evaluation [Evaluating]

## 824. MoC PHARM ANSWER: 1, 3, 4

1. **The HCP should be notified about the decreased DTRs because weakening of these may indicate magnesium sulfate toxicity.**

2. Increasing the magnesium sulfate dose would worsen the situation and could lead to a depressed respiratory rate.

3. **Any time the client is receiving a magnesium sulfate infusion, the nurse should be prepared for the possibility of needing the antidote, calcium gluconate.**

4. **The nurse should assess the client's vital signs and level of consciousness, as decreased level of consciousness and respiratory effort are serious side effects of magnesium sulfate.**

5. The nurse should ask the HCP about drawing a serum magnesium level (not a serum calcium level) to determine whether the client is experiencing magnesium toxicity.

▶ *Test-taking Tip:* Magnesium sulfate is used to prevent seizures in the client experiencing preeclampsia. Toxicity can result in absent DTRs.

**Content Area:** Childbearing; **Concept:** Pregnancy; Management; Medication; Integrated Processes: Nursing Process: Planning; **Client Needs:** Safe and Effective Care Environment: Management of Care; Physiological Integrity: Pharmacological and Parenteral Therapies; **Cognitive Level:** Analysis [Analyzing]

**825. ANSWER: 4**

1. Infection in the breast tissue results in flu-like symptoms and redness and tenderness of the breast. It is usually unilateral and does not cause bilateral breast enlargement.
2. Fluid is not retained during the postpartum period; rather, clients experience diuresis of the excess fluid volume accumulated during pregnancy.
3. Fullness in both breasts would not be the result of thrombi formation. Symptoms of thrombi include redness, pain, and increased skin temperature over the thrombi.
4. **Breast tissue increases as breast milk forms, so a bra that was adequate during pregnancy may no longer be adequate by the second or third postpartum day.**

▸ *Test-taking Tip: Generic signs of infection include inflammation and thrombosis. Eliminate Options 1 and 3, as bilateral breast fullness would not be caused by these conditions.*

Content Area: Childbearing; Concept: Pregnancy; Integrated Processes: Nursing Process: Planning; Client Needs: Physiological Integrity: Basic Care and Comfort; Cognitive Level: Application [Applying]

**826. ANSWER: 2**

1. Once the nurse has determined the length of time the pad has been in place, the nurse could decide if asking about uterine cramping is appropriate.
2. **The amount of lochia on a perineal pad is influenced by the individual client's pad changing practices. Thus the nurse should ask about the length of time the current pad has been in place before making a judgment about whether the amount is concerning.**
3. Although bladder incontinence could cause pad saturation, it is more important to ask about the length of time the pad has been in place. Based on the client's answer, the nurse could decide if asking about bladder urgency or frequency needs further assessment.
4. Passing clots may require more frequent pad change, but first the nurse should determine if the reason for the saturated pad is the length of time it has been in place.

▸ *Test-taking Tip: The key word is "first." Lochia amount should never exceed a moderate amount (less than a 6-inch stain on a perineal pad).*

Content Area: Childbearing; Concept: Assessment; Pregnancy; Integrated Processes: Nursing Process: Assessment; Client Needs: Physiological Integrity: Reduction of Risk Potential; Cognitive Level: Analysis [Analyzing]

**827. MoC ANSWER: 4**

1. A full bladder may displace the uterus, causing increased bleeding. However, a more complete assessment must be performed prior to getting the client out of bed to prevent increased bleeding and syncope.

2. Vigorously massaging the uterus may result in inversion of the uterus.
3. The client should not simply be reassured that heavy bleeding is expected because further assessment is necessary before concluding that the client's blood loss is WNL.
4. **The nurse's first action should be to support the lower uterine segment and to assess the fundus. Increased bleeding will occur if soft or "boggy." Failing to support the lower uterine segment may result in inversion of the uterus.**

▸ *Test-taking Tip: Use the nursing process. Assessment is the first step.*

Content Area: Childbearing; Concept: Pregnancy; Management; Integrated Processes: Nursing Process: Assessment; Client Needs: Safe and Effective Care Environment: Management of Care; Cognitive Level: Analysis [Analyzing]

**828. ANSWER: 1**

1. **Lochia normally pools in the vagina when the postpartum client remains in a recumbent position for any length of time. When the client then stands, gravity causes the blood to flow out. As long as the nurse knows the fundus is firm and not bleeding, a simple explanation to the client is all that is required.**
2. There is no reason to return the client to bed; the fundus is firm.
3. There is no reason to push the emergency call light. Increased bleeding is an expected response when standing for the first time.
4. There is no reason to call the HCP.

▸ *Test-taking Tip: Options 2, 3, and 4 are all interventions for a uterine hemorrhage. All of these interventions would be appropriate if the client were experiencing abnormal bleeding. Because all three cannot be selected, it would follow that the client in this situation is not hemorrhaging, therefore eliminating Options 2, 3, and 4.*

Content Area: Childbearing; Concept: Pregnancy; Integrated Processes: Nursing Process: Implementation; Client Needs: Health Promotion and Maintenance; Cognitive Level: Analysis [Analyzing]

**829. MoC ANSWER:**

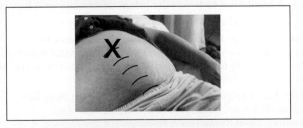

Six to 12 hours after birth, the fundus of the uterus rises to the level of the umbilicus due to blood and clots that remain within the uterus and changes in ligament support. Thus the RN should direct the LPN to locate the client's fundus at the level of the umbilicus.

♦ **Test-taking Tip:** *Focus on the time following delivery and think about the changes that occur due to ligament support and bleeding.*

**Content Area:** Childbearing; **Concept:** Assessment; Pregnancy; Management; **Integrated Processes:** Nursing Process: Assessment; **Client Needs:** Safe and Effective Care Environment: Management of Care; Physiological Integrity: Reduction of Risk Potential; **Cognitive Level:** Application [Applying]

## 830. ANSWER: 4

1. Seeking information about infant care is a sign that the mother is developing attachment to her infant.
2. Pointing out family traits or characteristics seen in the newborn is a sign that the mother is developing attachment.
3. Calling the infant by name is a sign that the mother is developing attachment to her infant.
4. **Attachment is demonstrated by expressing satisfaction with a baby's appearance and sex. Frequent expressions of dissatisfaction with the sex of the infant should be concerning and followed up.**

♦ **Test-taking Tip:** *The statement "the nurse becomes concerned" is a false-response item. Select the statement that describes incorrect attachment behaviors.*

**Content Area:** Childbearing; **Concept:** Nursing Roles; Family; Pregnancy; **Integrated Processes:** Nursing Process: Evaluation; Caring; **Client Needs:** Psychosocial Integrity; **Cognitive Level:** Evaluation [Evaluating]

## 831. ANSWER: 2

1. Not making face-to-face contact with the infant during communication demonstrates a lack of engrossment.
2. **Engrossment is demonstrated by the father touching the infant, making eye contact with the infant, and verbalizing awareness of features in the newborn that are similar to his and that validate his claim to that newborn.**
3. Feelings of frustration are not uncommon to fathers and are characteristic of the second stage, or reality stage, of the transition to fatherhood but are not a sign of engrossment.
4. A hesitation to touch the infant demonstrates a lack of engrossment.

♦ **Test-taking Tip:** *Paternal engrossment, like maternal attachment, involves making close physical contact with the infant. Eliminate Options 1 and 4, as these do not demonstrate that type of involvement.*

**Content Area:** Childbearing; **Concept:** Family; Diversity; Pregnancy; Integrated Processes: Nursing Process: Analysis; Culture and Spirituality; **Client Needs:** Health Promotion and Maintenance; **Cognitive Level:** Application [Applying]

## 832. ANSWER: 1, 2, 3

1. **Many women hesitate to ask for medication, as they believe their pain is expected. Thus the nurse should ask the client about pain and assure her that there are methods to decrease her pain.**

2. **During the initial postpartum "taking-in" phase, the client may have a great need to talk about her birthing experience and to ask questions for clarification as necessary. By encouraging this verbalization, the nurse helps the client to accept the experience and enables her to move to the next maternal phase.**
3. **Physical discomfort can be intense initially postpartum and can interfere with rest. Sleep is a major need and should be encouraged.**
4. Anxiety and preoccupation with her new role often narrow the client's perceptions, and information is not as easily assimilated at this time. Therefore attending education sessions should be delayed if possible until the mother has completed this "taking in" phase.
5. The client needs to suspend her involvement in every-day responsibilities during the "taking-in" phase, so writing birth announcements should be delayed until the mother has completed this phase.

♦ **Test-taking Tip:** *Three phases are evident as the mother adjusts to her maternal role after birth. The initial phase is the dependent, or "taking-in," phase, which can last up to 48 hours after birth. During this phase, the mother's dependency needs predominate, and, if these needs are met by others, the mother is eventually able to divert her energy to her infant. The mother needs "mothering" herself to enable her to mother her child. Select only the options that reflect this nurturing.*

**Content Area:** Childbearing; **Concept:** Pregnancy; **Integrated Processes:** Nursing Process: Implementation; **Client Needs:** Health Promotion and Maintenance; **Cognitive Level:** Analysis [Analyzing]

## 833. ANSWER: 1

1. **If perineal edema is present, ice packs should be applied for the first 24 hours. Ice reduces edema and vulvar irritation.**
2. The client should be taught to tighten, not relax, her buttocks when sitting. This compresses the buttocks and reduces pressure on the perineum.
3. After 24 hours, heat is recommended to increase circulation to the area.
4. Donut cushions should be avoided because they promote separation of the buttocks and decrease venous blood flow to the area, thus increasing pain.

♦ **Test-taking Tip:** *When selecting an option, recall basic initial first aid for any acute injury that results in edema.*

**Content Area:** Childbearing; **Concept:** Inflammation; Pregnancy; Integrated Processes: Nursing Process: Implementation; **Client Needs:** Physiological Integrity: Basic Care and Comfort; **Cognitive Level:** Application [Applying]

## 834. ANSWER: 2

1. Heat application to the abdomen should be avoided; it may cause uterine muscle relaxation.

2. **Multiparous women frequently experience intermittent uterine contractions called afterpains. Lying in a prone position applies pressure to the uterus, stimulating continuous uterine contraction. When the uterus maintains a state of contraction, the afterpains will cease.**

3. Ambulation has been shown to decrease muscle pain and should not be avoided.

4. Afterpains are not a symptom of potential postpartum hemorrhage.

▶ *Test-taking Tip: Relate the uterine cramping to the fact that the client is multiparous. This should identify that the pain is most likely afterpains. Then select the most appropriate treatment for afterpains.*

Content Area: Childbearing; Concept: Comfort; Pregnancy; Integrated Processes: Nursing Process: Implementation; Client Needs: Physiological Integrity: Basic Care and Comfort; Cognitive Level: Analysis [Analyzing]

## 835. ANSWER: 4

1. This graphic shows normal breasts.

2. This graphic shows the left breast with mastitis. Mastitis frequently presents as redness, warmth, and tenderness of the breast tissue, rather than the nipple.

3. This graphic shows engorged breasts.

4. **This graphic shows breasts that have reddened nipples, one of which is cracked. If proper latch is not obtained during breastfeeding, the newborn's sucking may cause nipple cracking, blistering, and bleeding.**

▶ *Test-taking Tip: When taking a test, remember to read/look at all options before deciding on an answer. Some options may be partially correct, but only one option will be the most correct.*

Content Area: Childbearing; Concept: Pregnancy; Integrated Processes: Nursing Process: Evaluation; Client Needs: Physiological Integrity: Basic Care and Comfort; Cognitive Level: Evaluation [Evaluating]

## 836. ANSWER: 3

1. In comparison studies between breast binders and bras, mothers using binders experienced more engorgement and discomfort.

2. Engorgement is not familial and not inevitable in bottle-feeding mothers.

3. **Wearing a supportive, well-fitting bra within 6 hours after birth can suppress lactation. The bra should be worn continuously, except for showering, until lactation is suppressed (usually 7 to 14 days).**

4. Signs of engorgement usually occur on the third to fifth postpartum day (not right after birth), and engorgement will spontaneously resolve by the tenth day postpartum.

▶ *Test-taking Tip: Breast emptying is required for continual milk production. Thus mechanically compressing the breast tissue would be the only way to suppress production. Eliminate Options 2 and 4, as these do not address breast tissue compression.*

Content Area: Childbearing; Concept: Pregnancy; Nursing Roles; Integrated Processes: Teaching/Learning; Client Needs: Physiological Integrity: Basic Care and Comfort; Cognitive Level: Analysis [Analyzing]

## 837. ANSWER: 2, 4, 5, 6

1. The peri-pad should be changed more frequently to reduce the risk of infection. Lochia amount should never exceed a moderate amount (less than a 6-inch stain on a perineal pad).

2. **A warm sitz bath is used after the first 24 hours to provide comfort, increase circulation to the area, and reduce the incidence of infection.**

3. Perineal lacerations are repaired with sutures that dissolve. Clients do not need to have perineal sutures removed.

4. **Cleansing the perineum after each void with the peri-bottle of water provides comfort and helps reduce the chance of infection.**

5. **Washing with mild soap and rinsing with water each 24 hours reduces the risk of infection.**

6. **Teaching the client to watch for signs and symptoms of infection is important and allows the client to be an active participant in her care.**

▶ *Test-taking Tip: Remember the basics of wound healing — cool for the first 24 hours, then move to warmth, keep clean, and monitor for signs and symptoms of infection.*

Content Area: Childbearing; Concept: Nursing Roles; Comfort; Pregnancy; Integrated Processes: Nursing Process: Implementation; Client Needs: Physiological Integrity: Basic Care and Comfort; Cognitive Level: Analysis [Analyzing]

## 838. ANSWER: 3

1. A decrease in lochia is expected after a cesarean birth; no further assessment is needed regarding the lochial amount unless it is totally absent.

2. A decrease in lochia is expected after a cesarean birth, not an increase.

3. **The client's lochial discharge is usually decreased after cesarean birth because the uterus is cleaned during surgery.**

4. The amount of lochia is not dependent on whether the surgery was emergent or planned because the uterus is cleaned during surgery in both situations.

▶ *Test-taking Tip: In a cesarean birth, after delivery of the placenta, the uterus is cleaned. Think about what effect this would have on the amount of lochia.*

Content Area: Childbearing; Concept: Pregnancy; Integrated Processes: Nursing Process: Planning; Client Needs: Physiological Integrity: Reduction of Risk Potential; Cognitive Level: Knowledge [Remembering]

## 839. ANSWER: 4

1. There is no need to be seen in the clinic; vaginal discharge that turns creamy white 10 days postpartum is normal.

2. The client does not have an infection, and no antibiotic is necessary.

3. There is no reason to take her temperature when the discharge is normal.

4. **Creamy white discharge 10 to 21 days postpartum is normal. Her lochia changed color on her 10th postpartum day.**

▶ *Test-taking Tip: The normal postpartum progression of lochia is red (rubra) for the first 1 to 3 days, pink (serosa) on days 3 to 10, and creamy white (alba) on days 10 to 21.*

Content Area: Childbearing; Concept: Pregnancy; Integrated Processes: Nursing Process: Evaluation; Client Needs: Health Promotion and Maintenance; Cognitive Level: Evaluation [Evaluating]

**840. MoC ANSWER: 1, 4, 3, 2**

1. **The client who had a normal, spontaneous vaginal delivery 30 minutes ago is priority. The first 2 hours after delivery is a time of transition, characterized by rapid changes in hemodynamic and physiological state for both the client and her newborn.**

4. **The client who delivered her newborn via scheduled C-section 8 hours ago and has a PCA pump with morphine for pain control should be assessed next. Although she is 8 hours postpartum and *probably* stable, she is receiving morphine, and her respiratory status should be monitored regularly.**

3. **The client who had a vaginal delivery 32 hours ago and is having difficulty breastfeeding should be assessed next. Newborn infants should successfully breastfeed every 2 to 3 hours. Failing to breastfeed with adequate amount and frequency may lead to newborn complications such as excessive weight loss and jaundice.**

2. **The client who had a cesarean section 48 hours ago and is bottle feeding her newborn infant should be seen last; there is nothing indicating urgency.**

▶ *Test-taking Tip: Select the client who would be most vulnerable to harm as the first client to assess and the one who has no problems indicating urgency as last. Once you have identified the first and the last client, it is easier to place the remaining two in the correct order for assessment.*

Content Area: Childbearing; Concept: Pregnancy; Integrated Processes: Nursing Process: Implementation; Client Needs: Safe and Effective Care Environment: Management of Care; Cognitive Level: Synthesis [Creating]

**841. MoC ANSWER: 2**

1. Although the client post–cesarean birth for a breech baby may be at risk for uterine atony and should be monitored, the client who delivered a macrosomic baby is more at risk.

2. **This client is the nurse's priority for monitoring for uterine atony. A macrosomic baby stretches the client's uterus, and thus the muscle fibers of the myometrium, beyond the usual pregnancy size. After delivery the muscles are unable to contract effectively.**

3. A firm fundus indicates that the client's uterine muscles are contracting.

4. Oxytocin (Pitocin) is being administered to increase uterine contractions. Although prolonged use of oxytocin can result in uterine exhaustion, 2 hours of use is not prolonged.

▶ *Test-taking Tip: A boggy or relaxed uterus is a sign of uterine atony.*

Content Area: Childbearing; Concept: Pregnancy; Integrated Processes: Nursing Process: Planning; Client Needs: Safe and Effective Care Environment: Management of Care; Cognitive Level: Application [Applying]

**842. ANSWER: 1**

1. **On the first postpartum day, the client should be taught to start abdominal breathing and pelvic rocking. Kegel exercises, which should have been taught during pregnancy, should be continued. Simple exercises should be added daily until, by 2 to 3 weeks postpartum, the mother should be able to do sit-ups and leg raises.**

2. Abdominal and pelvic exercises can begin right away and not wait for the 6-week postpartum checkup.

3. There is no reason for the client to wait until the lochia has stopped before beginning exercises.

4. There is no reason that a breastfeeding mother should not begin abdominal and pelvic exercises now.

▶ *Test-taking Tip: Think about the simple exercises that the client could begin after an uncomplicated vaginal birth.*

Content Area: Childbearing; Concept: Pregnancy; Integrated Processes: Teaching/Learning; Client Needs: Physiological Integrity: Basic Care and Comfort; Physiological Integrity: Physiological Adaptation; Cognitive Level: Application [Applying]

**843. ANSWER: 2**

1. Although the client needs information about incision care, the priority need is for assistance at home so that she can get the needed rest from multiple demands.

2. **Because the client has had a surgical procedure, the priority consideration is for the mother to plan for additional assistance at home. Without this assistance, it is difficult for the mother to get the rest she needs for healing, pain control, and appropriate infant care.**

3. Infant care is important, but having assistance at home after a surgical procedure is more important.

4. The need for increased rest is important, but she would not be able to obtain adequate rest without assistance at home.

▶ *Test-taking Tip: Think about which option if not accomplished would have a negative effect on the other options.*

Content Area: Childbearing; Concept: Nursing Roles; Pregnancy; Integrated Processes: Nursing Process: Implementation; Client Needs: Physiological Integrity: Basic Care and Comfort; Cognitive Level: Analysis [Analyzing]

## 844. ANSWER: 1

1. **Offering to order food later if the client changes her mind is the best response. Many clients have culturally based beliefs about food and beverages that should be consumed in the postpartum period. Unless contraindicated, nurses should support and encourage women to incorporate food preferences with cultural significance into their postpartum diet.**
2. Some breastfeeding infants are sensitive to certain flavors, seasonings, or foods, but there is no evidence to support maternal food restrictions unless the infant shows a sensitivity. If there is a strong family history of a food allergy that causes anaphylaxis, such as a peanut allergy, these foods may be avoided.
3. Many women would benefit from speaking to a dietician, but this client is not at any increased risk that would make a dietary consultation necessary.
4. There are no food restrictions 12 hours after delivery unless there have been complications.

▶ **Test-taking Tip:** *Failing to support cultural food preferences would lead to care that is not client centered.*

Content Area: Childbearing; Concept: Diversity; Pregnancy; Integrated Processes: Nursing Process: Implementation; Culture and Spirituality; Client Needs: Health Promotion and Maintenance; Cognitive Level: Analysis [Analyzing]

## 845. ANSWER: 1, 4, 5, 6

1. **If the latch is correct, the mother should feel only a firm tugging and not pain or pinching when the infant sucks.**
2. A smacking or clicking noise heard when the infant sucks is an indication that the latch is incorrect and that the infant's tongue may be inappropriately placed.
3. Sucking only on the mother's nipple will cause sore nipples, and milk will not be ejected from the milk ducts.
4. **When an infant is correctly latched to the breast, 2 to 3 centimeters (1/3 to 3/4 inch) of areola should be covered by the infant's mouth. If this occurs, it will result in the infant's nose, mouth, and chin touching the breast.**
5. **When the infant is latched correctly, the cheeks will be rounded rather than dimpled.**
6. **When the infant is latched correctly, the swallowing will be audible.**

▶ **Test-taking Tip:** *Eliminate options that would not promote optimum milk flow from the breast and sounds that would indicate latching is ineffective.*

Content Area: Childbearing; Concept: Pregnancy; Integrated Processes: Nursing Process: Evaluation; Client Needs: Physiological Integrity: Basic Care and Comfort; Cognitive Level: Evaluation [Evaluating]

## 846. ANSWER: 1

1. **In nonlactating women, the average time to first ovulation is 45 days, and the return of menstruation usually happens within 6 to 10 weeks postbirth.**
2. Most women can expect to have lochial discharge for up to 24 days. However, the cessation of discharge is not related to the return of menstruation.
3. The change in lochial color is not related to the return of menstruation.
4. The return of ovulation and menstruation is associated with a rise in serum progesterone levels. Bottle feeding does not affect when this change occurs in the client's body.

▶ **Test-taking Tip:** *Eliminate options that relate lochia to the return of menstruation.*

Content Area: Childbearing; Concept: Nursing Roles; Integrated Processes: Teaching/Learning; Client Needs: Health Promotion and Maintenance; Cognitive Level: Application [Applying]

## 847. ANSWER: 3

1. IUDs offer no protection against STIs. They are recommended for women who are in a stable, mutually monogamous relationship.
2. Depot-medroxyprogesterone acetate (Depo-Provera) is a long-acting progestin that is highly effective for birth control. A single injection will provide contraception for 3 months but does not offer protection against STIs.
3. **A female condom does provide protection against some of the pathogens that cause STIs, and it would be readily available over the counter.**
4. A diaphragm offers no protection against STIs.

▶ **Test-taking Tip:** *Note that only one option protects against STIs, which would be a necessary factor considering the client's lifestyle.*

Content Area: Childbearing; Concept: Pregnancy; Integrated Processes: Nursing Process: Analysis; Client Needs: Health Promotion and Maintenance; Cognitive Level: Analysis [Analyzing]

## 848. PHARM ANSWER: 3

1. Because a diaphragm must be fitted to the individual female cervix, the diaphragm must be rechecked for correct size after each childbirth; however, use of the diaphragm will not affect breast milk production.
2. An IUD will not affect breast milk production unless the IUD is inserted within the first 48 hours postpartum; insertion should be delayed until 4 weeks postpartum.

3. **Birth control pills containing progesterone and estrogen (COC) can cause a decrease in milk volume and may affect the quality of the breast milk.**
4. The progesterone-only mini pill may be used by breastfeeding clients because it does not interfere with breast milk production. However, it is recommended that the mother wait 6 to 8 weeks before starting this method of contraception.

▶ *Test-taking Tip: Eliminate Option 1, as a diaphragm is a barrier device inserted over the cervix. It would be impossible for this device to affect the breastfeeding process. To narrow the other options, think about the hormone that will affect milk production.*

Content Area: Childbearing; Concept: Pregnancy; Medication; Integrated Processes: Teaching/Learning; Client Needs: Health Promotion and Maintenance; Physiological Integrity: Pharmacological and Parenteral Therapies; Cognitive Level: Comprehension [Understanding]

## 849. ANSWER: 2, 4, 6

1. Moving the baby from the initial breast to the second breast during the feeding, before the initial breast is completely emptied, may result in neither breast being totally emptied and thus promote continued engorgement.
2. **Because engorgement is caused, in part, by swelling of the breast tissue surrounding the milk gland ducts, applying ice at intervals between feedings will help to decrease this swelling.**
3. Giving supplemental formula, thus limiting the time the baby nurses at the breast, prevents total emptying of the breast and promotes increased engorgement.
4. **Administering anti-inflammatory medication will decrease breast pain and inflammation.**
5. Because heat application increases blood flow, moist heat packs would exacerbate the engorgement.
6. **Pumping the breasts may be necessary if the infant is unable to completely empty both breasts at each feeding. Pumping at this time will not cause a problematic increase in breast milk production.**

▶ *Test-taking Tip: Heat and cold applications produce opposite physiological body responses, so eliminate one of these. Eliminate options that have the potential to increase engorgement rather than decrease it.*

Content Area: Childbearing; Concept: Pregnancy; Integrated Processes: Nursing Process: Implementation; Client Needs: Physiological Integrity: Basic Care and Comfort; Cognitive Level: Application [Applying]

## 850. ANSWER: 2

1. Oxytocin is released when the client has an orgasm and may cause breast milk to leak or squirt from the breasts. The production of breast milk may increase, not decrease.

2. **The nurse should inform the client that she may need lubrication with sexual intercourse because the low estrogen levels in the early postpartum period causes vaginal dryness.**
3. Women should refrain from sexual intercourse until lochia has ceased, which usually takes about 3 weeks. There is no need to wait two months if the lochia has ceased.
4. The client's HCP does not need to give approval to return to sexual activity.

▶ *Test-taking Tip: Hormones normally produced during the postpartum period influence decisions pertaining to sexual intercourse.*

Content Area: Childbearing; Concept: Pregnancy; Nursing Roles; Integrated Processes: Teaching/Learning; Communication and Documentation; Client Needs: Health Promotion and Maintenance; Cognitive Level: Application [Applying]

## 851. PHARM ANSWER: 3

1. The number of RhoGAM doses given in pregnancy does not affect whether or not the client receives a dose postpartum.
2. Both the client and newborn are Rh negative; no dose is required.
3. **Rh immune globulin (RhoGAM) is administered to women with Rh negative blood types at approximately 28 weeks of gestation and again after any trauma, such as a car accident or fall. After delivery, RhoGAM is only indicated if the newborn has a positive blood type; both the client and newborn are Rh negative.**
4. For postpartum clients who require RhoGAM, the dose is given within 72 hours of delivery. However, no dose is necessary because the client and newborn are both Rh negative.

▶ *Test-taking Tip: Read each question thoroughly before looking at the options. Some options may not be correct for the specific scenario in a question but might be correct in a different scenario.*

Content Area: Childbearing; Concept: Nursing Roles; Medication; Pregnancy; Integrated Processes: Teaching/Learning; Client Needs: Physiological Integrity: Pharmacological and Parenteral Therapies; Cognitive Level: Evaluation [Evaluating]

## 852. ANSWER: 1

1. **Continuing to breastfeed is recommended when the client has mastitis. If the breasts continue to be emptied by either breastfeeding or pumping, the duration of symptoms and the incidence of a breast abscess are decreased.**
2. Continuing to breastfeed will decrease the symptoms of mastitis; there is no need to wait for symptoms to decrease.
3. Usually an oral penicillinase-resistant penicillin or cephalosporin that is safe for the infant while breastfeeding is given to treat mastitis. There is no need for the client to stop breastfeeding for 24 hours.

4. The infant's nose and throat are the most common sources of the organism that causes mastitis. Infants of women with mastitis generally remain well; thus concern that the mother will infect the infant if she continues breastfeeding is unwarranted.

▶ *Test-taking Tip:* A major risk for mastitis development is poorly emptied breasts and plugged milk ducts. Discontinuing or decreasing breastfeeding would therefore be detrimental to the client with mastitis.

Content Area: Childbearing; Concept: Infection; Pregnancy; Integrated Processes: Nursing Process: Implementation; Client Needs: Physiological Integrity: Physiological Adaptation; Cognitive Level: Application [Applying]

## 853. ANSWER: 2, 3, 4, 6

1. Rest is important to promote healing. Bedrest may be initially prescribed for 24 hours.
2. **Treatment for mastitis includes administration of antibiotics to treat the infection.**
3. **Application of warm packs decreases pain and promotes milk flow and breast emptying.**
4. **Treatment for mastitis includes anti-inflammatory medications to treat fever and decrease breast inflammation.**
5. Increasing fluid intake to at least 2 to 3 liters is recommended, not limiting intake.
6. **If the breasts continue to be emptied by either breastfeeding or pumping, the duration of symptoms and the incidence of a breast abscess are decreased.**

▶ *Test-taking Tip:* Consider the options that will decrease infection and inflammation. Evaluate whether increased activity and limiting fluids promote healing.

Content Area: Childbearing; Concept: Infection; Pregnancy; Integrated Processes: Nursing Process: Planning; Client Needs: Physiological Integrity: Physiological Adaptation; Cognitive Level: Application [Applying]

## 854. ANSWER: 1, 2, 5

1. **Incorrect latch can cause nipple tissue to blister, crack, and bleed. These breaks in the tissue may serve as an entry point for pathogens.**
2. **Hand hygiene prior to breastfeeding reduces the number of pathogens available for invasion.**
3. While the infant's nose and throat are sources of pathogenic organisms that might cause mastitis, washing the infant's mouth would be difficult and would not provide adequate protection for the mother.
4. Wearing a tight bra, especially with an underwire, may restrict milk ducts, providing milk stasis and a medium for pathogenic growth.
5. **Allowing breasts to air-dry helps to reduce skin breakdown that might be caused by a moist, wet environment.**

▶ *Test-taking Tip:* Thinking about infection control measures will help you answer many questions, regardless of the infection type or location.

Content Area: Childbearing; Concept: Nursing Roles; Pregnancy; Integrated Processes: Nursing Process: Evaluation; Client Needs: Health Promotion and Maintenance; Cognitive Level: Evaluation [Evaluating]

## 855. ANSWER: 1

1. **While a constant trickle or oozing of lochia would indicate excessive bleeding, the nurse would need to first know how long the client had been wearing the peri-pad to evaluate whether the amount was excessive. The client should not be saturating a large peri-pad every hour. If the client had been wearing the same pad for 3 or 4 hours, it may indicate an expected amount of lochia.**
2. The nurse should not contact the client's HCP until further assessment and evaluation were complete.
3. While administering oxytocin (Pitocin) might be the correct action if the client is bleeding excessively as a result of a boggy uterus, the nurse should not administer the medication until further assessment and evaluation were complete.
4. Although the amount of bleeding may be normal for this client, the nurse would need further information before making this judgment and documenting the findings.

▶ *Test-taking Tip:* Think of the big picture rather than focusing on a snapshot of the client's situation. Use the first step in the nursing process, assessment, to answer this question.

Content Area: Childbearing; Concept: Critical Thinking; Pregnancy; Assessment; Integrated Processes: Nursing Process: Assessment; Client Needs: Physiological Integrity: Physiological Adaptation; Cognitive Level: Analysis [Analyzing]

## 856. ANSWER: 1

1. **Lochia rubra that persists for longer than 2 weeks is suggestive of subinvolution of the uterus, which is the most common cause of delayed postpartum hemorrhage. The client should be seen in the clinic immediately to determine what is causing her abnormal lochial discharge.**
2. Increased physical activity can lead to increased lochial discharge, but the client is reporting continuous lochia rubra, which is abnormal.
3. Lochia rubra is expected to last for up to 3 days after birth, not 20 days.
4. Waiting until next week to be seen only delays determining the cause for her abnormal bleeding and increases the risk of the client for other complications.

▶ *Test-taking Tip:* Lochia rubra should last only 3 days postpartum, and then the lochia becomes serosa and eventually alba.

Content Area: Childbearing; Concept: Pregnancy; Integrated Processes: Nursing Process: Analysis; Client Needs: Physiological Integrity: Reduction of Risk Potential; Cognitive Level: Analysis [Analyzing]

**857. ANSWER: 3, 5**

1. Activity should be increased, not decreased, to reduce the potential for constipation.
2. Fluids should be increased, not decreased, to reduce the potential for dehydration and constipation.
3. **The client with a fourth-degree perineal laceration should be instructed to increase dietary fiber to help maintain bowel continence and decrease perineal trauma from constipation.**
4. A perineal laceration will not affect the condition of the uterus; there is no need to increase uterine monitoring.
5. **The client with a fourth-degree perineal laceration should be given a stool softener bid to help maintain bowel continence and decrease perineal trauma from constipation.**

▸ *Test-taking Tip: A concern with a fourth-degree perineal laceration will be pain with having a bowel movement. Focus on options that include measures to prevent constipation.*

**Content Area:** Childbearing; **Concept:** Pregnancy; Integrated Processes: Nursing Process: Planning; **Client Needs:** Physiological Integrity: Reduction of Risk Potential; **Cognitive Level:** Synthesis [Creating]

**858. ANSWER: 2**

1. Reexamination of the perineum should be completed before calling the HCP to report the pain level.
2. **A forceps-assisted delivery can increase the risk of hematoma development. Rectal pressure and perineal pain can indicate a hematoma in the posterior vaginal wall. The nurse should closely examine the perineum and the vaginal introitus for ecchymosis and a bulging mass.**
3. Ambulation would not help the perineal pain.
4. A stool softener would be appropriate to avoid constipation but would not help the immediate problem.

▸ *Test-taking Tip: Managing pain is always a priority; however, complete assessment should be the initial approach to allow the gathering of enough data to determine the appropriate course of action.*

**Content Area:** Childbearing; **Concept:** Comfort; Pregnancy; Integrated Processes: Nursing Process: Analysis; **Client Needs:** Physiological Integrity: Reduction of Risk Potential; **Cognitive Level:** Analysis [Analyzing]

**859. MoC ANSWER: 1, 4**

1. **A temperature of 100. 4°F (38°C) or higher after 24 hours postpartum is associated with a puerperal infection.**
2. Telangiectasis is red, slightly raised vascular "spiders" that may appear during pregnancy over the neck, thorax, face, or arms and remain or fade during the postpartum period. It is not indicative of an infection.

3. Slight abdominal tenderness with palpation is a normal postpartum finding.
4. **Malodorous lochia is a common sign of a puerperal infection.**
5. A WBC count of 16,500 is normal for the postpartum client; labor produces a mild pro-inflammatory state.

▸ *Test-taking Tip: WBCs are normally elevated during the postpartum period and usually return to normal within a week. Eliminate other normal postpartum findings to arrive at the answer.*

**Content Area:** Childbearing; **Concept:** Pregnancy; Integrated Processes: Nursing Process: Evaluation; **Client Needs:** Safe and Effective Care Environment: Management of Care; **Cognitive Level:** Evaluation [Evaluating]

**860. ANSWER: 3**

1. The course of an endometrial infection is approximately 7 to 10 days, and thus standard precautions should be in place for that period of time even if the client has started antibiotics.
2. Puerperal infections are not spread by droplets, and thus a mask is not necessary.
3. **Other than hand hygiene, no additional precautions need to be taken by the client in her home.**
4. The client is able to provide care for her children, but hand washing is required before cares.

▸ *Test-taking Tip: Three options contain the absolute words "no," "always," and "all." Options with absolute words are usually not the answer.*

**Content Area:** Childbearing; **Concept:** Infection; Pregnancy; Integrated Processes: Teaching/Learning; **Client Needs:** Safe and Effective Care Environment: Safety and Infection Control; **Cognitive Level:** Application [Applying]

**861. MoC ANSWER: 1, 4, 5, 6**

1. **During pregnancy, fibrinogen levels increase, and this increase continues to be present in the postpartum period. The increased levels can contribute to clot formation.**
2. There is not a shift of fluid from the interstitial to the vascular spaces in the postpartum period. Actual blood volume increases during pregnancy and is further increased immediately after delivery. This fluid volume is eventually lost through diuresis during the first postpartum week.
3. Postpartum hormonal changes do occur, but they do not affect the vascular basement membranes.
4. **Elevation of the legs in stirrups during delivery leads to pooling of blood and vascular stasis.**
5. **Dilation of the veins in the lower extremities occurs during pregnancy and increases the risk of venous stasis.**
6. **Compression of the common iliac vein occurs during pregnancy due to an enlarging fetus and increases the risk of venous stasis.**

♦ **Test-taking Tip:** *Physiological causes of thrombophlebitis include blood stasis and increased blood coagulation. Use this information to select the correct options.*

**Content Area:** Childbearing; **Concept:** Clotting; Pregnancy; Integrated Processes: Teaching/Learning; **Client Needs:** Safe and Effective Care Environment: Management of Care; Physiological Integrity: Physiological Adaptation; **Cognitive Level:** Application [Applying]

### 862. ANSWER: 4

1. The client's support person should be given information about postpartum blues before the client is discharged from the hospital. However, contacting that individual should not be the first intervention.
2. Reminding the client that she has a healthy baby is a nontherapeutic communication technique that implies disapproval of the client's actions.
3. There is no need to notify the HCP, as postpartum blues is a common self-limiting postpartum occurrence.
4. **A key feature of postpartum blues is episodic tearfulness without an identifiable reason. Interventions for postpartum blues include allowing the client to relive her birth experience.**

♦ **Test-taking Tip:** *Nontherapeutic responses and an emergent intervention should be eliminated to narrow the options.*

**Content Area:** Childbearing; **Concept:** Mood; Pregnancy; Integrated Processes: Caring; **Client Needs:** Psychosocial Integrity; **Cognitive Level:** Application [Applying]

### 863. ANSWER: 1, 2

1. **SSRIs are first-line agents for treating moderate PPD.**
2. **Individual or group psychotherapy is a treatment for moderate PPD.**
3. If the client is displaying rejection of or aggression toward the infant, she should not be left alone with the infant, but the infant does not need to be removed from the home.
4. Hypnotic agents are medications that promote sleep, but they are not to be used during the postpartum period. If sleep deprivation is occurring, a TCA may be prescribed.
5. ECT would not be used in the initial treatment of moderate PPD. If puerperal psychosis develops, ECT is a treatment option.

♦ **Test-taking Tip:** *The key words are "initial treatment." PPD treatment is similar to depression occurring at any time in an individual's life.*

**Content Area:** Childbearing; **Concept:** Stress; Pregnancy; Integrated Processes: Nursing Process: Planning; **Client Needs:** Psychosocial Integrity; **Cognitive Level:** Synthesis [Creating]

### 864. ANSWER: 3

1. Lochia that is foul smelling could indicate that the client has a postpartum infection. The client needs to be seen by an HCP, but the safety of the infant is priority.
2. The presence of tender hemorrhoids may be uncomfortable and should be addressed, but this is not priority.
3. **It is inappropriate for the client to yell at her baby to stop crying. Verbal abuse can escalate to physical abuse. The safety of the infant should be the nurse's priority.**
4. Persistent crying is a sign of PPD and would be expected. However, persistent crying should be further explored because treatment may be ineffective.

♦ **Test-taking Tip:** *Safety of a vulnerable infant should be priority.*

**Content Area:** Childbearing; **Concept:** Safety; Pregnancy; Integrated Processes: Nursing Process: Planning; Caring; **Client Needs:** Safe and Effective Care Environment: Safety and Infection Control; **Cognitive Level:** Application [Applying]

### 865. ANSWER: 1

1. **The nurse should plan teaching about the use of tampons during postpartum. The tampon may irritate or dry the vagina, holds lochia in the body, and increases the risk of infection. The client should be instructed to wear a peri-pad.**
2. Loofas or bath sponges for bathing the body postpartum are not contraindicated.
3. While it is a good idea to hang towels neatly so that they dry more rapidly and reduce mold growth, this is not a priority for teaching.
4. The bathroom cleaner would be dangerous to an older child who is more mobile, but the client's parity is 1. The client would be wise to start considering safety issues by placing this out of reach, but this is not the priority teaching item.

♦ **Test-taking Tip:** *Remember that more than one option may be correct, but you are being asked to identify the most concerning item.*

**Content Area:** Childbearing; **Concept:** Pregnancy; Integrated Processes: Nursing Process: Analysis; **Client Needs:** Safe and Effective Care Environment: Safety and Infection Control; **Cognitive Level:** Analysis [Analyzing]

### 866. ANSWER: 1, 2, 4

1. **This is an appropriate statement. Sleeping while the infant sleeps will help the mother get the rest she needs.**
2. **This is an appropriate statement. The American Academy of Pediatricians recommends the supine position for infant sleeping to decrease the risk of SIDS.**

3. The mother should be in close proximity and ready to respond when the infant wakes and/or cries, but she does not need to sleep in the same room as the infant.

4. **This is an appropriate statement. While awake, the infant should be positioned prone and side-lying to help build neck muscles and decrease the chance of deformation plagiocephaly. Deformation plagiocephaly is a malformation of the skull caused by consistently lying on the back.**

5. A blanket, if used, should swaddle the infant rather than being draped over the infant. Swaddling helps prevent suffocation. Tucking the blanket sides under the mattress does not prevent suffocation.

▶ *Test-taking Tip: Statements with absolute words such as "always" are usually not correct. Using "best" when giving advice often is an incorrect statement.*

**Content Area:** Childbearing; **Concept:** Pregnancy; Integrated Processes: Teaching/Learning; Communication and Documentation; **Client Needs:** Safe and Effective Care Environment: Safety and Infection Control; Psychosocial Integrity; **Cognitive Level:** Analysis [Analyzing]

# Chapter Twenty-One

# Neonatal and High-Risk Neonatal Management

**867.** The nurse meets the frantic father at an ED door. He says he just delivered his wife's full-term newborn in the car when the temperature outside is only 10°F (–12.2°C). In response to the cold environment, the nurse knows that the infant's body will immediately begin to produce heat by which mechanism?

1. Shivering
2. Metabolizing body fat
3. Dilating surface blood vessels
4. Decreasing flexion of the extremities

**868.** The nurse has just assisted with the birth of a full-term infant. The nurse should take which measures immediately to promote parent-infant attachment? **Select all that apply.**

1. Have the mother nap before interacting with her newborn.
2. Dim the lights in the birthing room.
3. Place the newly delivered infant on the mother's abdomen.
4. Delay instilling the ophthalmic antibiotic for an hour.
5. Play loud music to keep the infant stimulated.
6. Ask the parents to delay phone calls for an hour after birth.

**869.** The agitated father of the 12-hour-old newborn reports that his baby's hands and feet are blue. After confirming the presence of acrocyanosis, what should the nurse do **next?**

1. Immediately stimulate the infant to cry.
2. Explain that this is normal in a newborn.
3. Assess the newborn's temperature.
4. Assess the newborn's cardiac status.

**870.** The nurse is completing the 1-minute Apgar assessment on the full-term newborn. The newborn's HR is 80 bpm. Which intervention should the nurse implement **next?**

1. Assign a 2 for the Apgar score that pertains to the HR.
2. Suction the excess secretions from the newborn's oral cavity.
3. Wrap in warm blankets and place on the mother's abdomen.
4. Begin immediate positive pressure ventilation on the newborn.

**871.** The client with oligohydramnios and possible intrauterine growth restriction gives birth. The newborn's 1-minute Apgar score was 6, and the 5-minute Apgar score is 7. Which conclusion should the nurse make from this information?

1. A low Apgar score at 1 minute correlates with infant mortality.
2. The 5-minute Apgar score of 7 is within normal parameters.
3. Neurological problems are unlikely with a 5-minute score of 7.
4. Oligohydramnios would not have affected the Apgar score.

**872.** The nurse finds documentation in the 4-hour-old newborn's medical record that states, "Clamping of the umbilical cord was delayed until cord pulsations ceased." When assessing and collecting additional information about the newborn, what effect should the nurse find as a result of the delayed cord clamping?

1. More rapid expulsion of meconium by the newborn
2. Increased level of newborn alertness after birth
3. An increase in the newborn's initial temperature
4. An increase in the newborn's hemoglobin and hematocrit

**873.** The nurse is caring for the newborn infant. Which **initial** measures should the nurse take to maintain the newborn's axillary body temperature between 97.7°F (36.5°C) and 98.9°F (37.2°C)? **Select all that apply.**

1. Carefully dry the infant immediately after birth.
2. Place the infant skin-to-skin with the mother.
3. Apply leggings to both of the newborn's legs.
4. Cover the infant's head with a stocking cap.
5. Place the infant in a bassinette close to the wall.

**874.** As the nurse prepares to administer prophylactic eye treatment to prevent gonorrheal conjunctivitis in the full-term newborn, the newborn's father asks if it is really necessary to put something into his baby's eyes. Which statement should be the basis for the nurse's response?

1. It is the law in the United States that newborns receive this prophylactic treatment.
2. This treatment is recommended but may be omitted at the parent's verbal request.
3. The antibiotic used for the treatment can be given orally at the parent's request.
4. The eye prophylaxis can be given any time up until the infant is 1 year old.

**875.** At a prenatal class, the nurse utilizes a picture of the fetal heart to explain that functional closure of the ductus arteriosus occurs within 15 hours after birth. Place an X at the location on the fetal heart illustrated where the nurse should be pointing to identify the ductus arteriosus.

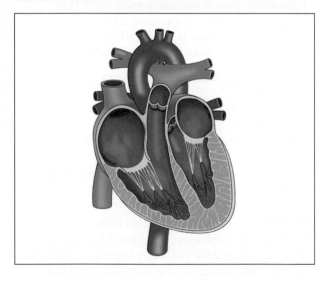

**876.** The nurse is measuring both the chest and head circumference during the full-term newborn's initial assessment. The newborn's father observes this and asks the nurse why both measurements are necessary. Which explanation is **most** accurate?

1. "Comparing the measurements helps determine if there are head or chest size abnormalities."
2. "Measuring the head circumference provides information about future intellectual ability."
3. "Measuring the newborn's chest provides needed information when assessing cardiac health."
4. "Comparing the head and chest measurements helps to determine future adult body size."

**877.** MoC  The nurse assesses that the 8-hour-old infant's axillary temperature is 97°F (36.1°C). Which intervention should the nurse implement **first?**

1. Document the findings as abnormal.
2. Place the infant under a radiant warmer.
3. Feed the infant formula that is warmed.
4. Call the HCP to report the temperature.

**878.** The nurse receives a laboratory report result showing that the blood glucose is 48 mg/dL for a full-term newborn. Which action should be taken by the nurse?

1. Have the mother breastfeed her newborn now.
2. Immediately feed the infant water with 10% dextrose.
3. Report the results immediately to the HCP.
4. Document the information in the newborn's medical record.

**879.** During an assessment of the full-term, 1-hour-old newborn, the nurse obtains an apical HR of 120 bpm and auscultates a soft murmur at the left sternal border, third intercostal space. In response to these assessment findings, which action should be taken by the nurse?

1. Immediately report the findings to the HCP.
2. Document the HR and murmur.
3. Recheck the murmur in the left side-lying position.
4. Stimulate crying and then reassess the cardiac status.

**880.** The nurse is assessing the full-term Caucasian infant who is 40 hours old. Which technique should the nurse use to evaluate the infant for jaundice?

1. Remove the infant's diaper and look at the color of the genitalia.
2. Apply pressure on the forehead for 3 seconds, release, and evaluate the skin color.
3. Assess the color of the palms and compare that skin color to the color of the soles.
4. Open the infant's mouth to assess the color of the infant's tongue and palate.

**881.** Calculating from the date of the mother's last menstrual period, the nurse determines that her newborn's gestational age is 40 weeks. Which normal findings should the nurse expect when assessing this newborn at birth? **Select all that apply.**

1. Hypertonic flexion of all extremities.
2. Sole creases on the anterior two-thirds of the sole.
3. Well-defined incurving of the entire ear pinna.
4. Presence of a prominent clitoris.
5. Infant is able to support the head momentarily when pulled to a sitting position.

**882.** MoC While supervising the LPN, the RN determines that the LPN needs additional instruction in newborn care. Which action by the LPN prompted the nurse's conclusion?

1. Assessed the newborn's HR apically
2. Covered the newborn's head with a stocking cap
3. Checked the newborn's temperature rectally
4. Positioned the newborn supine while sleeping

**883.** The first-time mother of the 2-hour-old full-term newborn worriedly tells the nurse, "Something black is coming out of my baby." After determining that the newborn has passed stool, which statement by the nurse is **most** appropriate?

1. "Black stools could be from bleeding. I will notify your provider now."
2. "Breastfeeding will cause all the baby's stools to be this dark in color."
3. "Babies normally pass this type of stool initially; it is called meconium."
4. "I'll check the baby's temperature; this occurs when babies need warming."

**884.** The nurse is admitting a neonate after delivery who is diagnosed with a myelomeningocele. Which intervention should the nurse implement immediately?

1. Positions the infant prone and covers the sac with sterile gauze
2. Notifies the surgeon on call that the infant is ready for surgery
3. Applies a pressure dressing to the sac and starts an intravenous access
4. Positions the infant prone, hips slightly flexed, and legs abducted

**885.** While performing an initial assessment on the full-term infant whose parents are Asian, the nurse notes the skin discoloration illustrated. What should be the nurse's interpretation of this finding?

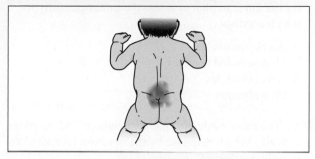

1. The infant was bruised during or after the delivery.
2. This is a normally occurring skin variation in newborns.
3. Hurriedly placing the infant supine can cause this bruising.
4. Seepage of blood from the intestine occurred during the birth process.

**886.** The nurse assesses that the full-term newborn's head has molding. Considering this finding, which information should the nurse expect to see on the mother's labor and delivery documentation?

1. Vaginal breech birth
2. Planned cesarean birth, no labor
3. Was in labor for 16 hours
4. Precipitous delivery after a 30-minute labor

**887.** The nurse is caring for the newborn infant. The nurse should prepare to assess the newborn's anterior fontanel by which method?

1. Lay the infant on his or her back.
2. Stimulate the infant to cry strongly.
3. Feel near the parietal and occipital bones.
4. Place the infant in a sitting position.

**888.** The nurse has provided the mother with information about her newborn's milia. The nurse evaluates that the mother understands information when the mother makes which statement?

1. "I will put lotion on my infant's nose in the morning and at night."
2. "I understand these raised white spots will clear up without treatment."
3. "I realize the baby will need surgery to remove these skin lesions."
4. "I will apply alcohol twice a day to the lesions until they disappear."

**889.** The nurse reviews the labor and delivery record of the 2-hour-old male newborn and sees this notation: "40 weeks' gestation, large for gestational (LGA) age." In response to this information, it is **most** important for the nurse to plan to assess the infant carefully for which condition?

1. Acrocyanosis
2. Undescended testicles
3. Intact clavicles
4. Hypothermia

**890.** The nurse evaluates that the newborn's Moro reflex is WNL. Which response by the newborn prompted the nurse's conclusion?

1. Straightens extremities and then flexes them in response to a loud noise
2. Right-side extremity extension when the head is quickly turned right
3. Turns the head toward the right side when the right cheek is touched
4. Attempts to walk when the sole of the foot touches a hard surface

**891.** The nurse completed discharge education to the Native American parents of a 48-hour-old, full-term infant. The nurse concludes that the mother needs additional teaching about jaundice when she makes which statement?

1. "I know keeping my baby warm will help to decrease jaundice."
2. "I know the jaundice should start to decrease after about 3 days."
3. "The bilirubin causing the jaundice is eliminated in my baby's stools."
4. "Feeding my baby frequently will help to decrease the jaundice."

**892.** MoC The client, who is a primiparous lesbian, delivered a term newborn. The client is in a monogamous relationship with a female partner and achieved her pregnancy via artificial insemination. Which intervention should the nurse add to the newborn's care plan?

1. Avoid acknowledging the client's lesbian relationship.
2. Encourage the client's partner to participate in newborn cares.
3. Ask the partner to leave the room when the newborn is present.
4. Avoid telling the newborn's caregivers about the client's situation.

**893.** MoC The nurse is preparing the parents of a full-term, 24-hour-old male newborn for discharge with their infant. Which are the expected discharge criteria that should be met before the infant leaves the hospital? **Select all that apply.**

1. Infant vital signs have been normal for the last 12 hours.
2. The infant has passed at least three meconium stools.
3. The infant has gained weight at the minimum 100 grams.
4. The circumcision has had no bleeding for the last 2 hours.
5. The infant has had six diaper changes in the last 24 hours.
6. The infant has completed two successful consecutive feedings.

**894.** The nurse is caring for the full-term newborn male who is 24 hours old and was circumcised with a Gomco clamp 30 minutes ago. Which interventions should the nurse plan for care of the newborn's circumcision? **Select all that apply.**

1. Monitor the newborn's penis hourly for 4 to 6 hours.
2. Observe for and document the first voiding after circumcision.
3. Use prepackaged commercial diaper wipes for perineal cleansing.
4. Apply petroleum ointment around the penis after each diaper change.
5. Apply a size-smaller diaper tightly to provide hemostasis.

**895.** MoC The nurse admits the term newborn, who is at risk to develop neonatal abstinence syndrome (NAS), to the newborn nursery. The nurse correctly places this infant in which location?

1. The general nursery with 15 other infants
2. A small, well-lit nursery with two other newborns
3. Alone in a small, darkened nursery room
4. Right next to the charge nurse's desk

**896.** When the nurse is preparing the 48-hour-old, full-term infant for discharge, the nurse learns that the couple has not named their infant. Which action should the nurse take in response to this information?

1. Ask the parents to choose a name before discharge.
2. Encourage other appropriate attachment behaviors.
3. Document the discharge and that the baby is unnamed.
4. Delay discharge until parental attachment is addressed.

**897.** The home-care nurse is educating the parents of a 1-week-old newborn. Which instruction should the nurse include about the care of the newborn's umbilical cord?

1. "Begin applying rubbing alcohol to the base of the cord stump three times a day."
2. "Attempt to gently dislodge the cord if it has not fallen off in the next week."
3. "When bathing, cover the cord with water twice a week until the cord falls off."
4. "Continue to place the diaper below the cord when diapering the infant."

**898.** The postpartum client (G2P2) asks the nurse for suggestions to help facilitate her 3-year-old's attachment and acceptance of their newborn. Which action should the nurse suggest?

1. Provide a doll for the 3-year-old to care for and nurture.
2. Avoid bringing the 3-year-old to the "scary" hospital.
3. Plan that dad cares for the 3-year-old and mom cares for the baby.
4. Encourage the child to be "grown up" and accept the newborn.

**899.** The nurse is caring for a 30-year-old, single female who delivered a term newborn. What is the **best** way for the nurse to assess the impact of the newborn on the client's lifestyle?

1. Observe how the client interacts with her hospital visitors.
2. Review the prenatal record for clues about the client's lifestyle.
3. Ask the client what plans she has made for newborn care at home.
4. Observe the relationship between the client and her newborn's father.

**900.** A new mother of a full-term, 7-lb newborn asks the nurse how to ensure that her baby is taking the correct amount of formula at each feeding. The nurse explains that the infant needs approximately 3 ounces of fluid per pound of body weight per day. How many ounces of formula should her infant be eating every 4 hours?

_____ ounces (Record your answer to the nearest tenth.)

**901.** The nurse completes teaching in preparation to discharge a mother and her 48-hour-old, full-term newborn. The nurse determines there is a need for further instruction about infant car safety when the newborn's father is overhead making which statement?

1. "We need to face the infant car seat toward the back of the car."
2. "I disarmed one front seat air bag so we can put the car seat in the front seat."
3. "Let's check the car seat to make sure it will position the baby at a 45-degree angle."
4. "I know the baby will need to be in the infant car seat until he is over 20 pounds."

**902.** A healthy postpartum mother who is breastfeeding her term infant states, "My roommate is feeding her newborn iron-enriched formula. Should I be giving my baby iron?" Which response by the nurse is correct?

1. "Your breast milk provides all the iron your baby needs."
2. "You, not your baby, will need an iron supplement daily."
3. "Your pediatrician will prescribe iron drops for your baby."
4. "You should feed your baby iron-fortified formula once daily."

**903.** The nurse and student nurse are caring for the postpartum client who delivered a term newborn 24 hours previously. The nurse recognizes that the student needs more information on newborn nutrition when making which statement?

1. About half of the baby's calorie needs are met by the fat in breast milk or formula.
2. Lactose is the primary source of carbohydrates in breast milk and formula.
3. Calcium supplements are not needed for the newborn regardless of the feeding method.
4. Supplemental water should be given to all infants daily, regardless of feeding method.

**904.** While preparing parents of a 2-day-old, bottle-feeding newborn for discharge, the nurse recognizes the parents' need for additional teaching about formula feeding. Which statement prompted the nurse's conclusion?

1. "We plan to clean our baby's bottles in the dishwasher."
2. "Placing the formula in a bowl of warm water will warm it."
3. "We will put the bottle of unfinished formula in the refrigerator."
4. "Using our city tap water to mix the powdered formula is safe."

**905.** A breastfeeding mother is being discharged with her 2-day-old, full-term newborn. The nurse recognizes that the mother understands how to determine if her newborn is getting enough breast milk when making which statement?

1. "He should have at least three wet diapers tomorrow."
2. "He should have one stool per day during the next week."
3. "At his 1-week checkup, he should weigh an additional 8 ounces."
4. "He should nurse for 5 minutes on each breast to get enough milk."

**906.** The nurse is about to perform a heel stick on a 32-weeks' gestation infant to obtain blood for a prescribed test. Which intervention should the nurse utilize to minimize the neonate's pain?

1. Apply an ice pack.
2. Apply a heel warmer.
3. Give morphine sulfate.
4. Give sucrose or Sweet-Ease.

**907.** The nurse is assessing the infant who may have FAS. Which findings, if observed, should the nurse associate with FAS? **Select all that apply.**

1. Broad nasal bridge and flat midface
2. Growth deficit in weight and length
3. Excessive irritability and hypotonia
4. Poor feeding and persistent vomiting
5. Large jaw and overdeveloped maxilla

**908.** The nurse is caring for the client who has just given birth. The mother is O negative. The nurse should assess for ABO incompatibility and hyperbilirubinemia if the infant's blood type is which type?

1. O positive
2. O negative
3. A negative
4. Any type

**909.** Before beginning a newborn's physical assessment, the nurse reviews the newborn's medical record and sees this notation: "31 weeks' gestation." Considering this information, the nurse determines that a physical assessment of the infant should reveal which finding?

1. Flexion of all four extremities
2. The ability to suck
3. The absence of lanugo
4. Vernix covering the infant

**910.** An infant had four wet diapers during the 8-hour shift. The weight of a dry diaper is 15 g. The four wet diapers weighed 30 g, 24 g, 21 g, and 25 g. What amount in milliliters should the nurse record for the total 8-hour urine?

_____ mL (Record your answer as a whole number.)

**911.** The nurse is preparing a bolus gavage feeding for the preterm infant who has a 5 French feeding tube already secured in the left naris. The nurse has aspirated the infant's stomach contents, noting color, amount, and consistency, and has reinserted the residual amount because it was less than one-fourth the previous feeding. Prioritize the remaining steps to complete this feeding.

1. Separate the barrel of the syringe from the plunger and connect the syringe barrel to the feeding tube.
2. Remove the syringe and clear the tubing with 2 to 3 mL of air.
3. Elevate the syringe 6 to 8 inches over the infant's head.
4. Position the infant on the right side.
5. Uncrimp the tubing and allow the feeding to flow by gravity at a slow rate.
6. Crimp the feeding tube and pour the specified amount of formula or breast milk into the barrel.
7. Cap the lavage feeding tube.

Answer: _____

**912.** The nurse evaluates a preterm infant after a gavage feeding. The nurse determines that feeding intolerance has developed when which finding is noted during assessment?

1. The infant immediately falls asleep after feeding.
2. The gastric residual is zero prior to the next feeding.
3. The infant's abdominal girth has increased in size.
4. The infant is having soft, loose stools.

**913.** The nurse completes teaching a new mother about swaddling her infant. Which illustration shows that the mother understood the teaching?

1.

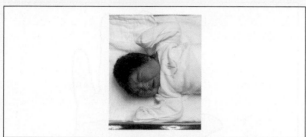

2.

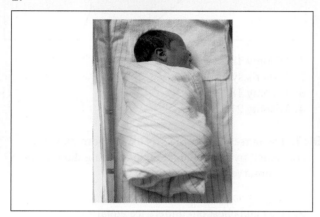

3.

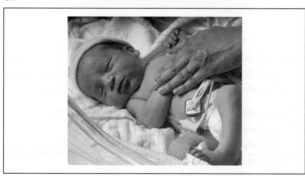

4.

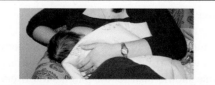

**914.** **PHARM** The nurse is administering surfactant via ET tube to a 48-hour-old preterm infant with respiratory distress syndrome (RDS). The father asks the nurse how this treatment will help his baby. The nurse should explain that the preterm infant is unable to produce adequate amounts of surfactant and that giving it to his baby will have what effect?

1. Increase $Paco_2$ levels in the bloodstream.
2. Prevent collapse of the alveoli.
3. Decrease $Pao_2$ levels in the bloodstream.
4. Prevent pleural effusion.

**915.** The nurse is caring for a preterm infant with respiratory distress syndrome (RDS). Which intervention should the nurse implement to maximize the infant's respiratory status?

1. Check blood glucose levels every 4 hours.
2. Cool and humidify all inspired gases.
3. Weigh the infant every other day.
4. Place the infant in a prone position.

**916.** The labor history of a postpartum mother states, "Mother positive for group B streptococcal (GBS) infection at 37 weeks' gestation. Membranes ruptured at home 14 hours before presentation to the hospital at 40 weeks' gestation. Precipitous labor, no antibiotic given." Considering this information, the nurse should observe the 15-hour-old newborn closely for which finding?

1. Temperature instability
2. Pink stains in the diaper
3. Meconium stools
4. Presence of erythema toxicum

**917.** **PHARM** The nurse is caring for the infant in the neonatal ICU who has an umbilical artery catheter (UAC) in place. To monitor for and prevent complications with this catheter, which actions should be planned by the nurse? **Select all that apply.**

1. Check the position marking on the catheter every shift.
2. Position the tubing close to the infant's lower limbs.
3. Check for erythema or discoloration of the abdominal wall.
4. Palpate for femoral, pedal, and tibial pulses every 2 to 4 hours.
5. Reposition the catheter tubing every hour.
6. Monitor blood glucose levels.

**918.** **MoC** While caring for the small-for-gestational-age newborn (SGA), the nurse notes slight tremors of the extremities, a high-pitched cry, and an exaggerated Moro reflex. In response to these assessment findings, what should be the nurse's **first** action?

1. Assess the infant's blood sugar level.
2. Document the findings in the infant's medical record.
3. Immediately inform the pediatrician of the symptoms.
4. Assess the infant's axillary temperature.

**919.** When assessing the infant undergoing phototherapy for hyperbilirubinemia, the nurse notes a maculopapular rash over the infant's buttocks and back. What action should the nurse take **next?**

1. Document the results in the newborn's record.
2. Call the HCP immediately to report this finding.
3. Discontinue the phototherapy immediately.
4. Assess the infant's axillary temperature.

**920.** The full-term newborn is placed under phototherapy lights to treat hyperbilirubinemia. The nurse should assess the newborn for dehydration due to which effect of phototherapy?

1. Decreases sodium absorption
2. Increases absorption of bilirubin
3. Decreases urinary output
4. Increases insensible water loss

**921.** The mother of a healthy 15-hour-old term newborn states, "We are going home. Should the PKU blood test be completed on my baby before we leave?" Which statement should be the basis for the nurse's response?

1. The PKU test must be completed when the infant is at least 1 month of age.
2. The parents must sign a consent form if the PKU test is completed before 24 hours of age.
3. The PKU test is best if completed after the infant is 24 hours old but before 7 days of age.
4. The PKU test is not needed if the infant is tolerating feedings without diarrhea or vomiting.

**922.** While assessing the full-term newborn, the nurse notes the abnormality illustrated in the infant's palm. The nurse should further assess the infant for signs and symptoms of which condition?

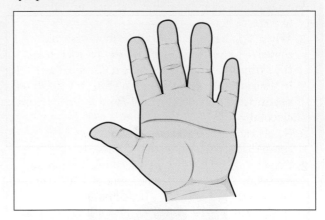

1. Trisomy 13
2. Turner's syndrome
3. Trisomy 18
4. Trisomy 21

**923.** The nurse is concerned that a newborn may have congenital hydrocephalus. Which finding did the nurse likely observe on assessment?

1. Bulging anterior fontanel
2. Head and chest circumference equal
3. A narrowed posterior fontanel
4. Low-set ears

**924.** After assisting in the delivery of a full-term infant with anencephaly, the parents ask the nurse to explain treatments that might be available for their infant. Which statement should be the basis for the nurse's response?

1. Immediate surgery is necessary to repair the congenital defect.
2. Anencephaly is incompatible with life; only palliative care should be provided.
3. A shunting procedure will be necessary initially to relieve intracranial pressure.
4. Antibiotics are needed initially before any treatment is started.

**925.** The nurse is discharging the 3-day-old term newborn with a right-sided cephalohematoma. The nurse should instruct the parents to observe their infant closely over the next week for the development of which problem associated with the cephalohematoma?

1. Jaundice
2. Difficulty feeding
3. Pale extremities
4. Bulging on the right side of the head with crying

## Answers and Rationales

**867. ANSWER: 2**

1. Shivering is rarely seen in newborns, and it does little to produce heat.

2. **When skin receptors of full-term newborns perceive a drop in environmental temperature, the sympathetic nervous system is stimulated. This in turn stimulates metabolism of brown fat, thus producing heat that is transferred to the peripheral circulation.**

3. Newborns are able to conserve body heat by constricting, not dilating, blood vessels.

4. Decreasing flexion promotes heat loss by exposing more skin surface to the environment. Full-term newborns normally maintain a flexed posture.

▸ *Test-taking Tip: Brown adipose tissue first appears in the fetus at 26 to 30 weeks' gestation. The ability to utilize brown adipose tissue (brown fat) to produce nonshivering thermogenesis is unique to full-term newborns.*

Content Area: Childbearing; Concept: Thermo-regulation; Pregnancy; Integrated Processes: Nursing Process: Analysis; Client Needs: Physiological Integrity: Physiological Adaptation; Cognitive Level: Knowledge [Remembering]

**868. ANSWER: 2, 3, 4, 6**

1. If the mother naps immediately after birth, the alert newborn period may be missed.

2. **Dimming the lights in the birthing room encourages the newborn to open his or her eyes. This in turn encourages eye contact between the parent and the newborn.**

3. **Skin-to-skin contact between mother and baby at birth improves mother-baby interaction.**

4. **Instillation of ophthalmic antibiotic ointment should be delayed for an hour because instilling it now may cause temporary blurred vision in the newborn. The temporary blurred vision can decrease the infant's ability to engage in eye-to-eye contact with the parents, thus affecting parent-infant attachment.**

5. Avoiding loud noises encourages parent-infant communication.

6. **The newborn is alert for up to 1 hour after birth. Parents should be encouraged to use this time for attachment and to delay phone calls.**

▸ *Test-taking Tip: The newborn has an alert period for up to 1 hour after birth. Eliminate options that would cause the parents to miss this time interacting with their newborn.*

Content Area: Childbearing; Concept: Nursing Roles; Pregnancy; Integrated Processes: Nursing Process: Implementation; Client Needs: Health Promotion and Maintenance; Cognitive Level: Application [Applying]

**869. ANSWER: 2**

1. It is unnecessary to stimulate the infant to cry because acrocyanosis is normal.

2. **Acrocyanosis, which is blueness of hands and feet, is a normal newborn phenomenon in the first 24 to 48 hours after birth. The nurse should explain this to the father to relieve his anxiety.**

3. It is unnecessary to assess the newborn's temperature because acrocyanosis is normal.

4. It is unnecessary to assess the newborn's cardiac status because acrocyanosis is normal.

▸ *Test-taking Tip: Peripheral circulation in newborns is immature.*

Content Area: Childbearing; Concept: Assessment; Pregnancy; Nursing Roles; Integrated Processes: Caring; Client Needs: Health Promotion and Maintenance; Cognitive Level: Application [Applying]

**870. ANSWER: 4**

1. To score a 2 on the HR criterion of the Apgar scoring, the newborn's HR must be above 100 bpm.

2. During birth, as soon as the head emerges, the newborn's mouth is suctioned first (because the newborn is an obligate nose breather) and then the nares with a bulb syringe to prevent aspiration of mucus, amniotic fluid, or meconium. Suctioning should be completed during the newborn's care, but there is no indication that this is needed.

3. The newborn would not be wrapped and placed on the mother's abdomen until the assessment is complete; the HR is only the first parameter to be scored on the Apgar scoring system.

4. **A newborn HR of less than 100 bpm scores as a 1 on the HR criterion and indicates a need to begin positive pressure ventilation by bag mask or Neopuff® ventilation.**

▸ *Test-taking Tip: The initial newborn apical pulse rate is between 110 and 160 bpm and somewhat irregular.*

Content Area: Childbearing; Concept: Assessment; Pregnancy; Critical Thinking; Integrated Processes: Nursing Process: Implementation; Client Needs: Physiological Integrity: Physiological Adaptation; Cognitive Level: Application [Applying]

**871. ANSWER: 2**

1. Whereas a low 1-minute Apgar score is not associated with infant mortality, a low 5-minute Apgar score is.

2. **A 5-minute Apgar score at or above 7 is considered normal.**

3. The Apgar score at 5 minutes in full-term infants is a poor predictor of neurological outcome.

4. Oligohydramnios is the presence of too little amniotic fluid. This as well as other variables such as gestational age, resuscitation measures, and medications can all affect the Apgar score.

▸ *Test-taking Tip: Three options concern medical diagnoses, and one option is different. Often the option that is different is the answer.*

Content Area: Childbearing; Concept: Assessment; Pregnancy; Integrated Processes: Nursing Process: Analysis; Client Needs: Physiological Integrity: Reduction of Risk Potential; Cognitive Level: Analysis [Analyzing]

### 872. ANSWER: 4

1. Full-term newborns normally pass meconium naturally within 8 to 24 hours after birth. Delayed clamping of the umbilical cord will not affect this process.
2. The healthy newborn is born awake and active. This alertness typically lasts for 30 minutes after birth and is known as the first period of reactivity. This will not be affected by delayed cord clamping.
3. At birth, the newborn's temperature may fall due to evaporative heat loss. Delayed cord clamping will not affect this evaporation process.
4. **Newborn Hgb and Hct values will be higher when placental transfusion, accomplished through delayed cord clamping, occurs at birth. Blood volume increases by up to 50% with delayed cord clamping.**

▶ *Test-taking Tip: Recall that blood travels from the mother to the fetus via the umbilical cord. Option 4 is most related to circulation and therefore would be the best selection.*

Content Area: Childbearing; Concept: Perfusion; Pregnancy; Integrated Processes: Nursing Process: Analysis; Client Needs: Physiological Integrity: Physiological Adaptation; Cognitive Level: Analysis [Analyzing]

### 873. ANSWER: 1, 2, 4

1. **Drying the newborn immediately after birth prevents heat loss through evaporation.**
2. **Skin-to-skin contact between mother and baby at birth assists to maintain newborn body temperature.**
3. If other appropriate warming measures are taken, there is no need to wrap the infant's legs in leggings.
4. **The newborn's head is dried first after birth, and a stocking cap is placed on the head to conserve heat.**
5. Placing the bassinette close to the wall will cause radiation heat loss because the wall is cooler in temperature than the newborn.

▶ *Test-taking Tip: Use the process of elimination to rule out Option 3 because it is not an initial measure, and Option 5 because a cool surface, such as a wall, would be detrimental to body warming.*

Content Area: Childbearing; Concept: Thermo-regulation; Pregnancy; Integrated Processes: Nursing Process: Implementation; Client Needs: Health Promotion and Maintenance; Cognitive Level: Application [Applying]

### 874. ANSWER: 1

1. **Currently every U.S. state requires that newborns receive prophylactic eye treatment against gonorrheal conjunctivitis.**

2. If a parent objects to the treatment, the parent will be asked to sign formal documentation of informed refusal.
3. The antibiotic can only be administered topically, not orally.
4. The eye prophylaxis must be administered within 1 hour of birth to be effective.

▶ *Test-taking Tip: Eliminate Option 3, as a medication to specifically prevent eye conjunctivitis would be unlikely to be effective if administered orally.*

Content Area: Childbearing; Concept: Legal; Infection; Pregnancy; Integrated Processes: Teaching/Learning; Client Needs: Safe and Effective Care Environment: Safety and Infection Control; Cognitive Level: Application [Applying]

### 875. ANSWER:

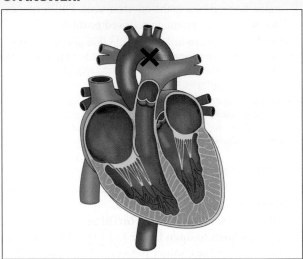

**The ductus arteriosus connects the pulmonary artery to the descending aorta (X) and acts as a shunt to carry blood directly from the right ventricle into the aorta. This should close within 15 hours after birth.**

▶ *Test-taking Tip: Focus on the term "ductus arteriosus," which indicates arterial connections; thus eliminate areas that pertain to veins and valves.*

Content Area: Childbearing; Concept: Development; Pregnancy; Nursing Roles; Integrated Processes: Teaching/Learning; Client Needs: Physiological Integrity: Physiological Adaptation; Cognitive Level: Comprehension [Understanding]

### 876. ANSWER: 1

1. **The circumference of the normal newborn's head is approximately 2 centimeters greater than the circumference of the newborn's chest at birth. Any extreme difference in head size may indicate microcephalus, hydrocephalus, or increased ICP.**
2. Head size is not related to intelligence. Heredity and interpersonal relationships play critical roles in intellectual development of the child.
3. Chest size does not provide information needed to assess cardiac status.

4. The relationship of the head and chest does not predict adult body size. Heredity, nutrition, and hormones are the major determinant of physical adult size.

▸ **Test-taking Tip:** *Eliminate Options 2 and 4, as these relate to future data. These parameters will be affected by different outside influences as the child grows and could not be predicted by simple newborn head and chest measurements.*

**Content Area:** Childbearing; **Concept:** Assessment; Pregnancy; Communication; **Integrated Processes:** Communication and Documentation; **Client Needs:** Health Promotion and Maintenance; **Cognitive Level:** Application [Applying]

## 877. MoC ANSWER: 2

1. Only after an intervention should the nurse document the findings because the temperature is abnormal.
2. **This infant's axillary temperature of 97°F (36.1°C) is below the normal range of 97.7°F (36.5°C) to 98.9°F (37.2°C). The infant should be gradually rewarmed under a temperature-controlled radiant warmer.**
3. Feeding warm formula is unnecessary and may affect the mother's breast milk production if she is breastfeeding.
4. There is no need to call the HCP unless the nurse is unable to warm the infant using appropriate interventions.

▸ **Test-taking Tip:** *The key word is "first." Consider that infants who become cold must increase their metabolic rate and thus their oxygen consumption to generate heat. This can lead to respiratory distress. Thus consider the ABC's when selecting the correct option.*

**Content Area:** Childbearing; **Concept:** Thermo-regulation; Pregnancy; Management; **Integrated Processes:** Nursing Process: Implementation; **Client Needs:** Safe and Effective Care Environment: Management of Care; **Cognitive Level:** Application [Applying]

## 878. ANSWER: 4

1. Although breast- or formula feeding helps to prevent hypoglycemia in newborns, feeding is not necessary because a blood sugar of 48 mg/dL is within normal parameters.
2. Oral glucose water can cause a rapid increase in glucose followed by an abrupt decrease and should not be given to treat hypoglycemia.
3. A blood sugar of 48 mg/dL is within normal parameters; there is no need to notify the HCP.
4. **Normal blood sugar values for a full-term newborn are 45 to 65 mg/dL. Therefore the only action required is to document the findings.**

▸ **Test-taking Tip:** *The normal blood sugar level for a full-term newborn is 45 to 65 mg/dL. Use this information to select the correct option.*

**Content Area:** Childbearing; **Concept:** Metabolism; Pregnancy; **Integrated Processes:** Nursing Process: Implementation; **Client Needs:** Health Promotion and Maintenance; **Cognitive Level:** Analysis [Analyzing]

## 879. ANSWER: 2

1. The assessment reveals normal findings so there is no need to notify the HCP.
2. **Documentation of the findings is all that is required. Both the HR and murmur are expected findings. The apical HR of the term newborn is normally between 100 and 160 bpm. A murmur heard at the sternal border, third intercostal space, is most likely caused by delayed closure of the foramen ovale, which functionally closes within 1 to 2 hours after birth. Permanent closure of the foramen ovale occurs within 6 months to 1 year after birth.**
3. A left side-lying position brings the heart closer to the chest wall to better hear a murmur, but this is not necessary because the presence of a murmur is expected.
4. There is no need to stimulate crying; crying will make it more difficult to hear heart sounds.

▸ **Test-taking Tip:** *In newborns, 90% of murmurs are transient and expected.*

**Content Area:** Childbearing; **Concept:** Assessment; Pregnancy; Communication; **Integrated Processes:** Communication and Documentation; **Client Needs:** Health Promotion and Maintenance; **Cognitive Level:** Application [Applying]

## 880. ANSWER: 2

1. Jaundice is generally first noticed in the head and then progresses gradually down the body; thus the change in skin color would not be evident as quickly in the genitalia.
2. **To differentiate cutaneous jaundice from normal skin color, the nurse should apply pressure with a finger over a bony area such as the forehead. If jaundice is present, the blanched area will look yellow before the capillaries refill.**
3. The change in skin color would not be evident as quickly in the extremities as in the head.
4. Because the tongue and palate are naturally darker in color than the rest of the skin, it is more difficult to determine jaundice by assessing in these areas.

▸ **Test-taking Tip:** *Think carefully about the color of the body in the different areas described in the options. Then elect the option with the area of the body with the lightest skin color.*

**Content Area:** Childbearing; **Concept:** Assessment; Pregnancy; Diversity; **Integrated Processes:** Nursing Process: Assessment; Culture and Spirituality; **Client Needs:** Health Promotion and Maintenance; **Cognitive Level:** Application [Applying]

## 881. ANSWER: 1, 3, 5

1. **As the fetal muscular tone matures, the posture becomes more flexed; thus the full-term newborn exhibits hypertonic flexion of all extremities.**
2. Sole creases over the anterior two-thirds of the sole indicate a gestational age of approximately 37 weeks.

3. **Cartilage gives the ear its shape. At full term, the newborn ear has enough cartilage to produce a well-defined incurving of the entire pinna.**

4. A prominent clitoris is found in a female infant whose gestational age is between 30 and 32 weeks. As the fetus matures, the labia majora become large enough to completely cover the clitoris and labia minora.

5. **The full-term infant has the muscle strength to momentarily support his or her head when pulled to a sitting position.**

▶ *Test-taking Tip: Muscle strength and resistance to positioning of arms and legs increase as gestational age increases. Eliminate any options suggesting a very immature infant because this infant is full term at 40 weeks' gestation.*

**Content Area:** Childbearing; **Concept:** Assessment; Pregnancy; **Integrated Processes:** Nursing Process: Assessment; **Client Needs:** Health Promotion and Maintenance; **Cognitive Level:** Analysis [Analyzing]

## 882. MoC ANSWER: 3

1. The newborn's HR should always be assessed apically because radial and temporal pulses are difficult to palpate.

2. A stocking cap is often utilized to conserve heat in newborns.

3. **The LPN needs additional instruction when observed monitoring the newborn's temperature rectally. Taking the temperature rectally may cause rectal mucosal irritation and increase the chances of rectal perforation.**

4. The American Academy of Pediatrics recommends that healthy full-term infants be placed on their backs to sleep because this has been found to reduce deaths from SIDS.

▶ *Test-taking Tip: The key words "needs more instruction" indicate that this question is a false-response item. Look for the incorrect statement. Consider which action could be unsafe.*

**Content Area:** Childbearing; **Concept:** Safety; Pregnancy; Management; **Integrated Processes:** Nursing Process: Evaluation; **Client Needs:** Safe and Effective Care Environment: Management of Care; **Cognitive Level:** Evaluation [Evaluating]

## 883. ANSWER: 3

1. This stool is normal and does not indicate that a newborn has active GI bleeding.

2. Stools of breastfed babies are usually pale yellow once the meconium has passed.

3. **The majority of full-term infants will normally pass the first meconium stool within 24 hours after birth. It is formed during fetal life from amniotic fluid and intestinal secretions and cells. It is greenish-black in color and normally contains occult blood.**

4. Being cold does not affect the passage of meconium. Exposure to cold will increase the infant's oxygen requirements, decrease glucose levels and surfactant production, and can eventually result in respiratory compromise.

▶ *Test-taking Tip: You should read the options carefully. Options with absolute words such as "all" are rarely correct. The nurse should not make a statement that would increase a mother's worry when she is already worried.*

**Content Area:** Childbearing; **Concept:** Bowel Elimination; Pregnancy; Nursing Roles; **Integrated Processes:** Teaching/ Learning; **Client Needs:** Physiological Integrity: Basic Care and Comfort; **Cognitive Level:** Application [Applying]

## 884. ANSWER: 4

1. Applying a dry gauze dressing would cause it to adhere to the sac and increase the risk of rupture of the sac when the gauze is removed. The sac should be covered with a dressing moistened with sterile saline to protect the integrity of the sac and decrease the risk for infection.

2. Preservation of the integrity of the sac is of primary concern, and surgical intervention will occur when the infant is stabilized and all appropriate measures are complete. Surgery usually occurs within the first few days of life.

3. A pressure dressing would increase the risk of rupturing the sac.

4. **Positioning the infant prone with hips slightly flexed and legs abducted helps to minimize tension and potential for rupture of the sac.**

▶ *Test-taking Tip: Myelomeningocele is a neural tube defect where there is an incomplete spinal canal because the spinal bones have not completely formed. This results in the meninges and spinal cord protruding "sac-like" from the infant's back. Consider options that would protect the integrity of the sac.*

**Content Area:** Childbearing; **Concept:** Pregnancy; Neurologic Regulation; **Integrated Processes:** Nursing Process: Implementation; **Client Needs:** Physiological Integrity: Reduction of Risk Potential; **Cognitive Level:** Application [Applying]

## 885. ANSWER: 2

1. Mongolian spots are not a result of injury during delivery; if it were bruising, bruising would not occur this rapidly.

2. **The image is illustrating Mongolian spots, a normal newborn skin variation.**

3. Mongolian spots are not a result of injury from improper handling of the infant; if it were bruising, bruising would not occur this rapidly.

4. Mongolian spots are not a result of intestinal bleeding.

▶ *Test-taking Tip: Mongolian spots are collections of pigmented cells that appear as slate-gray patches across the sacrum, buttocks, and, less commonly, arms and legs of newborns. These are more likely to occur in newborns of Asian, southern European, or African descent.*

**Content Area:** Childbearing; **Concept:** Assessment; Diversity; Pregnancy; **Integrated Processes:** Nursing Process: Analysis; Culture and Spirituality; **Client Needs:** Health Promotion and Maintenance; **Cognitive Level:** Application [Applying]

**886. ANSWER: 3**

1. No molding occurs when the fetus is breech because the buttocks, not the head, are the presenting part.
2. With planned cesarean section, the head is not pressed against the cervix because labor does not occur.
3. **A 16-hour labor will cause molding. Molding is a change in the shape of the fetal skull from the force of uterine contractions during labor pressing the vertex of the head against the cervix. The degree of molding varies with the amount and length of pressure exerted on the head. Thus a longer labor will increase molding.**
4. A precipitous delivery following only 30 minutes of labor would mean limited time for the vertex to be pressing against the cervix.

▸ **Test-taking Tip:** *Eliminate options where there is no or limited opportunity for the vertex to press against the cervix during birth.*

**Content Area:** Childbearing; **Concept:** Pregnancy; Communication; **Integrated Processes:** Nursing Process: Analysis; **Client Needs:** Safe and Effective Care Environment: Safety and Infection Control; **Cognitive Level:** Analysis [Analyzing]

**887. ANSWER: 4**

1. Laying the infant supine may cause bulging of the fontanel; assessing in this position is incorrect.
2. Crying may cause a temporary bulging of the fontanel and should not be stimulated.
3. Feeling near the parietal and occipital bones will locate the posterior and not anterior fontanel.
4. **To assess the anterior fontanel, the nurse should place the infant in a sitting position (45 to 90 degrees) so its location, size, and any abnormalities can be identified. If indented-appearing, it could indicate dehydration; if bulging, it could indicate increased ICP.**

▸ **Test-taking Tip:** *The anterior fontanel is located at the juncture of the frontal and two parietal bones.*

**Content Area:** Childbearing; **Concept:** Assessment; Pregnancy; **Integrated Processes:** Nursing Process: Assessment; **Client Needs:** Health Promotion and Maintenance; **Cognitive Level:** Application [Applying]

**888. ANSWER: 2**

1. Lotion may clog the exposed sebaceous glands.
2. **This statement indicates the mother understands information about milia. No treatment is necessary because it will clear spontaneously within the first month.**
3. Surgery is not necessary; these are not skin lesions but milia, which clear up within the first month.
4. Alcohol is drying and may aggravate milia.

▸ **Test-taking Tip:** *Milia are exposed sebaceous glands that appear as raised white spots on the face, usually the nose, of the newborn.*

**Content Area:** Childbearing; **Concept:** Pregnancy; Nursing Roles; **Integrated Processes:** Nursing Process: Evaluation; **Client Needs:** Health Promotion and Maintenance; **Cognitive Level:** Evaluation [Evaluating]

**889. ANSWER: 3**

1. Acrocyanosis is common after birth for full-term newborns due to poor peripheral circulation and is not particular to the infant that is LGA.
2. By full term, the testicles of the male newborn can be found in the lower scrotum. Undescended testicles are not unique to LGA infants.
3. **A major complication for LGA infants is birth trauma, such as a fractured clavicle, due to cephalopelvic disproportion from macrosomia.**
4. Hypothermia is always a concern with newborns; however, the increased amounts of subcutaneous fat in LGA infants provide added thermal protection.

▸ **Test-taking Tip:** *The key words are "most important." You should select the assessment that is most important with an LGA infant.*

**Content Area:** Childbearing; **Concept:** Development; Pregnancy; Assessment; **Integrated Processes:** Nursing Process: Planning; **Client Needs:** Physiological Integrity: Reduction of Risk Potential; **Cognitive Level:** Comprehension [Understanding]

**890. ANSWER: 1**

1. **An intact Moro reflex is demonstrated when the newborn straightens the extremities and then flexes them in response to a loud noise.**
2. Option 2 describes an intact tonic neck reflex.
3. Option 3 describes the rooting reflex.
4. Option 4 describes the stepping reflex.

▸ **Test-taking Tip:** *The Moro reflex is also known as the "startle" reflex.*

**Content Area:** Childbearing; **Concept:** Assessment; Pregnancy; **Integrated Processes:** Nursing Process: Evaluation; **Client Needs:** Health Promotion and Maintenance; **Cognitive Level:** Evaluation [Evaluating]

**891. ANSWER: 2**

1. The mother is correct to keep her baby warm, as cold stress can result in acidosis, which will decrease available serum albumin binding sites. This in turn will result in a decrease in unconjugated bilirubin being transported via albumin to the liver.
2. **Peak bilirubin levels are reached at 3 to 5 days of age for Caucasian infants. However, Native American babies have higher bilirubin levels than Caucasian babies, and the jaundice persists for longer periods with no apparent ill effects.**
3. Bilirubin is eliminated in the baby's stools; inadequate stooling may result in reabsorption of bilirubin.

4. Frequent feeding promotes intestinal elimination and provides protein intake necessary for the formation of hepatic binding proteins.

▸ **Test-taking Tip:** *You should note that three options include actions to decrease jaundice, but one option is different. Often the option that is different is the answer.*

**Content Area:** Childbearing; **Concept:** Nursing Roles; Diversity; Pregnancy; **Integrated Processes:** Nursing Process: Evaluation; Culture and Spirituality; **Client Needs:** Health Promotion and Maintenance; **Cognitive Level:** Evaluation [Evaluating]

## 892. MoC ANSWER: 2

1. To ensure that the needs and desires of the couple are recognized and met, the nurse will need to acknowledge the lesbian relationship with the client.
2. **The nurse should involve the partner in the newborn's care. This shows the partner the same respect, caring, and attention shown to the partners of heterosexual mothers.**
3. Asking the partner to leave the room is disrespectful and judgmental.
4. The nurse should ensure that the needs and desires of the couple are recognized and met by caregivers. To do so, the nurse needs to provide the information about the lesbian relationship to caregivers.

▸ **Test-taking Tip:** *Only one option represents a nonjudgmental, inclusive approach to client care.*

**Content Area:** Childbearing; **Concept:** Pregnancy; Diversity; Management; **Integrated Processes:** Nursing Process: Implementation; Culture and Spirituality; **Client Needs:** Safe and Effective Care Environment: Management of Care; Health Promotion and Maintenance; **Cognitive Level:** Synthesis [Creating]

## 893. MoC ANSWER: 1, 4, 6

1. **The American Academy of Pediatrics has determined that newborn discharge criteria include stable VS for 12 hours.**
2. One meconium stool, not three, is an expected discharge criterion.
3. There is no weight gain requirement for discharge; newborns are expected to lose weight during the first 3 to 4 days after birth.
4. **No bleeding from a circumcision for 2 hours is an expected discharge criterion.**
5. Discharge criteria include that the infant has urinated regularly. There is no specified number of diaper changes in a 24-hour period and no specified number of wet diapers.
6. **Completing two successful consecutive feedings is included in the discharge criteria. Successful feeding includes verification that the infant is able to coordinate sucking, swallowing, and breathing while feeding.**

▸ **Test-taking Tip:** *You should be sure to consider that newborns in the United States are usually discharged from the hospital within 48 hours after birth; if discharged earlier, the infant still needs to meet the discharge criteria. Consider what is applicable to a 48-hour-old infant.*

**Content Area:** Childbearing; **Concept:** Assessment; Pregnancy; **Integrated Processes:** Nursing Process: Evaluation; **Client Needs:** Safe and Effective Care Environment: Management of Care; Health Promotion and Maintenance; **Cognitive Level:** Evaluation [Evaluating]

## 894. ANSWER: 1, 2, 4

1. **After circumcision, the newborn's penis should be closely monitored, especially for swelling and bleeding.**
2. **To evaluate for urinary obstruction, the infant should be monitored frequently for the first urination postcircumcision, and this finding should be documented.**
3. Prepackaged commercial diaper wipes should be avoided because they may contain alcohol, which could be irritating.
4. **Petroleum and gauze should be applied to the circumcision site with each diaper change to prevent bleeding and to protect healing tissue.**
5. When diapering the newborn, the nurse should ensure that the diaper is not too tight or too small, which may cause pain. If too loose, it can cause rubbing with movement.

▸ **Test-taking Tip:** *You should eliminate options that could increase irritation and cause pain.*

**Content Area:** Childbearing; **Concept:** Skin Integrity; Pregnancy; **Integrated Processes:** Nursing Process: Planning; **Client Needs:** Physiological Integrity: Reduction of Risk Potential; **Cognitive Level:** Application [Applying]

## 895. MoC ANSWER: 3

1. Placing the newborn with NAS in with 15 other infants will be too stimulating due to increased noise from other infants.
2. The light of a well-lit nursery will be too stimulating for the newborn with NAS.
3. **The newborn with NAS will exhibit withdrawal behaviors due to exposure to chemical substances in utero. The nurse should place the newborn alone in a small, darkened nursery room to reduce environmental stimuli.**
4. Placing the newborn with NAS near the charge nurse's desk will be too stimulating due to environmental noise.

▸ **Test-taking Tip:** *Three options include stimulating environments, whereas one option is different. Often the option that is different is the answer.*

**Content Area:** Childbearing; **Concept:** Addiction; Safety; Pregnancy; **Integrated Processes:** Nursing Process: Planning; **Client Needs:** Safe and Effective Care Environment: Management of Care; Safe and Effective Care Environment: Safety and Infection Control; **Cognitive Level:** Application [Applying]

## 896. ANSWER: 3

1. It would be culturally inappropriate to ask the parents to choose a name before discharge.
2. It is always appropriate for the nurse to observe for and encourage attachment behaviors; however, in this situation, not naming the infant is not a sign of inappropriate attachment.
3. **In some cultures, the naming of a child is an important event, and the day is marked by a celebration. The naming of the child may not occur until the third day or later after birth. Thus the only response is to document this information.**
4. There is no need to delay discharge; not naming the infant is not a sign of inappropriate attachment.

▸ *Test-taking Tip: Consider cultural differences when answering the question.*

Content Area: Childbearing; Concept: Diversity; Pregnancy; Integrated Processes: Communication and Documentation; Culture and Spirituality; Client Needs: Psychosocial Integrity; Cognitive Level: Application [Applying]

## 897. ANSWER: 4

1. There is no evidence that applying alcohol to the cord keeps the baby's cord clean and dry.
2. The cord should never be pulled. The parents should be instructed not to attempt to remove the cord because this could lead to bleeding and infection.
3. Covering the cord when bathing would moisten the cord and delay separation, and should be avoided.
4. **Folding the diaper below the cord avoids cord contact with urine and stool. A wet, soiled environment slows drying and increases the risk of infection.**

▸ *Test-taking Tip: Keeping the cord dry and exposed to air promotes drying and eventual separation.*

Content Area: Childbearing; Concept: Nursing Roles; Pregnancy; Integrated Processes: Teaching/Learning; Client Needs: Health Promotion and Maintenance; Cognitive Level: Application [Applying]

## 898. ANSWER: 1

1. **Providing care to a doll encourages the 3-year-old to identify with the parents, which helps to decrease anger and regression to get attention.**
2. Bringing the 3-year-old to the hospital and pointing out similarities to the 3-year-old's birth is encouraged and increases the bond between the two children.
3. The 3-year-old needs individual attention from both parents to decrease jealousy, which may develop if the newborn is seen as taking all of the mother's time.
4. Regression is a common occurrence even in well-prepared siblings, and parents should be counseled to expect this and not become concerned.

▸ *Test-taking Tip: Think about the developmental needs of the preschool child. Select the option that would best reflect adaptation to those needs.*

Content Area: Childbearing; Concept: Family; Pregnancy; Integrated Processes: Teaching/Learning; Caring; Client Needs: Health Promotion and Maintenance; Cognitive Level: Application [Applying]

## 899. ANSWER: 3

1. Observing the mother's interaction with visitors and observing who visits will provide information about her social support system.
2. Reviewing the prenatal record will provide physical health information and information about attendance at prenatal visits. This may provide insight into the mother's commitment to the pregnancy and the newborn, but it will not provide information about the mother's postdelivery plans.
3. **Open-ended questions will encourage sharing of feelings and examination of available lifestyle options. A lower income and lack of a reliable backup person are common problems for the single parent.**
4. Single mothers do not always have an involved father; there is no indication that the father is involved.

▸ *Test-taking Tip: The key term is "best." Select the option that is most likely to provide the most information.*

Content Area: Childbearing; Concept: Assessment; Pregnancy; Communication; Integrated Processes: Nursing Process: Assessment; Client Needs: Safe and Effective Care Environment: Safety and Infection Control; Cognitive Level: Analysis [Analyzing]

## 900. ANSWER: 3.5

**Multiplying 3 oz by 7 (the weight of the baby) equals 21 oz needed per day. Dividing 21 oz by 6 (the number of feedings in 24 hours if the baby is fed every 4 hours) equals 3.5 oz per feeding.**

▸ *Test-taking Tip: Be sure you record your answer as the 4-hour feeding amount and not the daily total.*

Content Area: Childbearing; Concept: Nutrition; Pregnancy; Integrated Processes: Nursing Process: Analysis; Client Needs: Physiological Integrity: Basic Care and Comfort; Cognitive Level: Application [Applying]

## 901. ANSWER: 2

1. Children should face the rear of the vehicle in an infant car seat until they are at least 1 year of age.
2. **The parents should be advised not to disarm air bags and that the rear vehicle seat is the safest place for children of any age to ride.**
3. Infants should ride at approximately a 45-degree angle to prevent slumping and airway obstruction.
4. Children should remain in a car seat until they weigh at least 20 lb to decrease the risk of cervical spine injury in the event of a crash.

▸ *Test-taking Tip: The key words "a need for further instructions" indicate that this is a false-response item. Look for the incorrect statement.*

Content Area: Childbearing; Concept: Safety; Pregnancy; Integrated Processes: Nursing Process: Evaluation; Client Needs: Safe and Effective Care Environment: Safety and Infection Control; Cognitive Level: Evaluation [Evaluating]

## 902. ANSWER: 1

1. **It is unnecessary to provide iron supplementation to a breastfeeding infant. Although iron content in breast milk is much lower than in iron-fortified formulas, the iron in breast milk is much more completely absorbed.**
2. Taking an iron supplement does not influence the mineral content of breast milk.
3. It is unnecessary to provide an iron supplement to a breastfeeding infant when breast milk provides sufficient iron.
4. Supplementing a breastfed baby with formula decreases the amount of time the infant breastfeeds, thus decreasing breast milk supply. Using a bottle nipple for feeding also may cause nipple confusion in the newborn.

♦ **Test-taking Tip:** *Iron content in breast milk is much lower than in iron-fortified formulas (0.5–1 mg compared with 12 mg); however, the iron in breast milk is much more completely absorbed. The infant receiving breast milk absorbs 50% to 80% of the iron in breast milk compared with only 12% absorption of the iron in formula.*

Content Area: Childbearing; Concept: Nutrition; Pregnancy; Nursing Roles; Integrated Processes: Teaching/Learning; Client Needs: Physiological Integrity: Basic Care and Comfort; Cognitive Level: Application [Applying]

## 903. ANSWER: 4

1. Full-term infants do receive about half of their required calories from the fat in breast milk (52%) or formula (49%).
2. Lactose is the primary carbohydrate in both breast milk and formula, and its slow breakdown and absorption may increase calcium absorption.
3. Calcium levels are adequate in both types of milk for bone growth and prevention of tetany.
4. **Breast milk and formula contain almost 90% water, which meets the infant's water needs. Feeding supplemental water can cause hyponatremia and may result in seizures if water consumption is excessive.**

♦ **Test-taking Tip:** *Options that contain absolute words such as "all" are usually incorrect. The phrase "needs more information" indicates that you select a statement that is incorrect.*

Content Area: Childbearing; Concept: Nutrition; Pregnancy; Integrated Processes: Nursing Process: Evaluation; Client Needs: Physiological Integrity: Basic Care and Comfort; Cognitive Level: Evaluation [Evaluating]

## 904. ANSWER: 3

1. Bottles and nipples can be safely washed in the dishwasher with other family dishes.

2. If the formula has been refrigerated, it can be warmed to room temperature by placing it in a bowl of warm water. It should never be warmed in the microwave.
3. **The formula remaining in the bottle after feeding has mixed with the infant's saliva and should be discarded, not refrigerated; formula is a good medium for bacterial growth.**
4. Water from a municipal water supply is controlled by drinking water regulations and is safe for use with formula.

♦ **Test-taking Tip:** *Of the options, consider which has the greatest potential to make the formula unsafe.*

Content Area: Childbearing; Concept: Nursing Roles; Safety; Pregnancy; Integrated Processes: Nursing Process: Evaluation; Client Needs: Physiological Integrity: Basic Care and Comfort; Safe and Effective Care Environment: Safety and Infection Control; Cognitive Level: Evaluation [Evaluating]

## 905. ANSWER: 1

1. **This statement indicates the mother's understanding. A 3-day-old infant should produce at least three wet diapers. After 5 days of age, the newborn should produce six well-saturated diapers per day.**
2. Infants typically produce at least 3 to 4 stools per day, and it is not uncommon for a breastfed infant to have 10 stools per day for the first month of life.
3. It is expected that newborns, especially breastfed newborns, will lose from 5% to 10% of their birth weight during the first week after birth; therefore the mother should not expect an 8-ounce weight gain.
4. During a normal feeding session, the infant will nurse 10 to 20 minutes on the first breast, with feeding time on the second breast varying.

♦ **Test-taking Tip:** *Infants have a characteristic amount of output for their age if they are receiving sufficient intake.*

Content Area: Childbearing; Concept: Nutrition; Pregnancy; Integrated Processes: Nursing Process: Evaluation; Client Needs: Physiological Integrity: Basic Care and Comfort; Cognitive Level: Evaluation [Evaluating]

## 906. ANSWER: 4

1. The use of ice in preterm infants is contraindicated, as it may cause damage to their fragile skin and result in hypothermia.
2. A heel warmer may be used to improve blood flow to the extremity for easier and quicker collection of the specimen, but it does not alleviate pain.
3. Morphine sulfate is a potent opioid analgesic and is inappropriate for this procedure.
4. **Sucrose activates the endogenous opioid system through taste. It is given 2 minutes prior to a painful procedure and has an analgesic effect lasting about 3 to 5 minutes.**

▶ *Test-taking Tip: You should eliminate options that would be unsafe for a preterm infant and then one that does not provide pain relief but may make the heel stick easier.*

Content Area: Childbearing; Concept: Comfort; Pregnancy; Integrated Processes: Nursing Process: Implementation; Client Needs: Physiological Integrity: Reduction of Risk Potential; Cognitive Level: Application [Applying]

## 907. ANSWER: 1, 2, 3, 4

1. **Classic dysmorphic facial features such as a broad nasal bridge and flat midface are associated with FAS due to the effects of alcohol on the developing fetus.**
2. **Growth deficiency is associated with FAS due to the deprivation of nutrients needed for growth.**
3. **Various nervous system abnormalities including irritability and hypotonia are associated with FAS due to the effects of alcohol on the developing fetus.**
4. **Poor feeding and persistent vomiting are associated with FAS due to facial abnormalities and problems with digestion.**
5. With FAS, the infant's jaw may be abnormally small and the maxilla hypoplastic (under- and not overdeveloped).

▶ *Test-taking Tip: The infant with FAS may be underdeveloped and have abnormal structural development, CNS dysfunction, and classic dysmorphic facial features.*

Content Area: Childbearing; Concept: Development; Assessment; Pregnancy; Integrated Processes: Nursing Process: Assessment; Client Needs: Physiological Integrity: Physiological Adaptation; Cognitive Level: Application [Applying]

## 908. ANSWER: 3

1. If the infant's blood type is O positive, no ABO incompatibility will occur because there is no antigen on the RBCs and the plasma has A and B antibodies.
2. If the infant's blood type is O negative, no ABO incompatibility will occur because there is no antigen on the RBCs and the plasma has A and B antibodies.
3. **The nurse should assess for ABO incompatibility when the infant's blood type is A negative. The mother's type O blood has no antigens on the RBCs, whereas the infant has A antigens.**
4. ABO incompatibility is limited to mothers with O blood type who have infants with type A or B. The mother's O blood type has no RBC antigens, and the plasma has A and B antibodies. The plasma of the infant with A blood type will have only B antibodies, and the plasma of the infant with B blood type will have only A antibodies.

▶ *Test-taking Tip: If a mother is O negative, consider the absent RBC antigens and the presence of antibodies. Options 1 and 2 are opposites, so one or both of these can be eliminated as incorrect.*

Content Area: Childbearing; Concept: Assessment; Pregnancy; Integrated Processes: Nursing Process: Assessment; Client Needs: Physiological Integrity: Physiological Adaptation; Cognitive Level: Knowledge [Remembering]

## 909. ANSWER: 4

1. The preterm infant's posture is characterized by very little, if any, flexion of extremities.
2. The sucking and swallowing reflexes are absent in the infant younger than 33 weeks' gestation.
3. Lanugo is usually extensive in a 31-week infant, covering the back, forearms, forehead, and sides of the face.
4. **The preterm infant, 24 to 36 weeks' gestation, typically is covered with vernix caseosa—a waxy, white substance secreted by the fetus's sebaceous glands in utero.**

▶ *Test-taking Tip: At 31 weeks' gestation, the newborn is preterm. Think about how the physical characteristics of infants change as their gestational age progresses.*

Content Area: Childbearing; Concept: Development; Assessment; Pregnancy; Integrated Processes: Nursing Process: Analysis; Client Needs: Health Promotion and Maintenance; Physiological Integrity: Reduction of Risk Potential; Cognitive Level: Application [Applying]

## 910. ANSWER: 40

**If a dry diaper weighs 15 g, subtract that weight from the weight of each of the infant's diapers: 30 g – 15 g = 15 g; 24 g – 15 g = 9 g; 21 g – 15 g = 6 g; 25 g – 15 g = 10 g. Then add all of the totals: 15 g + 9 g + 6 g + 10 g = 40 g of fluid loss, which equals 40 mL of urine output.**

▶ *Test-taking Tip: One milliliter of urine output equals 1 gram.*

Content Area: Childbearing; Concept: Urinary Elimination; Pregnancy; Integrated Processes: Communication and Documentation; Client Needs: Physiological Integrity: Basic Care and Comfort; Cognitive Level: Application [Applying]

## 911. ANSWER: 4, 1, 6, 3, 5, 2, 7

4. **Position the infant on the right side. This decreases the risk of aspiration should emesis occurs.**
1. **Separate the barrel of the syringe from the plunger and connect the syringe barrel to the feeding tube. This allows the feeding to flow via gravity.**
6. **Crimp the feeding tube and pour the specified amount of formula or breast milk into the barrel. This prevents inadvertent flow of the feeding before the total amount is in the syringe barrel.**
3. **Elevate the syringe 6 to 8 inches over the infant's head. This allows for a slow gravity flow.**
5. **Uncrimp the tubing and allow the feeding to flow by gravity at a slow rate.**
2. **Remove the syringe and clear the tubing with 2 to 3 mL of air to make sure all the feeding is in the infant's stomach.**

7. **Cap the lavage feeding tube. Capping prevents contamination.**

▶ *Test-taking Tip: Visualize the step-by-step process that would be needed to administer a bolus feeding through a feeding tube before placing items in the correct sequence. Often selecting the first and last items makes it easier to place the remaining items in the correct sequence.*

**Content Area:** Childbearing; **Concept:** Nursing Roles; Pregnancy; **Integrated Processes:** Nursing Process: Implementation; **Client Needs:** Physiological Integrity: Basic Care and Comfort; **Cognitive Level:** Synthesis [Creating]

## 912. ANSWER: 3

1. Falling asleep after eating is a sign of feeding satisfaction.
2. Increasing gastric residual is a sign of feeding intolerance. No residual present prior to feeding indicates that the previous feeding has passed from the stomach into the intestines.
3. **Signs of feeding intolerance in preterm infants include increasing abdominal girth and abdominal distention. Feeding intolerance may indicate paralytic ileus or NEC.**
4. Soft, loose stools are expected in newborns.

▶ *Test-taking Tip: Be sure to read the stem correctly, noting "intolerance" and not reading it as "tolerance."*

**Content Area:** Childbearing; **Concept:** Nutrition; Pregnancy; **Integrated Processes:** Nursing Process: Evaluation; **Client Needs:** Physiological Integrity: Basic Care and Comfort; Physiological Integrity: Physiological Adaptation; **Cognitive Level:** Evaluation [Evaluating]

## 913. ANSWER: 2

1. Illustration 1 shows the newborn wearing a long-sleeved undershirt with hand covers. The hand covers help protect newborns' nails from scratching their sensitive skin.
2. **Illustration 2 shows swaddling. Swaddling is wrapping the blanket snugly around the newborn's body. This provides warmth and a sense of security for the newborn, which can have a calming effect.**
3. Illustration 3 shows the newborn being touched. Although touching is important for calming and providing comfort, it is not swaddling.
4. Illustration 4 shows the mother breastfeeding her newborn. Although the newborn is held snuggly against the mother's body with the blanket over the newborn's body, it is not swaddling.

▶ *Test-taking Tip: A blanket is folded in a particular way to swaddle the newborn.*

**Content Area:** Childbearing; **Concept:** Pregnancy; Nursing Roles; **Integrated Processes:** Nursing Process: Evaluation; **Client Needs:** Physiological Integrity: Basic Care and Comfort; **Cognitive Level:** Evaluation [Evaluating]

## 914. PHARM ANSWER: 2

1. Giving surfactant will prevent alveolar collapse and allow the exchange of gases and thus will cause a decrease, not an increase, in $Paco_2$.
2. **Surfactant replacement therapy decreases alveolar collapse that occurs with RDS and thus decreases the severity of RDS.**
3. Giving surfactant will prevent alveolar collapse and allow the exchange of gases and thus will cause an increase, not a decrease, in $Pao_2$.
4. Pleural effusion does not occur in RDS.

▶ *Test-taking Tip: RDS results from a primary absence, a deficiency, or an alteration in the production of pulmonary surfactant. Lack of surfactant in the preterm infant causes decreased lung compliance, resulting in increased inspiratory pressure needed to expand the alveoli and lungs with air. Increasing $Paco_2$ and decreasing $Pao_2$ would indicate increasing respiratory distress and would not be desired.*

**Content Area:** Childbearing; **Concept:** Oxygenation; Pregnancy; Medication; **Integrated Processes:** Nursing Process: Implementation; **Client Needs:** Physiological Integrity: Pharmacological and Parenteral Therapies; **Cognitive Level:** Analysis [Analyzing]

## 915. ANSWER: 4

1. While checking blood glucose levels is important, it will not assist in maximizing respiratory status.
2. All inspired gases should be warmed and humidified, as cold air or oxygen stimulates increased oxygen consumption by increasing the metabolic rate.
3. Infants should be weighed daily to monitor for fluid imbalances, which may adversely affect respiratory status.
4. **The prone position allows for better oxygenation of collapsed alveoli. Because the prone position is associated with sudden infant death, infants placed in this position should have continuous cardiorespiratory monitoring.**

▶ *Test-taking Tip: You should narrow the options to only those associated with respiratory status.*

**Content Area:** Childbearing; **Concept:** Oxygenation; Pregnancy; **Integrated Processes:** Nursing Process: Implementation; **Client Needs:** Physiological Integrity: Physiological Adaptation; **Cognitive Level:** Application [Applying]

## 916. ANSWER: 1

1. **The infant can be infected with GBS from the mother and may start to exhibit symptoms within the first 12 to 24 hours after birth. Temperature instability is one of the most common early symptoms.**
2. Pink stains in the diaper are caused by urates in the urine and are innocuous.
3. Meconium stools are expected within the first 24 hours after birth.
4. Erythema toxicum is a rash that is common to newborns and will disappear without treatment.

♦ **Test-taking Tip:** *GBS is a bacterial infection found in the mother's urogenital tract. It can be transmitted to the fetus during childbirth if the mother has the infection. The risk of infection is increased if the membranes are ruptured for more than 12 hours before birth occurs and if the mother is not given antibiotics during labor. Only one option is a symptom associated with an infection.*

**Content Area:** Childbearing; **Concept:** Infection; Pregnancy; **Integrated Processes:** Nursing Process: Planning; **Client Needs:** Physiological Integrity: Physiological Adaptation; **Cognitive Level:** Analysis [Analyzing]

### 917. PHARM ANSWER: 1, 3, 4, 6

1. **The nurse should verify that the catheter is secure and still at the prescribed, documented centimeter marking by examining the position of the centimeter marking on the catheter and comparing it to the mark recorded when the catheter was placed.**
2. The catheter should be positioned away from the infant's extremities to prevent the infant from accidentally dislocating or removing the catheter by toe or finger entrapment.
3. **After placement of a UAC, the nurse should perform abdominal assessments to monitor for intra-abdominal blood loss that may occur if an umbilical vessel becomes perforated.**
4. **At least every 2 to 4 hours, the nurse should systematically evaluate perfusion to the distal extremities. This includes examining the legs for color, temperature, and capillary refill, as well as assessing the extremity pulses.**
5. Frequent manipulation of the catheter is a contributing factor in catheter-related bloodstream infection; therefore manipulation of the catheter should be avoided unless necessary for medical procedures and assessments.
6. **Caregivers should monitor blood glucose levels and compare them to the amount of glucose the infant may be receiving. Abnormal values, especially hypoglycemia, may indicate that the catheter is out of position.**

♦ **Test-taking Tip:** *You should eliminate options that could increase catheter manipulation.*

**Content Area:** Childbearing; **Concept:** Nursing Roles; Pregnancy; **Integrated Processes:** Nursing Process: Planning; **Client Needs:** Physiological Integrity: Pharmacological and Parenteral Therapies; **Cognitive Level:** Application [Applying]

### 918. MoC ANSWER: 1

1. **The nurse should first check the infant's blood sugar level. SGA infants are at risk for hypoglycemia because they have poor hepatic glycogen stores and inadequate supplies of enzymes to activate gluconeogenesis.**
2. The nurse should recognize that these symptoms in an SGA infant necessitate action rather than just documentation.

3. The nurse should check the infant's blood glucose level first and then notify the HCP if the level is abnormal.
4. Assessing the infant's temperature should be completed, as a low temperature could contribute to hypoglycemia; however, this is not the first action.

♦ **Test-taking Tip:** *Symptoms of hypoglycemia in an SGA infant include tremors, high-pitched or weak cry, and exaggerated Moro reflex.*

**Content Area:** Childbearing; **Concept:** Metabolism; Pregnancy; Management; **Integrated Processes:** Nursing Process: Analysis; **Client Needs:** Safe and Effective Care Environment: Management of Care; Physiological Integrity: Reduction of Risk Potential; **Cognitive Level:** Analysis [Analyzing]

### 919. ANSWER: 1

1. **As a side effect of phototherapy, some newborns develop a transient maculopapular rash that does not require treatment. The only action required is to document the findings.**
2. There is no need to call the HCP because the rash does not require treatment.
3. There is no need to discontinue phototherapy; it is a transient rash.
4. Newborn temperatures should be monitored per agency standards when the infant is being treated with phototherapy.

♦ **Test-taking Tip:** *Some side effects of phototherapy do not require intervention.*

**Content Area:** Childbearing; **Concept:** Assessment; Pregnancy; Critical Thinking; **Integrated Processes:** Nursing Process: Implementation; **Client Needs:** Physiological Integrity: Basic Care and Comfort; **Cognitive Level:** Application [Applying]

### 920. ANSWER: 4

1. Phototherapy has no direct impact on sodium absorption.
2. Phototherapy is an intervention that breaks bilirubin down to be excreted in the stool.
3. The nurse should monitor the infant's I&O, but phototherapy by itself has no direct impact on urinary output.
4. **Insensible water losses (IWL) are significantly increased in infants who are treated with phototherapy. Additional water losses may occur with increased stooling associated with either the elimination of bilirubin or a temporary lactose intolerance resulting from exposure to phototherapy.**

♦ **Test-taking Tip:** *You should look for similar terms in the stem of the question and the options. Note that dehydration and loss are similar.*

**Content Area:** Childbearing; **Concept:** Fluid and Electrolyte Balance; Pregnancy; **Integrated Processes:** Nursing Process: Analysis; **Client Needs:** Physiological Integrity: Basic Care and Comfort; **Cognitive Level:** Application [Applying]

**921. ANSWER: 3**

1. The PKU test results will not be as accurate if the test is performed at 1 month because it is after the recommended time period.
2. If parents leave the hospital before their infant is 24 hours old, they are required to obtain the test within the first week after discharge; it cannot be completed now regardless whether the parents sign a consent form.
3. **The PKU test should be performed after 24 hours of life and before the infant is 7 days old. This allows for sufficient intake of protein for accurate results.**
4. The PKU test is needed even if the infant is tolerating feedings; it is part of mandatory newborn screening.

♦ *Test-taking Tip: Infants with PKU lack the ability to convert the amino acid phenylalanine to tyrosine. Phenylalanine accumulates in the blood and leads to progressive intellectual disability. Options 1 and 2 contain the absolute word "must." Usually options with absolute words are incorrect; thus eliminate these options. PKU testing is mandatory, thus eliminating Option 4.*

Content Area: Childbearing; Concept: Pregnancy; Safety; Integrated Processes: Nursing Process: Planning; Client Needs: Physiological Integrity: Reduction of Risk Potential; Cognitive Level: Application [Applying]

**922. ANSWER: 4**

1. Trisomy 13, or Patau syndrome, is a chromosomal condition associated with severe intellectual disability and physical abnormalities, but the abnormalities do not include a transverse palmar crease.
2. Turner syndrome is a chromosomal condition that affects development in females. A common feature is short stature. An infant with Turner's syndrome would not have a transverse palmar crease.
3. Trisomy 18, or Edwards's syndrome, is a chromosomal condition associated with multiple abnormalities and organ defects. The infant might have clenched fists with overlapping fingers, but the infant would not have a transverse palmar crease.
4. **A transverse palmar crease, also called a simian line, is a sign of trisomy 21 or Down's syndrome. The nurse should further assess for signs of Down's syndrome.**

♦ *Test-taking Tip: An infant with Down's syndrome will have a transverse palmar crease.*

Content Area: Childbearing; Concept: Assessment; Pregnancy; Integrated Processes: Nursing Process: Assessment; Client Needs: Physiological Integrity: Physiological Adaptation; Cognitive Level: Application [Applying]

**923. ANSWER: 1**

1. **A bulging anterior fontanel is an initial sign of congenital hydrocephalus.**
2. The head and chest circumferences of the full-term newborn should be very close to the same size, within 2 to 3 cm.
3. The posterior fontanel is normally smaller than the anterior fontanel, and molding may make it very narrow.
4. Low-set ears are a sign of trisomy 21.

♦ *Test-taking Tip: Hydrocephalus is an enlargement in the ventricles of the brain. Only one option is associated with enlargement.*

Content Area: Childbearing; Concept: Assessment; Pregnancy; Integrated Processes: Nursing Process: Assessment; Client Needs: Physiological Integrity: Physiological Adaptation; Cognitive Level: Application [Applying]

**924. ANSWER: 2**

1. Surgery will not repair anencephaly.
2. **Anencephaly is the absence of both cerebral hemispheres and of the overlying skull. It is a condition that is incompatible with life.**
3. Shunting will not repair anencephaly.
4. Antibiotics will not repair anencephaly.

♦ *Test-taking Tip: Three options address treatment, and one option is different. Often the option that is different is the answer.*

Content Area: Childbearing; Concept: Nursing Roles; Pregnancy; Integrated Processes: Nursing Process: Planning; Caring; Client Needs: Physiological Integrity: Physiological Adaptation; Cognitive Level: Application [Applying]

**925. ANSWER: 1**

1. **A cephalohematoma is the collection of blood between a skull bone and its periosteum. As the hematoma resolves, hemolysis of RBCs occurs, and jaundice may result. A cephalohematoma will resolve without treatment by 3 to 6 weeks.**
2. Difficulty feeding is not associated with a cephalohematoma.
3. With a cephalohematoma, bleeding stops spontaneously a few days after birth. Usually rebleeding does not recur, and there is no need for the parents to observe for paleness.
4. The hematoma does not bulge when the infant cries. The bleeding occurs from injury during the birth process, and all bleeding should stop by the second or third day after birth.

♦ *Test-taking Tip: A cephalohematoma is the collection of blood (hematoma) on the head (cephal). Consider what occurs with the breakdown of RBCs.*

Content Area: Childbearing; Concept: Neurologic Regulation; Pregnancy; Integrated Processes: Teaching/Learning; Client Needs: Physiological Integrity: Reduction of Risk Potential; Cognitive Level: Analysis [Analyzing]

## Chapter Twenty-Two

# Pharmacological and Parenteral Therapies During Childbearing

**926.** **PHARM** The nurse is assessing the female client who is taking clomiphene. Which finding should indicate to the nurse that the client is experiencing an adverse effect of the medication?

1. Pelvic pain
2. Nipple discharge
3. Weight gain
4. Watery diarrhea

**927.** **PHARM** The client who is 5 weeks pregnant asks the nurse for information about mifepristone use for medical abortion. Which statements, if made by the nurse, are accurate? **Select all that apply.**

1. "It must be taken immediately after your last menstrual cycle to be effective."
2. "It will block the action of progesterone on the uterus so that the fetus is aborted."
3. "Mifepristone must be followed up with a vaginal douche of vinegar and water."
4. "The success rate is very high, especially if taken within 42 days of conception."
5. "Mifepristone is given intravenously (IV) in the HCP's office."
6. "Many develop a transient temperature elevation after taking mifepristone."

**928.** **PHARM** The client has hyperemesis gravidarum. Which agents, if prescribed, should the nurse question? **Select all that apply.**

1. Pyridoxine (vitamin B₆) 50 mg oral daily
2. Promethazine 12.5 mg IV q4h
3. Dimenhydrinate 50 mg oral q4–6 h prn
4. Metoclopramide 100 mg IM q8h
5. Ginger capsule 1 g oral daily
6. Prochlorperazine 30 mg oral daily

**929.** **PHARM** The postpartum client with worsening HELLP syndrome (**h**emolysis, **e**levated **l**iver enzymes, and **l**ow **p**latelet count) is to receive platelets. The nurse reviews the client's laboratory results. Place an X next to each value that suggests HELLP syndrome.

| Serum Laboratory Test and Normal Values | Client's Value |
|---|---|
| Platelets (150,000–450,000/mm³) | 90,000 |
| Potassium (K) (3.5–5.5 mEq/L) | 3.4 mEq/L |
| RBC (4–6 m/mm³) | 2.9 |
| WBC (4500–11,000/mm³) | 12,000 |
| Albumin (3.2–4.6 gm/dL) | 2.8 |
| AST (15–40 units/L) | 65 |
| ALT (10–40 units/L) | 60 |
| ALP (35–142 units/L) | 160 |
| Total bilirubin (0.2–1.3 mg/dL) | 3.8 |

**930.** **PHARM** During a walk-in-clinic visit to receive vaccinations, the client states, "I think I may be pregnant." Which vaccine, if needed, should the nurse plan to give?

1. Rubella
2. Varicella
3. Hepatitis B
4. Mumps

**931.** PHARM The pregnant client who is prescribed supplemental vitamin D during pregnancy asks the nurse why vitamin D is so important. Which responses by the nurse are correct? **Select all that apply.**

1. "Almost 50% of pregnant women lack sufficient vitamin D levels during late pregnancy."
2. "A low level of vitamin D is associated with reduced bone-mineral accumulation during your child's growing years."
3. "A low level of vitamin D may predispose you to premature rupture of your membranes."
4. "A low level of vitamin D causes a breakdown of cervical collagen, causing early cervical dilation."
5. "Vitamin D supplements taken during pregnancy may reduce your child's risk for osteoporosis-related fractures."

**932.** PHARM The nurse is assessing a newly pregnant client. Which finding indicates that the client may need iron supplementation?

1. Gave birth a year ago
2. Over 35 years of age
3. First pregnancy
4. Primary infertility

**933.** PHARM The pregnant client presents to a clinic with a white, cottage cheese–like vaginal discharge, itching, and vulvar redness. The nurse should plan to teach about which correctly prescribed medication?

1. Metronidazole 250 mg orally bid for 1 week
2. Butoconazole vaginal cream once at bedtime
3. Imidazole vaginal cream daily for 1 week
4. Fluconazole 150 mg by mouth once

**934.** PHARM Benazepril is added to the antihypertensive medication regimen of an African American client who is 30 weeks pregnant. Which nursing intervention is **most** important?

1. Withhold the benazepril and contact the HCP.
2. Monitor for a diminished effect in lowering her BP.
3. Notify the HCP if the serum bilirubin level increases.
4. Notify the HCP if the serum potassium level increases.

**935.** PHARM The client, who is 8 weeks pregnant, tells the nurse that she wants to try an herbal remedy for treating her nausea. Which herb should the nurse suggest?

1. Ginger
2. Milk thistle
3. Black cohosh
4. Echinacea

**936.** PHARM The client who is 28 weeks pregnant and experiencing heartburn is prescribed to take omeprazole. In teaching the client, the nurse should explain that omeprazole reduces heartburn by which action?

1. Blocks the action of the enzyme that generates gastric acid
2. Blocks the $H_2$ receptor located on the parietal cells of the stomach
3. Neutralizes the gastric acid in the stomach
4. Coats the upper stomach and esophagus to decrease irritation from stomach acid

**937.** MoC PHARM The nurse receives medication orders for the client who is 28 weeks pregnant and experiencing CHF. Which medication should be clarified with the HCP before administration?

1. Furosemide 40 mg IV bid
2. Captopril 25 mg PO daily
3. Digoxin 0.125 mg IV daily
4. Metoprolol SR 50 mg PO daily

**938.** PHARM The pregnant client with HIV is receiving highly active antiretroviral therapy (HAART). The nurse should monitor the client for which potential pregnancy-related problems associated with HAART therapy? **Select all that apply.**

1. Preterm labor
2. Preeclampsia
3. Low birth weight
4. Gestational diabetes
5. Birth defects

**939.** MoC PHARM The nurse is checking the medical records of second-trimester clients for newly prescribed medications. Which prescription requires the nurse to contact the HCP?

1. Methyldopa 250 mg bid by mouth for elevated BP
2. $MgSO_4$ 5 g IM for BP >160/90 mm Hg × 2 readings
3. Terbutaline 5 mg q6h by mouth for preterm labor
4. Prenatal vitamins one tablet daily by mouth

**940.** PHARM The breastfeeding postpartum client is reporting afterpains and requests pain medication. Which medication is **best** for the nurse to select to prevent adverse effects on her breastfeeding infant?

1. Meperidine
2. Naproxen
3. Ibuprofen
4. Acetaminophen

**941.** **PHARM** The 28-year-old client at 28 weeks gestation presents with uterine contractions every 2 to 3 minutes. Which medications should the nurse prepare to administer for preterm labor? **Select all that apply.**

1. Terbutaline
2. Nifedipine
3. Magnesium sulfate
4. Atenolol
5. Oxytocin

**942.** **PHARM** The client, at 25.2 weeks' gestation in preterm labor, is given nifedipine and then magnesium sulfate to stop her contractions. When assessing the client, which findings indicate that she is experiencing an adverse effect from the magnesium sulfate? **Select all that apply.**

1. Shortness of breath
2. Flushing
3. Hypertension
4. Hyporeflexia
5. Insomnia

**943.** **PHARM** The nurse is caring for the client who is receiving magnesium sulfate IV to treat severe preeclampsia. When reviewing the client's serum magnesium levels, which value should the nurse conclude is therapeutic?

1. 0.5 mg/dL
2. 2 mg/dL
3. 6 mg/dL
4. 10.1 mg/dL

**944.** **PHARM** The client with severe preeclampsia has been receiving IV magnesium sulfate for 24 hours. Which nursing assessment finding indicates that the medication has been effective in treating preeclampsia?

1. An increase in BP
2. An increase in urine output
3. A decrease in platelet count
4. An increase in hematocrit

**945.** **PHARM** Prior to assisting with an external cephalic version on the client who is 38 weeks' gestation, the nurse is preparing to administer terbutaline sulfate subcutaneously. Which explanation should the nurse provide about terbutaline?

1. "Terbutaline will decrease uterine sensation."
2. "Terbutaline will relax your uterus."
3. "Terbutaline will cause you to feel sleepy."
4. "Terbutaline will stimulate labor contractions."

**946.** **PHARM** The client is to receive vaginal dinoprostone for cervical ripening. At which location should the nurse place the medication for correct administration?

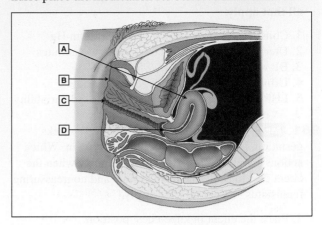

1. A
2. B
3. C
4. D

**947.** **PHARM** Four inpatient clients are prescribed dinoprostone for cervical ripening. The nurse should question the order for which client?

1. Client A, G1P0000, who is 41 weeks' gestation
2. Client B, G5P4004, who is at 40 and 4/7 weeks' gestation
3. Client C, G1P0000, type 1 diabetic who is 38 weeks' gestation and has fetal macrosomia
4. Client D, G2P1001, at 40 weeks' gestation delivering vaginally after a previous cesarean birth

**948.** **PHARM** The client who is at 40 weeks' gestation is prescribed misoprostol 25 mcg per vagina one time. Which question is **most** important for the nurse to ask this client before administering misoprostol?

1. At what time did you eat your breakfast?
2. Have you had a previous cesarean birth?
3. When did you last request an analgesic?
4. Have you emptied your bladder recently?

**949.** **PHARM** The nurse is caring for the postpartum client. Which assessment finding should prompt the nurse to conclude that the administration of carboprost tromethamine has been effective?

1. Reduction of fever
2. Stable BP
3. Increased comfort
4. Decreased lochia rubra

**950.** MoC PHARM The client is receiving IV oxytocin for labor induction. Which findings require the nurse to discontinue the IV infusion and notify the HCP? **Select all that apply.**

1. Consistent uterine resting tone of 18 mm Hg
2. Uterine contractions occurring every 4 minutes
3. BP was 100/60, now 130/85 mm Hg
4. Urine output of 60 mL for the past 2 hours
5. FHR 88 beats per minute with decreased variability

**951.** MoC PHARM The client, who is 40 weeks' gestation, is being induced with IV oxytocin. Which actions should the nurse take immediately when the client develops uterine tachysystole and nonreassuring fetal status? **Select all that apply.**

1. Place the client in knee-chest position.
2. Administer an intravenous fluid bolus.
3. Apply oxygen at 10 liters via facemask.
4. Stop the infusion of oxytocin promptly.
5. Notify the HCP regarding the client's status.

**952.** MoC PHARM While adding oxytocin to a solution bag, a 30-year-old nonpregnant female nurse pokes herself and injects oxytocin into her finger. When being seen in the agency's health service, which treatment should the nurse expect in addition to the care of the clean needlestick injury?

1. Subcutaneous terbutaline to relax her uterus
2. Ibuprofen for uterine cramping
3. No additional treatment measures
4. Teaching to limit free water intake for 24 hours

**953.** PHARM The client at 41 weeks' gestation is having labor induced by IV oxytocin. The nurse titrates the oxytocin to a rate of 4 milliunit/minute (mU/min). The oxytocin solution is labeled 10 units in 1000 mL of $D_5W$. At what rate, in mL per hour, is the IV pump currently programmed?

_____ mL/hr (Record your answer as a whole number.)

**954.** PHARM The nurse admits four clients to the labor and delivery unit. To which client should the nurse prepare to administer zolpidem tartrate?

1. The 40-week G2P1001 client; scheduled for a repeat cesarean section now
2. The 39-week G3P1102 client; 5 cm dilated, 80% effaced; contractions every 3 minutes
3. The 41-week G4P1112 client; admitted for induction of labor
4. The 40-week G1P0000 client; 1 cm dilated, 20% effaced; poor-quality uterine contractions

**955.** PHARM The pregnant client received a dinoprostone insert. The nurse determines that the client had the desired therapeutic response when obtaining which assessment finding?

1. Deep tendon reflexes of 2+
2. FHR of 130 beats per minute
3. Uterine contractions every 4 minutes
4. BP of 120/80 mm Hg

**956.** PHARM The laboring client is receiving bupivacaine per epidural route for analgesia. The nurse should closely monitor the client for which adverse effects of bupivacaine? **Select all that apply.**

1. Hypotension
2. Elevated temperature
3. Nausea
4. Urinary retention
5. Sedation

**957.** PHARM The laboring client is to receive nalbuphine hydrochloride 20 mg IM. Nalbuphine hydrochloride 10 mg/mL is available. The nurse should plan to administer how many milliliters?

_____ mL (Record your answer as a whole number.)

**958.** PHARM While the nurse is assessing the client in labor at 38 weeks' gestation, the client asks for pain medication. At which stage is it **most** appropriate for the nurse to administer narcotic analgesics?

1. Stage 1, first phase
2. Stage 1, second phase
3. Throughout Stage 2
4. Throughout Stage 3

**959.** PHARM MoC The client at 41 weeks' gestation has IV oxytocin infusing to induce labor. Prioritize the steps that the nurse should take when an indeterminate or abnormal FHR pattern is assessed.

1. Change the maternal position to lateral.
2. Administer fluid bolus of 500 mL lactated Ringer's solution.
3. Discontinue the oxytocin infusion.
4. Administer oxygen at 10 L/min via facemask.
5. Document the event and maternal/fetal response.
6. Notify the HCP.

Answer: _____

**960.** **PHARM** Prior to delivery, the client had prolonged rupture of her membranes. Since delivery 48 hours ago, she has been receiving IV cefotaxime. Which outcome is the **most** important for the nurse to establish?

1. Moderate amount of lochia rubra
2. Absence of high fever
3. Voiding in good quantities
4. Large, soft bowel movement

**961.** **PHARM** The HCP is preparing to administer sterile water injections to decrease the laboring client's back pain. The nurse would prepare the client to receive the injections by which administration route?

1. Intravenously into the lactated Ringer's solution
2. Subcutaneously into the tissue on her abdomen
3. Intradermally into her lower lumbar-sacral area
4. Intramuscularly into her posterior dorsal-gluteal muscle

**962.** **PHARM** The client, in labor at 39 weeks' gestation, is receiving epidural anesthesia. Which assessment findings require the nurse to intervene immediately because the client may be showing signs of IV injection?

1. Nausea and increased alertness
2. Irritability and hypotension
3. Tinnitus and a metallic taste
4. Headache and loss of hearing

**963.** **PHARM** The postpartum client, who just delivered a full-term infant, tells the nurse she is concerned about her Rh-negative status. She says that she received Rho(D) immune globulin (RhoGAM) during her pregnancy, and she wonders if she is going to need it again. Which statement, if made by the nurse, is correct?

1. "You will be given RhoGAM within the next 72 hours."
2. "You already had RhoGAM, so you won't need it again."
3. "One dose of RhoGAM will last you for your lifetime."
4. "You will need RhoGAM if your newborn is Rh-positive."

**964.** **PHARM** The nurse is caring for the client who is 1 hour postpartum. Which vital sign should the nurse check before administering methylergonovine IM?

1. Oral temperature
2. Respiratory rate
3. Apical heart rate
4. Blood pressure

**965.** **PHARM** The client who is 4 hours postpartum reports excessive bright red lochia rubra. Which medication, if prescribed, should the nurse plan to administer?

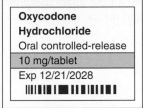

1.

| Ferrous Sulfate |
| Oral Tablet |
| 325 mg/tablet |
| Exp 12/21/2028 |

2.

| Methylergonovine Maleate Injection |
| For IV use only |
| 0.2 mg/1 mL |
| Exp 11/26/2028 |

3.

| Oxycodone Hydrochloride |
| Oral controlled-release |
| 10 mg/tablet |
| Exp 12/21/2028 |

4.

| Terbutaline Sulfate Subcutaneous Injection |
| 1 mg/1 mL |
| Exp 12/21/2028 |

**966.** **PHARM** The postpartum client experiencing uterine atony is to receive carboprost tromethamine. Due to the medication side effects, what should the nurse plan to give to the client?

1. A sedative
2. A stool softener
3. An antiemetic
4. Extra oral fluids

**967.** **PHARM** The client who is 2 days post–cesarean birth has all of following prn prescribed medications. Which medication should the nurse administer when the client reports painful ulcerations on the perineum?

1. Ritonavir
2. Zidovudine
3. Acyclovir
4. Lamivudine

**968.** **PHARM** The infant's mother tested positive for hepatitis B surface antigen. The nurse is preparing to administer the hepatitis B vaccine to the infant. To prevent infection, which medication should the nurse administer along with the hepatitis B vaccine?

1. Acyclovir
2. Ceftriaxone
3. Acetaminophen
4. Immune serum globulin (ISG)

**969.** PHARM The nurse in a large urban hospital is admitting a 2-hour-old infant whose mother is positive for HIV. The infant is to receive zidovudine. Which laboratory tests should the nurse analyze before administering the zidovudine?

1. Complete blood count (CBC) with differential and prothrombin time (PT)
2. Cluster of differentiation 4 (CD4) count, CBC, and lactate
3. CBC with differential and alanine aminotransferase (ALT)
4. CBC, CD4 count, ALT, and serum protein

**970.** PHARM The nurse is caring for the infant diagnosed with PDA. By which route should the nurse expect to administer indomethacin?

1. Intravenously (IV)
2. Orally
3. Rectally
4. Intramuscularly (IM)

**971.** PHARM The infant of a diabetic mother is receiving D10/0.2 NS IV through a peripheral vein to manage blood glucose levels. After examining the infant, the HCP tells the nurse to change the solution to D12.5/0.2 NS. Which action by the nurse is **most** important?

1. Telephone the pharmacy to get the newly prescribed IV solution.
2. Check a blood glucose level before starting the new solution.
3. Discuss the situation immediately with the HCP.
4. Increase the IV rate until the new bag is obtained from the pharmacy.

**972.** PHARM A 6-day-old infant is to receive nystatin to treat adherent white patches on the tongue, palate, and inner aspect of the cheeks. Which **most** important information should the nurse teach the parent about nystatin?

1. Look in the infant's mouth for signs of improvement.
2. Check the infant's skin for signs of contact dermatitis.
3. Have the infant "swish" nystatin before swallowing.
4. Adverse effects include nausea, vomiting, and diarrhea.

**973.** PHARM The nurse is caring for the infant who experienced asphyxiation at birth and is having seizure activity. The infant, weighing 4 kg, is to receive phenobarbital 4 mg/kg/day in divided doses q8h. To provide one dose, how many milligrams should the nurse administer?

_____ mg (Record your answer rounded to the nearest tenth.)

**974.** PHARM The nurse is caring for the newborn. Which assessment finding should the nurse expect after administering naloxone?

1. Decreased irritability
2. Meconium stool
3. Normal temperature
4. Improved respiratory effort

**975.** PHARM The newborn is prescribed to receive routine immunizations per written protocol. Which immunization should the nurse plan to give?

1. Mumps, measles, and rubella (MMR)
2. Influenza
3. Hepatitis B
4. Rotavirus

**976.** PHARM The nurse administers erythromycin ophthalmic solution to prevent ophthalmia neonatorum. Which actions should the nurse take after administration of the erythromycin? **Select all that apply.**

1. Gently massage the newborn's eyelids.
2. Immediately wipe away excess medication.
3. Clean the eyelids with a cotton swab and sterile water.
4. Provide comfort for the infant by swaddling.
5. Wait 1 minute to wipe excess medication.
6. Repeat the ophthalmic solution dose in 1 hour.

# Answers and Rationales

**926.** PHARM **ANSWER: 1**

1. **Pelvic pain may indicate ovarian enlargement from overstimulation of the ovary.**
2. Breast tenderness rather than nipple discharge may occur as an adverse effect of clomiphene.
3. Weight gain is not associated with the use of clomiphene.
4. Watery diarrhea is not associated with the use of clomiphene.

▶ *Test-taking Tip: Clomiphene (Clomid) is used in the treatment of infertility. It is an ovulation inducer that may lead to ovarian overstimulation and enlargement. The weight and size of the enlarged ovary may cause tissue displacement and partial torsion of the ovary. Focus on an option that can be the result of tissue displacement and ovarian enlargement and torsion.*

Content Area: Childbearing; Concept: Medication; Female Reproduction; Pregnancy; Integrated Processes: Nursing Process: Analysis; Client Needs: Physiological Integrity: Pharmacological and Parenteral Therapies; Cognitive Level: Comprehension [Understanding]

**927.** PHARM **ANSWER: 2, 4**

1. Mifepristone does not need to be taken immediately after the last menstrual cycle; however, to achieve a success rate at or above 91%, it should be taken within 49 days of conception.
2. **Mifepristone (Mifeprex) blocks the uterine progesterone receptors in the uterus, thereby altering the endometrium and causing the detachment of the conceptus.**
3. Douching is not required for abortion to occur with mifepristone.
4. **The abortion success rate for mifepristone is 96% to 98% when taken within 42 days of conception.**
5. Mifepristone is given orally, not intravenously.
6. Temperature elevation is a sign of infection and should be reported immediately to the HCP.

▶ *Test-taking Tip: Because most women do not realize they are pregnant until they have missed a menstrual period, it would be impossible to take the medication immediately after a menstrual cycle, thus eliminate Option 1. Douching is rarely recommended for any medical reason, thus eliminate Option 3. Of the remaining options, think about the usual route of medication administration and about signs of adverse effects to eliminate other options.*

Content Area: Childbearing; Concept: Pregnancy; Medication; Integrated Processes: Teaching/Learning; Client Needs: Physiological Integrity: Pharmacological and Parenteral Therapies; Cognitive Level: Application [Applying]

**928.** PHARM **ANSWER: 4, 6**

1. Pyridoxine has antiemetic effects and is used for treating nausea and vomiting in pregnancy. Its dose, route, and frequency are within the recommended range.
2. Promethazine (Phenergan) has antiemetic effects and is used for treating nausea and vomiting in pregnancy. Its dose, route, and frequency are within the recommended range.
3. Dimenhydrinate (Dramamine) has antiemetic effects and is used for treating nausea and vomiting in pregnancy. Its dose, route, and frequency are within the recommended range.
4. **The dose of metoclopramide (Reglan) is 10 times the usual dose; it should be 10 mg and not 100 mg.**
5. Ginger has antiemetic effects and is used for treating nausea and vomiting in pregnancy. Its dose, route, and frequency are within the recommended range.
6. **Prochlorperazine (Compazine) is also a pregnancy Category C drug, indicating that its safety has not been established for use during pregnancy.**

▶ *Test-taking Tip: All agents listed are used to treat nausea and vomiting. Eliminate any option that exceeds the recommended dosage range or is a pregnancy Category C drug.*

Content Area: Childbearing; Concept: Pregnancy; Medication; Integrated Processes: Nursing Process: Implementation; Communication and Documentation; Client Needs: Physiological Integrity: Pharmacological and Parenteral Therapies; Safe and Effective Care Environment: Safety and Infection Control; Cognitive Level: Analysis [Analyzing]

## 929. PHARM ANSWER:

**Hemolysis (low RBCs), elevated liver enzymes (albumin, AST, ALT, ALP, and total bilirubin), and a low platelet count are hallmarks of HELLP syndrome. The cause of HELLP syndrome is a genetic disorder of fatty acid oxidation in the fetus of the pregnant woman. Some women may experience worsening HELLP syndrome over the first 48-hour postpartum period. Although the WBCs are elevated and the serum potassium low, these are not associated with HELLP syndrome.**

| Serum Laboratory Test and Normal Values | Client's Value | |
| --- | --- | --- |
| Platelets (Plt) (150,000–450,000/mm³) | 90,000 | X |
| Potassium (K) (3.5–5.5 mEq/L) | 3.4 | |
| RBC (4–6 m/mm³) | 2.9 | X |
| WBC (4500–11,000/mm³) | 12,000 | |
| Albumin (3.2–4.6 gm/dL) | 2.8 | X |
| AST (15–40 units/L) | 65 | X |
| ALT (10–40 units/L) | 60 | X |
| ALP (35–142 units/L) | 160 | X |
| Total bilirubin (0.2–1.3 mg/dL) | 3.8 | X |

♦ *Test-taking Tip: A memory cue for the liver enzymes is to associate these with AA. Four liver enzymes begin with the letter a, and one liver enzyme begins with the letter b (the letter b follows the letter a).*

Content Area: Childbearing; Concept: Medication; Pregnancy; Integrated Processes: Nursing Process: Analysis; Client Needs: Physiological Integrity: Pharmacological and Parenteral Therapies; Physiological Integrity: Physiological Adaptation; Cognitive Level: Analysis [Analyzing]

## 930. PHARM ANSWER: 3

1. Rubella should not be administered to pregnant women because it contains live virus, which is contraindicated during pregnancy.
2. Varicella should not be administered to pregnant women because it contains live virus, which is contraindicated during pregnancy.
3. **Hepatitis B vaccination can be safely administered during pregnancy because it is a synthetically prepared or DNA-recombinant vaccine. The vaccine is made of noninfectious material and cannot cause hepatitis B infection. Hepatitis B may spread to the fetus if the mother is infected in the third trimester.**

4. Mumps should not be administered to pregnant women because it contains live virus, which is contraindicated during pregnancy.

♦ *Test-taking Tip: Identify which vaccinations are live. Live viruses should not be given in pregnancy. Use this information to rule out Options 1, 2, and 4.*

Content Area: Childbearing; Concept: Immunity; Pregnancy; Medication; Integrated Processes: Nursing Process: Implementation; Client Needs: Physiological Integrity: Pharmacological and Parenteral Therapies; Health Promotion and Maintenance; Cognitive Level: Comprehension [Understanding]

## 931. PHARM ANSWER: 1, 2, 5

1. **This response is correct. Research has shown that vitamin D levels during late pregnancy were insufficient in 31% and deficient in 18% of pregnant women.**
2. **This response is correct. A low level of vitamin D is associated with a child's reduced bone-mineral accumulation at age 9 years.**
3. A low level of vitamin C (not D) predisposes the client to premature rupture of the membranes.
4. The lack of vitamin C (not D) increases the rate of cervical collagen degradation. With decreased collagen, the cervix ripens more easily, prompting effacement and dilation.
5. **This response is correct. Supplements taken during pregnancy may reduce the child's risk for osteoporosis-related fractures.**

♦ *Test-taking Tip: Vitamin D is essential for the absorption of calcium. Use this information to eliminate options not related to bone growth.*

Content Area: Childbearing; Concept: Pregnancy; Medication; Evidence-based Practice; Integrated Processes: Nursing Process: Implementation; Client Needs: Physiological Integrity: Pharmacological and Parenteral Therapies; Cognitive Level: Application [Applying]

## 932. PHARM ANSWER: 1

1. **Pregnancy depletes iron stores, which are generally replaced with a well-balanced diet between gestation periods. When the second pregnancy is closely spaced, the iron stores have not been adequately replaced.**
2. Advanced maternal age is not associated with nutritional disorders.
3. A first pregnancy is not a nutritional risk factor, although pregnant adolescents are considered to be at nutritional risk.
4. Infertility is not usually associated with nutritional risk factors.

♦ *Test-taking Tip: Pregnancy places an increased demand on the body to produce more RBCs, thereby depleting iron stores. One factor that may place the pregnant client at risk for anemia includes closely spaced pregnancies.*

Content Area: Childbearing; Concept: Pregnancy; Medication; Integrated Processes: Nursing Process: Assessment; Client Needs: Physiological Integrity: Pharmacological and Parenteral Therapies; Cognitive Level: Application [Applying]

**933.** PHARM **ANSWER: 3**

1. Metronidazole (Flagyl) is used for the treatment of bacterial vaginosis, not *Candida albicans*, as the symptoms suggest.
2. Butoconazole (Gynazole) should not be used in pregnancy.
3. **The nurse should prepare to teach the client about the use of imidazole vaginal cream. It is indicated for the treatment of *Candida albicans,* and it is safe in pregnancy.**
4. One-time treatment with fluconazole (Diflucan) has not been well studied during pregnancy and therefore should not be used.

▶ *Test-taking Tip: Focus on the color of the discharge to recognize that this is caused by Candida albicans. Select the medication that would be most effective in treating a yeast infection and would not be contraindicated during pregnancy.*

**Content Area:** Childbearing; **Concept:** Infection; Medication; Pregnancy; **Integrated Processes:** Nursing Process: Evaluation; **Client Needs:** Physiological Integrity: Pharmacological and Parenteral Therapies; **Cognitive Level:** Evaluation [Evaluating]

**934.** PHARM **ANSWER: 1**

1. **Benazepril (Lotensin) may cause fetal injury and death. It is most important for the nurse to withhold the benazepril and contact the HCP.**
2. Although African American clients have a diminished therapeutic response to ACE inhibitors, benazepril should not be administered due to its teratogenic effects.
3. Although benazepril will increase serum bilirubin levels, withholding the benazepril is more important.
4. Although benazepril will increase serum potassium levels by inhibiting aldosterone secretion, withholding the benazepril is more important.

▶ *Test-taking Tip: You should be aware of medications that are contraindicated during pregnancy even though you may be drawn to Option 2 because it pertains to the African American client.*

**Content Area:** Childbearing; **Concept:** Pregnancy; Medication; Diversity; **Integrated Processes:** Nursing Process: Implementation; Culture and Spirituality; **Client Needs:** Physiological Integrity: Pharmacological and Parenteral Therapies; **Cognitive Level:** Analysis [Analyzing]

**935.** PHARM **ANSWER: 1**

1. **Ginger capsules of 250 mg taken four times a day have been demonstrated to be effective against nausea and vomiting associated with pregnancy, as well as hyperemesis. There is no evidence of significant side effects or adverse effects on pregnancy outcomes.**
2. Milk thistle does not have an effect on nausea. The seeds of the milk thistle plant exert hepatoprotective and antihepatotoxic action over liver toxins. Milk thistle also activates the liver's regenerative capacity, making this herb beneficial in the treatment of hepatitis.
3. Black cohosh is an herbal remedy used to treat menopausal and premenstrual syndrome symptoms but has no effect on nausea.
4. Echinacea is used to stimulate the immune system but has no effect on nausea.

▶ *Test-taking Tip: Ginger ale is often consumed by persons experiencing nausea. Use association between ginger and ginger ale to remember the herbal remedy for treating nausea and vomiting.*

**Content Area:** Childbearing; **Concept:** Pregnancy; Medication; **Integrated Processes:** Teaching/Learning; Caring; **Client Needs:** Physiological Integrity: Basic Care and Comfort; Physiological Integrity: Pharmacological and Parenteral Therapies; **Cognitive Level:** Application [Applying]

**936.** PHARM **ANSWER: 1**

1. **Omeprazole (Prilosec), a PPI, produces irreversible inhibition of $H^+$, $K^+$-ATPase, which is the enzyme that induces gastric acid production.**
2. Histamine blockers, such as ranitidine (Zantac), block the $H_2$ receptors located on the parietal cells of the stomach.
3. Antacids neutralize the gastric acid in the stomach.
4. Sucralfate (Carafate) coats the upper stomach and esophagus.

▶ *Test-taking Tip: The medication classification of omeprazole is a PPI. This should enable elimination of Options 2, 3, and 4.*

**Content Area:** Childbearing; **Concept:** Medication; Pregnancy; **Integrated Processes:** Teaching/Learning; **Client Needs:** Physiological Integrity: Pharmacological and Parenteral Therapies; **Cognitive Level:** Comprehension [Understanding]

**937.** MoC PHARM **ANSWER: 2**

1. Furosemide (Lasix), a diuretic, is a Category C medication. It has not been shown to cause fetal harm and may be administered in pregnancy.
2. **The nurse should clarify captopril (Capoten), an ACE inhibitor. ACE inhibitors are contraindicated in the second and third trimesters of pregnancy. They can cause oligohydramnios, intrauterine growth retardation (IUGR), congenital structural defects, and renal failure.**
3. Digoxin (Lanoxin) is a Category C medication but has not been shown to cause fetal harm. Digoxin exerts a positive inotropic action on the heart.
4. Metoprolol (Toprol XL) is a Category C medication but has not been shown to cause fetal harm. Metoprolol, which is a beta blocker, can improve left ventricular ejection fraction and slow the progression of heart failure.

▶ *Test-taking Tip: ACE inhibitors are contraindicated in the second and third trimesters of pregnancy. Only one medication is an ACE inhibitor.*

**Content Area:** Childbearing; **Concept:** Medication; Pregnancy; **Integrated Processes:** Nursing Process: Implementation; **Client Needs:** Safe and Effective Care Environment: Management of Care; Physiological Integrity: Pharmacological and Parenteral Therapies; **Cognitive Level:** Application [Applying]

**938.** PHARM **ANSWER: 1, 3, 4**

1. **Women receiving HAART during pregnancy are at higher risk for preterm labor.**
2. There is no known association between HAART and preeclampsia.
3. **Women receiving HAART during pregnancy are at higher risk for low-birth-weight babies.**
4. **Women receiving HAART during pregnancy are at higher risk for gestational diabetes.**
5. There is no known association between HAART and birth defects.

▸ *Test-taking Tip:* HAART use in pregnancy is associated with pregnancy-related problems, but preeclampsia and birth defects are not among these.

Content Area: Childbearing; **Concept:** Medication; Pregnancy; **Integrated Processes:** Nursing Process: Analysis; **Client Needs:** Physiological Integrity: Pharmacological and Parenteral Therapies; **Cognitive Level:** Application [Applying]

**939.** MoC PHARM **ANSWER: 2**

1. Methyldopa (Aldomet) 250 mg bid by mouth for elevated BP is correctly written.
2. **According to the Joint Commission, certain abbreviations should not be used because of different meanings. MgSO$_4$ (magnesium sulfate) can be confused with MSO$_4$ (morphine sulfate) and should be written out as magnesium sulfate. The > and < symbols may be added to the list in the near future and should also be avoided when writing orders or other medical documentation.**
3. Terbutaline (Brethine) is a bronchodilator that is used off-label to treat preterm labor and is correctly written.
4. Prenatal vitamins one tablet daily by mouth is correctly written.

▸ *Test-taking Tip:* Abbreviations used with medications have been demonstrated to contribute to medication errors. Select the option utilizing inappropriate abbreviations.

Content Area: Childbearing; **Concept:** Communication; Pregnancy; Medication; **Integrated Processes:** Communication and Documentation; **Client Needs:** Safe and Effective Care Environment: Management of Care; Physiological Integrity: Pharmacological and Parenteral Therapies; **Cognitive Level:** Evaluation [Evaluating]

**940.** PHARM **ANSWER: 4**

1. Meperidine (Demerol) is not the preferred analgesic for use in breastfeeding women because of the long half-life of its metabolite in infants.
2. Long half-life NSAIDs, such as naproxen (Naprosyn), can accumulate in the infant with prolonged use.
3. Although ibuprofen (Motrin), an NSAID, has poor transfer into milk and an occasional use of therapeutic dose is acceptable, prolonged use can cause accumulation in the infant. Thus it is not the best choice.

4. **Acetaminophen (Tylenol) is excreted in the breast milk in low concentrations, and no adverse infant effects have been reported. Acetaminophen is the analgesic of choice to decrease afterpains for breastfeeding women.**

▸ *Test-taking Tip:* Evaluate each medication relative to its concentration in breast milk and select the medication that is excreted in very low doses in breast milk.

Content Area: Childbearing; **Concept:** Medication; Pregnancy; **Integrated Processes:** Nursing Process: Planning; **Client Needs:** Physiological Integrity: Pharmacological and Parenteral Therapies; **Cognitive Level:** Application [Applying]

**941.** PHARM **ANSWER: 1, 2, 3**

1. **Terbutaline (Brethine) is a beta-adrenergic receptor agonist that causes relaxation of the uterus, stopping preterm labor.**
2. **Nifedipine (Procardia), a calcium channel blocker, is frequently used for the treatment of preterm labor by relaxing the smooth muscle in the uterus.**
3. **Magnesium sulfate (Sulfamag) is a tocolytic agent primarily used to treat preeclampsia and also commonly used to treat preterm labor.**
4. Atenolol (Tenormin), a beta blocker, is not used for the treatment of preterm labor. It is a Category D drug and should not be used during pregnancy.
5. Oxytocin (Pitocin) is used for labor induction and is contraindicated in this situation.

▸ *Test-taking Tip:* Identify which medications are contraindicated in pregnancy and eliminate those as potential options. From the medications that are listed after those options are deleted, select the ones that are used to treat preterm labor.

Content Area: Childbearing; **Concept:** Medication; Pregnancy; **Integrated Processes:** Nursing Process: Analysis; **Client Needs:** Physiological Integrity: Pharmacological and Parenteral Therapies; **Cognitive Level:** Application [Applying]

**942.** PHARM **ANSWER: 1, 2, 4**

1. **Shortness of breath is an adverse effect of magnesium sulfate (Citro Mag).**
2. **Flushing is an adverse effect of magnesium sulfate due to its direct dilating effects.**
3. Hypotension (not hypertension) is an adverse effect of magnesium sulfate due to its direct dilating effects.
4. **Hyporeflexia (flaccidity) is an adverse effect of magnesium sulfate due to its toxic effect on the CNS. The magnesium dose should be reduced or eliminated.**
5. Insomnia is not an adverse effect of magnesium sulfate.

▸ *Test-taking Tip:* You need to consider the effects of magnesium sulfate on the CNS. Adverse symptoms can occur when the dose is too high.

Content Area: Childbearing; **Concept:** Medication; Pregnancy; **Integrated Processes:** Nursing Process: Analysis; **Client Needs:** Physiological Integrity: Pharmacological and Parenteral Therapies; **Cognitive Level:** Application [Applying]

**943.** PHARM **ANSWER: 3**

1. A serum magnesium level of 0.5 mg/dL is subtherapeutic and below the normal serum magnesium level of 1.5 to 2.5 mg/dL for a healthy, nonpregnant person.
2. A serum magnesium level of 2 mg/dL is subtherapeutic for the pregnant client with preeclampsia. The level should be at least 4.8 mg/dL.
3. **A serum magnesium level of 6 mg/dL is therapeutic. The therapeutic magnesium level should be between 4.8 and 9.6 mg/dL to prevent seizure activity in the client with preeclampsia.**
4. A serum magnesium level of 10.1 mg/dL is a toxic level for the client with preeclampsia.

▶ *Test-taking Tip: The normal adult serum magnesium level is 1.5 to 2.5 mg/dL. A higher level would be needed to prevent seizure activity, but too high a level would be toxic.*

Content Area: Childbearing; Concept: Medication; Pregnancy; Integrated Processes: Nursing Process: Analysis; Client Needs: Physiological Integrity: Pharmacological and Parenteral Therapies; Physiological Integrity: Reduction of Risk Potential; Cognitive Level: Knowledge [Remembering]

**944.** PHARM **ANSWER: 2**

1. Women who develop preeclampsia become more sensitive to natural pressor agents. As the severity of the preeclampsia increases, the BP also increases. An increase in BP would indicate worsening preeclampsia and medication ineffectiveness.
2. **Diuresis within 24 to 48 hours is an excellent sign indicating that perfusion of the kidneys has improved as a result of the relaxation of arteriolar spasms. This finding indicates that the magnesium sulfate is effective in treating preeclampsia.**
3. Vasospasm occurs in preeclampsia and causes vascular damage that promotes platelet aggregation at the site of this damage. Decreasing platelet levels indicate more blood vessel damage, which could indicate worsening preeclampsia and medication ineffectiveness.
4. Vascular volume, which normally increases in pregnancy, may decrease with preeclampsia. This decrease in vascular volume will cause a corresponding increase in Hct. Increasing Hct is a concerning sign that could indicate worsening preeclampsia and medication ineffectiveness.

▶ *Test-taking Tip: Three options are signs indicating that preeclampsia is worsening and that the medication is ineffective in treating preeclampsia.*

Content Area: Childbearing; Concept: Medication; Pregnancy; Integrated Processes: Nursing Process: Evaluation; Client Needs: Physiological Integrity: Pharmacological and Parenteral Therapies; Cognitive Level: Evaluation [Evaluating]

**945.** PHARM **ANSWER: 2**

1. Terbutaline does not decrease the sensation in the uterus.
2. **Terbutaline (Brethaire) is a beta-adrenergic agonist that, in pregnant women, causes uterine relaxation. This greatly enhances the comfort of the women during the version and facilitates the maneuver.**
3. Terbutaline does not cause drowsiness.
4. Terbutaline does not stimulate contractions.

▶ *Test-taking Tip: An external cephalic version procedure is used to try to convert a breech presentation to a cephalic presentation. If unsure, consider the option that would make the version easier.*

Content Area: Childbearing; Concept: Medication; Pregnancy; Nursing Roles; Integrated Processes: Teaching/Learning; Client Needs: Physiological Integrity: Pharmacological and Parenteral Therapies; Cognitive Level: Application [Applying]

**946.** PHARM **ANSWER: 4**

1. Location A is the uterus; administration of the medication at the top of a pregnant uterus would not be possible.
2. Location B is the opening to the urethra and would not enhance cervical ripening.
3. Location C is the vaginal opening; this position would not introduce the medication for enough to enhance cervical ripening.
4. **Dinoprostone (Cervidil) is packaged as an intravaginal insert that resembles a 2-cm-square cardboard-like material. It should be placed transversely in the posterior fornix of the vagina (location D) and is left in place for 12 hours to provide a slow release of the medication. Cervical ripening may be necessary in the pregnant client or in the nulliparous nonpregnant client before insertion of an IUD.**

▶ *Test-taking Tip: The key words are "vaginal" and "cervical ripening." The medication should be placed in the vagina, and because it is being used for cervical ripening, logically it should be placed close to the cervix.*

Content Area: Childbearing; Concept: Medication; Pregnancy; Integrated Processes: Nursing Process: Implementation; Client Needs: Physiological Integrity: Pharmacological and Parenteral Therapies; Cognitive Level: Application [Applying]

**947.** PHARM **ANSWER: 4**

1. Prostaglandins can be given for cervical ripening to the primigravida client who is 41 weeks' gestation. Cervical ripening agents shorten labor and reduce the incidence of cesarean birth for this population.
2. Prostaglandins are not contraindicated in multiparous women until they have had six previous term vaginal births.
3. Macrosomia in the pregnant diabetic client may be an indication for early initiation of labor, and thus prostaglandins would be appropriate.

**4. The client with a previous uterine incision from a cesarean birth should not receive prostaglandin agents because the risk of uterine rupture is greatly increased. The nurse should question the order for this client.**

▶ *Test-taking Tip: The 5-digit system for summarizing the client's obstetric history uses the acronym GTPAL (gravidity, term, preterm, abortions, and living children). Dinoprostone (Prepidil) is a synthetically prepared prostaglandin. Cervical ripening will enhance labor. Of the clients, think about which would be at risk for uterine rupture if labor is enhanced.*

Content Area: Childbearing; Concept: Critical Thinking; Pregnancy; Medication; Integrated Processes: Nursing Process: Implementation; Client Needs: Safe and Effective Care Environment: Safety and Infection Control; Physiological Integrity: Pharmacological and Parenteral Therapies; Cognitive Level: Analysis [Analyzing]

### 948. PHARM ANSWER: 2

1. Misoprostol is administered vaginally. Whether or not the client has eaten should not influence its administration.
2. **The nurse should check the record and question the client for past history of cesarean birth. Misoprostol is contraindicated in clients with certain types of uterine scars because uterine rupture can occur.**
3. Lower abdominal pain from uterine contractions induced by misoprostol is common, and an analgesic may be necessary. However, this is not the most important question.
4. It is important to assess the client's bladder status in case of cesarean birth, but this is not the most important question to ask.

▶ *Test-taking Tip: Misoprostol is a prostaglandin that can cause uterine contractions and cervical ripening. Consider any contraindications to misoprostol use when reviewing the options.*

Content Area: Childbearing; Concept: Pregnancy; Medication; Integrated Processes: Nursing Process: Assessment; Client Needs: Physiological Integrity: Pharmacological and Parenteral Therapies; Cognitive Level: Application [Applying]

### 949. PHARM ANSWER: 4

1. Carboprost tromethamine is not used to decrease fever; a side effect of its use is fever.
2. Carboprost tromethamine is not used for BP control. It should be used with caution if the client has either hyper- or hypotension.
3. Carboprost tromethamine is not used to increase client comfort; a side effect of its use is abdominal pain.
4. **Carboprost tromethamine is given to reduce blood loss in uterine atony by stimulating myometrial contractions. Increased uterine tone results in decreased bleeding and a decrease in the amount of lochia rubra.**

▶ *Test-taking Tip: Carboprost tromethamine (Hemabate) is indicated for the control of increased postpartum bleeding. Think about the assessment finding that would indicate bleeding is controlled.*

Content Area: Childbearing; Concept: Pregnancy; Medication; Integrated Processes: Nursing Process: Evaluation; Client Needs: Physiological Integrity: Pharmacological and Parenteral Therapies; Cognitive Level: Evaluation [Evaluating]

### 950. MoC PHARM ANSWER: 1, 5

1. **IV oxytocin (Pitocin) should be discontinued and the HCP notified if there is insufficient uterine relaxation (resting tone) between contractions. Expected resting uterine tone is 10 to 12 mm Hg, not 18 mm Hg.**
2. The goal of induction with IV oxytocin is a uterine contraction pattern of three 40- to 60-second contractions in 10 minutes. Uterine contractions occurring every 4 minutes would indicate a need for a higher dose of oxytocin.
3. BP is expected to increase as much as 30% above baseline when oxytocin is given.
4. Larger doses of IV oxytocin exert an antidiuretic effect, causing a marked decrease in urine output. A urine output of 60 mL/hr or more is considered to be WNL and not a reason to stop oxytocin.
5. **The IV infusion should be discontinued if a nonreassuring fetal status develops. Fetal bradycardia is an FHR consistently below 90 bpm. When this is accompanied by decreased variability, it is considered an ominous sign of fetal distress.**

▶ *Test-taking Tip: Focus on concerning side effects of oxytocin. Eliminate options that describe expected responses to the use of oxytocin because these would be anticipated findings.*

Content Area: Childbearing; Concept: Assessment; Pregnancy; Medication; Integrated Processes: Nursing Process: Evaluation; Client Needs: Safe and Effective Care Environment: Management of Care; Physiological Integrity: Pharmacological and Parenteral Therapies; Cognitive Level: Evaluation [Evaluating]

### 951. MoC PHARM ANSWER: 2, 3, 4, 5

1. Placing the client in a side-lying position is indicated, not the knee-chest position.
2. **The IV fluids should be increased by at least giving a 500-mL bolus as an intrauterine resuscitation measure.**
3. **Oxygen at 10 liters via facemask is needed to increase oxygenation of the fetus.**
4. **Oxytocin (Pitocin) should be promptly stopped. Too high a dose of oxytocin or increasing the dose of oxytocin at incremental intervals less than 30 minutes can cause tachysystole.**
5. **The HCP should be advised of the client's status and the contraction pattern because intrauterine resuscitation measures are necessary.**

▶ *Test-taking Tip: Tachysystole is five or more uterine contractions (UC) in 10 minutes with less than 60 seconds of relaxation between UC, UC lasting 2 minutes or longer, or UC occurring within 1 minute of each other. Use the ABC's to identify emergency interventions.*

Content Area: Childbearing; Concept: Pregnancy; Medication; Integrated Processes: Nursing Process: Implementation; Client Needs: Physiological Integrity: Pharmacological and Parenteral Therapies; Safe and Effective Care Environment: Management of Care; Cognitive Level: Synthesis [Creating]

## 952. MoC PHARM ANSWER: 3

1. Terbutaline is not needed to relax her uterus because a nonpregnant uterus is fairly resistant to the effects of oxytocin.
2. There is no need for ibuprofen because there will be minimal, if any, cramping.
3. **In the nonpregnant uterus, smooth muscle cells have low strength, demonstrate asynchronous contractions, and are fairly resistant to the effects of the oxytocin. The oxytocin should have little or no effect on the nurse's uterus, so no additional treatment is needed.**
4. Oxytocin in larger doses does have an antidiuretic effect; however, because the dose received was relatively small, limiting free water intake is not necessary.

▶ *Test-taking Tip: Three options include effects of oxytocin (Pitocin) and interventions to treat the effects, whereas one option is different. Often the option that is different is the answer.*

Content Area: Childbearing; Concept: Safety; Medication; Pregnancy; Integrated Processes: Nursing Process: Planning; Client Needs: Safe and Effective Care Environment: Management of Care; Physiological Integrity: Pharmacological and Parenteral Therapies; Cognitive Level: Analysis [Analyzing]

## 953. PHARM ANSWER: 24

**Using dimensional analysis:**

$$X\,mL/h = \frac{1{,}000\ mL}{10\ units} \times \frac{4\ mU}{min} \times \frac{60\ min}{1\ h} = \frac{1\ unit}{1{,}000\ mU}$$

$$X\,mL/h = \frac{1{,}000\ mL}{10\ \cancel{units}} \times \frac{4\ \cancel{mU}}{\cancel{min}} \times \frac{60\ \cancel{min}}{1\ h} = \frac{1\ \cancel{unit}}{1{,}000\ \cancel{mU}} \quad \text{Cancel the units}$$

$$X\,mL/h = \frac{240{,}000}{10{,}000} \quad \text{Solve the equation}$$

$$X\,mL/h = 24$$

▶ *Test-taking Tip: Use the dimensional analysis method for medication and fluid administration. Leading zeros are required, and trailing zeros are NOT used. A calculator is required to find this answer. Be sure the answer is logical.*

Content Area: Childbearing; Concept: Medication; Pregnancy; Integrated Processes: Nursing Process: Planning; Client Needs: Physiological Integrity: Pharmacological and Parenteral Therapies; Cognitive Level: Analysis [Analyzing]

## 954. PHARM ANSWER: 4

1. A barbiturate should not be given to the client whose delivery is imminent via cesarean section because it can cause fetal depression.
2. A barbiturate should not be administered to the client in active labor because it can cause fetal depression.
3. The client admitted for induction of labor should be started on a medication to stimulate labor and should not be sedated.
4. **The client who is at 40 weeks' gestation, 1 cm dilated, and 20% effaced with poor-quality uterine contractions has hypertonic uterine dysfunction. Ineffectual uterine contractions are occurring in the latent phase of labor. Treatment is rest and sedation. Zolpidem tartrate is a sedative-hypnotic barbiturate that will produce sleep and maternal relaxation.**

▶ *Test-taking Tip: Zolpidem tartrate (Ambien) is a barbiturate medication that will produce sedation. Eliminate clients in which sedation would be harmful to the fetus or counterproductive.*

Content Area: Childbearing; Concept: Medication; Pregnancy; Integrated Processes: Nursing Process: Planning; Client Needs: Physiological Integrity: Pharmacological and Parenteral Therapies; Physiological Integrity: Physiological Adaptation; Cognitive Level: Analysis [Analyzing]

## 955. PHARM ANSWER: 3

1. Deep tendon reflexes of 2+ are a normal finding and are not the desired therapeutic response of dinoprostone use.
2. A fetal HR of 130 bpm is a normal finding and is not the desired therapeutic response of dinoprostone use.
3. **Dinoprostone inserts are placed vaginally near the cervix to produce cervical ripening prior to labor induction, and they induce uterine contractions. Uterine contractions every 4 minutes indicate that the client had the desired therapeutic response.**
4. BP of 120/80 mm Hg is a normal finding and is not the desired therapeutic response of dinoprostone use.

▶ *Test-taking Tip: Note that two options are maternal, and two are fetal. Use the medication's trade name (Cervidil) as a clue to the correct option.*

Content Area: Childbearing; Concept: Pregnancy; Medication; Integrated Processes: Nursing Process: Evaluation; Client Needs: Physiological Integrity: Pharmacological and Parenteral Therapies; Cognitive Level: Evaluation [Evaluating]

**956.** PHARM **ANSWER: 1, 2, 4**

1. **Bupivacaine (Marcaine) is a local anesthetic agent. The medication blocks sympathetic nerve fibers in the epidural space, which causes decreased peripheral resistance. This, in turn, causes hypotension.**
2. **Maternal temperature may be elevated to 100°F (37.8°C) or higher due to sympathetic blockage from bupivacaine that may decrease sweat production and diminish heat loss.**
3. Nausea is not a side effect of bupivacaine.
4. **Bupivacaine alters transmission of impulses to the bladder, thus causing urinary retention.**
5. Sedation is not a side effect of bupivacaine.

▶ *Test-taking Tip: The suffix of the medication "-caine" is common for local anesthetic agents. Select options that would be related to this type of pain control.*

Content Area: Childbearing; Concept: Medication; Pregnancy; Integrated Processes: Nursing Process: Implementation; Client Needs: Physiological Integrity: Pharmacological and Parenteral Therapies; Cognitive Level: Application [Applying]

**957.** PHARM **ANSWER: 2**

Use a proportion to determine the amount in milliliters. Multiply the extremes, then the means, and solve for $X$.

$10 \text{ mg} : 1 \text{ mL} :: 20 \text{ mg} : X \text{ mL}; 10X = 20; X = 20 \div 10; X = 2$

▶ *Test-taking Tip: Because the ordered dose of nalbuphine hydrochloride (Nubain) is greater than 10 mg, the amount to give should be greater than 1 mL. Use the formula dose needed/dose on hand or a proportion formula.*

Content Area: Childbearing; Concept: Medication; Pregnancy; Integrated Processes: Nursing Process: Implementation; Client Needs: Physiological Integrity: Pharmacological and Parenteral Therapies; Cognitive Level: Application [Applying]

**958.** PHARM **ANSWER: 2**

1. Stage 1, first phase generally does not require medication, nor is it indicated.
2. **Cervical effacement and dilation occur during Stage 1 of labor. The second phase of Stage 1 occurs when the cervix dilates from 3 to 7 cm. Narcotic analgesia is given during this phase to assist the client to relax and better tolerate the discomfort. When analgesia is given too close to birth, the newborn can have a higher serum drug concentration.**
3. During Stage 2 the fetus is expelled. Pain management for this stage is by regional anesthesia, rather than narcotic analgesia use.
4. During Stage 3 the placenta is expelled. Pain management for this stage is by regional anesthesia, rather than narcotic analgesia use.

▶ *Test-taking Tip: Thinking about the potential adverse effects of narcotic analgesics on the fetus and newborn, you should be able to eliminate the last two stages. Then, of the remaining options, think about when narcotic use would be most effective.*

Content Area: Childbearing; Concept: Comfort; Pregnancy; Medication; Integrated Processes: Nursing Process: Planning; Caring; Client Needs: Physiological Integrity: Pharmacological and Parenteral Therapies; Psychosocial Integrity; Cognitive Level: Application [Applying]

**959.** MoC PHARM **ANSWER: 3, 4, 1, 2, 6, 5**

3. **Discontinue the oxytocin infusion. This allows the uterus to relax, thereby increasing blood flow to the fetus.**
4. **Administer oxygen at 10 L/min via facemask. Oxygen increases the oxygen concentration in the maternal blood.**
1. **Change maternal position to lateral. A side-lying position increases blood flow to the uterus.**
2. **Administer fluid bolus of 500 mL lactated Ringer's solution. A bolus of fluid will help to increase blood flow and perfusion. This will take longer to prepare than applying oxygen and repositioning the client.**
6. **Notify the HCP after initiating interventions per protocol.**
5. **Document the event and maternal/fetal response. Client care should be provided prior to documentation.**

▶ *Test-taking Tip: The nurse must recognize high-alert drugs such as oxytocin. The ABC's can be helpful in deciding the priorities and actions to be taken to optimize fetal circulation.*

Content Area: Childbearing; Concept: Medication; Pregnancy; Integrated Processes: Nursing Process: Implementation; Caring; Client Needs: Safe and Effective Care Environment: Management of Care; Physiological Integrity: Pharmacological and Parenteral Therapies; Cognitive Level: Synthesis [Creating]

**960.** PHARM **ANSWER: 2**

1. Moderate lochia rubra is expected by postpartum day 2 but is not related to the use of cefotaxime and not most important.
2. **Cefotaxime is indicated for intra-abdominal or pelvic infection and septicemia. Absence of high fever indicates resolving infection.**
3. Voiding in good quantities is an expectation by postpartum day 2 but is not related to the use of cefotaxime.
4. Bowel patterns may not have returned to normal by day 2 and would not be the result of cefotaxime, which could cause diarrhea.

▶ *Test-taking Tip: Prolonged rupture of membranes is associated with an increased risk of chorioamnionitis and intrauterine infection. Cefotaxime (Claforan) is a third-generation cephalosporin used to treat severe infections. The only answer related to infection is fever.*

Content Area: Childbearing; Concept: Infection; Pregnancy; Medication; Integrated Processes: Nursing Process: Planning; Client Needs: Physiological Integrity: Pharmacological and Parenteral Therapies; Cognitive Level: Application [Applying]

**961.** PHARM **ANSWER: 3**

1. There would be no benefit to adding sterile water to an existing IV solution.
2. Administering the sterile water into the abdomen will not affect the back pain.
3. **Injection of a small amount of sterile water into the intradermal layer of skin in the lumbar-sacral region of the back produces hyperstimulation of the large inhibitory nerve fibers. The onset of pain relief usually occurs within a few minutes and can last 1 to 2 hours. The treatment can be repeated several times.**
4. Injections into the posterior dorsal-gluteal muscle are not recommended due to possible sciatic nerve injury.

◗ *Test-taking Tip: You should associate key words in the stem with similar words in the options. The lumbar-sacral region is in the back.*

Content Area: Childbearing; **Concept:** Comfort; Pregnancy; Medication; **Integrated Processes:** Nursing Process: Implementation; **Client Needs:** Physiological Integrity: Pharmacological and Parenteral Therapies; Physiological Integrity: Basic Care and Comfort; **Cognitive Level:** Application [Applying]

**962.** PHARM **ANSWER: 3**

1. Nausea is not a finding associated with intravascular injection of epidural anesthesia; a loss of consciousness, not increased alertness, may occur.
2. Irritability is not a finding associated with intravascular injection of epidural anesthesia. Hypertension, not hypotension, may occur.
3. **Tinnitus and a metallic taste in the mouth are associated with IV injection of epidural anesthesia. Other findings include hypertension, maternal tachy- or bradycardia, dizziness, and loss of consciousness.**
4. Headache is not a finding associated with IV injection of epidural anesthesia. Tinnitus, rather than a loss of hearing, may occur.

◗ *Test-taking Tip: IV injection of epidural anesthesia produces some unusual symptoms. Use this information to select the option with the most unusual symptoms.*

Content Area: Childbearing; **Concept:** Medication; Pregnancy; **Integrated Processes:** Nursing Process: Analysis; **Client Needs:** Physiological Integrity: Pharmacological and Parenteral Therapies; **Cognitive Level:** Application [Applying]

**963.** PHARM **ANSWER: 4**

1. The mother will only be given RhoGAM within 72 hours if her newborn is Rh-positive.
2. The mother will need to receive RhoGAM with each subsequent pregnancy, pregnancy trauma, or pregnancy loss.
3. RhoGAM does not last for a lifetime.

4. **RhoGAM is given in the postpartum period to Rh-negative women who have delivered Rh-positive newborns. RhoGAM is usually given within 72 hours. It prevents the mother from becoming sensitized from the fetomaternal transfusion of Rh-positive blood that occurred at delivery.**

◗ *Test-taking Tip: Recall that Rho(D) immune globulin is an immune globulin that provides passive immunity to a foreign protein. Think of the Rh protein as a foreign protein for Rh-negative women, and select the option that best demonstrates that concept.*

Content Area: Childbearing; **Concept:** Immunity; Pregnancy; Medication; Nursing Roles; **Integrated Processes:** Teaching/Learning; **Client Needs:** Physiological Integrity: Pharmacological and Parenteral Therapies; **Cognitive Level:** Application [Applying]

**964.** PHARM **ANSWER: 4**

1. Methylergonovine is not contraindicated in, nor does it have any adverse effects in, clients with altered body temperature.
2. Methylergonovine is not contraindicated in, nor does it have any adverse effects in, clients with altered respiratory rates.
3. Methylergonovine is not contraindicated in, nor does it have any adverse effects in, clients with altered HR.
4. **The nurse should check the BP because hypertension is a contraindication to, and an adverse effect of, methylergonovine.**

◗ *Test-taking Tip: You should focus on contraindications to and adverse effects of methylergonovine (Methergine). Fever and respiratory rate are expected to be normal soon after delivery, and these can be eliminated. Using the ABC's, consider which vital sign would affect perfusion the most.*

Content Area: Childbearing; **Concept:** Pregnancy; Medication; **Integrated Processes:** Nursing Process: Assessment; **Client Needs:** Physiological Integrity: Pharmacological and Parenteral Therapies; **Cognitive Level:** Application [Applying]

**965.** PHARM **ANSWER: 2**

1. Ferrous sulfate is indicated for anemia that may result from excessive blood loss but would not be administered at this time.
2. **The nurse should administer methylergonovine (Methergine); excessive amounts of bright red lochia rubra indicate potential postpartum hemorrhage. Methylergonovine, an ergot alkaloid, stimulates uterine contractions to help reduce blood loss after delivery.**
3. Oxycodone (OxyContin) is indicated for pain.
4. Terbutaline is a tocolytic agent used to prevent uterine contractions and delay preterm labor.

◗ *Test-taking Tip: You should select a medication that produces tectonic contractions of uterine smooth muscles, thereby increasing uterine tone and decreasing the amount of bleeding.*

Content Area: Childbearing; **Concept:** Pregnancy; Medication; **Integrated Processes:** Nursing Process: Planning; **Client Needs:** Physiological Integrity: Pharmacological and Parenteral Therapies; **Cognitive Level:** Application [Applying]

**966.** PHARM **ANSWER: 3**

1. Carboprost tromethamine does not cause restlessness, agitation, or sleeplessness; therefore a sedative would not be required.
2. Carboprost tromethamine causes diarrhea; a stool softener would be contraindicated.
3. **Carboprost tromethamine is a synthetic analog of naturally occurring prostaglandin F$_2$ alpha, which stimulates myometrial contractions and is used to treat postpartum hemorrhage caused by uterine atony. As a synthetic prostaglandin, it also stimulates the smooth muscle of the GI tract, causing nausea and diarrhea. An antiemetic should be given.**
4. Oral fluids would be difficult to tolerate because carboprost tromethamine causes nausea and vomiting.

♦ *Test-taking Tip: Carboprost tromethamine (Hemabate) is a synthetic prostaglandin. Select the option that best treats the common side effects of prostaglandins. If unsure, consider that nausea is a common side effect for many medications.*

Content Area: Childbearing; Concept: Medication; Pregnancy; Integrated Processes: Nursing Process: Planning; Client Needs: Physiological Integrity: Pharmacological and Parenteral Therapies; Cognitive Level: Application [Applying]

**967.** PHARM **ANSWER: 3**

1. Ritonavir (Norvir) is used as a component of highly active retroviral therapy (HAART) in people who are HIV positive or who have AIDS.
2. Zidovudine (Retrovir) is used as a component of HAART in people who are HIV positive or who have AIDS.
3. **The nurse should administer acyclovir (Zovirax); it is indicated for genital herpes.**
4. Lamivudine (Epivir) is used as a component of HAART in people who are HIV positive or who have AIDS.

♦ *Test-taking Tip: You should recognize that three of the medications are components of HAART used in the treatment of people who are HIV positive or who have AIDS, and these options can be eliminated. The painful ulcerative lesions on the genitalia (perineum) are indicative of a herpes outbreak. The remaining medication is an antiviral used in its treatment.*

Content Area: Childbearing; Concept: Pregnancy; Medication; Integrated Processes: Nursing Process: Planning; Client Needs: Physiological Integrity: Pharmacological and Parenteral Therapies; Cognitive Level: Application [Applying]

**968.** PHARM **ANSWER: 4**

1. Acyclovir (Zovirax), an antiviral medication, is not used at this age to treat hepatitis B.
2. Ceftriaxone (Rocephin) is used to treat a bacterial infection.
3. Acetaminophen (Tylenol) could be administered if the infant is uncomfortable or in pain, but it does not decrease the risk of an infection.

4. **An infant born to a mother who is hepatitis B surface antigen–positive should receive both the hepatitis B vaccine and 0.5 mL of hepatitis B immune globulin (HBIG) within 12 hours of birth. This combination has a greater effect on reducing the risk of developing hepatitis B than the vaccine alone.**

♦ *Test-taking Tip: You should eliminate medications based on their classifications. The medication you select should be one that helps prevent the infant from contracting hepatitis B from the mother.*

Content Area: Childbearing; Concept: Infection; Pregnancy; Integrated Processes: Nursing Process: Implementation; Client Needs: Physiological Integrity: Pharmacological and Parenteral Therapies; Cognitive Level: Application [Applying]

**969.** PHARM **ANSWER: 3**

1. Zidovudine does not affect coagulation; a PT would not be available.
2. Serum lactate is completed only if the infant develops severe clinical symptoms of unknown etiology. Zidovudine (Retrovir) would be initiated regardless of the CD4 values.
3. **The nurse should analyze the CBC with differential and ALT to obtain the newborn's baseline Hgb and liver function and to identify if significant anemia or alteration in liver function is present before initiating therapy.**
4. Serum protein values are unnecessary. Zidovudine (Retrovir) would be initiated regardless of the CD4 values.

♦ *Test-taking Tip: ALT is a liver function test, and CD4 cells are a type of lymphocyte. Knowing this, you should consider the laboratory test results that could be affected by an antiviral medication that affects the liver and can cause anemia.*

Content Area: Childbearing; Concept: Infection; Pregnancy; Integrated Processes: Nursing Process: Implementation; Client Needs: Physiological Integrity: Reduction of Risk Potential; Physiological Integrity: Pharmacological and Parenteral Therapies; Cognitive Level: Analysis [Analyzing]

**970.** PHARM **ANSWER: 1**

1. **The preferred administration route of indomethacin (Indocin) for treatment of a PDA is IV so the medication can quickly enter the vascular system. Indomethacin is given to infants with PDA to stimulate closure of the defect.**
2. Although indomethacin can be administered orally, the onset of action is delayed.
3. Although indomethacin can be administered rectally, the onset of action is delayed.
4. Indomethacin is not administered IM.

♦ *Test-taking Tip: Focusing on the point of impact for which the medication is being given will help you identify the preferred route.*

Content Area: Childbearing; **Concept:** Medication; Pregnancy; **Integrated Processes:** Nursing Process: Planning; **Client Needs:** Physiological Integrity: Pharmacological and Parenteral Therapies; **Cognitive Level:** Application [Applying]

## 971. PHARM ANSWER: 3

1. The nurse should not call the pharmacy for the solution because D12.5/0.2 NS should not be administered until a central line is placed.
2. While obtaining blood glucose is acceptable, D12.5/0.2 NS should not be started yet.
3. **The nurse should discuss the situation immediately with the HCP; the infant's IV access is in a peripheral vein. A neonate can have D10 in peripheral veins for short periods of time, but solutions with higher concentrations of dextrose should be given through a central line. The HCP should either place a central line or prescribe insertion of a PICC.**
4. The nurse should be concerned about fluid balance and should not adjust the rate to increase dextrose administration, especially when a rate adjustment has not been prescribed.

▶ **Test-taking Tip:** *Recognize that there is a difference between what has been prescribed and what has been infusing. Determine if the solution change is appropriate.*

Content Area: Childbearing; **Concept:** Communication; Medication; Pregnancy; **Integrated Processes:** Communication and Documentation; **Client Needs:** Physiological Integrity: Pharmacological and Parenteral Therapies; **Cognitive Level:** Analysis [Analyzing]

## 972. PHARM ANSWER: 1

1. **The most important information for use of nystatin (Mycostatin) is whether the oral area is improving. Thrush can be self-limiting and can have a spontaneous resolution, although it could take up to 2 months; it is much quicker with nystatin (Mycostatin) use.**
2. Monitoring for signs of contact dermatitis is correct for topical application, but the infant is receiving nystatin (Mycostatin) to treat thrush.
3. "Swish and swallow" administration is appropriate for an older person, but this is a 6-day-old infant.
4. Adverse effects occur in less than 1% of the population and need not be stated at this time.

▶ **Test-taking Tip:** *Identify related words used in the scenario and an option to select the answer.*

Content Area: Childbearing; **Concept:** Nursing Roles; Medication; Pregnancy; **Integrated Processes:** Nursing Process: Implementation; **Client Needs:** Physiological Integrity: Pharmacological and Parenteral Therapies; **Cognitive Level:** Application [Applying]

## 973. PHARM ANSWER: 5.3

**Multiply the dose (4 mg) by kilograms (4 kg) and divide it by 3.**

$$4 \times 4 = 16; 16 \div 3 = 5.3$$

▶ **Test-taking Tip:** *Be sure to recognize that the 4 mg/kg/day is the total dose and that divided doses should be administered every 8 hours for a total of three doses.*

Content Area: Childbearing; **Concept:** Medication; Pregnancy; **Integrated Processes:** Nursing Process: Planning; **Client Needs:** Physiological Integrity: Pharmacological and Parenteral Therapies; Physiological Integrity: Reduction of Risk Potential; **Cognitive Level:** Application [Applying]

## 974. PHARM ANSWER: 4

1. Naloxone is not used to decrease irritability.
2. Naloxone is not used to promote a bowel movement.
3. Naloxone is not used to increase or decrease a temperature.
4. **Naloxone (Narcan) is an opioid antagonist that is given to reverse the CNS and respiratory depression associated with opioid overdose.**

▶ **Test-taking Tip:** *Use the ABC's to select an answer.*

Content Area: Childbearing; **Concept:** Oxygenation; Medication; Pregnancy; **Integrated Processes:** Nursing Process: Evaluation; **Client Needs:** Physiological Integrity: Pharmacological and Parenteral Therapies; **Cognitive Level:** Evaluation [Evaluating]

## 975. PHARM ANSWER: 3

1. The first dose of MMR vaccine, a live virus, is recommended to be given at 12 months of age but can be given at 6 months if traveling internationally.
2. The influenza vaccine annual dose is recommended to be given at 6 months of age.
3. **The first dose of hepatitis B vaccine is recommended for newborns and should be given prior to hospital discharge.**
4. The first dose of the rotavirus vaccine is recommended to be given at 2 months of age.

▶ **Test-taking Tip:** *A vaccine that protects against a blood-borne virus is recommended to be given at birth. A live virus vaccine is not given until on or after the first birthday.*

Content Area: Childbearing; **Concept:** Promoting Health; Medication; Pregnancy; **Integrated Processes:** Nursing Process: Planning; **Client Needs:** Physiological Integrity: Pharmacological and Parenteral Therapies; **Cognitive Level:** Application [Applying]

**976.** **PHARM** **ANSWER: 1, 4, 5**

1. Once the erythromycin ophthalmic solution has been instilled, the nurse should gently massage the eyelids to ensure the spreading of the medication.
2. The lids should be wiped 1 minute, and not immediately, after application.
3. Cleaning the eyelids is completed prior to administering the medication.
4. After any procedure, the psychological needs of the infant should be a focus by the nurse; swaddling is a comforting technique.
5. The nurse should wait 1 minute and then wipe away excess medication with a sterile cotton swab.
6. The dose is not repeated.

▶ *Test-taking Tip: The key words in the stem are "after administration." Options 2 and 5 are similar but with different time periods. Both of these cannot be correct.*

Content Area: Childbearing; Concept: Medication; Clotting; Pregnancy; Integrated Processes: Nursing Process: Implementation; Caring; Client Needs: Physiological Integrity: Pharmacological and Parenteral Therapies; Psychosocial Integrity; Cognitive Level: Application [Applying]

# Chapter Twenty-Three

# Adult and Older Adult Development

**977.** The unsteady 20-year-old client persists in ambulating to the bathroom alone despite being reminded to call for assistance. The nurse concludes that, according to Havighurst's developmental tasks, this behavior reflects which need of the client?

1. Adjusting to physiological changes
2. Independence
3. Industry
4. Integrity

**978.** The nurse is completing an assessment on the 19-year-old female who participates in strenuous physical activities many hours daily. Which nursing assessment is **most** important?

1. Check for the presence of lordosis.
2. Look for signs of an eating disorder.
3. Examine muscles for increased mass.
4. Ask about excessive bleeding with menses.

**979.** The nurse is assessing the chest of a healthy adult male client without chest abnormalities. Which chest curvature illustrated should the nurse expect to observe?

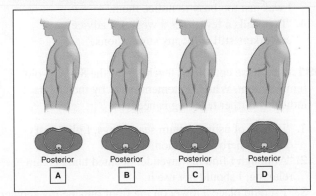

1. Illustration A
2. Illustration B
3. Illustration C
4. Illustration D

**980.** The nurse is collecting information from the young adult client. Which psychosocial questions should the nurse ask during the admission assessment? **Select all that apply.**

1. "Do you have any pets?"
2. "How many hours of sleep do you get?"
3. "When was your last bowel movement?"
4. "How much alcohol do you drink?"
5. "Can you describe your sexual activity?"

**981.** The nurse assesses that a hospitalized 20-year-old college student is anxious and not able to concentrate when given self-care instructions. Which intervention should the nurse implement to assist the client to deal with the stress of hospitalization?

1. Have one parent stay in the room when the client is anxious.
2. Encourage using a cell phone or Internet to talk with friends.
3. Contact psychiatry to discuss treatments for depression.
4. Reinforce multiple times how best to perform self-care.

**982.** The nurse is caring for the middle-aged client. Which client behavior should indicate to the nurse that the client may have difficulty achieving Erikson's developmental stage of generativity?

1. Talks about accomplishments that made the workplace a better place to work
2. Volunteers at the local nursing home reading to residents 1 day a week
3. Focuses conversation on self and displays disinterest in the activities of others
4. Shows pictures of the client's grandchildren and the client at various sports events

**983.** The nurse is assessing a healthy middle-aged adult. Which finding should the nurse expect?

1. Weight gain of 20 pounds in the past year
2. Tactile fremitus is absent at the apex of the lungs
3. Counts backward from 100 subtracting 7 each time
4. Percussion shows heart is larger than at last checkup

**984.** The nurse is assessing the 50-year-old female client who is hospitalized. The nurse should assess the client for which physical changes associated with aging? **Select all that apply.**

1. Increased sweat gland activity
2. Decreased ability to read smaller print
3. Weight loss due to hypermetabolism
4. Increased sebaceous gland activity
5. Absence of a menstrual cycle

**985.** The home-care nurse assesses the middle-aged client who is disabled after a recent accident. The client has few interests, spends most days watching TV, and has become estranged from the family. Which of Erikson's developmental stages should the nurse conclude that the client is not meeting?

1. Industry versus inferiority
2. Initiative versus guilt
3. Generativity versus stagnation
4. Intimacy versus isolation

**986.** MoC The nurse is caring for the hospitalized 60-year-old client who emigrated from Asia. Which statement, if made by the client, correctly reflects cultural beliefs and should alert the nurse that intervention is needed?

1. "Since 60 is considered old age, I retired as expected. I'm now worried about insurance."
2. "Value is on youth and beauty; so little attention is paid to problems of the elderly."
3. "Fathers are expected to continue to contribute financially even for their adult children."
4. "Grandchildren are raised by the grandparents until school age, so we have a full house."

**987.** The nurse is caring for the chronically ill middle-aged adult who has had numerous hospitalizations. Which behaviors may interfere with the client's achievement of the developmental task associated with middle adulthood? **Select all that apply.**

1. Writes thank-you notes to friends
2. Stays at home and refuses visitors
3. Self-absorbed in own psychological needs
4. Attempts to perform own personal cares
5. Continually relays feelings of inadequacy

**988.** The nurse plans to teach the client progressive muscle relaxation. Prioritize the steps that the nurse should teach to correctly perform progressive muscle relaxation.

1. Relax the feet, imagining the tension flowing out with each exhalation.
2. Lie down in a quiet place where you are undisturbed.
3. Contract the muscles of your feet first as you inhale and hold the contraction briefly.
4. Relax your body, allowing it to feel heavy.
5. Lie still for a few minutes after the contraction and relaxation of all muscles.
6. Imagine the tension flowing out with each breath you take.
7. Move up the body, contracting then relaxing each muscle.

Answer: _____

**989.** MoC The nurse is reviewing a laboratory report for a 61-year-old client. Which finding is **most** important for the nurse to address with the HCP?

1. Total cholesterol 180 mg/dL; was 140 at age 50
2. Erythrocyte sedimentation rate (ESR) increased
3. Alkaline phosphatase increased
4. AST, ALT, and serum bilirubin increased

**990.** The 66-year-old client recently retired after working 30 years as a bank manager. Which statement to the nurse during a clinic visit **best** suggests that the client is achieving the developmental stage of "integrity versus despair"?

1. "Now that I have some free time, I want to treat my wife to a trip to Hawaii."
2. "I seem to be staying in bed longer and longer each day. There isn't a reason to get up now."
3. "I am noticing the little aches and pains more; before I was just too busy to notice them."
4. "I get calls a few times a week for advice; my coworkers still value my suggestions."

**991.** The nurse completes teaching for the 80-year-old female client. Which statement made by the client indicates further teaching is needed?

1. "Instead of using sodium seasonings, I plan to try one with herbs and lemon."
2. "Although I find my lavender-scented hand cream relaxing, I should not use it."
3. "I should place a towel on the floor outside my shower so I don't slip when getting out."
4. "Rather than relying on laxatives, I should increase my intake of fruits and vegetables."

**992.** The 87-year-old hospitalized client is noted to have normal skin changes of senile purpura, but no other skin abnormalities. When assessing the client, which skin change illustrated should the nurse expect to find?

1.

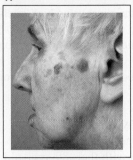

2.

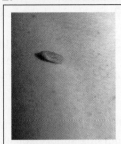

3.

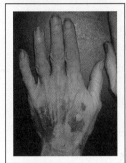

4.

**993.** The nurse overhears a person say, "I'm having a senior moment because I forgot ..." How should the nurse interpret this statement?

1. This phrase is a comical statement without age bias and is acceptable to others.
2. This phrase is a stereotypical reference to older adults that can be termed ageism.
3. This phrase admits that the older adult's ability to learn new information is limited.
4. This phrase recognizes that all older adults have short- and long-term memory issues.

**994.** When the office nurse completes height measurement for the 72-year-old female, the client says that she lost half an inch. Which explanation by the nurse is **most** accurate?

1. "As we age, we lose muscle mass."
2. "Bone loss is due to lack of exercise."
3. "As we age, we lose knee and hip cartilage."
4. "The vertebral column shortens with aging."

**995.** A 72-year-old woman reports she is sexually active. It is **most** important for the nurse to follow up by asking which question?

1. "Can you tell me more about your sexual partners?"
2. "Have you tried artificial water-based lubricants?"
3. "Are any medications having any drying effects?"
4. "Do you need to use different sexual positions?"

**996.** **PHARM** The nurse is interviewing a family member of the hospitalized 90-year-old client to assess for common problems associated with an increased risk for falling. Which questions should the nurse ask? **Select all that apply.**

1. "Has your mother fallen within the past year?"
2. "Has your mother had her annual influenza vaccine?"
3. "When was the last time your mother took a pain pill?"
4. "Does your mother have any problems with urination?"
5. "Does your mother have difficulty falling asleep at night?"

**997.** The nurse is teaching newly hired NAs in a long-term care facility. What information about skin care for older adults should the nurse emphasize?

1. Avoid skin products purchased for the resident by family that contain alcohol.
2. Apply perfumed skin lotions after the resident's bath when the skin is still moist.
3. When taking residents outdoors, apply sunscreen with a sun protection factor of 8.
4. Apply a strong detergent to clothing with food stains before sending to laundry.

**998.** **MoC** The nurse manager is observing care for the older adult client. Which observations require the nurse manager to intervene because it increases the client's risk for developing skin breakdown? **Select all that apply.**

1. The NA applies a perfumed lotion to the client's skin.
2. Two NAs are elevating the client's heels off the bed.
3. A family member brings the client custard from home.
4. The nurse applies an alcohol-based hand wash to the client's hands.
5. The nurse tells the client to push with the heels to move up in bed.

**999.** CJ The nurse walks into a room after the NA has helped to reposition the client (see illustration). The nurse identifies five safety concerns that increase the client's risk for a fall. Place an X on each item that poses a safety concern identified by the nurse.

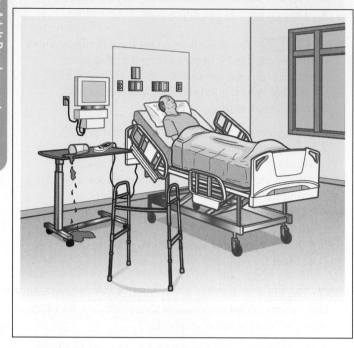

**1000.** The nurse is assessing the older adult client experiencing problems sleeping. Which statements, if made by the client, indicate that the client may benefit from teaching? **Select all that apply.**

1. "I am so tired that I need to take a nap in the middle of the day."
2. "My routine includes a glass of warm chocolate milk at bedtime."
3. "I installed room-darkening shades after my doctor advised these."
4. "I'm in my bed a lot; it is the most comfortable place in my home."
5. "I often take my pain pill for my leg pain just before going to bed."

**1001.** MoC The nurse is admitting the older adult client to a nursing home. Which is the nurse's **best** approach when obtaining information during the admission interview?

1. Direct questions to the family member accompanying the client.
2. Speak clearly and slowly to the client using high-pitched vocal tones.
3. Take the client and family members to a private room without distractions.
4. Speak to the client loudly about familiar topics before asking questions.

**1002.** MoC The client's family approaches the nursing supervisor with a complaint about the NA's inappropriate communication with their 89-year-old father. When evaluating the NA's communication, which statements does the nurse determine **most** likely caused the family's complaint? **Select all that apply.**

1. "Are you ready for the nurse to give you your medicine?"
2. "Would you like to go to breakfast now, Grandpa?"
3. "Would you prefer to wear the brown socks today?"
4. "Your family will be visiting today. Isn't that nice?"
5. "Honey, this is your bath day. Are you ready to go?"

**1003.** The older adult client is experiencing relocation stress after being admitted to a nursing home. Which intervention is **best** for the nurse to implement?

1. Ask family members to explore placing the client in another nursing home.
2. Change the client's room every week until a compatible roommate is found.
3. Place the client's favorite items, such as a family picture, at the client's bedside.
4. Ask that family members avoid talking to the client about being in the nursing home.

**1004.** MoC The nurse observes the NA providing a stuffed animal to the hospitalized older adult client who is experiencing delirium. Which action by the nurse is **most** appropriate?

1. Reprimand the NA for treating the client like a child.
2. Remove the stuffed animal before anyone else sees it.
3. Report the NA's action to the unit's nurse manager.
4. Thank the NA for providing it for the client's fidgeting.

**1005.** The home health nurse suspects elder mistreatment of the 93-year-old client by the live-in caregiver. Which findings support the nurse's conclusion? **Select all that apply.**

1. The client has urine burns.
2. The client has wrist bruises.
3. The client states that there have been some unexplained financial expenditures.
4. The client is more talkative than during previous home visits.
5. The smell of alcohol is noted on the live-in caregiver's breath.

**1006.** During a nursing home visit, the son notices multiple healing bruises on his father's arms and legs and calls a friend who is a nurse. Which **initial** recommendations should the nurse provide to the son? **Select all that apply.**

1. "Ask your father how the bruises occurred and whether he was abused."
2. "Contact Adult Protective Services immediately to report the abuse."
3. "Verify with the nursing staff whether your father is on anticoagulants."
4. "Inform the agency's nursing supervisor that your father is being abused."
5. "Contact the state ombudsman who can help you make an anonymous report."

**1007.** The nurse assesses the 84-year-old client during a routine health examination. Which finding should the nurse plan to investigate **first?**

1. Decreased force of cough
2. Impaired swallowing
3. Urine light yellow in color
4. Height decreased by one-half inch

**1008.** MoC The experienced nurse is observing the new nurse recommend screening tests to the 80-year-old female client. Which recommendation made by the new nurse should the experienced nurse correct?

1. Hearing screen annually
2. Colonoscopy every 10 years
3. Pneumococcal vaccine annually
4. Mammogram every 1 to 2 years

**INSTRUCTIONS:** The clinic nurse is reviewing the client's medical record. Use the information provided to answer Questions 1009, 1010, and 1011.

| Client | 62-year-old African American female |
| --- | --- |
| Allergies | Pollen (hay fever); no known drug allergies |
| Medical History | Graves' disease; depression; osteoporosis; hay fever |
| Past Surgical Procedures | Total abdominal hysterectomy with bilateral S&O at age 45 |
| Current Vital Signs | BP 96/64; pulse 118; respirations 20; oral temperature 98.8°F (37.1°C); wt. 110 lbs (8 lb weight loss in last 3 months); BMI 19 |
| Significant Assessment Data | *Neurologic:* Alert & oriented; responds appropriately, clearly to questions *Fatigue:* Tired a lot; states does not go out much, but able to get around the house *Skin:* Paper thin *Psychosocial:* Denies psychological issues |
| Medications | *Aspirin* 75 mg oral taken daily for past 4 years *Budesonide* nostril spray bid taken daily for past 10 years *Escitalopram* 5 mg oral taken daily for past 7 months *Levothyroxine* 100 mcg oral taken daily for last 5 years after treatment for Graves' disease *Multivitamin* 1 tab oral taken daily for many years |
| Serum Laboratory Results | *TSH:* 3.75 UIU/mL (range = 0.47–5.00 UIU/mL) *Free T4*: 1.0 ng/dL (range = 0.7–2.0 ng/dL) |
| Radiologic Results | *Bone Density Scan:* 10 years ago; T-score of –1.0 signifying osteopenia |

**1009.** `CJ` `PHARM` `MoC` Which medication is **most** important for the nurse to bring to the attention of the HCP because it may have contributed to the client's osteoporosis? Write your answer in the box provided.

```



```

**1010.** `CJ` `MoC` The nurse consults the HCP about scheduling another bone density scan. Which risk factors influenced the nurse's recommendation? **Select all that apply.**

1. Hyperthyroidism
2. Postmenopausal
3. Overweight
4. African American
5. 62-year-old female

**1011.** `CJ` The nurse completes the Geriatric Mini Nutrition Assessment. What score should the nurse assign for this client?

_____ (Record your answer as a whole number.)

| Geriatric Mini Nutrition Assessment | Score |
|---|---|
| Has food intake declined over the past 3 months due to loss of appetite, digestive problems, or chewing or swallowing difficulties? <br> 0 = severe loss of appetite <br> 1 = moderate 2 = no loss | |
| Weight loss during past 3 months <br> 0 = >3 kg 1 = unknown 2 = 1–3 kg <br> 3 = no weight loss | |
| Mobility <br> 0 = bed- or chair-bound 1 = able to get out of bed/chair but does not go out 2 = goes out | |
| Psychological stress or acute disease in past 3 months <br> 0 = yes 2 = no | |
| Neuropsychological problems <br> 0 = severe dementia or depression <br> 1 = mild dementia 2 = no psychological problems | |
| BMI <br> 0 = <19   1 = 19–20.9   2 = 21–22.9 <br> 3 = 23 or more | |
| Score (max. 14): 12 or more = normal; 11 or less = possible malnutrition, continue assessing | |

Source: Rubenstein, 2001.

# Answers and Rationales

## 977. ANSWER: 2

1. Adjusting to physiological changes is a developmental task of middle age.
2. **The client is attempting to perform self-care and to demonstrate the ability to be self-sufficient and independent from other adults.**
3. Industry is one of Erikson's developmental tasks, not Havighurst's. Industry versus inferiority occurs from ages 6 to 12 years.
4. Integrity is one of Erikson's developmental tasks, not Havighurst's. Integrity versus despair occurs at 65 years and older.

▶ *Test-taking Tip: Narrow the options by eliminating those pertaining to Erikson's developmental tasks. Of the two remaining options, focus on the age of the client.*

Content Area: Adult; Concept: Promoting Health; Integrated Processes: Nursing Process: Analysis; Client Needs: Health Promotion and Maintenance; Cognitive Level: Knowledge [Remembering]

## 978. ANSWER: 2

1. Strenuous physical activity does not cause lordosis (excessive inward curvature of the spine in the lower back). Lordosis is common in children before age 5.
2. **Females who participate in strenuous physical activities are at risk for eating disorders.**
3. An increase in muscle mass is expected with physical activity; thus it would not be the most important assessment.
4. Delayed menses, not excessive bleeding, would be a concern with strenuous physical activity.

▶ *Test-taking Tip: Note the key phrase "most important." You need to consider the risks associated with participating in strenuous physical activities many hours daily and why a female young adult might participate in these.*

Content Area: Adult; Concept: Promoting Health; Assessment; Integrated Processes: Nursing Process: Assessment; Client Needs: Health Promotion and Maintenance; Cognitive Level: Application [Applying]

## 979. ANSWER: 3

1. Illustration A is pectus excavatum, or funnel chest, caused by sternal retraction.
2. Illustration B is pectus carinatum, or pigeon breast, with sternal bulging.
3. **The normal adult chest has an anteroposterior-to-lateral ratio of approximately 1:2 and a costal angle less than 90 degrees. There should be no sternal or intercostal retractions or bulging at rest.**
4. Illustration D is barrel chest with increased anteroposterior diameter of the chest, with near-parallel rib sloping and a costal angle greater than 90 degrees. Barrel chest occurs with COPD.

▶ *Test-taking Tip: Note that the illustration shows four chest curvatures. You can easily eliminate both extremes and then decide between the two middle illustrations.*

Content Area: Adult; Concept: Promoting Health; Assessment; Integrated Processes: Nursing Process: Assessment; Client Needs: Health Promotion and Maintenance; Cognitive Level: Application [Applying]

## 980. ANSWER: 1, 2, 4, 5

1. **The nurse should ask about pets. Pets can enhance mental well-being and promote responsibility.**
2. **The nurse should ask about sleep. Insufficient amounts of sleep and rest can decrease coping and impair the immune system.**
3. Asking for the date of the last bowel movement relates to physiological functions.
4. **The nurse should ask about alcohol use. Regular consumption of three or more alcoholic drinks a day increases the risk of hypertension and decreases immune competence.**
5. **The nurse should ask about sexual activity. Multiple sex partners and anal sex are risk factors for STIs and HIV.**

▶ *Test-taking Tip: Focus on the key word "psychosocial" and eliminate any options that relate to only physiological functioning.*

Content Area: Adult; Concept: Promoting Health; Integrated Processes: Nursing Process: Assessment; Client Needs: Health Promotion and Maintenance; Psychosocial Integrity; Cognitive Level: Analysis [Analyzing]

## 981. ANSWER: 2

1. A young adult is not in need of constant accompaniment of a parent and may find this intrusive.
2. **To enhance coping, the nurse should focus on the developmental needs of a young adult, which include interaction with peers. Finding ways to help the client communicate with friends, such as using a cell phone or the Internet, may assist in dealing with the stress of the hospitalization and trauma.**
3. The client's behavior does not indicate depression.
4. Reinforcing information focuses on the injuries and self-care and not on the emotional needs of the client for stress management.

▶ *Test-taking Tip: Life span development is an important aspect of coping with hospitalization. Only Option 2 focuses on the developmental needs of a young adult.*

Content Area: Adult; Concept: Stress; Integrated Processes: Caring; Nursing Process: Implementation; Client Needs: Psychosocial Integrity; Cognitive Level: Application [Applying]

## 982. ANSWER: 3

1. Making the workplace a better place to work suggests that the client has an interest in future generations and is in the stage of generativity.
2. Volunteering shows interest in others and in making a contribution to the community; it is in the stage of generativity.
3. **Having a self-focus and displaying a disinterest in the activities of others suggest self-absorption and an inability to play a role in the development of the next generation; this can result in stagnation.**
4. Pictures showing the client involved with the grandchildren demonstrate the client's interest in future generations and the stage of generativity.

♦ *Test-taking Tip: According to Erik Erikson's psychosocial development theory, middle-aged adults achieve generativity by contributing to future generations through parenthood, teaching, community involvement, or contributing to positive changes that benefit others. Three options are similar, and one is different. Often the option that is different is the answer.*

**Content Area:** Adult; **Concept:** Promoting Health; **Integrated Processes:** Nursing Process: Analysis; **Client Needs:** Health Promotion and Maintenance; **Cognitive Level:** Analysis [Analyzing]

## 983. ANSWER: 3

1. Although muscle is replaced by adipose tissue as a person ages, a weight gain of 20 lb in a year is excessive.
2. Tactile fremitus (the vibrations felt when the hand is held against the client's chest and the client is speaking) is a normal finding; it is decreased or absent with a pneumothorax.
3. **The nurse should expect that the middle-aged adult should be able to focus on a mental task such as subtraction.**
4. Percussion that indicates the heart is enlarged indicates that a medical problem has occurred since the last examination. If no disease is present, the heart stays the same size during middle age.

♦ *Test-taking Tip: You should be eliminating abnormal findings on assessment of a middle-aged adult.*

**Content Area:** Adult; **Concept:** Promoting Health; Assessment; **Integrated Processes:** Nursing Process: Assessment; **Client Needs:** Health Promotion and Maintenance; **Cognitive Level:** Comprehension [Understanding]

## 984. ANSWER: 2, 5

1. Sweat gland activity decreases, not increases, with aging.
2. **Visual acuity declines in middle-aged adults, often by the late 40s, especially near vision.**
3. Weight gain, and not weight loss, occurs due to a slowing of metabolism occurring with aging.
4. Sebaceous gland activity decreases, not increases, with aging.
5. **Hormonal changes result in menopause, most commonly between ages 40 and 55 years.**

♦ *Test-taking Tip: Aging is associated with a decline in many physiological processes. Thus focus on options that show a decline when selecting the answers.*

**Content Area:** Adult; **Concept:** Promoting Health; **Integrated Processes:** Nursing Process: Assessment; **Client Needs:** Health Promotion and Maintenance; **Cognitive Level:** Analysis [Analyzing]

## 985. ANSWER: 3

1. "Industry versus inferiority" is the developmental stage for the school-age child, 6 to 12 years.
2. "Initiative versus guilt" is the developmental stage for the preschool-age child, 3 to 5 years.
3. **The central task of adulthood is "generativity versus stagnation." The client has indicators of negative resolution of this developmental stage.**
4. "Intimacy versus isolation" is the developmental task for young adulthood, 18 to 25 years.

♦ *Test-taking Tip: Use cues of inactivity in the stem and associate these with a word in one of the options.*

**Content Area:** Adult; **Concept:** Promoting Health; **Integrated Processes:** Nursing Process: Analysis; **Client Needs:** Health Promotion and Maintenance; **Cognitive Level:** Analysis [Analyzing]

## 986. MoC ANSWER: 1

1. **In some cultures, 60 is considered old age, and elders are expected to retire. At a retirement age of 60, the client does not yet qualify for Medicare insurance coverage in the United States. A social worker consult may be needed to discuss insurance options.**
2. Some cultures focus on youth and beauty, but this is of lesser importance than the financial needs of the client.
3. Giving money to adult children is not an expectation of any one culture specifically.
4. In some cultures grandchildren are raised by grandparents, and they offer economic support, but there is no indication that the client cannot meet the financial obligations.

♦ *Test-taking Tip: You need to consider when to consult a social worker due to financial concerns.*

**Content Area:** Adult; **Concept:** Diversity; **Integrated Processes:** Nursing Process: Analysis; Culture and Spirituality; **Client Needs:** Safe and Effective Care Environment: Management of Care; **Cognitive Level:** Analysis [Analyzing]

## 987. ANSWER: 2, 3, 5

1. Writing thank-you notes to friends indicates that the client is trying to maintain social relationships, which is one of the developmental tasks of middle adulthood.
2. **Stays at home and refuses visitors may interfere with maintaining social relationships, which is one of the developmental tasks of middle adulthood.**
3. **Self-absorption may interfere with maintaining social relationships, which is one of the developmental tasks of middle adulthood.**

4. Attempting to perform self-care activities shows initiative and interest in improving one's health and will not interfere with the developmental tasks associated with middle adulthood.

5. **Continually relaying feelings of inadequacy may interfere with the client's ability to improve his or her health status and to resume a career. This may interfere with achieving the developmental tasks of middle adulthood.**

▸ *Test-taking Tip: The key word is "interfere." Thus you should select options that have a negative undertone.*

Content Area: Adult; Concept: Promoting Health; Integrated Processes: Nursing Process: Analysis; Client Needs: Health Promotion and Maintenance; Cognitive Level: Analysis [Analyzing]

## 988. ANSWER: 2, 4, 6, 3, 1, 7, 5

2. **Lie down in a quiet place where you are undisturbed. A quiet place is needed so the client can focus on the muscle relaxation techniques.**

4. **Relax your body, allowing it to feel heavy. The feeling of heaviness before beginning muscle tension and relaxation helps the client to monitor the state of muscle contraction and relaxation as the steps progress.**

6. **Imagine the tension flowing out with each breath you take. Focusing on breathing allows for further muscle relaxation.**

3. **Contract the muscles of your feet first as you inhale and hold the contraction briefly. Tensing the muscles in a particular area should occur before relaxation of those muscles.**

1. **Relax the feet, imagining the tension flowing out with each exhalation. Relaxation should occur after muscle tension.**

7. **Move up the body, contracting then relaxing each muscle. Progressive muscle relaxation can occur from the feet up or the head down. In this scenario, the feet were first.**

5. **Lie still for a few minutes after the contraction and relaxation of all muscles. The last step is to lie still so the person can monitor what muscles feel like when they are relaxed after performing the steps.**

▸ *Test-taking Tip: Read all options first. You should note that the progressive muscle relaxation is moving up the body. Options 2 and 5 include "lie" as the first word; one must be first and the other last.*

Content Area: Adult; Concept: Nursing Roles; Promoting Health; Stress; Integrated Processes: Teaching/Learning; Client Needs: Psychosocial Integrity; Physiological Integrity: Basic Care and Comfort; Cognitive Level: Synthesis [Creating]

## 989. MoC ANSWER: 4

1. Total cholesterol increases by 30 to 40 mg/dL with aging. This value is still less than 200 mg/dL.

2. ESR increases with aging for unknown reasons.

3. Alkaline phosphatase is an enzyme found throughout the body that increases with aging.

4. **It is most important for the nurse to notify the HCP if liver function tests are elevated. AST, ALT, and serum bilirubin are liver function tests that are unchanged with age.**

▸ *Test-taking Tip: Certain laboratory values increase or decrease with aging, but liver function tests, coagulation tests, ABG, renal function tests (serum creatinine), thyroid function test (T4), and completed blood count (Hct, Hgb, erythrocytes) are unchanged with age.*

Content Area: Adult; Concept: Management; Integrated Processes: Nursing Process: Implementation; Client Needs: Safe and Effective Care Environment: Management of Care; Cognitive Level: Analysis [Analyzing]

## 990. ANSWER: 4

1. Making plans to stay active in retirement reflects positive resolution of generativity versus stagnation and shows concern for others.

2. Not having a reason to get out of bed indicates that the client is experiencing difficulty achieving the developmental stage of "integrity versus despair."

3. Staying busy and not focusing on physical issues are not reflective of any stage.

4. **"Integrity versus despair" is Erikson's stage of development from 65 years of age and older. Indicators of positive resolution include statements of acceptance of worth and uniqueness of one's own life.**

▸ *Test-taking Tip: Note the key word "best." Focus on the defining characteristics for a positive or negative resolution of the developmental stage integrity versus despair, which occurs from 65 years to death.*

Content Area: Adult; Concept: Promoting Health; Integrated Processes: Nursing Process: Evaluation; Communication and Documentation; Caring; Client Needs: Health Promotion and Maintenance; Psychosocial Integrity; Cognitive Level: Evaluation [Evaluating]

## 991. ANSWER: 3

1. Nonsodium seasonings such as herbs, garlic, and lemon are recommended to prevent hypertension.

2. Scented lotions increase skin irritation and the risk for skin breakdown; their use should be avoided in older adult clients.

3. **Placing a towel outside the shower on the floor can increase the client's risk for a fall. A slip-resistant mat should be used and the towel placed within reach without bending.**

4. Older adults have decreased GI motility, and laxatives can be overused by those who are constipated; roughage from fruits and vegetables will decrease constipation and the need for laxatives.

▸ *Test-taking Tip: The key phrase is "further teaching is needed." You should be selecting a statement that is incorrect. Use Maslow's Hierarchy of Needs to recognize the need for safety.*

Content Area: Adult; **Concept:** Nursing Roles; Safety; **Integrated Processes:** Teaching/Learning; **Client Needs:** Safe and Effective Care Environment: Safety and Infection Control; **Cognitive Level:** Application [Applying]

## 992. ANSWER: 3

1. Seborrheic keratosis is a benign pigmented lesion with a waxy surface on the face and trunk.
2. Acrochordon is a small, benign polyp growth also known as a skin tag.
3. **Senile purpura is characterized by areas of ecchymosis and petechiae found on the hands, arms, and legs caused by frail capillaries and decreased collagen support. It is a common skin lesion associated with aging.**
4. Urticaria is an abnormal lesion that can occur anywhere on the body from an allergic reaction.

▶ *Test-taking Tip: "Purpura" relates to vascular; thus eliminate Options 1 and 2. Eliminate Option 4 because it is an abnormal finding.*

Content Area: Adult; **Concept:** Skin Integrity; Assessment; **Integrated Processes:** Nursing Process: Assessment; **Client Needs:** Health Promotion and Maintenance; **Cognitive Level:** Application [Applying]

## 993. ANSWER: 2

1. The statement is biased against older adults.
2. **This statement is a form of ageism, which comprises the prejudices and stereotypes that are applied to older people and perpetuate negativism against them.**
3. In older adulthood, the processes of learning new information and recalling old information slow down somewhat, but the overall ability to learn and remember is not significantly affected in healthy older people.
4. Although short-term memory may decline with age, not all older adults are affected with short- and long-term memory loss.

▶ *Test-taking Tip: Focus on "interpret." Look for a nonbiased interpretative statement.*

Content Area: Adult; **Concept:** Communication; **Integrated Processes:** Nursing Process: Analysis; Culture/Spirituality; **Client Needs:** Health Promotion and Maintenance; Psychosocial Integrity; **Cognitive Level:** Analysis [Analyzing]

## 994. ANSWER: 4

1. Loss of muscle mass does not affect height.
2. Bone loss can be due to lack of exercise, but it can also result from aging. There is no indication that the client lacks exercise.
3. Although there is loss of cartilage in joints, this does not affect height.
4. **With aging, there is shortening and thinning of the vertebral column due to loss of water and bone density, causing compression resulting in decreased height.**

▶ *Test-taking Tip: Two options are potentially correct, but one is better than the other. Avoid reading into the question stem.*

Content Area: Adult; **Concept:** Nursing Roles; Promoting Health; **Integrated Processes:** Teaching/Learning; **Client Needs:** Physiological Integrity: Physiological Adaptation; **Cognitive Level:** Application [Applying]

## 995. ANSWER: 1

1. **It is important to assess the types of sexual relationships in which the client is engaged and whether the relationship is monogamous. The incidence of HIV and AIDS infection and other STIs is rising among older adults.**
2. Water-based lubricants can decrease discomfort, but it is more important to assess the risk for transmission of STIs.
3. Some medications dry vaginal secretions, but it is more important to assess the risk for transmission of STIs.
4. Different sexual positions, aids to increase stimulation, and lubrication can all enhance sexual activity and comfort, but it is more important to assess the risk for transmission of STIs.

▶ *Test-taking Tip: The key words "most important" indicate that more than one response may be correct and that you will need to determine which question is the most important to ask. Focus on using therapeutic communication techniques to elicit information other than a yes-or-no response.*

Content Area: Adult; **Concept:** Promoting Health; **Integrated Processes:** Nursing Process: Assessment; **Client Needs:** Health Promotion and Maintenance; **Cognitive Level:** Application [Applying]

## 996. PHARM ANSWER: 1, 3, 4, 5

1. **Asking if the client has fallen in the last year will help determine if the client has a history of falls and the risk level for a fall.**
2. Having an influenza vaccination is not a problem that can increase the client's risk for falling.
3. **Analgesics can contribute to dizziness and increase the risk for falling.**
4. **Asking about elimination will help determine if the client has problems with incontinence or urgency. Needing to hurriedly use the bathroom can increase the risk for falling.**
5. **Asking about the client's nighttime sleep will help determine if the client has any sleep disorders that could contribute to night-time wandering and the risk for falling.**

▶ *Test-taking Tip: The key word is "falling." All options are similar except one. With multiple-response items, similar options are likely to be the answers.*

Content Area: Adult; **Concept:** Safety; **Integrated Processes:** Nursing Process: Assessment; **Client Needs:** Safe and Effective Care Environment: Safety and Infection Control; Physiological Integrity: Pharmacological and Parenteral Therapies; **Cognitive Level:** Application [Applying]

**997. ANSWER: 1**

1. **The nurse should emphasize avoiding skin products containing alcohol, which is drying to the skin. Age-related skin changes of the elderly include dry and fragile skin.**
2. Perfume-free (not perfumed) skin lotions should be used because perfumed lotions increase skin irritation.
3. Sunscreen should have an SPF of 15 (not an SPF of 8) or greater to protect against sunburn.
4. Strong laundry detergents should be avoided (not used) because of skin irritation and the risk of skin breakdown.

♦ *Test-taking Tip: If unsure, note the key word "avoid" in Option 1, which is an opposite action as compared to the other options. Often the option that is different is the answer.*

**Content Area:** Adult; **Concept:** Safety; **Integrated Processes:** Teaching/Learning; **Client Needs:** Health Promotion and Maintenance; **Cognitive Level:** Application [Applying]

**998. MoC ANSWER: 1, 4, 5**

1. **Perfumed lotion increases skin irritation and can lead to skin breakdown.**
2. Elevating the heels off the bed will reduce pressure on bony prominences and skin breakdown.
3. Adequate nutrition promotes tissue repair and maintains healthy tissues.
4. **Alcohol-based hand wash is drying and can increase skin irritation and lead to skin breakdown.**
5. **Using the heels to reposition in bed causes friction and sheer and increases the risk for skin breakdown.**

♦ *Test-taking Tip: Skin breakdown and pressure ulcers are major concerns among hospitalized older adults and those in nursing homes. Friction, sheer, alcohol-based products, and perfumed lotions all can cause skin irritation and can increase the risk for skin breakdown.*

**Content Area:** Adult; **Concept:** Skin Integrity; **Integrated Processes:** Nursing Process: Evaluation; **Client Needs:** Safe and Effective Care Environment: Management of Care; Safe and Effective Care Environment: Safety and Infection Control; **Cognitive Level:** Evaluation [Evaluating]

**999. CJ ANSWER:**

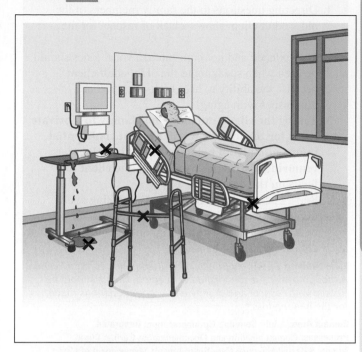

**A side rail left down, the bed left in high position, the bedside table positioned away from the client, the walker away from the client all increase the client's risk for a fall. Because the call light is out of reach, the client is unable to alert the nurse for help. Water on the floor increases the risk for slipping.**

♦ *Test-taking Tip: Five items should be identified. Think about the safety of the client and others who enter the client's room.*

**Content Area:** Adult; **Concept:** Safety; **Integrated Processes:** Nursing Process: Analysis; **Client Needs:** Safe and Effective Care Environment: Safety and Infection Control; **Cognitive Level:** Application [Applying]

**1000. ANSWER: 1, 2, 4**

1. **The client with sleep problems could benefit from teaching because daytime napping can result in nighttime wakefulness.**
2. **The client with sleep problems could benefit from teaching because chocolate milk is a caffeinated beverage that can increase alertness and cause difficulty falling asleep.**
3. Reducing lighting decreases sensory stimulation and can help promote sleep.
4. **The client with sleep problems could benefit from teaching about using the bedroom only for sexual activity and sleeping.**
5. Taking analgesics at bedtime will prevent interruption of sleep from pain.

♦ *Test-taking Tip: The client experiencing sleep problems can benefit from teaching when either environmental factors or the client's actions can delay or interrupt sleep.*

**Content Area:** Adult; **Concept:** Nursing Roles; Sleep, Rest, and Activity; **Integrated Processes:** Teaching/Learning; **Client Needs:** Physiological Integrity: Basic Care and Comfort; **Cognitive Level:** Analysis [Analyzing]

## 1001. MoC ANSWER: 3

1. Directing questions to the family members of the older adult client shows a lack of respect for the client.
2. Low-pitched and not high-pitched vocal tones should be used when speaking to the older adult client because the ability to hear high-pitched tones diminishes with aging.
3. **Taking the client and his or her family to a private room for the interview will prevent confidential information from being overhead by others; removing distractions will allow the client to focus on the questions.**
4. Some clients may be put at ease by talking about familiar topics first, but not everyone. Although hearing diminishes with aging, not all older adult clients are hard of hearing.

▸ *Test-taking Tip: Apply principles of therapeutic communication. Although hearing is diminished with aging, clients should be treated with respect and dignity and accommodations made for the hearing loss.*

Content Area: Adult; Concept: Communication; Integrated Processes: Communication and Documentation; Caring; Client Needs: Safe and Effective Care Environment: Management of Care; Cognitive Level: Application [Applying]

## 1002. MoC ANSWER: 2, 4, 5

1. Asking the client questions is appropriate communication.
2. **"Grandpa" is a diminutive, or an inappropriate intimate term of endearment, implying a parent–child relationship.**
3. Asking the client questions is appropriate communication.
4. **The statement "Isn't that nice?" uses a cliché that can block the feelings and thoughts of the client. It could be interpreted as infantilizing the client.**
5. **"Honey" is a diminutive, or an inappropriate intimate term of endearment.**

▸ *Test-taking Tip: Note the key words "inappropriate communication." Select options that use inappropriate intimate terms of endearment or that are diminutive.*

Content Area: Adult; Concept: Communication; Management; Integrated Processes: Communication and Documentation; Client Needs: Safe and Effective Care Environment: Management of Care; Psychosocial Integrity; Cognitive Level: Analysis [Analyzing]

## 1003. ANSWER: 3

1. Moving to another nursing home may increase the client's stress.
2. There is no indication that the client has an incompatible roommate. Changing rooms frequently can increase the client's stress.
3. **Having familiar objects nearby can help to minimize the effects of relocation stress.**
4. Avoiding talking about the nursing home placement may increase the client's stress.

▸ *Test-taking Tip: Relocation stress syndrome is a physical and emotional distress experienced by a person when moving from one setting to another. Interventions should be implemented to minimize the effects of relocation stress.*

Content Area: Adult; Concept: Stress; Integrated Processes: Nursing Process: Implementation; Client Needs: Psychosocial Integrity; Cognitive Level: Application [Applying]

## 1004. MoC ANSWER: 4

1. Providing an object to the delirious client has been shown to reduce the incidence of accidental removal of IV lines or drains by the client; the NA should not be reprimanded.
2. The stuffed animal should not be removed; it may be comforting and beneficial to the delirious client.
3. It is unnecessary to report the NA's actions to the nurse manager because providing a stuffed animal may be beneficial to the delirious client.
4. **Having a stuffed animal may occupy the hands and fingers of the delirious client and prevent the client's accidental removal of lines or drains. Thanking the NA is appropriate.**

▸ *Test-taking Tip: Older adults may experience confusion and acute delirium when hospitalized. Measures should be implemented that protect the client from self-harm.*

Content Area: Adult; Concept: Safety; Cognition; Management; Integrated Processes: Nursing Process: Implementation; Client Needs: Safe and Effective Care Environment: Management of Care; Cognitive Level: Analysis [Analyzing]

## 1005. ANSWER: 1, 2, 3, 5

1. **Urine burns suggest caregiver neglect by not assisting the client to the toilet or changing the client if incontinent.**
2. **Wrist bruises suggest physical abuse that may be caused by physically restraining the client.**
3. **Unexplained financial expenditures suggest financial exploitation and use of funds for personal use by the caregiver.**
4. The more withdrawn client, rather than the more talkative one, suggests psychological or emotional abuse.
5. **Substance abuse is an abuser characteristic.**

▸ *Test-taking Tip: Elder mistreatment is an umbrella term for abuse, exploitation, and neglect.*

Content Area: Adult; Concept: Violence; Safety; Integrated Processes: Nursing Process: Analysis; Client Needs: Psychosocial Integrity; Physiological Integrity: Physiological Adaptation; Cognitive Level: Analysis [Analyzing]

## 1006. ANSWER: 1, 3

1. **More information is needed about the healing bruises before abuse should be considered.**
2. Contacting Adult Protective Services is an appropriate recommendation when abuse is suspected. More information is needed before considering if these are due to abuse.
3. **The nurse should initially recommend exploring whether the client is receiving any anticoagulants such as warfarin or aspirin. Their use, frequent blood draws, and bumping of the arms and legs can cause the client to bruise easily.**
4. Nurses are mandatory reporters and are required to report allegations and/or suspicions of abuse, but more information is needed before considering if these are due to abuse.
5. Although a report to the state ombudsman will be investigated, more information is needed before considering if the bruises are due to abuse.

▶ **Test-taking Tip:** *Do not read into the question. The scenario does not indicate the size or number of bruises; nor does it provide any other information that might indicate abuse. Use the nursing process step of assessment to collect more information. Allegations of abuse should not be made based on casual suspicion but on solid evidence.*

**Content Area:** Adult; **Concept:** Safety; Medication; **Integrated Processes:** Nursing Process: Implementation; **Client Needs:** Psychosocial Integrity; **Cognitive Level:** Application [Applying]

## 1007. ANSWER: 2

1. Decreased force of cough is an age-related change. Although important to investigate further to rule out an underlying respiratory condition, this is not priority.
2. **Gastric motility decreases with aging, but impaired swallowing can be due to other conditions and increases the client's risk for aspiration. This should be investigated first.**
3. Decreased urine concentration is an age-related change. Although important to investigate further to rule out an underlying renal condition, this is not priority.
4. Height decreases with aging. Although important to investigate further to rule out an underlying medical condition, this is not priority.

▶ **Test-taking Tip:** *Use the ABC's to establish the finding that should be further investigated first. Airway compromise is priority.*

**Content Area:** Adult; **Concept:** Promoting Health; **Integrated Processes:** Nursing Process: Planning; **Client Needs:** Physiological Integrity: Reduction of Risk Potential; **Cognitive Level:** Analysis [Analyzing]

## 1008. MoC ANSWER: 3

1. Hearing screen should be performed annually for older adults because hearing loss occurs with aging.

2. Colonoscopy should be performed every 10 years unless the client is at high risk; there is no indication of this in the question stem.
3. **Pneumococcal vaccine is administered at age 65 and every 10 years, not annually. An influenza vaccine should be administered annually.**
4. Mammogram should be performed every 1 to 2 years to rule out the presence of a breast mass.

▶ **Test-taking Tip:** *When supervising the new nurse, the experienced nurse should correct incorrect information provided by the new nurse. A pneumococcal and an influenza vaccine are different.*

**Content Area:** Adult; **Concept:** Promoting Health; **Integrated Processes:** Nursing Process: Evaluation; **Client Needs:** Safe and Effective Care Environment: Management of Care; **Cognitive Level:** Synthesis [Creating]

## 1009. MoC PHARM CJ ANSWER:

> **Budesonide (Pulmicort) nasal spray**

**Long-term use of corticosteroids, such as budesonide (Pulmicort), should be brought to the attention of the HCP because it is a risk factor for osteoporosis development.**

Aspirin, used for its cardioprotective effect, **has not been identified to cause bone loss (osteoporosis).**

Escitalopram (Lexapro), an antidepressant, **has not been identified to cause bone loss (osteoporosis).**

Having thyroid disease can be a contributing factor to osteoporosis, but the client is receiving treatment with levothyroxine. The laboratory data indicate that the dose is therapeutic.

**The calcium and vitamin D supplement in multivitamins is helpful in preventing bone loss.**

▶ **Test-taking Tip:** *The use of corticosteroids is a risk factor for osteoporosis.*

**Content Area:** Adult; **Concept:** Medication; Management; **Integrated Processes:** Nursing Process: Analysis; **Client Needs:** Safe and Effective Care Environment: Management of Care; Physiological Integrity: Pharmacological and Parenteral Therapies; **Cognitive Level:** Analysis [Analyzing]

## 1010. MoC CJ ANSWER: 1, 2, 5

1. **Too much thyroid hormone can cause bone loss.**
2. **Estrogen levels decrease at menopause; this decrease is one of the strongest risk factors for osteoporosis.**
3. The client has a low BMI and is underweight. Being overweight is a risk factor for osteoporosis and can contribute to the development of OA.

4. Major risk factors for osteoporosis include white or Asian race, not African American.

5. **Advancing age and being female are both risk factors for osteoporosis.**

▶ *Test-taking Tip:* You need to identify the risk factors for bone loss.

**Content Area:** Adult; **Concept:** Assessment; Management; Diversity; **Integrated Processes:** Nursing Process: Evaluation; Culture and Spirituality; **Client Needs:** Safe and Effective Care Environment: Management of Care; **Cognitive Level:** Evaluation [Evaluating]

**1011.** **CJ** **ANSWER: 4**

**The nurse should give a score of 4 on the Geriatric Mini Nutrition Assessment. Severe loss of appetite = 0; 8–lb (3.6 kg) weight loss during last 3 months is >3 kg = 0; able to get out of bed/chair but does not go out = 1; acute disease (cancer) in past 3 months = 0; no psychological problems = 2; and BMI 19 = 1.**

▶ *Test-taking Tip:* Carefully read the client's information in the situation. Remember to convert pounds to kilograms for weight loss (2.2 lb = 1 kg).

**Content Area:** Adult; **Concept:** Assessment; Safety; **Integrated Processes:** Nursing Process: Analysis; **Client Needs:** Physiological Integrity: Basic Care and Comfort; **Cognitive Level:** Analysis [Analyzing]

# Chapter Twenty-Four

# Cardiovascular Management

**1012.** The clinic nurse is teaching the client at risk for arteriosclerosis. The nurse should teach the client that the dietary therapy to decrease homocysteine levels includes eating foods rich in which nutrient?

1. Monosaturated fats
2. B complex vitamins
3. Vitamin C
4. Calcium

**1013.** The nurse is taking the client's BP at a screening clinic. Which statement demonstrates the client's awareness of having a risk factor for hypertension?

1. "My doctor told me my body mass index is 23 and my blood pressure is 118/70."
2. "I usually have a glass of wine to unwind when I come home from work."
3. "I plan to get my blood pressure checked more often, as I am African American."
4. "I have colds during the winter, so I plan to get the influenza vaccine every year."

**1014.** The nurse is assessing the dark-skinned client who has a perfusion problem. Which findings support the nurse's conclusion of cyanosis? **Select all that apply.**

1. Bluish appearing nail beds
2. Grayish-green skin tone
3. Blue color in the soles of the feet
4. Whitish color around the mouth
5. Yellow-colored oral mucous membranes
6. Grayish-colored conjunctivae

**1015.** PHARM The nurse has prepared medications for a 75-year-old client with hypertension. The nurse notes that the client has an elevated serum potassium level. Which medication is **most** important for the nurse to address with the HCP before administration?

1.

| **Lisinopril** |
| 40 mg Oral Tablet |
| Exp 10/21/2022 |
| ‖‖‖‖‖▌‖▌‖‖‖▌‖ |

2.

| **Metoprolol** |
| 25 mg Oral tablet |
| Exp 10/21/2022 |
| ‖‖‖‖‖▌‖▌‖‖‖▌‖ |

3.

| **Atorvastatin** |
| 20 mg Oral tablet |
| Exp 12/21/2022 |
| ‖‖‖‖‖▌‖▌‖‖‖▌‖ |

4.

| **Sertraline** |
| 25 mg Oral tablet |
| Exp 12/21/2022 |
| ‖‖‖‖‖▌‖▌‖‖‖▌‖ |

**1016.** The nurse completes discharge teaching for the client with chronic stage 2 hypertension. Which statement by the client indicates that teaching was effective?

1. "I will limit my intake of potassium."
2. "I will start a rigorous exercise program now."
3. "I will call my provider if my vision blurs."
4. "I will strive to maintain my BMI at 32."

**1017.** MoC The nurse is taking the BP on multiple clients. Which reading warrants the nurse notifying the HCP because the client's MAP is abnormal?

1. 94/60 mm Hg
2. 98/36 mm Hg
3. 110/50 mm Hg
4. 140/78 mm Hg

**1018.** The nurse is assessing the client. At which area should the nurse place the stethoscope to **best** auscultate the client's murmur associated with mitral regurgitation?

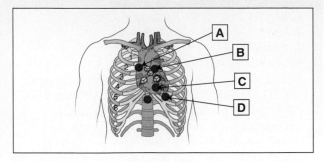

1. Line A
2. Line B
3. Line C
4. Line D

**1019.** The new nurse is experiencing difficulty auscultating the client's heart sounds and consults an experienced nurse. Which techniques should the experienced nurse recommend? **Select all that apply.**

1. Auscultate over the client's gown.
2. Auscultate from the left side of the client.
3. Ask the client to sit and lean forward.
4. Feel the radial pulse while listening to heart sounds.
5. Turn the client to the left side-lying position.

**1020.** MoC At 0745 hours, the nurse is informed by the HCP that a cardiac catheterization is to be completed on the client at 1400 hours. Which intervention should be the nurse's **priority**?

1. Place the client on nothing per mouth status.
2. Teach about the cardiac catheterization.
3. Start an intravenous infusion of 0.9% NaCl.
4. Witness the client's signature on the consent.

**1021.** The nurse completes teaching the client with a newly inserted ICD. Which statement, if made by the client, indicates that further teaching is needed?

1. "The ICD will give me a shock if my heart goes into ventricular fibrillation again."
2. "When I feel the first shock, my family should start CPR immediately and call 911."
3. "I'm afraid of my first shock; my friend stated his shock felt like a blow to the chest."
4. "Some states do not allow driving until there is a 6-month discharge-free period."

**1022.** MoC The nurse reviews the client's laboratory results exhibited. Which findings, indicative of an MI, should the nurse report to the HCP? Place an X on each laboratory finding indicative of an MI.

| Laboratory Tests | Client Results |
|---|---|
| SCr (0.4–1.4 mg/dL) | 1.8 |
| BUN (10–20 mg/dL) | 30 |
| Potassium (3.8–5.3 mEq/L) | 5.8 |
| Mg (1.7–2.2 mg/dL) | 1.6 |
| CK-MB (0–16 units/L) | 32 |
| Troponin T (cTnT) (0.0–0.4 ng/mL) | 34 |
| WBC (3.9–11.9 K/microL or mm³) | 14 |
| Platelets (Plt 179– 450 K/microL or mm³) | 175 |
| PT (9.2–11.9 sec) | 22 |
| INR (0.9–1.1 sec) | 2.2 |

**1023.** The client is admitted with an ACS. Which should be the nurse's **priority** assessment?

1. Pain
2. Blood pressure
3. Heart rate
4. Respiratory rate

**1024.** MoC The client with a left anterior descending (LAD) 90% blockage has crushing chest pain that is unrelieved by taking sublingual nitroglycerin. Which **most** concerning ECG finding should the nurse report to the HCP STAT?

1. Q waves
2. Flipped T waves
3. Peaked T waves
4. ST segment elevation

**1025.** MoC The nurse observes sinus tachycardia with new-onset ST segment elevation on the ECG monitor of the client reporting chest pain. Which should be the nurse's **priority** intervention?

1. Draw blood for cardiac enzymes STAT.
2. Call the cardiac catheterization laboratory.
3. Apply 1 inch of nitroglycerin paste topically.
4. Apply 4 liters of oxygen via nasal cannula.

**1026.** PHARM The nurse is to administer 40 mg of furosemide to the client. The prefilled syringe reads 100 mg/mL. How many milliliters should the nurse administer to the client?

_____ mL. (Record your answer rounded to the nearest tenth.)

**1027.** The nurse assesses the client returning from a coronary angiogram in which the femoral artery approach was used. The client's baseline BP during the procedure was 130/72 mm Hg, and the cardiac rhythm was sinus rhythm. Which finding should alert the nurse to a potential complication?

1. BP 154/78 mm Hg
2. Pedal pulses palpable at +1
3. Left groin soft to palpation with 1 cm ecchymotic area
4. Apical pulse 132 beats per minute (bpm) with an irregular–irregular rhythm

**1028.** **MoC** The client, returning from a coronary catheterization in which the femoral artery approach was used, sneezes. Which should be the nurse's **priority** intervention?

1. Palpate pedal pulses.
2. Measure vital signs.
3. Assess for urticaria.
4. Check the insertion site.

**1029.** **PHARM** The client being admitted has a new diagnosis of persistent atrial fibrillation with rapid ventricular response. The client has been in atrial fibrillation for more than 2 days and has had no previous cardiac problems. Which **initial** interventions should the nurse anticipate? **Select all that apply.**

1. Ablation of the AV node
2. Immediate cardioversion
3. Oxygen 2 liters per nasal cannula
4. Heparin IV infusion
5. Amiodarone IV infusion
6. Diltiazem IV infusion

**1030.** **MoC** **PHARM** The client is having sharp chest pains that radiate to the left shoulder and calls for the nurse. Which prescribed intervention should the nurse implement **first**?

1. STAT 12-lead electrocardiogram (ECG)
2. Oxygen 4 liters by nasal cannula
3. Nitroglycerin 0.4 mg sublingual
4. Morphine sulfate 2–4 mg IV prn

**1031.** The nurse obtains the client's cardiac monitor printout illustrated. What should be the nurse's interpretation of the client's rhythm?

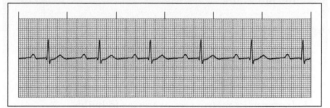

1. Atrial flutter
2. Atrial fibrillation
3. Sinus bradycardia
4. Sinus rhythm with premature atrial contractions (PACs)

**1032.** **PHARM** The client with atrial flutter is receiving a continuous infusion of 25,000 units of heparin in 500 mL of 5% dextrose at a rate of 12 mL per hour. The aPTT laboratory result is 92 seconds. According to the heparin infusion protocol, the nurse should administer the heparin infusion at a rate of how many mL per hour?

_____ mL/hr (Record your answer as a whole number.)

## Heparin Infusion Protocol Adjustment Table

| aPTT Results | Bolus Dose | Stop Infusion | Rate Change | Repeat aPTT |
| --- | --- | --- | --- | --- |
| Less than 50 | 5000 units | 0 minutes | +3 mL/hr | 6 hr |
| 50–59 | 0 | 0 minutes | +2 mL/hr | 6 hr |
| 60–85 | 0 | 0 minutes | No change | Next a.m. |
| 86–100 | 0 | 0 minutes | –1 mL/hr | Next a.m. |
| 101–120 | 0 | 30 minutes | –2 mL/hr | 6 hr |
| 120–150 | 0 | 60 minutes | –3 mL/hr | 6 hr |
| Greater than 150 | 0 | 60 minutes | –5 mL/hr | 6 hr |

**1033.** MoC The client arrives to the unit following insertion of a permanent pacemaker via the right subclavian vein approach. Which intervention should the nurse include in the client's plan of care to **best** prevent pacemaker lead dislodgement?

1. Inspect the incision for approximation and bleeding.
2. Prevent the right arm from going above shoulder level.
3. Assist the client with using a walker when out of bed.
4. Request a STAT chest x-ray upon return from the procedure.

**1034.** The nurse is teaching the client newly diagnosed with chronic stable angina. Which instructions on measures to prevent future angina should the nurse incorporate? **Select all that apply.**

1. Increase isometric arm exercises to build endurance.
2. Wear a facemask when outdoors in cold weather.
3. Take nitroglycerin before a stressful event even if pain-free.
4. Perform most exertional activities in the morning.
5. Take a daily laxative to avoid straining with bowel movements.
6. Discontinue use of all tobacco products if you use these.

**1035.** PHARM The nurse collects the following assessment data on the client who has no known health problems: BP 135/89 mm Hg; BMI 23; waist circumference 34 inches; serum creatinine 0.9 mg/dL; serum potassium 4.0 mEq/L; LDL cholesterol 200 mg/dL; HDL cholesterol 25 mg/dL; and triglycerides 180 mg/dL. Which intervention should the nurse anticipate?

1. A low-calorie regular diet
2. A statin antilipidemic medication
3. A thiazide diuretic medication
4. Low-salt, low-saturated-fat, low-potassium diet

**1036.** The nurse increases activity for the client diagnosed with ACS. Which client finding **best** supports that the client is not tolerating the activity?

1. Pulse rate increased by 15 beats per minute during activity
2. BP 130/86 mm Hg before activity; 108/66 mm Hg during activity
3. Increased dyspnea and diaphoresis relieved when sitting in a chair
4. A mean arterial pressure (MAP) of 80 following activity

**1037.** The nurse is assessing the client following an inferior-septal wall MI. Which potential complication should the nurse further explore when noting that the client has jugular venous distention (JVD) and ascites?

1. Left-sided heart failure
2. Pulmonic valve malfunction
3. Right-sided heart failure
4. Ruptured septum

**1038.** MoC The client newly diagnosed with HF has an ejection fraction of 20%. Which criteria should the nurse use to evaluate the client's readiness for discharge to home? **Select all that apply.**

1. There is a scale in the client's home.
2. The client started ambulating 24 hours ago.
3. The client is receiving furosemide IV 20 mg bid.
4. A smoking cessation consult is scheduled for 2 days after discharge.
5. A home-care nurse is scheduled to see the client 3 days after discharge.

**1039.** The nurse observes that the client, 3 days post-MI, seems unusually fatigued. Upon assessment, the client is dyspneic with activity, has sinus tachycardia, and has generalized edema. Which action by the nurse is **most** appropriate?

1. Administer high-flow oxygen.
2. Encourage the client to rest more.
3. Continue to monitor the client's heart rhythm.
4. Compare the admission and current weight.

**1040.** The 20-year-old is diagnosed with hypertrophic cardiomyopathy. Knowing that the client is on the college soccer team, which information should be the nurse's **priority** when planning to teach?

1. Provide pamphlets on genetic testing to avoid passing on an inherited disease.
2. Reinforce the need to continue exercise with soccer to strengthen the heart.
3. Provide information about CPR to persons living with the client.
4. Counsel on foods for consuming on a low-fat, low-cholesterol diet.

**1041.** The client with class II HF according to the New York Heart Association Functional Classification has been taught about the initial treatment plan for this disease. The nurse determines that the client needs additional teaching if the client states that the treatment plan includes which component?

1. Diuretics
2. A low-sodium diet
3. Home oxygen therapy
4. Angiotensin-converting enzyme (ACE) inhibitors

**1042.** The nurse is assessing the client following cardiac surgery. Which assessment findings should be of the greatest concern to the nurse?

1. Jugular vein distention, muffled heart sounds, and BP 84/48
2. Temperature 96.4°F (35.8°C), HR 58 bpm, and s hivering
3. Increased HR, audible S1 and S2, and pain rated at a 5
4. Central venous pressure (CVP) 4 mm Hg, urine output 30 mL/hr, and sinus rhythm with a few PVCs

**1043.** The nurse completes discharge teaching to the client following aortic valve replacement surgery with a synthetic valve. The nurse evaluates that the client understands the teaching when the client states plans to take which action? **Select all that apply.**

1. Use a soft toothbrush for dental hygiene.
2. Floss teeth daily to prevent plaque.
3. Wear loose-fitting T-shirts or tops.
4. Use an electric razor for shaving.
5. Consume foods high in vitamin K.

**1044.** PHARM The client who had a synthetic valve replacement a year ago is hospitalized with unstable angina. Heparin and nitroglycerin IV infusions were started, but then nitroglycerin was discontinued after the client's pain resolved. The HCP prescribes oral warfarin 5 mg to start at 1700 hours. Which is the nurse's **best** action?

1. Administer the warfarin as prescribed.
2. Call the HCP to question starting warfarin.
3. Discontinue heparin and then give warfarin.
4. Hold warfarin until heparin is discontinued.

**1045.** PHARM The client is scheduled for a coronary artery bypass graft in 1 week. Which instructions should the nurse provide to the client? **Select all that apply.**

1. Stop taking aspirin now and any products containing aspirin.
2. Do perform aerobic exercises 30 minutes daily before surgery.
3. Use the prescribed antimicrobial soap before hospital arrival.
4. Shave your chest and legs and then shower to remove the hair.
5. Resume normal activities when discharged from the hospital.

**1046.** MoC The nurse, caring for the client following an anterior MI, obtains the assessment findings illustrated. On the basis of these findings, the nurse should immediately notify the HCP and plan which intervention?

| TIME | 7:00 | 8:00 | 8:30 | 9:00 |
|---|---|---|---|---|
| Temp | | | | |
| Tm=Tympanic O=Oral R=Rectal Ax=Axillary | | 98.6 (O) | | |
| Pulse | | 96 | 104 | 118 |
| Resp | | 22 | 28 | 32 |
| BP mm Hg | | 116 80 | 102 56 | 85 48 |
| POx | | 94 | | 89 |
| O₂ L/M/NC | | 2 | | 4 |
| Pain Rating: Numeric 0-10 | | 0 | | 4 |

| INTAKE AND OUTPUT | 7:00 | 8:00 | 8:30 | 9:00 | 9:30 |
|---|---|---|---|---|---|
| IVPB | | | | | |
| Oral Intake | | | | | |
| Urine Output | | 30 mL | | 20 mL | |

1. Administer an IV fluid bolus of 0.9% NaCl; the client is in right heart failure.
2. Initiate an IV infusion of dopamine; the client is in cardiogenic shock.
3. Prepare the client for pericardiocentesis; the findings support cardiac tamponade.
4. Notify radiology for a STAT chest x-ray to rule out pulmonary embolism (PE).

**1047.** MoC PHARM The cardiac monitor of the client diagnosed with Prinzmetal's angina shows a PR interval of 0.32 seconds. Which prescribed medication should the nurse withhold and consult with the HCP?

1. Isosorbide mononitrate 20 mg oral daily
2. Amlodipine 10 mg oral daily
3. Nitroglycerin 0.4 mg sublingual prn
4. Atenolol 50 mg oral daily

**1048.** MoC The nurse receives a serum laboratory report for six clients with admitting diagnoses of chest pain. Prioritize the order in which the nurse should address each client's laboratory result.

1. Troponin T 42 ng/mL (0.0–0.4 ng/mL)
2. WBC 11,000/mm³
3. Hgb 7.2 g/dL
4. SCr 2.2 mg/dL
5. K 2.2 mEq/L
6. Total cholesterol 430 mg/dL

Answer: _____

**1049.** MoC PHARM The CXR results of the client who had cardiac surgery is WNL. The nurse plans to remove the client's chest tubes as prescribed. Which is the nurse's **priority** intervention?

1. Auscultate the client's lung sounds.
2. Administer 2 mg morphine sulfate intravenously.
3. Turn off the suction to the chest drainage system.
4. Put the needed supplies at the client's bedside.

**1050.** MoC The nurse who is beginning a shift on a cardiac step-down unit receives shift report for four clients. Prioritize the order, from most urgent to least urgent, that the nurse should assess the clients.

1. The 56-year-old client who was admitted 1 day ago with chest pain receiving intravenous heparin and has a partial thromboplastin time (PTT) due back in 30 minutes
2. The 62-year-old client with end-stage cardiomyopathy, BP of 78/50 mm Hg, 20 mL/hr urine output, and a "Do Not Resuscitate" order whose family has just arrived
3. The 72-year-old client who was transferred 2 hours ago from the ICU following a coronary artery bypass graft and has new-onset atrial fibrillation with rapid ventricular response
4. The 38-year-old postoperative client who had an aortic valve replacement 2 days ago, BP 114/72 mm Hg, HR 100 beats/min, RR 28 breaths/min, and temperature 101.2°F (38.4°C)

Answer: _____

**1051.** The nurse is assessing the client following a coronary artery bypass graft. Which finding in the immediate postoperative period should be **most** concerning to the nurse?

1. Copious chest tube output; now none for 1 hour
2. Current core temperature of 101.3°F (38.5°C)
3. pH 7.32; Paco$_2$ 48; HCO$_3$ 28; Pao$_2$ 80
4. Urine output 160 mL in the last 4 hours

**1052.** MoC The nurse, assessing the client hospitalized following an MI, obtains these VS: BP 78/38 mm Hg, HR 128, RR 32. The nurse notifies the HCP concerned that the client may be experiencing which **most** life-threatening complication?

1. Pulmonary embolism
2. Cardiac tamponade
3. Cardiomyopathy
4. Cardiogenic shock

**1053.** MoC The RN and the NA are caring for four clients, all in need of immediate attention. The NA is a senior nursing student who has been giving medications and performing procedures on clients as a student nurse. The unit charge nurse determines that care is appropriate when the RN working with the NA delegates which actions? **Select all that apply.**

1. Give acetaminophen to the client with a high temperature.
2. Take vital signs on the client newly admitted with heart failure.
3. Discuss the pacemaker discharge handout so this client can go home.
4. Change this client's chest tube dressing; it got wet with drinking water.
5. Provide a sponge bath for the client with the increased temperature.

**1054.** The nurse is assessing the client with an 8-cm AAA. Which finding should the nurse expect?

1. Report of persistent nagging pain in the upper anterior chest
2. Systolic bruit palpated over the upper abdomen
3. Edema of the face and neck with distended neck veins
4. A pulsating mass in the mid to upper abdomen

**1055.** MoC The nurse is assessing the client who had an AAA repair with graft placement 30 minutes ago. The nurse is unable to palpate the posterior tibial pulse of one leg that was palpable 15 minutes earlier. What should be the nurse's **priority**?

1. Recheck the pulse in 5 minutes.
2. Reposition the affected leg.
3. Notify the surgeon of the finding.
4. Document that the pulse is absent.

**1056.** MoC The client who had a femoral-popliteal bypass graft 3 days ago summons the nurse because of throbbing pain in the surgical extremity. Which action should the nurse take **first**?

1. Explain that the throbbing pain is from the increased blood flow.
2. Check the dressings for an increase in the amount of drainage.
3. Assess the dorsalis pedis and posterior tibial pulses in the surgical extremity.
4. Ask the client to rate the level of pain on the pain scale.

**1057.** The client is discovered to have a popliteal aneurysm. Because of the aneurysm, the nurse should closely monitor the client for which associated problem?

1. Thoracic outlet syndrome
2. Ischemia in the lower limb
3. Pulmonary embolism
4. Raynaud's phenomenon

**1058.** The nurse is admitting the client with a thoracic aortic aneurysm. Which intervention should the nurse plan to include?

1. Administering antihypertensive medications
2. Palpating the abdomen to determine the aneurysm's size
3. Inserting a nasogastric tube set to moderate suction
4. Teaching about a diet high in potassium and low in sodium

**1059.** The nurse is preparing the client for a thoracic aneurysm repair. Which assessment findings should prompt the nurse to conclude that a rupture may have occurred? **Select all that apply.**

1. Oliguria
2. Dyspnea
3. Hypotension
4. Abdominal distention
5. Severe chest pain radiating to the back

**1060.** The nurse notes the wound illustrated when assessing the client who has distal foot pain due to vascular insufficiency. Which notation is the nurse likely to find in the client's medical record?

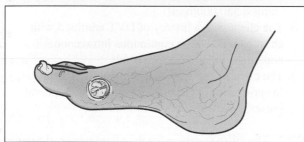

1. Venous ulcer on left foot
2. Arterial ulcer on right foot
3. Diabetic ulcer on left foot
4. Stress ulcer on right foot

**1061.** The nurse is completing a home visit with the client who has an arterial ulcer secondary to PAD. Which statement by the client warrants immediate intervention by the nurse?

1. "I soak my feet daily to warm them and keep them soft."
2. "I cover the sore on my foot with sterile gauze to protect it."
3. "I use a pillow under my calves to keep my heels off the bed."
4. "I lubricate my feet daily to prevent them from cracking."

**1062.** Two days ago the client underwent femoral-popliteal artery bypass graft surgery. What should be the nurse's **priority** at this time?

1. Monitor intake and output every 4 hours.
2. Report any edema that develops in the operative leg.
3. Place the client in a 60-degree sitting position when in bed.
4. Check pedal and post-tibial pulses bilaterally every 4 hours.

**1063.** The nurse reviews symptoms of acute graft occlusion with the client who has had a revascularization graft procedure of the lower extremity. Which symptom of acute arterial occlusion stated by the client indicates the need for further teaching?

1. Severe pain
2. Paresthesia
3. Warm and red incisions
4. Inability to move the foot

**1064.** The client with symptoms of intermittent claudication receives treatment with a peripheral percutaneous transluminal angioplasty procedure with placement of an endovascular stent. Which statements, if made by the client, support the home-care nurse's conclusion that the client is making lifestyle changes to decrease the likelihood of restenosis and arterial occlusion? **Select all that apply.**

1. "I have been doing exercises twice daily."
2. "All nicotine products were thrown away."
3. "These support hose keep my legs warm."
4. "I see a podiatrist tomorrow for foot care."
5. "I'm following a low-saturated-fat diet."
6. "I now take rosuvastatin calcium."

**1065.** PHARM The nurse assesses the client at a vascular clinic after being treated with pentoxifylline for 6 weeks. The nurse determines that pentoxifylline has been effective when noting that the client has which finding?

1. A decrease in lower-extremity edema
2. No symptoms of withdrawal after quitting smoking
3. A venous ulcer on the ankle that has decreased in size
4. The ability to walk a longer distance without claudication

**1066.** The client, who is a 15-pack-year cigarette smoker, has painful fingers and toes and is diagnosed with Buerger's disease (thromboangiitis obliterans). Which measure to prevent disease progression should be the nurse's **initial** focus when teaching the client?

1. Avoid exposure to cold temperatures.
2. Maintain meticulous hygiene.
3. Abstain from all tobacco products.
4. Follow a low-saturated-fat diet.

**1067.** PHARM The client with Raynaud's disease is seen in a vascular clinic 6 weeks after nifedipine has been prescribed. The nurse evaluates that the medication has been effective when which findings are noted?

1. The client's BP is 110/68 mm Hg.
2. The client states experiencing less pain and numbness.
3. The client states that tolerance to heat is improved.
4. The client walks without intermittent claudication.

**1068.** The nurse is discussing healthy lifestyle practices with the client who has chronic venous insufficiency. Which practices should be emphasized with this client? **Select all that apply.**

1. Avoid eating an excess of dark green vegetables.
2. Take rests and elevate the legs while sitting.
3. Wear graduated compression stockings, removing them at night.
4. Increase standing time and shift weight when upright.
5. Sleep with legs elevated above the level of the heart.

**1069.** MoC The client states to the clinic nurse, "I had pain in the left calf for a few days earlier in the week, but I am pain free now." The nurse's assessment findings include: dorsalis pedis pulses palpable, no pain upon dorsiflexion bilaterally, a few visible varicose veins in each leg, and slight swelling in only the left leg. Which is the nurse's **best** action?

1. Ask if the client has been walking more lately.
2. Inform the HCP of the assessment findings.
3. Ask if the client has considered taking a baby aspirin daily.
4. Explain to the client that there are no significant findings.

**1070.** The nurse is caring for the client with varicose veins. Which action should indicate to the nurse that an expected outcome has been met?

1. States will walk daily to promote venous return
2. Reports decreased need for compression stockings
3. States can finally stand for prolonged periods of time
4. Chooses diet high in potassium and low in magnesium

**1071.** The nurse is caring for multiple clients. Which client should the nurse identify as having the greatest risk for developing a DVT?

1. The client with an area of slight induration at the peripheral IV site with a PT of 25 seconds, INR of 2.5
2. The client postoperative hip arthroplasty who has venous insufficiency and is immobile; platelet count = 550,000/mm³
3. The client with a history of DVT admitted with chest pain and has a continuous intravenous heparin drip; PTT of 55 seconds
4. The client with dependent rubor, pallor upon lower-extremity elevation, and absent peripheral pulses; platelet count of 350,000/mm³

**1072.** The nurse is caring for the client who had a cardiac valve replacement. To decrease the risk of DVT and PE, which interventions should the nurse plan to include? **Select all that apply.**

1. Apply a pneumatic compression device.
2. Administer a heparin infusion intravenously.
3. Encourage coughing and deep breathing hourly.
4. Teach about performing isometric leg exercises.
5. Avoid the use of graded compression elastic stockings.

**1073.** The client is admitted with acute infective endocarditis (IE). Which assessment findings should the nurse associate with IE? **Select all that apply.**

1. Skin petechiae
2. Crackles in lung bases
3. Peripheral edema
4. Murmur
5. Arthralgia
6. Hemangioma

**1074.** The client returns to a hospital unit after undergoing placement of a vena cava filter. Which intervention should the nurse implement?

1. Restart heparin therapy as soon as possible.
2. Reinforce the abdominal incision dressing.
3. Inspect the groin insertion site for bleeding.
4. Increase fluids to promote excretion of the dye.

**1075.** The client asks the nurse what can be done to alleviate the pain and discomfort associated with varicose veins. Which response by the nurse is **best?**

1. "Dangle your legs off the side of the bed as often as possible to alleviate the pain."
2. "There isn't much you can do about the pain except have surgery to remove the veins."
3. "You should wear long pants to hide bulging veins; this will help your self-confidence."
4. "Wear elastic stockings to promote venous return; these will also help reduce discomfort."

**INSTRUCTIONS:** Read the case study illustrated, noting the times and the nurse's assessment and intervention over time. Refer to the case study to answer Questions 1076 and 1077.

| Client | 72-year-old male |
|---|---|
| Allergies | Sulfonamide antibiotics |
| Admitting Diagnosis | Left ventricular heart failure |
| Diagnostic Results | *Echocardiogram*: Ejection fraction 20%; heart enlarged |

| Time | Assessment | Interventions |
|---|---|---|
| 0800 | Alert and oriented; BP 110/68, P. 118, RR 28; Dyspnea at rest; crackles bil. bases; oxygen at 2L/NC; fatigue; ECG: PR = 0.32; QRS = 0.10; QT = 0.40; HR 122; sinus tachycardia | Positioned in chair for breakfast Gave prescribed carvedilol 25 mg and captopril 25 mg oral tabs with food; and furosemide 10 mg IV. |
| 0900 | Serum lab results: K 4.9 mEq/L; creatinine 1.1 mg/dL; Mag 1.6 mg/dL; Na 138 mEq/L; Hgb 11.8 g/dL | Initiated prescribed electrolyte protocol for magnesium sulfate 1 g in 0.9% NaCl 50 mL IV piggyback infusing over 1 hr |
| 0930 | Diaphoretic; pale; states not feeling well. BP: 87/48, P. 44, RR 28, oxygen saturation at 85%; ECG monitor: sinus bradycardia with 1st-degree heart block | Applied nonrebreather mask with oxygen flow at 15 L; Notified HCP; Called for 12-lead ECG stat as prescribed |
| 0935 | Diaphoretic, states feeling dizzy. BP: 92/50, P. 30, RR 30, Oxygen saturation at 89%. 12-lead ECG: 3rd-degree heart block | External transcutaneous pacemaker pads applied; pacing initiated with capture. Plan for transfer to coronary care unit per HCP. |

**1076.** MoC CJ PHARM At which time did the nurse intervene incorrectly?

1. 0800
2. 0900
3. 0930
4. 0935

**1077.** MoC CJ PHARM Which intervention should the nurse have performed instead? Enter the information into the box below.

# Answers and Rationales

## 1012. ANSWER: 2

1. Monosaturated fats are included in a healthy diet but have not been found to affect the homocysteine levels.
2. **Homocysteine interferes with the elasticity of the endothelial layer in blood vessels. Foods rich in B-complex vitamins, especially folic acid, have been found to lower serum homocysteine levels.**
3. Vitamin C is included in a healthy diet and enhances immune system functions but has not been found to affect the homocysteine levels.
4. Calcium is important for bone health but has not been found to affect the homocysteine levels.

▸ *Test-taking Tip: B vitamins help the body use homocysteine.*

Content Area: Adult; Concept: Promoting Health; Nutrition; Integrated Processes: Teaching/Learning; Client Needs: Health Promotion and Maintenance; Physiological Integrity: Basic Care and Comfort; Cognitive Level: Application [Applying]

## 1013. ANSWER: 3

1. A BMI of 25 or higher is considered a risk factor for hypertension. A BMI of 23 is normal. A BP of 118/70 is within normal range for an adult.
2. Excessive alcohol intake is a risk factor for hypertension; consuming two glasses of wine daily increases the risk for hypertension.
3. **Being African American is a known risk factor for hypertension. Starting to have the BP taken more often demonstrates awareness of having a risk factor for hypertension.**
4. Having frequent colds and taking the influenza vaccine does not increase the risk for hypertension. Medications for treating colds, if taken frequently, can increase the risk for hypertension.

▸ *Test-taking Tip: You should associate hypertension in the stem with BP in the options. Eliminate Option 1 because the BMI and BP are normal.*

Content Area: Adult; Concept: Promoting Health; Diversity; Perfusion; Integrated Processes: Communication and Documentation; Culture and Spirituality; Client Needs: Health Promotion and Maintenance; Cognitive Level: Application [Applying]

## 1014. ANSWER: 1, 3, 4, 6

1. **Blue-colored nail beds may indicate cyanosis in a dark-skinned client.**
2. A client with yellowish skin, but not dark skin, may have a grayish-green skin tone with cyanosis.
3. **The soles of the feet of a dark-skinned client will have a blue color due to diminished blood supply.**
4. **A whitish color around the mouth of a dark-skinned client may indicate cyanosis due to diminished blood supply.**
5. Jaundice and not cyanosis appears as a yellow color in oral mucous membranes.
6. **In dark-skinned clients, cyanosis may present as gray- or bluish-colored conjunctivae.**

▸ *Test-taking Tip: To assess cyanosis in a dark-skinned client, the nurse should assess for a gray or whitish color around the mouth and tongue, blue color in nail beds, palms, and soles, and pallor, gray, or bluish color in the conjunctiva.*

Content Area: Adult; Concept: Perfusion; Integrated Processes: Nursing Process: Analysis; Culture and Spirituality; Client Needs: Physiological Integrity: Reduction of Risk Potential; Cognitive Level: Analysis [Analyzing]

## 1015. PHARM ANSWER: 1

1. **Hyperkalemia can occur as a side effect to lisinopril (Prinivil, Zestril), an ACE inhibitor. The HCP should be notified prior to administration. The drug or dose may need to be changed; 40 mg is the maximum daily dose for an elderly client.**
2. Metoprolol (Lopressor), a beta adrenergic blocker, can increase serum creatinine and BUN levels and cause hypoglycemia. There is no information in the stem about these levels.
3. Atorvastatin (Lipitor), an antilipidemic agent, lowers LDL levels; it has no effect on serum potassium levels.
4. Sertraline (Zoloft), an SSRI, is used in treating anxiety or depression. Is has no effect on serum potassium levels. It may produce hyponatremia in older adults.

▸ *Test-taking Tip: If uncertain, narrow the options to the medication with the higher doses. Then think about the action of these medications.*

Content Area: Adult; Concept: Nursing Roles; Medication; Perfusion; Integrated Processes: Nursing Process: Implementation; Client Needs: Safe and Effective Care Environment: Safety and Infection Control; Physiological Integrity: Pharmacological and Parenteral Therapies; Cognitive Level: Application [Applying]

## 1016. ANSWER: 3

1. Reduced intake of dietary potassium is a contributory factor associated with malignant hypertension and should not be limited unless serum potassium levels are elevated. Sodium, not potassium, should be limited with hypertension.
2. Clients with hypertension are advised to gradually increase to regular physical activity, and should avoid sudden rigorous exercise programs.

3. **Teaching is effective if the client states to call the HCP immediately if experiencing vision changes. Sudden vision changes may be associated with stroke, a complication of hypertension.**

4. A BMI of 32 is obese. Obesity is a contributing factor of hypertension and is defined as a BMI greater than 30.

▶ *Test-taking Tip: Read each option carefully. Rule out Option 1 because clients with hypertension should avoid sodium, not potassium. Options with extremes words, such as "rigorous," should usually be eliminated. Knowing that the normal BMI is between 18.5 and 24.9 should lead you to eliminate Option 4. This leaves only Option 3, which is the answer.*

Content Area: Adult; Concept: Nursing Roles; Perfusion; Integrated Processes: Teaching/Learning; Nursing Process: Evaluation; Client Needs: Physiological Integrity: Physiological Adaptation; Cognitive Level: Evaluation [Evaluating]

## 1017. MoC ANSWER: 2

1. The MAP of 94/60 is 71.3.
2. **A MAP of less than 60 mm Hg indicates that there is inadequate perfusion to organs. The MAP is calculated by the sum of the SBP + 2DBP and then dividing by 3 [MAP = (SBP + 2DBP)/3]. Thus the MAP of 98/36 mm Hg is (98 + 72)/3 = 170/3 = 56.7.**
3. The MAP of 110/50 is 70.
4. The MAP of 140/78 is 98.7.

▶ *Test-taking Tip: Normal MAP is 70 to 100. Use the formula for calculating the MAP of each BP reading to arrive at the answer: [MAP = (SBP + 2DBP) ÷ 3]*

Content Area: Adult; Concept: Perfusion; Management; Integrated Processes: Nursing Process: Analysis; Client Needs: Safe and Effective Care Environment: Management of Care; Cognitive Level: Analysis [Analyzing]

## 1018. ANSWER: 4

1. Line A points to the aortic valve and would be associated with aortic stenosis, not mitral regurgitation.
2. Line B points to the pulmonic valve and is not the valve to assess for mitral regurgitation.
3. Line C points to the tricuspid valve and is not the valve to assess for mitral regurgitation.
4. **Mitral regurgitation is heard at the location of the mitral valve (line D) and should be auscultated with the bell of the stethoscope at the fifth intercostal space, left midclavicular line. The bell is used to auscultate low-pitched sounds.**

▶ *Test-taking Tip: A mnemonic for remembering the auscultation points and the location of the heart valves is: "All Points To Monitor." The first letter of each word represents the auscultation point: aortic valve, pulmonic valve, tricuspid valve, and mitral valve.*

Content Area: Adult; Concept: Assessment; Perfusion; Integrated Processes: Nursing Process: Assessment; Client Needs: Physiological Integrity: Reduction of Risk Potential; Cognitive Level: Application [Applying]

## 1019. ANSWER: 3, 4, 5

1. Heart sounds are more difficult to auscultate through clothing; auscultate only under the gown.
2. Auscultating from the right side, not the left, allows stretching of the stethoscope across the chest and reduces interference from the tubing.
3. **The experienced nurse should recommend having the client lean forward during auscultation because this position brings the heart closer to the chest wall and accentuates sounds from the aortic and pulmonic areas.**
4. **The experienced nurse should recommend feeling the pulse beat and listening at the same time because it helps to focus on the rhythm and sounds and aids in filtering extraneous stimuli.**
5. **The experienced nurse should recommend a left side-lying position during auscultation of heart sounds; this brings the heart closer to the chest wall and accentuates sounds produced at the mitral area.**

▶ *Test-taking Tip: Visualize each of the options to determine if the action would help or hinder hearing the heart sounds.*

Content Area: Adult; Concept: Assessment; Perfusion; Management; Integrated Processes: Nursing Process: Assessment; Client Needs: Health Promotion and Maintenance; Cognitive Level: Analysis [Analyzing]

## 1020. MoC ANSWER: 1

1. **A cardiac catheterization is an invasive procedure requiring the client to lie still in a supine position. The client is usually sedated with medication, such as midazolam, during the procedure. To avoid aspiration, the client should be NPO 6 to 12 hours before the procedure.**
2. Because of the time element, NPO status should be initiated first, and then teaching should occur.
3. To avoid administering too much fluid to the cardiac client, the saline infusion is usually only started just before the client leaving the unit for the procedure.
4. A consent form should be signed after the cardiologist has spoken with the client.

▶ *Test-taking Tip: Cardiac catheterization is an invasive procedure that has the potential to cause aspiration from sedation. Use the ABC's to determine which action should be first. Any action that pertains to maintaining a patent airway should be first.*

Content Area: Adult; Concept: Critical Thinking; Perfusion; Management; Integrated Processes: Nursing Process: Implementation; Client Needs: Safe and Effective Care Environment: Management of Care; Cognitive Level: Analysis [Analyzing]

## 1021. ANSWER: 2

1. The ICD monitors the client's HR and rhythm, identifies ventricular tachycardia or ventricular fibrillation, and delivers a 25-joule or less shock if a lethal rhythm is detected.

2. **CPR should only be initiated if the client is unresponsive and pulseless. EMS should be called if there is more than one shock. This statement indicates further teaching is needed.**

3. Various sensations have been described when the device delivers a shock, including a blow to or kick in the chest.

4. State laws vary regarding drivers with ICDs. The decision regarding driving is also based on whether dysrhythmias are present, the frequency of firing, and the client's overall health.

▸ *Test-taking Tip: The key phrase "further teaching is needed" indicates a false-response item. Select the client's statement that is not correct.*

Content Area: Adult; Concept: Nursing Roles; Perfusion; Integrated Processes: Teaching/Learning; Nursing Process: Evaluation; Client Needs: Physiological Integrity: Reduction of Risk Potential; Cognitive Level: Analysis [Analyzing]

## 1022. MoC ANSWER:

| Laboratory Tests | Client Results |
|---|---|
| CK-MB (0–16 units/L) | X |
| Troponin T (cTnT) (0.0–0.4 ng/mL) | X |

**The CK-MB band is specific to myocardial cells and increases with myocardial injury. Cardiospecific troponins (troponin T [cTnT] and troponin I [cTnI]) are released into circulation after myocardial injury, are highly specific indicators of MI, and have greater sensitivity and specificity than CK-MB.**

▸ *Test-taking Tip: Although all abnormal values should be reported to the HCP, the issue of the question is laboratory values specific for MI.*

Content Area: Adult; Concept: Management; Perfusion Integrated Processes: Nursing Process: Implementation; Client Needs: Safe and Effective Care Environment: Management of Care; Cognitive Level: Analysis [Analyzing]

## 1023. ANSWER: 1

1. **The nurse's priority assessment in ACS is the client's pain; pain indicates that the heart is not receiving adequate oxygen and blood flow (perfusion).**

2. BP is a response stemming from the lack of perfusion but is not the priority assessment.

3. HR is a response stemming from the lack of perfusion but is not the priority assessment.

4. RR is a response stemming from the lack of perfusion but is not the priority assessment.

▸ *Test-taking Tip: Remember that when a muscle is ischemic (not receiving adequate oxygen), pain occurs as a result. By eliminating the pain in cardiac conditions, the sympathetic nervous system will stop trying to compensate for lack of perfusion.*

Content Area: Adult; Concept: Perfusion; Comfort; Integrated Processes: Nursing Process: Assessment; Client Needs: Physiological Integrity: Reduction of Risk Potential; Cognitive Level: Application [Applying]

## 1024. MoC ANSWER: 4

1. The presence of Q waves indicates an MI over 24 hours old.

2. Flipped T waves indicate myocardial ischemia.

3. Peaked T waves may indicate hyperkalemia and are concerning, but ST-segment elevation is more concerning.

4. **The nurse should be most concerned about ST elevation because it indicates an evolving MI.**

▸ *Test-taking Tip: Recognize that the LAD vessel supplies blood to much of the left ventricle and that unrelieved chest pain indicates decreased perfusion. The ECG change associated with cardiac injury is ST-segment elevation.*

Content Area: Adult; Concept: Perfusion; Management; Integrated Processes: Nursing Process: Analysis; Client Needs: Safe and Effective Care Environment: Management of Care; Physiological Integrity: Reduction of Risk Potential; Cognitive Level: Application [Applying]

## 1025. MoC ANSWER: 4

1. Cardiac enzymes would be a likely intervention but the second intervention.

2. Cardiac catheterization would be a likely intervention but the third intervention.

3. Topical nitroglycerin is never given in an acute situation because its route has a much slower rate of absorption.

4. **The nurse's priority intervention should be to increase oxygen to the heart muscle.**

▸ *Test-taking Tip: Key phrases include chest pain and new ST elevation, which should indicate cardiac ischemia and potential acute MI. Applying oxygen is necessary to increase oxygenation to cardiac tissue and can be quickly performed.*

Content Area: Adult; Concept: Perfusion; Management; Integrated Processes: Nursing Process: Implementation; Client Needs: Safe and Effective Care Environment: Management of Care; Cognitive Level: Application [Applying]

## 1026. PHARM ANSWER: 0.4

**Use a proportion formula and multiply the extremes (outside values) and the means (inside values); then solve for X.**

**100 mg : 1 mL :: 40 mg : X mL; 100X = 40; X = 40 ÷ 100; X = 0.4**

**The nurse should administer 0.4 mL of furosemide (Lasix).**

▸ *Test-taking Tip: In this medication calculation problem, first determine the dose on hand; then determine the dose needed. Calculate the amount that should be administered. Recheck your answer using a calculator.*

Content Area: Adult; Concept: Medication; Perfusion; Integrated Processes: Nursing Process: Implementation; Client Needs: Physiological Integrity: Pharmacological and Parenteral Therapies; Cognitive Level: Application [Applying]

**1027. ANSWER: 4**

1. A slight elevation of BP could be related to pain at the incision site. It is not indicative of a complication without additional information.
2. Usually pulses are palpable at +2, but without additional baseline information on the client's pulses, this warrants monitoring but is not indicative in itself of a complication.
3. A soft groin area where the puncture site is located is a normal finding. Ecchymosis (bruising) does not indicate a complication.
4. **An apical pulse of 132 bpm with an irregular–irregular rhythm could indicate atrial fibrillation or a rhythm with premature beats. Dysrhythmias are a complication that can occur following coronary angiogram.**

▶ **Test-taking Tip:** Three options warrant nothing more than monitoring. Select the option that is the most concerning. Dysrhythmias are a complication following a coronary angiogram.

**Content Area:** Adult; **Concept:** Assessment; Perfusion; **Integrated Processes:** Nursing Process: Evaluation; **Client Needs:** Physiological Integrity: Physiological Adaptation; **Cognitive Level:** Evaluation [Evaluating]

**1028. MoC ANSWER: 4**

1. Sneezing would not affect the pedal pulses.
2. Although the BP could decrease if the client were bleeding, this is not the priority.
3. Sneezing can be an early sign of an allergic reaction to the contrast but is a minor sign compared with the potential loss of blood.
4. **Checking the insertion site is priority. Sneezing increases intra-abdominal pressure and increases the risk for clot disruption and bleeding from the femoral artery.**

▶ **Test-taking Tip:** The key word is "sneeze," which increases the risk for bleeding due to rupture of the newly formed clot at the insertion site. This should direct you to consider Option 4 as the priority.

**Content Area:** Adult; **Concept:** Clotting; Perfusion; **Integrated Processes:** Nursing Process: Implementation; **Client Needs:** Safe and Effective Care Environment: Management of Care; **Cognitive Level:** Application [Applying]

**1029. PHARM ANSWER: 3, 4, 5, 6**

1. Ablation of the AV node would only be considered if medications were ineffective in controlling the client's HR.
2. Cardioversion would only be considered if medications were ineffective in converting the client's rhythm and only after the presence of an atrial clot has been ruled out.
3. **The ineffective atrial contractions or loss of atrial kick with atrial fibrillation can decrease cardiac output. Administering oxygen enhances tissue oxygenation.**
4. **The client is at risk for thrombi in the atria from stasis. Anticoagulant therapy is used to prevent thromboembolism.**
5. **Amiodarone (Cordarone) is used for pharmacological cardioversion of the atrial fibrillation rhythm.**
6. **Diltiazem (Cardizem), a calcium channel antagonist, is prescribed to slow the ventricular response to atrial fibrillation. An alternative to a calcium channel antagonist would be the use of a beta blocker, such as esmolol, metoprolol, or propranolol.**

▶ **Test-taking Tip:** The key word is "initial." The nurse should direct interventions at the client's potential complications from the arrhythmia. Pharmacological therapies are usually tried before more invasive procedures.

**Content Area:** Adult; **Concept:** Nursing Roles; Perfusion; Medication; **Integrated Processes:** Nursing Process: Planning; **Client Needs:** Physiological Integrity: Pharmacological and Parenteral Therapies; Physiological Integrity: Reduction of Risk Potential; **Cognitive Level:** Application [Applying]

**1030. MoC PHARM ANSWER: 2**

1. Although a STAT 12-lead ECG is needed to identify ischemia or infarct location, the first action is to treat the client's pain.
2. **Oxygen should be available in the room and should be initiated first to enhance oxygen flow to the myocardium.**
3. Sublingual nitroglycerin dilates coronary arteries and will enhance blood flow to the myocardium. Once oxygen is in place and the VS known, nitroglycerin should be given.
4. Morphine sulfate is a narcotic analgesic used for pain control and anxiety reduction. Because it is a controlled substance, extra steps are needed to retrieve the medication from a secure source, so this is not the first action.

▶ **Test-taking Tip:** Use the ABC's. Improving oxygen flow to the myocardium is priority.

**Content Area:** Adult; **Concept:** Critical Thinking; Perfusion; Medication; **Integrated Processes:** Nursing Process: Implementation; **Client Needs:** Safe and Effective Care Environment: Management of Care; Physiological Integrity: Pharmacological and Parenteral Therapies; **Cognitive Level:** Application [Applying]

**1031. ANSWER: 3**

1. Atrial flutter is either a regular or an irregular rhythm with multiple discernible P waves prior to each QRS complex and no measurable PR interval.
2. Atrial fibrillation is an irregular rhythm with multiple nondiscernible fibrillatory P waves prior to each QRS and no measurable PR interval.
3. **Sinus bradycardia is a regular rhythm with a ventricular rate less than 60 bpm and one discernable P wave prior to each QRS.**

4. Sinus rhythm with PACs is an irregular rhythm with a ventricular rate between 60 and 100 bpm, one discernable P wave prior to each QRS, and a PR interval between 0.12 and 0.20 second, with the presence of premature atrial beats that occur early in the cardiac cycle. The PACs also have one discernible P wave prior to each QRS and a PR interval between 0.08 to 0.20 second.

▶ *Test-taking Tip: Use the steps in interpreting an ECG rhythm to select the correct option. Note that the rhythm is regular, so eliminate Option 4, which is an irregular rhythm. Recall that atrial fibrillation and atrial flutter do not have a measurable PR interval, so eliminate Options 1 and 2.*

**Content Area:** Adult; **Concept:** Nursing Roles; Perfusion; **Integrated Processes:** Nursing Process: Analysis; **Client Needs:** Physiological Integrity: Physiological Adaptation; **Cognitive Level:** Application [Applying]

## 1032. PHARM ANSWER: 11

**According to the protocol, with an aPTT value of 92 seconds, the rate should be decreased by 1 mL per hour. If the infusion was previously infusing at 12 mL per hour, the new rate is 11 mL/hr.**

▶ *Test-taking Tip: Read the information carefully and follow the directions of the heparin infusion protocol to determine the new rate.*

**Content Area:** Adult; **Concept:** Medication; Perfusion; **Integrated Processes:** Nursing Process: Implementation; **Client Needs:** Physiological Integrity: Pharmacological and Parenteral Therapies; **Cognitive Level:** Analysis [Analyzing]

## 1033. MoC ANSWER: 2

1. The dressing should not be removed to check the incision immediately after insertion but should be checked for bleeding to monitor for potential complications.
2. **Limiting arm and shoulder activity initially and up to 24 hours after the pacing leads are implanted helps prevent lead dislodgement. Often an arm sling is used as a reminder to the client to limit arm activity.**
3. The nurse should assist the client the first time out of bed following a pacemaker implant, but the client should not use a walker for 24 hours after the procedure, and out-of-bed activity would not resume until the client is stable.
4. A postinsertion CXR is completed to check lead placement and to rule out a pneumothorax. It does not promote the intactness of pacing leads.

▶ *Test-taking Tip: Focus on the issue of the question: measures to promote intactness of the pacing leads. Eliminate Options 1, 3, and 4 because these actions do not pertain to the intactness of the pacing leads.*

**Content Area:** Adult; **Concept:** Safety; Management; Perfusion; **Integrated Processes:** Nursing Process: Planning; **Client Needs:** Safe and Effective Care Environment: Management of Care; Physiological Integrity: Reduction of Risk Potential; **Cognitive Level:** Synthesis [Creating]

## 1034. ANSWER: 2, 3, 6

1. Isometric exercise of the arms can cause exertional angina.
2. **Blood vessels constrict in response to cold and increase the workload of the heart.**
3. **Nitroglycerin produces vasodilation and improves blood flow to the coronary arteries and should be taken before exertional or stressful activities.**
4. Exertional activity increases the HR. This reduces the time the heart is in diastole when blood flow to the coronary arteries is the greatest. A period of rest should occur between activities, and activities should be spaced.
5. Straining at stool increases sympathetic stimulation and cardiac workload, and it should be avoided. However, a daily laxative should not be taken; it may result in diarrhea.
6. **Nicotine stimulates catecholamine release, producing vasoconstriction and an increased HR.**

▶ *Test-taking Tip: The key phrase is "measures to prevent future angina." Consider if each option could potentially increase myocardial oxygen demand or decrease available oxygen, either of which could precipitate angina.*

**Content Area:** Adult; **Concept:** Perfusion; Nursing Roles; **Integrated Processes:** Teaching/Learning; **Client Needs:** Physiological Integrity: Physiological Adaptation; **Cognitive Level:** Application [Applying]

## 1035. PHARM ANSWER: 2

1. A low-calorie diet is not indicated. The normal BMI is 18.5 to 24.9.
2. **A statin antilipidemic should be prescribed to manage the client's hypercholesterolemia. It will lower the LDL cholesterol and triglycerides and increase the HDL cholesterol.**
3. The client's BP is slightly elevated but would be initially treated with lifestyle changes, not a diuretic.
4. Although a low-saturated-fat diet is indicated, a low-potassium diet is not because the serum potassium of 4.0 mEq/L is normal.

▶ *Test-taking Tip: Focus on the data provided in the situation and identify the abnormal findings. Note that the client's serum cholesterol level analysis includes more data. Conclude that these are abnormal and then use "lipids" as a key to identifying the correct option.*

**Content Area:** Adult; **Concept:** Critical Thinking; Nursing Roles; Perfusion; Medication; **Integrated Processes:** Nursing Process: Planning; **Client Needs:** Physiological Integrity: Pharmacological and Parenteral Therapies; Physiological Integrity: Reduction of Risk Potential; **Cognitive Level:** Analysis [Analyzing]

## 1036. ANSWER: 2

1. An increased HR during activity indicates that the heart is able to adapt.
2. **A drop in BP of 20 mm Hg from the baseline indicates that the client's heart is unable to adapt to the increased energy and oxygen demands of the activity. The client is not tolerating the activity; the length of time or the intensity should be reduced.**
3. The relief of dyspnea and diaphoresis with rest indicates the heart is able to adapt.
4. A MAP of 80 is normal.

▸ **Test-taking Tip:** The key words are "best supports." Select the option that is most abnormal.

Content Area: Adult; Concept: Perfusion; Integrated Processes: Nursing Process: Evaluation; Client Needs: Physiological Integrity: Physiological Adaptation; Cognitive Level: Evaluation [Evaluating]

## 1037. ANSWER: 3

1. Left-sided HF produces signs of pulmonary congestion, including crackles, S3 and S4 heart sounds, and pleural effusion.
2. A characteristic finding of pulmonic valve malfunction would be a murmur.
3. **Right-sided HF produces venous congestion in the systemic circulation, resulting in JVD and ascites (from vascular congestion in the GI tract). Additional signs include hepatomegaly, splenomegaly, and peripheral edema.**
4. A murmur would be auscultated with a ruptured septum, and the client would experience signs of cardiogenic shock; these findings are not present.

▸ **Test-taking Tip:** Note that Options 1 and 3 focus on different types of HF; either one or both of these must be wrong. Venous blood returns to the right side of the heart.

Content Area: Adult; Concept: Assessment; Perfusion; Integrated Processes: Nursing Process: Analysis; Client Needs: Physiological Integrity: Reduction of Risk Potential; Cognitive Level: Analysis [Analyzing]

## 1038. MoC ANSWER: 1, 2, 5

1. **A scale is needed to monitor a change in fluid status and weight gain.**
2. **The client should be ambulating 24 hours preceding discharge to determine functional capability.**
3. Oral diuretic agents such as furosemide (Lasix) should be administered 24 hours prior to discharge to monitor effectiveness.
4. Smoking cessation should be initiated prior to, not after, discharge.
5. **The client should have the home-care nurse visit or provide telephonic assistance within the first 3 days of discharge.**

▸ **Test-taking Tip:** Look for key words in options that would make the option incorrect. "Intravenous" in Option 3 and "after discharge" in Option 4 make these options incorrect, and these should be eliminated.

Content Area: Adult; Concept: Management; Perfusion; Integrated Processes: Nursing Process: Analysis; Caring; Client Needs: Safe and Effective Care Environment: Management of Care; Psychosocial Integrity; Cognitive Level: Application [Applying]

## 1039. ANSWER: 4

1. There is no indication that the client is hypoxic and in need of high-flow oxygen. To treat the dyspnea, oxygen by nasal cannula would be appropriate.
2. The fatigue is caused by decreased cardiac output, impaired perfusion to vital organs, decreased tissue oxygenation, and anemia. Rest alone will not relieve the fatigue. Interventions are needed to improve cardiac output and tissue oxygenation.
3. Continuing to monitor the client's heart rhythm, without further assessment, will delay an appropriate intervention.
4. **A complication of MI is HF. Signs of HF include fatigue, dyspnea, tachycardia, edema, and weight gain. Other signs include nocturia, skin changes, behavioral changes, and chest pain.**

▸ **Test-taking Tip:** Use the nursing process to determine the next action. The symptoms together imply HF. Further data collection is needed to confirm the problem.

Content Area: Adult; Concept: Assessment; Perfusion; Integrated Processes: Nursing Process: Assessment; Client Needs: Physiological Integrity: Reduction of Risk Potential; Cognitive Level: Analysis [Analyzing]

## 1040. ANSWER: 3

1. Only half of the clients with hypertrophic cardiomyopathy have this autosomal dominant disorder. Genetic testing may be important to include but is not a priority over the lifesaving measures of CPR.
2. Strenuous exercise is restricted in clients with hypertrophic cardiomyopathy.
3. **Because sudden cardiac death is a large risk factor for those under 30 years of age, the nurse should provide information about having others living with the client trained in CPR as a preventative measure.**
4. Although consuming a low-fat, low-cholesterol diet is a good lifestyle choice, no specific diet will prevent or reverse symptoms of hypertrophic cardiomyopathy.

▸ **Test-taking Tip:** Use the ABC's to answer this question. Lifesaving preventative measures are priority.

Content Area: Adult; Concept: Nursing Roles; Perfusion; Integrated Processes: Nursing Process: Implementation; Teaching/Learning; Client Needs: Safe and Effective Care Environment: Safety and Infection Control; Psychosocial Integrity; Cognitive Level: Analysis [Analyzing]

## 1041. ANSWER: 3

1. Diuretics mobilize edematous fluid, act on the kidneys to promote excretion of sodium and water, and reduce preload and pulmonary venous pressure.
2. Dietary restriction of sodium aids in reducing edema.
3. **In class II HF, normal physical activity results in fatigue, dyspnea, palpitations, or anginal pain. The symptoms are absent at rest. Home oxygen therapy is unnecessary unless there are other comorbid conditions.**
4. ACE inhibitors block the conversion of angiotensin I to the vasoconstrictor angiotensin II, prevent the degradation of bradykinin and other vasodilatory prostaglandins, and increase plasma renin levels and reduce aldosterone levels. The net result is systemic vasodilation, reduced SVR, and improved cardiac output.

♦ *Test-taking Tip: The key phrase "needs additional teaching" indicates that this is a false-response item. Select the option that is incorrect for treating class II HF.*

Content Area: Adult; Concept: Nursing Roles; Perfusion; Medication; Integrated Processes: Teaching/Learning; Client Needs: Physiological Integrity: Physiological Adaptation; Cognitive Level: Analysis [Analyzing]

## 1042. ANSWER: 1

1. **The nurse should be most concerned with JVD, muffled heart sounds, and hypotension (Beck's Triad). This is a life-threatening event suggesting cardiac tamponade.**
2. These are expected findings postsurgery, although efforts should be made to rewarm the client and prevent shivering.
3. An increased HR can occur with a pain rated at 5; these are expected findings postsurgery.
4. The CVP, urine output measurement, and cardiac rhythm are within normal findings. A urine output of 30 mL is the minimum hourly urine output. A urine output of less than 30 mL/hr is indicative of decreased perfusion and needs further follow-up. If PVCs are frequent and cause symptoms, follow-up is needed.

♦ *Test-taking Tip: Poor perfusion (hypotension) is normally a late sign and cause for alarm.*

Content Area: Adult; Concept: Assessment; Perfusion; Integrated Processes: Nursing Process: Evaluation; Client Needs: Physiological Integrity: Physiological Adaptation; Cognitive Level: Evaluation [Evaluating]

## 1043. ANSWER: 1, 3, 4

1. **Using a soft toothbrush reduces the risk for bleeding when taking anticoagulants that are prescribed when the client has a synthetic heart valve.**

2. Flossing should be avoided because it causes tissue trauma, increases the risk of bleeding, and increases the risk of infective endocarditis.
3. **Loose-fitting clothing, such as T-shirts, will avoid friction on the sternal incision.**
4. **An electric razor is safer than a straightedge or disposable razor in preventing nicks or cuts when shaving. The client will be on anticoagulants that increase the risk for bleeding.**
5. The diet should contain normal amounts of vitamin K; excessive amounts antagonize the effects of the anticoagulant.

♦ *Test-taking Tip: Anticoagulation is prescribed when the client has a synthetic valve. You should select options that include bleeding precautions.*

Content Area: Adult; Concept: Clotting; Perfusion; Integrated Processes: Teaching/Learning; Nursing Process: Evaluation; Client Needs: Physiological Integrity: Reduction of Risk Potential; Cognitive Level: Evaluation [Evaluating]

## 1044. PHARM ANSWER: 1

1. **Both heparin and warfarin (Coumadin) are anticoagulants, but their actions are different. Oral warfarin requires 3 to 5 days to reach effective levels. It is usually begun while the client is still on heparin. Warfarin should be given as prescribed.**
2. Calling the HCP is unnecessary because warfarin is indicated with a synthetic valve replacement and should be given as prescribed.
3. The nurse should not discontinue the heparin without its being prescribed.
4. The nurse should not hold the warfarin without its being prescribed to be held.

♦ *Test-taking Tip: Narrow the options by eliminating those not within the nurse's scope of practice. Of the two remaining options, consider that the actions of heparin and warfarin are different.*

Content Area: Adult; Concept: Medication; Perfusion; Integrated Processes: Nursing Process: Implementation; Client Needs: Physiological Integrity: Pharmacological and Parenteral Therapies; Cognitive Level: Application [Applying]

## 1045. PHARM ANSWER: 1, 3

1. **Aspirin decreases platelet aggregation and increases the risk of bleeding. It is usually discontinued a week before surgery.**
2. Aerobic exercises before surgery may be too strenuous and increase oxygen demand. A postoperative cardiac rehabilitation program is begun usually on the second postoperative day and includes exercises while being monitored.
3. **The client should use an antimicrobial soap when showering or bathing as prescribed, usually a day or two before and the day of surgery, to decrease the risk of infection.**

CHAPTER 24 Cardiovascular Management **419**

24 Cardiovascular Management
Answers and Rationales

4. Although the client's skin will be shaved, this will be completed just prior to surgery to avoid nicks and decrease the risk of infection.

5. Activities that stress the sternum, such as lifting, driving, and overhead reaching, will be restricted after surgery.

▶ *Test-taking Tip: Read the options carefully for key words that would increase surgical risk and the risk of complications after surgery, and eliminate these options.*

Content Area: Adult; Concept: Nursing Roles; Perfusion; Integrated Processes: Teaching/Learning; Client Needs: Physiological Integrity: Reduction of Risk Potential; Physiological Integrity: Pharmacological and Parenteral Therapies; Cognitive Level: Analysis [Analyzing]

**1046.** MoC **ANSWER: 2**

1. IV fluids may be administered if the client is showing signs of dehydration. However, the client is not experiencing right-sided HF. Right HF produces signs of venous congestion, including jugular venous distention, hepatomegaly, splenomegaly, and ascites.

2. **Complications of an anterior MI are left ventricular failure, reduced cardiac output, and cardiogenic shock. The client's MAP is 55 (MAP = [Systolic BP + Diastolic BP + Diastolic BP]/3 or 85 + 40 + 40 = 165/3 = 55). Hypotension, tachycardia, tachypnea, a low MAP, and decreasing urine output are classic signs of cardiogenic shock. Dopamine (Intropin) is administered in cardiogenic shock to increase cardiac output.**

3. Although symptoms of cardiac tamponade do include hypotension, tachycardia, and tachypnea, other signs include muffled heart sounds. Appropriate treatment for cardiac tamponade is pericardiocentesis.

4. A CXR is used to diagnose PE, but the data do not suggest PE. The signs of PE can be subtle and nonspecific but most commonly present with dyspnea, tachycardia, tachypnea, and/or chest pain.

▶ *Test-taking Tip: Focus on the client's vital sign changes and decreased urine output. Calculate the MAP. Complications of an anterior MI include left ventricular failure, reduced cardiac output, and cardiogenic shock. Use this information to rule out options.*

Content Area: Adult; Concept: Perfusion; Medication; Integrated Processes: Nursing Process: Analysis; Client Needs: Safe and Effective Care Environment: Management of Care; Physiological Integrity: Reduction of Risk Potential; Cognitive Level: Application [Applying]

**1047.** MoC PHARM **ANSWER: 4**

1. Isosorbide mononitrate (Imdur), a nitrate, causes vasodilatation of the large coronary arteries. Nitrates act as an exogenous source of nitric oxide, which causes vascular smooth muscle relaxation, resulting in decreased myocardial oxygen consumption and a possible modest effect on platelet aggregation and thrombosis. It will not prolong the PR interval further.

2. Amlodipine (Norvasc), a calcium channel blocker, relaxes coronary smooth muscle and produces coronary vasodilation. This in turn improves myocardial oxygen delivery. It will not further prolong the PR interval.

3. Nitroglycerin (Nitrostat) sublingual effectively treats episodes of angina and myocardial ischemia within minutes of administration. It will not prolong the PR interval further.

4. **Atenolol (Tenormin), a beta blocker, blocks stimulation of beta1 (myocardial)-adrenergic receptors, causing a reduction in BP and HR. A side effect of the atenolol is a prolongation of the PR interval (normal PR interval is 0.12 to 0.20 second). Continued use of the drug can result in heart block. The nurse should consult with the HCP.**

▶ *Test-taking Tip: The focus of the question is a medication contraindicated with a prolonged PR interval. Think about the action of the medications prescribed. The generic names of the beta blockers end in "-lol."*

Content Area: Adult; Concept: Medication; Perfusion; Integrated Processes: Nursing Process: Analysis; Client Needs: Safe and Effective Care Environment: Management of Care; Physiological Integrity: Pharmacological and Parenteral Therapies; Cognitive Level: Analysis [Analyzing]

**1048.** MoC **ANSWER: 1, 5, 3, 4, 6, 2**

1. **Troponin T 42 ng/mL (Normal = 0.0 to 0.4 ng/mL). The nurse should address the elevated troponin level first. Cardiospecific troponins (troponin T [cTnT] and troponin I [cTnI]) are released into circulation after myocardial injury and are highly specific indicators of MI. Because "time is muscle," the HCP should be notified and the client treated immediately to prevent extension of the infarct and possible death.**

5. **K 2.2 mEq/L. The nurse should address the decreased serum potassium level (K) second. The normal serum K level is 3.5 to 5.8 mEq/L. A low serum level can cause life-threatening dysrhythmias.**

3. **Hgb 7.2 g/dL. The normal Hgb is 13.1 to 17.1 g/dL. A low Hgb can contribute to inadequate tissue perfusion and contribute to myocardial ischemia.**

4. SCr 2.2 mg/dL. The normal serum creatinine (SCr) is 0.4 to 1.4 mg/dL. Impaired circulation may be causing this alteration, and further client assessment is needed. Medication doses may need to be adjusted with impaired renal perfusion.

6. Total cholesterol 430 mg/dL. The normal total serum cholesterol should be less than 200 mg/dL. This is a risk factor for development of CAD. The client needs teaching.

2. WBC 11,000/mm³. The normal WBC count is 3900 to 11,900 cells/mm³. Because the finding is normal, it can be addressed last.

▶ *Test-taking Tip:* Knowledge of the normal ranges and the significance for critical laboratory values is expected on the NCLEX-RN®. Use the ABC's to determine priority. Of the laboratory values, determine those that are related to tissue perfusion (circulation), and then determine which value is most life-threatening.

Content Area: Adult; Concept: Critical Thinking; Perfusion; Integrated Processes: Nursing Process: Implementation; Client Needs: Safe and Effective Care Environment: Management of Care; Cognitive Level: Synthesis [Creating]

## 1049. MoC PHARM ANSWER: 2

1. Auscultating the client's lungs before and after the procedure is necessary to ensure that an air leak did not occur with removal, but administering the analgesic should be first.

2. **Because the peak action of morphine sulfate is 10 to 15 minutes, this should be administered first.**

3. Turning off the suction is necessary, but administering the analgesic should be first.

4. Assembling the dressing supplies is necessary, but administering the analgesic should be first.

▶ *Test-taking Tip:* Focusing on the client should be the priority.

Content Area: Adult; Concept: Critical Thinking; Comfort; Medication; Integrated Processes: Nursing Process: Planning; Client Needs: Physiological Integrity: Pharmacological and Parenteral Therapies; Safe and Effective Care Environment: Management of Care; Cognitive Level: Application [Applying]

## 1050. MoC ANSWER: 3, 4, 1, 2

3. **The 72-year-old client who was transferred 2 hours ago from the ICU following a coronary artery bypass graft and has new-onset atrial fibrillation with rapid ventricular response. This client should be assessed first because the client is most unstable and the rhythm most life-threatening.**

4. **The 38-year-old postoperative client who had an aortic valve replacement 2 days ago, BP 114/72 mm Hg, HR 100 bpm, RR 28 breaths/min, and T 101.2°F (38.4°C). This postoperative client is assessed next because the elevated temperature, RR, and HR increase the demands on the heart and could be a sign of pulmonary complications.**

1. **The 56-year-old client who was admitted 1 day ago with chest pain receiving IV heparin and has a PTT due back in 30 minutes. The nurse should assess this client next. PTT results should be back, and the dose may require adjustment.**

2. **The 62-year-old client with end-stage cardiomyopathy, BP of 78/50 mm Hg, 20 mL/hr urine output, and a "Do Not Resuscitate" order; whose family has just arrived. This client can be assessed last. The family members will have had time alone with the client, and the client and family may need emotional support.**

▶ *Test-taking Tip:* When establishing priorities, first determine life-threatening situations and then prioritize remaining clients by using the ABC's. Recall from Maslow's Hierarchy of Needs that physiological problems are priority over psychosocial issues; thus the client with end-stage cardiomyopathy should be assessed last.

Content Area: Adult; Concept: Critical Thinking; Perfusion; Integrated Processes: Nursing Process: Planning; Client Needs: Safe and Effective Care Environment: Management of Care; Cognitive Level: Synthesis [Creating]

## 1051. ANSWER: 1

1. **A copiously draining chest tube that is no longer draining indicates an obstruction. It should be most concerning because there is an increased risk for cardiac tamponade or pleural effusion.**

2. A slight elevation in temperature could be the effect of rewarming or inflammation after surgery. This should continue to be monitored but is not immediately concerning. Core temperature is one degree higher than an oral temperature.

3. The ABG results show compensated respiratory acidosis. Although the pH is low and the $PaCO_2$ is high, the kidneys are compensating by conserving $HCO_3$. Normal pH is 7.35 to 7.45, $PaCO_2$ is 32 to 42 mm Hg, $HCO_3$ is 20 to 24 mmol/L, and $PaO_2$ is 75 to 100 mm Hg.

4. A urine output of 160 mL/4 h is equivalent to 40 mL/h, which is adequate, but it warrants continued monitoring. Less than 30 mL/h indicates decreased renal function.

▶ *Test-taking Tip:* The key phrase in the question is "most concerning." Use the process of elimination and eliminate Options 3 and 4 because these are normal findings. Of Options 1 and 2, determine which option has the most concerning information.

Content Area: Adult; Concept: Assessment; Perfusion; Integrated Processes: Nursing Process: Evaluation; Client Needs: Physiological Integrity: Reduction of Risk Potential; Cognitive Level: Evaluation [Evaluating]

**1052.** MoC **ANSWER: 4**

1. Pulmonary embolism is a cause of cardiogenic shock and could occur after an MI, but it is not the most life-threatening complication.
2. Cardiac tamponade is a cause of cardiogenic shock, but cardiac tamponade would not be expected after an MI.
3. Cardiomyopathy may be an underlying cause of the MI, but it would not be an immediate complication following an MI.
4. **The symptoms are indicative of cardiogenic shock (decreased cardiac output leading to inadequate tissue perfusion and initiation of the shock syndrome).**

▶ *Test-taking Tip: The key word is "most life-threatening," indicating that more than one option may be correct. Select the most global option.*

Content Area: Adult; **Concept:** Assessment; Perfusion; Management; **Integrated Processes:** Nursing Process: Assessment; **Client Needs:** Safe and Effective Care Environment: Management of Care; **Cognitive Level:** Analysis [Analyzing]

**1053.** MoC **ANSWER: 2, 5**

1. Medication administration is not within the NA's scope of practice.
2. **The RN delegates appropriately when having the NA take the VS.**
3. Teaching is not within the NA's scope of practice.
4. Performing a chest tube dressing change where there is the potential for introducing air during the procedure is not within the NA's scope of practice.
5. **The RN delegates appropriately when having the NA perform a sponge bath.**

▶ *Test-taking Tip: Legally, the student nurse employed as an NA in a facility is only allowed to perform tasks listed in the job description of an NA, even though the student nurse has received instruction and acquired competence in administering medications and performing sterile procedures.*

Content Area: Adult; **Concept:** Safety; Legal; Regulations; **Integrated Processes:** Nursing Process: Evaluation; **Client Needs:** Safe and Effective Care Environment: Management of Care; **Cognitive Level:** Evaluation [Evaluating]

**1054. ANSWER: 4**

1. The client with an AAA typically reports persistent nagging pain in the abdomen, flank, and/or back, not the anterior upper chest.
2. A systolic bruit (swishing-like sound) may be auscultated over the abdominal aneurysm; a bruit is not palpated.
3. Edema of the face and neck with distended neck veins is associated with thoracic aortic aneurysms, not AAA.
4. **Throbbing or pulsating in the abdomen is the sign most indicative of an AAA.**

▶ *Test-taking Tip: Narrow the options to only those pertaining to the abdomen.*

Content Area: Adult; **Concept:** Perfusion; **Integrated Processes:** Nursing Process: Assessment; **Client Needs:** Physiological Integrity: Reduction of Risk Potential; Physiological Integrity: Physiological Adaptation; **Cognitive Level:** Comprehension [Understanding]

**1055.** MoC **ANSWER: 3**

1. Rechecking the pulse in 5 minutes could allow ischemia to progress.
2. The leg should already be in an appropriate position, so repositioning is not indicated.
3. **The nurse should notify the surgeon immediately to reassess the client. The loss of the pulse could signify graft occlusion or embolization.**
4. Although the nurse should document the finding, this is not the priority.

▶ *Test-taking Tip: Use the ABC's to establish that circulation is a priority concern. Thus notifying the surgeon would be the most immediate action so that the impaired circulation can be corrected.*

Content Area: Adult; **Concept:** Perfusion; **Integrated Processes:** Nursing Process: Implementation; **Client Needs:** Safe and Effective Care Environment: Management of Care; Physiological Integrity: Physiological Adaptation; **Cognitive Level:** Analysis [Analyzing]

**1056.** MoC **ANSWER: 3**

1. Throbbing pain can be due to improved blood flow, but it is also a sign of graft occlusion. Assessment of the pulses should occur first to rule out graft occlusion.
2. Assessing the dressing is important if bleeding were a concern, but it is more important to assess the pulses first.
3. **Pain is the first sign of graft occlusion, but it can also be due to improved blood flow after the bypass. The nurse must first assess that the graft is still patent by assessing distal pulses.**
4. Having the client rate the level of pain is important for adequate dosing of analgesics but is not the priority.

▶ *Test-taking Tip: Use ABC's (airway, breathing, circulation). Select the option that addresses the priority concern of maintaining graft patency—circulation.*

Content Area: Adult; **Concept:** Perfusion; **Integrated Processes:** Nursing Process: Implementation; **Client Needs:** Safe and Effective Care Environment: Management of Care; Physiological Integrity: Physiological Adaptation; **Cognitive Level:** Analysis [Analyzing]

**1057. ANSWER: 2**

1. Thoracic outlet syndrome is compression of the subclavian artery due to anatomic structures, leading to pain and ischemia in the arm.
2. **A popliteal aneurysm (located in the space behind the knee) may cause ischemia in the leg distal to the aneurysm due to thrombus forming inside the aneurysm and potential emboli.**

3. Pulmonary embolism develops from deep venous thrombosis in the leg or pelvic veins.

4. Raynaud's phenomenon consists of vasospasms in small arteries of the extremities, causing intermittent ischemia.

▶ *Test-taking Tip: Apply knowledge of medical terminology (popliteal) and note the relationship to one of the options.*

**Content Area:** Adult; **Concept:** Assessment; Perfusion; **Integrated Processes:** Nursing Process: Assessment; **Client Needs:** Physiological Integrity: Reduction of Risk Potential; **Cognitive Level:** Application [Applying]

## 1058. ANSWER: 1

1. **The nurse should include administering antihypertensive medications to the client with a thoracic aortic aneurysm; controlling HR and BP is important to decrease the risk of aneurysm rupture.**

2. The ribs would prevent palpation of the aneurysm; palpation of any aneurysm is contraindicated due to the risk of plaque breaking loose or aneurysm rupture.

3. An NG tube is not indicated for this client with only the information presented.

4. There is no indication that the client should be receiving a high-potassium and low-sodium diet.

▶ *Test-taking Tip: You should apply the pathophysiological concept that an increase in pressure can cause an aneurysm to rupture.*

**Content Area:** Adult; **Concept:** Perfusion; Medication; **Integrated Processes:** Nursing Process: Planning; **Client Needs:** Physiological Integrity: Physiological Adaptation; **Cognitive Level:** Application [Applying]

## 1059. ANSWER: 1, 2, 3, 5

1. **Blood loss will lead to low BP and scant urinary output due to decreased renal perfusion.**

2. **The pressure from the hemorrhage will interfere with the client's breathing, causing dyspnea.**

3. **Blood loss will lead to low BP (hypotension).**

4. A thoracic aneurysm does not cause abdominal distention because the bleeding is in the thoracic area.

5. **A thoracic aneurysm that ruptures will cause pain in the thoracic area.**

▶ *Test-taking Tip: Think about each option and its relationship to loss of blood volume and to bleeding into the thoracic cavity.*

**Content Area:** Adult; **Concept:** Assessment; Perfusion; **Integrated Processes:** Nursing Process: Analysis; **Client Needs:** Physiological Integrity: Physiological Adaptation; **Cognitive Level:** Application [Applying]

## 1060. ANSWER: 2

1. Venous ulcers typically occur at the ankle area with ankle discoloration; they have a pink ulcer bed with granulation tissue and are typically superficial with uneven, undefined edges.

2. **The nurse should find a notation of an arterial ulcer on the right foot. Arterial ulcers typically occur on the feet; they are deep, and the ulcer bed is pale with even, defined edges and limited granulation tissue.**

3. Diabetic ulcers are typically seen on the plantar area of the foot and are painless; there is no indication that this client has diabetes.

4. A stress ulcer occurs in the gastric mucosa and not on the lower extremities; a pressure ulcer may be found on bony prominences.

▶ *Test-taking Tip: If uncertain of the information, you can narrow the options by looking at the illustration and using the right or left foot stated in the option.*

**Content Area:** Adult; **Concept:** Perfusion; Communication; **Integrated Processes:** Communication and Documentation; **Client Needs:** Physiological Integrity: Physiological Adaptation; **Cognitive Level:** Analysis [Analyzing]

## 1061. ANSWER: 1

1. **The nurse should immediately intervene when the client states soaking feet daily; foot soaks when the client has PAD can cause maceration (tissue breakdown).**

2. Covering a sore with sterile gauze is an appropriate action for the client with a peripheral ulcer from PAD and does not require that the nurse intervene.

3. Using a pillow under the knees will keep the heels from having pressure areas; it is an appropriate action for the client with PAD and does not require that the nurse intervene.

4. Daily foot lubrication prevents cracking and infection and is an appropriate action for the client with PAD and does not require that the nurse intervene.

▶ *Test-taking Tip: The phrase "warrants immediate intervention" indicates an action that would be inappropriate for the client with PAD. Of the options, you need to consider that only one option would increase the client's risk for injury.*

**Content Area:** Adult; **Concept:** Perfusion; **Integrated Processes:** Nursing Process: Implementation; **Client Needs:** Physiological Integrity: Physiological Adaptation; **Cognitive Level:** Application [Applying]

## 1062. ANSWER: 4

1. I&O is important to monitor for fluid retention, dehydration, or renal function, but is not the priority.

2. Edema in the operative leg is expected from the surgical procedure and improved circulation.

3. Bending from the hip or knee should be limited to avoid graft occlusion.

4. The priority nursing action should be to monitor the pulses in the feet to detect graft occlusion. Checking both sides allows for comparison.

▶ *Test-taking Tip:* Use the ABC's to select the priority action of circulation.

Content Area: Adult; Concept: Perfusion; Integrated Processes: Nursing Process: Implementation; Client Needs: Physiological Integrity: Reduction of Risk Potential; Cognitive Level: Application [Applying]

## 1063. ANSWER: 3

1. Lack of blood supply to a body extremity may result in pain, pallor, pulselessness, paresthesia (numbness and tingling), paresis (decreased ability to move), and poikilothermia (coolness).
2. Lack of blood supply to a body extremity may result in paresthesia (numbness and tingling).
3. **Redness and warmth along the incision line are associated with inflammation or infection, not graft occlusion.**
4. Lack of blood supply to a body extremity may result in paresis (weakness) or paralysis (inability to move the foot).

▶ *Test-taking Tip:* Focus on the symptoms associated with decreased circulation. The symptoms can be remembered by six words, each beginning with the letter "P": pain, pallor, pulselessness, paresthesia (numbness and tingling), paresis (decreased ability to move), and poikilothermia (coolness).

Content Area: Adult; Concept: Perfusion; Clotting; Integrated Processes: Teaching/Learning; Client Needs: Physiological Integrity: Reduction of Risk Potential; Cognitive Level: Application [Applying]

## 1064. ANSWER: 1, 2, 5, 6

1. **Exercising promotes collateral circulation.**
2. **Discontinuing the use of nicotine products deters the arteriosclerotic process.**
3. Wearing support hose may impede circulation and increase the risk of restenosis.
4. Receiving professional foot care is a positive factor but does not prevent the progressive nature of peripheral arterial disease.
5. **A low-saturated-fat diet deters the arteriosclerotic process.**
6. **Taking cholesterol-lowering medications such as rosuvastatin calcium (Crestor) deters the arteriosclerotic process.**

▶ *Test-taking Tip:* Eliminate options that do not reduce the client's risk for developing atherosclerosis.

Content Area: Adult; Concept: Promoting Health; Perfusion; Integrated Processes: Nursing Process: Evaluation; Client Needs: Physiological Integrity: Basic Care and Comfort; Health Promotion and Maintenance; Cognitive Level: Evaluation [Evaluating]

## 1065. PHARM ANSWER: 4

1. A diuretic medication is used to decrease edema.
2. Pentoxifylline is not prescribed for smoking cessation. Nicotine substitutes are commonly prescribed to control nicotine withdrawal symptoms.

3. Venous ulcers resulting from prolonged venous hypertension are not treated with pentoxifylline.
4. **Pentoxifylline (Trental) is thought to act by improving capillary blood flow and is prescribed to decrease intermittent claudication. Effects are usually seen in 2 to 4 weeks.**

▶ *Test-taking Tip:* Consider that the action of the pentoxifylline is to improve circulation, and then use the process of elimination.

Content Area: Adult; Concept: Medication; Perfusion; Integrated Processes: Nursing Process: Evaluation; Client Needs: Physiological Integrity: Pharmacological and Parenteral Therapies; Cognitive Level: Evaluation [Evaluating]

## 1066. ANSWER: 3

1. Avoiding exposure to cold will reduce the pain but is not the nurse's initial focus.
2. Maintaining meticulous hygiene is a positive action to follow but is not the nurse's initial focus.
3. **Buerger's disease is an uncommon vascular occlusive disease that affects the medial and small arteries and veins, initially in the distal limbs. It is strongly associated with tobacco use, which causes vasoconstriction. The most important action to communicate to the client is that he must abstain from tobacco in all forms to prevent progression of the disease.**
4. A low-saturated-fat diet is a healthy diet but is not the nurse's initial focus.

▶ *Test-taking Tip:* You should look for related words in the stem and the options to arrive at the answer.

Content Area: Adult; Concept: Perfusion; Nursing Roles; Integrated Processes: Teaching/Learning; Client Needs: Safe and Effective Care Environment: Safety and Infection Control; Physiological Integrity: Physiological Adaptation; Cognitive Level: Application [Applying]

## 1067. PHARM ANSWER: 2

1. Nifedipine is used as an antihypertensive agent, but that is not the purpose with Raynaud's disease. The client is at risk to develop hypotension as an adverse effect.
2. **Raynaud's disease is a disease in which cutaneous arteries in the extremities have recurrent episodes of vasospasm that result in pain and numbness. Nifedipine (Procardia), a calcium-channel blocker, causes vasodilation, thus reducing pain and numbness.**
3. Tolerance to cold, not heat, should improve.
4. Claudication is not associated with Raynaud's disease but is associated with arteriosclerotic changes in the larger arteries.

▶ *Test-taking Tip:* Nifedipine has multiple uses; you need to relate its use to relieving the symptoms of Raynaud's disease.

Content Area: Adult; Concept: Medication; Perfusion; Integrated Processes: Nursing Process: Evaluation; Client Needs: Physiological Integrity: Pharmacological and Parenteral Therapies; Cognitive Level: Evaluation [Evaluating]

**1068. ANSWER: 2, 3, 5**

1. Eating excessive amounts of dark green vegetables could affect the anticoagulant effect of warfarin, but there is no indication the client is taking an anticoagulant.
2. **Elevating the legs when sitting promotes venous return and reduces edema.**
3. **Wearing graduated compression stockings promotes venous return and reduces edema.**
4. Clients who have chronic venous insufficiency should avoid prolonged standing.
5. **Elevating the legs when sleeping increases venous return and reduces edema.**

▶ *Test-taking Tip:* Chronic venous insufficiency develops because of damaged valves in the veins, resulting in venous hypertension and impairment of blood return to the heart. Select options that will improve venous return.

Content Area: Adult; Concept: Perfusion; Integrated Processes: Teaching/Learning; Client Needs: Physiological Integrity: Basic Care and Comfort; Cognitive Level: Analysis [Analyzing]

**1069. MoC ANSWER: 2**

1. With the unilateral leg swelling, the nurse does not need additional assessment data about activity.
2. **The nurse should inform the HCP about the assessment findings. A possible DVT is taken seriously because it can lead to PE. Unilateral swelling of one leg is a classic symptom of DVT.**
3. Advising aspirin is not within the scope of nursing practice and has possible negative consequences.
4. Findings are significant and should be reported to the HCP.

▶ *Test-taking Tip:* You should eliminate options that are not within the nurse's scope of practice. Research has shown that the Homans' sign is not an accurate indicator of the presence of a DVT.

Content Area: Adult; Concept: Perfusion; Clotting; Management; Integrated Processes: Nursing Process: Implementation; Client Needs: Safe and Effective Care Environment: Management of Care; Physiological Integrity: Reduction of Risk Potential; Cognitive Level: Analysis [Analyzing]

**1070. ANSWER: 1**

1. **Walking promotes venous return; verbalizing intent to increase activity indicates that an expected outcome has been met for the client with varicose veins.**
2. Compression stockings should be worn often to promote venous return and prevent further varicosities, rather than decreasing their use.
3. Standing for a prolonged period of time should be avoided.
4. Choosing a diet high in potassium and low in magnesium does not apply to the client with varicose veins.

▶ *Test-taking Tip:* Using clues such as "vein" in the stem and finding similar words in the options often will help you to find the answer.

Content Area: Adult; Concept: Perfusion; Integrated Processes: Nursing Process: Evaluation; Client Needs: Physiological Integrity: Physiological Adaptation; Cognitive Level: Evaluation [Evaluating]

**1071. ANSWER: 2**

1. A PT of 25 seconds and INR of 2.5 are prolonged and do not indicate hypercoagulability.
2. **Blood stasis (immobility), endothelial injury (postoperative client), and hypercoagulability (platelet count increased) suggest Virchow's triad, which is associated with an increased risk of DVT.**
3. The client's PTT of 55 seconds is prolonged and does not indicate hypercoagulability.
4. This client has arterial insufficiency, not a venous disorder; the platelet count of $350,000/mm^3$ is within the normal range.

▶ *Test-taking Tip:* When presented with a question about risk factors, count the number of risk factors for the condition in each of the options. The client with the greatest number of risk factors for DVT development is the answer.

Content Area: Adult; Concept: Perfusion; Integrated Processes: Nursing Process: Analysis; Client Needs: Physiological Integrity: Reduction of Risk Potential; Cognitive Level: Analysis [Analyzing]

**1072. ANSWER: 1, 4**

1. **A pneumatic compression device applies pulsing pressures similar to those that occur during normal walking. They can help reduce the risk of DVT and PE.**
2. Although giving heparin intravenously will achieve anticoagulation, a subcutaneous injection of low-dose unfractionated or low-molecular-weight heparin is usually prescribed.
3. Coughing and deep breathing promote lung expansion and help prevent pulmonary complications after surgery, but this does not decrease the risk for DVT or PE.
4. **Isometric exercises are muscle-strengthening exercises that also compress vessels and thus decrease the risk for DVT and PE.**
5. Graded compression elastic stockings should be worn to improve venous return and prevent thrombi formation. Their use is avoided if peripheral arterial disease is present.

▶ *Test-taking Tip:* Focus on actions to decrease the risk for deep venous thrombosis and pulmonary embolism. Evaluate each option to determine its effect on improving circulation and reducing hypercoagulation.

Content Area: Adult; Concept: Perfusion; Clotting; Integrated Processes: Nursing Process: Planning; Client Needs: Physiological Integrity: Reduction of Risk Potential; Cognitive Level: Application [Applying]

**1073. ANSWER: 1, 2, 3, 4, 5**

1. A vascular sign of microembolism is skin petechiae.
2. Crackles occur due to HF secondary to IE.
3. Peripheral edema occurs due to HF secondary to IE.
4. **Vegetations that adhere to the heart valves can break off into the circulation, causing embolism, valve incompetence, and a murmur.**
5. **Arthralgia (joint pain) can occur from microembolism and inadequate perfusion.**
6. Hemangioma is a benign vascular tumor of dilated blood vessels; it is not associated with IE.

▶ *Test-taking Tip: In IE, microorganisms and debris from the inflammatory process can adhere to heart valves. Select signs and symptoms indicating that the heart valves are affected and also those that can occur if portions of the vegetation should break off into the circulation.*

Content Area: Adult; Concept: Infection; Perfusion; Integrated Processes: Nursing Process: Assessment; Client Needs: Physiological Integrity: Reduction of Risk Potential; Cognitive Level: Knowledge [Remembering]

**1074. ANSWER: 3**

1. Anticoagulation is not necessary if a vena cava filter is in place.
2. There is no abdominal incision with the percutaneous approach.
3. **The procedure for placement of a vena cava filter is done percutaneously, usually through the subclavian or femoral vein approach. The nurse should check the groin insertion site for bleeding.**
4. Dye is not used during placement of a vena cava filter.

▶ *Test-taking Tip: A percutaneous approach is used to place a vena cava filter.*

Content Area: Adult; Concept: Nursing Roles; Perfusion; Integrated Processes: Nursing Process: Implementation; Client Needs: Physiological Integrity: Reduction of Risk Potential; Cognitive Level: Application [Applying]

**1075. ANSWER: 4**

1. Dangling legs in a dependent position decreases venous return and will increase pain and discomfort.
2. There *are* nonsurgical management options for treating varicose veins.
3. Telling the client to wear long pants implies judgment of the client's perception of the varicose veins; it also does not address the question of pain and discomfort associated with varicose veins.
4. **The best response to alleviate pain and discomfort associated with varicose veins includes application of elastic stockings and elevating the lower extremities. These promote venous return.**

▶ *Test-taking Tip: Consider nonsurgical options to alleviate the pain and discomfort associated with varicose veins. Remember that veins promote venous return to the heart; you should be drawn to Option 4.*

Content Area: Adult; Concept: Perfusion; Integrated Processes: Teaching/Learning; Communication and Documentation; Client Needs: Physiological Integrity: Basic Care and Comfort; Psychosocial Integrity; Cognitive Level: Application [Applying]

**1076. MoC PHARM CJ ANSWER: 1**

1. **The client's PR interval was prolonged (normal is 0.12–0.20 seconds). Carvedilol (Coreg) is a beta blocker that can further lengthen the PR internal, resulting in heart block.**
2. The client's serum magnesium level of 1.6 mg/dL is low (normal range is 1.8–2.6 mg/dL). The dosing and rate of administration for magnesium replacement is correct. A sulfate can be safely given when a person has a sulfonamide allergy.
3. Interventions are correct. An oxygen saturation at 85% is below the expected range of 92% to 100%. A nonrebreather mask with an oxygen flow at 15 L can deliver an $F_{IO2}$ of 100%.
4. Interventions are correct. An external pacemaker will deliver a pacing impulse to increase the client's HR.

▶ *Test-taking Tip: The normal PR interval is 0.12 to 0.20 seconds.*

Content Area: Adult; Concept: Medication; Management; Perfusion; Integrated Processes: Nursing Process: Evaluation; Client Needs: Safe and Effective Care Environment: Management of Care; Physiological Integrity: Pharmacological and Parenteral Therapies; Cognitive Level: Evaluation [Evaluating]

**1077. MoC PHARM CJ ANSWER:**

> **Withheld the carvedilol (Coreg) and notified the HCP**

▶ *Test-taking Tip: When a medication will have an adverse effect, the nurse should withhold the medication and notify the HCP.*

Content Area: Adult; Concept: Medication; Management; Perfusion; Integrated Processes: Nursing Process: Evaluation; Client Needs: Safe and Effective Care Environment: Management of Care; Physiological Integrity: Pharmacological and Parenteral Therapies; Cognitive Level: Evaluation [Evaluating]

## Chapter Twenty-Five

# Endocrine Management

**1078.** The nurse is interviewing four clients. Which client is at the greatest risk for developing type 2 DM?

1. The 56-year-old Hispanic female
2. The 40-year-old Asian American female
3. The 25-year-old obese Caucasian male
4. The 38-year-old Native American male

**1079.** **PHARM** The nurse obtains a fingerstick blood glucose reading of 48 mg/dL for the client with type 1 DM. The client is to receive 6 units of regular and 10 units of NPH insulin now. Which is the nurse's **best** immediate intervention?

1. Administer the insulin that is due now.
2. Call the lab for a STAT serum glucose level.
3. Have the client choose foods for a meal now.
4. Provide juice with 15 grams of carbohydrates.

**1080.** **MoC** The nurse is reviewing serum laboratory results for four female clients. Place an X on the client requiring the most immediate assessment.

| Client | Lab Test | Result | Normal Ranges |
|--------|----------|--------|---------------|
| A | Thyroid-stimulating hormone (TSH) level | 5.2 mIU/L | 0.4–4.2 mIU/L |
| | Free thyroxine (T4) | 0.8 ng/dL | 0.8–2.7 ng/dL |
| B | Growth hormone (GH) | 23 µg/L | 8–18 µg/L |
| | Insulin-like growth factor I (IGF-I) | 490 ng/mL | 105–441 ng/mL |
| C | Free thyroxine (T4) | 7.0 ng/dL | 0.8–2.7 ng/dL |
| | Thyroid-stimulating hormone (TSH) level | 0.1 mIU/L | 0.4–4.2 mIU/L |
| D | Fasting glucose | 140 mg/dL | 70–110 mg/dL |
| | Hgb A$_{1c}$ | 6.9% | Less than 6% |

**1081.** The clinic nurse is evaluating the client with type 1 DM who intends to enroll in a tennis class. Which statement made by the client indicates that the client understands the effects of exercise on insulin demand?

1. "I will carry a high-fat, high-calorie food, such as a cookie."
2. "I will administer 1 unit of lispro insulin prior to playing tennis."
3. "I will eat a 15-gram carbohydrate snack before playing tennis."
4. "If I feel sweaty or shaky during tennis, my blood sugar is too high."

**1082.** PHARM The client taking NPH insulin at 0800 reports feeling anxious and shaky in the midafternoon. Which intervention is **best** for the nurse to initiate?

1. Have the client rate the level of anxiety.
2. Give the client's prn dose of lorazepam.
3. Check the client's fingerstick blood glucose level.
4. Advise the client to sit in a recliner to relax.

**1083.** MoC The nurse is caring for multiple clients with DM. It is **most** important for the nurse to initiate a referral to a diabetes educator for which client?

1. The client who states diabetes is well controlled with diet and exercise; Hgb $A_{1c}$ is 11%.
2. The client requesting diabetes information; fingerstick glucose is 132 mg/dL, Hgb $A_{1c}$ is 5.6%.
3. The client who states perfect compliance with diet, exercise, and meds; Hgb $A_{1c}$ is 7%.
4. The client with short-term memory loss; fingerstick glucose is 110 mg/dL, Hgb $A_{1c}$ is 4.5%.

**1084.** The nurse is reviewing information for the client with type 1 DM. The nurse concludes that the client may be experiencing the Somogyi phenomenon, as evidenced by which finding?

1. 0200 blood glucose between 80–110 mg/dL and morning levels between 80–100 mg/dL
2. 0200 blood glucose between 50–60 mg/dL and morning levels between 48–62 mg/dL
3. 0200 blood glucose between 130–140 mg/dL and morning levels between 180–200 mg/dL
4. 0200 blood glucose between 45–62 mg/dL and morning levels between 200–305 mg/dL

**1085.** MoC The nurse is planning to complete noon assessments for four assigned clients with type 1 DM. All of the clients received subcutaneous insulin aspart at 0800 hours. Place the clients in the order of priority for the nurse's assessment.

1. The 60-year-old client who is nauseated and has just vomited for the second time
2. The 45-year-old client who is dyspneic and has chest pressure and new-onset atrial fibrillation
3. The 75-year-old client with a fingerstick blood glucose level of 300 mg/dL
4. The 50-year-old client with a fingerstick blood glucose level of 70 mg/dL

Answer: _____

**1086.** PHARM The client with DM is to receive insulin IV at 1.5 units/hr. The insulin bag contains 10 units of insulin in 100 mL of NS. At what rate in mL/hr should the nurse set the infusion pump?

_____ mL/hr (Record your answer rounded to the nearest tenth.)

**1087.** PHARM The client ate 45 g of carbohydrate (carb) with the dinner meal. The client is to receive 2 units of aspart insulin subcutaneously for each carb choice (CHO) eaten (1 carb choice = 15 g). Which syringe shows the correct amount of insulin that the nurse should administer?

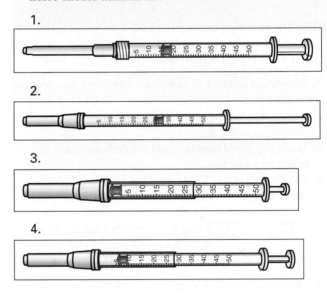

1.

2.

3.

4.

**1088.** MoC The client with type 1 DM is scheduled for major surgery in the morning. The nurse on the night shift observes that the client's daily insulin dose remains the same as previously given. Which nursing action is **most** appropriate?

1. Notify the prescribing HCP about the client's surgery and ask about any insulin changes.
2. Write an order to decrease the morning insulin dose by one-half of the prescribed dose.
3. Do nothing; the HCP would want the client to receive the usual insulin dose prior to surgery.
4. Have the day shift nurse check a morning glucose level and, if normal, hold the insulin dose.

**1089.** PHARM The nurse administers a usual morning dose of 4 units of regular insulin and 8 units of NPH insulin at 7:30 a.m. to the client with a blood glucose level of 110 mg/dL. Which statements regarding the client's insulin are correct?

1. The onset of the regular insulin will be at 7:45 a.m. and the peak at 1:00 p.m.
2. The onset of the regular insulin will be at 8:00 a.m. and the peak at 10:00 a.m.
4. The onset of the NPH insulin will be at 8:00 a.m. and the peak at 10:00 a.m.
6. The onset of the NPH insulin will be at 12:30 p.m. and the peak at 11:30 p.m.

**1090.** The nurse is planning to address diabetic meal planning with the client recently diagnosed with type 1 DM. Which action should the nurse take **first**?

1. Encourage use of non-nutritive sweeteners that contain no calories.
2. Emphasize the importance of keeping regular mealtimes every day.
3. Teach the client how to count the carbohydrates in meals and snacks.
4. Ask the client to identify favorite foods and the client's usual mealtimes.

**1091.** MoC PHARM The nurse reviews the HCP's orders for the newly admitted client who has DKA. Which order should the nurse question?

1. Start intravenous $D_5W$ at 125 mL/hr.
2. Give KCL 10 mEq in 100 mL NaCl IV now.
3. Give sodium bicarbonate IV per pharmacy dosing if arterial pH is less than 7.0.
4. Start regular insulin infusion per protocol; titrate based on hourly glucose level.

**1092.** The nurse evaluates the client who is being treated for DKA. Which finding indicates that the client is responding to the treatment plan?

1. Eyes sunken and skin flushed
2. Skin moist with rapid elastic recoil
3. Serum potassium level is 3.3 mEq/L
4. ABG results are pH 7.25, $Paco_2$ 30, $HCO_3$ 17

**1093.** The client with type 2 DM is scheduled for cardiac rehabilitation exercises (cardiac rehab). The nurse notes that the client's blood glucose level is 300 mg/dL and that the urine is positive for ketones. How should the nurse proceed?

1. Send the client to cardiac rehab; exercise will lower the client's glucose level.
2. Give insulin; send the client for exercises with a 15-gram carbohydrate snack.
3. Delay cardiac rehab; blood glucose levels will decrease too much with exercise.
4. Cancel cardiac rehab; blood glucose levels will increase further with exercise.

**1094.** The client residing in a long-term care facility has type 2 DM and is sick with influenza. The client's blood glucose is 245 mg/dL. Which action should the nurse take **next**?

1. Check the client's urine for ketones.
2. Keep the client NPO until glucose levels decline.
3. Immediately contact the client's HCP.
4. Monitor blood glucose levels every 6 hours.

**1095.** The nurse is teaching the client newly diagnosed with type 2 DM. Which information should the nurse emphasize in the session?

1. Use the arm when self-administering insulin.
2. Exercise for 30 minutes daily after a meal.
3. Get 30% of daily calories from protein foods.
4. Eat a 30-gram carbohydrate snack prior to strenuous activity.

**1096.** The nurse is assessing the client who has type 2 DM. Which findings indicate to the nurse that the client is experiencing HHNS? **Select all that apply.**

1. Serum osmolality 364 mOsm/kg
2. Blood glucose level 160 mg/dL
3. Very dry mucous membranes
4. BP of 90/42 mm Hg
5. Urine output 500 mL past 8 hours

**1097.** The nurse determined that the client's fluid volume deficit from HHNS has resolved. Which serum laboratory finding led to the nurse's conclusion?

1. Decreased glucose
2. Decreased sodium
3. Decreased osmolality
4. Decreased potassium

**1098.** The elderly Hispanic client, newly diagnosed with type 2 DM, has been instructed on self-administering NPH and regular insulin in the morning and at suppertime. When completing teaching during a home visit, what information should the nurse reinforce? **Select all that apply.**

1. Inspect the feet and between the toes daily.
2. Use magnifying devices to read small print.
3. Perform a hemoglobin $A_{1c}$ test once a week.
4. Eat a 15-gram carbohydrate snack at bedtime.
5. Inject 1 unit of NPH insulin after eating a snack.

**1099.** The nurse is caring for the client with type 2 DM. Which instructions should the nurse provide to the client regarding diabetes management during stress or illness? **Select all that apply.**

1. Notify the HCP if unable to keep fluids or foods down.
2. Test fingerstick glucose levels and urine ketones daily and keep a record.
3. Continue to take oral hypoglycemic medications and/or insulin as prescribed.
4. Supplement food intake with carbohydrate-containing fluids, such as juices or soups.
5. When on an oral agent, administer insulin in addition to the oral agent during the illness.

**1100.** **PHARM** The nurse is caring for the client diagnosed with DI. Which nursing actions are **most** appropriate? **Select all that apply.**

1. Monitoring hourly urine output and daily weights
2. Checking urine osmolality and urine ketones
3. Giving desmopressin acetate as prescribed
4. Checking glucose levels before meals and at bedtime
5. Monitoring for signs or symptoms of hyperkalemia

**1101.** The client develops SIADH secondary to a pituitary tumor. The client's assessment findings include thirst, weight gain, fatigue, and a serum sodium of 127 mEq/L. Which intervention, if prescribed, should the nurse implement to treat SIADH?

1. Elevate the head of the bed 30 degrees.
2. Administer vasopressin intravenously (IV).
3. Restrict fluids to 800 to 1000 mL per day.
4. Give 0.3% sodium chloride IV infusion.

**1102.** The nurse is collecting information about the client who underwent a transsphenoidal removal of a pituitary tumor. Which findings should indicate to the nurse that the client is experiencing DI? **Select all that apply.**

1. Serum osmolality 310 mOsm/kg
2. Weight increased 2 kg in 24 hours
3. Experiencing an extreme thirst
4. Urine output 4200 mL in 24 hours
5. BP averaging 164/92 mm Hg or higher

**1103.** **MoC** The client had a hypophysectomy via the transsphenoidal approach 12 hours ago. Which action by a new nurse would require the observing nurse to intervene?

1. Elevates the head of the client's bed to 30 degrees
2. Gathers supplies to replace the bloody nasal packing
3. Moisturizes the client's oral mucous membranes
4. Places a cold washcloth over the client's swollen eyes

**1104.** The nurse is caring for the client with SIADH. Which of the following should the nurse plan to implement? **Select all that apply.**

1. Obtain the weight near the same time each morning.
2. Place on a fluid-restricted diet as prescribed.
3. Prepare to give an IV fluid bolus of 500-mL NaCl.
4. Administer furosemide IV as prescribed.
5. Monitor for hyperactive reflexes and heightened alertness.

**1105.** **MoC** The client taking thyroid replacement hormone is hospitalized, and a thyroid replacement hormone is not prescribed. A week after being hospitalized, the nurse assesses that the client is becoming increasingly lethargic and has a decreased BP, RR, temperature, and pulse. Which actions should be taken by the nurse? Place each nursing action in the order of priority.

1. Warm the client.
2. Administer intravenous fluids.
3. Assist in ventilatory support.
4. Administer thyroxine as prescribed.

Answer: _____

**1106.** The nurse assesses the client following a total thyroidectomy. Which finding indicates that the client has a positive Trousseau's sign?

1.

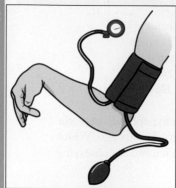

2.

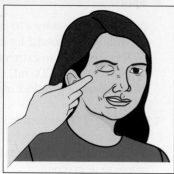

3.

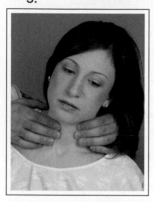

4.

**1107.** The client newly diagnosed with hyperthyroidism has a fever of 101.3°F (38.5°C). Which additional assessment findings should the nurse identify as those associated with thyroid storm? **Select all that apply.**

1. Hypoventilation
2. HR 140 bpm
3. Diarrhea lasting 4 days
4. Periorbital edema
5. Recent tooth extraction

**1108.** MoC The agitated client is hospitalized with tachycardia, dyspnea, and intermittent chest palpitations. The client's BP is 170/110 mm Hg, and HR is 130 bpm. The client's health history reveals thinning hair, recent 10-lb weight loss, increased appetite, fine hand and tongue tremors, hyperreflexic tendon reflexes, and smooth, moist skin. Which prescribed intervention should be the nurse's **priority**?

1. Do 12-lead electrocardiogram (ECG) and cardiac enzyme levels.
2. Obtain thyroid-stimulating hormone (TSH) and free $T_4$ levels.
3. Give propranolol 2 mg IV q15 min or until symptoms are controlled.
4. Give propylthiouracil 600-mg oral loading dose; then 200 mg orally q4h.

**1109.** PHARM A clinic nurse is teaching the client newly diagnosed with hypothyroidism. Which instructions should the nurse provide about taking levothyroxine sodium? **Select all that apply.**

1. Take the medication 1 hour before or 2 hours after breakfast.
2. Call the clinic if the pulse before taking the medication is greater than 100 beats per minute.
3. Report adverse drug effects, including weight gain, cold intolerance, and alopecia.
4. Take this drug as prescribed; it replaces thyroid hormone that is diminished or absent.
5. Have frequent laboratory monitoring to be sure your levels of $T_3$ and $T_4$ decrease.

**INSTRUCTIONS:** Refer to the information provided to answer Questions 1110 and 1111.

**1110.** `PHARM` `CJ` The nurse is caring for the client who had a thyroidectomy 2 days ago. Based on the findings of the client's serum laboratory report, which medication should the nurse plan to administer **first?**

| Serum Lab Test | Client's Value | Normal |
|---|---|---|
| BUN | 24 mg/dL | 5–25 mg/dL |
| Creatinine | 1.2 mg/dL | 0.5–1.5 mg/dL |
| Na | 138 mEq/L | 135–145 mEq/L |
| K | 3.4 mEq/L | 3.5–5.3 mEq/L |
| Calcium | 6 mg/dL | 9–11 mg/dL |
| Hgb | 10.0 g/dL | 13.5–17 g/dL |
| Hct | 38% | 40%–54% |

1. Potassium chloride 20 mEq oral bid
2. Calcium gluconate 4.5 mEq IV once
3. Dolasetron 12.5 mg IV as needed
4. Levothyroxine 50 mcg oral daily

**1111.** `PHARM` `CJ` One month after discharge, the clinic nurse assesses the client. The nurse evaluates that the client's levothyroxine dose is too low when which findings are noted on assessment? **Select all that apply.**

1. Increased appetite
2. Decreased sweating
3. Apathy and fatigue
4. Paresthesias
5. Finger and tongue tremors
6. Slowed mental processes

**1112.** The female client is to receive radioactive iodine (RAI) therapy for an enlarged thyroid gland. The client asks, "Are there precautions with this therapy?" Which is the nurse's **best** response?

1. "No precautions are necessary. The radiation in the form of an oral capsule will target and destroy thyroid tissue only."
2. "Use contraceptives or abstain from intercourse to avoid conceiving during and for 6 months after treatment."
3. "Discontinue taking the antithyroid medication and propranolol; results are seen immediately with RAI therapy."
4. "Some people need a thyroid hormone replacement, but it is not necessary when the thyroid gland is enlarged."

**1113.** The nurse is teaching the client who lacks parathyroid hormone (PTH) about foods to consume. Which items should be included on a list of appropriate foods for the client?

1. Dark green vegetables, soybeans, and tofu
2. Spinach, strawberries, and yogurt
3. Whole grain bread, milk, and liver
4. Rhubarb, yellow vegetables, and fish

**1114.** The client is hospitalized with possible Cushing's syndrome. Which laboratory results should the nurse expect if the diagnosis of Cushing's syndrome is confirmed? **Select all that apply.**

1. Hyperglycemia
2. Eosinophilia
3. Hypocalcemia
4. Hypokalemia
5. Thrombocytopenia
6. Elevated serum cortisol

**1115.** `MoC` The nurse assesses that the client diagnosed with Cushing's syndrome has an irregular HR, right arm ecchymosis, 4+ pitting edema in the legs, and a blood glucose of 140 mg/dL. Which action should be the nurse's **priority**?

1. Weigh the client again.
2. Administer insulin as prescribed.
3. Notify the HCP.
4. Measure the client's abdominal girth.

**1116.** `PHARM` The nurse completes teaching the client with Cushing's disease. Which statement demonstrates that the client understands measures to prevent bone resorption from corticosteroid therapy?

1. "I will increase calcium in my diet to 3000 mg daily."
2. "I should participate in daily weight-bearing exercises."
3. "I should limit my dietary intake of sodium and vitamin D."
4. "I plan to rise slowly from a bed or chair to avoid falling."

**1117.** The client diagnosed with Cushing's syndrome is admitted with fluid volume overload. The client weighed 190 lb on admission and 179 lb after treatment. The nurse estimates that the amount of fluid the client lost was how many milliliters?

_____ mL (Record your answer as a whole number.)

**1118.** The nurse is preparing to care for the stable client with Addison's disease. Which skin appearance should the nurse expect when performing an assessment?

1. Very white, dry, and scaly
2. Bronzed and suntanned hue
3. Diaphoretic and cyanotic
4. Puffy and butterfly-like rash

**1119.** The nurse is providing teaching to multiple clients. Which client should the nurse determine would benefit if the following illustration were utilized when teaching?

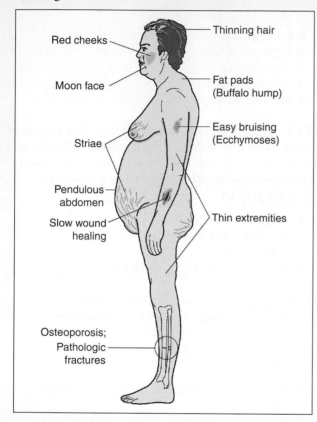

Red cheeks
Moon face
Striae
Pendulous abdomen
Slow wound healing
Osteoporosis; Pathologic fractures

Thinning hair
Fat pads (Buffalo hump)
Easy bruising (Ecchymoses)
Thin extremities

1. The client with hyperthyroidism
2. The client with diabetes mellitus
3. The client with Addison's disease
4. The client with Cushing's syndrome

**1120.** **PHARM** The nurse is caring for the client admitted in Addisonian crisis. Which medication, if prescribed, should the nurse plan to administer?

1. Regular insulin
2. Ketoconazole
3. Sodium nitroprusside
4. Hydrocortisone

**1121.** **MoC** The nurse is reviewing the serum laboratory report for the hospitalized client who has adrenocortical insufficiency. The nurse should immediately notify the HCP about which value?

1. White blood cells 11,000/mm³
2. Glucose 138 mg/dL
3. Sodium 148 mEq/L
4. Potassium 6.2 mEq/L

**1122.** The nurse receives orders for the newly admitted client with Addison's disease. Which orders should the nurse question with the HCP? **Select all that apply.**

1. Potassium 20 mEq oral now
2. Sodium-restricted diet of 1000 mg
3. Serum cortisol level in early a.m.
4. Obtain serum glucose level now
5. 5% dextrose in NS at 100 mL/hr

**1123.** **PHARM** The nurse is caring for the client with Addisonian crisis. Which clinical change should indicate to the nurse that the therapy is effective?

1. Increase of 25 mm Hg in the client's BP
2. Decrease of 25 mm Hg in the systolic BP
3. Increase in serum potassium from 3.4 to 5.8 mEq/dL
4. Decrease in serum sodium from 146 to 136 mEq/L

**1124.** **MoC** The nurse is admitting the client tentatively diagnosed with possible hyperaldosteronism. What should be the nurse's **priority?**

1. Prepare for a computed tomography (CT) scan.
2. Give prn prescribed analgesic to treat headache.
3. Obtain an ECG to evaluate for dysrhythmias.
4. Assess for generalized weakness and fatigue.

**1125.** The nurse is preparing to discharge the client following a unilateral adrenalectomy to treat hyperaldosteronism caused by an adenoma. Which instruction should be included in this client's discharge teaching?

1. Avoid foods high in potassium.
2. Self-monitor BP daily.
3. Stop drugs taken before adrenalectomy.
4. Carry epinephrine for emergency use.

**1126.** PHARM The nurse is caring for the client who is experiencing symptoms associated with pheochromocytoma. Which intervention should be included in the plan of care for this client?

1. Offer distractions such as television or music.
2. Encourage family and friends to visit often.
3. Assist with ambulation at least three times a day.
4. Administer nicardipine for hypertension.

**1127.** MoC The nurse is preparing to care for four clients. In which order should the nurse plan to attend to the clients?

1. The client following a thyroidectomy who has hoarseness and an SaO₂ of 86%
2. The client with hyperparathyroidism with a serum calcium level of 10.1 mg/dL
3. The client with diabetes insipidus drinking frequently and asking for more cold water
4. The client with hyperthyroidism who has a temperature of 102.2°F (39°C) and tachycardia

Answer: _____

# Answers and Rationales

## 1078. ANSWER: 4

1. Although the incidence of DM is higher among Hispanics than Caucasians, Native Americans have the highest risk.
2. The incidence of DM is low among Asian Americans.
3. The young client who is obese does have an increased risk and should be explored for DM, but the Native American client is at greatest risk. The incidence of DM is higher among Native Americans than Caucasians, and the Native American client is older.
4. **The nurse should further explore whether the Native American male client has developed DM. Research has shown that the highest incidence of DM is among Native Americans.**

▶ *Test-taking Tip: When the stem includes the word "most," more than one option could be correct, but one option is more important than the other.*

Content Area: Adult; Concept: Diversity; Metabolism; Integrated Processes: Nursing Process: Assessment; Culture and Spirituality; Client Needs: Health Promotion and Maintenance; Cognitive Level: Knowledge [Remembering]

## 1079. PHARM ANSWER: 4

1. Administering insulin when hypoglycemia is already present could cause unconsciousness and death.
2. Calling the lab to obtain a STAT serum glucose level will delay the client's treatment for hypoglycemia.
3. Having the client choose foods for a meal will delay the client's treatment for hypoglycemia.
4. **Normal blood glucose level is 70–110 mg/dL. Hypoglycemia is treated with 15 to 20 g of a simple (fast-acting) carbohydrate, such as 4 to 6 oz of fruit juice or 8 oz of low-fat milk.**

▶ *Test-taking Tip: Focus on the issue: interventions for a low blood sugar reading. Insulin is contraindicated when hypoglycemia exists. Knowledge of critical lab values, such as the normal blood glucose range of 70–110 mg/dL, is tested on the NCLEX-RN® examination.*

Content Area: Adult; Concept: Metabolism; Integrated Processes: Nursing Process: Implementation; Client Needs: Physiological Integrity: Physiological Adaptation; Physiological Integrity: Pharmacological and Parenteral Therapies; Cognitive Level: Application [Applying]

## 1080. MoC ANSWER:

| | | | |
|---|---|---|---|
| C | Free thyrox-ine (T4) | 7.0 ng/dL | 0.8–2.7 ng/dL |
| X | Thyroid-stimulating hormone (TSH) level | 0.1 mIU/L | 0.4–4.2 mIU/L |

**Client C has an elevated T4 and decreased TSH, indicating an excess of thyroid hormone. This client has life-threatening results that can produce severe hypertension and tachycardia. The client should be assessed for impending thyroid storm.**

Client A has an elevated TSH level indicating hypothyroidism. TSH is needed to ensure proper synthesis and secretion of the thyroid hormones, which are essential for life. Although it should be addressed, this client is not in need of immediate assessment because an elevated TSH and normal T4 indicate mild hypothyroidism.

Client B has elevated growth hormone (GH) and insulin-like growth factor 1(IGF-I), which are associated with acromegaly. Bone and soft tissue deformities and enlarged viscera can occur. The HCP should be aware of this level, but the client does not need immediate assessment.

Client D has elevated glucose and Hgb A$_{1c}$ levels, which are associated with DM. These levels are not life-threatening, requiring immediate assessment, or intervention.

♦ *Test-taking Tip: Focus on the laboratory values and the normal ranges. Think about the functions of the hormones and the values that would be most life-threatening to establish priority.*

Content Area: Adult; Concept: Critical Thinking; Assessment; Metabolism; Management; Integrated Processes: Nursing Process: Analysis; Client Needs: Safe and Effective Care Environment: Management of Care; Cognitive Level: Analysis [Analyzing]

## 1081. ANSWER: 3

1. The food should be a simple sugar food because the fat content of a high-fat food will delay the absorption of the glucose in the food.
2. Taking insulin prior to activity will lower the blood glucose level such that hypoglycemia can occur.
3. **Excessive exercise without sufficient carbohydrates can result in unexpected hypoglycemia.**
4. Feeling sweaty or shaky during exercise indicates hypoglycemia, not hyperglycemia.

♦ *Test-taking Tip: Recall that type 1 DM requires daily insulin administration and that activity increases energy expenditure and glucose demand.*

Content Area: Adult; Concept: Metabolism; Integrated Processes: Nursing Process: Evaluation; Client Needs: Physiological Integrity: Physiological Adaptation; Cognitive Level: Evaluation [Evaluating]

## 1082. PHARM ANSWER: 3

1. Having the client rate the level of anxiety will delay obtaining a fingerstick blood glucose; the problem may not be anxiety but hypoglycemia.
2. The problem may not be anxiety but hypoglycemia; administering lorazepam (Ativan) should not be considered until hypoglycemia is ruled out.
3. **The best intervention is to check a fingerstick blood glucose level because anxiety and shakiness in the midafternoon when taking NPH insulin (Humulin N) could indicate hypoglycemia; NPH insulin peaks in 6 to 8 hours after administration.**
4. The problem may not be anxiety but hypoglycemia; having the client sit in a recliner to relax should not be considered until hypoglycemia is ruled out.

♦ *Test-taking Tip: Options 1, 2, and 4 focus on treating the anxiety, and Option 3 is different. Often the option that is different is the answer. Remember to collect sufficient information prior to initiating an intervention.*

Content Area: Adult; Concept: Metabolism; Integrated Processes: Nursing Process: Implementation; Client Needs: Physiological Integrity: Pharmacological and Parenteral Therapies; Cognitive Level: Application [Applying]

## 1083. MoC ANSWER: 1

1. **It is most important for the nurse to initiate a referral for clients who falsely think their diabetes is well controlled. The client's Hgb A$_{1c}$, which measures average blood glucose over the previous 3 months, is 11%, indicating that the diabetes is not well controlled. The Hgb A$_{1c}$ goal is less than 7%.**
2. The client who wants more information about DM does not need a referral because the client's Hgb A$_{1c}$ is less than 7%. The nurse can provide resources for additional information.
3. Although this client states perfect compliance, the client could benefit from a referral due to Hgb A$_{1c}$ of 7%. However, this client's DM is better controlled than that of the client in Option 1.
4. This client does not need a referral for a diabetes educator because the fingerstick glucose and the Hgb A$_{1c}$ are both within normal ranges. A referral to a neurologist may be indicated.

♦ *Test-taking Tip: Hgb A$_{1c}$ is the best indicator of compliance with DM management. The client with the highest Hgb A$_{1c}$ is most in need of a referral for diabetes education.*

Content Area: Adult; Concept: Management; Metabolism; Integrated Processes: Nursing Process: Planning; Communication and Documentation; Client Needs: Safe and Effective Care Environment: Management of Care; Cognitive Level: Analysis [Analyzing]

## 1084. ANSWER: 4

1. Both the middle-of-the-night and morning blood glucose readings are within normal ranges.
2. A middle-of-the-night blood glucose between 50 and 60 mg/dL and a morning level of 48 and 62 mg/dL both indicate hypoglycemia.
3. The above-normal blood glucose in the middle of the night and morning hyperglycemia are signs of Dawn phenomenon.
4. **The nurse should conclude that the low blood glucose in the middle of the night (45–62 mg/dL) and a rebound morning hyperglycemia (200–305 mg/dL) are signs of Somogyi phenomenon, also known as Somogyi effect.**

♦ *Test-taking Tip: To narrow the options, associate Somogyi with a rebound effect (a low, then a high). You can remember this by thinking about a gym when you see the word "somogyi."*

Content Area: Adult; Concept: Metabolism; Integrated Processes: Nursing Process: Evaluation; Client Needs: Physiological Integrity: Physiological Adaptation; Cognitive Level: Analysis [Analyzing]

**1085.** MoC **ANSWER: 2, 1, 3, 4**

2. **The 45-year-old client who is dyspneic and has chest pressure and new-onset atrial fibrillation should be assessed first. Diabetes increases the risk of CAD and MI.**

1. **The 60-year-old client who is nauseated and has just vomited for the second time should be next. If breakfast was undigested, the client's blood glucose level could be low.**

3. **The 75-year-old client with a fingerstick blood glucose level of 300 mg/dL should be assessed third. This blood glucose level is not immediately life-threatening but needs to be lowered as soon as possible.**

4. **The 50-year-old client with a fingerstick blood glucose level of 70 mg/dL can be assessed last because this is a normal blood glucose level.**

♦ *Test-taking Tip: Use the ABC's to establish the priority client. Then look at the information provided for each client to determine the next priority. Consider that all clients received insulin at 0800.*

Content Area: Adult; Concept: Critical Thinking; Metabolism; Integrated Processes: Nursing Process: Assessment; Client Needs: Safe and Effective Care Environment: Management of Care; Cognitive Level: Synthesis [Creating]

**1086.** PHARM **ANSWER: 15**

10 units : 100 mL :: 1.5 units : $X$ mL
$10X = 100 \times 1.5$; $10X = 150$; $X = 150 \div 10$;
$X = 15$

♦ *Test-taking Tip: Use a drug calculation formula and the onscreen calculator and double-check the answer if it seems unusually large.*

Content Area: Adult; Concept: Medication; Metabolism; Integrated Processes: Nursing Process: Analysis; Client Needs: Physiological Integrity: Pharmacological and Parenteral Therapies; Cognitive Level: Analysis [Analyzing]

**1087.** PHARM **ANSWER: 4**

1. Illustration 1 shows 16 units of insulin, which is too much.

2. Illustration 2 shows 29 units of insulin, which is too much.

3. Illustration 3 shows 1 unit of insulin, which is too little.

4. **The client should receive 6 units of insulin (Illustration 4). Eating 45 g of carbohydrates equals 3 CHOs. If the client is to receive 2 units of insulin for each CHO, the total amount of aspart insulin is 3 CHO times 2 units per CHO = 6 units.**

♦ *Test-taking Tip: Read the information in the question carefully. Calculate the amount of insulin the client should receive prior to making the selection.*

Content Area: Adult; Concept: Medication; Metabolism; Integrated Processes: Nursing Process: Implementation; Client Needs: Physiological Integrity: Pharmacological and Parenteral Therapies; Cognitive Level: Analysis [Analyzing]

**1088.** MoC **ANSWER: 1**

1. **Because the client will be NPO for surgery, the nurse should verify the insulin type and dose to be administered to prevent a hypoglycemic reaction.**

2. An RN is unable to prescribe medications. The nurse could write the order based on protocol or standing orders, but this is not noted in the option.

3. Doing nothing could cause a hypoglycemic reaction because the client will be NPO for surgery.

4. Holding the morning dose of insulin can cause hyperglycemia, leading to DKA. Even without food, glucose levels increase from hepatic glucose production. Clients with type 1 DM require insulin 24 hours a day.

♦ *Test-taking Tip: The nurse must function within the scope of practice. The scope of practice does not include prescribing medications or altering medication orders without first consulting the HCP.*

Content Area: Adult; Concept: Medication; Metabolism; Safety; Management; Integrated Processes: Nursing Process: Implementation; Client Needs: Safe and Effective Care Environment: Management of Care; Cognitive Level: Application [Applying]

**1089.** PHARM **ANSWER: 2**

1. The onset of regular insulin (short acting) is one-half to 1 hour, not 15 minutes; its peak is 2 to 3 hours, not 5.5 hours.

2. **The onset of regular insulin (short acting) is one-half to 1 hour, and the peak is 2 to 3 hours. The onset of NPH insulin (intermediate acting) is 2 to 4 hours, and the peak is 4 to 12 hours.**

3. The onset of NPH insulin (intermediate acting) is 2 to 4 hours, not 30 minutes; its peak is 4 to 12 hours, not 2.5 hours.

4. The onset of NPH insulin (intermediate acting) is 2 to 4 hours, not 5 hours; the peak is 4 hours, which is within the normal peak time of 4 to 12 hours.

♦ *Test-taking Tip: Regular insulin is rapid acting, whereas NPH is intermediate-acting insulin.*

Content Area: Adult; Concept: Medication; Metabolism; Integrated Processes: Nursing Process: Evaluation; Client Needs: Physiological Integrity: Pharmacological and Parenteral Therapies; Cognitive Level: Evaluation [Evaluating]

**1090. ANSWER: 4**

1. Addressing nutritive and non-nutritive sweeteners with the client is important because nutritive sweeteners contain calories and non-nutritive sweeteners are calorie free; however, this is an intervention; assessment is first.

2. If the client is taking insulin, keeping regular mealtimes will help to cover the peak times of insulin. This is important to address but is an intervention; assessment is first.

3. One method for dosing insulin is based on the number of carbohydrates consumed. This is important to address but is an intervention; assessment is first.

4. **Asking about favorite foods and usual mealtimes is an assessment question used in obtaining a thorough diet history; the nurse should take this action first prior to beginning teaching.**

▶ *Test-taking Tip: Assessment is the first step in the nursing process and should be accomplished first.*

Content Area: Adult; Concept: Metabolism; Integrated Processes: Nursing Process: Assessment; Client Needs: Physiological Integrity: Basic Care and Comfort; Physiological Integrity: Reduction of Risk Potential; Cognitive Level: Application [Applying]

### 1091. MoC PHARM ANSWER: 1

1. **In DKA, the blood glucose level is above 300 mg/dL. Additional glucose will increase the glucose level further. Initially 0.45% or 0.9% sodium chloride (NaCl) is administered for fluid resuscitation. Glucose may be added when blood glucose levels approach 250 mg/dL.**

2. Insulin will drive potassium into the cells, so potassium chloride (KCL) is administered to prevent life-threatening hypokalemia.

3. Normal arterial pH is 7.35 to 7.45. Sodium bicarbonate will reverse the severe acidosis.

4. IV insulin will correct the hyperglycemia and hyperketonemia. Tight glucose control can be maintained by hourly glucose checks and adjusting the insulin infusion dose.

▶ *Test-taking Tip: Note the key word "question." Select the option that would not be included in the treatment of the client with DKA and could result in further hyperglycemia.*

Content Area: Adult; Concept: Medication; Metabolism; Safety; Collaboration; Integrated Processes: Nursing Process: Analysis; Communication and Documentation; Client Needs: Safe and Effective Care Environment: Management of Care; Physiological Integrity: Pharmacological and Parenteral Therapies; Cognitive Level: Application [Applying]

### 1092. ANSWER: 2

1. Sunken eyes and flushing are signs of dehydration.

2. **Moist skin and good skin turgor indicate that dehydration secondary to hyperglycemia is resolving.**

3. Normal serum potassium levels are 3.5 to 5.0 mEq/L; a level of 3.3 mEq/L is low.

4. The abnormal ABGs indicate compensating metabolic acidosis; the pH, $Paco_2$, and $HCO_3$ are all low.

▶ *Test-taking Tip: Note the key phrase "responding to treatment." Select the option that is a normal finding.*

Content Area: Adult; Concept: Fluid and Electrolyte Balance; Metabolism; Integrated Processes: Nursing Process: Evaluation; Client Needs: Physiological Integrity: Physiological Adaptation; Cognitive Level: Evaluation [Evaluating]

### 1093. ANSWER: 4

1. Exercise in the presence of hyperglycemia does not lower the blood glucose level.

2. Administering insulin may be an option, but the blood glucose level should be known before sending the client to cardiac rehab.

3. Exercise, even if delayed, will not lower the blood glucose level in the presence of hyperglycemia.

4. **Exercising with blood glucose levels exceeding 250 mg/dL and ketonuria increases the secretion of glucagon, growth hormone, and catecholamines, causing the liver to release more glucose.**

▶ *Test-taking Tip: Think about the physiological effects of stress on blood glucose levels. You need to decide which action is safest for the client.*

Content Area: Adult; Concept: Metabolism; Safety; Integrated Processes: Nursing Process: Planning; Client Needs: Physiological Integrity: Basic Care and Comfort; Cognitive Level: Analysis [Analyzing]

### 1094. ANSWER: 1

1. **The nurse should check the client's urine for ketones whenever the blood glucose level is greater than 240 mg/dL.**

2. The client should continue to eat meals as tolerated and not be placed on NPO. If a regular diabetic diet is not tolerated, easily digested foods and regular soda can be substituted.

3. The ketone should be known before contacting the HCP; some agencies have protocols in place for treating elevated glucose levels when the client with diabetes is ill.

4. Sick-day management of the client with diabetes includes more frequent monitoring of blood glucose levels to at least every 2 to 4 hours, not every 6 hours.

▶ *Test-taking Tip: Utilize the nursing process. Additional assessment is needed before taking further action.*

Content Area: Adult; Concept: Metabolism; Integrated Processes: Nursing Process: Planning; Client Needs: Physiological Integrity: Physiological Adaptation; Cognitive Level: Application [Applying]

### 1095. ANSWER: 2

1. Usually type 2 DM is controlled with oral hypoglycemic agents. If insulin is needed, sites should be rotated.

2. **Exercise increases insulin receptor sites in the tissue and can have a direct effect on lowering blood glucose levels. Exercise contributes to weight loss, which also decreases insulin resistance.**

3. For those with DM, protein should contribute less than 10% of the total energy consumed.

4. Strenuous activity can be perceived by the body as a stressor, causing a release of counter-regulatory hormones that subsequently increase blood glucose. Hyperglycemia can result from the combination of strenuous activity and extra carbohydrates.

▶ *Test-taking Tip: Clients with type 2 DM will produce some insulin, and often weight reduction, calorie reduction, and exercise will help to normalize glucose levels so that insulin is not needed; clients may still need an oral antidiabetic agent.*

Content Area: Adult; Concept: Nursing Roles; Metabolism; Integrated Processes: Teaching/Learning; Client Needs: Physiological Integrity: Physiological Adaptation; Cognitive Level: Analysis [Analyzing]

## 1096. ANSWER: 1, 3, 4

1. **A serum osmolality of 364 mOsm/kg is elevated (normal 275–295 mOsm/kg); the extremely high blood glucose levels in HHNS increase serum osmolality.**

2. Although a blood glucose level of 160 mg/dL is elevated, the blood glucose levels in HHNS are extremely elevated, usually 600 to 1200 mg/dL.

3. **Very dry mucous membranes indicate dehydration. Persistent hyperglycemia in HHNS causes osmotic diuresis, a loss of water and electrolytes, and extreme dehydration.**

4. **A BP of 90/42 indicates hypotension from loss of water and electrolytes in HHNS.**

5. Urine output of 500 mL in 8 hours is normal; in HHNS polyuria occurs from the high glucose levels and osmotic diuresis.

▶ *Test-taking Tip: Look for key words in the stem to select and eliminate options. Hyperglycemic hyperosmolar should help you to select Option 1. Then thinking about the physiology associated with hyperosmolar, you should be able to select Options 3 and 4, then eliminate Option 5. Finally, consider that while blood glucose of 160 mg/dL is elevated, it would not cause the serum to be hyperosmolar enough to result in HHNS.*

Content Area: Adult; Concept: Metabolism; Integrated Processes: Nursing Process: Assessment; Client Needs: Physiological Integrity: Physiological Adaptation; Cognitive Level: Application [Applying]

## 1097. ANSWER: 3

1. A decrease in serum glucose indicates that the hyperglycemia is resolving, but not the fluid volume deficit.

2. Serum sodium values should increase, not decrease, with treatment.

3. **Extreme hyperglycemia produces severe osmotic diuresis; loss of sodium, potassium, and phosphorus; and profound dehydration. Consequently, hyperosmolality occurs. A normalizing of the serum osmolality indicates that the fluid volume deficit is resolving.**

4. Potassium values should increase, not decrease, with treatment.

▶ *Test-taking Tip: Focus on the issue, deficient fluid volume; look for similar words in the question and the options.*

Content Area: Adult; Concept: Fluid and Electrolyte Balance; Metabolism; Integrated Processes: Nursing Process: Evaluation; Client Needs: Physiological Integrity: Reduction of Risk Potential; Cognitive Level: Evaluation [Evaluating]

## 1098. ANSWER: 1, 2, 4

1. **Diabetes, diabetic complications, and increased mortality have been reported to occur at a higher rate in Hispanics compared with non-Hispanic whites of the same age. Therefore, careful daily skin assessment is necessary. Neuropathy, PVD, and immunocompromise can result in diabetic foot ulcer and complications.**

2. **Magnifying devices are available if the client is unable to read small print to prevent dosing errors.**

3. Blood is drawn in the laboratory to check the $A_{1c}$.

4. **Regular insulin peaks in 2 to 3 hours, and NPH insulin peaks in 4 to 12 hours after administration. A bedtime snack will cover the insulin peak to prevent hypoglycemia.**

5. Only short-acting (regular) or rapid-acting insulin (aspart or lispro), not NPH insulin, would be administered to cover for additional carbohydrates if the client were on a carbohydrate-counting regimen with insulin coverage. This would be prescribed by the HCP.

▶ *Test-taking Tip: Carefully read the scenario and the options. Avoid reading information into the scenario.*

Content Area: Adult; Concept: Nursing Roles; Metabolism; Diversity; Integrated Processes: Teaching/Learning; Culture and Spirituality; Caring; Client Needs: Physiological Integrity: Physiological Adaptation; Psychosocial Integrity; Cognitive Level: Application [Applying]

## 1099. ANSWER: 1, 3

1. **If the client is unable to eat due to nausea and vomiting, dehydration can occur from hyperglycemia and the lack of fluid intake. The HCP should be notified.**

2. Blood glucose should be checked every 4 hours when ill (not daily) and the ketones tested every 3 to 4 hours if the glucose is greater than 240 mg/dL.

3. **An acute or minor illness can evoke a counter-regulatory hormone response, resulting in hyperglycemia; thus the client should continue medications as prescribed.**

4. The client should supplement the diet with carbohydrate-containing fluids only if eating less than normal due to the illness.

5. Insulin may or may not be necessary; it is based on the client's blood glucose level.

▶ **Test-taking Tip:** *Recall that hyperglycemia occurs during an illness. Use this information to narrow the Options to 1 and 3.*

**Content Area:** Adult; **Concept:** Nursing Roles; Metabolism; **Integrated Processes:** Teaching/Learning; **Client Needs:** Physiological Integrity: Physiological Adaptation; **Cognitive Level:** Application [Applying]

## 1100. PHARM ANSWER: 1, 3

1. **A decreased production of ADH results in increased urine output and increased plasma osmolality. Thus urine output should be monitored hourly. Daily weights should be monitored because weight loss is associated with DI, and weight gain is associated with receiving DDAVP.**
2. Urine osmolality may be monitored, but checking urine ketones is unnecessary.
3. **DDAVP, administered orally, by IV, or nasally, is an analog of ADH for ADH replacement. The client should be monitored for weight gain, hyponatremia, and water intoxication when taking DDAVP.**
4. Elevated blood glucose levels are associated with DM, not DI.
5. Hypernatremia, not hyperkalemia, is associated with DI.

▶ **Test-taking Tip:** *DI is associated with decreased production and secretion of ADH. You should eliminate options pertaining to DM. Carefully consider the electrolyte imbalances that occur with fluid loss.*

**Content Area:** Adult; **Concept:** Fluid and Electrolyte Balance; Metabolism; Medication; **Integrated Processes:** Nursing Process: Implementation; **Client Needs:** Physiological Integrity: Physiological Adaptation; Physiological Integrity: Pharmacological and Parenteral Therapies; **Cognitive Level:** Application [Applying]

## 1101. ANSWER: 3

1. The bed should be positioned flat or with no more than 10 degrees of elevation to enhance venous return to the heart and increase left atrial filling pressure, reducing ADH release.
2. Vasopressin is an ADH; thus it will aggravate the client's problem.
3. **If symptoms are mild and serum sodium is greater than 125 mEq/L (125 mmol/L), treatment includes fluid restriction to 800 to 1000 mL per day and discontinuation of medications that stimulate the release of ADH. The fluid restriction should result in a progressive rise in serum sodium concentration and osmolality and symptomatic improvement.**
4. Hypertonic saline (3% to 5%) should be administered if hyponatremia is severe (less than 120 mEq/L; normal serum sodium levels are 136–146 mEq/L). Hypertonic solutions cause fluid to be drawn into the vascular system.

▶ **Test-taking Tip:** *Note that the client's symptoms are mild, but the serum sodium is low. Treatment is initially conservative.*

**Content Area:** Adult; **Concept:** Fluid and Electrolyte Balance; Cellular Regulation; Metabolism; **Integrated Processes:** Nursing Process: Planning; **Client Needs:** Physiological Integrity: Physiological Adaptation; **Cognitive Level:** Application [Applying]

## 1102. ANSWER: 1, 3, 4

1. **The serum osmolality of 310 mOsm/kg is elevated; this finding should indicate to the nurse that the client is experiencing DI because fluid loss with DI increases serum osmolality.**
2. The client's weight has increased; a decreased weight occurs in DI due to excessive diuresis.
3. **Excessive thirst occurs with DI due to excessive diuresis; this finding should indicate to the nurse that the client is experiencing DI.**
4. **Urine output of 4200 mL in 24 hours is excessive and occurs in DI from a deficiency of ADH, resulting in an inadequate reabsorption of water by the kidney tubules; this finding should indicate to the nurse that the client is experiencing DI.**
5. A BP averaging 164/92 or higher indicates hypertension; DI produces hypotension from fluid loss by the kidneys.

▶ **Test-taking Tip:** *Associate DI with diuresis to select the correct options. Recall that when intravascular fluid is lost, serum osmolality increases, and the client is thirsty.*

**Content Area:** Adult; **Concept:** Fluid and Electrolyte Balance; Metabolism; Cellular Regulation; **Integrated Processes:** Nursing Process: Analysis; **Client Needs:** Physiological Integrity: Reduction of Risk Potential; **Cognitive Level:** Analysis [Analyzing]

## 1103. MoC ANSWER: 2

1. Elevating the head of the client's bed to 30 degrees is an appropriate action because it will promote cerebral venous drainage and prevent pressure on the sella turcica.
2. **The nurse should intervene when observing the nurse prepare to replace the nasal packing. The nasal packing and "mustache dressing" under the nose to collect drips are left in place for 3 to 4 days; these are not changed without an HCP order.**
3. Moisturize oral mucous membrane is an appropriate action because the nasal packing produces the need for mouth-breathing.
4. Placing a cold washcloth over the client's swollen eyes is an appropriate action because cold will help to reduce swelling and provide comfort.

▶ **Test-taking Tip:** *This is an "except" question, meaning all of the options except one option are correct actions.*

**Content Area:** Adult; **Concept:** Safety; Metabolism; Management; **Integrated Processes:** Nursing Process: Evaluation; **Client Needs:** Safe and Effective Care Environment: Management of Care; **Cognitive Level:** Evaluation [Evaluating]

**1104. ANSWER: 1, 2, 4**

1. **Weight gain occurs because of fluid retention in SIADH. The nurse should weigh the client at the same time each day and using the same scale to evaluate treatment effectiveness.**
2. **Manifestations of SIADH include hyponatremia (sodium <134 mEq/L). The nurse should place the client on fluid restrictions.**
3. Fluid volume overload occurs in SIADH, and fluids are restricted. A 3% NaCl IV solution may be administered to treat hyponatremia.
4. **The nurse should administer the loop diuretic furosemide (Lasix) to treat fluid retention.**
5. The nurse should monitor for hypoactive (not hyperactive) reflexes and lethargy (not heightened alertness), which are symptoms of cerebral edema from fluid overload.

▶ *Test-taking Tip: You should look for similarities in options. Options 2 and 4 will manage fluid retention, and Option 1 will help monitor the effectiveness of interventions. Options 1 and 5 are unrelated to these options.*

**Content Area:** Adult; **Concept:** Nursing Roles; Metabolism; Fluid and Electrolyte Balance; **Integrated Processes:** Nursing Process: Implementation; **Client Needs:** Physiological Integrity: Physiological Adaptation; **Cognitive Level:** Application [Applying]

**1105. MoC ANSWER: 3, 2, 1, 4**

3. **Assist in ventilatory support first because the RR is decreased and the client is lethargic.**
2. **Administer intravenous fluids next because of hypotension.**
1. **Warm the client to prevent an increase in metabolic demand.**
4. **Administer thyroxine as prescribed. It should be administered cautiously because the decreased metabolic rate and atherosclerosis of myxedema may result in angina.**

▶ *Test-taking Tip: The client is experiencing myxedema coma. Use the ABC's to establish priority and then order the remaining actions.*

**Content Area:** Adult; **Concept:** Critical Thinking; Metabolism; Safety; Management; **Integrated Processes:** Nursing Process: Implementation; **Client Needs:** Safe and Effective Care Environment: Management of Care; **Cognitive Level:** Synthesis [Creating]

**1106. ANSWER: 1**

1. **Trousseau's sign (Illustration 1) is carpal spasm as a result of hypocalcemia. During thyroid surgery, the parathyroid glands can be injured or removed, affecting calcium metabolism and resulting in hypocalcemia, nerve hyperirritability, and spasms.**
2. Chvostek's sign (Illustration 2) is muscle twitching of the client's cheek when the facial nerve in front of the ear is tapped.
3. Illustration 3 shows the method to palpate the thyroid gland using the posterior approach.

4. Illustration 4 shows the red reflex over the pupil when performing an ophthalmic examination.

▶ *Test-taking Tip: Trousseau's sign involves spasms of the thumb, and Chvostek's sign involves spasms of the cheek. Remember these signs by associating the first letter of the name of the sign with the first letter of the involved area.*

**Content Area:** Adult; **Concept:** Assessment; Metabolism; Fluid and Electrolyte Balance; **Integrated Processes:** Nursing Process: Assessment; **Client Needs:** Physiological Integrity: Physiological Adaptation; **Cognitive Level:** Application [Applying]

**1107. ANSWER: 2, 3, 5**

1. Hypoventilation occurs with hypothyroidism and myxedema coma, not thyroid storm.
2. **The nurse should identify tachycardia as a symptom associated with thyroid storm. Tachycardia results from excessive secretion of thyroid hormone and the increased response to circulating catecholamines (epinephrine and norepinephrine).**
3. **Thyroid storm can produce exaggerated symptoms of hyperthyroidism in major body systems including the GI system. The diarrhea could also be caused from an illness that can be a precipitating factor of thyroid storm.**
4. Periorbital edema occurs with hypothyroidism and myxedema coma, not thyroid storm.
5. **The stress of a recent tooth extraction can be a precipitating event to thyroid storm.**

▶ *Test-taking Tip: Focus on the issue: thyroid storm, which is the same as thyrotoxic crisis. The client has too much circulating thyroid hormone. Think about the effects of the thyroid hormone on increasing metabolism and sympathetic stimulation.*

**Content Area:** Adult; **Concept:** Metabolism; **Integrated Processes:** Nursing Process: Assessment; **Client Needs:** Physiological Integrity: Physiological Adaptation; **Cognitive Level:** Application [Applying]

**1108. MoC ANSWER: 3**

1. An ECG and cardiac enzymes will aid in the diagnosis, but are not the priority. Dysrhythmias can occur from beta-adrenergic receptor stimulation caused by excess thyroid hormone or following an ACS. Cardiac enzymes, if elevated, confirm ACS.
2. These aid in diagnosis but do not immediately treat the client. Decreased TSH and elevated free $T_4$ confirm the diagnosis of hyperthyroidism.
3. **Treatment of the client should be first. Propranolol (Inderal) is a beta-adrenergic blocker for symptomatic relief of thyrotoxicosis and decreasing peripheral conversion of $T_4$ to $T_3$. It controls cardiac and psychomotor manifestations within minutes. A beta blocker is also a first-line treatment for the client with ACS.**

4. Propylthiouracil (PTU) will inhibit the synthesis of thyroid hormone. Clinical effects may be seen as soon as 1 hour after administration, thus is not the priority.

▶ *Test-taking Tip: Use the ABC's to establish priority. Treatment of the client by controlling the client's BP and HR is priority.*

**Content Area:** Adult; **Concept:** Critical Thinking; Metabolism; Medication; **Integrated Processes:** Nursing Process: Implementation; Caring; **Client Needs:** Safe and Effective Care Environment: Management of Care; **Cognitive Level:** Analysis [Analyzing]

**1109.** PHARM **ANSWER: 1, 2, 4**

1. **Taking the medication on an empty stomach promotes regular absorption. It should be taken in the morning to mimic normal hormone release and prevent insomnia.**
2. **During initial dosage adjustment, tachycardia could indicate a dose that is too high; the clinic should be notified if the HR is high.**
3. Weight gain and cold intolerance could indicate that the dose is too low; these do not indicate adverse effects.
4. **The drug should be taken as prescribed; it is a replacement hormone used in primary or secondary atrophy of the gland, after thyroidectomy, after excessive thyroid radiation, after the administration of antithyroid medications, or in congenital thyroid defects.**
5. Alopecia may indicate that the dose is too high. $T_3$ and $T_4$ should rise, not decrease, with treatment.

▶ *Test-taking Tip: Carefully read options that suggest that the medication dose is too high or too low.*

**Content Area:** Adult; **Concept:** Medication; Metabolism; **Integrated Processes:** Teaching/Learning; **Client Needs:** Physiological Integrity: Pharmacological and Parenteral Therapies; **Cognitive Level:** Application [Applying]

**1110.** PHARM CJ **ANSWER: 2**

1. Although the serum potassium is low, it is not as critically low as the serum calcium level.
2. **The nurse should administer calcium gluconate first. The serum calcium is critically low. Damage or removal of the parathyroid glands during surgery leads to hypocalcemia and tetany.**
3. Dolasetron (Anzemet) is an antiemetic. There is no indication from the lab analysis that the medication is needed at this time.
4. Giving levothyroxine (Synthroid), a thyroid hormone, is usually avoided immediately after surgery because the remaining thyroid tissue hypertrophies, recovering the capacity to produce sufficient hormone. Exogenous hormone inhibits pituitary production of TSH and delays or prevents the restoration of thyroid tissue regeneration and function.

▶ *Test-taking Tip: The key word is "first." Analyze the laboratory report for critically low values. Use the name of the critically low value as a key to the medication that should be priority.*

**Content Area:** Adult; **Concept:** Medication; Metabolism; Fluid and Electrolyte Balance; **Integrated Processes:** Nursing Process: Planning; **Client Needs:** Physiological Integrity: Pharmacological and Parenteral Therapies; **Cognitive Level:** Analysis [Analyzing]

**1111.** PHARM CJ **ANSWER: 2, 3, 4, 6**

1. Increased appetite is a sign of hyperthyroidism and can indicate the dose is too high.
2. **Symptoms of hypothyroidism appear if the dose is too low and include decreased sweating.**
3. **Symptoms of hypothyroidism appear if the dose is too low and include apathy and fatigue.**
4. **Symptoms of hypothyroidism appear if the dose is too low and include paresthesias.**
5. Tremors are a sign of hyperthyroidism and can indicate the dose is too high.
6. **Symptoms of hypothyroidism appear if the dose is too low and include slowed mental processes.**

▶ *Test-taking Tip: Levothyroxine (Synthroid) is used in treating hypothyroidism. Hypothyroidism is characterized by a slowing of body processes. Eliminate options that reflect increased sympathetic stimulation.*

**Content Area:** Adult; **Concept:** Medication; Metabolism; **Integrated Processes:** Nursing Process: Assessment; **Client Needs:** Physiological Integrity: Pharmacological and Parenteral Therapies; **Cognitive Level:** Application [Applying]

**1112. ANSWER: 2**

1. Precautions about avoiding pregnancy should be advised.
2. **Pregnancy should be postponed for at least 6 months after treatment because RAI crosses the placenta. Approximately 5% of individuals require more than one dose to destroy overactive thyroid cells.**
3. Effects of RAI therapy are not immediate. Symptoms of hyperthyroidism may subside in 3 to 4 weeks, but the maximum effects may not be seen for 3 to 4 months. Some individuals require a second treatment. Clients should continue (not discontinue) taking the antithyroid medication and propranolol.
4. Almost 80% of individuals experience posttreatment hypothyroidism and require thyroid hormone replacement after therapy is completed.

▶ *Test-taking Tip: The key word is "precaution." The best option is the one that directly answers the client's question. Options with absolute words are usually incorrect.*

**Content Area:** Adult; **Concept:** Safety; Metabolism; Sexuality; Communication; **Integrated Processes:** Communication and Documentation; Caring; **Client Needs:** Safe and Effective Care Environment: Safety and Infection Control; Psychosocial Integrity; **Cognitive Level:** Analysis [Analyzing]

## 1113. ANSWER: 1

1. **Appropriate foods on the list should be those high in calcium because hypoparathyroidism from lack of PTH produces chronic hypocalcemia. High-calcium foods include dark green vegetables, soybeans, and tofu.**
2. Foods containing oxalic acid (spinach) reduce calcium absorption.
3. Foods containing phytic acid (whole grain bread) reduce calcium absorption.
4. Foods containing oxalic acid (rhubarb) reduce calcium absorption.

▶ *Test-taking Tip: A lack of PTH will result in chronic hypocalcemia. Eliminate options that reduce calcium absorption.*

Content Area: Adult; Concept: Nutrition; Metabolism; Fluid and Electrolyte Balance; Integrated Processes: Teaching/Learning; Client Needs: Physiological Integrity: Basic Care and Comfort; Cognitive Level: Application [Applying]

## 1114. ANSWER: 1, 4, 6

1. **Cushing's syndrome results from excessive adrenocortical activity producing hyperglycemia.**
2. A decrease of eosinophils, rather than an increase, is associated with Cushing's syndrome.
3. Hypercalcemia (high serum calcium levels), rather than hypocalcemia, is associated with Cushing's syndrome.
4. **Cushing's syndrome results from excessive adrenocortical activity producing hypokalemia.**
5. Thrombocytopenia (low platelets) is not associated with the disorder.
6. **Cushing's syndrome results from excessive adrenocortical activity producing elevated serum cortisol, and elevated ACTH levels.**

▶ *Test-taking Tip: Focus on the effects of excess glucocorticoids and mineralocorticoids on the body.*

Content Area: Adult; Concept: Metabolism; Integrated Processes: Nursing Process: Analysis; Client Needs: Physiological Integrity: Reduction of Risk Potential; Cognitive Level: Analysis [Analyzing]

## 1115. MoC ANSWER: 3

1. The weight of the client should be known because the client has signs of fluid retention, but notifying the HCP is priority because the HR is irregular.
2. Although the blood glucose level is elevated and the client is to receive insulin, the nurse's priority is to notify the HCP first. It may take a while for the HCP to respond.
3. **The HCP should be notified immediately to obtain serum laboratory studies and to treat the irregular HR and hypokalemia if present. An irregular HR can occur from hypokalemia. Cushing's syndrome causes overproduction of aldosterone, retention of sodium and water, and excretion of potassium.**

4. Knowing the abdominal girth provides additional information about fluid retention but is not the priority.

▶ *Test-taking Tip: The key word is "priority." The priority should address the client's major problem to prevent complications. Use the ABC's to determine the client's major problem.*

Content Area: Adult; Concept: Critical Thinking; Metabolism; Management; Integrated Processes: Nursing Process: Implementation; Client Needs: Safe and Effective Care Environment: Management of Care; Cognitive Level: Analysis [Analyzing]

## 1116. PHARM ANSWER: 2

1. A calcium intake of 3000 mg is excessive; calcium is released into the vascular system with bone resorption, and hypocalcemia can result.
2. **Daily weight-bearing exercises can help prevent bone loss and strengthen bones and muscles. This statement indicates the client understands the teaching.**
3. Vitamin D is needed for absorption of calcium and should not be limited.
4. Rising slowly will help prevent falls, but it will not affect bone resorption.

▶ *Test-taking Tip: Bone resorption is a process in which bone is broken down within the body. You should focus on selecting a statement about a measure that will help prevent bone loss.*

Content Area: Adult; Concept: Metabolism; Fluid and Electrolyte Balance; Medication; Integrated Processes: Nursing Process: Evaluation; Client Needs: Physiological Integrity: Pharmacological and Parenteral Therapies; Cognitive Level: Evaluation [Evaluating]

## 1117. ANSWER: 5000

**First, determine the amount of weight loss (190 lb – 179 lb = 11 lb).**
**Because 1 liter of fluid (1000 mL) weighs approximately 2.2 lb, divide 11 lb by 2.2 lb/L (11 lb ÷ 2.2 lb/L = 5 L). To obtain mL of fluid loss, multiply: 5 L × 1000 ml/L to arrive at 5000 mL.**

▶ *Test-taking Tip: Recall that 1 L of fluid is approximately equal to 2.2 lb. The question is asking for mL of fluid loss, and 1 L = 1000 mL.*

Content Area: Adult; Concept: Fluid and Electrolyte Balance; Metabolism; Integrated Processes: Nursing Process: Analysis; Client Needs: Physiological Integrity: Physiological Adaptation; Cognitive Level: Analysis [Analyzing]

## 1118. ANSWER: 2

1. The depletion of sodium and water causes dehydration that results in dry and scaly skin, but the skin will be pigmented in Addison's disease and not white.
2. **The nurse should expect a bronzed, suntanned hue with the pigmentation changes occurring in Addison's disease; this occurs from an increase in the melanocyte-stimulating hormone.**
3. Diaphoresis and cyanosis can occur in Addisonian crisis and shock, but this client is stable.

4. A butterfly-like rash occurs with systemic lupus erythematous and not Addison's disease.

▶ *Test-taking Tip: Narrow the options by noting that all options but one contain multiple descriptors, whereas one option pertains only to the hue of the skin.*

**Content Area:** Adult; **Concept:** Critical Thinking; Assessment; Metabolism; **Integrated Processes:** Nursing Process: Assessment; **Client Needs:** Physiological Integrity: Physiological Adaptation; **Cognitive Level:** Application [Applying]

### 1119. ANSWER: 4

1. The classic manifestations of hyperthyroidism include tremors, weight loss, heat intolerance, tachycardia, and hypertension, none of which are present in the illustration.
2. The classic manifestations of DM include polydipsia, polyphagia, and polyuria due to hyperglycemia, none of which are present in the illustration.
3. The classic manifestations of Addison's disease include muscle weakness, anorexia, fatigue, emaciation, dark pigmentation, and hypotension, none of which are present in the illustration.
4. **The nurse should determine that the client with Cushing's syndrome would benefit by utilizing the illustration during a teaching session. Clinical manifestations of Cushing's syndrome include moon face, red cheeks, thinning hair, fat pads, slow wound healing, and others that are present in the illustration.**

▶ *Test-taking Tip: Focus on the signs and symptoms shown in the illustration to select the correct option.*

**Content Area:** Adult; **Concept:** Nursing Roles; Metabolism; **Integrated Processes:** Teaching/Learning; **Client Needs:** Physiological Integrity: Physiological Adaptation; **Cognitive Level:** Comprehension [Understanding]

### 1120. PHARM ANSWER: 4

1. Hypoglycemia, not hyperglycemia, is associated with Addisonian crisis.
2. Ketoconazole (Nizoral) is a systemic antifungal that has an unlabeled use in treating Cushing's syndrome as an adrenal enzyme inhibitor.
3. Addisonian crisis produces severe hypotension; sodium nitroprusside (Nipride) is used to treat severe hypertension.
4. **Addisonian crisis results from insufficient secretion of glucocorticoids and mineralocorticoids from the adrenal cortex. Hydrocortisone (Solu Cortef) is a corticosteroid used in the absence of sufficient glucocorticoid production.**

▶ *Test-taking Tip: Focus on the hormones secreted by the adrenal cortex to answer this question.*

**Content Area:** Adult; **Concept:** Medication; Metabolism; **Integrated Processes:** Nursing Process: Planning; **Client Needs:** Physiological Integrity: Pharmacological and Parenteral Therapies; **Cognitive Level:** Application [Applying]

### 1121. MoC ANSWER: 4

1. An acute infection can precipitate Addisonian crisis, but the WBC count is on the high side of normal.
2. Hypoglycemia, not hyperglycemia, is associated with adrenocortical insufficiency. The serum glucose is slightly elevated, but not alarmingly. Normal serum glucose is 70–110 mg/dL.
3. Hyponatremia, not hypernatremia, is associated with adrenocortical insufficiency. The serum sodium is slightly elevated, but not alarmingly. Normal serum sodium is 136–146 mEq/L.
4. **The nurse should immediately notify the HCP regarding the serum potassium of 6.2 mEq/L (normal is 3.8–5.0 mEq/L). Adrenocortical insufficiency causes excessive potassium reabsorption, producing hyperkalemia. Hyperkalemia can result in dysrhythmias and cardiac arrest if not treated promptly.**

▶ *Test-taking Tip: Focus on the lab value that is most life-threatening.*

**Content Area:** Adult; **Concept:** Fluid and Electrolyte Balance; Metabolism; Management; **Integrated Processes:** Nursing Process: Implementation; **Client Needs:** Safe and Effective Care Environment: Management of Care; **Cognitive Level:** Application [Applying]

### 1122. ANSWER: 1, 2

1. **The nurse should question administration of potassium. The client with Addison's disease presents with hyperkalemia.**
2. **The nurse should question a sodium-restricted diet. The client with Addison's disease presents with hyponatremia (low serum sodium).**
3. In Addison's disease, the adrenal glands produce too little cortisol; obtaining a serum cortisol level is appropriate.
4. In Addison's disease, the adrenal glands produce too little cortisol; obtaining a serum glucose level now is appropriate.
5. The client with Addison's disease needs fluid replacement to treat hypotension and glucose to treat hypoglycemia. The order of 5% dextrose in 0.9% NaCl is appropriate.

▶ *Test-taking Tip: The nurse should question orders that are inappropriate for treating the client's condition. The nurse is legally liable if the client was harmed by the implementation of an inappropriate order.*

**Content Area:** Adult; **Concept:** Collaboration; Metabolism; Management; **Integrated Processes:** Nursing Process: Evaluation; **Client Needs:** Safe and Effective Care Environment: Safety and Infection Control; **Cognitive Level:** Evaluation [Evaluating]

**1123.** PHARM **ANSWER: 1**

1. **An increase in BP is indicative of effective therapy. Addisonian crisis is caused by adrenocortical insufficiency with disturbances of sodium and potassium metabolism resulting in hyponatremia, hyperkalemia, dehydration, and hypotension.**
2. A decrease of 25 mm Hg in the client's systolic BP indicates therapy is not effective. In Addisonian crisis, the depletion of sodium and water causes severe dehydration and hypotension. An increase in BP would be expected.
3. Effective therapy would lower potassium levels. A serum potassium level of 3.4 to 5.8 mEq/dL shows an increase in the level beyond the normal range.
4. In Addisonian crisis, there is sodium depletion. The serum sodium is within the normal range before and after treatment. An increase in serum sodium would be expected.

▶ *Test-taking Tip: The key word is "effective." Select the option that would show improvement for the client in Addisonian crisis. Use the ABC's to select an answer.*

**Content Area:** Adult; **Concept:** Fluid and Electrolyte Balance; Metabolism; Medication; **Integrated Processes:** Nursing Process: Evaluation; **Client Needs:** Physiological Integrity: Pharmacological and Parenteral Therapies; **Cognitive Level:** Evaluation [Evaluating]

**1124.** MoC **ANSWER: 3**

1. Adenomas can be localized by a CT scan, but this is not priority. Assessing for life-threatening conditions is priority.
2. Headache occurs from hypertension and should be treated, but this is not priority.
3. **Obtaining an ECG is priority. The excessive aldosterone secretion of hyperaldosteronism causes sodium retention and potassium and hydrogen ion excretion. The potassium wasting produces hypokalemia, which can cause life-threatening dysrhythmias.**
4. Hypokalemia produces generalized muscle weakness and fatigue, which can predispose the client to falls. Assessing for these is important, but this is not priority.

▶ *Test-taking Tip: The key word is "priority." Use the ABC's and nursing process to establish the priority.*

**Content Area:** Adult; **Concept:** Critical Thinking; Assessment; Metabolism; **Integrated Processes:** Nursing Process: Implementation; **Client Needs:** Safe and Effective Care Environment: Management of Care; **Cognitive Level:** Analysis [Analyzing]

**1125. ANSWER: 2**

1. There are no dietary potassium restrictions after adrenalectomy. Hypokalemia occurs with hyperaldosteronism and resolves after surgery.
2. **Unilateral adrenalectomy is successful in controlling hypertension in only 80% of clients with adenoma, so the client should continue to self-monitor the BP.**
3. The nurse should not inform the client to stop medications. The client may still need medications to treat hypertension and hyperaldosteronism after adrenalectomy.
4. There is no reason for the client with hyperaldosteronism to carry epinephrine.

▶ *Test-taking Tip: Excessive production of aldosterone occurs in hyperaldosteronism. Excess aldosterone causes increased renal reabsorption of sodium, an increase in extracellular fluids and BP, and a profound decline in serum potassium (hypokalemia) and hydrogen ions (alkalosis). Serum sodium levels may be high or normal, depending on the amount of water reabsorbed with the sodium.*

**Content Area:** Adult; **Concept:** Nursing Roles; Metabolism; Fluid and Electrolyte Balance; **Integrated Processes:** Teaching/Learning; **Client Needs:** Health Promotion and Maintenance; Physiological Integrity: Physiological Adaptation; **Cognitive Level:** Application [Applying]

**1126.** PHARM **ANSWER: 4**

1. A calm environment is needed to prevent hypertensive crisis. Noise can increase sympathetic nervous system (SNS) stimulation, inducing hypertension and an anxiety attack.
2. A calm environment is needed to prevent hypertensive crisis. Too many visitors and noise can increase SNS stimulation.
3. Reduced activity, not ambulation three times daily or more, is needed to prevent hypertensive crisis.
4. **Until the tumor can be surgically removed, calcium channel blockers such as nicardipine (Cardene) are used to control BP and other excess catecholamine symptoms.**

▶ *Test-taking Tip: Recall that "-oma" refers to tumor. Pheochromocytoma is characterized by a tumor of the adrenal medulla that produces excessive catecholamines (epinephrine and norepinephrine). The increased catecholamines result in hypertension.*

**Content Area:** Adult; **Concept:** Perfusion; Metabolism; Medication; **Integrated Processes:** Nursing Process: Planning; **Client Needs:** Physiological Integrity: Pharmacological and Parenteral Therapies; Psychosocial Integrity; **Cognitive Level:** Application [Applying]

**1127.** MoC **ANSWER: 1, 4, 3, 2**

1. Client following a thyroidectomy who has hoarseness and an SaO$_2$ of 86%. This client should be attended to first because the client has a life-threatening respiratory issue. Swelling in the neck after a thyroidectomy can compromise the airway.

4. Client with hyperthyroidism who has a temperature of 102.2°F (39°C) and tachycardia. This client should be next because an elevated temperature and tachycardia could indicate thyroid storm, a life-threatening condition.

3. Client with DI drinking frequently and asking for more cold water. This client is next because large volumes of urine output with DI place the client at risk for dehydration.

2. Client with hyperparathyroidism with a serum calcium level of 10.1 mg/dL. This client can be last because a serum calcium level of 10.1 mg/dL is WNL (8.2–10.2 mg/dL), indicating that treatment is effective and this client is stabilizing.

▶ **Test-taking Tip:** Apply the ABC's to establish priority. The client with a life-threatening condition should be assessed first. The stable client can be assessed last.

**Content Area:** Adult; **Concept:** Critical Thinking; Metabolism; Management; **Integrated Processes:** Nursing Process: Planning; **Client Needs:** Safe and Effective Care Environment: Management of Care; **Cognitive Level:** Evaluation [Evaluating]

## Chapter Twenty-Six

# Gastrointestinal Management

**1128.** **MoC** The nurse is assigned to four clients who were diagnosed with gastric ulcers. Which client should be the nurse's **priority** when monitoring for GI bleeding?

1. The 40-year-old client who is positive for *Helicobacter pylori* (*H. pylori*)
2. The 45-year-old client who drinks 4 ounces of alcohol a day
3. The 70-year-old client who takes daily baby aspirin of 81 mg
4. The 30-year-old pregnant client taking acetaminophen prn

**1129.** The nurse is assessing the client who is 24 hours post–GI hemorrhage. The findings include BUN of 40 mg/dL and serum creatinine of 0.8 mg/dL. Which action should be taken by the nurse?

1. Call the HCP to report these results.
2. Monitor urine output; these suggest renal failure.
3. Document the findings and continue monitoring.
4. Encourage limiting intake of dietary protein.

**1130.** The experienced nurse is instructing the new nurse. The experienced nurse explains that the definitive diagnosis of PUD involves which test?

1. A urea breath test
2. Upper GI endoscopy with biopsy
3. Barium contrast studies
4. The string test

**1131.** **MoC** The client with a history of a duodenal ulcer is hospitalized with upper abdominal discomfort and projectile vomiting that has a foul odor. The nurse immediately notifies the HCP, concluding that the client may have developed which complication?

1. Gastric perforation
2. Gastrointestinal hemorrhage
3. Gastric outlet obstruction
4. *Helicobacter pylori* infection

**1132.** The nurse is completing the client's hospital admission history. Which statement should prompt the nurse to further question the client about symptoms associated with GERD?

1. "I have been experiencing headaches immediately after eating."
2. "Lately, I wake up at night with a burning feeling in my chest."
3. "I have been waking up at night sweating and wet all over."
4. "Immediately after eating I feel sleepy and want to go to bed."

**1133.** The nurse is preparing to care for the client who has hepatitis A. Which interventions should the nurse plan to implement?

1. Teach the client to limit use of alcohol and drugs containing acetaminophen.
2. Provide a high-protein, high-carbohydrate diet with three large meals per day.
3. Wear gloves, mask, and gown when providing the client's personal cares.
4. Provide rest periods, alternating this with moderate activity during the day.

**1134.** **PHARM** The home health nurse is assessing the client who is taking interferon alpha-2b for treatment of chronic hepatitis B. Which client comment requires further follow-up by the nurse?

1. "My clothes are tight; I gained 2 pounds this month."
2. "Whenever I lightly bump into something, I get a bruise."
3. "I've been staying home and avoiding large crowds."
4. "I get tired easily, so I just take my time with things."

**1135.** The nurse is helping the client to manage and decrease the sensation of nausea. Which intervention should the nurse recommend?

1. Sipping tea made from ginger root
2. Changing positions more rapidly
3. Decreasing intake of solid food
4. Playing stimulating classical music

**1136.** The nurse is caring for the client who had a vertical banded gastroplasty. The nurse teaches that nausea can occur after this surgery from which situation?

1. The stomach pouch becomes overfilled.
2. The lower half of the stomach becomes spastic.
3. The duodenum incision becomes inflamed.
4. The dumping syndrome that occurs from a high-protein meal.

**1137.** The nurse is discharging the client after Billroth II surgery (gastrojejunostomy). To assist the client to control dumping syndrome, what information will the nurse include in the discharge instructions?

1. Drink plenty of fluids with all your meals.
2. Eat a high-carbohydrate, low-protein diet.
3. Wait to eat at least 5 hours between meals.
4. Lie down for 20 to 30 minutes after meals.

**1138.** After Billroth II surgery (gastrojejunostomy), the client experiences weakness, diaphoresis, anxiety, and palpitations 2 hours after a high-carbohydrate meal. The nurse should interpret that these symptoms indicate the development of which problem?

1. Steatorrhea
2. Duodenal reflux
3. Hypervolemic fluid overload
4. Postprandial hypoglycemia

**1139.** MoC The nurse is caring for the postoperative client who underwent an open Roux-en-Y gastric bypass. The charge nurse should intervene if which observation is made?

1. The nursing care plan for postoperative day one indicates restricting fluids to 30–60 mL per hour of clear liquids.
2. The nurse is instructing the licensed practical nurse (LPN) to remove the client's urinary catheter 24 hours after surgery.
3. The client is wearing a bilevel positive airway pressure (BiPAP) mask when sleeping during the day.
4. A bottle of saline and 60-mL catheter-tip syringe are on the bedside table for NG tube irrigation.

**1140.** The nurse is performing an initial postoperative assessment on the client following upper GI surgery. The client has an NG tube to low intermittent suction. To best assess for the presence of bowel sounds, what should the nurse do?

1. Start auscultating to the left of the umbilicus.
2. Turn off the NG suction before auscultation.
3. Use the bell of the stethoscope for auscultation.
4. Empty the drainage canister before auscultation.

**1141.** While performing a home visit, the nurse observes that the client's head of the bed is raised on 6-in. blocks. The nurse should question the client for a history of which conditions? **Select all that apply.**

1. Hiatal hernia
2. Dumping syndrome
3. Crohn's disease
4. Gastroesophageal reflux disease
5. Gastritis

**1142.** MoC The nurse is caring for the client with a Zenker's diverticulum. Which problem should be the nurse's **priority?**

1. Pain related to heartburn from gastric reflux
2. Aspiration related to regurgitation of food accumulated in the diverticula
3. Constipation related to anatomical changes of the sigmoid colon
4. Altered nutrition, less than body requirements related to dysphagia

**1143.** During a clinic visit the client provides all of the following health history information. Which client statement should be **most** concerning to the nurse because it could describe a symptom of esophageal cancer?

1. "I have been having a lot of indigestion lately."
2. "When I eat meat, it seems to get stuck halfway down."
3. "I have been waking up at night lately with chest pain."
4. "I gained weight, even though I have not changed my diet."

**1144.** Following an esophagectomy with colon interposition (esophagoenterostomy) for esophageal cancer, the client is beginning to eat oral foods. The nurse monitors for aspiration because the client no longer has which structure?

1. A stomach
2. A pyloric sphincter
3. A pharynx
4. A lower esophageal sphincter

**1145.** **MoC** The client had Billroth II surgery 24 hours ago. The client's son approaches the nurse in the hallway and asks for information regarding his father's condition. The wife is listed as the designated contact person. Which nurse response is **best?**

1. "What has the surgeon told you about your father's condition?"
2. "Let's both go into your father's room and ask him how he feels."
3. "Let's go to a more private place to discuss your father's condition."
4. "Let's review your father's medical record information together."

**1146.** The nurse is admitting the client with gastric cancer to an oncology unit for treatment. Which assessment finding should prompt the nurse to review the medical record to determine whether the cancer may have metastasized to the peritoneal cavity?

1. The client is reporting nausea.
2. Grey Turner's sign is present.
3. The client reports a rapid weight loss.
4. Ascites is evident in the abdomen.

**1147.** The serum ammonia level of the client with cirrhosis is elevated. What should the nurse do?

1. Monitor for temperature elevation.
2. Observe for increasing confusion.
3. Measure the urine specific gravity.
4. Restrict the intake of oral fluids.

**1148.** **PHARM** When admitting the hospitalized client, the client's daughter presents the medication list illustrated. After reviewing the list, which nursing action is **most** appropriate?

| Medications |
| --- |
| Lactulose, 30 mL oral, every 6 hours |
| Pantoprazole, 40 mg oral, daily |
| Propranolol, 20 mg oral, twice daily |
| Rifaximin, 400 mg oral, three times daily |
| Furosemide, 20 mg oral, twice daily; a.m. and suppertime |
| Phytonadione (Vitamin K), 10 mg oral, daily |
| Spironolactone, 300 mg oral, daily |
| Thiamine (Vitamin B$_1$), 100 mg, oral daily |
| Diphenhydramine, 50 mg oral, as needed at night for itching |

1. Ask about a history of PUD and infections.
2. Assess abdominal pain and palpate the abdomen.
3. Teach and initiate droplet isolation precautions.
4. Assess orientation and measure abdominal girth.

**1149.** **MoC** The client is hospitalized for conservative treatment of cirrhosis. Which intervention should the nurse anticipate in the plan of care?

1. Monitor the blood sugar level.
2. Keep on nothing per mouth status.
3. Administer intravenous antibiotics.
4. Encourage ambulation every 4 hours.

**1150.** The nurse is reviewing the health history of the client hospitalized with nonalcoholic fatty liver disease (NAFLD). Which finding should the nurse associate with this disease process?

1. 70 years of age at diagnosis
2. Body mass index of 35
3. History of recent antibiotic use
4. Living in a colder climate

**1151.** The client with cirrhosis is scheduled for a transjugular intrahepatic portosystemic shunt (TIPS) placement. The nurse realizes the client does not understand the procedure when the client makes which statement?

1. "I hope the abdominal incision heals fast after this procedure so I can return home."
2. "My risk of bleeding from my esophagus again should be decreased after this procedure."
3. "The shunt they are placing could become occluded in the future; I hope it doesn't happen."
4. "This procedure should keep me from getting so much fluid buildup in my abdomen."

**1152.** **PHARM** The nurse is caring for the client diagnosed with cirrhosis. After completing discharge education, the nurse recognizes the need for further teaching when the client makes which statement?

1. "My cirrhosis was caused from too much alcohol; I plan to stop drinking."
2. "I need to rest more; I plan on only going to work on a part-time basis."
3. "Propranolol has been ordered to decrease my blood pressure."
4. "Furosemide will help to reduce the amount of abdominal fluid."

**1153.** The client is scheduled for a percutaneous liver biopsy. Place an X in the quadrant where the nurse should tell the client that the needle will be inserted.

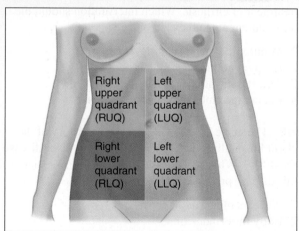

**1154.** The client is admitted with upper right-side abdominal pain. The nurse is concerned that the client may have liver cancer when which serum laboratory test results are elevated?

1. Creatinine and BUN
2. α-fetoprotein (AFP)
3. Phosphorus levels
4. CA-125 levels

**1155.** **MoC** After receiving the shift report, the nurse is planning care for four clients. Prioritize the order in which the nurse should plan to attend to the clients.

1. The client with ascites who is having mild dyspnea with activity
2. The client with a peptic ulcer who now has severe vomiting
3. The client who had a colonoscopy and is having diarrheal stools.
4. The client with Crohn's disease who received an initial dose of certolizumab is having generalized rashes

Answer: _____

**1156.** **MoC** The student nurse is caring for the client following a liver biopsy. Which observation of the student nurse's care demonstrates to the RN that the student understands the postprocedure care?

1. Takes the client's vital signs every hour
2. Walks the client 1 hour postprocedure
3. Positions the client onto the right side
4. Has the client cough and deep-breathe hourly

**1157.** The nurse is taking a hospital admission history for the 40-year-old client. The nurse is concerned about possible acute pancreatitis when the client makes which statement?

1. "I have sudden-onset intense pain in my upper left abdomen that goes to my back."
2. "I had persistent lower abdominal pain that now shifted to the lower right quadrant."
3. "My stools are loose and bloody, and I have cramping abdominal pain with spasms."
4. "I have this mild pain in my upper abdomen, but I have been vomiting forcefully a lot."

**1158.** **MoC** The nurse is caring for the newly admitted client with acute necrotizing pancreatitis. Which interventions, if prescribed, should the nurse implement? **Select all that apply.**

1. NS 1000 mL IV over 1 hour, then IV fluids at 250 mL/hour
2. Initiate nasojejunal enteral feedings with a low-fat formula
3. Imipenem-cilastatin 500 mg IV every 6 hours
4. Up to chair for meals and ambulate four times daily
5. Position left side-lying with head of bed elevated 30 degrees
6. Insert a urinary catheter; monitor urine output every 2 hours

**1159.** While assessing the client with acute pancreatitis, the nurse sees the skin appearance illustrated. What should be the nurse's interpretation of this finding?

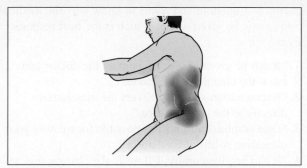

1. Portal hypertension has developed from the acute pancreatitis.
2. Seepage of blood-stained exudates from the pancreas has occurred.
3. Pancreatitis resulted in stomach bleeding, and the blood is now in the interstitial tissue.
4. Increased vascular pressure from pancreatic inflammation caused an intestinal obstruction.

**1160.** The client recovering from acute pancreatitis who has been NPO asks, "When can I start eating again?" Which response by the nurse is **most** accurate?

1. "As soon as you start to feel hungry you can begin eating."
2. "When I hear that your bowel sounds are active and you are passing flatus."
3. "When your pain is controlled and your serum lipase level has decreased."
4. "You will be NPO for at least more 2 weeks; oral intake stimulates the pancreas."

**1161.** PHARM The client who has chronic pancreatitis is concerned about pain control. Which **initial** plan for chronic pancreatic pain control should the nurse explain to the client?

1. Opioid analgesics, such as morphine sulfate
2. Nonsteroidal anti-inflammatory drugs (NSAIDS)
3. Pancreatic enzymes with H2 blocker medications
4. Injection of medication directly into the nerves

**1162.** MoC The nurse is preparing to care for the client who just had a Whipple procedure. What should the nurse include in the **immediate** plan of care?

1. Monitor blood glucose levels.
2. Initiate enteral feedings.
3. Irrigate the NG tube with 30 mL of saline.
4. Remove the epidural line and start IV analgesics.

**1163.** MoC The nurse has been assigned to care for four clients. Which client should the nurse plan to assess **first?**

1. The 50-year-old client who has chronic pancreatitis and is reporting a pain level of 6 out of 10 on a numerical scale
2. The 47-year-old client with esophageal varices who has influenza and has been coughing for the last 30 minutes
3. The 60-year-old client who had an open cholecystectomy 15 hours ago and has been stable through the night
4. The 54-year-old client with cirrhosis and jaundice who is reporting having itching all over the body

**1164.** The client has diarrhea that has been cultured positive for *Clostridium difficile (C. diff).* To prevent the spread of infection, the nurse should perform which intervention?

1. Wear an isolation gown, gloves, and mask when providing care.
2. Perform vigorous hand hygiene using only soap and water.
3. Place the client in a private room with negative-pressure airflow.
4. Instruct visitors to use the alcohol-based hand wash for self-protection.

**1165.** The client has diarrhea and refuses to drink the prescribed oral hydration solution, insisting on having chicken broth instead due to cultural beliefs. Which statement **best** describes the possible reason for the client's request for chicken broth?

1. The chicken broth has yang qualities.
2. Extra protein in the chicken broth reduces the diarrhea.
3. The high sodium in the broth is needed to treat diarrhea.
4. Modern medicine cannot be trusted; broth is needed to treat disease.

**1166.** MoC The nurse is caring for the client who is 6 hours post–open cholecystectomy. The client's T-tube drainage bag is empty, and the nurse notes slight jaundice of the sclera. Which action by the nurse is **most** important?

1. Reposition the client to promote T-tube drainage.
2. Telephone the surgeon to report these findings.
3. Ask the NA to obtain a BP.
4. Record the findings and continue to monitor the client.

**1167.** **PHARM** The nurse is caring for the client with acute cholecystitis. The nurse anticipates that conservative treatment will include which component?

1. Providing a low-texture bland diet
2. Giving anticholinergic medications
3. Positioning so the head of the bed is flat
4. Administering laxatives to clear the bowel

**1168.** The HCP writes the following admission orders for the client with possible appendicitis. Which order should the nurse question?

1. Place on NPO (nothing per mouth) status.
2. No analgesics until diagnosis is confirmed.
3. Apply heat to abdomen to decrease pain.
4. Start IV lactated Ringer's at 125 mL/hr.

**1169.** The nurse is taking a hospital admission history of the client. The nurse considers that the client may have IBS when the client makes which statement?

1. "I am having a lot of bloody diarrhea."
2. "I have been vomiting for 2 days."
3. "I have lost 10 pounds in the last month."
4. "I have noticed mucus in my stools."

**1170.** **PHARM** The nurse is preparing to give amitriptyline 10 mg orally to the client diagnosed with IBS. The client states, "I don't need this. I'm not depressed." Which response by the nurse is **best?**

1. "The medication is working. People with chronic diseases typically also suffer from depression."
2. "People with IBS have difficulty returning to sleep after walking to the bathroom. It will help you get adequate rest."
3. "The anticholinergic side effects of the drug will help prevent bowel irritability and constipation."
4. "Tricyclic antidepressants reduce abdominal pain by affecting the communication from the bowel to the brain."

**1171.** The nurse is reviewing the history and physical (H&P) of a teenager hospitalized with ulcerative colitis. Based on this diagnosis, which information should the nurse expect to see on this client's H&P?

1. Heartburn and regurgitation
2. Abdominal pain and bloody diarrhea
3. Weight gain and elevated blood glucose
4. Abdominal distention and hypoactive bowel sounds

**1172.** **PHARM** The 25-year-old client, hospitalized with an exacerbation of distal ulcerative colitis, is prescribed mesalamine rectally via enema. The client states that an enema is disgusting and wants to know why the medication cannot be given orally. Which is the **best** response by the nurse?

1. "It can be given orally; I'll contact the doctor and see if the change can be made."
2. "Rectal administration delivers the mesalamine directly to the affected area."
3. "Oral administration is not possible for treating your ulcerative colitis exacerbation."
4. "It can be given orally; I'll make the change, and we'll tell the doctor in the morning."

**1173.** The client is 6 days post-total proctocolectomy with ileostomy creation for ulcerative colitis. The client's ileostomy is draining large amounts of liquid stool, and the client has dizziness with ambulation. Which parameters should the nurse assess immediately? **Select all that apply.**

1. Pulse rate for the last 24 hours
2. Urine output for the last 24 hours
3. Weight over the last 3 days
4. Ability to move the lower extremities
5. Temperature readings for the last 24 hours

**1174.** The client with Crohn's disease has undergone a barium enema that showed strictures in the ileum. Based on this finding, the nurse should monitor the client closely for signs of which complication?

1. Peritonitis
2. Obstruction
3. Malabsorption
4. Fluid imbalance

**1175.** **MoC** The 20-year-old female is being admitted to the hospital with exacerbation of Crohn's disease. The client is alert and oriented, and has been taking azathioprine for disease control. Into which room should the charge nurse place the client?

1. Private room across from the nurse's station
2. Room with a female who has Crohn's disease
3. Private room that has a private attached bathroom
4. Room with an elderly female who is on bedrest

**1176.** **PHARM** The client is prescribed infliximab 5 mg/kg every 8 weeks to treat Crohn's disease. The client weighs 116 lb. How many milligrams (mg) should the nurse administer?

_____ mg (Record the answer as a whole number.)

**1177.** The nurse is completing a home visit with the client who had a partial resection of the ileum for Crohn's disease 4 weeks previously. The nurse should collect additional information when the client makes which statement?

1. "My stools float and seem to have fat in them."
2. "I have gained 5 pounds since I left the hospital."
3. "I am still avoiding milk and milk products."
4. "I am having only two formed stools per day."

**1178.** The nurse assesses the client previously diagnosed as having an inguinal hernia. The nurse considers that the client's hernia may be strangulated when which assessment findings are noted? **Select all that apply.**

1. Abdominal distention
2. Dyspnea with exertion
3. Severe abdominal pain
4. No stool for the past week
5. Hyperactive bowel sounds

**1179.** The nurse is reviewing the health history of the client receiving treatment for hemorrhoids. Which information, related to the development of hemorrhoids, should the nurse expect to find in the client's medical history? **Select all that apply.**

1. Body mass index of 18
2. Chronic constipation
3. Nulliparous female
4. Works as a salesperson
5. Taking iron supplements

**1180.** The client is being admitted to a postsurgical unit following anorectal surgery. The nurse reviews the following postoperative orders from the surgeon. Which order should the nurse question?

1. Give morphine sulfate per IV bolus before the first defecation.
2. Have the client take a sitz bath after each defecation.
3. Begin high-fiber diet as soon as client can tolerate oral intake.
4. Position supine with the head of the bed elevated to 30 degrees.

**1181.** The nurse is caring for the client with diverticulitis. The nurse should plan to instruct the client to avoid which food during an episode of diverticulitis?

1. White bread
2. Ripe banana
3. Cooked oatmeal
4. Iceberg lettuce

**1182.** The client is admitted to a hospital for medical management of acute diverticulitis. The nurse should anticipate that this client's plan of care will include which components? **Select all that apply.**

1. NPO status
2. Frequent ambulation
3. Prescribed antibiotics
4. Antiemetic medication
5. Deep breathing every 2 hours

**1183.** The nurse is caring for the client with acute diverticulitis. Which finding should **most** prompt the nurse to consider that the client has developed an intestinal perforation?

1. White blood cells (WBCs) elevated
2. Temperature of 101°F (38.3°C)
3. Bowel sounds are absent
4. Reports intense abdominal pain

**1184.** The nurse is caring for the client who has a temporary colostomy following surgery for colon cancer. The nurse assesses that the client's colostomy bag is empty and that there has been no stool since surgery 24 hours ago. What should the nurse do?

1. Call the surgeon immediately.
2. Place the client left side-lying.
3. Document these findings.
4. Give a bulk-forming laxative.

**1185.** The nurse is caring for clients with different types of ostomies. The nurse should teach that the client with which type of ostomy would most benefit from the procedure illustrated to control bowel evacuation?

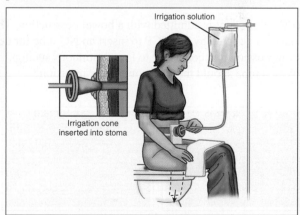

1. Ascending colostomy
2. Double-barreled colostomy
3. Transverse colostomy
4. Sigmoid colostomy

**1186.** The client is scheduled for an abdominal-perineal resection for cancer of the rectum. Which components should the nurse include in the client's preoperative education? **Select all that apply.**

1. The enterostomal nurse will be visiting the client prior to surgery.
2. After surgery rectal suppositories will be given to prevent straining and stress.
3. The bowel will be cleansed before surgery with a laxative, enema, or whole-gut lavage.
4. Oral or intravenous (IV) antibiotics will be prescribed to be given preoperatively.
5. A member of the surgical team will discuss the risk of postoperative sexual dysfunction.

**1187.** MoC The nurse is caring for the surgical client during the first 24 hours after an abdominal-perineal resection. Which action should have **priority?**

1. Provide a diet that is low in residue.
2. Check the colostomy bag for stool amount.
3. Assess the perineal dressing for drainage.
4. Encourage the client to see the colostomy site.

**1188.** The nurse is preparing to admit the hospitalized client diagnosed with peritonitis. Which collaborative interventions should the nurse anticipate? **Select all that apply.**

1. Intravenous fluids
2. Oral or IV antibiotics
3. NPO status
4. Analgesic medications
5. Supine positioning
6. NG tube to suction

**1189.** The client is admitted with a bowel obstruction. The nurse is directed by the HCP to insert an NG tube for decompression and connect it to low continuous suction. Which tube should the nurse obtain for insertion?

1.
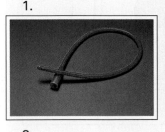

2.
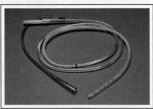

3.
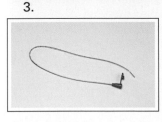

4.
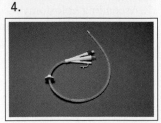

**1190.** The client is hospitalized with a large bowel obstruction resulting in massive abdominal distention. Which assessment findings should be **most** concerning to the nurse?

1. Urine specific gravity value of 1.020
2. High-pitched and tinkling bowel sounds
3. Decreased lung sounds in both lung bases
4. Client describes abdominal pain as colicky

**INSTRUCTIONS:** Read the case study illustrated, and then refer to the case study to answer Questions 1191 and 1192.

| Client | 65-year old |
|---|---|
| **Allergies** | Cephalosporin antibiotics |
| **Admitting Diagnosis** | Colon Cancer |

| Serum Lab Test | Client Value | Normal Values |
|---|---|---|
| BUN | 30 | 5–25 mg |
| Creatinine | 2.0 | 0.5–1.5 mg/dL |
| Na | 133 | 135–145 mEq/L |
| K | 4.5 | 3.5–5.3 mEq/L |
| Cl | 92 | 95–105 mEq/L |
| CO$_2$ | 23 | 22–30 mEq/L |
| Hgb/Hct | 10/32% | 13.5–17 g/dL, 40%–54% |
| WBC | 12,000 | 4500–10,000/mm³ |
| Neutrophils | 87% | 50%–70% |
| Albumin | 2.5 | 3.5–5.0 g/dL |
| Alkaline phosphatase (ALP) | 500 | 42–136 unit/L |
| AST | 76 | 8–38 unit/L |
| Calcium | 3.0 | 4.5–5.5 mEq/L |
| Phosphorus | 3.5 | 1.7–2.6 mg/dL |
| Procalcitonin | 1.9 | <0.15 ng/mL |
| CRP | 262 | <3.0 mg/dL |

**1191.** CJ What should the nurse do **immediately** after reviewing the client's laboratory results? Enter the information into the box below.

1192. **CJ** After examining the client's laboratory results, the nurse thinks that the client's colon cancer may have metastasized to the liver. Which laboratory findings led the nurse to this conclusion?

1. AST and ALP
2. BUN and creatinine
3. Albumin and calcium
4. WBCs and neutrophils

# Answers and Rationales

## 1128. MoC ANSWER: 3

1. The presence of *H. pylori* has not been proven to predispose to GI bleeding.
2. Although alcohol is associated with gastric mucosal injury, its causative role in bleeding is unclear.
3. **It is most important for the nurse to monitor the 70-year-old client who is taking aspirin. The client has two risk factors for GI bleeding: age and taking aspirin.**
4. Pregnancy and acetaminophen usage do not predispose to GI bleeding.

▶ *Test-taking Tip: Examine each option and count the number of risk factors for bleeding. The client with the most risk factors should be selected as the answer.*

Content Area: Adult; Concept: Management; Digestion; Integrated Processes: Nursing Process: Analysis; Client Needs: Safe and Effective Care Environment: Management of Care; Cognitive Level: Analysis [Analyzing]

## 1129. ANSWER: 3

1. No treatment is required; it is unnecessary to call the HCP.
2. If acute kidney failure is present, both the BUN and creatinine would be elevated.
3. **The findings should be documented. The BUN can be elevated after a significant GI hemorrhage from the breakdown of blood proteins. The protein breakdown releases nitrogen that is then converted to urea.**
4. Limiting protein intake in the presence of healthy kidneys is unnecessary.

▶ *Test-taking Tip: Focus on the situation: 24 hours post–GI hemorrhage. The serum creatinine is within the normal range. Use this information to eliminate Options 2 and 4. Although the BUN is elevated, this is expected following any type of hemorrhage. Thus eliminate Option 1.*

Content Area: Adult; Concept: Digestion; Critical Thinking; Communication; Integrated Processes: Communication and Documentation; Client Needs: Physiological Integrity: Physiological Adaptation; Cognitive Level: Analysis [Analyzing]

## 1130. ANSWER: 2

1. A urea breath test only tests for the presence of *Helicobacter pylori (H. pylori)*.
2. **The gastric mucosa can be visualized with an endoscope. A biopsy is possible to differentiate PUD from gastric cancer and to obtain tissue specimens to identify *H. pylori*. These are used to make a definitive diagnosis of PUD.**
3. Barium studies do not provide an opportunity for biopsy and *H. pylori* testing.
4. A urea breath test and a string test only test for the presence of *H. pylori*.

▶ *Test-taking Tip: The key words are "definitive diagnosis." This positive diagnosis usually involves actually viewing the tissue or taking biopsies.*

Content Area: Adult; Concept: Assessment; Collaboration; Digestion; Integrated Processes: Teaching/Learning; Client Needs: Physiological Integrity: Reduction of Risk Potential; Cognitive Level: Knowledge [Remembering]

## 1131. MoC ANSWER: 3

1. Symptoms of perforation include severe abdominal pain; vomiting usually does not occur.
2. The client with GI hemorrhage would have bright red or coffee-ground-colored emesis.
3. **Symptoms of gastric outlet obstruction include abdominal pain and projectile vomiting when the stomach fills enough to stimulate afferent nerve fibers relaying information to the vomiting center in the brain. The emesis may have a foul odor or contain food particles if the contents have been dormant in the stomach for a prolonged time period.**
4. Infection with *H. pylori* is not a complication of PUD; rather, it is a major cause of peptic ulcers.

▶ *Test-taking Tip: Note the symptoms presented in the stem, especially the foul odor of the emesis, and compare them to the symptoms of the answer options.*

Content Area: Adult; Concept: Digestion; Collaboration; Integrated Processes: Nursing Process: Analysis; Client Needs: Physiological Integrity: Reduction of Risk Potential; Safe and Effective Care Environment: Management of Care; Cognitive Level: Analysis [Analyzing]

## 1132. ANSWER: 2

1. Headaches are a symptom not related to GERD.
2. **Heartburn, which is described as a burning, tight sensation in the lower sternum, is the most common symptom of GERD. It will often wake the client from sleep.**
3. Night sweats are a symptom not related to GERD.
4. Postprandial sleepiness is a symptom not related to GERD.

♦ *Test-taking Tip: Examine Options 2 and 3 first because these have duplicate information (waking up at night). Of these, select Option 2 because it is associated with the GI system.*

Content Area: Adult; Concept: Assessment; Digestion; Integrated Processes: Nursing Process: Assessment; Client Needs: Physiological Integrity: Reduction of Risk Potential; Cognitive Level: Analysis [Analyzing]

## 1133. ANSWER: 4

1. Clients with viral hepatitis should avoid all alcohol and all medications containing acetaminophen, not just limit their use.
2. Clients should eat small, frequent meals with a high-carbohydrate, moderate-fat, and moderate-protein content.
3. It is not necessary to wear a mask when caring for an individual with hepatitis A. A gown and gloves should be worn when in contact with blood and body fluids.
4. **Rest is an essential intervention to decrease the liver's metabolic demands and increase its blood supply. Rest should be alternated with periods of activity to prevent complications and to restore health.**

♦ *Test-taking Tip: If an option contains multiple parts, each part must be correct. Examine options for key words that make the option incorrect.*

Content Area: Adult; Concept: Nutrition; Infection; Integrated Processes: Nursing Process: Planning; Client Needs: Physiological Integrity: Physiological Adaptation; Psychosocial Integrity; Cognitive Level: Application [Applying]

## 1134. PHARM ANSWER: 2

1. Anorexia is commonly seen with hepatitis B. A weight gain of 2 lb in 1 month would typically not be a cause for concern.
2. **Bruising can indicate thrombocytopenia, which is an adverse effect of treatment. Thrombocytopenia can also occur from liver dysfunction.**
3. Avoiding large crowds is appropriate; the client will be at increased risk for infection while taking interferon alpha-2b.
4. Fatigue is commonly associated with chronic hepatitis B.

♦ *Test-taking Tip: Remember to assess for symptoms associated with liver dysfunction.*

Content Area: Adult; Concept: Medication; Infection; Integrated Processes: Nursing Process: Analysis; Client Needs: Physiological Integrity: Pharmacological and Parenteral Therapies; Cognitive Level: Application [Applying]

## 1135. ANSWER: 1

1. **Ginger has demonstrated antiemetic properties as well as analgesic and sedative effects on GI motility.**
2. Avoidance of sudden changes in position and decreasing activity are recommended to control nausea.
3. All food should be stopped when nausea is present to prevent stomach stretching and stimulation of the afferent nerve fibers.
4. A quiet, calm environment, rather than one that is stimulating, is recommended to decrease nausea.

♦ *Test-taking Tip: Focus on selecting an option that would reduce GI stimulation. Eliminate Options 2 and 4 because they can be stimulating in general.*

Content Area: Adult; Concept: Nursing Roles; Nutrition; Digestion; Integrated Processes: Nursing Process: Implementation; Client Needs: Physiological Integrity: Basic Care and Comfort; Cognitive Level: Application [Applying]

## 1136. ANSWER: 1

1. **A small pouch (15–20 mL capacity) is constructed in the upper part of the stomach during vertical banded gastroplasty. Overfilling of this pouch stimulates afferent nerve fibers, which relay information to the chemoreceptor trigger zone in the brain, causing nausea.**
2. The function of the lower half of the stomach is not affected with a vertical banded gastroplasty.
3. The duodenum is not incised during a vertical banded gastroplasty.
4. Dumping syndrome is more likely to occur from a meal high in simple carbohydrates, not protein.

♦ *Test-taking Tip: Narrow the options by looking for associated words in the stem (gastro-) and options (stomach).*

Content Area: Adult; Concept: Nutrition; Digestion; Nursing Roles; Integrated Processes: Teaching/Learning; Client Needs: Physiological Integrity: Reduction of Risk Potential; Cognitive Level: Application [Applying]

## 1137. ANSWER: 4

1. Drinking fluids at mealtime increases the size of the food bolus that enters the stomach.
2. Carbohydrates are more rapidly digested than fats and proteins and would cause the food bolus to pass quickly into the intestine, increasing the likelihood that dumping syndrome would occur. Meals high in carbohydrates result in postprandial hypoglycemia, which is considered a variant of dumping syndrome.
3. Small, frequent meals are recommended to decrease dumping syndrome.
4. **Lying down after meals slows the passage of the food bolus into the intestine and helps to control dumping syndrome.**

♦ *Test-taking Tip: Focus on the anatomical changes that cause dumping syndrome. Select the option that slows peristalsis and eliminate other options.*

Content Area: Adult; Concept: Nursing Roles; Nutrition; Digestion;
Integrated Processes: Teaching/Learning; Client Needs: Physiological
Integrity: Reduction of Risk Potential; Health Promotion and Maintenance;
Cognitive Level: Application [Applying]

## 1138. ANSWER: 4

1. Although steatorrhea may occur after gastric resection, the symptoms of steatorrhea include fatty stools with a foul odor, not these symptoms.
2. The symptoms of duodenal reflux are abdominal pain and vomiting, not these symptoms. Duodenal reflux is not associated with food intake.
3. Symptoms of fluid overload would include increased BP, edema, and weight gain, not these symptoms.
4. **When eating large amounts of carbohydrates at a meal, the rapid glucose absorption from the chime results in hyperglycemia. This elevated glucose stimulates insulin production, which then causes an abrupt lowering of the blood glucose level. Hypoglycemic symptoms of weakness, diaphoresis, anxiety, and palpitations occur.**

▸ **Test-taking Tip:** *Focus on the symptoms that are characteristic of hypoglycemia. Rule out options that are not associated with high-carbohydrate intake.*

Content Area: Adult; Concept: Nutrition; Metabolism; Digestion;
Integrated Processes: Nursing Process: Analysis; Client Needs:
Physiological Integrity: Reduction of Risk Potential; Cognitive
Level: Analysis [Analyzing]

## 1139. MoC ANSWER: 4

1. For the first 24 to 48 hours postoperatively, the client sips small amounts of clear liquids to avoid nausea, vomiting, and distention and stress on the suture line.
2. If used, urinary catheters should be removed within 24 hours after surgery to prevent UTIs and to encourage mobility. The nurse may delegate this task to an LPN.
3. The BiPAP mask is used to keep the airway open and should be worn whenever the client is sleeping.
4. **A bottle of saline and a large-sized syringe may indicate that the client's NG tube has been or will be irrigated. Manipulating or irrigating an NG tube with too much solution can lead to disruption of the anastomosis in gastric surgeries. If an NG tube is present, the surgeon should be consulted before irrigating the tube.**

▸ **Test-taking Tip:** *Consider which observation indicates an unsafe action or situation. Think about the size of the stomach after gastric bypass surgery.*

Content Area: Adult; Concept: Safety; Management; Digestion; Integrated
Processes: Nursing Process: Analysis; Client Needs: Safe and Effective
Care Environment: Management of Care; Cognitive Level: Analysis
[Analyzing]

## 1140. ANSWER: 2

1. When the client has hypoactive bowel sounds, which would be expected in a postsurgical client, the nurse should begin listening over the ileocecal valve in the right lower abdominal quadrant rather than to the left of the umbilicus. The ileocecal valve normally is a very active area.
2. **When listening for bowel sounds on the client who has an NG tube to suction, the nurse should turn off the suction during auscultation to prevent mistaking the suction sound for bowel sounds.**
3. The diaphragm of the stethoscope should be utilized for bowel sounds. The bell of the stethoscope should be utilized for abdominal vascular sounds, such as bruits.
4. There is no reason to empty the canister before auscultation.

▸ **Test-taking Tip:** *Focus on the presence of the NG tube attached to suction, as this will alter the assessment procedure.*

Content Area: Adult; Concept: Assessment; Digestion; Integrated
Processes: Nursing Process: Assessment; Client Needs: Physiological
Integrity: Reduction of Risk Potential; Cognitive Level: Application
[Applying]

## 1141. ANSWER: 1, 4

1. **Clients with a hiatal hernia are encouraged to sleep with the HOB elevated on 4- to 6-in. blocks to reduce intraabdominal pressure and to foster esophageal emptying.**
2. Dumping syndrome occurs after surgery when the stomach no longer has control over the amount of chime that enters the small intestine. Clients are encouraged to lie flat after a meal.
3. Crohn's disease is an inflammatory disease of the bowel. Positioning interventions do not decrease symptoms.
4. **Clients with GERD are encouraged to sleep with the HOB elevated on 4- to 6-in. blocks to reduce intraabdominal pressure and to foster esophageal emptying.**
5. Gastritis is inflammation of the gastric mucosa. Positioning interventions do not decrease symptoms.

▸ **Test-taking Tip:** *When the HOB is elevated, gravity is used to move contents more quickly through the stomach. Evaluate each option and consider whether this intervention would be appropriate for the condition.*

Content Area: Adult; Concept: Digestion; Assessment; Integrated
Processes: Nursing Process: Assessment; Client Needs: Physiological
Integrity: Physiological Adaptation; Cognitive Level: Application
[Applying]

## 1142. MoC ANSWER: 2

1. The client may have difficulty with heartburn, but this does not have priority over aspiration.

2. **Zenker's diverticulum is an outpouching of the esophagus near the hypopharyngeal sphincter. Food can become trapped in the diverticula and cause aspiration.**

3. Constipation is not a concern with Zenker's diverticulum.

4. The client may have weight loss, but this does not have priority over aspiration.

▶ *Test-taking Tip: Use the ABC's to identify the priority.*

**Content Area:** Adult; **Concept:** Critical Thinking; Oxygenation; Digestion; **Integrated Processes:** Nursing Process: Analysis; **Client Needs:** Safe and Effective Care Environment: Management of Care; **Cognitive Level:** Application [Applying]

### 1143. ANSWER: 2

1. Indigestion is not a symptom of esophageal cancer.

2. **Progressive dysphagia is the most common symptom associated with esophageal cancer, and it is initially experienced when eating meat. It is often described as a feeling that food is not passing.**

3. Chest pain is not a symptom of esophageal cancer.

4. Weight loss rather than gain is a symptom of esophageal cancer.

▶ *Test-taking Tip: Eliminate options not associated with esophageal cancer.*

**Content Area:** Adult; **Concept:** Assessment; Cellular Regulation; Digestion; **Integrated Processes:** Nursing Process: Assessment; Communication and Documentation; **Client Needs:** Physiological Integrity: Reduction of Risk Potential; **Cognitive Level:** Application [Applying]

### 1144. ANSWER: 4

1. All or part of the stomach will remain intact following an esophagoenterostomy.

2. The pyloric sphincter will remain intact following an esophagoenterostomy.

3. The pharynx will remain intact following an esophagoenterostomy.

4. **An esophagectomy for cancer involves removal of the lower esophageal sphincter, which normally functions to keep food from refluxing back into the esophagus. The absence of the lower esophageal sphincter places the client at risk for aspiration.**

▶ *Test-taking Tip: Focus on the esophagectomy with colon interposition surgical procedure, specifically what organs and tissues that are removed to treat the cancer. Associate the prefix "esopha-" in the stem of the question with one of the options.*

**Content Area:** Adult; **Concept:** Nutrition; Oxygenation; Digestion; **Integrated Processes:** Nursing Process: Analysis; **Client Needs:** Physiological Integrity: Physiological Adaptation; **Cognitive Level:** Comprehension [Understanding]

### 1145. MoC ANSWER: 2

1. Discussing client information in a hospital hallway is inappropriate; individuals passing by could overhear confidential client information.

2. **Going into the client's room together allows the client to determine if he wants to disclose information and how much information he wants to disclose.**

3. Even if in a private location, the nurse should not share confidential client information with anyone unless the client has specifically given permission.

4. The nurse should not review the medical record of the client with a family member without permission. Some facilities require the client to complete a form requesting permission to review his or her own medical records.

▶ *Test-taking Tip: The topic of this question is maintaining confidentiality of client information. The key word is "best."*

**Content Area:** Adult; **Concept:** Legal; Digestion; Management; **Integrated Processes:** Caring; **Client Needs:** Safe and Effective Care Environment: Management of Care; Psychosocial Integrity; **Cognitive Level:** Application [Applying]

### 1146. ANSWER: 4

1. Nausea is a sign of gastric outlet obstruction or impending hemorrhage.

2. Grey Turner's sign is a symptom of pancreatitis, not metastasis.

3. Weight loss is an initial sign associated with cancer.

4. **The presence of ascites indicates seeding of the tumor in the peritoneal cavity.**

▶ *Test-taking Tip: Look for words in the stem of the question ("peritoneal") that are related to a word in one of the options ("abdomen").*

**Content Area:** Adult; **Concept:** Assessment; Cellular Regulation; Digestion; **Integrated Processes:** Nursing Process: Assessment; **Client Needs:** Physiological Integrity: Physiological Adaptation; **Cognitive Level:** Application [Applying]

### 1147. ANSWER: 2

1. The client's temperature will not be affected.

2. **Elevated serum ammonia levels may cause neurological changes, such as confusion.**

3. The client's urine specific gravity will not be affected.

4. Oral fluid intake should be encouraged if tolerated by the client.

▶ *Test-taking Tip: Focus on the symptoms of hepatic encephalopathy, which is caused by increased circulating ammonia levels. If uncertain of the answer, use Maslow's Hierarchy of Needs theory to establish priority. Option 2 is a safety need.*

**Content Area:** Adult; **Concept:** Neurologic Regulation; Digestion; **Integrated Processes:** Nursing Process: Planning; **Client Needs:** Physiological Integrity: Reduction of Risk Potential; **Cognitive Level:** Application [Applying]

**1148.** PHARM **ANSWER: 4**

1. Antibiotics and acid-reducing medications are expected with the treatment of PUD, but propranolol (Inderal) would not be expected. Although these medications may cue the nurse to further explore a history of PUD, this is not the most likely conclusion.
2. There is no indication that the client has abdominal pain, and the medication list does not include an analgesic.
3. There is no indication that the client has an infectious condition necessitating airborne precautions.
4. **All medications listed are used to treat liver cirrhosis and its complications of portal hypertension and hepatic encephalopathy. The antibiotic rifaximin (Xifaxan) and the laxative lactulose (Cephulac) are used for treating hepatic encephalopathy. Thus assessing the client's orientation and measuring abdominal girth are most important.**

▸ *Test-taking Tip: Review the entire list of medications to determine if some medications are specific for one condition. Use the nursing process to narrow the options; assessment should be the first action.*

Content Area: Adult; Concept: Inflammation; Digestion; Medication; Integrated Processes: Nursing Process: Implementation; Client Needs: Physiological Integrity: Pharmacological and Parenteral Therapies; Cognitive Level: Analysis [Analyzing]

**1149.** MoC **ANSWER: 1**

1. **The nurse should prepare to monitor the client's blood sugar level. The client with cirrhosis may develop insulin resistance. Impaired glucose tolerance is common with cirrhosis, and about 20% to 40% of clients also have diabetes. Hypoglycemia may occur during fasting because of decreased hepatic glycogen reserves and decreased gluconeogenesis.**
2. The client with cirrhosis would not be NPO but should receive a high-protein diet unless hepatic encephalopathy is present.
3. Antibiotics are not part of the treatment plan of cirrhosis because it is not caused by microorganisms.
4. The client with cirrhosis requires rest; thus ambulation should not be encouraged every 4 hours.

▸ *Test-taking Tip: Focus on the location of the liver in relation to other body organs and its pathophysiology to select the correct option.*

Content Area: Adult; Concept: Metabolism; Digestion; Integrated Processes: Nursing Process: Planning; Client Needs: Safe and Effective Care Environment: Management of Care; Physiological Integrity: Physiological Adaptation; Cognitive Level: Synthesis [Creating]

**1150. ANSWER: 2**

1. Adults in their forties are most at risk for NAFLD, not someone 70 years of age.

2. **The client's BMI is 35; a BMI of greater than 30 indicates obesity. The risk for developing NAFLD is directly related to body weight and is a major complication of obesity.**
3. Antibiotic use has no influence on NAFLD development.
4. Climate has no influence on NAFLD development.

▸ *Test-taking Tip: The topic of the question is risk factors associated with NAFLD. Note that the stem addresses "fatty liver" and that Option 2 is "obese."*

Content Area: Adult; Concept: Assessment; Nutrition; Digestion; Integrated Processes: Nursing Process: Assessment; Client Needs: Physiological Integrity: Physiological Adaptation; Cognitive Level: Application [Applying]

**1151. ANSWER: 1**

1. **This statement indicates the client does not understand the procedure. There is no need for an abdominal incision. The TIPS is placed through the jugular vein and threaded down to the hepatic vein.**
2. The TIPS procedure will decrease pressure in the portal vein and thus decrease the risk of bleeding from esophageal varices.
3. There is a risk that the stent that is placed will become occluded.
4. The shunt will decrease ascites formation.

▸ *Test-taking Tip: The statement "does not understand the procedure" indicates a false-response item. Select the incorrect statement.*

Content Area: Adult; Concept: Nursing Roles; Digestion; Integrated Processes: Nursing Process: Evaluation; Client Needs: Physiological Integrity: Basic Care and Comfort; Cognitive Level: Evaluation [Evaluating]

**1152.** PHARM **ANSWER: 3**

1. Alcohol intake is a major cause of cirrhosis and must be eliminated from the client's diet.
2. Rest may enable the liver to restore itself and should be encouraged.
3. **Although propranolol (Inderal) does decrease BP, it is not ordered for this purpose in treating cirrhosis. Prophylactic treatment with a nonselective beta blocker like propranolol has been shown to reduce the risk of bleeding from esophageal varices and to reduce bleeding-related deaths.**
4. Furosemide (Lasix) is used in combination with potassium-sparing diuretics to decrease ascites.

▸ *Test-taking Tip: The statement "need for further teaching" indicates an item with incorrect information. Select the statement that is not consistent with the diagnosis.*

Content Area: Adult; Concept: Nursing Roles; Digestion; Medication; Integrated Processes: Nursing Process: Evaluation; Teaching/Learning; Client Needs: Physiological Integrity: Physiological Adaptation; Physiological Integrity: Pharmacological and Parenteral Therapies; Health Promotion and Maintenance; Cognitive Level: Evaluation [Evaluating]

## 1153. ANSWER:

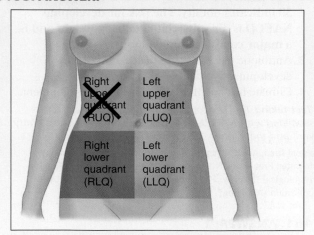

**The right upper quadrant is the site used for a percutaneous liver biopsy. The liver is located under the right diaphragm and extends just below the right costal margin. The client will be asked to sustain exhalation during the biopsy to reduce the possibility of a pneumothorax.**

▶ *Test-taking Tip: Recall normal anatomy and the location of the liver. A percutaneous biopsy means a needle is inserted through the skin (cutaneous) for the purpose of removing cells or tissues for examination.*

Content Area: Adult; Concept: Nursing Roles; Digestion; Integrated Processes: Teaching/Learning; Client Needs: Physiological Integrity: Reduction of Risk Potential; Cognitive Level: Application [Applying]

## 1154. ANSWER: 2

1. Elevated serum creatinine and BUN are associated with renal problems.
2. **Serum a-fetoprotein is a major serum protein synthesized by fetal liver cells, by yolk track cells, and in small amounts by the fetal GI system. Reappearance of AFP in adults signals pathological problems. In 50% to 75% of clients with liver cancer, serum AFP levels are elevated.**
3. Elevated serum phosphorus is associated with renal and many other diseases and is not specific to liver cancer.
4. CA-125 is a tumor marker for ovarian cancer.

▶ *Test-taking Tip: Recall that cancer tumor markers are usually proteins that are not normally present in the adult body. With this knowledge, eliminate Options 1 and 3.*

Content Area: Adult; Concept: Digestion; Cellular Regulation; Integrated Processes: Nursing Process: Analysis; Client Needs: Physiological Integrity: Reduction of Risk Potential; Cognitive Level: Application [Applying]

## 1155. MoC ANSWER: 4, 2, 3, 1

4. **The client with Crohn's disease who received an initial dose of certolizumab (Cimzia) and is having generalized rashes should be attended to first. Generalized rash indicates an allergic reaction. This could develop into an anaphylactic reaction.**

2. **The client with a peptic ulcer who now has severe vomiting should be attended to second. Vomiting in PUD may indicate a complication such as mechanical obstruction from scarring.**
3. **The client who had a colonoscopy and is having diarrheal stools should be attended to third. Diarrhea may have been the indication for the client's colonoscopy or a side effect of the bowel prep.**
1. **The client with ascites who is having mild dyspnea with activity can be attended to last. The dyspnea is usually due to the enlarged abdomen.**

▶ *Test-taking Tip: Use the ABC's to establish priority. Assign a low level of priority to options where the presenting problem is already expected due to the client's condition.*

Content Area: Adult; Concept: Medication; Infection; Management; Digestion; Integrated Processes: Nursing Process: Analysis; Client Needs: Safe and Effective Care Environment: Management of Care; Cognitive Level: Synthesis [Creating]

## 1156. MoC ANSWER: 3

1. After a liver biopsy VS should be assessed every 15 minutes times two, every 30 minutes times four, and then every hour times four to monitor for shock, peritonitis, and pneumothorax.
2. The client should be kept flat in bed for 12 to 14 hours following the procedure to prevent the risk of bleeding.
3. **Positioning the client on the right side after a liver biopsy splints the puncture site to prevent and decrease bleeding.**
4. The client should be cautioned to avoid coughing, which could precipitate bleeding.

▶ *Test-taking Tip: Recall that the liver is very vascular. Select the option that would decrease bleeding by pressure following the biopsy procedure. Eliminate options that increase the risk of bleeding.*

Content Area: Adult; Concept: Management; Digestion; Integrated Processes: Nursing Process: Evaluation; Client Needs: Safe and Effective Care Environment: Management of Care; Physiological Integrity: Reduction of Risk Potential; Cognitive Level: Evaluation [Evaluating]

## 1157. ANSWER: 1

1. **The predominant symptom of acute pancreatitis is severe, deep or piercing, continuous or steady abdominal pain in the upper left quadrant. The pain may radiate to the back because of the retroperitoneal location of the pancreas. Middle-aged individuals are at increased risk for developing acute pancreatitis.**
2. Abdominal pain located mainly in the right lower quadrant may be a symptom of appendicitis (not pancreatitis). Appendicitis is more common in younger adults.
3. Bloody diarrhea and colicky abdominal pain are symptoms of IBD, also more common in young adults.
4. Upper abdominal pain and projectile vomiting are symptoms of gastric outlet obstruction or another GI disorder and not pancreatitis.

▸ *Test-taking Tip: Think of the location of the pancreas. Look for key words in the location of each option and use the process of elimination.*

**Content Area:** Adult; **Concept:** Critical Thinking; Digestion; Inflammation; **Integrated Processes:** Nursing Process: Analysis; **Client Needs:** Physiological Integrity: Reduction of Risk Potential; **Cognitive Level:** Application [Applying]

**1158.** MoC **ANSWER: 1, 2, 3, 6**

1. **Giving an IV bolus followed by fluids at 250 mL/hour should be implemented. A large amount of fluids is lost due to third spacing into the retroperitoneum and intraabdominal area. Fluids are needed to prevent hypovolemia and maintain hemodynamic stability.**
2. **Nasojejunal enteral feedings with a low-fat formula should be initiated to decrease the secretion of secretin, meet caloric needs, and maintain a positive nitrogen balance.**
3. **Antibiotics, usually medications of the imipenem class such as imipenem/cilastatin (Primaxin), are used when pancreatitis is complicated by infected pancreatic necrosis. They have greater potency and a broader antimicrobial spectrum than other beta-lactam antibiotics.**
4. The client should be maintained on bedrest to decrease the metabolic rate and therefore reduce pancreatic secretions.
5. Discomfort frequently improves with the client in the supine position rather than side-lying.
6. **A urinary catheter should be inserted to closely monitor urine output for circulating fluid volume status and to monitor for complications.**

▸ *Test-taking Tip: Use knowledge of generic treatment of inflammatory body conditions, which requires resting of the inflamed body part, to eliminate Option 4. Thinking about the location of the pancreas should allow elimination of Option 5.*

**Content Area:** Adult; **Concept:** Fluid and Electrolyte Balance; Nutrition; Digestion; Medication; **Integrated Processes:** Nursing Process: Implementation; **Client Needs:** Safe and Effective Care Environment: Management of Care; **Cognitive Level:** Analysis [Analyzing]

**1159. ANSWER: 2**

1. Portal hypertension is related to cirrhosis, not pancreatitis.
2. **The bluish flank discoloration (Grey Turner's sign) indicates blood-stained exudates have seeped from the pancreas due to the severity of the disease process.**
3. Pancreatitis will not cause stomach bleeding.
4. Pancreatitis will not cause intestinal obstruction.

▸ *Test-taking Tip: To arrive at the answer, eliminate options involving other organs and not the pancreas.*

**Content Area:** Adult; **Concept:** Inflammation; Digestion; **Integrated Processes:** Nursing Process: Analysis; **Client Needs:** Physiological Integrity: Reduction of Risk Potential; **Cognitive Level:** Analysis [Analyzing]

**1160. ANSWER: 3**

1. Regaining appetite is a positive sign, but it must be accompanied by a decrease in pain before the client is allowed to take food orally.
2. Intestinal peristalsis may be slowed due to inflammation associated with acute pancreatitis, but the return of bowel sounds and flatus is not used to determine when to begin oral intake.
3. **This response is correct. Once pain is controlled and the serum enzyme levels begin to decrease, the client can begin oral intake. These are signs that the pancreas is healing.**
4. There is no specific time limit for being NPO.

▸ *Test-taking Tip: Recall that severe pain and elevated serum amylase and lipase are the main symptoms of pancreatitis. A decrease in these symptoms indicates healing.*

**Content Area:** Adult; **Concept:** Nutrition; Digestion; **Integrated Processes:** Nursing Process: Evaluation; Communication and Documentation; **Client Needs:** Physiological Integrity: Physiological Adaptation; **Cognitive Level:** Evaluation [Evaluating]

**1161.** PHARM **ANSWER: 3**

1. Opioid analgesics may be prescribed if pancreatic enzymes do not relieve pain.
2. NSAIDS, such as ibuprofen, may be used to treat chronic pancreatic pain, but they are not the initial treatment and are usually not sufficient to control the pain.
3. **The initial pain control measures include exogenous pancreatic enzymes because pancreatic stimulation by food is thought to cause pain. Pancreatic enzymes are coupled with H2 blockers, which block the action of histamine on parietal cells in the stomach. H2 blockers are used because gastric acid destroys the lipase needed to break down fats.**
4. A nerve block relieves pain in about 50% of people who undergo the procedure, but this is not the initial measure for pain control.

▸ *Test-taking Tip: The key word is "initial." Use similar words in the stem and the options to select the answer.*

**Content Area:** Adult; **Concept:** Comfort; Medication; Nutrition; Digestion; **Integrated Processes:** Nursing Process: Implementation; **Client Needs:** Physiological Integrity: Pharmacological and Parenteral Therapies; **Cognitive Level:** Application [Applying]

**1162.** MoC **ANSWER: 1**

1. **The Whipple procedure induces insulin-dependent diabetes because the proximal pancreas is resected. Thus the blood glucose levels should be monitored closely starting immediately after surgery.**
2. Parenteral (not enteral) feedings are the method of choice for providing nutrition immediately after surgery.
3. The NG tube is strategically placed during surgery and should not be irrigated without a surgeon's order. With an order, gentle irrigation with 10 to 20 mL of NS is appropriate.

4. Pancreaticoduodenectomy (Whipple procedure) involves removal of the head of the pancreas, the duodenum, the gallbladder and the bile duct, and is consider a major abdominal surgery. Epidural analgesia is given for pain control.

▶ *Test-taking Tip: The Whipple procedure entails resection of the proximal pancreas, the adjoining duodenum, the distal portion of the stomach, and the distal segment of the common bile duct. The pancreatic duct, common bile duct, and stomach are then anastomosed to the jejunum. Eliminate options that pertain to the GI tract.*

Content Area: Adult; Concept: Metabolism; Management; Digestion; Integrated Processes: Nursing Process: Planning; Client Needs: Safe and Effective Care Environment: Management of Care; Physiological Integrity: Physiological Adaptation; Cognitive Level: Synthesis [Creating]

## 1163. MoC ANSWER: 2

1. The client with a pain rating of 6 out of 10 on a numerical scale needs attention, but the pain is not a life-threatening concern.
2. **Bleeding esophageal varices are the most life-threatening complication of cirrhosis. Coughing can precipitate a bleeding episode. The nurse should assess this client first.**
3. The client who is postcholecystectomy is reported as being stable and could be assessed last.
4. The client reporting itching needs attention, but the itching is not a life-threatening concern.

▶ *Test-taking Tip: Use prioritization criteria: life-threatening concerns must be addressed first; client safety concerns second; and concerns essential to the plan of care third. Use the ABC's to determine priority.*

Content Area: Adult; Concept: Critical Thinking; Nutrition; Digestion; Management; Integrated Processes: Nursing Process: Planning; Caring; Client Needs: Safe and Effective Care Environment: Management of Care; Cognitive Level: Analysis [Analyzing]

## 1164. ANSWER: 2

1. The nurse does not need to wear a mask when caring for the client; the bacterium is transmitted through direct contact.
2. **Hand washing with soap and water is performed instead of using alcohol-based hand cleaners; alcohol-based cleaners lack sporicidal activity. Even vigorous scrubbing with soap and water does not kill all of the spores.**
3. The client should be in a private room but does not need a flow pressure room. Flow pressure rooms are used with airborne diseases.
4. The spores of *Clostridium difficile* can survive on inanimate objects such as tables and bedrails. For self-protection, visitors should be instructed to wash vigorously with soap and water and not to use the alcohol-based hand wash.

▶ *Test-taking Tip: Use information in the stem to narrow the options. Clostridium difficile is a spore-forming microbe that is not transmitted through the air.*

Content Area: Adult; Concept: Safety; Infection; Integrated Processes: Nursing Process: Implementation; Client Needs: Safe and Effective Care Environment: Safety and Infection Control; Cognitive Level: Application [Applying]

## 1165. ANSWER: 1

1. **Loose stools are a yin symptom, which should be treated with foods that have yang qualities, one of which is chicken.**
2. A high-protein diet can cause gastric distress and diarrhea.
3. There is no indication that the chicken broth is high in sodium.
4. Although the client may distrust Western medicine, there is a stronger association between chicken broth and diarrhea when considering the yang qualities of chicken.

▶ *Test-taking Tip: Some cultures believe in the balance between yin and yang.*

Content Area: Adult; Concept: Diversity; Bowel Elimination; Nutrition; Integrated Processes: Nursing Process: Analysis; Culture and Spirituality; Client Needs: Psychosocial Integrity; Physiological Integrity: Physiological Adaptation; Cognitive Level: Application [Applying]

## 1166. MoC ANSWER: 2

1. Repositioning the client might promote bile flow into the T-tube if the client were lying on the tube. However, the jaundice indicates that the problem is internal.
2. **The T-tube is placed in the common bile duct to ensure patency of the duct. Lack of bile draining into the T-tube and jaundiced sclera are signs of an obstruction to the bile flow. This is most important to report to the surgeon.**
3. The client's BP would not be affected by this situation.
4. Recording the findings and continuing to monitor the client are inappropriate because the client is experiencing signs of a complication.

▶ *Test-taking Tip: The presence of jaundice and the absence of T-tube drainage after biliary surgery are signs of a possible complication. Select the option that reflects the urgency of the situation.*

Content Area: Adult; Concept: Critical Thinking; Nutrition; Digestion; Management; Integrated Processes: Nursing Process: Implementation; Client Needs: Safe and Effective Care Environment: Management of Care; Cognitive Level: Analysis [Analyzing]

## 1167. PHARM ANSWER: 2

1. The client should be NPO rather than be given a bland diet to decrease gallbladder stimulation.
2. **The nurse should anticipate giving anticholinergic medications to decrease secretions and counteract smooth muscle spasms.**
3. The client should be positioned with the head of the bed elevated (not flat) to decrease the pressure of the abdominal contents on the diaphragm and to improve ventilation.
4. Laxatives would increase GI stimulation unnecessarily.

▶ *Test-taking Tip: Generic treatment of inflammation is to rest the involved body part. Knowing this, Options 1 and 4 should be eliminated.*

Content Area: Adult; Concept: Inflammation; Nutrition; Digestion; Medication; Integrated Processes: Nursing Process: Planning; Client Needs: Physiological Integrity: Pharmacological and Parenteral Therapies; Cognitive Level: Application [Applying]

## 1168. ANSWER: 3

1. Clients are kept NPO in case surgery is needed.
2. Analgesic medications are usually withheld until a definitive diagnosis is established to avoid masking critical symptom changes.
3. **The nurse should question applying heat to the abdomen when appendicitis is suspected. Heat is contraindicated because it increases circulation, which, in turn, could cause the appendix to rupture.**
4. Isotonic IV fluids are initiated to replace lost body fluid and prevent dehydration.

▶ *Test-taking Tip: The question is a false-response item. Select the incorrect statement.*

Content Area: Adult; Concept: Inflammation; Safety; Bowel Elimination; Management; Integrated Processes: Nursing Process: Implementation; Client Needs: Safe and Effective Care Environment: Safety and Infection Control; Cognitive Level: Analysis [Analyzing]

## 1169. ANSWER: 4

1. Clients with IBS may have diarrhea, but it is not bloody.
2. Vomiting is not a symptom of IBS.
3. Clients with IBS do not have unintentional weight loss.
4. **Mucus in the stools is a sign of IBS.**

▶ *Test-taking Tip: Narrow the options to the two associated with the bowel.*

Content Area: Adult; Concept: Assessment; Bowel Elimination; Integrated Processes: Nursing Process: Analysis; Client Needs: Physiological Integrity: Physiological Adaptation; Cognitive Level: Application [Applying]

## 1170. PHARM ANSWER: 4

1. Not all clients with chronic diseases suffer from depression. The response does not address the primary reason for the use of a TCA such as amitriptyline (Elavil) in IBS.
2. A common response to TCAs is sedation; however, this medication is not given for this reason.
3. TCAs do have anticholinergic side effects and can cause (not prevent) constipation. Clients with IBS can have constipation or diarrhea.
4. **Evidence supports that TCAs, such as amitriptyline (Elavil), can reduce abdominal pain, and this benefit is unrelated to whether or not the client is being treated for depression.**

▶ *Test-taking Tip: The key word "best" suggests that more than one option may be correct but that one option is better than the other. Focus on the reason that this particular category of medication is used for this client.*

Content Area: Adult; Concept: Bowel Elimination: Evidence-based Practice; Nursing Roles; Integrated Processes: Teaching/Learning; Client Needs: Physiological Integrity: Pharmacological and Parenteral Therapies; Cognitive Level: Application [Applying]

## 1171. ANSWER: 2

1. Heartburn and regurgitation are not symptoms of ulcerative colitis.
2. **The nurse should expect to read about the primary symptoms of ulcerative colitis, which are bloody diarrhea and abdominal pain.**
3. Weight loss, not weight gain, often occurs in severe cases of ulcerative colitis.
4. Bowel sounds are often hyperactive rather than hypoactive in ulcerative colitis.

▶ *Test-taking Tip: Narrow the options to those only associated with the colon. Of the two remaining options, consider the effects of ulceration.*

Content Area: Adult; Concept: Assessment; Bowel Elimination; Communication; Integrated Processes: Nursing Process: Assessment; Communication and Documentation; Client Needs: Physiological Integrity: Physiological Adaptation; Cognitive Level: Application [Applying]

## 1172. PHARM ANSWER: 2

1. If the client still desires a change in medication route after the rationale for rectal administration is explained, the HCP should be consulted.
2. **This is the nurse's best response because it explains the purpose for administration via enema. This route delivers mesalamine (Asacol) directly to the affected area, thus maximizing effectiveness and minimizing side effects.**
3. Oral administration is possible, but rectal administration is preferred in distal colitis.
4. Nurses cannot order medications or change medication routes without specific approval by the HCP, who is licensed to prescribe medications.

▶ *Test-taking Tip: The key word is "best." Eliminate any options that are not within the nurse's legal scope of practice. Treatment of IBD often involves topical application of medication directly to the tissue involved.*

Content Area: Adult; Concept: Medication; Bowel Elimination; Communication; Integrated Processes: Nursing Process: Implementation; Communication and Documentation; Client Needs: Physiological Integrity: Pharmacological and Parenteral Therapies; Cognitive Level: Analysis [Analyzing]

## 1173. ANSWER: 1, 2, 3, 5

1. **The nurse should assess for increasing pulse rate over time because it is a sign of dehydration; large amounts of ileostomy output can result in dehydration, and the dizziness with ambulation could be from dehydration.**
2. **The nurse should assess for decreasing urine output because it is a sign of dehydration; large amounts of ileostomy output can result in dehydration, and the dizziness with ambulation could be from dehydration.**

3. **The nurse should assess for decreasing weight because it is a sign of dehydration; large amounts of ileostomy output can result in dehydration, and the dizziness with ambulation could be from dehydration.**

4. The ability to move the lower extremities is not related to dehydration.

5. **The nurse should assess the temperature readings because a low-grade temperature is a sign of dehydration; large amounts of ileostomy output can result in dehydration, and the dizziness with ambulation could be from dehydration.**

▶ *Test-taking Tip: Concentrate on the symptoms presented in the stem of the question: large ileostomy output and dizziness with ambulation. These should be recognized as signs of dehydration. Choose options that would provide more information about the client's fluid balance and pattern of temperature elevations.*

**Content Area:** Adult; **Concept:** Fluid and Electrolyte Balance; Bowel Elimination; **Integrated Processes:** Nursing Process: Analysis; **Client Needs:** Physiological Integrity: Physiological Adaptation; **Cognitive Level:** Analysis [Analyzing]

### 1174. ANSWER: 2

1. Peritonitis would not be an expected consequence of a bowel stricture.

2. **The nurse should monitor for signs of a bowel obstruction. Bowel strictures are a common complication of Crohn's disease and can result in an acute bowel obstruction.**

3. Malabsorption would not be an expected consequence of a bowel stricture.

4. Fluid balance would be affected once total obstruction develops.

▶ *Test-taking Tip: Focus on what can be expected if the bowel is narrowed in a specific area. This would help to eliminate Options 3 and 4.*

**Content Area:** Adult; **Concept:** Assessment; Bowel Elimination; **Integrated Processes:** Nursing Process: Assessment; **Client Needs:** Physiological Integrity: Reduction of Risk Potential; **Cognitive Level:** Application [Applying]

### 1175. MoC ANSWER: 3

1. The client is alert and oriented; there is no need to be near the nurse's station.

2. The client is at an increased risk for infection and should have a private room rather than rooming with another female with Crohn's disease.

3. **The client should be in a private room with a private bathroom due to an increased risk for infection with azathioprine (Imuran). Azathioprine suppresses cell-mediated immune responses and may cause bone marrow suppression. It is also a biohazard medication.**

4. The client is at an increased risk for infection and should have a private room rather than rooming with another female.

▶ *Test-taking Tip: Options 1 and 3 have "private room." Think of azathioprine's adverse effects of bone marrow suppression when selecting an option.*

**Content Area:** Adult; **Concept:** Inflammation; Bowel Elimination; Management; **Integrated Processes:** Nursing Process: Planning; **Client Needs:** Safe and Effective Care Environment: Management of Care; **Cognitive Level:** Application [Applying]

### 1176. PHARM ANSWER: 264

**First, the client's weight should be converted to kg. Formula:**
**Weight in lb ÷ 2.2 kg = kg wt. Thus 116 lb ÷ 2.2 lb/kg = 52.7 kg**
**Next, multiply the weight in kg by 5; 52.7 kg × 5 mg/kg = 263.6 mg or 264 mg**
**The nurse should administer 264 mg infliximab (Remicade).**

▶ *Test-taking Tip: Recall that 1 kg = 2.2 lb. Use this information to convert pounds to kilograms.*

**Content Area:** Adult; **Concept:** Medication; Bowel Elimination; **Integrated Processes:** Nursing Process: Implementation; **Client Needs:** Physiological Integrity: Pharmacological and Parenteral Therapies; **Cognitive Level:** Application [Applying]

### 1177. ANSWER: 1

1. **The nurse should collect additional information when the client states having stools that float and have fat in them. Bile salts are absorbed in the terminal ileum. Disease in this area or resection of the ileum can result in poor fat absorption and loss of fat in the stool. The presence of bile salts leads to diarrhea.**

2. Weight gain is a positive sign after small bowel resection for Crohn's disease.

3. Many clients with Crohn's disease develop lactose intolerance and therefore should avoid milk products.

4. Formed stools are a positive sign after small bowel resection for Crohn's disease.

▶ *Test-taking Tip: Focus on the digestive process, on what actually happens in the ileum, and on what problems might develop if the ileum were resected.*

**Content Area:** Adult; **Concept:** Bowel Elimination; Assessment; **Integrated Processes:** Nursing Process: Evaluation; **Client Needs:** Physiological Integrity: Basic Care and Comfort; **Cognitive Level:** Evaluation [Evaluating]

### 1178. ANSWER: 1, 3, 4

1. **Abdominal distention occurs because the bowel is obstructed when the hernia is strangulated.**

2. Dyspnea with exertion is not associated with strangulation of an inguinal hernia.

3. **Lack of blood supply from strangulation causes severe abdominal pain.**

4. **A bowel obstruction prevents the passage of stool.**

5. Bowel sounds with strangulation and bowel obstruction would be hypoactive or absent, not hyperactive.

▶ **Test-taking Tip:** *When a hernia is irreducible and intestinal flow and blood supply are obstructed, the hernia is strangulated. Focus on the body response when blood supply to intestinal tissue is reduced.*

**Content Area:** Adult; **Concept:** Assessment; Bowel Elimination; **Integrated Processes:** Nursing Process: Analysis; **Client Needs:** Physiological Integrity: Reduction of Risk Potential; **Cognitive Level:** Application [Applying]

## 1179. ANSWER: 2, 5

1. Clients who are thin (BMI = 18) would have a decreased risk of hemorrhoid development. Obesity is a risk factor for hemorrhoid development.
2. **Prolonged constipation is a risk factor for development of hemorrhoids.**
3. Because pregnancy is a common cause of constipation, nulliparous women would have a decreased risk of hemorrhoid development.
4. Sedentary rather than active occupations have an increased risk of hemorrhoid development.
5. **Iron supplements can lead to constipation and straining, which can precipitate hemorrhoid development.**

▶ **Test-taking Tip:** *Hemorrhoids are swollen or distended veins in the anorectal area. Consider the risk for developing hemorrhoids with each option.*

**Content Area:** Adult; **Concept:** Assessment; Bowel Elimination; **Integrated Processes:** Nursing Process: Assessment; **Client Needs:** Physiological Integrity: Reduction of Risk Potential; **Cognitive Level:** Application [Applying]

## 1180. ANSWER: 4

1. Pain medication is recommended before the first defecation to avoid straining.
2. A sitz bath is encouraged for rectal cleansing after defecation.
3. A high-fiber diet prevents constipation.
4. **After anorectal surgery, the client should be positioned in a side-lying (not supine) position to decrease rectal edema and client discomfort.**

▶ **Test-taking Tip:** *This item is a false-response question. You should select the incorrect statement.*

**Content Area:** Adult; **Concept:** Collaboration; Bowel Elimination; **Integrated Processes:** Communication and Documentation; **Client Needs:** Safe and Effective Care Environment: Safety and Infection Control; **Cognitive Level:** Analysis [Analyzing]

## 1181. ANSWER: 3

1. White bread is a recommended food for fiber-restricted diets. It contains less than 1 g fiber per ounce.
2. Ripe bananas, canned soft fruits, and most well-cooked vegetables without seeds or skins are recommended for fiber-restricted diets.
3. **Cooked oatmeal contains 4 g of fiber per serving. Foods high in fiber should be avoided during an episode of diverticulitis, and foods should be restricted to low fiber or clear liquids. Once diverticulitis is resolved, the client should return to a high-fiber diet.**
4. Iceberg lettuce contains less than 1 g of fiber.

▶ **Test-taking Tip:** *Note the "-itis" ending in diverticulitis, which indicates an inflammatory condition. During an inflammatory period, rest of the colon is indicated. Look for commonalities in the answers. Only one food is a high-fiber food.*

**Content Area:** Adult; **Concept:** Nutrition; Digestion; Inflammation; **Integrated Processes:** Nursing Process: Planning; **Client Needs:** Physiological Integrity: Basic Care and Comfort; Health Promotion and Maintenance; **Cognitive Level:** Application [Applying]

## 1182. ANSWER: 1, 3

1. **The nurse should plan for the client to be NPO. Medical management for diverticulitis includes resting the bowel. NPO status will help to achieve this.**
2. Ambulation is not encouraged; resting the body promotes bowel rest.
3. **Broad-spectrum antibiotics effective against known enteric pathogens are used in treating every stage of diverticulitis.**
4. Nausea is not a concern with diverticulitis.
5. The client did not have surgery; there is no need for deep breathing every 2 hours.

▶ **Test-taking Tip:** *Focus on basic treatment for any inflamed body part to eliminate options that do not promote resting the body part. Of the remaining options, consider the location of diverticula.*

**Content Area:** Adult; **Concept:** Inflammation; Bowel Elimination; **Integrated Processes:** Nursing Process: Planning; **Client Needs:** Physiological Integrity: Physiological Adaptation; **Cognitive Level:** Synthesis [Creating]

## 1183. ANSWER: 3

1. Elevated WBCs are a symptom of acute diverticulitis.
2. Increased temperature is a symptom of acute diverticulitis.
3. **Clients with intestinal perforation develop paralytic ileus. Bowel sounds would be absent.**
4. Abdominal pain is a symptom of acute diverticulitis that may worsen with intestinal perforation, but the most significant finding would be absent bowel sounds.

▶ **Test-taking Tip:** *The key word is "most." Select the option that is most likely to indicate intestinal perforation. Focus on symptoms of peritonitis and eliminate these.*

**Content Area:** Adult; **Concept:** Assessment; Inflammation; Bowel Elimination; **Integrated Processes:** Nursing Process: Evaluation; **Client Needs:** Physiological Integrity: Reduction of Risk Potential; **Cognitive Level:** Evaluation [Evaluating]

## 1184. ANSWER: 3

1. The absence of stool is an expected finding; there is no need to call the surgeon.
2. A left side-lying position will not produce stool if peristalsis has not yet returned.
3. **The nurse should document the findings; the absence of stool is expected 24 hours postsurgery.**
4. A laxative is unnecessary.

▶ **Test-taking Tip:** *After abdominal surgery, peristalsis in the large intestine may not return for 3 to 5 days.*

Content Area: Adult; Concept: Bowel Elimination; Cellular Regulation; Integrated Processes: Communication and Documentation; Client Needs: Physiological Integrity: Basic Care and Comfort; Cognitive Level: Analysis [Analyzing]

### 1185. ANSWER: 4

1. Ascending colostomies contain liquid stool that cannot be controlled with colonic irrigation.
2. A double-barreled colostomy is a temporary colostomy. It can be located anywhere along the large intestine and thus may or may not be appropriate to irrigate.
3. Transverse colostomies contain stool that is too loose to benefit from colostomy irrigation.
4. **Stool is most formed with a sigmoid colostomy. Thus the client with this type of colostomy would benefit the most from colonic irrigation to control evacuation.**

▶ *Test-taking Tip:* Look at key words "most benefit." Review each option to determine the location of the ostomy and typical stool consistency.

Content Area: Fundamentals; Concept: Bowel Elimination; Integrated Processes: Teaching/Learning; Client Needs: Physiological Integrity: Basic Care and Comfort; Health Promotion and Maintenance; Cognitive Level: Application [Applying]

### 1186. ANSWER: 1, 3, 4, 5

1. **An abdominal-perineal resection removes the sigmoid colon, rectum, and anus. As a result, the client will have a permanent colostomy. The enterostomal nurse will identify and mark an appropriate stoma location after considering the client's skinfolds, clothing preferences, and the level of the colostomy.**
2. After an abdominal-perineal resection the client needs to avoid rectal temperatures, suppositories, or other rectal procedures. These interventions may damage the anal suture line, cause bleeding, or impair healing.
3. **The bowel is cleansed preoperatively to reduce the risk of peritoneal contamination by bowel contents during surgery.**
4. **Antibiotics are prescribed to be given preoperatively to reduce the risk of peritoneal contamination by bowel contents during surgery.**
5. **Postoperatively the client with an abdominal-perineal resection is at risk for sexual dysfunction and urinary incontinence as a result of nerve damage. This needs to be discussed with the client prior to surgery by the surgeon or a member of the surgical team.**

▶ *Test-taking Tip:* As you go through each option, ask if this option is correct and should be included in the preoperative education of the client who will be experiencing an abdominal-perineal resection.

Content Area: Adult; Concept: Cellular Regulation; Bowel Elimination; Nursing Roles; Integrated Processes: Teaching/Learning; Client Needs: Physiological Integrity: Reduction of Risk Potential; Cognitive Level: Application [Applying]

### 1187. MoC ANSWER: 3

1. After bowel surgery, a temporary ileus is expected; thus the client would be NPO (nothing per mouth) initially.
2. There would not be stool coming from the colostomy until bowel peristalsis returns.
3. **The perineal incision must be examined frequently to assess for drainage and the need for dressing changes.**
4. The client's physiological needs in the early postoperative period take precedence over the integration of the body image change into the client's self-concept.

▶ *Test-taking Tip:* After an abdominal-perineal resection, the client will have two incisions—one in the abdomen and one in the perineal area. Apply the nursing process and Maslow's Hierarchy of Needs theory to narrow the options. Assessment has priority.

Content Area: Adult; Concept: Bowel Elimination; Management; Integrated Processes: Nursing Process: Implementation; Client Needs: Safe and Effective Care Environment: Management of Care; Cognitive Level: Application [Applying]

### 1188. ANSWER: 1, 3, 4, 6

1. **IV fluids are given to replace fluids shifting in the peritoneum and bowel from the inflammatory process.**
2. Appropriate antibiotics are given, but these would only be by the IV route because the client should be NPO.
3. **NPO status will rest the bowel.**
4. **Analgesics are utilized for pain control.**
5. The client can assume any position that promotes comfort; a supine position is not required.
6. **NG suction decompresses the stomach and intestine and rests the GI tract.**

▶ *Test-taking Tip:* Initial interventions for peritonitis are supportive and include fluid replacement and resting the GI tract.

Content Area: Adult; Concept: Inflammation; Infection; Integrated Processes: Nursing Process: Implementation; Client Needs: Physiological Integrity: Physiological Adaptation; Cognitive Level: Application [Applying]

### 1189. ANSWER: 2

1. The red tube is a single-lumen tube and comes in varying lengths that can be used for NG suction, postpyloric feedings, or urinary catheterizations. Single-lumen tubes should not be used with continuous suction.
2. **The nurse should obtain a double-lumen NG tube with an air vent for continuous suction. The pigtail (air vent) helps to keep the tube away from the stomach wall so that it is not damaged.**
3. This is a single-lumen feeding tube. It should not be used for GI suctioning.
4. This is a gastrostomy tube. It is commonly inserted endoscopically into the stomach; it is unnecessary to have this invasive procedure for gastric decompression.

▶ **Test-taking Tip:** *Note which tube (double lumen) is different from the other three tubes (single lumen). You might also recognize the smaller size of some of the tubes. Typically a larger-size tube, 14 or 16 Fr, is used in the adult to decompress the stomach and prevent plugging.*

**Content Area:** Adult; **Concept:** Nursing Roles; Bowel Elimination; **Integrated Processes:** Nursing Process: Planning; **Client Needs:** Physiological Integrity: Reduction of Risk Potential; **Cognitive Level:** Application [Applying]

## 1190. ANSWER: 3

1. A specific gravity value of 1.020 is normal. The nurse would expect to see an increase in specific gravity due to sequestering of fluids in the abdomen.
2. High-pitched bowel sounds are expected with a bowel obstruction.
3. **Decreased lung sounds are the most concerning finding because it can be life-threatening. Massive distention can impair function of the diaphragm, which in turn leads to atelectasis and compromised respiratory function.**
4. Pain that is colicky in nature is a usual manifestation of the obstruction. If the pain is deep and cramping or continuous, the bowel may be ischemic or possibly perforated.

▶ **Test-taking Tip:** *A complication of the disease process should be the most concerning finding. Eliminate options that are expected as part of the disease process. Use the ABC's to identify the most concerning finding.*

**Content Area:** Adult; **Concept:** Oxygenation; Bowel Elimination; **Integrated Processes:** Nursing Process: Assessment; **Client Needs:** Physiological Integrity: Reduction of Risk Potential; **Cognitive Level:** Analysis [Analyzing]

## 1191. CJ MoC PHARM ANSWER:

> **Check whether the client is receiving any antibiotics and contact the HCP.**

**The elevated WBCs and neutrophils suggest an infection. The elevated procalcitonin and CRP indicates that the client may be septic. The client should be placed on antibiotics, if not already receiving these, and treated for sepsis.**

▶ **Test-taking Tip:** *You need to consider that elevated WBCs and neutrophils indicate an acute infection.*

**Content Area:** Adult; **Concept:** Cellular Regulation; Bowel Elimination; Medication; **Integrated Processes:** Nursing Process: Analysis; **Client Needs:** Safe and Effective Care Environment: Management of Care; Physiological Integrity: Pharmacological and Parenteral Therapies; **Cognitive Level:** Analysis [Analyzing]

## 1192. CJ ANSWER: 1

1. **ALP is an enzyme produced in the bone and liver, and AST is an enzyme produced in the heart and liver. Both are elevated when liver cancer is present.**
2. Elevated BUN and Cr could indicate kidney involvement.
3. Decreased albumin and calcium could be related to the kidney or to poor nutrition.
4. Elevated WBCs and neutrophils would indicate an acute inflammatory/infectious process.

▶ **Test-taking Tip:** *A cue to remember the liver enzymes is to consider that a common cause of liver failure is alcoholism. Many alcoholics attend AA. Use AA to remember that the liver enzymes that are elevated with liver disorders begin with the letter A.*

**Content Area:** Adult; **Concept:** Cellular Regulation; Bowel Elimination; **Integrated Processes:** Nursing Process: Analysis; **Client Needs:** Physiological Integrity: Reduction of Risk Potential; **Cognitive Level:** Analysis [Analyzing]

## Chapter Twenty-Seven

# Hematological and Oncological Management

**1193.** The nurse is discussing prevention of liver cancer with the client. Which vaccine should the nurse recommend?

1. Varicella vaccine
2. Hepatitis A vaccine
3. Meningococcal vaccine
4. Hepatitis B vaccine

**1194.** MoC The nurse is preparing the client for a bone marrow biopsy of the iliac crest. Place the nurse's actions in order of priority.

1. Premedicate with lorazepam.
2. Obtain a signed informed consent.
3. Position prone and provide emotional support.
4. Verify that the HCP has explained the procedure.
5. Check for signs of bleeding every 2 hours for 24 hours.
6. Teach what may be expected during the procedure.

Answer: _____

**1195.** Laboratory tests are prescribed for the client who has a smooth and reddened tongue and ulcers at the corners of the mouth. Which result would the nurse find if the client has iron-deficiency anemia?

1. Low hemoglobin and hematocrit
2. Elevated red blood cells (RBCs)
3. Prolonged prothrombin time (PT)
4. Elevated white blood cells (WBCs)

**1196.** The nurse is teaching the client who is a strict vegetarian how to decrease the risk of developing megaloblastic anemia. Which information should the nurse provide?

1. Undergo an annual Schilling test.
2. Increase intake of foods high in iron.
3. Supplement the diet with vitamin $B_{12}$.
4. Have a hemoglobin level drawn monthly.

**1197.** The nurse assesses that the client with hemolytic anemia has weakness, fatigue, malaise, and skin and mucous membrane pallor. Which finding should the nurse also associate with hemolytic anemia?

1. Scleral jaundice
2. A smooth, red tongue
3. A craving for ice to chew
4. A poor intake of fresh vegetables

**1198.** MoC The nurse is caring for multiple 25-year-old female clients. The nurse should plan to consult the HCP about a referral for genetic counseling and family planning for which clients? **Select all that apply.**

1. The client diagnosed with thalassemia major
2. The client diagnosed with sickle cell anemia
3. The client diagnosed with hemophilia A
4. The client diagnosed with autoimmune hemolytic anemia
5. The client diagnosed with hemophilia B

**1199.** The client is hospitalized with a diagnosis of sickle cell crisis. Which findings should prompt the nurse to consider that the client is ready for discharge? **Select all that apply.**

1. Leukocyte count is at 7500/mm$^3$
2. Describes the importance of keeping warm
3. Pain controlled at 2 on a 0 to 10 scale with analgesics
4. Has not had chest pain or dyspnea for past 24 hours
5. Blood transfusions effective in diminishing cell sickling
6. Hydroxyurea effective in suppressing leukocyte formation

**1200.** The client with COPD has developed polycythemia vera, and the nurse completes teaching on measures to prevent complications. During a home visit, the nurse evaluates that the client is correctly following the teaching when which actions are noted? **Select all that apply.**

1. Tells the nurse about discontinuing iron supplements
2. States increasing alcohol intake to decrease blood viscosity
3. Presents a record that shows a daily fluid intake of 3000 mL
4. Discusses yesterday's phlebotomy treatment to remove blood
5. Shows the nurse a menu plan for eating three large meals daily
6. Wears antiembolic stockings and sits in a recliner with legs uncrossed

**1201.** MoC The nurse assesses the client diagnosed with acute myeloid leukemia. Which finding should be the nurse's **priority** for implementing interventions?

1. Pain from mucositis and oral tissue injury
2. Weakness and fatigue with slight activity
3. T 99°F (37.2°C), P 100, R 22, BP 132/64
4. Ecchymosis and petechiae noted on arms

**1202.** MoC The new nurse requests information about chronic lymphocytic leukemia (CLL). Which statements should an experienced nurse include? **Select all that apply.**

1. CLL is a malignancy of activated B lymphocytes.
2. CLL is the most common malignancy of older adults.
3. CLL is unresponsive to chemotherapy treatment.
4. Clients are monitored in its early stages and often not treated.
5. In CLL immature lymphocytes accumulate in the bone marrow.
6. Clients with CLL often have no symptoms of the disorder.

**1203.** PHARM MoC The nurse receives orders after notifying an HCP about the client who has tachycardia, diaphoresis, and an elevated temperature after treatments for ALL. Which order should be the nurse's **priority?**

1. Portable chest x-ray in the client's room
2. Urine culture, and blood cultures × 2
3. Vancomycin 500 mg IV q6h
4. Filgrastim 0.3 mg subcut daily

**1204.** The nurse is analyzing the serum laboratory report illustrated for the client with acute myeloid leukemia (AML). Based on the findings of the serum laboratory report, which nursing action is **most** appropriate?

| Serum Laboratory Test | Client's Value | Normal Values (Conventional Units) |
| --- | --- | --- |
| WBC ($\times 10^3$) | 15 | $4.5–11.1 \times 10^3$/microL |
| Neutrophils | 40% | 40%–43% |
| Lymphocytes | 47% | 16%–49% |
| Monocytes | 11% | 2%–13% |
| EOS | 2% | 0%–2% |
| Basophils | 0% | 0%–2% |
| RBC ($\times 10^6$) | 2.1 | Male: $5.21–5.81 \times 10^6$ cells/microL<br>Female: $3.91–5.11 \times 10^6$ cells/microL |
| Hgb | 9.5 | Male: 13.5–17.3 g/dL<br>Female: 11.7–15.5 g/dL |
| Hct | 30.5% | Male: 38–51%<br>Female: 33%–45% |
| Platelets ($\times 10^3$) | 98 | $150–450 \times 10^3$/mcL |

1. Instruct on eating high-iron foods.
2. Assess for an allergic reaction.
3. Place on neutropenic precautions.
4. Teach to use an electric razor for shaving.

**1205.** The client with multiple myeloma has a total serum calcium level of 13.2 mEq/L. Which interventions, if prescribed, should the nurse plan to implement? **Select all that apply.**

1. Encourage fluid intake.
2. Maintain strict bedrest.
3. Administer furosemide IV.
4. Give allopurinol by mouth.
5. Offer foods high in calcium.

**1206.** MoC Following morning shift report, the nurse identifies care needs for four clients. Which client should be the nurse's **priority?**

1. The client with lung cancer who is to receive ondansetron 8 mg IV 30 minutes prior to chemotherapy
2. The client with an absolute neutrophil count of 98/mm$^3$ who needs to be placed on neutropenic precautions
3. The client who is stable but has breast cancer and is scheduled for external beam radiation in 15 minutes
4. The client with stomatitis from radiation for tonsillar cancer who is to receive a gastrostomy tube feeding

**1207.** The client's lymph node biopsy revealed Hodgkin's lymphoma. When teaching the client, the nurse should obtain the educational brochure that explains which information?

1. Elevated reticulocyte counts
2. CA-125 tumor markers
3. Elevated WBC counts
4. Reed-Sternberg cells

**1208.** PHARM The client undergoing intensive chemotherapy for Hodgkin's lymphoma is hospitalized with fever and a depressed immune system. The nurse is administering filgrastim subcutaneously daily. Which laboratory value should the nurse monitor to determine the medication's effectiveness?

1. Hemoglobin
2. Platelet count
3. Absolute neutrophil count (ANC)
4. Reed-Sternberg cells

**1209.** The nurse is teaching the client hospitalized with ITP. What information should the nurse plan to include? **Select all that apply.**

1. "Use dental floss after brushing your teeth."
2. "Use only an electric razor when shaving."
3. "Remove throw rugs and avoid clutter."
4. "Increase dietary fiber and drink lots of liquids."
5. "Schedule monthly platelet transfusions."

**1210.** The nurse is planning to check the lymph nodes for the client with possible Hodgkin's lymphoma. On the illustration shown, which area should the nurse first examine if starting at the location where the disease usually originates?

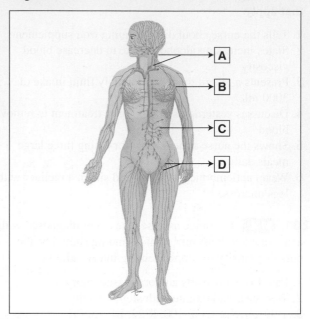

1. A
2. B
3. C
4. D

**1211.** PHARM The nurse teaches a coworker about the treatment for hemophilia. The nurse instructs that the treatment will likely include periodic self-administration of which component?

1. Platelets
2. Whole blood
3. Factor concentrates
4. Fresh frozen plasma

**1212.** The client diagnosed with von Willebrand's disease calls a clinic after experiencing hemarthrosis. The client states that factor concentrate is infusing. Which intervention should the nurse recommend **now**?

1. "Take two 325-mg aspirin tablets every 4 hours for pain."
2. "Apply a cold pack to the area for 30 minutes every 1 to 2 hours."
3. "Come to the clinic; you need an infusion of fresh frozen plasma."
4. "If wearing a splint, remove it to avoid compartment syndrome."

**1213.** **PHARM** The client has a blood type of B negative. The client's family asks if they can donate blood for the client. The nurse informs the family that they would need to be of which blood type to be considered for a directed donation of RBCs for this client? **Select all that apply.**

1. Type A positive
2. Type B positive
3. Type B negative
4. Type O positive
5. Type O negative
6. Type AB positive

**1214.** The nurse is caring for the client placed on neutropenic precautions. Which interventions should the nurse implement? **Select all that apply.**

1. Apply pressure for at least 5 minutes to any site that is bleeding.
2. Prevent anyone from bringing fresh flowers into the client's room.
3. Teach the client to avoid eating unwashed fruits and vegetables.
4. Perform hand hygiene before touching any of the client's belongings.
5. Inform the client that fresh water will be delivered every 2 hours.
6. Stop visitors from entering the room if observed to be coughing.

**1215.** **PHARM** The client is symptomatic with a Hgb of 7.8 g/dL, but refuses blood and blood products transfusions for religious reasons. The nurse should prepare the client that the HCP may prescribe which alternatives? **Select all that apply.**

1. Epoetin alfa
2. Folic acid
3. Albumin
4. Platelets
5. Fresh frozen plasma
6. Granulocytes

**1216.** **PHARM** The client who received 50 mL from a unit of whole blood has new onset low back pain. What should the nurse do **first?**

1. Reposition the client.
2. Assess the pain further.
3. Administer an analgesic.
4. Stop the blood transfusion.

**1217.** **PHARM** At 1000 hours, the nurse is documenting the administration of 275 mL of compatible platelets, unit number XR123. Which information should the nurse document? **Select all that apply.**

1. One unit blood was administered over 4 hours
2. Platelet XR123 double-checked before infusion
3. No transfusion reactions noted during infusion
4. $D_5W$ infused with platelets to prevent clumping
5. Infused 275 mL of platelets started at 0830

**1218.** **PHARM** The client diagnosed with acute myeloid leukemia receives a bone marrow transplant. Which medication to prevent graft-versus-host disease (GVHD) should the nurse plan to administer?

1. A cephalosporin antibiotic, such as ceftazidime
2. An immunosuppressant, such as cyclosporine
3. A chemotherapeutic agent, such as cisplatin
4. Peginterferon alfa-2a for prevention and treatment of hepatitis

**1219.** The nurse completed teaching the client who had a bone marrow transplant (BMT). Which statement by the client indicates the client **misunderstood** the expected changes following a BMT?

1. "I may gain weight from my immunosuppressant medication."
2. "Sterility can occur from the chemotherapy and radiation."
3. "I may have vision changes from the total body irradiation."
4. "Changes to my mouth could include a white, patchy tongue."

**1220.** The nurse is caring for the client experiencing superior vena cava syndrome secondary to lung cancer. Which problem should be the nurse's **priority?**

1. Ineffective breathing pattern
2. Ineffective tissue perfusion
3. Risk for infection
4. Impaired skin integrity

**1221.** The nurse explains "watchful waiting" (ongoing visits to a HCP for observation of signs and symptoms without treatment) to the client with prostate cancer. Which client is a candidate for "watchful waiting"?

1. The 50-year-old with prostate cancer that has metastasized to the bone
2. The 75-year-old who is expected to live 5 years and has low-grade disease
3. The 45-year-old who has extension of the tumor outside of the prostate
4. The 59-year-old who is asymptomatic with an elevated prostate-specific antigen

**1222.** **PHARM** The nurse is preparing to administer cisplatin IV to the client with ovarian cancer. The dose is 100 mg/m² in 2 liters of $D_5W$ given over 8 hours. What is the rate in milliliters (mL) per hour that the nurse should set the infusion pump?

_____ mL/hr (Record your answer as a whole number.)

**1223.** The nurse is teaching the client about breast self-examination and discusses where breast cancer commonly occurs. Place an X on the area that the nurse should identify as the most frequent location for breast cancer occurrence.

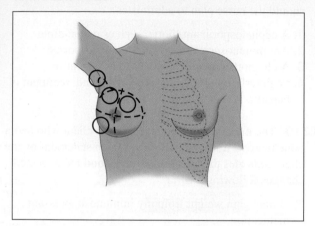

**1224.** The nurse is caring for the client who had a left modified radical mastectomy (a total mastectomy with axillary node dissection and removal of the lining over the pectoralis major muscle). Which action by the nurse is appropriate?

1. Have the client elevate the left arm above the head.
2. Ensure that IV access sites are only on the right side.
3. Have the client view the incision site as soon as possible.
4. Initiate left arm strengthening within 24 hours of surgery.

**1225.** **MoC** The client, who underwent a right mastectomy with lymph node dissection, is being admitted to a nursing unit from the PACU. When settling the client in bed, which action by the NA requires the nurse to intervene?

1. Placing a BP cuff on the left arm for vital signs
2. Taping a sign to the side rail stating no IVs or lab draws on the right
3. Elevating the bed to 90 degrees and keeping the right arm dependent
4. Asking if the client feels ready to allow family to enter the room

**1226.** The nurse is planning care for the client who is to receive an internal radiation implant later in the day. In preparing the client's room, which sign should the nurse plan to post outside the client's room?

1.
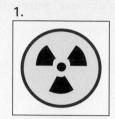

2.

3.
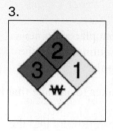

4.

**1227.** The nurse discusses the self-care guidelines to minimize the side effects of radiation on the skin. Which actions to reduce radiation skin reactions should the nurse explain to the client? **Select all that apply.**

1. Wear loose-fitting, soft clothing over the treated skin.
2. Use a straight-edged razor to shave hair in the treated area.
3. Swim only in swimming pools to avoid stagnant water.
4. Use only skin-care products suggested by the radiation staff.
5. Apply skin products immediately after radiation treatment.
6. Wash treated area gently with lukewarm water and mild soap.

**1228.** The nurse is discussing the prevention of bladder cancer with the client. Which factors that increase the client's risk for bladder cancer should the nurse emphasize? **Select all that apply.**

1. Consuming caffeine beverages
2. Smoking tobacco products
3. Consuming multivitamins daily
4. Prolonged exposure to paint smells
5. Prolonged exposure to rubber smells

**1229.** The client with Hodgkin's lymphoma receives radiation. The nurse should monitor the client for which specific symptoms of radiation pneumonitis?

1. Tachypnea, hypotension, and fever
2. Cough, elevated temperature, and dyspnea
3. Bradypnea, cough, and decreased urine output
4. Cough, tachycardia, and altered mental status

**1230.** PHARM The nurse is administering vesicant chemotherapy medications such as doxorubicin hydrochloride to clients. Which nursing actions should the nurse implement to prevent extravasation? **Select all that apply.**

1. Give through an IV catheter in a large peripheral vein if infusing in less than 60 minutes.
2. Check patency every 5 to 10 minutes during infusion and ask about IV site discomfort.
3. Check the IV pump and alarm for indications of an infiltration of the medication.
4. Check for blood return in a central venous catheter prior to administration of the vesicant.
5. Use small-gauged syringes with small barrels when flushing any access devices with saline.

**1231.** PHARM The nurse is caring for the client receiving combination chemotherapy of oxaliplatin, fluorouracil, and leucovorin. The nurse should assess the client for which common side effects of this chemotherapy regimen?

1. Neurotoxicity and diarrhea
2. Cardiomyopathy and dysphagia
3. Renal insufficiency and gastritis
4. Photophobia and stomatitis

**1232.** PHARM The client who has renal cancer that has metastasized rates pain at a 9 on a 0 to 10 pain scale. Which medication should the nurse plan to administer now and then schedule to be administered at the prescribed dosing interval?

1. Meperidine
2. Propoxyphene
3. Pentazocine
4. Oxycodone

**1233.** MoC PHARM The nurse is preparing epoetin alfa for the client who has chemotherapy-associated anemia. The nurse recognizes the need to consult with the HCP before administration when the client makes which statements? **Select all that apply.**

1. "I spend most of my days lying on the couch."
2. "I usually eat a lot of salads for my main meals."
3. "I seem to have an aversion to eating eggs right now."
4. "I developed a blood clot in my leg on my last admission."
5. "I hope this helps so I don't have to have a blood transfusion."

**1234.** The nurse is collecting data from the client undergoing testing for possible basal cell carcinoma (BCC). Which information in the client's health history should the nurse identify as risk factors for BCC? **Select all that apply.**

1. Taking immune-suppressing medications
2. 10-pack-year history of cigarette smoking
3. Has fair skin color, red hair, and blue eyes
4. Had home exposure to high radon gas levels
5. Works as a laborer in road construction

**1235.** The client asks the nurse to look at a lesion on the client's body. Which characteristics should prompt the nurse to consider that the client may have a basal cell carcinoma (BCC)?

1. Nodular in appearance, depression in the center, and has a "pearly" characteristic
2. Irregular color, surface, and border, less than one centimeter, and appears eroded
3. Dry, hyperkeratotic scaly-like papule and has the appearance similar to a wart
4. Vesiculopustular lesion with a thick, honey-colored crust and pruritic in nature

**1236.** The client had basal cell carcinoma lesions excised 24 hours ago at an outpatient clinic. The client telephones concerned that the wounds are draining watery, pale pink fluid and that the small dressing is leaking. What should the nurse recommend?

1. Apply ice to the area.
2. Contact the surgeon.
3. Take pain medication.
4. Change the dressings.

**1237.** MoC When reviewing the client's medical record, the experienced nurse discovers that the client's breast cancer is staged as T4 N3 M1. Which comment made by the experienced nurse to the new nurse is correct?

1. "This client has a 3-cm breast tumor that has spread to only one lymph node."
2. "The TNM system is used to classify solid tumors by size and degree of spread."
3. "The higher the number in the TNM system, the better the chances are for a cure."
4. "This TNM system helps to classify tumors as either well- or poorly differentiated."

**1238.** The nurse is teaching the client who is to undergo diagnostic testing for possible gastric cancer. Teaching the client about which specific diagnostic test would be **most** helpful?

1. Bronchoscopy
2. Sigmoid colonoscopy
3. Esophagogastroduodenoscopy
4. Multigated acquisition (MUGA) scan

**1239.** The recently admitted client with gastric cancer is pale and states feeling fatigued. In reviewing the client's CBC results, which component should the nurse **most** associate with the client's gastric cancer and the reason for the fatigue?

1. White blood cell 12,200/mm³
2. Hemoglobin 7.9 g/dL
3. Serum protein 5.9 g/dL
4. Blood urea nitrogen 22 mg/dL

**1240.** The client is admitted with a diagnosis of colon cancer. The nurse considers that the client's cancer may be in the descending colon when collecting which information?

1. Pain in the lower abdomen
2. Change in bowel habits
3. Bright red blood in the stool
4. Nausea and vomiting

**1241.** MoC The client diagnosed with esophageal cancer is having work-related problems that are interfering with the client's treatment. Which organization should the nurse advise the client to contact for assistance with these issues?

1. National Cancer Institute
2. Leukemia Society of America
3. Corporate Angel Network
4. Patient Advocate Foundation

**1242.** MoC The nurse is caring for the client following a total laryngectomy for treatment of laryngeal cancer. The nurse should plan consultations with which members of the multidisciplinary team? **Select all that apply.**

1. Physical therapist
2. Dietitian
3. Speech therapist
4. Dentist
5. Occupational therapist
6. Social worker

**1243.** MoC In which order should the nurse address the assessment findings for the client who has undergone a total laryngectomy? Place the findings in the order of priority.

1. Copious oral secretions and nasal mucus draining from the nose
2. Restless and has a mucus plug in the tracheostomy
3. NG tube used for intermittent feedings pulled halfway out
4. Oozing serosanguineous drainage around the tracheostomy tube and dressing saturated

Answer: _____

**1244.** MoC PHARM A home-care nurse is following up with the client who was diagnosed with liver cancer 3 months ago. Which assessment information should the nurse communicate immediately to the HCP?

1. Weak and pale; remained in bed during the visit.
2. Weight is unchanged since the previous visit.
3. Itching is less with diphenhydramine cream use
4. Pain level averages a 7 on a 0 to 10 scale with scheduled opioids.

**1245.** The client hospitalized with cervical cancer is receiving radiation therapy via a temporary radioactive cervical implant. Which nursing actions would be appropriate for this client? **Select all that apply.**

1. Minimize anxiety and confusion by telling the client the reason for the time and distance limitations.
2. Utilize the unit's common film badge that indicates the cumulative radiation exposure while caring for the client.
3. Organize cares to limit the amount of time spent in direct contact with the client receiving internal radiation.
4. Use shielding if delivering care within close proximity to the client, such as checking placement of the implant.
5. Encourage frequent oral care with warm saline rinses to help with irritation of oral mucosa.

**1246.** The nurse is assessing the client newly diagnosed with endometrial cancer. Which common findings would the nurse expect?

1. Abnormal vaginal bleeding and pain in the pelvic area
2. Weight loss and profuse sweating, especially at night
3. Anorexia and enlarged supraclavicular lymph nodes
4. Unexplained spikes in temperature and splenomegaly

**1247.** The nurse assesses that the client who is receiving radiation for cervical cancer continues to have diarrhea. Which nursing advice is **most** appropriate?

1. Eat a low-residue diet and take sitz baths twice daily.
2. Drink fluids low in potassium and take frequent tub baths.
3. Consume more milk products and take frequent showers.
4. Drink high-sodium fluids and apply hydrocolloid pads to rectum.

**1248.** When assessing the client who is recovering from a radical hysterectomy with vulvectomy, the nurse notes lymphedema of the lower extremities. Which interventions should the nurse implement? **Select all that apply.**

1. Elevate the head of the bed to 45 degrees.
2. Offer more fluids high in sodium.
3. Instruct on exercising the lower extremities.
4. Apply splints to both lower extremities.
5. Consult the HCP about compression stockings.

**1249.** PHARM The client is experiencing pain due to cancer treatment. The client tells the nurse, "Methadone has always worked well for me in the past." Which effects of methadone should the nurse consider when administering methadone?

1. Has a long half-life and high level of potency
2. May cause an increase in BP and confusion
3. Causes severe allergic reactions and liver failure
4. Has active metabolites, but it is well tolerated

**1250.** The nurse is totaling the 8-hour fluid intake for the client with cancer who has hypercalcemia. The client's intake includes: 1 L pitcher of water, bowl of oatmeal, 8-oz cup of decaffeinated coffee for breakfast and lunch, 90 mL apple juice, 120 mL ice cream, 180 mL chicken broth, mashed potatoes, few bites of chicken, bowl of carrots, 240 mL milk, and 90 mL gelatin. How many milliliters should the nurse record for the client's 8-hour fluid intake?

_____ mL (Record your answer as a whole number.)

**1251.** PHARM The client on hospice care has cancer pain and requires coanalgesics in addition to the prescribed opioids. Which medication should the nurse ask the HCP to prescribe?

1. Promethazine
2. Gabapentin
3. Diphenhydramine
4. Droperidol

**1252.** MoC The client has acute myeloid leukemia (AML). Which **most** important assessment finding warrants the nurse's immediate notification of the HCP?

1. Temperature 101.2°F (38.4°C)
2. Platelet count 9500/mm$^3$
3. Neutrophils count 2250/mm$^3$
4. Bone pain rated at 9 on a 0 to 10 scale

# Answers and Rationales

**1193. ANSWER: 4**

1. The varicella vaccine is a live (attenuated) virus administered to protect against chicken pox. There is no evidence that it has an effect on preventing liver cancer.
2. Hepatitis A vaccine is given to protect against hepatitis A virus (HAV). HAV can be spread by stool, blood, or food and water that is infected with HAV. There is no evidence that it has an effect on preventing liver cancer.
3. Meningococcal vaccine is used to prevent meningitis caused by *Neisseria meningitides*. There is no evidence that it has an effect on preventing liver cancer.
4. **Hepatitis B vaccine dramatically reduces the incidence of hepatitis B virus (HBV) and, in turn, prevents liver cancer. HBV is transmitted through contact with blood or body fluids of an infected person, and it can survive outside the body for at least 7 days.**

♦ **Test-taking Tip:** Narrow the options to those associated with the liver. Of the remaining options, consider which virus is most prevalent.

Content Area: Adult; Concept: Promoting Health; Cellular Regulation; Integrated Processes: Teaching/Learning; Client Needs: Health Promotion and Maintenance; Cognitive Level: Comprehension [Understanding]

**1194.** MoC **ANSWER: 4, 6, 2, 1, 3, 5**

4. **Verify that the HCP has explained the procedure. The HCP should include the purpose, intended outcomes, and potential complications.**
6. **Teach what may be expected during the procedure, including that pressure or discomfort may be experienced.**
2. **Obtain a signed informed consent. This is obtained only after the HCP has met with the client and teaching is completed.**

1. **Premedicate with lorazepam (Ativan). Midazolam (Versed) is another option for sedation. A local anesthetic is used at the site, and some clients may not need sedation.**
3. **Position prone and provide emotional support. The client should be prone because the iliac crest is the site being used for this biopsy, but the position will vary with the site. Holding the client's hand and using guided imagery help support the client.**
5. **Check for signs of bleeding every 2 hours for 24 hours. A pressure dressing is applied by the HCP after the procedure. Ice can be applied to reduce bruising and for comfort.**

▶ *Test-taking Tip: Visualize how to prepare and monitor the client for a bone marrow biopsy before prioritizing the nurse's actions. Often selecting the first and last actions helps to place the other actions in the correct sequence more quickly.*

**Content Area:** Adult; **Concept:** Nursing Roles; Cellular Regulation; Management; **Integrated Processes:** Nursing Process: Implementation; **Client Needs:** Physiological Integrity: Reduction of Risk Potential; Safe and Effective Care Environment: Management of Care; **Cognitive Level:** Synthesis [Creating]

## 1195. ANSWER: 1

1. **A smooth, red tongue, ulcers at the corners of the mouth (angular cheilosis), and a low Hgb are signs of iron-deficiency anemia.**
2. Excess RBCs are associated with polycythemia vera.
3. Prolonged PT is seen with clients taking anticoagulants or experiencing a coagulation disorder.
4. Elevated WBCs are not associated with iron-deficiency anemia but with an infection. Ulcers, if infected, would elevate the WBCs.

▶ *Test-taking Tip: Think about the conditions that would produce the altered lab values in each option before answering the question.*

**Content Area:** Adult; **Concept:** Hematologic Regulation; **Integrated Processes:** Nursing Process: Analysis; **Client Needs:** Physiological Integrity: Reduction of Risk Potential; **Cognitive Level:** Analysis [Analyzing]

## 1196. ANSWER: 3

1. The Schilling test is used to diagnose vitamin $B_{12}$ deficiency; it is not necessary to have this completed annually.
2. Consuming foods high in iron will prevent iron-deficiency, not megaloblastic, anemia.
3. **The client consuming a vegetarian diet can prevent megaloblastic anemia from a vitamin $B_{12}$ deficiency with oral vitamin supplements or fortified soy milk.**
4. Monthly lab work is unnecessary and costly.

▶ *Test-taking Tip: Differentiate between iron-deficiency and megaloblastic anemia to select the answer. Megaloblastic anemia is caused by deficiency of vitamin $B_{12}$ or folic acid.*

**Content Area:** Adult; **Concept:** Nutrition; Hematologic Regulation; **Integrated Processes:** Teaching/Learning; **Client Needs:** Physiological Integrity: Basic Care and Comfort; **Cognitive Level:** Application [Applying]

## 1197. ANSWER: 1

1. **Jaundice occurs in hemolytic anemia from the shortened life span of the RBC and the breakdown of Hgb. About 80% of heme is converted to bilirubin, conjugated in the liver, and excreted in the bile. The increased bilirubin in the blood causes the jaundice.**
2. A smooth, red tongue is seen with iron-deficiency anemia.
3. A craving for ice is seen with iron-deficiency anemia.
4. Folate deficiency occurs in people who rarely eat fresh vegetables.

▶ *Test-taking Tip: Use knowledge of medical terminology, recalling that "-lytic" is "destruction of" and "heme-" pertains to the blood.*

**Content Area:** Adult; **Concept:** Assessment; Hematologic Regulation; **Integrated Processes:** Nursing Process: Assessment; **Client Needs:** Physiological Integrity: Reduction of Risk Potential; **Cognitive Level:** Comprehension [Understanding]

## 1198. MoC ANSWER: 1, 2, 3, 5

1. **Thalassemia is a hereditary disorder; the client could benefit from a referral for genetic counseling.**
2. **Sickle cell anemia is a hereditary disorder; the client could benefit from a referral for genetic counseling.**
3. **Hemophilia A is a hereditary disorder; the client could benefit from a referral for genetic counseling.**
4. Autoimmune hemolytic anemia is an acquired hemolytic anemia.
5. **Hemophilia B is a hereditary disorder; the client could benefit from a referral for genetic counseling.**

▶ *Test-taking Tip: The key words are "genetic counseling." Select only hereditary disorders.*

**Content Area:** Adult; **Concept:** Female Reproduction; Hematologic Regulation; Management; **Integrated Processes:** Nursing Process: Planning; **Client Needs:** Safe and Effective Care Environment: Management of Care; **Cognitive Level:** Application [Applying]

## 1199. ANSWER: 1, 2, 3, 4

1. **A leukocyte count of 7500/mm³ is within normal range (5000 to 10,000/mm³ indicates the absence of an infection).**
2. **Keeping warm and avoiding chills will help to prevent infection. Cold causes vasoconstriction, slowing blood flow and aggravating the sickling process.**
3. **Acute pain is due to tissue hypoxia from the agglutination of sickled cells within blood vessels. Pain controlled at 2 indicates readiness for discharge.**
4. **The absence of symptoms of complication such as acute chest syndrome and pulmonary hypertension indicates readiness for discharge.**
5. RBC transfusions may help to prevent complications, but transfusions do not alter the person's body from producing the deformed erythrocytes.

6. Hydroxyurea (Hydrea) can decrease the permanent formation of sickled cells. A side effect (not therapeutic effect) of hydroxyurea is suppression of leukocyte formation.

▸ *Test-takingTip: The key phrase is "ready for discharge." Select the options with normal findings. Be sure to read options for incorrect information.*

**Content Area:** Adult; **Concept:** Hematologic Regulation; **Integrated Processes:** Nursing Process: Evaluation; **Client Needs:** Physiological Integrity: Physiological Adaptation; **Cognitive Level:** Evaluation [Evaluating]

## 1200. ANSWER: 1, 3, 4, 6

1. **Iron supplements, including those in multivitamins, should be avoided because the iron stimulates RBC production.**
2. Alcohol increases the risk of bleeding.
3. **Increasing fluid intake to 3000 mL daily will help decrease blood viscosity.**
4. **Phlebotomy is performed on a routine or intermittent basis to diminish blood viscosity, deplete iron stores, and decrease the client's ability to manufacture excess erythrocytes.**
5. Frequent, small meals are better tolerated, especially if the liver is involved.
6. **Elevating the legs, avoiding constriction or crossing the legs, and wearing antiembolic stockings help prevent DVT.**

▸ *Test-takingTip: RBC production and blood viscosity are increased in polycythemia vera. Select options that decrease the number of RBCs, decrease blood viscosity, and prevent DVTs.*

**Content Area:** Adult; **Concept:** Hematologic Regulation; **Integrated Processes:** Teaching/Learning; **Client Needs:** Health Promotion and Maintenance; Physiological Integrity: Basic Care and Comfort; **Cognitive Level:** Analysis [Analyzing]

## 1201. MoC ANSWER: 1

1. **Pain control is priority. The altered VS (other than temperature) could be related to pain.**
2. Weakness and fatigue are due to anemia and also the disease process. It is important to allow rest, but if pain is not controlled the client may not be able to rest.
3. The temperature warrants further monitoring because it could indicate a developing infection; the other VS may decrease if pain is controlled.
4. Ecchymosis and petechiae are associated with low platelets counts. The nurse should check the laboratory report for the platelet level, but this is an assessment and not an intervention.

▸ *Test-takingTip: Use the ABC's to determine priority. In the absence of life-threatening findings, pain control should be priority.*

**Content Area:** Adult; **Concept:** Comfort; Hematologic Regulation; **Integrated Processes:** Nursing Process: Implementation; **Client Needs:** Safe and Effective Care Environment: Management of Care; Physiological Integrity: Physiological Adaptation; **Cognitive Level:** Analysis [Analyzing]

## 1202. MoC ANSWER: 1, 2, 4, 6

1. **CLL derives from a malignant clone of B lymphocytes. T-lymphocytic CLL is rare.**
2. **Two-thirds of all persons with CLL are older than 60 years at diagnosis.**
3. Treatment for CLL includes chemotherapy with fludarabine (Fludara), but a major side effect is prolonged bone marrow suppression.
4. **Clients with CLL are monitored, and treatment is initiated when symptoms are severe (night sweats, painful lymphadenopathy) or the disease progresses to later stages.**
5. In CLL there is an accumulation of mature-appearing but functionally inactive lymphocytes, and not immature lymphocytes. Excessive accumulation of immature lymphocytes occurs in ALL.
6. **Because many persons are asymptomatic, it is often diagnosed during a routine physical or during treatment for another condition.**

▸ *Test-takingTip: ALL frequently occurs in children, whereas CLL frequently occurs in adults. A mnemonic for differentiating CLL from ALL can be used to select the answers: "**B**e **o**lder and **m**ature" (B = B lymphocytes; o = older adult; a = asymptomatic; m = mature but inactive lymphocytes).*

**Content Area:** Adult; **Concept:** Cellular Regulation; Hematologic Regulation; Nursing Roles; **Integrated Processes:** Teaching/Learning; **Client Needs:** Safe and Effective Care Environment: Management of Care; Physiological Integrity: Physiological Adaptation; **Cognitive Level:** Knowledge [Remembering]

## 1203. MoC PHARM ANSWER: 2

1. The results of the portable CXR will help determine if the cause is a respiratory infection. It will not change the treatment.
2. **Urine and blood cultures are priority; these should be obtained before antibiotics are administered.**
3. National recommendations are to administer broad-spectrum antibiotics such as vancomycin (Vancocin) within 1 hour of a suspected infection diagnosis. The antibiotics may be changed after culture and sensitivity reports are available (usually 24 to 48 hours).
4. It takes 4 days for filgrastim (Neupogen) to return the neutrophil count to baseline, so this is not priority. Filgrastim should not be given within 24 hours of cytotoxic chemotherapy.

▸ *Test-takingTip: Consider the effects of administering an antibiotic if another intervention does not occur first.*

**Content Area:** Adult; **Concept:** Critical Thinking; Hematologic Regulation; Medication; Management; **Integrated Processes:** Nursing Process: Implementation; **Client Needs:** Safe and Effective Care Environment: Management of Care; Physiological Integrity: Pharmacological and Parenteral Therapies; **Cognitive Level:** Analysis [Analyzing]

## 1204. ANSWER: 4

1. Although the Hgb is low, the anemia that occurs in AML is unrelated to iron-deficiency anemia, so foods high in iron will not treat the anemia.

2. The eosinophils (EOS) are in the normal range, so the client is not experiencing an allergic reaction.

3. The neutrophils are within the normal range, so it is unnecessary to place the client on neutropenic precautions.

4. **The client is at risk for bleeding due to thrombocytopenia (platelet count less than 100,000/mm³). Other bleeding precautions include a soft toothbrush; avoiding dental flossing, rectal temperatures, suppositories, and enemas; using stool softeners; and holding pressure to venipuncture sites for 5 minutes.**

♦ *Test-takingTip: First focus on the laboratory values that are abnormal. Eliminate Options 2 and 3 because the laboratory values associated with these actions are normal. If unsure between Options 1 and 4, note that the laboratory value associated with the intervention in Option 4 is very abnormal.*

**Content Area:** Adult; **Concept:** Perfusion; Hematologic Regulation; **Integrated Processes:** Nursing Process: Implementation; **Client Needs:** Physiological Integrity: Reduction of Risk Potential; Physiological Integrity: Physiological Adaptation; **Cognitive Level:** Analysis [Analyzing]

### 1205. ANSWER: 1, 3

1. **Adequate hydration dilutes calcium and prevents precipitates from causing renal tubular obstruction.**

2. The client with multiple myeloma is encouraged to ambulate because weight-bearing activities can help the bone resorb some calcium as well as prevent thrombosis that can accompany immobility.

3. **Furosemide (Lasix) given IV can promote the excretion of calcium when hypercalcemia exists due to multiple myeloma.**

4. Allopurinol (Zyloprim) may be administered to reduce the hyperuricemia that can accompany multiple myeloma, not the hypercalcemia.

5. The serum calcium level is elevated (normal is 9–10.5 mg/dL). Foods high in calcium would not be offered. However, limiting the intake of foods high in calcium will not make any difference to the elevated calcium level that is caused by cancer.

♦ *Test-takingTip: Focus on treatment for hypercalcemia.*

**Content Area:** Adult; **Concept:** Fluid and Electrolyte Balance; Cellular Regulation; **Integrated Processes:** Nursing Process: Implementation; **Client Needs:** Safe and Effective Care Environment: Safety and Infection Control; **Cognitive Level:** Application [Applying]

### 1206. MoC ANSWER: 2

1. No time is noted for the administration of ondansetron (Zofran) prior to chemotherapy treatment; this client is not the nurse's priority.

2. **The client with neutropenia should be the nurse's priority. If seen first, microorganisms from other clients would be less likely to be transmitted to the client. This client is at risk for infection and severe sepsis because the absolute neutrophil count is less than 100/mm³ (normal = 1500 to 8000/mm³).**

3. This client is stable; another person can take this client to radiation therapy, and the nurse's assessment can wait until the client returns.

4. The tube feeding can be initiated after the needs of the most critical client are met.

♦ *Test-takingTip: The most critical client should be the nurse's priority.*

**Content Area:** Adult; **Concept:** Critical Thinking; Cellular Regulation; Management; **Integrated Processes:** Nursing Process: Assessment; Caring; **Client Needs:** Safe and Effective Care Environment: Management of Care; Safe and Effective Care Environment: Safety and Infection Control; **Cognitive Level:** Analysis [Analyzing]

### 1207. ANSWER: 4

1. Reticulocytes are found in a CBC, not from a lymph node biopsy, and are not indicative of either Hodgkin's or non-Hodgkin's lymphoma.

2. CA-125 tumor markers are sometimes used in the management of ovarian cancer.

3. WBCs are collected from a complete blood panel, not a lymph node biopsy, and could be indicative of other lymphomas and/or leukemia.

4. **The nurse should obtain the brochure that explains about Reed-Sternberg cells. The main diagnostic feature of Hodgkin's lymphoma is the presence of Reed-Sternberg cells in a lymph node biopsy.**

♦ *Test-takingTip: Think about the cell types that can be collected from a lymph node biopsy versus a serum laboratory report. If uncertain, narrow the options by eliminating those that are common cell types in a CBC. Of the two remaining options, determine which can be obtained from a lymph node biopsy.*

**Content Area:** Adult; **Concept:** Cellular Regulation; **Integrated Processes:** Nursing Process: Analysis; **Client Needs:** Physiological Integrity: Physiological Adaptation; **Cognitive Level:** Analysis [Analyzing]

### 1208. PHARM ANSWER: 3

1. Epoetin alfa, not filgrastim, is used to treat anemia that is associated with cancer, and its effectiveness would be reflected in the Hgb values.

2. Oprelvekin (Neumega), not filgrastim, enhances the synthesis of platelets.

3. **The nurse should monitor the ANC. Filgrastim (Neupogen) is usually discontinued when the client's absolute neutrophil count (ANC) is above 1000 cells/mm³. Filgrastim, a granulocyte colony-stimulating factor (G-CSF) analog, is used to stimulate the proliferation and differentiation of granulocytes and treat neutropenia.**

4. Reed-Sternberg cells are found in lymph node biopsy cells and are indicative of Hodgkin's lymphoma; they are not monitored to determine the effectiveness of filgrastim, which is used to treat neutropenia.

♦ *Test-takingTip: The focus of the question is expected effects of filgrastim (Neupogen). If uncertain, use the trade name of Neupogen as a clue to the laboratory value to monitor.*

Content Area: Adult; Concept: Cellular Regulation; Medication; Integrated Processes: Nursing Process: Evaluation; Client Needs: Physiological Integrity: Pharmacological and Parenteral Therapies; Cognitive Level: Evaluation [Evaluating]

### 1209. ANSWER: 2, 3, 4

1. Dental floss can traumatize the gums and increase the risk for bleeding.
2. **Because the client is at risk for bleeding due to low platelets counts, measures to decrease the risk of bleeding should be implemented, such as using an electric razor.**
3. **Throw rugs and clutter increase the risk for falls with subsequent bleeding.**
4. **Fiber and fluids help prevent constipation. Constipation can lead to hemorrhoids and increase the risk for bleeding.**
5. Platelet transfusions are usually avoided because the person's antiplatelet antibodies bind with the transfused platelets, causing them to be destroyed.

▶ *Test-takingTip: If unsure of ITP, recall that purpura is caused from bleeding into the tissues. Select the options that would prevent bleeding.*

Content Area: Adult; Concept: Hematologic Regulation; Integrated Processes: Nursing Process: Planning; Client Needs: Safe and Effective Care Environment: Safety and Infection Control; Cognitive Level: Application [Applying]

### 1210. ANSWER: 1

1. **Line A is pointing to the cervical lymph nodes. Hodgkin's lymphoma usually begins with a painless enlargement of one or more lymph nodes on one side of the neck (cervical or supraclavicular).**
2. Line B is pointing to the axillary nodes.
3. Line C is pointing to the spleen.
4. Line D is pointing to the inguinal nodes. The most common sites for lymphadenopathy are the cervical, supraclavicular, and mediastinal nodes; involvement of the iliac or inguinal nodes or spleen is much less common.

▶ *Test-takingTip: If uncertain, select the option that allows for examination from "head to toe."*

Content Area: Adult; Concept: Assessment; Cellular Regulation; Integrated Processes: Nursing Process: Planning; Client Needs: Physiological Integrity: Reduction of Risk Potential; Health Promotion and Maintenance; Cognitive Level: Application [Applying]

### 1211. PHARM ANSWER: 3

1. Platelets do not contain the deficient clotting factors.
2. Although whole blood contains the deficient factors, periodic administration of factor concentrates are safer.
3. **A person with hemophilia A is deficient in factor VIII; hemophilia B, factor IX; and von Willebrand's hemophilia, the von Willebrand's factor and factor VIII. Recombinant forms of the factors are available for the client to self-administer intravenously at home.**

4. Although fresh frozen plasma contains the deficient factors, periodic administration of factor concentrates are safer.

▶ *Test-takingTip: Persons with hemophilia are deficient in one or more clotting factors. You should narrow the options to the least global option.*

Content Area: Adult; Concept: Hematologic Regulation; Nursing Roles; Integrated Processes: Teaching/Learning; Client Needs: Physiological Integrity: Pharmacological and Parenteral Therapies; Cognitive Level: Application [Applying]

### 1212. ANSWER: 2

1. Aspirin (Ecotrin) and NSAIDs are contraindicated because they interfere with platelet aggregation.
2. **Hemarthrosis is bleeding into the joint. The pressure of the ice pack and cold will reduce the bleeding and swelling. The ice pack should be covered with a cloth.**
3. The client and family are usually taught how to administer factor concentrates at home at the first sign of bleeding.
4. The splint should be left on initially to control bleeding. The client should be instructed on how to assess for adequate tissue perfusion.

▶ *Test-takingTip: If unsure of the meaning of hemarthrosis, apply knowledge of medical terminology. "Heme-" refers to blood, and "arthrosis" refers to joints. Remember that cold reduces bleeding.*

Content Area: Adult; Concept: Hematologic Regulation; Nursing Roles; Integrated Processes: Nursing Process: Implementation; Client Needs: Physiological Integrity: Reduction of Risk Potential; Cognitive Level: Application [Applying]

### 1213. PHARM ANSWER: 3, 5

1. Blood type A positive has the D antigen on the RBC, making it incompatible with blood type B negative.
2. Blood type B positive has the D antigen on the RBC, making it incompatible with blood type B negative.
3. **The client with B negative blood type has B antigen on the RBC and does not have an Rh (or D) antigen on the cell. Because the client can receive RBCs of the same blood type, a person with type B negative blood could be considered for a directed donation.**
4. Blood type O positive has the D antigen, making it incompatible with blood type B negative.
5. **Type O negative has no antigens on the RBC so a directed donation from a person with type O negative blood could also be considered.**
6. Blood type AB positive has the D antigen on the RBC, making it incompatible with blood type B negative.

▶ *Test-takingTip: The ABO system identifies the type of antigen present on the person's erythrocyte (RBC) membrane: A, B, both A and B, or neither A or B (type O). Persons with positive blood type have an Rh (or D) antigen on the cell, whereas Rh negative does not have a D antigen on the cell. Eliminate options in which the blood type is Rh positive because the client is Rh negative.*

Content Area: Adult; **Concept:** Safety; Hematologic Regulation; Medication; **Integrated Processes:** Nursing Process: Implementation; **Client Needs:** Physiological Integrity: Pharmacological and Parenteral Therapies; **Cognitive Level:** Application [Applying]

## 1214. ANSWER: 2, 3, 4, 6

1. Pressure should be applied to an area that is bleeding when the client has thrombocytopenia, not neutropenia.
2. **Fresh flowers harbor microorganisms that can cause an infection.**
3. **Unwashed fruits and vegetables have been found to be colonized with various bacteria, particularly gram-negative enteric organisms, as well as pseudomonas and fungi. Recent research indicates that well-washed fresh fruits and vegetables may be eaten.**
4. **Hand hygiene reduces microbial counts on hands and helps to prevent the transmission of microorganisms to the client's belongings.**
5. The client should not consume any liquids that have been standing at room temperature for longer than an hour due to risk of microbial colonization.
6. **Visitors with a transmittable infection place the client at a high risk for becoming infected due to the client's depressed immune system.**

▶ *Test-taking Tip: Neutropenia places the client at risk for an infection.*

Content Area: Adult; **Concept:** Nursing Roles; Cellular Regulation; **Integrated Processes:** Nursing Process: Implementation; **Client Needs:** Physiological Integrity: Reduction of Risk Potential; **Cognitive Level:** Application [Applying]

## 1215. PHARM ANSWER: 1, 2

1. **Epoetin alfa (erythropoietin growth factor; Procrit) promotes erythropoiesis (production of RBCs), thus decreasing the need for transfusions.**
2. **Folic acid promotes erythropoiesis and production of WBCs and platelets.**
3. Albumin is a blood product.
4. Platelets are blood products.
5. Plasma is a blood product.
6. Granulocytes are blood products.

▶ *Test-taking Tip: Evidence supports the use of either transfusion or erythropoietic growth factor in persons with Hgb of less than 8 g/dL. Eliminate options that are blood products.*

Content Area: Adult; **Concept:** Hematologic Regulation; Diversity; Medication; **Integrated Processes:** Nursing Process: Planning; Culture and Spirituality; **Client Needs:** Physiological Integrity: Pharmacological and Parenteral Therapies; **Cognitive Level:** Application [Applying]

## 1216. PHARM ANSWER: 4

1. Repositioning focuses on treating the client's back pain and not on the blood transfusion, which could be the cause of the back pain.
2. Further assessment should occur after stopping the blood transfusion.

3. The client may need an analgesic for pain control, but this should occur after stopping the blood transfusion.
4. **Low back pain is a symptom of a potentially life-threatening acute hemolytic reaction. The pain is caused from agglutination of RBCs in the kidneys and renal vasoconstriction. Hemolytic reactions occur most often within the first 50 mL of the infusion.**

▶ *Test-taking Tip: When a question asks for the first action, all other actions may also be correct, but the answer is the option that should be first. Use the nursing process. With a possible life-threatening situation, the action should be an intervention.*

Content Area: Adult; **Concept:** Safety; Hematologic Regulation; Medication; **Integrated Processes:** Nursing Process: Implementation; **Client Needs:** Physiological Integrity: Pharmacological and Parenteral Therapies; **Cognitive Level:** Application [Applying]

## 1217. PHARM ANSWER: 2, 3, 5

1. This documents an incomplete blood type, and platelets are unlikely to be administered over 4 hours.
2. **Documentation should include the type of product infused (platelets), product number (compatible platelets were ordered), and that it was double-checked.**
3. **Documentation should include any adverse reactions.**
4. Only 0.9% NaCl should be used when administering blood or blood products, and usually only to purge the line before and after administration.
5. **Documentation should include volume infused. Platelets should be infused as fast as the client can tolerate the infusion to diminish clumping.**

▶ *Test-taking Tip: Platelets are a blood component; protocols for administration of blood products should be followed when administering platelets.*

Content Area: Adult; **Concept:** Hematologic Regulation; Communication; **Integrated Processes:** Communication and Documentation; **Client Needs:** Physiological Integrity: Pharmacological and Parenteral Therapies; **Cognitive Level:** Analysis [Analyzing]

## 1218. ANSWER: 2

1. Antibiotics such as ceftazidime (Fortaz) are administered to prevent infection.
2. **GVHD occurs when the T lymphocytes proliferate from the transplanted donor marrow and mount an immune response against the recipient's tissues. An immunosuppressant such as cyclosporine (Neoral) prevents the immune response.**
3. Cisplatin (Platinol A Q) is administered mainly to treat metastatic testicular, ovarian, and cervical carcinoma; advanced bladder cancer; and head and neck cancer.
4. Interferons such as peginterferon alfa-2a (Pegasys) have antiviral activity, which decrease the progression of hepatic damage associated with hepatitis A and B. This would only be administered if the transplanted cells transmitted the disease. The biological agent interferon is used to treat follicular low-grade lymphomas.

▶ *Test-takingTip: You should select a medication that prevents the body from rejecting the donor cells.*

Content Area: Adult; Concept: Medication; Cellular Regulation; Integrated Processes: Nursing Process: Planning; Client Needs: Physiological Integrity: Pharmacological and Parenteral Therapies; Cognitive Level: Application [Applying]

## 1219. ANSWER: 4

1. A common side effect of immunosuppressant medications is weight gain.
2. Sterility can occur as a result of chemotherapy and the total body irradiation after BMT.
3. Changes in vision are common as a result of the total body irradiation after BMT.
4. **A white, patchy tongue is a sign of a fungal infection with *Candidiasis albicans* and would not be an expected change.**

▶ *Test-takingTip: Note the key words "expected change" and "misunderstood." Look for the option that would not be an expected change.*

Content Area: Adult; Concept: Nursing Roles; Hematologic Regulation; Integrated Processes: Teaching/Learning; Client Needs: Physiological Integrity: Physiological Adaptation; Cognitive Level: Application [Applying]

## 1220. ANSWER: 1

1. **Ineffective breathing pattern occurs with superior vena cava syndrome because the superior vena cava is located next to the main stem bronchus and causes compression of the intrathoracic structures.**
2. Ineffective tissue perfusion may occur with superior vena cava syndrome, but ineffective breathing pattern is priority.
3. Risk for infection occurs with chemotherapy treatment and not from superior vena cava syndrome.
4. Impaired skin integrity occurs with malignant skin conditions and usually not from lung cancer.

▶ *Test-takingTip: Use the ABC's to establish priority.*

Content Area: Adult; Concept: Oxygenation; Cellular Regulation; Integrated Processes: Nursing Process: Analysis; Client Needs: Physiological Integrity: Physiological Adaptation; Cognitive Level: Analysis [Analyzing]

## 1221. ANSWER: 2

1. The client with prostate cancer that has metastasized to the bone generally requires aggressive therapy.
2. **The client is a candidate for "watchful waiting" when older than age 70 with a life expectancy of less than 10 years and with low-grade disease.**
3. The client with extension of the tumor outside of the prostate generally requires aggressive therapy.
4. The client who is asymptomatic with an elevated prostate-specific antigen generally requires aggressive therapy.

▶ *Test-takingTip: Focus on the meaning of "watchful waiting" to identify the answer. Three clients have evidence of advanced cancer. Often the option that is different is the correct one.*

Content Area: Adult; Concept: Cellular Regulation; Management; Integrated Processes: Nursing Process: Implementation; Client Needs: Physiological Integrity: Physiological Adaptation Management; Cognitive Level: Application [Applying]

## 1222. PHARM ANSWER: 250

**First convert liters to milliliters. 1000 mL = 1 L; Then use the proportion formula: 1000 mL: 1 L :: X mL: 2 L. Multiple inside values and outside values and solve for X.**

**$X = 1000 \times 2$; $X = 2000$ mL. Next, calculate the mL per hour. 2000 mL ÷ 8 hours = 250 mL/hour.**

▶ *Test-takingTip: Use knowledge of conversion and IV rate dosage calculation to answer the question.*

Content Area: Adult; Concept: Cellular Regulation; Medication; Integrated Processes: Nursing Process: Implementation; Client Needs: Physiological Integrity: Pharmacological and Parenteral Therapies; Cognitive Level: Application [Applying]

## 1223. ANSWER:

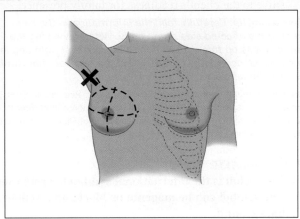

**Breast cancer lesions are frequently found in the upper outer quadrant, near the axilla known as the tail of Spence. Breast cancer lesions can occur anywhere in the breast, including the upper and lower margins, but they are less frequent in these locations than near the axilla.**

▶ *Test-takingTip: The phrases "breast cancer" and "most frequently" are key phrases in the stem. Recall that lymph tissue from the breast empties into the lymph drainage system in the axilla.*

Content Area: Adult; Concept: Promoting Health; Nursing Roles; Integrated Processes: Teaching/Learning; Client Needs: Health Promotion and Maintenance; Cognitive Level: Application [Applying]

## 1224. ANSWER: 2

1. The arm on the operative side should be elevated on a pillow but not above the head.
2. **All IV access sites should be located on the nonoperative side to prevent circulatory impairment.**
3. Having the client look at the incision should be at the client's readiness, not as soon as possible.
4. Only ROM to the lower arm should be carried out for the first few days after surgery, with exercises and ROM to the shoulder after the drains are removed.

▶ *Test-takingTip:* When reviewing the options, consider which options could cause harm to the client and eliminate these.

**Content Area:** Adult; **Concept:** Safety; Cellular Regulation; **Integrated Processes:** Nursing Process: Implementation; **Client Needs:** Physiological Integrity: Reduction of Risk Potential; **Cognitive Level:** Application [Applying]

### 1225. MoC ANSWER: 3

1. BPs, venipunctures, and injections should not be done on the affected arm, so taking the BP on the left arm would be appropriate.
2. It would be appropriate for the NA to tape a sign at the side rail to remind others of the restrictions following a mastectomy.
3. **The client should be placed in a semi-Fowler's position with the arm on the affected side elevated on a pillow to promote restoring arm function and to prevent arm edema.**
4. It would be beneficial for the NA and nurse to be sensitive to the client's readiness for family presence.

▶ *Test-takingTip:* Carefully read the information in the stem and note the affected side of the body. When reviewing the options, focus on this information to be sure that right and left are not used incorrectly. Consider also the position that would ensure lymphatic drainage and venous return.

**Content Area:** Adult; **Concept:** Management; Cellular Regulation; Safety; **Integrated Processes:** Nursing Process: Implementation; **Client Needs:** Safe and Effective Care Environment: Management of Care; Psychosocial Integrity; **Cognitive Level:** Analysis [Analyzing]

### 1226. ANSWER: 1

1. **The trefoil is the international symbol for radiation. The symbol can be magenta or black, on a yellow background.**
2. This is a universal biohazard symbol indicating a potentially infectious specimen.
3. This symbol is used to identify the hazard of a chemical using the NFPA diamond. None of the diamonds are specific for radiation.
4. This is the Mr. Yuk symbol indicating that a substance is a poison.

▶ *Test-takingTip:* To answer items in the graphic format, identify key words in the stem, such as "radiation." Next, focus on the various graphics provided and eliminate options by deciphering the meaning of each graphic.

**Content Area:** Adult; **Concept:** Cellular Regulation; Safety; **Integrated Processes:** Nursing Process: Planning; **Client Needs:** Safe and Effective Care Environment: Safety and Infection Control; **Cognitive Level:** Application [Applying]

### 1227. ANSWER: 1, 4, 6

1. **Wearing loose-fitting, soft clothing over the treated skin is a recommended skin-care activity to reduce radiation skin reactions.**
2. The use of an electric, not a straight-edged, razor for shaving a treated area is recommended.
3. Clients are advised to avoid swimming in chlorinated water.

4. **Using only skin-care products suggested by the radiation staff is a recommended skin-care activity to reduce radiation skin reactions.**
5. Clients are advised to delay the application of skin-care products within 4 hours of radiation treatment.
6. **Washing the treated area gently with lukewarm water and mild soap is a recommended skin-care activity to reduce radiation skin reactions.**

▶ *Test-takingTip:* Options that can have negative effects on the skin should be eliminated.

**Content Area:** Adult; **Concept:** Cellular Regulation; Skin Integrity; Nursing Roles; **Integrated Processes:** Teaching/Learning; **Client Needs:** Safe and Effective Care Environment: Safety and Infection Control; **Cognitive Level:** Application [Applying]

### 1228. ANSWER: 2, 4, 5

1. Consumption of caffeine is not associated with an increased risk for bladder cancer.
2. **Smoking is the number one cause of bladder cancer in the world.**
3. Studies show a protective effect with an increased intake of vitamins A, B$_6$, and E.
4. **Exposure to aromatic amines in the textile and paint industries is clearly associated with bladder cancer.**
5. **Exposure to aromatic amines in the rubber industry is clearly associated with bladder cancer.**

▶ *Test-takingTip:* Research has shown that there is a strong association between inhalation of carcinogens and bladder cancer. Narrow the options to those that pertain to inhalation.

**Content Area:** Adult; **Concept:** Promoting Health; Cellular Regulation; **Integrated Processes:** Teaching/Learning; **Client Needs:** Health Promotion and Maintenance; **Cognitive Level:** Application [Applying]

### 1229. ANSWER: 2

1. Hypotension is a symptom that is not common in radiation pneumonitis.
2. **Cough, fever, and dyspnea are classic symptoms in radiation pneumonitis due to a decrease in the surfactant in the lung.**
3. Decreased urine output is a symptom that is not common in radiation pneumonitis.
4. Altered mental status is a symptom that is not common in radiation pneumonitis.

▶ *Test-takingTip:* Narrow the options to those most associated with the respiratory system.

**Content Area:** Adult; **Concept:** Assessment; Cellular Regulation; **Integrated Processes:** Nursing Process: Assessment; **Client Needs:** Physiological Integrity: Reduction of Risk Potential; **Cognitive Level:** Analysis [Analyzing]

### 1230. PHARM ANSWER: 1, 2, 4

1. **A peripheral IV catheter may be used for a vesicant if administration time is less than 60 minutes, a large vein is used, and there is careful monitoring of the IV site.**

2. **Checking for patency and asking about discomfort at the IV site will help prevent an infiltration.**
3. IV pumps and alarms cannot be relied upon to detect extravasation because infiltration usually does not cause sufficient pressure to trigger an alarm.
4. **Checking for blood return in the central venous catheter prior to administration will help ensure that the medication is being administered into a vessel and not into tissues.**
5. Small-gauge syringes with small barrels produce high pressures and may cause injury to the blood vessel or may damage a central line catheter and should not be used.

▶ *Test-takingTip: Extravasation is the unintentional administration of IV medications into the tissue around the infusion site. Eliminate options that increase the risk of extravasation.*

Content Area: Adult; **Concept:** Safety; Medication; Integrated Processes: Nursing Process: Implementation; **Client Needs:** Safe and Effective Care Environment: Safety and Infection Control; Physiological Integrity: Pharmacological and Parenteral Therapies; **Cognitive Level:** Application [Applying]

### 1231. PHARM ANSWER: 1

1. **Neurotoxicity and diarrhea occur frequently in clients receiving the medication regimen of oxaliplatin (Eloxatin), fluorouracil (5-FU), and leucovorin (Wellcovorin).**
2. Cardiomyopathy and dysphagia are not common side effects of these chemotherapy agents.
3. Renal insufficiency and gastritis are not common side effects of these chemotherapy agents.
4. Photophobia and stomatitis are not common side effects of these chemotherapy agents.

▶ *Test-takingTip: If unsure, consider a side effect that is common to many medications.*

Content Area: Adult; **Concept:** Medication; Cellular Regulation; Integrated Processes: Nursing Process: Analysis; **Client Needs:** Physiological Integrity: Pharmacological and Parenteral Therapies; **Cognitive Level:** Analysis [Analyzing]

### 1232. PHARM ANSWER: 4

1. Meperidine (Demerol) is not recommended because it causes CNS toxicity from metabolites. It should not be used for the treatment of chronic pain.
2. Propoxyphene (Darvon) is best used for moderate to severe pain; a rating of 9 is severe pain.
3. Pentazocine (Talwin) is used for moderate pain only, and it can cause confusion and hallucinations in older adults and clients with renal impairment.
4. **Opioids, such as oxycodone (OxyContin), remain the most frequently prescribed analgesic for severe cancer pain. To help with pain control, the nurse should plan to administer it now and then again at the prescribed dosing interval.**

▶ *Test-takingTip: Consider the side effects of each medication and which would provide the best pain control while minimizing side effects.*

Content Area: Adult; **Concept:** Medication; Cellular Regulation; Integrated Processes: Nursing Process: Planning; **Client Needs:** Physiological Integrity: Pharmacological and Parenteral Therapies; **Cognitive Level:** Analysis [Analyzing]

### 1233. MoC PHARM ANSWER: 1, 4

1. **Erythropoiesis-stimulating agents, such as epoetin alfa (Epogen), can cause thromboembolic events. It would be concerning if the client had limited activity because this could further increase the client's risk of a thromboembolic event. The HCP should be consulted.**
2. Dark green, leafy vegetables are high in iron and help with Hgb synthesis and therefore would be beneficial.
3. Eggs are high in iron, but there are other food sources high in iron that the client can consume if an aversion exists.
4. **A history of a thromboembolic event and use of epoetin alfa increase the client's risk for another thromboembolic event. The HCP should be consulted.**
5. The use of epoetin alfa is recommended as a treatment option for clients with chemotherapy-associated anemia and an Hgb concentration that is approaching, or has fallen below, 10 g/dL, to increase the Hgb level and decrease the need for a transfusion.

▶ *Test-takingTip: A side effect of epoetin alfa (Epogen) is an increase in thromboembolic events. Consider options that will increase this risk and eliminate the other options.*

Content Area: Adult; **Concept:** Clotting; Cellular Regulation; Management; **Integrated Processes:** Communication and Documentation; **Client Needs:** Physiological Integrity: Pharmacological and Parenteral Therapies; Safe and Effective Care Environment: Management of Care; **Cognitive Level:** Application [Applying]

### 1234. ANSWER: 1, 3, 5

1. **Immune-suppressing drugs weaken the immune system, and cellular changes can occur more aggressively.**
2. Smoking history is a risk factor for lung cancer, not BCC.
3. **Persons with fair skin, blond or red hair, and blue, green, or gray eyes have a higher risk for BCC due to the ease of sunburn with sun exposure if the skin is not protected.**
4. Exposure to indoor radon gas is a risk factor for lung cancer, not BCC. Radon is a radioactive colorless, odorless, tasteless, and chemically inert gas. It is formed by the natural radioactive decay of uranium in rock, soil, and water.
5. **Frequent participation in outdoor activities with exposure to sunlight is a risk factor for BCC due to the damage caused by UV light. UV light damages DNA.**

▶ *Test-takingTip: Focus on the type of cancer (skin) and whether there is a relationship between each option and the skin or basal cells.*

Content Area: Adult; **Concept:** Assessment; Cellular Regulation; **Integrated Processes:** Nursing Process: Assessment; **Client Needs:** Physiological Integrity: Physiological Adaptation; **Cognitive Level:** Analysis [Analyzing]

## 1235. ANSWER: 1

1. **BCC is nodular and ulcerative. Clinical manifestations include small, slowly enlarging papule; borders are translucent or "pearly" with overlying telangiectasia; erosion, ulceration, and depression of center.**
2. Clinical manifestations of malignant melanoma (not BCC) include irregular color, surface, and border; variegation of color including red, white, blue, black, gray, brown; flat or elevated; eroded or ulcerated.
3. Actinic keratosis (not BCC) is characterized by being horny and "wartlike."
4. Impetigo is characterized by thick, honey-colored crusts and is treated with antibiotics and topical treatment.

▶ **Test-taking Tip:** Use nursing knowledge of the different manifestations of skin cancers and infection and their treatment modalities.

Content Area: Adult; **Concept:** Cellular Regulation; **Integrated Processes:** Nursing Process: Assessment; **Client Needs:** Physiological Integrity: Physiological Adaptation; **Cognitive Level:** Application [Applying]

## 1236. ANSWER: 4

1. Applying ice to the area is not necessary because the client did not mention swelling.
2. Because the wounds do not drain purulent material, contacting the physician is not necessary.
3. Because the client is not experiencing pain, pain medication is not needed.
4. **The nurse should recommend changing the dressing because a small amount of serosanguineous drainage is a normal response to surgical removal of a lesion.**

▶ **Test-taking Tip:** When selecting an option, you should consider that "serosanguineous fluid" is watery and pale pink and is an expected finding. Consider also that the dressing is "small."

Content Area: Adult; **Concept:** Skin Integrity; Cellular Regulation; **Integrated Processes:** Nursing Process: Analysis; **Client Needs:** Physiological Integrity: Reduction of Risk Potential; **Cognitive Level:** Application [Applying]

## 1237. MoC ANSWER: 2

1. The T4 N3 M1 indicates that the client's primary tumor is very large, involves three lymph nodes, with distant metastasis (T is the size and extent and ranges from 1-4; N is number of nodes involved, and M1 indicates metastasis).
2. **This statement is correct. The tumor-node-metastasis (TNM) system classifies solid tumors by size and degree of spread. It is an international system that allows comparison of statistics among cancer centers.**

3. A higher number means that a more serious situation exists.
4. A different rating system is used to define the cell types of tumors as well differentiated (closely resembles normal tissue) or poorly differentiated (tumor that contains some normal cells, but most cells are abnormal).

▶ **Test-taking Tip:** In the TNM classification system, T indicates the primary tumor size and extent, N is regional lymph node involvement, and M is distant metastasis. Identify the option that best fits with this information.

Content Area: Adult; **Concept:** Nursing Roles; Cellular Regulation; Communication; Management; **Integrated Processes:** Teaching/Learning; **Client Needs:** Safe and Effective Care Environment: Management of Care; **Cognitive Level:** Application [Applying]

## 1238. ANSWER: 3

1. Bronchoscopy includes insertion of a bronchoscope to examine the lungs.
2. Colonoscopy is used to inspect the large intestines.
3. **EGD is an invasive procedure in which a lighted instrument (scope) is lowered into the stomach and duodenum to examine gastric tissues and obtain biopsies for cancer cell analysis. Because it is the preferred test to diagnose gastric cancer, the nurse should teach the client about this test.**
4. A MUGA scan creates video images of the ventricles of the heart to evaluate their correct function in pumping blood. A person who is to receive chemotherapy for cancer treatment may have a MUGA scan completed to identify preexisting heart conditions.

▶ **Test-taking Tip:** Identifying similar words or portions of a word between the stem of the question and the options is often helpful in identifying the answer.

Content Area: Adult; **Concept:** Nursing Roles; Cellular Regulation; **Integrated Processes:** Teaching/Learning; **Client Needs:** Physiological Integrity: Reduction of Risk Potential; **Cognitive Level:** Application [Applying]

## 1239. ANSWER: 2

1. The elevation in the WBC to 12,200/mm$^3$ (normal is 4500–10,000/mm$^3$ or microL) is concerning because it could indicate an infection, but the elevation would not necessarily be related to the gastric cancer.
2. **The presenting symptoms are indicative of anemia, which is common in gastric cancer due to chronic blood loss, or because of pernicious anemia (due to loss of intrinsic factor). The low Hgb of 7.9 g/dL (normal is 12–15 g/dL) may be the causative factor for the fatigue.**
3. The serum protein of 5.9 g/dL is slightly low (normal is 6.0–8.0 g/dL) and could be indicative of nutritional problems associated with the gastric cancer, but it is not specific to the signs and symptoms described in the question, and it is not part of a CBC.
4. The BUN of 22 mg/dL (normal is 5–25 mg/dL) is within normal parameters and is measuring kidney function or hydration status. It is not part of the CBC.

▶ *Test-takingTip: When reviewing laboratory results, eliminate options that are within normal ranges. Be careful reading information. This question is asking about laboratory results in a CBC. Serum protein and BUN are not part of the CBC.*

**Content Area:** Adult; **Concept:** Hematologic Regulation; Cellular Regulation; **Integrated Processes:** Nursing Process: Analysis; **Client Needs:** Physiological Integrity: Physiological Adaptation; **Cognitive Level:** Application [Applying]

## 1240. ANSWER: 3

1. Pain may be a symptom of a tumor located on the left side of the colon, but it is not exclusive and could be a symptom of a tumor elsewhere in the colon.
2. Change of bowel habits may be a symptom of a tumor located on the left side of the colon, but this is not exclusive and could be a symptom of a tumor elsewhere in the colon.
3. **Bright red blood in the stool is a sign or symptom of a colorectal tumor located in the descending colon.**
4. Nausea and vomiting are not symptoms specific to colon cancer.

▶ *Test-takingTip: Eliminate the options that are more general, or vague, and that could be attributed to a variety of conditions.*

**Content Area:** Adult; **Concept:** Cellular Regulation; **Integrated Processes:** Nursing Process: Assessment; **Client Needs:** Physiological Integrity: Physiological Adaptation; **Cognitive Level:** Application [Applying]

## 1241. MoC ANSWER: 4

1. The National Cancer Institute answers questions and has free information about cancer.
2. The Leukemia Society of America provides education regarding leukemia.
3. The Corporate Angel Network provides free plane transportation for cancer clients going to and from treatment centers.
4. **The Patient Advocate Foundation provides counseling to resolve job-related problems.**

▶ *Test-takingTip: The key word is "assistance." The client needs someone who can speak on the client's behalf.*

**Content Area:** Adult; **Concept:** Collaboration; Cellular Regulation; **Integrated Processes:** Caring; **Client Needs:** Safe and Effective Care Environment: Management of Care; **Cognitive Level:** Application [Applying]

## 1242. MoC ANSWER: 1, 2, 3, 6

1. **Total laryngectomy is removal of the entire larynx as well as the hyoid bone, the true vocal cords, the false vocal cords, the epiglottis, the cricoid cartilage, and two to three tracheal rings. The physical therapist is needed for neck exercises.**
2. **The dietitian is needed to ensure adequacy of oral intake.**
3. **The speech therapist is needed for other forms of communication and swallowing.**
4. The dentist is not routinely consulted when caring for a laryngectomy client.
5. An occupational therapist is not routinely consulted when caring for a laryngectomy client.

6. **The social worker is needed for contact with outside resources to assist the client in ongoing needs.**

▶ *Test-takingTip: Knowing that a total laryngectomy involves the removal of the voice box and the excision of the neck muscles, and that swallowing is affected and that outside resources may be needed, should direct you to the correct options.*

**Content Area:** Adult; **Concept:** Collaboration; Cellular Regulation; Management; **Integrated Processes:** Nursing Process: Planning; **Client Needs:** Safe and Effective Care Environment: Management of Care; **Cognitive Level:** Analysis [Analyzing]

## 1243. MoC ANSWER: 2, 1, 4, 3

2. **Restless and has a mucus plug in the tracheostomy is priority requiring immediate attention due to the negative impact on air exchange. The client needs immediate suctioning.**
1. **Copious oral secretions and nasal mucus draining from the nose should be next. After a total laryngectomy the mouth does not communicate with the trachea, so copious oral secretions and nasal drainage would not influence air exchange, but these create a source of discomfort for the client.**
4. **Oozing serosanguineous drainage around the tracheostomy tube and saturated dressing should be addressed third. Changing the dressing now would allow the nurse to inspect the site and ensure tube patency.**
3. **NG tube used for intermittent feedings pulled halfway out can be addressed last. There is no indication that a tube feeding is infusing. The HCP should be contacted to reinsert the NG tube to prevent disruption of the suture line in the esophagus.**

▶ *Test-takingTip: The words "total laryngectomy" and "immediate attention" are key words in the stem, and the nurse needs to think about the ABC's to prioritize the options.*

**Content Area:** Adult; **Concept:** Critical Thinking; Oxygenation; Cellular Regulation; Management; **Integrated Processes:** Nursing Process: Implementation; **Client Needs:** Safe and Effective Care Environment: Management of Care; **Cognitive Level:** Synthesis [Creating]

## 1244. MoC PHARM ANSWER: 4

1. Finding that the client with liver cancer is weak and pale would be important to document, but it does not warrant immediate communication to the HCP because it may be expected.
2. The client's weight being stable would not necessitate communication to the HCP, but a significant decrease would.
3. Abdominal itching may occur with liver cancer, but the fact that it is less with diphenhydramine (Benadryl) use is positive and would not necessitate a call to the HCP.
4. **The client's pain level is high and does not seem to be controlled with the current opioid schedule. The nurse should notify the HCP to request a change in analgesic medication, dosing schedule, or administration route.**

▶ *Test-takingTip:* Eliminate options that are expected findings for the client diagnosed with liver cancer or findings that are being controlled.

**Content Area:** Adult; **Concept:** Comfort; Cellular Regulation; Medication; **Integrated Processes:** Communication and Documentation; **Client Needs:** Physiological Integrity: Pharmacological and Parenteral Therapies; Safe and Effective Care Environment: Management of Care; **Cognitive Level:** Application [Applying]

## 1245. ANSWER: 1, 3, 4

1. **Safety measures for caring for someone undergoing internal radiation therapy include limiting time, distance, and shielding. It would be important to make the client aware of the time and distance limitations to help ease anxiety.**
2. A personal, not shared, film badge should be worn so cumulative radiation exposure can be measured accurately.
3. **Organizing care would be appropriate to limit the exposure to radiation.**
4. **Shielding is important for keeping caregivers safe from potential radiation exposure.**
5. The implant is placed in the vaginal canal and has no impact on oral mucosa.

▶ *Test-takingTip:* Eliminate Option 2 because it would pose a safety risk. Focus on the fact that the client is receiving radiation through a temporary cervical implant and eliminate Option 5, which would pertain to chemotherapy treatment or radiation to the head or neck.

**Content Area:** Adult; **Concept:** Safety; Cellular Regulation; **Integrated Processes:** Nursing Process: Implementation; **Client Needs:** Safe and Effective Care Environment: Safety and Infection Control; **Cognitive Level:** Application [Applying]

## 1246. ANSWER: 1

1. **Abnormal vaginal bleeding and pain in the pelvic region appear as the most common presenting symptoms in the client with endometrial cancer.**
2. Weight loss is not a common presenting symptom unless the cancer is advanced. Night sweats may occur with hormone changes.
3. Supraclavicular lymph nodes are located just above the clavicle, lateral to where it joins the sternum, and not near the uterus.
4. Unexplained temperature spikes and splenomegaly are not common presenting symptoms.

▶ *Test-takingTip:* The key word is "newly." Endometrial cancer starts in the inner lining of the uterus. Relate this area to one of the options.

**Content Area:** Adult; **Concept:** Assessment; Cellular Regulation; **Integrated Processes:** Nursing Process: Assessment; **Client Needs:** Physiological Integrity: Physiological Adaptation; **Cognitive Level:** Comprehension [Understanding]

## 1247. ANSWER: 1

1. **The client with diarrhea should eat a low-residue diet to decrease roughage and bowel irritability and take sitz (or tub) baths twice daily to increase comfort.**

2. Intake of fluids that are high in potassium (not low) is recommended to replace electrolytes lost through diarrhea.
3. Milk products are discouraged because they increase bowel irritability.
4. Intake of fluids high in sodium should be avoided because it contributes to water retention, but hydrocolloid pads may be used on reddened areas to promote healing.

▶ *Test-takingTip:* When options contain more than one part, both parts must be correct for the option to be the answer.

**Content Area:** Adult; **Concept:** Cellular Regulation; Bowel Elimination; **Integrated Processes:** Teaching/Learning; **Client Needs:** Physiological Integrity: Basic Care and Comfort; **Cognitive Level:** Application [Applying]

## 1248. ANSWER: 3, 5

1. Elevating the head of the bed to a 45-degree angle may increase lymphedema of the lower extremities.
2. Intake of fluids high in sodium will cause fluid retention.
3. **Leg exercises will improve drainage when lymphedema is present.**
4. Lower-extremity splints can cause skin breakdown of edematous tissue.
5. **Compression stocking enhance the flow of the lymph fluid out of the affected limbs.**

▶ *Test-takingTip:* Lymphedema is the accumulation of lymph fluid in the tissues of the lower extremities. Eliminate options that would have no therapeutic benefit or that could cause tissue damage.

**Content Area:** Adult; **Concept:** Fluid and Electrolyte Balance; Cellular Regulation; **Integrated Processes:** Nursing Process: Implementation; **Client Needs:** Physiological Integrity: Basic Care and Comfort; **Cognitive Level:** Application [Applying]

## 1249. PHARM ANSWER: 1

1. **Methadone (Dolophine) does have a long half-life of 15 to 25 hours and high potency. The nurse should consider that a longer administration interval is needed.**
2. Methadone may cause a transient fall in BP (not increase) and confusion.
3. Methadone has no greater incidence of allergic reactions than other medications. Liver failure is not an adverse effect, but the medication should be used cautiously with those who have liver dysfunction.
4. Methadone has no known active metabolites. Recent evidence indicates it is well tolerated in the management of cancer pain due to its prolonged duration of action, resulting in longer administration intervals.

▶ *Test-takingTip:* Focus on the word "administration" in the question stem. Think about which option would require longer administration intervals.

**Content Area:** Adult; **Concept:** Medication; Cellular Regulation; **Integrated Processes:** Nursing Process: Assessment; **Client Needs:** Physiological Integrity: Pharmacological and Parenteral Therapies; **Cognitive Level:** Analysis [Analyzing]

**1250. ANSWER: 2200**

**First convert to milliliters: 1 L = 1000 mL; 1 oz = 30 mL**

**Next add the values for fluids: 1000 mL + 240 mL + 240 mL + 90 mL + 120 mL + 180 mL + 240 mL + 90 mL = 2200 mL**

▶ *Test-taking Tip: Remember that 1 L equals 1000 mL. Be sure you record only fluid intake.*

Content Area: Adult; Concept: Nutrition; Fluid and Electrolyte Balance: Cellular Regulation; Integrated Processes: Communication and Documentation; Client Needs: Physiological Integrity: Basic Care and Comfort; Cognitive Level: Application [Applying]

**1251. PHARM ANSWER: 2**

1. Promethazine (Phenergan) is given with pain medications, but it treats nausea and vomiting, not pain.
2. **Gabapentin (Neurontin) is often administered with opioid pain medications because of its efficacy in relieving neuropathic pain and its limited adverse effects.**
3. Diphenhydramine (Benadryl) is not a coanalgesic but an antihistamine.
4. Droperidol (Inapsine) is not a coanalgesic but an antiemetic to control nausea and vomiting.

▶ *Test-taking Tip: Focus on the key word "coanalgesic" (action is for treating pain along with the main medication). Eliminate medications that do not have pain-relieving actions.*

Content Area: Adult; Concept: Medication; Cellular Regulation; Integrated Processes: Nursing Process: Analysis; Client Needs: Physiological Integrity: Pharmacological and Parenteral Therapies; Cognitive Level: Analysis [Analyzing]

**1252. MoC ANSWER: 2**

1. Fever and infection are common signs of AML.
2. **The platelet count of 9500/mm³ is dangerously low, and the client is at risk for hemorrhaging when platelets are less than 10,000/mm³.**
3. A normal neutrophil count is greater than 2000/mm³.
4. Bone pain is a sign of AML that results from expansion of the bone marrow from the proliferation of leukemic cells.

▶ *Test-taking Tip: The key word is "immediately." Use the ABC's to select the most critical abnormal finding.*

Content Area: Adult; Concept: Hematologic Regulation; Clotting; Integrated Processes: Nursing Process: Analysis; Client Needs: Safe and Effective Care Environment: Management of Care; Cognitive Level: Analysis [Analyzing]

## Chapter Twenty-Eight

# Integumentary Management

**1253.** Three days ago, the client received circumferential, partial, and full-thickness burns to 30% of the total body surface area of the chest and abdomen. The nurse monitors the client for restricted breathing due to which physiological response?

1. Development of a layer of eschar
2. Loss of elastin and collagen in the tissues
3. Hypoxia and ischemia of the lungs' alveoli
4. Fluid overload in the alveoli of the lungs

**1254.** The client telephones the ED asking for advice for singed fingers. Which initial statement by the nurse is **most** appropriate?

1. "Wrap ice in a washcloth and put it on the burn area."
2. "Come to the ED so a doctor can assess your fingers."
3. "Run cool water over the burned area on your fingers."
4. "Apply an antibiotic skin ointment to prevent infection."

**1255.** The nurse assesses that the client with partial-thickness burns over 50% of the total body surface area (TBSA) has gained weight and has generalized edema after the first 24 hours. The nurse should consider that the edema and weight gain are most likely related to which physiological processes?

1. Elevated serum sodium and potassium levels
2. Increased hemoglobin and hematocrit levels
3. Excess intravenous fluid volume replacement
4. Leakage of plasma into the interstitial space

**1256.** **PHARM** The nurse is determining the IV fluid needs for the 110-lb client with partial-thickness burns to 40% of the total body surface area (TBSA). Using the Parkland formula (4 mL × weight in kg × % TBSA burn = 24-hour IV fluid volume replacement; half given in first 8 hours), how many mL of IV fluid are needed during the first 8 hours?

_____ mL of IV fluid (Record your answer as a whole number.)

**1257.** When assessing a burn victim's skin, the nurse notices the entire right and left upper extremities are red, moist, weeping, and blistered. How should the nurse document the degree and total body surface area (TBSA) burned?

1. First-degree burn on 9% TBSA
2. Partial-thickness burn on 18% TBSA
3. Partial-thickness burn on 27% TBSA
4. Full-thickness burn on 36% TBSA

**1258.** **PHARM** The nurse completes teaching the client with a second-degree burn about silver sulfadiazine. Which client statements should indicate to the nurse that the teaching was effective? **Select all that apply.**

1. "I apply the cream only to the opened areas of the burned area."
2. "Silver sulfadiazine will prevent an infection of the burned area."
3. "I never should apply a dressing after applying silver sulfadiazine."
4. "I use a tongue blade to remove the old ointment before reapplying."
5. "The cream is dark-colored and cannot be removed with water."

**1259.** The nurse is providing postoperative care for the client with a split-thickness skin graft on the burn wound at the sole of the right foot. Which plan is appropriate for this client?

1. Immobilization of the graft site
2. Weight-bearing exercises to the graft site
3. Assist client out of bed as much as tolerated
4. Maintain right leg in a dependent position

**1260.** **PHARM** The nurse is caring for clients with second- and third-degree burns. Which medication, if prescribed, should the nurse plan to apply topically to treat bacterial and yeast infections?

1. Bismuth subsalicylate
2. Gold sodium thiomalate
3. Silver sulfadiazine
4. Arsenic trioxide

**1261.** The nurse is caring for the client with problems of anxiety and confusion in the critical phase of burn injury. Which interventions should the nurse implement? **Select all that apply.**

1. Repeat orientation statements of person, place, and time.
2. Turn and reposition the client at least every 2 hours.
3. Place familiar objects from home near the client.
4. Implement a schedule for regular sleep-wake cycles.
5. Control distractions by keeping the room door closed.
6. Encourage the client to write notes to family members.

**1262.** **MoC** The client sustained partial- and full-thickness burns to the anterior left and right arms, anterior chest and abdominal area, and anterior left leg. Using the Rule of Nines, what is the estimated extent of this injury that the ED nurse should relay to the HCP?

_____ % (Record your answer as a whole number.)

**1263.** **MoC** The nurse is assessing the client with a burn injury. Which findings should prompt the nurse to notify the HCP with a concern about sepsis?

1. $Paco_2$ 35 mm Hg and blood glucose level 250
2. Bleeding from IV site and blood glucose level 55
3. Temperature 103.2°F (39.6°C) and HR 120 bpm
4. RR 34 breaths/min and WBC 10,000/mm³

**1264.** The nurse is caring for the client with a large, open sternal wound resulting from a burn injury. The client is receiving enteral feeding, Oxepa (an anti-inflammatory, pulmonary 1.5 Cal/mL formula), at 25 mL/hour. Which laboratory result **best** indicates that the client's nutrition is **inadequate?**

| Serum Lab Test | Client's Value | Normals |
|---|---|---|
| Phosphorus | 2.0 | 2.5–4.5 mg/dL |
| Platelets (×10³) | 110 | 150–450 × 10³/microL |
| Prealbumin | 10 | 12–42 mg/dL |
| Potassium | 3.1 | 3.5–5.0 mEq/L |

1. Phosphorus
2. Platelets
3. Prealbumin
4. Potassium

**1265.** **PHARM** The client experiences local burning and stinging when mafenide cream is applied to a burn. What should the nurse do now?

1. Remove any mafenide that has been applied.
2. Immediately notify the HCP.
3. Double-check the concentration of mafenide.
4. Inform the client that this is a normal response.

**1266.** The nurse is irrigating the arm of the client with an acid burn. Which factors should prompt the nurse to continue with the irrigation? **Select all that apply.**

1. Burning sensation is felt in the affected arm.
2. Pain is reduced from 5 to 2 on a 0 to 10 scale.
3. Irrigation runoff solution pH measures 7.0.
4. Pain is absent in the arm with the acid burn.
5. Affected arm skin surface pH measures 4.8.

**1267.** **MoC** The client is admitted to the ED after a house fire. Place the client's problems in the order of priority for the nurse to address.

1. Has 48% partial- and full-thickness burn injury
2. Laceration on the face that has stopped bleeding
3. Inhalation injury from smoke
4. History of hypertension

Answer: _____

**1268.** The client has an entrance wound on the right hand and an exit wound on the left hand after contact with a high-power electrical line. Considering the nature and trajectory of the electrical current, which nursing action is **priority**?

1. Obtain a 12-lead ECG.
2. Check pupil size and reaction.
3. Auscultate both lung fields.
4. Check arm range of motion.

**1269.** MoC The client is scheduled for application of a cadaver homograph to a burn on the forearm. Which comment by the client demonstrates an accurate understanding of this procedure?

1. "The graft donor site from my right upper thigh shouldn't take too long to heal."
2. "I know this graft will only be a temporary measure to protect and help heal my arm."
3. "I am glad that there is no risk of me getting a blood-borne disease with this type of graft."
4. "If this graft doesn't permanently take, then I'll need to select another graft donor site."

**1270.** The nurse is assessing the client's grafted wound following a skin graft. Which information provided during shift report should prompt the nurse to carefully assess if the client has a wound infection?

1. WBC at 9900/microL
2. Serosanguineous drainage
3. Temperature 103°F (39.4°C)
4. Urine output 100 mL past 4 hours

**1271.** The client has a split-thickness skin graft taken from the thigh to cover a burn on the back. Which intervention should the nurse implement to help reduce the risk of infection at the donor and graft site?

1. Obtain serial wound cultures of the donor site.
2. Eliminate plants and flowers in the client's room.
3. Use clean technique for all wound care procedures.
4. Give a continual low dose of an IV antibiotic.

**1272.** The nurse is planning care for the client with a Stage II pressure ulcer on the ball of the right foot. Which interventions should the nurse include in this client's plan of care? **Select all that apply.**

1. Obtain cultures of the wound daily.
2. Clean vigorously to remove dead tissue.
3. Cover with a protective dressing.
4. Reposition at least every 2 hours.
5. Elevate the right heel completely off the bed.

**1273.** The nurse is caring for the client with the pressure ulcer illustrated. Which stage should the nurse document?

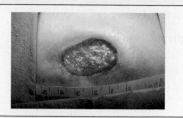

1. Stage I pressure ulcer
2. Stage II pressure ulcer
3. Stage III pressure ulcer
4. Stage IV pressure ulcer

**1274.** The nurse is caring for the client at increased risk for developing pressure ulcers. Which measure should the nurse take to limit shearing forces?

1. Padding the client's sacrum and heels
2. Obtaining an alternating air pressure mattress
3. Using a lifting device when turning the client
4. Keeping the head of bed lower than 30 degrees

**1275.** The nurse is caring for the immobile client who is at risk for developing pressure ulcers. Which food should the nurse recommend?

1. Assorted fruit salad
2. Oatmeal with raisins
3. Baked chicken breast
4. Lettuce and tomato salad

**1276.** The nurse is concerned that a very dark-skinned African American client may be developing a pressure injury on the heel. What should the nurse do to assess for the presence of pressure injury?

1. Turn on all of the fluorescent lights in the client's room before inspection.
2. Apply pressure to the heel, remove the pressure, and observe for blanching.
3. Check to see if the area of pressure appears darker than the surrounding skin.
4. Ask about pain and check the heel for redness, edema, and cracks in the tissue.

**1277.** The client receives treatment for uncomplicated lower-extremity cellulitis. The nurse notes improvement in the client's condition when which observation is noted on assessment?

1. Decreased swelling in the lower extremity
2. Strong dorsalis pedis pulses felt bilaterally
3. Increased erythema in the lower extremity
4. White blood cell (WBC) count 14,000/mm³

**1278.** While the nurse is assessing the client hospitalized with recurrent lower-extremity cellulitis, the client states, "I have athlete's foot; do you want to check it?" The nurse concludes that this information is significant for what reason?

1. Cellulitis is commonly caused by a similar fungal infection.
2. Both infections should resolve with topical fungicide therapy.
3. Painful neuralgia can occur after the cellulitis infection has resolved.
4. The skin disruption with tinea pedis may be the cause of the cellulitis.

**1279.** The nurse is assessing the client. Which findings should the nurse associate with herpes zoster?

1. Serous drainage and pus
2. Nodular lesions and burning
3. Painful vesicles and pruritus
4. Macule lesions and petechiae

**1280.** The nurse is assessing the client newly diagnosed with psoriasis. Which findings should the nurse expect? **Select all that apply.**

1. Pruritus at the affected areas
2. Nailbeds that are pink and clear
3. Stringy, oily hair that falls out in clumps
4. Lesions appear as red plaques with silvery scales
5. Affected areas at elbows, knees, scalp, palms, or soles

**1281.** PHARM The client is receiving UV light treatments for psoriasis along with methoxsalen, a photosensitizing agent. What precaution should be followed the first day after treatment?

1. Wear ultraviolet B–protective sunglasses.
2. Avoid applying skin ointments and lotions.
3. Check for elevated temperature every 4 hours.
4. Stop treatments if skin redness or erythema occurs.

**1282.** PHARM The nurse is caring for the client with psoriasis taking methotrexate. Which laboratory tests are **most** important for the nurse to monitor? **Select all that apply.**

1. Serum potassium level
2. Liver function tests
3. Serum glucose level
4. Arterial blood gases
5. White blood cells

**1283.** PHARM The client with the condition illustrated is prescribed adapalene topical daily to the affected areas. Which information should the nurse **exclude** when planning client education?

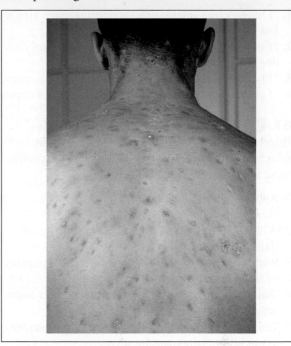

1. "You are receiving adapalene for acne vulgaris."
2. "Apply adapalene once daily to your entire back."
3. "Exposure to the sun after use will help drying."
4. "Apply a thin film to clean affected skin areas."

**1284.** PHARM The nurse is teaching a 24-year-old female with severe cystic acne who is prescribed a systemic retinoic acid drug. Which question has **priority**?

1. "Are you sexually active?"
2. "Are you allergic to vitamin A?"
3. "Is your skin dry or sensitive?"
4. "Can you take the drug as scheduled?"

**1285.** The nurse is explaining facelift (rhytidectomy) surgery to the client and describing the site where the incision is most commonly made. Place an X on the site where the incision most commonly used for rhytidectomy is made.

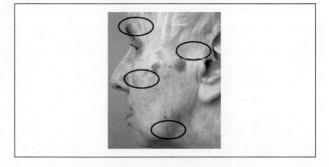

**1286.** The nurse is obtaining a preoperative health history on the client scheduled for revision of facial scars. Which client comment indicates an increased risk for a poor cosmetic outcome?

1. "I haven't had anything to eat or drink since 10 p.m. last night."
2. "I'm nervous about surgery; what if the surgery doesn't work?"
3. "My high blood pressure is controlled with lisinopril."
4. "I plan to continue taking diclofenac for pain control."

**1287.** **MoC** **PHARM** The experienced nurse is observing the new nurse administer medications. Which actions by the new nurse require the experienced nurse to intervene? **Select all that apply.**

1. Applies tretinoin to an open wound on the face of the client with acne
2. Withholds isotretinoin until the client's pregnancy status is known
3. Withholds fluorouracil because the client's papules of actinic keratosis are worse
4. Waits 2 hours after the client bathes and uses lotion before applying tacrolimus
5. Tells the client, who is taking acitretin for psoriasis, to not become pregnant for a year

**1288.** **MoC** The experienced nurse is supervising the new nurse. The nurse should intervene if observing the new nurse performing which intervention?

1. Applying skin lotion to the face, feet, and hands of the client with pemphigus
2. Applying a skin emollient to the arms and legs of the client with scleroderma
3. Informing the client with herpes simplex that the lesions are contagious until crusted
4. Telling the client that ultraviolet light therapy is one option for treating acne vulgaris

**1289.** **PHARM** The nurse is planning teaching for the client who is using miconazole cream topically for tinea pedis. Which instruction should the nurse include?

1. Cover the treated area with an occlusive dressing.
2. Avoid washing the area prior to applying the cream.
3. Massage miconazole into the affected area of the foot.
4. Once symptoms resolve, discontinue using miconazole.

**1290.** The nurse is assessing the client with atopic dermatitis. Which finding should the nurse expect?

1.

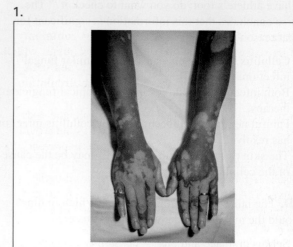

2.

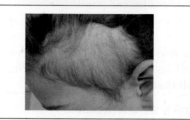

3.

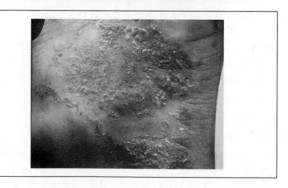

4.

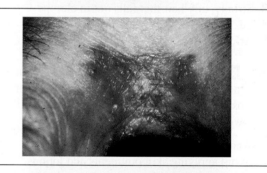

**1291.** The nurse is assessing the client for possible scabies infestation. Which findings should the nurse expect?

1. Serosanguineous drainage and fever
2. Malaise and local edema
3. Itching and papule-like rash
4. Macule rash and blisters

# Answers and Rationales

## 1253. ANSWER: 1

1. **A layer of eschar or devitalized tissue commonly forms over partial- and full-thickness burns, which, when circumferential and when combined with increased fluid retention, can restrict circulation and lung expansion.**
2. Loss of tissue containing elastin and collagen does occur in partial- and full-thickness burns but would not be a source of constriction that would prevent lung expansion.
3. Ischemia and hypoxia may be experienced in the alveoli due to inhalation burns; however, restricted breathing (a mechanical process) is more of a risk due to circumferential eschar formation.
4. Although fluid overload is a possibility, it is not likely to restrict breathing unless it is combined with eschar formation.

▶ **Test-taking Tip:** *Key information in the stem is the character of the burn, its depth, extent, and the fact that it is circumferential. Eschar is devitalized tissue. Consider how this could restrict breathing.*

**Content Area:** Adult; **Concept:** Skin Integrity; Critical Thinking; **Integrated Processes:** Nursing Process: Analysis; **Client Needs:** Physiological Integrity: Reduction of Risk Potential; **Cognitive Level:** Analysis [Analyzing]

## 1254. ANSWER: 3

1. Ice causes vasoconstriction and can worsen the tissue damage.
2. The nurse should collect additional information before advising that the client be seen in the ED. A first-degree burn ordinarily does not require medical care.
3. **Cool water will minimize skin redness, pain, and swelling and limit tissue damage.**
4. Applying a skin ointment as an initial intervention can trap heat in the tissues; if it has an oily base, it can prevent healing.

▶ **Test-taking Tip:** *The key word is "singed," indicating that the burn is superficial. Consider actions for a first-degree burn.*

**Content Area:** Adult; **Concept:** Skin Integrity; Communication; **Integrated Processes:** Communication and Documentation; **Client Needs:** Physiological Integrity: Reduction of Risk Potential; **Cognitive Level:** Application [Applying]

## 1255. ANSWER: 4

1. Sodium is lost due to diuresis, and existing sodium tends to be diluted by an influx of fluid, so serum sodium levels will be decreased, not increased. Potassium may initially increase due to massive cellular destruction and release of intracellular potassium.
2. Hgb and Hct levels may change in severe burns, but they are the result of the fluid shift, not the cause.

3. Fluid volume deficit (not excess) is a major risk during this phase; therefore large amounts of IV fluids are administered. However, this does not explain the underlying physiological processes that cause the edema.
4. **Initially after a severe burn injury there is a loss of capillary integrity and a shift of fluid, sodium, and protein from the intravascular to the interstitial spaces. The body compensates for this interstitial hemoconcentration by retaining more fluid.**

▶ **Test-taking Tip:** *Visualize the damage to the cellular structures from a burn and how this would affect fluid balance.*

**Content Area:** Adult; **Concept:** Fluid and Electrolyte Balance; Skin Integrity; **Integrated Processes:** Nursing Process: Analysis; **Client Needs:** Physiological Integrity: Physiological Adaptation; **Cognitive Level:** Comprehension [Understanding]

## 1256. PHARM ANSWER: 4000

**Convert lb to kg (110 ÷ 2.2 – 50 kg). Then, use the Parkland formula provided: 4.0 mL × 50 kg = 200 mL; 200 mL × 40% TBSA burn = 8000 mL. Half of 8000 mL, or 4000 mL, is given in the first 8 hours after the burn.**

▶ **Test-taking Tip:** *Convert lb to kg. Read the formula carefully; then plug the values into the formula. If you change 40% to a decimal, you will get the wrong amount.*

**Content Area:** Adult; **Concept:** Fluid and Electrolyte Balance; Skin Integrity; **Integrated Processes:** Nursing Process: Planning; **Client Needs:** Physiological Integrity: Pharmacological and Parenteral Therapies; **Cognitive Level:** Application [Applying]

## 1257. ANSWER: 2

1. This is not a first-degree burn. In a first-degree burn the skin may appear red but intact, no weeping, and no blistering. In an adult, one upper extremity is approximately 9% of the TBSA. However, in this example both upper extremities are burned, which equals 18% TBSA.
2. **Partial-thickness burns damage the dermis and epidermis, often resulting in loss of epidermis and/or blistering. Each entire upper extremity is blistered. Approximately 18% of the TBSA has a partial-thickness burn (9% TBSA per each upper extremity).**
3. With full-thickness burns there would be loss of tissue and a black or white charred/waxy appearance to the remaining tissues. In addition, the % TBSA is too high for a burn affecting only the upper extremities.
4. With full-thickness burns there would also be loss of tissue and a black or white charred/waxy appearance. In addition, the % TBSA is too high for a burn affecting only the upper extremities.

▶ *Test-taking Tip:* To calculate % TBSA, use the palmar rule, where the client's palm size equals 1%; or apply the Rule of Nines for calculating, where each upper extremity equals 9%; or visualize the body and estimate the % TBSA for both upper extremities. Pick the option that is closest to your estimate.

**Content Area:** Adult; **Concept:** Skin Integrity; Communication; **Integrated Processes:** Communication and Documentation; **Client Needs:** Physiological Integrity: Physiological Adaptation; **Cognitive Level:** Analysis [Analyzing]

## 1258. PHARM ANSWER: 1, 2

1. **Silver sulfadiazine (Silvadene) is only applied to opened areas; this statement indicates client understanding of the instructions.**
2. **Silver sulfadiazine is used to reduce/prevent bacterial growth and thus an infection; this statement indicates client understanding of the instructions.**
3. Dressings can be applied but are not necessary; this statement does not indicate client understanding.
4. Removal of old ointment with a tongue blade can damage new granulation tissue; this statement does not indicate client understanding.
5. The cream is white in color and water-soluble; if it darkens it should not be used; this statement does not indicate client understanding.

▶ *Test-taking Tip:* Options with absolute words such as "never" are usually incorrect.

**Content Area:** Adult; **Concept:** Skin Integrity; Nursing Roles; **Integrated Processes:** Nursing Process: Evaluation; **Client Needs:** Physiological Integrity: Pharmacological and Parenteral Therapies; **Cognitive Level:** Evaluation [Evaluating]

## 1259. ANSWER: 1

1. **The graft must be immobilized so that it can remain in place and be able to revascularize.**
2. The client cannot place weight on the graft site. Bearing weight causes trauma.
3. The graft site has to stay immobile. There can be no weight on the graft site.
4. A dependent position impairs circulation and may cause further tissue injury.

▶ *Test-taking Tip:* Anything that may loosen the graft should be avoided.

**Content Area:** Adult; **Concept:** Skin Integrity; Perioperative; **Integrated Processes:** Nursing Process: Planning; **Client Needs:** Physiological Integrity: Reduction of Risk Potential; **Cognitive Level:** Application [Applying]

## 1260. PHARM ANSWER: 3

1. Bismuth subsalicylate (Kaopectate) is an antidiarrheal medication.
2. Gold sodium thiomalate (Aurolate) is used to treat rheumatoid arthritis resistant to conventional therapy.
3. **Silver sulfadiazine (Silvadene) is a topical anti-infective agent for prevention and treatment of wound infection in second- and third-degree burn clients.**
4. Arsenic trioxide (Trisenox) is an antineoplastic.

▶ *Test-taking Tip:* Note the key word "topically" in the stem. Only one option is a topical medication.

**Content Area:** Adult; **Concept:** Medication; Infection; Skin Integrity; **Integrated Processes:** Nursing Process: Planning; **Client Needs:** Physiological Integrity: Pharmacological and Parenteral Therapies; **Cognitive Level:** Application [Applying]

## 1261. ANSWER: 1, 3, 4

1. **Reiterating statements of orientation to the client decreases confusion.**
2. Turning and repositioning improves circulation and aeration but does not affect confusion. Turning can increase the client's anxiety.
3. **Familiar objects reduce anxiety when clients are in unfamiliar surroundings.**
4. **Employing a regular schedule for sleep-wake cycles assists in decreasing confusion and anxiety.**
5. Closing the door of the room may increase client anxiety.
6. In the acute phase of burns, the client is too ill to write notes to family members.

▶ *Test-taking Tip:* Note the key phrase "anxiety and confusion" and focus on interventions that can decrease these symptoms. You should be alert that the client is critical.

**Content Area:** Adult; **Concept:** Stress; Sensory Perception; Skin Integrity; **Integrated Processes:** Nursing Process: Implementation; Caring; **Client Needs:** Physiological Integrity: Basic Care and Comfort; Psychosocial Integrity; **Cognitive Level:** Application [Applying]

## 1262. MoC ANSWER: 36

**According to the Rule of Nines, this client sustained injuries on about 36% of the body surface: right arm is 4.5%; left arm is 4.5%; left leg is 9%; anterior chest and abdomen are 18%.**

▶ *Test-taking Tip:* Use the Rule of Nines. The body is divided into areas of multiples of 9% with the perineal area being 1%. The palm of the client's hand is approximately equal to 1%.

**Content Area:** Adult; **Concept:** Skin Integrity; Communication; **Integrated Processes:** Communication and Documentation; **Client Needs:** Safe and Effective Care Environment: Management of Care; Physiological Integrity: Reduction of Risk Potential; **Cognitive Level:** Analysis [Analyzing]

## 1263. MoC ANSWER: 3

1. A $Paco_2$ 35 mm Hg is WNL. Hyperglycemia does occur in sepsis.
2. Abnormal clotting may occur with sepsis, but hypoglycemia does not.
3. **T 103.2°F (39.6°C) and HR 120 bpm may indicate that the client has sepsis.**
4. An RR of 34 breaths/min may indicate sepsis, but the WBC is WNL.

▶ *Test-taking Tip:* Two or more of the following clinical signs and symptoms suggest sepsis: T >38°C (100.4°F) or <36°C (96.8°F); HR >90 bpm; RR >30 breaths/min; $Paco_2$ <32 mm Hg; WBC count >12,000 cells/mm³, <4000 cells/mm³, or >10% immature WBCs (bands); hyperglycemia; and abnormal clotting and bleeding.

## 1264. ANSWER: 3

1. The phosphorus level decreases in malnutrition as well as other conditions, but this is not the best indicator of inadequate nutrition.
2. The platelets are essential to blood clotting and may or may not be altered with inadequate nutrition.
3. **Prealbumin is used to evaluate nutritional status. A low level of prealbumin indicates inadequate nutrition. Prealbumin has a half-life of 2 days and reflects changes in serum protein stores more rapidly than other indices.**
4. Potassium is the major cation within the cell and may be low due to renal failure or GI disorders. It may or may not be altered with inadequate nutrition.

♦ **Test-taking Tip:** Note the key words "inadequate nutrition" and focus on what this means. Eliminate options that do not measure protein stores.

## 1265. PHARM ANSWER: 4

1. Removal of mafenide is unnecessary because burning and stinging with application is a normal response.
2. Notifying the HCP is unnecessary because burning and stinging with application is a normal response.
3. Mafenide cream is supplied in 11.2% cream; there are no other concentrations available.
4. **Burning or stinging with application of mafenide (Sulfamylon) is a normal response. Mafenide is bacteriostatic and used to reduce gram-negative and gram-positive organisms present in burned tissues.**

♦ **Test-taking Tip:** Think about your normal response when medication is applied to damaged tissue.

## 1266. ANSWER: 1, 2, 5

1. **The presence of a burning sensation may indicate that some acid remains on the skin and additional irrigation is needed.**
2. **The presence of pain, even though reduced, could indicate that not all of the acid has been removed from the skin.**
3. A pH of 7.0 indicates a nonacidic status, which would be a positive finding.
4. The absence of pain would indicate that all acid was removed before it could damage the skin.

5. **A pH of 4.8 is acidic and indicates there is still acid residue that needs to be removed.**

♦ **Test-taking Tip:** The key word is "continue." Consider which options require continued treatment. An acid has a low pH value. Use this information to narrow the options.

## 1267. MoC ANSWER: 3, 1, 2, 4

3. **Inhalation injury from smoke is the priority problem that should be addressed first to ensure that the client has a patent airway.**
1. **The 48% partial- and full-thickness burn injury should be addressed next. Fluid loss will occur from the exposed tissues, and the client will have pain that should be treated.**
2. **Laceration on the face that has stopped bleeding should be addressed third. The laceration may require suturing.**
4. **The history of hypertension can be addressed last. With fluid shifts and loss from the burn, the client's BP is likely to be low.**

♦ **Test-taking Tip:** Use the ABC's to establish priority.

## 1268. ANSWER: 1

1. **Electrical current will follow through the path of least resistance in the body, which is the bloodstream. The heart could have been damaged by the electrical current. Therefore obtaining a 12-lead ECG is priority.**
2. Pupil checks may be indicated if there was a fall or period of unconsciousness, but this information was not provided in the stem.
3. Lung sounds should be assessed eventually, but electrical current will follow through the path of least resistance in the body, which is the bloodstream. Therefore the heart warrants priority assessment.
4. ROM may be assessed eventually, but it is not a priority based on the ABC's of medical emergencies.

♦ **Test-taking Tip:** Use the ABC's to identify priority areas to assess. Electricity follows the path of least resistance in the body (the bloodstream).

**1269.** MoC **ANSWER: 2**

1. A cadaver skin graft does not use the client's own skin, so the client will not have a donor site.
2. **A cadaver skin graft is a type of temporary graft, also called a biological dressing, and it is used to protect the damaged skin and promote healing and epithelialization.**
3. Cadaver skin grafts use human skin, so there is the risk of transmitting blood-borne infections and diseases.
4. A cadaver skin graft is a temporary measure to promote healing; it is not permanent.

▶ *Test-taking Tip: The key word is "cadaver." Use this to eliminate options.*

Content Area: Adult; Concept: Skin Integrity; Nursing Roles; Management; Integrated Processes: Nursing Process: Evaluation; Client Needs: Safe and Effective Care Environment: Management of Care; Cognitive Level: Evaluation [Evaluating]

**1270. ANSWER: 3**

1. Normal WBC is 4500 to 11,100 microL. When reported in microL, 1 microL equals 1 $mm^3$. The normal WBC can also be reported as $4.5–11.1 \times 10^3$/microL.
2. Clean wounds have serosanguineous drainage.
3. **An elevated temperature could be a sign of an infection.**
4. Decreased urine output can indicate dehydration or renal failure.

▶ *Test-taking Tip: Focus on the general signs of an infection. Think about yourself when you have an infection and the common symptom experienced.*

Content Area: Adult; Concept: Assessment; Infection; Skin Integrity; Integrated Processes: Nursing Process: Assessment; Client Needs: Physiological Integrity: Reduction of Risk Potential; Cognitive Level: Application [Applying]

**1271. ANSWER: 2**

1. Wound cultures are used to confirm an infection but do not prevent one.
2. **Pseudomonas has been found in plants and flowers, which may be a source of wound infection.**
3. The use of clean technique may be used instead of sterile technique in certain burn units. However, the use of sterile technique would eliminate additional sources of infection during wound care.
4. Due to an increased metabolism, clients with burns typically require higher than normal doses of antibiotics to maintain effective blood levels. Continual low-dose infusions would not be effective.

▶ *Test-taking Tip: One option is different from the others. Often the option that is different is the answer.*

Content Area: Adult; Concept: Infection; Skin Integrity; Integrated Processes: Nursing Process: Implementation; Client Needs: Safe and Effective Care Environment: Safety and Infection Control; Cognitive Level: Application [Applying]

**1272. ANSWER: 3, 4, 5**

1. Daily wound cultures are unnecessary, as all wounds contain bacteria.
2. The wound should be cleansed gently to prevent further tissue trauma.
3. **The dressing protects the underlying wound and provides a moist environment for healing. Pressure ulcers left open to air are exposed to more contamination and potential injury.**
4. **The client should be repositioned at least every 2 hours and more often if the client has less tissue tolerance (e.g., elderly client).**
5. **Positioning devices are utilized to keep the load or pressure off the wound.**

▶ *Test-taking Tip: The goal of care is to promote tissue repair and regeneration. Eliminate options that are unnecessary or cause further tissue trauma.*

Content Area: Adult; Concept: Skin Integrity; Integrated Processes: Nursing Process: Planning; Client Needs: Physiological Integrity: Physiological Adaptation; Cognitive Level: Synthesis [Creating]

**1273. ANSWER: 3**

1. Stage I pressure ulcer is skin that is intact but red and nonblanching.
2. Stage II pressure ulcer involves a break in the skin with partial-thickness skin loss of epidermis or dermis.
3. **Stage III pressure ulcer is full-thickness skin loss that extends to the subcutaneous fat, but not fascia; bone, tendon, and muscle are not visible.**
4. Stage IV pressure ulcer is full-thickness skin loss with exposed muscle and bone.

▶ *Test-taking Tip: Narrow the options to Stage II and III because Stage I would not have a break in the skin, and Stage IV would be the worst and include exposed muscle and bone.*

Content Area: Adult; Concept: Skin Integrity; Communication; Integrated Processes: Communication and Documentation; Client Needs: Physiological Integrity: Physiological Adaptation; Cognitive Level: Analysis [Analyzing]

**1274. ANSWER: 4**

1. Applying padding helps reduce tissue pressure that restricts blood flow but does not limit shearing forces.
2. Obtaining an air pressure mattress helps reduce tissue pressure that restricts blood flow but does not limit shearing forces.
3. Using a lift sheet helps reduce friction but does not limit shearing forces.
4. **Keeping the HOB higher than 30 degrees increases the shearing forces to the shoulders, sacrum, and heels. When higher than 30 degrees, the client's skin layers in these areas are pulled away from underlying tissue, and blood vessels may become pinched.**

▶ *Test-taking Tip: Shearing forces are those that cause the skin to be pulled away from underlying tissue.*

Content Area: Adult; Concept: Skin Integrity; Integrated Processes: Nursing Process: Implementation; Client Needs: Physiological Integrity: Basic Care and Comfort; Cognitive Level: Application [Applying]

## 1275. ANSWER: 3

1. Fruit salad is composed of complex carbohydrates and is a high-fiber food. Adequate protein is needed to prevent the development of pressure ulcers.
2. Oatmeal is a grain, a high-fiber food. Adequate protein is needed to help prevent the development of pressure ulcers.
3. **Chicken is a high-protein food. Proteins are needed to help meet the body's needs for tissue repair and to maintain skin integrity.**
4. A lettuce and tomato salad is composed of complex carbohydrates and is high-fiber food. Adequate protein is needed to help prevent the development of pressure ulcers.

▶ *Test-taking Tip: Three options are similar, and one is different. Often the option that is different is the answer.*

Content Area: Adult; Concept: Nutrition; Skin Integrity; Nursing Roles; Integrated Processes: Teaching/Learning; Client Needs: Physiological Integrity: Basic Care and Comfort; Health Promotion and Maintenance; Cognitive Level: Application [Applying]

## 1276. ANSWER: 3

1. Natural light or a halogen light should be used. Fluorescent light produces a bluish tone to the dark skin, making it more difficult to see skin changes.
2. Dark skin does not blanch (turn white) when pressure is applied.
3. **In a dark-skinned client, injured skin may appear darker than surrounding skin.**
4. Red tones are absent in very dark-skinned persons. Areas of inflammation may appear purplish-blue or violet rather than appearing erythematous.

▶ *Test-taking Tip: Remember that signs of inflammation and tissue injury are different for dark-skinned clients. Only one option focuses on the difference in skin appearance between dark-skinned and light-skinned persons.*

Content Area: Adult; Concept: Skin Integrity; Diversity; Assessment; Integrated Processes: Nursing Process: Assessment; Culture and Spirituality; Client Needs: Physiological Integrity: Reduction of Risk Potential; Cognitive Level: Application [Applying]

## 1277. ANSWER: 1

1. **Cellulitis is an infection with diffuse inflammation occurring in the tissue just under the skin. Observing a decrease in swelling is evidence of improvement.**
2. Circulation is not involved with cellulitis, so there should be no change in the intensity of pedal pulses.
3. Increased erythema (redness) indicates that cellulitis is worsening, not improving.
4. The WBC of 14,000/mm$^3$ is elevated, indicating an infection is present. Normal WBC is 4500 to 11,100/mm$^3$ or /microL.

▶ *Test-taking Tip: The suffix "-itis" indicates inflammation. Only one option is associated with inflammation.*

Content Area: Adult; Concept: Infection; Skin Integrity; Integrated Processes: Nursing Process: Evaluation; Client Needs: Physiological Integrity: Physiological Adaptation; Cognitive Level: Evaluation [Evaluating]

## 1278. ANSWER: 4

1. Cellulitis is caused by a bacterial (not fungal) infection, most commonly *Streptococcus pyogenes*.
2. Cellulitis is treated with antibiotics, not a topical fungicide.
3. Herpes zoster (shingles) infection is sometimes complicated by neuralgic pain after the acute infection and not cellulitis or tinea pedis.
4. **Cellulitis is an infection with diffuse inflammation occurring in the tissue just under the skin. Chronic athlete's foot causes minute breaks in the skin, allowing bacteria on the skin to enter the tissue and cause the infectious process.**

▶ *Test-taking Tip: Tinea pedis is athlete's foot. Consider the effects from the loss of skin integrity occurring with athlete's foot.*

Content Area: Adult; Concept: Infection; Skin Integrity; Integrated Processes: Nursing Process: Analysis; Client Needs: Physiological Integrity: Physiological Adaptation; Cognitive Level: Analysis [Analyzing]

## 1279. ANSWER: 3

1. Serous drainage and pus are associated with infection and would only be present if the vesicles were infected.
2. Nodular lesions are not associated with a herpes zoster infection, but a burning sensation may be present.
3. **The nurse should associate pain and pruritus (itching) with herpes zoster. Herpes zoster follows the path of peripheral sensory nerves; symptoms come from the nerve involvement.**
4. Macule lesions may occur early in the condition, but petechiae are not associated with herpes zoster.

▶ *Test-taking Tip: Use the letter P as a cue to remember the different signs and symptoms of herpes zoster; pain, pruritus, and paresthesias are common symptoms associated with herpes zoster. Both factors in the option must be correct for the option to be the answer.*

Content Area: Adult; Concept: Skin Integrity; Assessment; Integrated Processes: Nursing Process: Assessment; Client Needs: Physiological Integrity: Physiological Adaptation; Cognitive Level: Application [Applying]

## 1280. ANSWER: 1, 4, 5

1. **Itching is a common symptom of psoriasis.**
2. Nail involvement may include thickening, discoloration, and pitting; pink and clear describes normal nailbeds.
3. Hair is dry and brittle, not oily.
4. **Psoriatic patches are red, scaly plaques with silvery scales.**
5. **Psoriatic patches occur most often on elbows, knees, scalp, palms, and soles.**

▶ *Test-taking Tip:* First narrow the options by eliminating options with normal findings. Then eliminate the one option that is inconsistent with the other options (e.g., dry versus oily).

**Content Area:** Adult; **Concept:** Skin Integrity; Assessment; **Integrated Processes:** Nursing Process: Assessment; **Client Needs:** Physiological Integrity: Physiological Adaptation; **Cognitive Level:** Knowledge [Remembering]

## 1281. PHARM ANSWER: 1

1. **Treatment with methoxsalen (Uvadex) enhances sensitivity of the eyes to the sunlight. Sunglasses that provide UVB protection need to be worn for at least 24 hours following treatments.**
2. Certain skin ointments may be prescribed as part of the therapeutic regimen for the client receiving UV light treatments for psoriasis.
3. Temperature is monitored to detect infection, hyperthermia, or hypothermia, none of which are risks for this client.
4. Redness and erythema are normal responses to this treatment, and treatment should not be stopped if these occur.

▶ *Test-taking Tip:* The key words are "UV" and "precaution." Focus on the option that uses the same or similar words as the stem.

**Content Area:** Adult; **Concept:** Nursing Roles; Skin Integrity; Medication; **Integrated Processes:** Teaching/Learning; **Client Needs:** Safe and Effective Care Environment: Safety and Infection Control; Physiological Integrity: Pharmacological and Parenteral Therapies; **Cognitive Level:** Application [Applying]

## 1282. PHARM ANSWER: 2, 5

1. Methotrexate has no effect on serum potassium levels unless complications arise; routine monitoring is unnecessary.
2. **The nurse should monitor liver function tests because methotrexate (Trexall) is metabolized by the liver, and a side effect of methotrexate is hepatotoxicity.**
3. If the client is a diabetic, the blood glucose should be monitored; there is no indication that the client is a diabetic.
4. Obtaining ABGs is an invasive test and would not be prescribed for routine monitoring of methotrexate use.
5. **The nurse should monitor WBCs because a side effect of methotrexate use is leukopenia.**

▶ *Test-taking Tip:* To narrow the options, consider that methotrexate is cytotoxic and affects cells. Only Options 2 and 5 pertain to cells.

**Content Area:** Adult; **Concept:** Medication; Skin Integrity; **Integrated Processes:** Nursing Process: Assessment; **Client Needs:** Physiological Integrity: Reduction of Risk Potential; Physiological Integrity: Pharmacological and Parenteral Therapies; **Cognitive Level:** Application [Applying]

## 1283. PHARM ANSWER: 3

1. The client has acne vulgaris, an inflammatory disease involving the sebaceous glands of the skin characterized by papules or pustules or comedones.
2. Adapalene should be applied once daily in the evening.
3. **The nurse should exclude exposing the back to the sun after adapalene (Differin) is applied. This increases the risk for sunburn. Adapalene should also not be applied to sunburned areas.**
4. Only a thin film of adapalene should be applied. Excessive application will not result in faster healing but will cause marked redness, peeling, and discomfort.

▶ *Test-taking Tip:* The key word is "exclude."

**Content Area:** Adult; **Concept:** Skin Integrity; Medication; Nursing Roles; **Integrated Processes:** Teaching/Learning; **Client Needs:** Physiological Integrity: Pharmacological and Parenteral Therapies; **Cognitive Level:** Analysis [Analyzing]

## 1284. PHARM ANSWER: 1

1. **A systemic retinoic acid drug is teratogenic. A sexually active female must be instructed to practice birth control while taking this class of drugs, to avoid pregnancy.**
2. Asking allergy questions is important, but they should have been asked before the medication was prescribed.
3. Asking about skin dryness and sensitivity is important but not the priority.
4. Taking the medication as scheduled is important to prevent complications but is not the priority.

▶ *Test-taking Tip:* Rule out options that do not address a serious complication.

**Content Area:** Adult; **Concept:** Skin Integrity; Medication; Assessment; **Integrated Processes:** Nursing Process: Assessment; Caring; **Client Needs:** Physiological Integrity: Pharmacological and Parenteral Therapies; Health Promotion and Maintenance; **Cognitive Level:** Application [Applying]

## 1285. ANSWER:

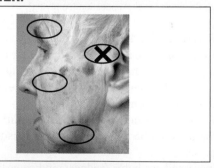

An incision either in front or behind the ear is made during rhytidectomy to remove excess skin and treat muscle laxity of the face. Incisions are made in the forehead and periorbital area for blepharoplasty and browlift. Head and neck reconstruction utilizes the chin site.

♦ **Test-taking Tip:** *Focus on the key word "facelift." If unsure, think about the area for the incision that would best pull the skin upward.*

**Content Area:** Adult; **Concept:** Nursing Roles; Skin Integrity; **Integrated Processes:** Teaching/Learning; **Client Needs:** Physiological Integrity: Reduction of Risk Potential; **Cognitive Level:** Application [Applying]

## 1286. ANSWER: 4

1. Fasting before surgery is a standard practice and poses no significant risk to the client.
2. This comment indicates uncertainty, but reassurance and explanations can help the client cope. The comment does not pose a direct risk in terms of obtaining an optimal cosmetic outcome.
3. High BP that is controlled with medication such as lisinopril (Prinivil) poses no significant risk to the client and would not adversely affect the cosmetic outcome.
4. **Diclofenac (Voltaren) is an NSAID; increased bleeding tendency and increased sensitivity to sunlight are side effects that may inhibit achieving optimal cosmetic outcomes.**

♦ **Test-taking Tip:** *When reviewing the options, consider the side effects of NSAIDS.*

**Content Area:** Adult; **Concept:** Skin Integrity; Nursing Roles; Medication; **Integrated Processes:** Nursing Process: Evaluation; **Client Needs:** Physiological Integrity: Reduction of Risk Potential; Psychosocial Integrity; **Cognitive Level:** Evaluation [Evaluating]

## 1287. MoC PHARM ANSWER: 1, 3, 5

1. **Tretinoin (Retin-A) should not be applied to open wounds; the experienced nurse should intervene.**
2. Isotretinoin (Amnesteem) is teratogenic and a pregnancy category X, indicating it should not be used in pregnancy. Withholding isotretinoin until the pregnancy test results are available and the pregnancy status is known is appropriate.
3. **Actinic keratosis is rough, sandpaper-like red or brown papules from excessive sun exposure. Treatment using fluorouracil (Carac) causes the affected area to become worse before getting better; the medication should not be withheld, and the nurse should intervene.**
4. Tacrolimus (Protopic) should not be applied within 2 hours of emollient or lotion application. This client just applied lotion, so it is appropriate to wait 2 hours to apply the medication; the nurse should also document the reason that the medication was delayed.
5. **When taking acitretin (Soriatane), the client should not become pregnant for 3 years following treatment; the experienced nurse should intervene to correct this information.**

♦ **Test-taking Tip:** *The experienced nurse should intervene when observing the less-experienced nurse performing actions incorrectly.*

**Content Area:** Adult; **Concept:** Management; Skin Integrity; Medication; **Integrated Processes:** Nursing Process: Implementation; **Client Needs:** Safe and Effective Care Environment: Management of Care; Physiological Integrity: Pharmacological and Parenteral Therapies; **Cognitive Level:** Analysis [Analyzing]

## 1288. MoC ANSWER: 1

1. **The skin of a person with pemphigus is so fragile that touching the skin can cause it to tear; the experienced nurse should intervene.**
2. In scleroderma, the skin is dry and itching. These can be relieved by emollient application.
3. Lesions of herpes simplex are contagious for approximately 2 to 4 days until dry crusts form.
4. Ultraviolet light with or without photosensitizing agents is a treatment option for acne vulgaris.

♦ **Test-taking Tip:** *When reviewing the options, think about the option that could cause harm for the client with the diagnosis indicated. The option that could cause harm would be the answer.*

**Content Area:** Adult; **Concept:** Skin Integrity; Management; **Integrated Processes:** Nursing Process: Evaluation; **Client Needs:** Safe and Effective Care Environment: Management of Care; **Cognitive Level:** Evaluation [Evaluating]

## 1289. PHARM ANSWER: 3

1. Occlusive dressings should be avoided to prevent systemic absorption.
2. The affected area should be washed and dried prior to application of miconazole.
3. **Tinea pedis is athlete's foot. Miconazole (Lotrimin AF) should be massaged into the affected area.**
4. Miconazole should be continued for the full course of therapy, not discontinued when symptoms resolve.

♦ **Test-taking Tip:** *Pedis pertains to foot. Use this as a clue to narrow the options to those that identify the foot.*

**Content Area:** Adult; **Concept:** Nursing Roles; Skin Integrity; Medication; **Integrated Processes:** Teaching/Learning; **Client Needs:** Physiological Integrity: Pharmacological and Parenteral Therapies; Health Promotion and Maintenance; **Cognitive Level:** Application [Applying]

## 1290. ANSWER: 4

1. Image 1 shows patchy loss of skin pigmentation called vitiligo.
2. Image 2 shows trichotillomania, a type of hair loss from compulsive pulling and/or twisting of the hair.
3. Image 3 shows blistering, redness, and a white patch between the fingers, characteristic of candidiasis.
4. **Image 4 shows atopic dermatitis, which is characterized by redness and irregular, scaly lesions.**

♦ **Test-taking Tip:** *Break down the word dermatitis; "derm-" refers to skin and the suffix "-itis" means inflammation. Rule out options that do not show signs of inflammation.*

**Content Area:** Adult; **Concept:** Skin Integrity; Assessment; **Integrated Processes:** Nursing Process: Assessment; **Client Needs:** Physiological Integrity: Reduction of Risk Potential; **Cognitive Level:** Application [Applying]

## 1291. ANSWER: 3

1. Serosanguineous drainage occurs with normal-healing wounds. Fever occurs with wound infections.
2. Malaise and local edema occur with wound infections.
3. **The most common symptoms of a scabies infestation are itching and papule rash.**
4. Macule rash and blisters may occur with allergic reactions.

▶ *Test-taking Tip: A papule is a small, solid circumscribed bump in the skin, whereas a macule is a flat, circumscribed area of the skin that is discolored. Use this information to narrow the options.*

**Content Area:** Adult; **Concept:** Infection; Skin Integrity; Assessment; **Integrated Processes:** Nursing Process: Assessment; **Client Needs:** Physiological Integrity: Physiological Adaptation; **Cognitive Level:** Application [Applying]

## Chapter Twenty-Nine

# Musculoskeletal Management

**1292.** The nurse is caring for the client following a knee arthroscopy. What information should the nurse teach? **Select all that apply.**

1. Elevate the involved extremity on pillows for 24 to 48 hours.
2. Apply an ice pack continually to the involved joint for 24 hours.
3. Report severe joint pain immediately to the HCP.
4. Resume usual activities to minimize joint stiffness and swelling.
5. Treat pain with a mild analgesic such as acetaminophen.

**1293.** The client is being seen in the clinic for a second-degree ankle sprain. Which treatments should the nurse plan?

1. Rest, elevate the extremity, apply ice intermittently, and apply a compression bandage.
2. Do range of motion to determine the extent of injury, apply heat, and check circulation.
3. Use moist heat and then apply ice; check circulation, motion, and sensation; and elevate.
4. Refer to an orthopedic surgeon, apply ice, give an analgesic, elevate, and encourage rest.

**1294.** The nurse is assessing the client who is to have a closed reduction for a right elbow dislocation. Which should be the nurse's **priority?**

1. Presence of bruising to the right elbow
2. Pain level rating on a 0 to 10 scale
3. Sensation and pulse of the right forearm
4. Left-handed or right-handed

**1295.** The client has an external fixator for reduction of a tibia fracture. The nurse is evaluating the client's effectiveness in ambulating with crutches. Place an X on each of the three areas where the client should be bearing weight when crutch walking.

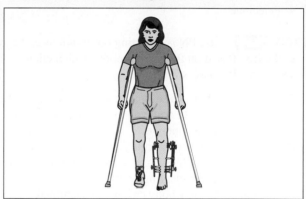

**1296.** MoC  An hour ago, the HCP split the client's forearm cast due to severe arm pain, throbbing, and tingling. When the client's symptoms return, which nursing action is **most** important?

1. Administer an intravenous pain medication.
2. Notify the HCP immediately.
3. Cut the cast padding and spread the cast further.
4. Elevate the arm on pillows above heart level.

**1297.** MoC  The nurse is caring for the client involved in an MVA who sustained an unstable pelvic fracture. Which HCP order should be the nurse's **priority?**

1. Do urinalysis and urine culture and sensitivity.
2. Do blood alcohol level and toxicology screen.
3. Have CT scan of the pelvis completed.
4. Give two units of cross-matched whole blood.

**1298.** The nurse is teaching the client who has a lower leg plaster of Paris cast. Which self-care instructions should the nurse include? **Select all that apply.**

1. Sprinkle powder in the cast to decrease moisture from sweating.
2. Direct cool air from a hair dryer into the cast to relieve itching.
3. Cover the cast with a plastic wrap before bathing in a tub.
4. Use hot, soapy water to wash the cast if it becomes very soiled.
5. Avoid the cast's contact with hard surfaces while it is drying

**1299.** The client with a pelvic fracture developed a fat embolism. The nurse should assess the client for which specific sign?

1. Dyspnea
2. Chest pain
3. Delirium
4. Petechiae

**1300.** MoC The LPN is reporting observations and cares to the RN. Based on the LPN's report, which client should the RN assess immediately?

1. The client, 2 hours post–total knee replacement, who has 100 mL bloody drainage in the autotransfusion drainage system container
2. The client with a crush injury to the arm who was given another analgesic and a skeletal muscle relaxant for throbbing, unrelenting pain
3. The client in a new body cast who was turned every 2 hours and is being supported with waterproof pillows
4. The client with a left leg external fixator who has serous drainage from the pin sites, and pulses are present by Doppler

**1301.** The nurse assesses that the client has some finger swelling of a newly casted right arm fracture with no other abnormal findings. Which is the nurse's **priority** action?

1. Notify the HCP immediately.
2. Split the cast to prevent constriction.
3. Elevate the casted arm on pillows.
4. Document the degree of finger swelling.

**1302.** The nurse is reviewing the laboratory results of the client with DM prior to surgical removal of pins used to stabilize a compound ankle fracture. Based on the results, which action should the nurse take?

| Client's Serum Lab | Client's Value |
| --- | --- |
| Creatinine (SCr) | 1.1 mg/dL |
| Potassium | 4.1 mEq/L |
| Glucose | 79 mg/dL |
| WBC | 17,900/mm³ |
| Hgb | 14.1 g/dL |
| Hct | 40% |

1. Notify the surgeon because the white blood cell count is elevated.
2. Notify the anesthesiologist because multiple lab values are abnormal.
3. Give potassium chloride 10 mEq in 100 mL NaCl per agency protocol.
4. Continue to prepare the client for the scheduled pin removal surgery.

**1303.** The clinic nurse completed teaching the client with a rotator cuff tear who is being treated conservatively. Which client statement indicates that further teaching is needed?

1. "I received a corticosteroid injection in my shoulder to reduce the inflammation and pain."
2. "Now that the pain is controlled, I can do progressive stretching and strengthening exercises."
3. "I will continue to take ibuprofen for pain control, but I should take it with food."
4. "I will need an open acromioplasty to repair the torn cuff after the swelling is reduced."

**1304.** The client, admitted to the ED, verbalizes extreme shoulder pain. The nurse sees that the client's right arm is shorter than the left. What should the nurse do **initially? Select all that apply.**

1. Lift the right arm to support it with a pillow.
2. Apply a covered ice pack to the left shoulder.
3. Prepare the client for immediate surgical repair.
4. Check the pulses and sensation of the right arm.
5. Prepare to administer an analgesic as prescribed.

**1305.** The nurse is assessing the client diagnosed with a left femoral neck fracture. Which findings should the nurse expect? **Select all that apply.**

1. Left leg is in an abducted position.
2. Left leg is externally rotated.
3. Left leg is shorter than the right.
4. Pain is in the lateral left knee.
5. Pain is in the groin area.

**1306.** MoC The client with DM is admitted with possible osteomyelitis secondary to an ankle wound. The client's ankle is painful, red, swollen, and warm, and the wound is persistently draining. The client's temperature is 102.2°F (39°C). Based on the client's status, which HCP order should the nurse plan to defer until later?

1. Obtain a culture of the ankle wound.
2. Administer ceftriaxone 1 g IV q12h.
3. Apply splint to immobilize the ankle.
4. Teach on IV antibiotic self-administration.

**1307.** PHARM The nurse is to administer nafcillin 500 mg intravenously to the client with osteomyelitis. A vial of 1 g of powdered nafcillin is to be reconstituted with 3.4 mL of 0.9% NaCl. How many mL should the nurse plan to administer?

_____ mL (Round your answer to tenths.)

**1308.** The client has Buck's traction to temporarily immobilize a fracture of the proximal femur prior to surgery. Which assessment finding requires the nurse to intervene **immediately?**

1. Reddened area at the client's coccygeal area
2. Voiding concentrated urine at 50 mL/hr
3. Capillary refill 3 seconds, pedal pulses palpable
4. Ropes, pulleys intact; 5-lb weight hangs freely

**1309.** MoC The client has been in a body cast for the past 2 days to treat numerous broken vertebrae from a fall. The client is reporting dyspnea, vomiting, epigastric pain, and abdominal distention. Which action demonstrates the nurse's **best** clinical judgment?

1. Immediately notify the HCP.
2. Initiate oxygen at 2 liters per nasal cannula.
3. Place ice packs around the outside of the cast.
4. Administer ondansetron prescribed q6h prn.

**1310.** MoC The experienced nurse observes the new nurse caring for the client who is in skeletal traction to stabilize a proximal femur fracture prior to surgery. Which observation by the experienced nurse indicates the new nurse needs additional orientation?

1. Positions the client so the client's feet stay clear of the bottom of the bed
2. Checks ropes so that they are positioned in the wheel groves of the pulleys
3. Removes weights from ropes until the weights hang free of the bed frame
4. Performs pin site care with chlorhexidine solution once during the 8-hour shift

**1311.** The new NA assists the client who just had a left THR with repositioning in bed. The client hears a "pop" and has severe left groin and hip pain. Which is the most appropriate **initial** action by the nurse?

1. Check the position of the left leg.
2. Elevate the head of the client's bed.
3. Adjust the pillow used for abduction.
4. Give the prescribed pain medication.

**1312.** PHARM The client is 2 days post–right THR in which the traditional posterior approach was used. Which interventions should the nurse implement?

1. Checks that an elevated toilet seat is in place and assists the client to the bathroom using a walker
2. Removes the wedge pillow at the client's request and places pillows to maintain right leg adduction
3. Reinfuses 400-mL autotransfusion wound drainage returns from the past 24 hours
4. Assists the client to get out of bed on the left side so the client can stand to place and use the urinal

**1313.** The nurse is caring for the client 24 hours following total hip arthroplasty using the traditional posterior approach. Which interventions should the nurse plan to implement? **Select all that apply.**

1. Place pillows or a wedge pillow between the client's legs to keep them abducted.
2. Have the client flex the unaffected hip and use the trapeze to help move up in bed.
3. Raise the head of the bed to no more than 90 degrees when the bed is placed contour.
4. Place a pillow between the client's knees when initially assisting the client out of bed.
5. Apply antiembolism stockings that should be kept on for 24 hours postoperatively.

**1314.** The home health nurse is caring for clients who had a THR through the posterior surgical approach 2 weeks ago. It is most important for the nurse to intervene **immediately** for which client?

1.

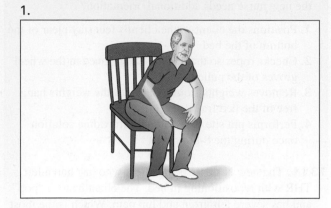

2.

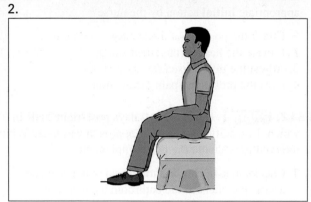

3.

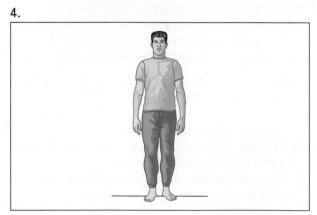

4.

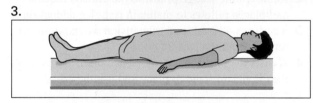

**1315.** **MoC** The nurse, caring for the client who had bilateral THRs 2 days ago, determines that the client will need a referral to manage exercises and stairs when at home. The nurse should plan to initiate a referral with which interdisciplinary team member?

1. Occupational therapist
2. Social worker
3. Physical therapist
4. Health care provider

**1316.** **MoC** The client, who is diagnosed with OA, tells the clinic nurse about the inability to ambulate and about staying on bedrest due to hip stiffness. In addition to teaching the client measures to reduce joint stiffness, which referral for the client should the nurse plan to discuss with the HCP?

1. Psychiatrist
2. Social worker
3. Physical therapist
4. Arthritis Foundation

**1317.** The client has had a right TKR. To prevent circulatory complications, the nurse should ensure that the client is performing which action?

1. Flexing both feet and exercising uninvolved joints every hour while awake
2. Using the continuous passive motion device (CPM) every 2 hours for 30 minutes
3. Being assisted up to a chair as soon as the effects of anesthesia have worn off
4. Using the trapeze to lift off the bed and then rotating each leg intermittently

**1318.** The nurse assesses the client 4 hours following a left TKR. The client has a knee immobilizer in place with medial and lateral packs that are warm. An autotransfusion wound drainage system has 350 mL collected. The client has not voided since before surgery but does not express a need. Which interventions should the nurse plan to implement at this time? **Select all that apply.**

1. Reinfuse the salvaged blood from the wound drainage system.
2. Remove the immobilizer to place the knee in 90-degree flexion.
3. Stand the client at the bedside to facilitate bladder emptying.
4. Place the left leg in a continuous passive motion device (CPM).
5. Replace the warm packs in the knee immobilizer with ice packs.

**1319.** MoC The nursing student is caring for the client who had a right TKR 1 day ago. Which action by the student requires the nurse to intervene?

1. Hands the client the control for the continuous passive motion (CPM) machine
2. Offers the client an analgesic when pain is rated at 3 on a 0 to 10 scale
3. Repositions the leg to insert an abductor pillow between the client's legs
4. Places an ice pack wrapped within a towel on the client's operative knee

**1320.** The nurse is assessing the client immediately following a C5–C6 anterior cervical discectomy. Which potential problem should be the nurse's **priority?**

1. Altered breathing pattern
2. Impaired tissue perfusion
3. Altered mobility
4. Impaired skin integrity

**1321.** PHARM The HCP prescribes cyclobenzaprine 30 mg orally tid for the client hospitalized with acute cervical neck pain. The pharmacy supplied 10-mg tablets. Which action by the nurse is **best?**

1. Administer three 10-mg tablets with food.
2. Call the HCP to question the dose prescribed.
3. Observe for drowsiness after administration.
4. Also give prn prescribed morphine sulfate IV.

**1322.** The college student consults the clinic nurse for advice on managing lower back pain. Which instructions should the nurse include? **Select all that apply.**

1. Continue routine activity within your pain tolerance while paying attention to correct posture.
2. Temporarily avoid lifting and other activities that increase mechanical stress on your spine.
3. When sleeping on your side, flex your hips and knees and place a pillow between your knees.
4. Stay at home for 2 weeks on bedrest to minimize physical activity and straining your back.
5. Stand intermittently during classes, and sit with a soft support at the small of your back.

**1323.** MoC The nurse assesses the client 6 hours following a lumbar spinal fusion. The client has a throbbing headache, but VS and CMS of the lower extremities are WNL. The lungs have fine basilar crackles. The back dressing has a dime-sized bloody spot surrounded by clear yellow drainage. Which nursing action demonstrates the nurse's **best** clinical judgment?

1. Give prescribed morphine sulfate IV.
2. Have the client cough and deep breathe.
3. Reinforce the incisional dressing.
4. Notify the HCP.

**1324.** The nurse is caring for the client who had a surgical repair of a right Dupuytren's contracture. Which intervention should the nurse plan?

1. Elevate the right lower extremity above the level of the heart.
2. Assist the client with bathing, dressing, grooming, and toileting.
3. Instruct about wearing low-heeled and properly fitting shoes.
4. Frequently rewrap the elastic bandage on the right extremity.

**1325.** The nurse is teaching the client with carpal tunnel syndrome how best to utilize a wrist splint. Which statement is **most** appropriate for the nurse to include in the teaching?

1. Leave the splint in place even when bathing.
2. Wear the splint as tight as can be tolerated.
3. Remove the splint intermittently throughout the day.
4. Only wear the splint when doing work that stresses the fingers.

**1326.** The client is to be discharged after receiving treatment for right shoulder tendonitis. Which actions indicate to the nurse that the client is ready for discharge? **Select all that apply.**

1. Discusses plan to resume normal activities in 1 to 2 days
2. Demonstrates proper use of an arm sling and the need to wear it during sleep
3. Verbalizes to keep the arm extended and flat on the mattress when lying in bed
4. Demonstrates how to properly apply the ice packs on the shoulder joint
5. States will take ibuprofen every 4 to 6 hours as needed for pain

**1327.** The nurse is assessing the client 3 months following a left shoulder arthroplasty. Which assessment findings should prompt the nurse to consider that the client may have developed osteomyelitis? **Select all that apply.**

1. Sudden onset of chills
2. Temperature 103°F (39.4°C)
3. Sudden onset of bradycardia
4. Pulsating shoulder pain that is worsening
5. Painful, swollen area on the left shoulder

**1328.** MoC The client is hospitalized following surgical repair of a hip fracture. The client informs the nurse about wishing to observe Ramadan, which is occurring now. Which statement by the nurse demonstrates an understanding of Ramadan?

1. "I'm going to uncover your hip and leg now to check the incision and your pulses."
2. "A dietitian helps to plan your meals so that meat and dairy products are not together."
3. "I've asked that physical therapy be postponed until around 3 p.m., when Ramadan ends."
4. "I should let the care team know not to bring food or beverages from sunrise to sunset."

**1329.** CJ The nurse is planning to teach the client about performing adduction of the right arm. Place an X at the location where the nurse should start the exercise and an arrow in the direction that the arm should move.

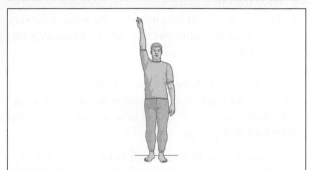

**1330.** The 25-year-old male has hypercalcemia. Further work-up revealed osteosarcoma of the distal femur. Which statement indicates the nurse's correct understanding of the client's diagnosis?

1. The tumor originated in the client's vascular system and metastasized to the bone.
2. Osteosarcoma is the most common and most often fatal primary malignant bone tumor.
3. The only treatment for osteosarcoma is a leg amputation well above the tumor growth.
4. The tumor is nonmalignant; it can be excised and the bone replaced with a bone graft.

**1331.** The client continues to have phantom limb pain following an AKA, despite receiving the prescribed morphine sulfate and using distraction. Which interventions, if prescribed, should the nurse plan to implement? **Select all that apply.**

1. Apply lidocaine patch 5% to the residual limb.
2. Start transcutaneous electrical nerve stimulation.
3. Give atenolol 12.5 mg orally bid with food.
4. Give oxcarbazepine 300 mg orally bid.
5. Limit activity until the sensations resolve.

**1332.** MoC The client with a lower leg amputation has edema, so the NA elevates the client's residual left limb on pillows. What is the **most** appropriate action by the nurse when observing that the client's leg has been elevated?

1. Thank the NA for being so observant and intervening appropriately to treat the client's edema of the residual limb.
2. Remove the pillows, raise the foot of the bed, and inform the NA that the limb should not be elevated on pillows because it could cause a flexion contracture.
3. Inform the NA that this was the correct action at this time in the client's recovery, but once the client's incision heals, the leg should not be elevated.
4. Report the incident to the surgeon and tell the NA to complete a variance report because the client's leg should not have been elevated.

**1333.** MoC The nurse starting the shift is determining priorities for the day. Prioritize the order that the nurse should plan to assess the four clients.

1. The client who had a left BKA and has left foot pain of 6 on a 0 to 10 scale
2. The client who has a right lower leg cast whose right foot is cold to the touch
3. The client who had a THR and 200-mL wound drain output during the past 8 hours
4. The client who had a spinal fusion and has not voided since the urinary catheter removal 4 hours ago

Answer: _____

**1334.** MoC While caring for multiple clients, the nurse delegates client skin care to the UAP on a musculoskeletal unit. Which client is **most** appropriate for the nurse to delegate skin care to the UAP?

1. The client with osteomyelitis of the tibia who needs a wound dressing change
2. The client with an inoperable hip fracture who is in Buck's traction
3. The client with a pelvic fracture who is in skeletal traction
4. The client with a femur fracture who has an external fixator in place

## *Answers and Rationales*

**1292. ANSWER: 1, 3, 5**

1. **Elevation will help to decrease edema.**
2. Ice should be applied intermittently (usually 20 to 30 minutes with 10- to 15-minute warming periods between applications). Hypothermia causes vasoconstriction and decreased circulation to the area.
3. **Severe joint pain may indicate a possible complication and should be reported immediately.**
4. Activity is initially limited and slowly progressed.
5. **Usually a mild analgesic such as acetaminophen (Tylenol) is sufficient for pain control following a diagnostic arthroscopy.**

♦ **Test-taking Tip:** *During a knee arthroscopy a scope is inserted through small incisions to visualize and examine the knee joint. Eliminate options that are unsafe following this procedure.*

**Content Area:** Adult; **Concept:** Promoting Health; Perioperative; Mobility; **Integrated Processes:** Teaching/Learning; **Client Needs:** Health Promotion and Maintenance; **Cognitive Level:** Application [Applying]

**1293. ANSWER: 1**

1. **Rest prevents further injury and promotes healing. Ice and elevation control swelling. Compression with an elastic bandage controls bleeding, reduces edema, and provides support for injured tissues.**
2. Performing ROM would be contraindicated initially because it causes pain and possible further injury. Heat causes vasodilation, increasing edema, and should not be used if swelling is present.
3. Heat causes vasodilation, increasing edema, and should not be used if swelling is present.
4. Immediate orthopedic referral is reserved for emergent, frequently open, injuries.

♦ **Test-taking Tip:** *A second-degree ankle sprain involves the tearing of ligament fibers, thus producing edema, tenderness, pain with motion, joint instability, and partial loss of normal joint function. To identify treatments, use the acronym RICE— rest, ice, compression, and elevation.*

**Content Area:** Adult; **Concept:** Critical Thinking; Mobility; Inflammation; **Integrated Processes:** Nursing Process: Planning; **Client Needs:** Physiological Integrity: Reduction of Risk Potential; **Cognitive Level:** Application [Applying]

**1294. ANSWER: 3**

1. Bruising is a common finding with dislocation. It can indicate bleeding in the tissue due to trauma, but that would not affect neurovascular status of the extremity.
2. Pain is expected with a dislocation; the client should be medicated before the procedure regardless of current pain level. After the procedure, pain management is a nursing priority but not as urgent as other assessments.

3. **Impairment of the neurovascular system is a priority. The closed reduction could cause further damage, which would be noted distal to the injury. Sensation and pulses are part of a neurovascular assessment to an extremity.**
4. Dominant hand is important to address in discharge instructions; this is not a priority before the reduction.

♦ **Test-taking Tip:** *The priority is to obtain baseline information that could indicate if serious complications are present prior to the procedure. You should use the ABC's to determine that circulation is a priority assessment.*

**Content Area:** Adult; **Concept:** Mobility; Assessment; **Integrated Processes:** Nursing Process: Assessment; **Client Needs:** Physiological Integrity: Reduction of Risk Potential; **Cognitive Level:** Application [Applying]

**1295. ANSWER:**

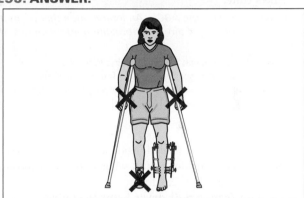

**The client should be bearing weight on the hand grips when bringing legs forward. When moving crutches, the weight should be borne on the unaffected leg.**

♦ **Test-taking Tip:** *Visualize crutch walking without bearing weight on the affected extremity.*

**Content Area:** Adult; **Concept:** Mobility; Nursing Roles; **Integrated Processes:** Nursing Process: Evaluation; **Client Needs:** Physiological Integrity: Basic Care and Comfort; **Cognitive Level:** Evaluation [Evaluating]

**1296.** MoC **ANSWER: 2**

1. Although an analgesic should be administered, it is more important to notify the HCP because these symptoms suggest compartment syndrome.
2. **The nurse should notify the HCP immediately because these symptoms suggest compartment syndrome, which is a medical emergency.**
3. Bivalving the cast further may not relieve the pressure area, and further intervention such as cast removal may now be required.
4. The nurse should elevate the arm to prevent edema and compartment syndrome; once compartment syndrome occurs, elevation is contraindicated because it further reduces perfusion to the extremity.

▶ *Test-taking Tip: When a question asks for the **most important** action when the client is experiencing a complication, the most important action is to notify the HCP.*

**Content Area:** Adult; **Concept:** Mobility; Safety; Management; **Integrated Processes:** Nursing Process: Implementation; Communication and Documentation; **Client Needs:** Safe and Effective Care Environment: Management of Care; **Cognitive Level:** Analysis [Analyzing]

## 1297. MoC ANSWER: 4

1. The client is at risk for fat emboli. Free fat may show in the urine, but this does not have priority.
2. The administration of analgesics and anesthetics is affected by blood alcohol and toxicology results, but this does not have priority.
3. CT of the pelvis will determine the extent of the fracture but does not have priority.
4. **Significant blood loss occurs because the pelvis is a highly vascular area. A type and cross-match must be completed prior to administering blood, which takes time.**

▶ *Test-taking Tip: Use the ABC's. An intervention that promotes circulation has priority if airway or breathing interventions are not indicated.*

**Content Area:** Adult; **Concept:** Safety; Mobility; Perfusion; Management; **Integrated Processes:** Nursing Process: Analysis; **Client Needs:** Safe and Effective Care Environment: Management of Care; **Cognitive Level:** Analysis [Analyzing]

## 1298. ANSWER: 2, 5

1. Nothing should be placed inside a cast; powder may become pasty inside the cast when exposed to moisture and increase skin breakdown.
2. **Cool air from a hair dryer helps to control itching on the skin within a cast. Hot air is not recommended because it could burn the skin.**
3. A plaster of Paris cast should not be submerged in water. A fiberglass cast may get wet.
4. A plaster of Paris cast should be kept dry and should not be washed with soap and water.
5. **The cast's contact with hard or sharp surfaces while it is wet can cause dents in the cast. These dents can cause pressure areas on the underlying extremity.**

▶ *Test-taking Tip: Focus on safety. Think about the type of cast to determine whether or not it can get wet and how fast it dries. There is a difference in care between a plaster of Paris and a fiberglass cast.*

**Content Area:** Adult; **Concept:** Mobility; Nursing Roles; **Integrated Processes:** Teaching/Learning; Caring; **Client Needs:** Physiological Integrity: Basic Care and Comfort; Health Promotion and Maintenance; **Cognitive Level:** Application [Applying]

## 1299. ANSWER: 4

1. Dyspnea can occur when pulmonary or cardiac vessels are occluded.
2. Chest pain can occur when pulmonary or cardiac vessels are occluded.
3. Cerebral disturbances, due to hypoxia and the lodging of emboli in the brain, vary from headache and mild agitation to delirium.

4. **The nurse should assess for petechiae. Petechiae (small purplish hemorrhagic spots on the skin) are thought to be due to transient thrombocytopenia. They can occur over the chest, anterior axillary folds, hard palate, buccal membranes, and conjunctival sacs.**

▶ *Test-taking Tip: Eliminate symptoms associated with blood emboli.*

**Content Area:** Adult; **Concept:** Assessment; Mobility; **Integrated Processes:** Nursing Process: Assessment; **Client Needs:** Physiological Integrity: Physiological Adaptation; **Cognitive Level:** Comprehension [Understanding]

## 1300. MoC ANSWER: 2

1. Postoperative drainage from a TKR ranges from 200 to 400 mL during the first 24 hours. This amount is neither alarming nor sufficient enough to autotransfuse.
2. **The RN should assess this client immediately. Throbbing, unrelenting pain could be the first sign of compartment syndrome. The neurovascular status of the extremity should be assessed. Unrelieved pressure can lead to compromised circulation and avascular necrosis.**
3. The client in a body cast should be turned every 2 hours to promote drying of the cast. To avoid cracking or denting of the cast, the client is supported with waterproof pillows next to each other without open spaces.
4. Some serous drainage, which is due to tissue trauma and edema, is expected from pin sites of an external fixator. The pulses obtainable by Doppler are concerning, but the client with unrelenting pain is priority.

▶ *Test-taking Tip: Focus on the issue, the client who needs immediate assessment, and use the ABC's. Throbbing, unrelenting pain could indicate that circulation is compromised.*

**Content Area:** Adult; **Concept:** Critical Thinking; Mobility; Perfusion; **Integrated Processes:** Nursing Process: Analysis; **Client Needs:** Safe and Effective Care Environment: Management of Care; Physiological Integrity: Physiological Adaptation; **Cognitive Level:** Analysis [Analyzing]

## 1301. ANSWER: 3

1. There is no indication of a complication, so it is unnecessary to notify the HCP.
2. There is no indication of a complication, so it is unnecessary to cut the cast open.
3. **Swelling is an expected finding; elevating the extremity decreases edema.**
4. Findings should be documented, but this is not the priority action.

▶ *Test-taking Tip: You should select an intervention that will decrease edema.*

**Content Area:** Adult; **Concept:** Mobility; Safety; **Integrated Processes:** Nursing Process: Implementation; **Client Needs:** Physiological Integrity: Basic Care and Comfort; **Cognitive Level:** Application [Applying]

**1302. ANSWER: 1**

1. **The elevated WBC indicates that the client may have an infection, which increases the risk of developing osteomyelitis. DM and a compound fracture also increase the client's risk for osteomyelitis.**
2. Only the WBC is elevated, not multiple lab values.
3. Potassium chloride would not be administered when the potassium is WNL of 3.5–5.5 mEq/L.
4. The nurse should notify the surgeon because surgery may need to be postponed.

♦ *Test-taking Tip: Look at each option and then look at the lab values. Knowing the ranges for these critical values is expected on the NCLEX-RN® examination.*

Content Area: Adult; Concept: Infection; Mobility; Management; Integrated Processes: Nursing Process: Analysis; Client Needs: Physiological Integrity: Reduction of Risk Potential; Cognitive Level: Analysis [Analyzing]

**1303. ANSWER: 4**

1. Initial conservative treatment includes corticosteroid injections to reduce inflammation and pain.
2. Initial conservative treatment includes rest with modified activities and progressive exercises.
3. Initial conservative treatment includes NSAIDs such as ibuprofen (Advil).
4. **Surgery is not a conservative treatment. However, some rotator cuff tears do require arthroscopic débridement or an open acromioplasty with tendon repair.**

♦ *Test-taking Tip: Focus on the key words "conservatively" and "further teaching." This is a false-response item. Select the client statement that is incorrect.*

Content Area: Adult; Concept: Nursing Roles; Mobility; Integrated Processes: Teaching/Learning; Nursing Process: Evaluation; Client Needs: Physiological Integrity: Reduction of Risk Potential; Cognitive Level: Evaluation [Evaluating]

**1304. ANSWER: 4, 5**

1. Movement should be restricted with a possible shoulder dislocation.
2. Ice will constrict blood vessels and reduce inflammation. However, the right shoulder is affected, not the left.
3. Usually the HCP can manipulate the shoulder to realign the bones (shoulder reduction) without surgical repair.
4. **Assessment of pulses and sensation is important because compression of nerves and blood vessels can occur with shoulder dislocation. A shortened arm on the right indicates that the right shoulder is affected.**
5. **The client is in severe pain and requires pain control.**

♦ *Test-taking Tip: Extreme shoulder pain and an arm that is shorter than the other suggest a shoulder dislocation on that side.*

Content Area: Adult; Concept: Mobility; Safety; Integrated Processes: Nursing Process: Planning; Client Needs: Physiological Integrity: Basic Care and Comfort; Safe and Effective Care Environment: Safety and Infection Control; Cognitive Level: Application [Applying]

**1305. ANSWER: 2, 3, 5**

1. With a left femoral neck fracture, the leg is adducted (not abducted).
2. **With a left femoral neck fracture, the leg is externally rotated.**
3. **With a left femoral neck fracture, the leg is shortened.**
4. With a left femoral neck fracture, pain is in the medial (not lateral) side of the knee and hip.
5. **With a left femoral neck fracture, pain is experienced in the groin area.**

♦ *Test-taking Tip: Visualize the fracture before selecting the options.*

Content Area: Adult; Concept: Assessment; Mobility; Integrated Processes: Nursing Process: Assessment; Client Needs: Physiological Integrity: Reduction of Risk Potential; Cognitive Level: Application [Applying]

**1306. MoC ANSWER: 4**

1. The wound culture should be obtained before antibiotics are started. Ceftriaxone is a third-generation cephalosporin used in treating bone infections.
2. The order is correct. The usual dose of ceftriaxone (Rocephin) ranges from 1 to 2 g every 12 or 24 hours.
3. Immobilizing with a splint helps to decrease pain and muscle spasms.
4. **The nurse should defer teaching. Pain and an elevated temperature are barriers to learning.**

♦ *Test-taking Tip: You need to consider the client's readiness for learning when selecting the correct option.*

Content Area: Adult; Concept: Infection; Mobility; Integrated Processes: Nursing Process: Analysis; Client Needs: Physiological Integrity: Physiological Adaptation; Safe and Effective Care Environment: Management of Care; Cognitive Level: Analysis [Analyzing]

**1307. PHARM ANSWER: 1.7**

$$\frac{500 \text{ mg}}{1} \times \frac{3.4 \text{ mL}}{1,000 \text{ mg}} = \frac{1,700 \text{ mL}}{1,000} = 1.7 \text{ mL}$$

**The nurse should prepare 1.7 mL nafcillin (Nallpen).**

♦ *Test-taking Tip: You should convert 1 g to 1000 mg. Then determine how many mLs are in a 500-mg dose using dimensional analysis.*

Content Area: Adult; Concept: Critical Thinking; Medication; Mobility; Integrated Processes: Nursing Process: Implementation; Client Needs: Physiological Integrity: Pharmacological and Parenteral Therapies; Cognitive Level: Application [Applying]

## 1308. ANSWER: 1

1. **A reddened sacrum is the first sign of a pressure ulcer that is caused by pressure or friction and shear. Shear results from the weight of the skin traction pulling the client to the foot of the bed and then sliding back up in bed. Immediate interventions are required before it develops into a stage II ulcer.**
2. The 50-mL/hr output is adequate, although the nurse should evaluate the client's amount of intake.
3. These findings are normal.
4. Buck's traction is skeletal traction. Traction (usually 5 to 8 lb) is applied either to a boot in which the client's lower extremity is secured or to traction tapes applied to the client's extremity.

▶ **Test-taking Tip:** The key word is "immediately." Eliminate options with normal findings.

**Content Area:** Adult; **Concept:** Skin Integrity; Mobility; **Integrated Processes:** Nursing Process: Analysis; **Client Needs:** Physiological Integrity: Reduction of Risk Potential; **Cognitive Level:** Application [Applying]

## 1309. MoC ANSWER: 1

1. **The nurse should immediately notify the HCP. A window in the abdominal portion of the cast or bivalving is needed to relieve the pressure.**
2. The action of initiating oxygen at 2 liters per nasal cannula to relieve the dyspnea should also be implemented, but Option 1 demonstrates the nurse's best clinical judgment of suspecting cast syndrome.
3. The action of placing ice packs around the cast to reduce the abdominal distention should also be implemented, but Option 1 demonstrates the nurse's best clinical judgment of suspecting cast syndrome.
4. Ondansetron (Zofran) should be given, but Option 1 demonstrates the nurse's best clinical judgment of suspecting cast syndrome.

▶ **Test-taking Tip:** Note the key words "best clinical judgment." Vomiting, epigastric pain, and abdominal distention are classic symptoms of cast syndrome with partial or complete upper intestinal obstruction from compression of the duodenum between the superior mesenteric artery and the aorta. Use this information to select the correct option.

**Content Area:** Adult; **Concept:** Safety, Critical Thinking; Mobility; Management; **Integrated Processes:** Nursing Process: Analysis; **Client Needs:** Safe and Effective Care Environment: Management of Care; **Cognitive Level:** Analysis [Analyzing]

## 1310. MoC ANSWER: 3

1. The client's feet need to stay clear of the bottom of the bed for the traction to be effective.
2. Ropes should be correctly positioned in the pulleys for the traction to be effective.

3. **Weights should be hanging freely, but weights should never be removed (unless a life-threatening situation occurs) because removal could result in injury and defeats the purpose of the traction. The lengths of the ropes need to be adjusted so the weights do not rest on the bed frame.**
4. Chlorhexidine is recommended by some as the most effective cleansing solution. Water and saline are alternate choices.

▶ **Test-taking Tip:** Note the key words "needs additional orientation." Select the option that is incorrect.

**Content Area:** Adult; **Concept:** Safety; Mobility; Management; **Integrated Processes:** Nursing Process: Evaluation; **Client Needs:** Safe and Effective Care Environment: Management of Care; **Cognitive Level:** Evaluation [Evaluating]

## 1311. ANSWER: 1

1. **The nurse's initial action should be to check the extremity's position. Improper movement and repositioning can cause prosthesis dislocation; an audible pop and increased pain are signs of possible dislocation.**
2. The nurse should not raise the head of the bed until the cause of the pain is determined.
3. Adjusting the abduction pillow may increase comfort, but the cause of the pain should be determined first.
4. The nurse should not medicate for pain before determining the cause of the pain.

▶ **Test-taking Tip:** You should use the nursing process to determine the first action. Assessment should be the first action. Select the only option that relates to assessment.

**Content Area:** Adult; **Concept:** Mobility; Safety; Assessment; **Integrated Processes:** Nursing Process: Assessment; **Client Needs:** Safe and Effective Care Environment: Safety and Infection Control; **Cognitive Level:** Application [Applying]

## 1312. PHARM ANSWER: 1

1. **The client should be able to ambulate with the use of a walker. An elevated toilet seat is used to prevent hip flexion of greater than 90 degrees when the client sits.**
2. The wedge pillow maintains the client's legs in abduction; using pillows for adduction could cause dislocation.
3. Drainage from a wound drain reinfusion system would not be used after 6 hours postoperatively because the drainage would primarily be fluid and debris and not blood. Not every client may have a wound drainage system following a THR.
4. The best side for the client to get out of bed is the affected side. This allows the client to shift position to the edge of the bed by using the good leg and the trapeze. As the client lowers the affected leg over the edge of the bed, the nurse can assist the client to turn to a sitting position without exceeding the 90-degree hip flexion.

▶ *Test-taking Tip: Focus on the actions that would promote client safety. Hip precautions are necessary when the posterior approach is used for a THR because the muscle has been excised.*

Content Area: Adult; Concept: Nursing Roles; Mobility; Perioperative; Integrated Processes: Nursing Process: Implementation; Client Needs: Physiological Integrity: Basic Care and Comfort; Physiological Integrity: Pharmacological and Parenteral Therapies; Cognitive Level: Analysis [Analyzing]

## 1313. ANSWER: 1, 2, 4

1. **A pillow should be used to maintain abduction to prevent dislocation.**
2. **Using the trapeze and flexing the unaffected legs while keeping the affected leg straight help prevent flexion with position changes. The client's hip should not be flexed more than 90 degrees.**
3. Elevating the head of the bed to no more than 90 degrees when the bed is in a contour position will result in a greater than 90-degree hip flexion.
4. **In initial transfers, a pillow is used to remind the client to maintain abduction and prevent internal and external hip rotation.**
5. Antiembolic stockings should be removed twice daily to prevent skin breakdown.

▶ *Test-taking Tip: Total hip precautions when the posterior approach is used for THR include protecting the hip from adduction, flexion, internal or external rotation, and excessive weight-bearing.*

Content Area: Adult; Concept: Mobility; Perioperative; Integrated Processes: Nursing Process: Planning; Client Needs: Physiological Integrity: Reduction of Risk Potential; Cognitive Level: Application [Applying]

## 1314. ANSWER: 1

1. **After a THR, the client should not flex the hip greater than 90 degrees or have adduction of the hip because it can cause hip dislocation. Wearing socks that do not have grippers on the bottom increases the client's risk for a fall.**
2. After a THR the client may sit at 90 degrees.
3. After a THR the client may lie supine.
4. After a THR the client may be up. However, this client should be wearing shoes or gripper socks or slippers to prevent a fall. Although the nurse should intervene, it is more important for the nurse to intervene with Client 1.

▶ *Test-taking Tip: You should select the position that places the client at risk for hip dislocation.*

Content Area: Adult; Concept: Mobility; Safety; Perioperative; Integrated Processes: Nursing Process: Implementation; Client Needs: Physiological Integrity: Reduction of Risk Potential; Cognitive Level: Analysis [Analyzing]

## 1315. MoC ANSWER: 3

1. The occupational therapist can assist the client with activities of daily living such as bathing, dressing, and meal preparation.
2. The social worker assists the client with acquiring resources needed for continuation of care.
3. **The physical therapist is the team member with expertise to assist in exercises and ambulating with assistive devices.**
4. The HCP is responsible for the medical management and overall treatment plan for the client.

▶ *Test-taking Tip: You should use the terminology in the options to determine the answer. Because the client's needs relate to mobility, "physical" should be a clue to the correct interdisciplinary team member to assist the client.*

Content Area: Adult; Concept: Collaboration; Mobility; Integrated Processes: Nursing Process: Planning; Client Needs: Safe and Effective Care Environment: Management of Care; Cognitive Level: Application [Applying]

## 1316. MoC ANSWER: 3

1. A psychiatrist would assist the client in dealing with the mental health aspects related to the disease, such as ineffective coping, loss, or anger. There is no evidence that the client has mental health issues.
2. The social worker would address issues such as finances, home assistance, placement, or acquiring assistive devices.
3. **The nurse should plan to discuss a referral to a physical therapist (PT). The PT can assist the client in adopting self-management strategies and teach isometric, postural, and aerobic exercises that prevent joint overuse.**
4. The Arthritis Foundation provides a wealth of information to the client, but a referral is not necessary. The client can initiate the contact.

▶ *Test-taking Tip: Focus on the issue, joint stiffness, and the specialty that can best assist the client to regain mobility.*

Content Area: Adult; Concept: Collaboration; Mobility; Integrated Processes: Nursing Process: Planning; Client Needs: Safe and Effective Care Environment: Management of Care; Cognitive Level: Application [Applying]

## 1317. ANSWER: 1

1. **Dorsiflexion of the foot promotes muscle contraction, which compresses veins. This reduces venous stasis and risk of thrombus formation. It should be performed every hour while awake.**
2. The CPM device may or may not be prescribed. If prescribed, it should be on and used most of the time.
3. The client may be up the evening of surgery or the following day; the client may not be stable immediately after the anesthesia has worn off.
4. Rotating the right knee could result in dislocation of the knee prosthesis. The knee should be kept in a neutral position.

▶ *Test-taking Tip: Visualize each of the activities and determine if they would be safe following a TKR.*

Content Area: Adult; Concept: Mobility; Safety; Perioperative; Integrated Processes: Nursing Process: Implementation; Client Needs: Physiological Integrity: Reduction of Risk Potential; Cognitive Level: Application [Applying]

### 1318. ANSWER: 1, 5

1. **An autotransfusion drainage system is used in the immediate postoperative period if extensive bleeding is anticipated. Collected drainage can be reinfused up to 6 hours postoperative.**
2. Flexing the knee to 90 degrees staunches excessive bleeding, but this is not necessary because 350 mL is an acceptable amount.
3. The client's bladder should first be scanned using a bedside bladder ultrasound device to determine the amount of urine in the bladder.
4. The client's leg would not begin cycling in the CPM machine until the amount of drainage decreases.
5. **Ice packs, used to reduce swelling and control bleeding, are replaced every 2 hours. If they have warmed, they need to be replaced.**

♦ *Test-taking Tip: Focus on the situation and the data that would be expected 4 hours following a TKR.*

Content Area: Adult; Concept: Critical Thinking; Mobility; Perioperative; Integrated Processes: Nursing Process: Planning; Client Needs: Physiological Integrity: Physiological Adaptation; Cognitive Level: Analysis [Analyzing]

### 1319. MoC ANSWER: 3

1. The client should have the control to the CPM machine to stop the machine when indicated.
2. Most clients who have had a TKR will have pain. A level of 3 may indicate the need for an analgesic before the pain intensifies.
3. **Attempting to insert an abductor pillow may cause knee misalignment. An abductor pillow may be used for the client following a THR.**
4. An ice pack is applied to the operative site to decrease swelling.

♦ *Test-taking Tip: You should focus on the surgical procedure of a TKR and recognize that Option 3 pertains to the care following a total hip and not a total knee replacement.*

Content Area: Adult; Concept: Safety; Mobility; Perioperative; Integrated Processes: Nursing Process: Implementation; Client Needs: Safe and Effective Care Environment: Safety and Infection Control; Safe and Effective Care Environment: Management of Care; Cognitive Level: Evaluation [Evaluating]

### 1320. ANSWER: 1

1. **Retractors used during surgery can injure the recurrent laryngeal nerve, resulting in the inability to cough effectively to clear secretions. Edema and bleeding can also compromise the airway and compress the spinal cord.**
2. Bleeding from the surgical incision can place the client at risk for impaired tissue perfusion, but the airway is priority.
3. After a cervical discectomy, the client should prevent neck flexion, but this is not the priority.
4. The surgical incision alters skin integrity, but this is not the priority.

♦ *Test-taking Tip: Focus on the ABC's. Assessment of the client's airway is priority.*

Content Area: Adult; Concept: Critical Thinking; Oxygenation; Mobility; Perioperative; Integrated Processes: Nursing Process: Analysis; Client Needs: Physiological Integrity: Reduction of Risk Potential; Cognitive Level: Application [Applying]

### 1321. PHARM ANSWER: 2

1. Cyclobenzaprine can be given with food to decrease gastric distress, but 30 mg is too high a dose.
2. **The nurse should call the HCP to question the dose. If carried out as prescribed, the client would receive a total daily dose of 90 mg of cyclobenzaprine (Flexeril). The total daily dose should not exceed 60 mg.**
3. Although drowsiness is a side effect and should be assessed by the nurse, the dose is excessive.
4. The nurse should consider immediate pain control measures because the onset of action is 1 hour, but the dose of cyclobenzaprine is excessive and should not be given.

♦ *Test-taking Tip: The key word is "best." Cyclobenzaprine (Flexeril) is a centrally acting skeletal muscle relaxant.*

Content Area: Adult; Concept: Medication; Comfort; Mobility; Integrated Processes: Nursing Process: Implementation; Client Needs: Physiological Integrity: Pharmacological and Parenteral Therapies; Safe and Effective Care Environment: Safety and Infection Control; Cognitive Level: Analysis [Analyzing]

### 1322. ANSWER: 1, 2, 3, 5

1. **Remaining active is best and promotes coping. Using good posture will minimize back strain.**
2. **Mechanical stress can increase pain. Prolonged unsupported sitting, heavy lifting, and bending or twisting the back, especially while lifting, should be avoided.**
3. **Using pillows and hip and knee flexion promotes lumbar flexion and back alignment.**
4. Prolonged bedrest is not recommended because it contributes to deconditioning.
5. **Prolonged sitting should be avoided because fatigue contributes to spasm of the back muscles. Lordosis can be decreased by using a soft support at the small of the back.**

♦ *Test-taking Tip: Note the time frame of "2 weeks" in the incorrect option.*

Content Area: Adult; Concept: Promoting Health; Mobility; Nursing Roles; Integrated Processes: Teaching/Learning; Client Needs: Safe and Effective Care Environment: Safety and Infection Control; Physiological Integrity: Reduction of Risk Potential; Psychosocial Integrity; Cognitive Level: Application [Applying]

### 1323. MoC ANSWER: 4

1. The nurse should administer morphine sulfate because the client has pain, but this does not demonstrate the nurse's best clinical judgment.

2. Encouraging coughing and deep breathing is correct because the client has crackles, but this does not demonstrate the nurse's best clinical judgment.

3. Reinforcing the incisional dressing is correct because there is drainage, but this does not demonstrate the nurse's best clinical judgment.

4. **A bloody area surrounded by clear yellowish fluid on the dressing and the client's headache suggest a CSF leak. The nurse should notify the HCP.**

▶ *Test-taking Tip: A complication following spinal fusion is a CSF leak. The client may need to be kept on bedrest for a few days while the dural tear heals or may need a blood patch to seal the leak because the client is at risk for a CNS infection.*

Content Area: Adult; Concept: Critical Thinking; Mobility; Management; Integrated Processes: Nursing Process: Implementation; Client Needs: Safe and Effective Care Environment: Management of Care; Cognitive Level: Analysis [Analyzing]

## 1324. ANSWER: 2

1. Dupuytren's contracture involves the palm and fingers, not the lower extremity.

2. **Independent self-care is impaired for a few days after surgery because the hand is bandaged. The nurse should plan that the client receive assistance with personal care and ADLs.**

3. Dupuytren's contracture involves the palm and fingers, not the foot.

4. The elastic bandage should be kept clean and dry and removed only by the surgeon.

▶ *Test-taking Tip: Dupuytren's contracture is a slowly progressive contracture of the palmar fascia that severely impairs function of the fourth, fifth, and sometimes middle fingers.*

Content Area: Adult; Concept: Nursing Roles; Mobility; Integrated Processes: Nursing Process: Planning; Client Needs: Physiological Integrity: Basic Care and Comfort; Physiological Integrity: Physiological Adaptation; Cognitive Level: Analysis [Analyzing]

## 1325. ANSWER: 3

1. The splint should be removed for bathing and intermittently during the day to exercise the wrist.

2. The splint should not be overly tight, as it can impair circulation to the hand.

3. **Although the splint decreases swelling and promotes healing and is necessary in the management of the pain with carpal tunnel syndrome, it should be removed intermittently during the day to exercise the wrist and bathe.**

4. The splint is used to protect the wrist and not the fingers.

▶ *Test-taking Tip: Remember that treatment with a splint for carpal tunnel syndrome protects the wrist from overuse. Its purpose is not to immobilize the joint.*

Content Area: Adult; Concept: Mobility; Nursing Roles; Integrated Processes: Teaching/Learning; Client Needs: Physiological Integrity: Basic Care and Comfort; Health Promotion and Maintenance; Cognitive Level: Application [Applying]

## 1326. ANSWER: 2, 4, 5

1. With tendonitis, the joint should be rested until inflammation and pain have decreased. Resting 1 to 2 days is an insufficient amount of time.

2. **An arm sling helps to rest the joint and keep it stabilized, especially during sleep. The client should demonstrate proper application and use.**

3. The affected joint in tendonitis should be elevated as often as possible to promote a decrease in inflammation; lying with the head and arm elevated (not flat) would decrease inflammation.

4. **Ice application reduces joint inflammation and pain associated with tendonitis. The client should demonstrate proper application.**

5. **NSAIDs such as ibuprofen (Motrin) are effective for controlling pain and reducing inflammation with tendonitis.**

▶ *Test-taking Tip: Tendonitis is inflammation of the joint and pain resulting from overuse. The client will need to demonstrate understanding of appropriate care for the shoulder.*

Content Area: Adult; Concept: Mobility; Inflammation; Integrated Processes: Nursing Process: Evaluation; Client Needs: Physiological Integrity: Physiological Adaptation; Cognitive Level: Evaluation [Evaluating]

## 1327. ANSWER: 1, 2, 4, 5

1. **A sudden onset of chills suggests the infection of osteomyelitis is blood-borne.**

2. **A high fever suggests the infection of osteomyelitis is blood-borne.**

3. Tachycardia, not bradycardia, would be present from the pain associated with osteomyelitis.

4. **The pulsating shoulder pain is caused from the pressure of the collecting pus.**

5. **The infected area becomes swollen, painful, and extremely tender.**

▶ *Test-taking Tip: Osteomyelitis is an infection of the bone.*

Content Area: Adult; Concept: Infection; Mobility; Integrated Processes: Nursing Process: Analysis; Client Needs: Physiological Integrity: Reduction of Risk Potential; Cognitive Level: Application [Applying]

## 1328. MoC ANSWER: 4

1. The nurse should first request permission of any client before uncovering any part of the body.

2. A kosher meal would not have meat and dairy products at the same meal. This does not describe Ramadan.

3. Fasting occurs from sunrise to sunset during Ramadan, and the client's fall risk increases if fasting, so delaying physical therapy is appropriate. However, Ramadan ends at sundown and not at a specific time.

4. **Some people do not eat or drink from sunrise to sunset during Ramadan.**

▶ *Test-taking Tip: Fasting is a fundamental principle of Islam. Use this information to narrow the options.*

Content Area: Adult; Concept: Diversity; Mobility; Perioperative; Management; Integrated Processes: Culture and Spirituality; Communication and Documentation; Client Needs: Safe and Effective Care Environment: Management of Care; Cognitive Level: Application [Applying]

### 1329. CJ ANSWER:

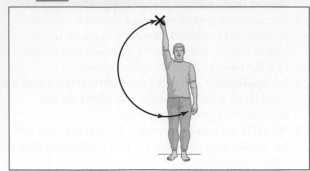

**In adduction, the arm is moved downward from a position next to the head to across the front of the body as far as possible.**

▶ *Test-taking Tip: Use the "add-" in adduction to remember that you move it toward, or add it to, the body.*

Content Area: Adult; Concept: Mobility; Integrated Processes: Teaching/Learning; Client Needs: Physiological Integrity: Physiological Adaptation; Cognitive Level: Application [Applying]

### 1330. ANSWER: 2

1. Osteosarcoma does not originate elsewhere in the client's body. The hypercalcemia is due to an increased release of calcium from the bones.
2. **Osteosarcoma is a malignant primary tumor of the bone, appearing most frequently in males between 10 and 25 years (when bones grow rapidly). Prognosis depends on whether the tumor has metastasized to the lungs, but it is often fatal.**
3. Treatment includes combined chemotherapy that is started before and continued after surgery.
4. Osteosarcoma is a primary malignant tumor.

▶ *Test-taking Tip: Apply knowledge of medical terminology; "sarcoma" is cancer arising from underlying tissue, and "osteo-" is bone. Thus eliminate Options 1 and 4. If uncertain, the "only" in Option 3 should lead to eliminating this option.*

Content Area: Adult; Concept: Cellular Regulation; Mobility; Integrated Processes: Nursing Process: Evaluation; Client Needs: Physiological Integrity: Physiological Adaptation; Cognitive Level: Evaluation [Evaluating]

### 1331. ANSWER: 1, 2, 3, 4

1. **A local anesthetic provides pain relief for some with phantom limb pain.**
2. **A TENS unit sends stimulating pulses across the skin surface and along the nerve to help prevent pain signals from reaching the brain.**
3. **Beta blockers such as atenolol (Tenormin) may relieve dull, burning discomfort.**

4. **Antiseizure medication such as oxcarbazepine (Trileptal) has been shown to control stabbing and cramping pain.**
5. Increasing, not decreasing, the client's activity helps to reduce the occurrence of phantom limb pain.

▶ *Test-taking Tip: Focus on the issue: controlling phantom limb pain.*

Content Area: Adult; Concept: Sensory Perception; Mobility; Comfort; Integrated Processes: Nursing Process: Planning; Client Needs: Physiological Integrity: Physiological Adaptation; Cognitive Level: Application [Applying]

### 1332. MoC ANSWER: 2

1. Thanking the NA for being so observant and intervening appropriately is inappropriate since the action was incorrect.
2. **The nurse should perform this action. Flexion, abduction, and external rotation of the residual lower limb are avoided to prevent hip contracture.**
3. The NA should not have elevated the client's residual limb at this time in the client's recovery.
4. It is unnecessary for the nurse to report the incident to the surgeon and to complete a variance report unless the client was in the position for an extended period of time.

▶ *Test-taking Tip: Options 1 and 3 suggest the NA's action is correct. Because these are similar, both should be eliminated. Eliminate Option 4 because it is an extreme measure.*

Content Area: Adult; Concept: Safety; Mobility; Integrated Processes: Nursing Process: Evaluation; Client Needs: Safe and Effective Care Environment: Management of Care; Cognitive Level: Evaluation [Evaluating]

### 1333. MoC ANSWER: 2, 1, 4, 3

2. **The client who has a right lower leg cast whose right foot is cold to the touch should be assessed first. The data could indicate compartment syndrome, which is an emergent condition.**
1. **The client who had a left BKA and has left foot pain of 6 on a 0 to 10 scale should be assessed second because pain is a priority in a postoperative client and should be addressed in a timely manner, but this is not an emergent situation.**
4. **The client who had a spinal fusion and has not voided since the urinary catheter removal 4 hours ago should be assessed third for the presence of urinary retention. Usually the client should void within 6 hours after the urinary catheter was removed.**
3. **The client who had a THR and 200-mL wound drain output during the past 8 hours should be assessed last. This amount of output is a common finding following a THR due to the vascular nature of the operative site.**

▶ *Test-taking Tip: In setting priorities for assessing the clients, you should first identify the client who is unstable or has life-threatening/limb-threatening conditions. Then evaluate the other clients for normal versus abnormal findings for the client's condition. The most stable client should be assessed last.*

**Content Area:** Adult; **Concept:** Critical Thinking; Mobility; Nursing Roles; **Integrated Processes:** Nursing Process: Planning; **Client Needs:** Safe and Effective Care Environment: Management of Care; **Cognitive Level:** Synthesis [Creating]

**1334.** MoC **ANSWER: 2**

1. Osteomyelitis is a bone infection that requires specific wound care and careful assessment. This skin care would not be appropriate to delegate.
2. **Buck's traction is skin traction. Because there is no open site that needs care with this type of traction, it would be appropriate to delegate skin care.**
3. Skeletal traction has pins that enter the skin. The nurse should perform the pin site care and carefully assess the pin sites for infection.
4. An external fixator has pin sites that need to be cleaned and carefully assessed. This type of skin care would not be appropriate to delegate.

▶ *Test-taking Tip: You should look for the similarities in the options. Options 3 and 4 involve pin sites, and Option 1 involves a wound. Option 3 is different. Often the option that is different is the answer.*

**Content Area:** Adult; **Concept:** Nursing Roles; Mobility; **Integrated Processes:** Nursing Process: Implementation; **Client Needs:** Safe and Effective Care Environment: Management of Care; **Cognitive Level:** Evaluation [Evaluating]

## Chapter Thirty

# Neurological Management

**1335.** The nurse is teaching the client who is scheduled for an outpatient EEG. Which instruction should the nurse include?

1. Remove all hairpins before coming in for the EEG test.
2. Avoid eating or drinking at least 6 hours prior to the test.
3. Some hair will be removed with a razor to place electrodes.
4. Have blood drawn for a glucose level 2 hours before the test.

**1336.** The client, who has type 1 DM, is scheduled for an MRI of the brain after an MVA. Which intervention should the nurse implement to prepare the client for the test?

1. Make the client NPO for 6 hours before the MRI and hold the morning insulin dose.
2. Inform the client that the machine is noisy and earplugs can be worn during the test.
3. Explain that the extremity used for injection must remain straight for a few hours after MRI.
4. Ensure that the serum BUN and creatinine levels are obtained and evaluated prior to the MRI.

**1337.** The nurse is assessing the client after sustaining a closed head injury. When applying nailbed pressure, the client's body suddenly stiffens, the eyes roll upward, and there is increased salivation and a loss of swallowing reflex. Which observation should the nurse document?

1. Decerebrate posturing observed
2. Decorticate posturing observed
3. Positive Kernig's sign observed
4. Tonic seizure activity observed

**1338.** The nurse is assessing the client with a tentative diagnosis of meningitis. Which findings should the nurse associate with meningitis? **Select all that apply.**

1. Nuchal rigidity
2. Severe headache
3. Pill-rolling tremor
4. Photophobia
5. Lethargy

**1339.** The client is at risk for septic emboli after being diagnosed with meningococcal meningitis. Which action by the nurse directly addresses this risk?

1. Monitoring vital signs and oxygen saturation levels hourly
2. Planning to give meningococcal polysaccharide vaccine
3. Assessing neurological function with the Glasgow Coma Scale q2h
4. Completing a thorough vascular assessment of all extremities q2h

**1340.** MoC After receiving report, the nurse working on the step-down neurological unit begins care for four clients. Prioritize the order in which the nurse should plan to assess the four clients.

1. The 78-year-old who underwent evacuation of a chronic subdural hematoma 24 hours earlier and is recovering
2. The 30-year-old who was diagnosed with viral meningitis 2 days earlier and wants to talk with the HCP
3. The 24-year-old who had been unconscious at the scene of an MVA and is being admitted from the ED for observation
4. The 40-year-old with Guillain-Barré who is currently receiving a third bedside plasmapheresis treatment being administered by another nurse

Answer: _____

**1341.** The client has an intraventricular catheter for ICP monitoring and CSF drainage based on the client's CSF pressure. The stopcock to the drain has been open, and the nurse is assessing the CSF output hourly. Place an X at the location where the nurse should check now for the CSF output for the past hour.

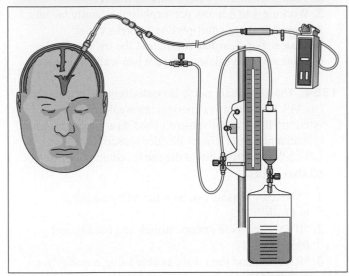

**1342.** The nurse in the ED documents that the newly admitted client who sustained a TBI is "postictal upon transfer." What did the nurse observe?

1. Yellowing of the skin due to a liver condition
2. Drowsy or confused state following a seizure
3. Severe itching of the eyes from an allergic reaction
4. Abnormal sensations including tingling of the skin

**1343.** **PHARM** The client is prescribed a loading dose of phenytoin of 15 mg/kg IV for seizure activity, then 100 mg IV tid. The client weighs 198 lb. How many milligrams should the nurse administer for the loading dose?

_____ mg (Record your answer as a whole number.)

**1344.** A hospitalized client diagnosed with seizures has a vagus nerve stimulation (VNS) device implanted. The nurse determines that the VNS is working properly when making which observation?

1. It stimulated a heartbeat when bradycardia occurred during a seizure.
2. It defibrillated a lethal rhythm that occurred during the client's seizure.
3. The client activates the VNS device to stop a seizure from occurring.
4. The client activates the device at seizure onset to prevent aspiration.

**1345.** **PHARM** **MoC** The client is in status epilepticus. Which interventions, if prescribed, should be included in this client's immediate treatment? **Select all that apply.**

1. Administer dexamethasone intravenously.
2. Give oxygen and prepare for endotracheal intubation.
3. Obtain a defibrillator and prepare to use it immediately.
4. Remove nearby objects to protect the client from injury.
5. Administer lorazepam intravenously STAT.

**1346.** The client has a neck injury after an MVA. EMS initiates spinal precautions because a cervical fracture has not been ruled out. Which action is the nurse's **priority** when receiving the client in the ED?

1. Assessing the client using the Glasgow Coma Scale (GCS)
2. Assessing the level of sensation in the client's extremities
3. Checking that the cervical collar was correctly placed by EMS
4. Applying antiembolism hose to the client's lower extremities

**1347.** The nurse assesses the client injured in a diving accident 2 hours earlier. The client breathes independently but has no movement or muscle tone below the injured area. A CT scan reveals a C4 cervical vertebra fracture. The nurse should plan interventions for which problem?

1. Complete spinal cord transection
2. Spinal shock
3. An upper motor neuron injury
4. Quadriplegia

**1348.** The client hospitalized with a vertebral fracture has a halo external fixation device in place. Which intervention should the nurse plan?

1. Ensure the traction weight hangs freely.
2. Remove the vest from the device at bedtime.
3. Cleanse sites where the pins enter the skull.
4. Screw the pins in the skull daily to tighten.

**1349.** The nurse is caring for the client with a C6 SCI. Which findings support the nurse's conclusion that the client may be experiencing autonomic dysreflexia? **Select all that apply.**

1. Blurred vision
2. BP 198/102 mm Hg
3. HR 150 bpm
4. Extreme headache
5. Sweaty face and arms

**1350.** The nurse is assisting the client who sustained a C5 SCI to cough using the quad coughing technique. The nurse correctly demonstrates quad coughing with which actions? **Select all that apply.**

1. Places a suction catheter in the client's oral cavity to stimulate the cough reflex
2. Puts hands on the upper abdomen, has client inhale; pushes upward during a cough
3. Cups the hands and percusses the client's anterior, lateral, and posterior lung fields
4. Hyperoxygenates the client by using a resuscitation bag to deliver 100% oxygen
5. Elevates the head of the bed to a high Fowler's position if the client is sitting in bed

**1351.** The client with a T2 SCI is dysreflexic and has a BP of 170/90 mm Hg. Place the nurse's interventions in the order that these should be performed.

1. Lower the end of the bed so feet are dependent.
2. Remove elastic stocking and other constricting devices; assess below the level of injury.
3. Elevate the HOB to 90 degrees.
4. Inform the HCP of the incident, measures taken, and client response.
5. Perform digital removal of impacted stool (last BM found to be 10 days ago).
6. Administer a prn prescribed sublingual nifedipine for continued elevated BP.
7. Retake the BP after being upright for 2 to 3 minutes.

Answer: _____

**1352.** The female client with an incomplete T6 spinal cord transection asks the nurse for sexual health advice and the possibility of ever conceiving. Which statements by the nurse will be helpful to the client? **Select all that apply.**

1. "You need to continue to use contraceptives if you do not wish to have children."
2. "Unfortunately, your injury prevents you from being able to conceive children."
3. "Because feeling is affected, it is not likely that you will be able to deliver a baby."
4. "Sexual intercourse is generally prohibited because it can worsen your condition."
5. "You can engage in sexual intimacy, but you may not be able to feel an orgasm."

**1353.** The client with MS tells the nurse about extreme fatigue. Which assessment findings should the nurse identify as contributing to the client's fatigue? **Select all that apply.**

1. Hemoglobin 9.5 g/dL and hematocrit is 31.8%
2. Taking baclofen 15 mg 3 times per day
3. Working 4 to 8 hours per week in the family business
4. Stopped taking amitriptyline 8 weeks earlier
5. Presence of a cardiac murmur at the tricuspid valve
6. Bilateral leg weakness noted when walking in room

**1354.** The home-care nurse is counseling the client who has MS. The client is experiencing weakness, ataxia, intermittent adductor spasms of the hips, and occasional incontinence from loss of bladder sensation. Which self-care measures should the nurse recommend? **Select all that apply.**

1. "Adductor spasms can be relieved by taking a hot bath."
2. "If a muscle is in spasm, stretch and hold it, and then relax."
3. "Rest first and then walk as able using a walker for support."
4. "When walking, keep feet close together, legs slightly bent."
5. "Set an alarm to remind you to void 30 minutes after fluid intake."

**1355.** The nurse is caring for the client who has Guillain-Barré syndrome (GBS). It is **most** important for the nurse to monitor for which complication?

1. Autonomic dysreflexia
2. Septic emboli
3. Cardiac dysrhythmias
4. Respiratory failure

**1356.** The nurse is caring for the client who has severe craniocerebral trauma. Which finding indicates that the client is developing DI?

1. Blood glucose level at 230 mg/dL
2. Urinary output 1500 mL over 4 hours
3. Urine specific gravity at 1.042
4. Somnolent when previously alert

**1357.** The nurse plans to show the spouse of the client with a suspected epidural hematoma where the epidural hematoma occurs in the brain. Which illustration should the nurse select when teaching the client's spouse?

1.

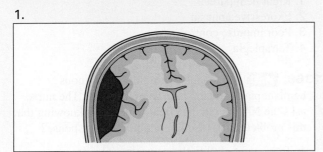

2.

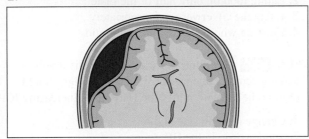

3.

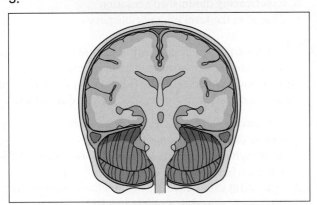

4.

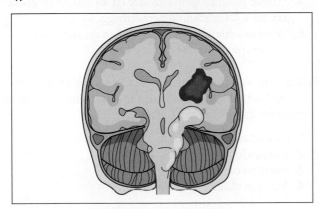

**1358.** **PHARM** The nurse is administering mannitol IV to decrease the client's ICP following a craniotomy. Which laboratory test result should the nurse monitor during the client's treatment with mannitol?

1. Serum osmolarity
2. White blood cell count
3. Serum cholesterol
4. Erythrocyte sedimentation rate (ESR)

**1359.** The nurse is caring for the client who, 6 weeks after an MVA, was diagnosed with a mild TBI. Which information in the client's history of the injury should the nurse associate with the TBI? **Select all that apply.**

1. The client has had no episodes of vomiting after the accident.
2. The client remembers events before and right after the accident.
3. The client has had headache and dizziness daily since the accident.
4. The client has difficulty concentrating and focusing while at work.
5. The client lost consciousness momentarily at the time of the injury.

**1360.** The nurse is implementing interventions for the client who has increased ICP. The nurse knows that which result will occur if the increased ICP is left untreated?

1. Displacement of brain tissue
2. Increase in cerebral perfusion
3. Increase in the serum pH level
4. Leakage of cerebrospinal fluid

**1361.** **PHARM** The client, diagnosed with an ischemic stroke, is being evaluated for thrombolytic therapy. Which assessment finding should prompt the nurse to withhold thrombolytic therapy?

1. Brain CT scan results show no bleeding.
2. The client had a serious head injury 4 weeks ago.
3. The client has a history of type 1 diabetes mellitus.
4. Neurological deficits started 2 hours ago.

**1362.** The client who has expressive aphasia is having difficulty communicating with the nurse. Which action by the nurse would be **most** helpful?

1. Position the client facing the nurse.
2. Enunciate directions very slowly.
3. Use gestures and body language.
4. Ask the client to point to needed objects.

**1363.** The client being monitored while receiving tissue plasminogen activator (tPA) following an ischemic stroke opens both eyes spontaneously, mumbles inappropriate words in response to orientation questions, has no ability to move any extremities, and has decerebrate posturing in response to nailbed pressure. On the basis of the chart illustrated, what is the client's Glasgow Coma Scale (GCS) score?

_____ GCS score (Record your answer as a whole number.)

| Glasgow Coma Scale | | |
|---|---|---|
| **Category** | **Score** | **Response** |
| Eye Opening | 4 | Spontaneous |
| | 3 | To speech |
| | 2 | To pain |
| | 1 | None |
| Best Verbal Response | 5 | Oriented |
| | 4 | Confused |
| | 3 | Inappropriate words |
| | 2 | Incomprehensible |
| | 1 | None |
| Best Motor Response | 6 | Obeys commands |
| | 5 | Localizes to pain |
| | 4 | Withdraws from pain |
| | 3 | Abnormal flexion |
| | 2 | Extension |
| | 1 | None |

**1364.** An unconscious client has left-sided paralysis. Which intervention should the nurse implement to **best** prevent foot drop?

1. Ensure that the feet are firmly against the footboard.
2. Use pillows to elevate the legs and support the soles.
3. Perform range of motion to the legs and feet daily.
4. Apply a foot boot brace, 2 hours on and 2 hours off.

**1365.** The nurse is caring for the client who had a stroke affecting the right hemisphere of the brain. The nurse should **initially** assess for which problem?

1. Right hemiparesis
2. Expressive aphasia
3. Poor impulse control
4. Tetraplegia

**1366.** MoC The client has right homonymous hemianopia following an ischemic stroke. The nurse asks the NA to help the client with meals knowing that this problem may result in which client response?

1. Tendency to fall to the contralateral side
2. Eating food on only half of the plate
3. Using the silverware inappropriately
4. Choking when swallowing any liquids

**1367.** MoC The nurse is caring for the client with a leaking cerebral aneurysm. Which early sign should prompt the nurse to notify the HCP of an increasing ICP?

1. Change in pupil size and reaction
2. Sudden drop in the BP
3. Experiencing diminished sensation
4. Change in the level of consciousness

**1368.** The experienced nurse is instructing the new nurse on subarachnoid hemorrhage. The nurse evaluates that the new nurse understands the information when the new nurse makes which statements? **Select all that apply.**

1. "Subarachnoid hemorrhage is often associated with a rupture of a cerebral aneurysm."
2. "Subarachnoid hemorrhage occurs during sleep and is noticed when the client awakens."
3. "The client experiencing a subarachnoid hemorrhage may describe having a severe headache."
4. "Tissue plasminogen activator (tPA) should be given to treat a subarachnoid hemorrhage."
5. "A subarachnoid hemorrhage often results in the cerebrospinal fluid appearing bloody."

**1369.** The nurse is caring for the older adult client with normal pressure hydrocephalus (NPH). Which treatment measure should the nurse anticipate?

1. Carotid endarterectomy
2. Ventriculoperitoneal shunt
3. Insertion of a lumbar drain
4. Anticonvulsant medications

**1370.** The client, who has a deteriorating status after having a stroke, has a rectal temperature of 102.3°F (39.1°C). Which should be the nurse's rationale for initiating interventions to bring the temperature to a normal level?

1. A normal temperature will strengthen the client's immune system.
2. A hypothermic state may increase the client's chance of survival.
3. A normal temperature will decrease the Glasgow Coma Scale score.
4. Hyperthermia increases the likelihood of a larger area of brain infarct.

**1371.** ☐ **CJ** The nurse is checking the client's pupillary reaction to light. Place an X at the location where the nurse should place the flashlight initially and then a line in the direction that the nurse should move the flashlight to check the client's right pupil.

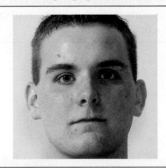

**1372.** The client, undergoing testing for a possible brain tumor, asks the nurse about treatment options. The nurse's response should be based on knowing that treatment of a brain tumor depends on which factors? **Select all that apply.**

1. How rapidly the tumor is growing
2. Whether the tumor is malignant or benign
3. Cell type from which the tumor originates
4. Where the tumor is located within the brain
5. The client's age and type of insurance

**1373.** The nurse is monitoring clients for complications. Which client would be the nurse's **lowest** priority for monitoring for a brain abscess?

1. The client with endocarditis
2. The client with idiopathic epilepsy
3. The client who had a liver transplant
4. The client with meningitis

**1374.** The client with PD has a new surgically implanted DBS. After the stimulator is operational, which criterion should the nurse use to evaluate that the DBS is effective?

1. The client has cogwheel rigidity when moving the upper extremities.
2. The client has a decrease in the frequency and severity of tremors.
3. The client has less facial pain and converses with more facial expression.
4. The client no longer experiences auras or a severe frontal headache.

**1375.** **PHARM** An older adult with PD is prescribed levodopa and carbidopa. What information should the nurse include when teaching the client and spouse?

1. The client has an increased risk for falls.
2. The client should stop taking multiple vitamins.
3. The medication should not be taken with food.
4. The medication has very few adverse effects.

**1376.** The client with muscle weakness asks the nurse during the initial assessment if the symptoms suggest "Lou Gehrig's disease." Which is the nurse's **most** appropriate response?

1. "Muscle weakness can occur from working too much. Avoid thinking the worst."
2. "Tell me what has you thinking that you might have Lou Gehrig's disease."
3. "Have you been having trouble remembering things along with this weakness?"
4. "That is a good question. We will be doing tests to figure out what is going on."

**1377.** The nurse assessed the client newly diagnosed with MG. Which finding should the nurse recognize as being **unrelated** to the diagnosis?

1. Drooping eyelids
2. Slurred speech
3. Weak lower extremities
4. Circumoral tingling

**1378.** The client has had recurrent episodes of low back pain. Which statement indicates that the client has incorporated positive lifestyle changes to decrease the incidence of future back problems?

1. "I stoop and avoid bending and twisting when lifting objects."
2. "I can walk farther if I wear my old comfortable shoes."
3. "I can walk only on weekends but walk 5 miles each day."
4. "I sit for 2 to 3 hours with my legs elevated for pain control."

**INSTRUCTIONS:** Refer to the information provided to answer Question 1379.

**1379.** MoC PHARM CJ The nurse reviews the medical record of the client illustrated. Which information is **most** important for the nurse to discuss with the HCP?

| Client: 48-year-old, single Somali female | Allergies: Penicillin | Diagnosis: Sacral ulcer; T12 SCI 12 years ago |
|---|---|---|
| Tab 1 | Tab 2 | Tab 3 |
| Assessment | Serum Laboratory Results | Prescribed Medications |
| • BP (mm Hg): Lying: 102/62<br>• Pulse: 100 bpm<br>• Resp: 20 bpm<br>• Temp: 100°F (37.8°C)<br>• Exaggerated spasticity<br>• Muscle rigidity<br>• Tinnitus<br>• Stage 2 sacral ulcer | • WBC 4900/mm³<br>• AST 15 units/L<br>• Alkaline phosphatase 100 units/L<br>• Glucose 180 mg/dL | • aspirin 81 mg oral daily<br>• baclofen 800 mcg/day per intrathecal pump<br>• bisacodyl 10 mg supp qod<br>• enoxaparin sodium 40 mg daily subq<br>• magnesium citrate 1 bottle oral qod<br>• oxybutynin 5 mg oral tid<br>• paroxetine 20 mg oral daily<br>• polyethylene glycol 1 packet oral daily<br>• sennosides 2 tab oral bid<br>• sulfamethoxazole/trimethoprim 1 tab oral daily |

1. Assessment findings
2. Bowel elimination meds
3. Laboratory test results
4. Medication allergies

# Answers and Rationales

**1335. ANSWER: 1**

1. **In an EEG, electrodes are placed on the scalp over multiple areas of the brain to detect and record patterns of electrical activity. Preparation includes clean hair without any objects in the hair to prevent inaccurate test results.**
2. The client should not be NPO because a typical glucose level is important for normal brain functioning.
3. The scalp will not be shaved; the electrodes are applied with paste.
4. There is no indication to have a serum glucose drawn before the test.

▶ *Test-taking Tip: The question calls for a true response. The prefix "cephalo-" in electroencephalogram refers to head, so the test involves the head. Consider each option separately and use the process of elimination.*

**Content Area:** Adult; **Concept:** Critical Thinking; Neurologic Regulation; Nursing Roles; **Integrated Processes:** Teaching/Learning; **Client Needs:** Physiological Integrity: Reduction of Risk Potential; Physiological Integrity: Basic Care and Comfort; **Cognitive Level:** Application [Applying]

**1336. ANSWER: 2**

1. Clients undergoing positron emission tomography (PET) scans, but not those undergoing MRI, are made NPO and have insulin held.
2. **Clients are given earplugs to wear while undergoing the test because the machine makes a loud clanging noise that is unpleasant.**
3. Clients undergoing cerebral angiography, not MRI, must be on bedrest with the extremity used for injection held straight for several hours after the test.
4. Serum BUN and creatinine levels to assess renal function are required before CT scans or other tests involving contrast material to prevent renal complications.

▶ *Test-taking Tip: You should consider that the MRI uses magnetic fields to produce images to evaluate brain structures and not function. It is noninvasive, and no contrast material is used.*

**Content Area:** Adult; **Concept:** Safety; Neurologic Regulation; Metabolism; **Integrated Processes:** Nursing Process: Implementation; **Client Needs:** Physiological Integrity: Reduction of Risk Potential; **Cognitive Level:** Application [Applying]

**1337. ANSWER: 4**

1. Decerebrate posture involves rigid extension of the arms and legs, downward pointing of the toes, and backward arching of the head.
2. Decorticate posture involves rigidity, flexion of the arms toward the body with the wrists and fingers clenched and held on the chest, and extended legs.
3. A positive Kernig's sign is flexing the leg at the hip and then raising the leg into extension. Severe head and neck pain occurs.
4. **Body stiffening, eyes rolled upward, increase in salivation, and a loss of swallowing reflex are signs consistent with the tonic phase of a tonic-clonic seizure. This phase is followed by the clonic phase with violent muscle contractions.**

▶ *Test-taking Tip: A noxious stimuli can be a precipitating event for a seizure. Use this information to select the correct option.*

Content Area: Adult; Concept: Neurologic Regulation; Communication; Integrated Processes: Communication and Documentation; Client Needs: Physiological Integrity: Physiological Adaptation; Cognitive Level: Application [Applying]

**1338. ANSWER: 1, 2, 4, 5**

1. **Irritation of the meninges causes nuchal rigidity (stiff neck).**
2. **Irritation of the meninges causes severe headache.**
3. Pill-rolling tremors are associated with PD.
4. **Irritation of the meninges causes photophobia (light irritates the eyes).**
5. **Lethargy, pathological state of sleepiness or unresponsiveness, indicates a decreased level of consciousness, which is associated with meningitis.**

▶ *Test-taking Tip: The "meninges" include the dura mater, arachnoid, and the pia mater. Meningitis is an inflammation affecting the arachnoid and pia mater that cover the brain and spinal cord. Evaluate whether each option can result from irritation of the meninges.*

Content Area: Adult; Concept: Infection; Neurologic Regulation; Integrated Processes: Nursing Process: Analysis; Client Needs: Physiological Integrity: Physiological Adaptation; Cognitive Level: Knowledge [Remembering]

**1339. ANSWER: 4**

1. Monitoring VS is indicated but does not address the complication of septic emboli.
2. Immunization with the meningococcal polysaccharide vaccine (Menomune) is a preventive measure against meningitis and would not be included in treatment.
3. Frequent neurological assessments are indicated but do not address the complication of septic emboli.
4. **Frequent vascular assessments will detect vascular compromise secondary to septic emboli. Early detection allows for interventions that will prevent gangrene and possible loss of limb.**

▶ *Test-taking Tip: The word "emboli" suggests a vascular concern. You should eliminate Options 2 and 3 and then decide which remaining option is best.*

Content Area: Adult; Concept: Assessment; Neurologic Regulation; Infection; Integrated Processes: Nursing Process: Assessment; Client Needs: Physiological Integrity: Reduction of Risk Potential; Cognitive Level: Analysis [Analyzing]

**1340. MoC ANSWER: 3, 1, 2, 4**

3. **The 24-year-old who had been unconscious at the scene of an MVA and is being admitted from the ED for observation. The nurse should assess the newly admitted client first to determine whether there are changes in the client's level of consciousness and any early signs of increased ICP.**
1. **The 78-year-old who underwent evacuation of a chronic subdural hematoma 24 hours earlier and is recovering. This client should be assessed next because the client is postoperative day 1, but stable.**
2. **The 30-year-old who was diagnosed with viral meningitis 2 days earlier and wants to talk with the HCP. This client has a self-limiting condition and likely wants to be discharged; thus, he or she should be assessed third.**
4. **The 40-year-old with Guillain-Barré who is currently receiving a third bedside plasmapheresis treatment being administered by another nurse. This client can be assessed last because another nurse is in the room with the client administering the plasmapheresis treatment.**

▶ *Test-taking Tip: Read each option and determine which client is most unstable and in need of assessment first. Proceed to assess the least stable client first. You should note that the client with Guillain-Barré has another nurse in attendance.*

Content Area: Adult; Concept: Safety; Neurologic Regulation; Management; Integrated Processes: Nursing Process: Planning; Client Needs: Safe and Effective Care Environment: Management of Care; Cognitive Level: Synthesis [Creating]

**1341. ANSWER:**

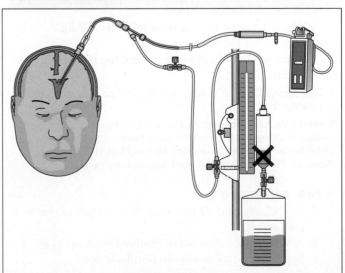

The smaller drainage container should be checked for the CSF drainage for the past hour. Once the volume is documented, the nurse closes the stopcock to the intraventricular catheter and opens the stopcock from the small drainage container into the larger bag. Once drained, the stopcock to the larger bag is closed, and the stopcock from the intraventricular catheter to the small drainage container is opened.

♦ *Test-taking Tip: If unsure of which container should be checked, think about the volume in each container and the expected output after only an hour.*

Content Area: Adult; Concept: Assessment; Neurologic Regulation; Integrated Processes: Nursing Process: Analysis; Client Needs: Physiological Integrity: Reduction of Risk Potential; Cognitive Level: Analysis [Analyzing]

### 1342. ANSWER: 2

1. Jaundice and icterus are terms for yellowing of the skin.
2. **The client had experienced a tonic-clonic seizure recently and is now in a state of deep relaxation and is breathing quietly. During this period, the client may be unconscious or awaken gradually but is often confused and disoriented. Often the client is amnesic regarding the seizure.**
3. Pruritus is a term for itching.
4. Paresthesia is the term for abnormal sensations such as tingling and burning of the skin.

♦ *Test-taking Tip: The term "postictal" can be broken down into the prefix "post-," which means "after," and "-ictal," which means attack. The correct answer describes a medical event that could merit a visit to an ED.*

Content Area: Adult; Concept: Assessment; Neurologic Regulation; Integrated Processes: Communication and Documentation; Client Needs: Physiological Integrity: Reduction of Risk Potential; Cognitive Level: Application [Applying]

### 1343. PHARM ANSWER: 1350

**Convert pounds to kilograms: 198 lb = 90 kg**
**(198 lb ÷ 2.2 lb/kg = 90 kg)**
**Then, determine the mg to administer: 90 kg ×**
**15 mg/kg = 1350 mg**
**The nurse should administer 1350 mg phenytoin (Dilantin).**

♦ *Test-taking Tip: You should first convert pounds to kilograms; 1 kg = 2.2 lb.*

Content Area: Adult; Concept: Medication; Neurologic Regulation; Integrated Processes: Nursing Process: Planning; Client Needs: Physiological Integrity: Pharmacological and Parenteral Therapies; Cognitive Level: Application [Applying]

### 1344. ANSWER 3

1. A VNS device does not stimulate the heart to beat as a pacemaker.
2. A VNS device does not defibrillate the heart as an implantable cardioverter/defibrillator does.

3. A VNS is a medical device that is implanted in the chest and stimulates the vagus nerve to control seizures unresponsive to medical treatment. Clients who experience auras before a seizure use a magnet to activate the VNS to stop the seizure.
4. The device does not have an effect on the airway or secretions.

♦ *Test-taking Tip: A VNS device is a treatment option used for clients with seizures who do not respond to treatment with anticonvulsant medications. The client can activate the device during an aura. Eliminate Options 1 and 2 because they relate to the heart.*

Content Area: Adult; Concept: Management; Neurologic Regulation; Integrated Processes: Nursing Process: Evaluation; Client Needs: Safe and Effective Care Environment: Safety and Infection Control; Physiological Integrity: Reduction of Risk Potential; Cognitive Level: Application [Applying]

### 1345. MoC PHARM ANSWER: 2, 4, 5

1. Anticonvulsant medications such as phenytoin (Dilantin), and not anti-inflammatory medications such as dexamethasone (Decadron), are administered IV to control seizure activity.
2. **Status epilepticus is a medical emergency. The client is at risk for brain hypoxia and permanent brain damage. The client needs additional oxygen, and intubation will secure the airway.**
3. Defibrillation is treatment for ventricular fibrillation, a lethal heart dysrhythmia.
4. **Care is taken to protect the client from injury during the seizure.**
5. **Either lorazepam (Ativan) or diazepam (Valium) is administered initially to terminate the seizure because they can be administered more rapidly than phenytoin.**

♦ *Test-taking Tip: Status epilepticus is consecutive seizures lasting longer than 5 minutes. You should apply the ABC's to identify airway and oxygen as priority interventions. Use Maslow's Hierarchy of Needs to include protection from injury.*

Content Area: Adult; Concept: Safety; Neurologic Regulation; Management; Medication; Integrated Processes: Nursing Process: Implementation; Client Needs: Safe and Effective Care Environment: Management of Care; Physiological Integrity: Pharmacological and Parenteral Therapies; Physiological Integrity: Physiological Adaptation; Cognitive Level: Analysis [Analyzing]

### 1346. ANSWER: 3

1. The nurse should determine the neurological status using the GCS, but this is not the priority.
2. The nurse should assess sensation status at intervals to determine neurological injury progression, but this is not the priority.
3. **Maintaining the correct placement of the cervical collar will keep the client's head and neck in a neutral position and prevent further injury if a spinal fracture or SCI is present. Because ensuring that the cervical collar is correctly placed will prevent further injury, it is priority.**

4. Applying antiembolism hose is an intervention to prevent thromboembolic complications, but this is not the priority.

▶ *Test-taking Tip: You need to focus on an action that will prevent further injury to the client.*

Content Area: Adult; Concept: Neurologic Regulation; Mobility; Integrated Processes: Nursing Process: Implementation; Client Needs: Physiological Integrity: Reduction of Risk Potential; Safe and Effective Care Environment: Safety and Infection Control; Cognitive Level: Application [Applying]

## 1347. ANSWER: 2

1. A complete spinal cord transection results in no reflexes or movement distal to the injury. With a C4 injury, the client initially would have some difficulty breathing due to edema of the spinal cord that occurs above the level of the injury.
2. **The client is experiencing spinal shock that manifests within a few hours after the injury. Hypotension, flaccid paralysis, and absence of muscle contractions occur. Spinal shock lasts 7 to 20 days, and the SCI cannot be classified accurately until spinal shock resolves.**
3. An injury of the upper motor neuron results in spastic paralysis.
4. Quadriplegia, now termed tetraplegia, is paralysis involving all four extremities.

▶ *Test-taking Tip: Focus on the client's symptoms, location of the fracture, and the time of the accident to select the answer. SCI cannot be accurately classified until edema resolves.*

Content Area: Adult; Concept: Assessment; Neurologic Regulation; Mobility; Integrated Processes: Nursing Process: Analysis; Client Needs: Physiological Integrity: Reduction of Risk Potential; Cognitive Level: Analysis [Analyzing]

## 1348. ANSWER: 3

1. Neither traction nor weights are part of the halo device.
2. The halo external fixation device includes a vest that is worn continuously and should not be removed. The neurosurgeon will discontinue it when the injury has stabilized and sufficient healing has occurred.
3. **A halo external fixation device is a static device that consists of a "halo" that is screwed into the skull by four pins. It is attached to a vest that the client wears. The device provides immobilization and stability to the spinal cord while healing occurs with or without surgical intervention. Care includes inspection and cleansing of the pin sites.**
4. The nurse should not tighten the pins. These are secured in the skull to maintain alignment of the cervical vertebrae. If loose, the nurse should contact the HCP for tightening.

▶ *Test-taking Tip: You should recall that external fixation devices are attached to bones with pins. Pin site care is needed to prevent an infection.*

Content Area: Adult; Concept: Critical Thinking; Neurologic Regulation; Integrated Processes: Nursing Process: Planning; Client Needs: Physiological Integrity: Reduction of Risk Potential; Physiological Integrity: Basic Care and Comfort; Safe and Effective Care Environment: Safety and Infection Control; Cognitive Level: Application [Applying]

## 1349. ANSWER: 1, 2, 4, 5

1. **Blurred vision results from the hypertension occurring with autonomic dysreflexia.**
2. **Hypertension is a symptom of autonomic dysreflexia from overstimulation of the sympathetic nervous system (SNS).**
3. Bradycardia (not tachycardia) results from autonomic dysreflexia; the parasympathetic nervous system attempts to maintain homeostasis by slowing down the HR.
4. **Headache results from the hypertension occurring with autonomic dysreflexia.**
5. **Sweating results from the sympathetic stimulation above the level of injury.**

▶ *Test-taking Tip: Autonomic dysreflexia is overstimulation of the sympathetic nervous system that cannot be resolved by the parasympathetic system due to a blockage in the spinal cord from an injury at or above T6. You need to select options that result from SNS stimulation. Then select the options associated with severe hypertension.*

Content Area: Adult; Concept: Neurologic Regulation; Mobility; Integrated Processes: Nursing Process: Analysis; Client Needs: Physiological Integrity: Physiological Adaptation; Cognitive Level: Evaluation [Evaluating]

## 1350. ANSWER: 2, 5

1. Stimulating a cough with a suction catheter is not associated with the quad cough technique, and it may cause regurgitation.
2. **The nurse's hand placement and pushing upward during a cough help to overcome the impaired diaphragmatic function that occurs with a C5 SCI.**
3. Cupping the hands and percussing the lung fields is a technique to loosen secretions but is not the quad coughing technique.
4. Hyperoxygenating the client is a measure to prevent hypoxia associated with suctioning but is not included in the quad coughing technique.
5. **Elevating the head of the bed will promote lung expansion, thus enabling a stronger cough.**

▶ *Test-taking Tip: Family members can be taught to perform a quad cough. Eliminate options that are likely to be performed by health care professionals for other reasons.*

Content Area: Adult; Concept: Neurologic Regulation; Oxygenation; Mobility; Integrated Processes: Nursing Process: Implementation; Client Needs: Physiological Integrity: Reduction of Risk Potential; Cognitive Level: Application [Applying]

**1351. ANSWER: 3, 1, 2, 7, 6, 5, 4**

3. **Elevate the HOB to 90 degrees. This initial quick action may help lower the client's BP.**

1. **Lower the end of the bed so feet are dependent. Placing the feet lower than the head will help decrease blood return and may help lower the BP.**

2. **Remove elastic stocking and other constricting devices; assess below the level of injury. Anything constricting below the level of injury can be the stimulus that precipitates autonomic dysreflexia. The nurse can assess for other precipitating factors, such as a full bladder, while removing constricting devices.**

7. **Retake the BP after being upright for 2 to 3 minutes. Elevating the HOB, lowering the feet, and removing constricting devices may have lowered the BP. If not, further interventions are needed.**

6. **Administer a prn prescribed sublingual nifedipine for continued elevated BP. If the BP remains elevated, the prescribed antihypertensive medication, such as nifedipine (Procardia), should be given next to quickly lower the BP.**

5. **Perform digital removal of impacted stool (last BM found to be 10 days ago). Digitally removing stool impaction may cause a further spike in BP, so removal of the stool impaction should be completed after the BP medication is given.**

4. **Inform the HCP of the incident, measures taken, and client response. This is last because a prn antihypertensive medication had already been prescribed. Care of the client is priority.**

▶ *Test-taking Tip: Autonomic dysreflexia is overstimulation of the sympathetic nervous system that cannot be resolved by the parasympathetic system due to a blockage in the spinal cord from an injury at or above T6. If medications for hypertension are already prescribed, treating the client should occur before notifying the HCP.*

**Content Area:** Adult; **Concept:** Neurologic Regulation; Mobility; **Integrated Processes:** Nursing Process: Implementation; **Client Needs:** Safe and Effective Care Environment: Safety and Infection Control; Physiological Integrity: Physiological Adaptation; **Cognitive Level:** Synthesis [Creating]

**1352. ANSWER: 1, 5**

1. **Although the client has an incomplete T6 SCI, the woman is still capable of becoming pregnant.**

2. The client with an incomplete T6 SCI is able to get pregnant.

3. Although the client may not feel the onset of labor, she may still be able to deliver the baby vaginally or via cesarean section.

4. Sexual intercourse is allowable and would not worsen the client's condition. The female may not be able to feel an orgasm.

5. **The client may not be able to feel an orgasm after an incomplete T6 SCI.**

▶ *Test-taking Tip: An SCI at this level does not affect fertility and pregnancy. However, when selecting options you need to consider that with the loss of nerve function with a complete cord transection, sensation and motor function below the level of the injury are affected.*

**Content Area:** Adult; **Concept:** Neurologic Regulation; Mobility; Communication; **Integrated Processes:** Communication and Documentation; Caring; **Client Needs:** Physiological Integrity: Physiological Adaptation; Psychosocial Integrity; **Cognitive Level:** Application [Applying]

**1353. ANSWER: 1, 2, 4, 5, 6**

1. **The lower-than-normal Hgb and Hct indicate anemia. Inadequate cell oxygenation contributes to fatigue.**

2. **Baclofen (Lioresal), a skeletal muscle relaxant used to relieve spasms, has the adverse effects of drowsiness and fatigue.**

3. Working 4 to 8 hours per week is a limited number of hours and should not contribute to the client's fatigue.

4. **The client has stopped amitriptyline (Elavil), an antidepressant, and may be clinically depressed. Fatigue is a major symptom of depression.**

5. **A tricuspid murmur indicates an incompetent cardiac valve, which will decrease the amount of oxygenated blood reaching the tissues.**

6. **The increased energy expenditure with ambulation can increase fatigue.**

▶ *Test-taking Tip: You need to consider that abnormal laboratory values, medication adverse effects, and the primary and other conditions can all contribute to fatigue.*

**Content Area:** Adult; **Concept:** Sensory Perception; Neurologic Regulation; Mobility; **Integrated Processes:** Nursing Process: Analysis; **Client Needs:** Physiological Integrity: Reduction of Risk Potential; **Cognitive Level:** Evaluation [Evaluating]

**1354. ANSWER: 2, 3, 5**

1. Hot baths should be avoided; increasing the body temperature can exacerbate symptoms. Burns can occur with sensory loss associated with MS.

2. **A stretch–hold–relax routine is often helpful for relaxing the muscle and treating muscle spasms.**

3. **Walking will help improve the gait, strengthen weakened muscles, and help relieve spasticity in the legs. If a muscle group is irreversibly affected by MS, other muscles can learn to compensate. A walker should be used for safety to help prevent falling.**

4. Widening the base of support increases walking stability, especially if ataxia (incoordination) is present; if feet are close together it increases the risk for a fall.

5. **Drinking fluids and then using an alarm to void 30 minutes later may be helpful in reducing incontinence from loss of bladder sensation.**

▶ *Test-taking Tip: Relate information in the stem about the client's problems to terms in the options. Eliminate options that increase the client's risk for injury.*

Content Area: Adult; Concept: Sensory Perception; Neurologic Regulation; Mobility; Integrated Processes: Nursing Process: Implementation; Client Needs: Safe and Effective Care Environment: Safety and Infection Control; Physiological Integrity: Reduction of Risk Potential; Cognitive Level: Analysis [Analyzing]

## 1355. ANSWER: 4

1. The client with SCI, not GBS, should be monitored for autonomic dysreflexia.
2. The client who has bacterial meningitis should be monitored for septic emboli.
3. Although the client with GBS should be monitored for cardiac dysrhythmias, it is most important to monitor for respiratory failure.
4. **It is most important for the nurse to monitor for respiratory failure. Ascending paralysis that occurs in GBS can affect the innervation of the muscles used in respiration, leading to respiratory failure.**

▶ *Test-taking Tip: You should consider that GBS can lead to muscular paralysis, so select the most serious complication.*

Content Area: Adult; Concept: Oxygenation; Neurologic Regulation; Integrated Processes: Nursing Process: Assessment; Client Needs: Physiological Integrity: Reduction of Risk Potential; Cognitive Level: Application [Applying]

## 1356. ANSWER: 2

1. Elevated glucose levels are not associated with DI.
2. **The lack of ADH that occurs in DI results in excreting a large amount of pale, dilute urine.**
3. The urine of clients with DI is very dilute and therefore has a very low, not high, specific gravity.
4. Decrease in level of consciousness is not directly associated with DI but rather with craniocerebral swelling or bleeding from the trauma.

▶ *Test-taking Tip: Craniocerebral trauma can result in compression of the pituitary gland and loss of ADH production. You should note that large amounts of urine output and a high specific gravity are not usually associated together, so one of these options must be incorrect.*

Content Area: Adult; Concept: Fluid and Electrolyte Balance; Neurologic Regulation; Metabolism; Integrated Processes: Nursing Process: Analysis; Client Needs: Physiological Integrity: Reduction of Risk Potential; Cognitive Level: Analysis [Analyzing]

## 1357. ANSWER: 2

1. This illustration shows a subdural hematoma, which occurs below the dura.
2. **This illustration shows an epidural hematoma, which occurs between the skull and the dura.**
3. This illustration shows normal brain structures.
4. An intracerebral hematoma occurs within the brain tissue and can result in brain herniation as shown in this illustration.

▶ *Test-taking Tip: The word "epi-" means above, so an epidural hematoma is blood accumulation "above the dura."*

Content Area: Adult; Concept: Neurologic Regulation; Nursing Roles; Integrated Processes: Teaching/Learning; Client Needs: Physiological Integrity: Physiological Adaptation; Cognitive Level: Application [Applying]

## 1358. PHARM ANSWER: 1

1. **Mannitol (Osmitrol), an osmotic diuretic, increases the serum osmolarity and pulls fluid from the tissues, thus decreasing cerebral edema postoperatively. Serum osmolarity levels should be assessed as a parameter to determine proper dosage.**
2. The WBC count is not affected by mannitol.
3. Serum cholesterol is not affected by mannitol.
4. ESR is not affected by mannitol.

▶ *Test-taking Tip: The brand name Osmitrol suggests that the medication acts by regulation of osmosis. Use this information to narrow the options.*

Content Area: Adult; Concept: Medication; Neurologic Regulation; Integrated Processes: Nursing Process: Implementation; Client Needs: Physiological Integrity: Pharmacological and Parenteral Therapies; Physiological Integrity: Reduction of Risk Potential; Cognitive Level: Application [Applying]

## 1359. PHARM ANSWER: 3, 4, 5

1. The client with mild TBI usually experiences symptoms commonly associated with mild concussion, such as vomiting.
2. The client with mild TBI usually experiences amnesia and is unable to recall events regarding the accident.
3. **Recurrent problems with headache and dizziness are the most prominent symptoms of mild TBI.**
4. **Cognitive difficulties, including inability to concentrate and forgetfulness, occur with mild TBI.**
5. **At the time of the accident, the person with mild TBI may experience a loss of consciousness for a few seconds or minutes.**

▶ *Test-taking Tip: Symptoms of mild TBI result from axonal or neuronal and glial cell injury. You should eliminate options with normal findings.*

Content Area: Adult; Concept: Assessment; Neurologic Regulation; Trauma; Sensory; Integrated Processes: Nursing Process: Analysis; Client Needs: Physiological Integrity: Physiological Adaptation; Psychosocial Integrity; Cognitive Level: Analysis [Analyzing]

## 1360. ANSWER: 1

1. **If untreated, increased ICP causes a shift in brain tissue and can result in irreversible brain damage and possibly death.**
2. ICP compresses structures within the cranium and leads to a decrease in cerebral perfusion, not increased perfusion.
3. ICP compresses structures within the cranium and leads to acidosis; the pH level is decreased in acidosis.
4. Leakage of CSF could occur if there were an opening in the subarachnoid space that could occur with trauma, but there is no indication that the increased ICP is due to trauma.

▶ *Test-taking Tip: You need to avoid reading into the question. There is no indication in the question as to what is causing the increased ICP.*

Content Area: Adult; Concept: Neurologic Regulation; Integrated Processes: Nursing Process: Analysis; Client Needs: Physiological Integrity: Physiological Adaptation; Cognitive Level: Comprehension [Understanding]

### 1361. PHARM ANSWER: 2

1. A negative CT scan is a criterion for administering the thrombolytic therapy.
2. **Contraindications to thrombolytic therapy for the client with an ischemic stroke include a serious head injury within the previous 3 months. This would put the client at risk of developing serious bleeding problems, specifically cerebral hemorrhage.**
3. History of type 1 DM is not a contraindication for thrombolytic therapy.
4. The onset of neurological deficits within 3 hours is a criterion for administering thrombolytic therapy.

▶ *Test-taking Tip: The word "thrombolytic" means breakdown of a blood clot, so a risk associated with the thrombolytic therapy is bleeding. Read each option carefully and select the option that relates to bleeding.*

Content Area: Adult; Concept: Medication; Neurologic Regulation; Integrated Processes: Nursing Process: Analysis; Client Needs: Physiological Integrity: Pharmacological and Parenteral Therapies; Physiological Integrity: Reduction of Risk Potential; Cognitive Level: Application [Applying]

### 1362. ANSWER: 4

1. Having the client face the nurse will not aid the client in expressing his or her needs.
2. The nurse's slow enunciation of directions will not aid the client in expressing his or her needs.
3. Using gestures and body language will not aid the client in expressing his or her needs.
4. **Asking the client to point to needed objects would be most helpful when the client is having difficulty communicating with the nurse.**

▶ *Test-taking Tip: Three options are similar, and one is different. Often the option that is different is the answer. The client with expressive aphasia understands what the nurse is saying but has difficulty finding the correct words.*

Content Area: Adult; Concept: Neurologic Regulation; Communication; Integrated Processes: Communication and Documentation; Client Needs: Physiological Integrity: Physiological Adaptation; Psychosocial Integrity; Cognitive Level: Application [Applying]

### 1363. ANSWER: 9

**Spontaneous eye opening is scored as 4; the best verbal response of inappropriate words is scored as 3, and the best motor response of decerebrate posturing is scored as 2.**

▶ *Test-taking Tip: The best score on the Glasgow Coma Scale is 15. You can remember the scoring by remembering 4, 5, 6. The best score for eye opening is 4, for verbal response is 5, and motor response is 6. The lowest score in each category is 1, which is no response.*

Content Area: Adult; Concept: Neurologic Regulation; Integrated Processes: Nursing Process: Analysis; Client Needs: Physiological Integrity: Physiological Adaptation; Cognitive Level: Application [Applying]

### 1364. ANSWER: 4

1. Pressure exerted on the soles of the feet when placed firmly against the footboard can impair circulation and lead to skin breakdown.
2. Pillows provide inadequate support to prevent plantar flexion (foot drop).
3. Performing ROM daily helps to maintain muscle tone, but it is inadequate to prevent plantar flexion when the client is in bed.
4. **Applying a foot boot brace provides good support to prevent foot drop. Removing and reapplying it every 2 hours allows for pressure reduction and promotes circulation.**

▶ *Test-taking Tip: The key word is "best." You should consider the option that best prevents plantar flexion.*

Content Area: Adult; Concept: Neurologic Regulation; Mobility; Integrated Processes: Nursing Process: Implementation; Client Needs: Physiological Integrity: Reduction of Risk Potential; Physiological Integrity: Basic Care and Comfort; Cognitive Level: Application [Applying]

### 1365. ANSWER: 3

1. A stroke affecting the right hemisphere may produce left, not right hemiparesis. Motor fibers in the brain cross over in the medulla before entering the spinal column.
2. This client may or may not have aphasia because the center for language is located on the left side of the brain in 75% to 80% of the population; this client had a stroke involving the right hemisphere. Even though the client may have expressive aphasia, it is more important to assess for poor impulse control due to the risk for injury.
3. **The client with a stroke affecting the right side of the brain often exhibits impulsive behavior and is unaware of the neurological deficits. Poor impulse control increases the client's risk for injury.**
4. Tetraplegia (quadriplegia) is associated with an SCI; tetraplegia usually does not occur from a stroke.

▶ *Test-taking Tip: You should eliminate options knowing that the nerves cross over at the medulla, which produces contralateral effects from the stroke. You should consider an option that increases the client's risk for injury.*

Content Area: Adult; Concept: Neurologic Regulation; Safety; Integrated Processes: Nursing Process: Assessment; Client Needs: Physiological Integrity: Physiological Adaptation; Cognitive Level: Analysis [Analyzing]

### 1366. MoC ANSWER: 2

1. Tendency to fall to the contralateral side would be a concern if the client were weak or paralyzed.
2. **Homonymous hemianopia (hemianopsia) is a visual field abnormality that results in blindness in half of the visual field in the same side of both eyes. It results from damage to the optic tract or occipital lobe.**

3. Using the silverware inappropriately is a concern if the client has agnosia.
4. Choking when swallowing any liquids is a concern if the client has dysphagia.

▸ *Test-taking Tip: The prefix "hemi-" means half; only one option contains the word half.*

Content Area: Adult; **Concept:** Neurologic Regulation; Nutrition; Management; **Integrated Processes:** Nursing Process: Implementation; **Client Needs:** Safe and Effective Care Environment: Management of Care; **Cognitive Level:** Application [Applying]

## 1367. MoC ANSWER: 4

1. Pupillary changes may occur with ICP as it progresses, but they are not an early sign of developing ICP.
2. A drop in BP is not directly associated with neurological deterioration. A BP with a wide pulse pressure is a late sign of increased ICP.
3. Diminished sensation may occur with increased ICP, but it is not the earliest sign.
4. **A change in the level of consciousness is the first sign of neurological deterioration and is often associated with the development of increased ICP.**

▸ *Test-taking Tip: The key words are "earliest sign of ICP." Consider that the earliest sign may be the subtlest change.*

Content Area: Adult; **Concept:** Neurologic Regulation; Management; Assessment; **Integrated Processes:** Nursing Process: Assessment; **Client Needs:** Safe and Effective Care Environment: Management of Care; Physiological Integrity: Reduction of Risk Potential; **Cognitive Level:** Application [Applying]

## 1368. ANSWER: 1, 3, 5

1. **A subarachnoid hemorrhage is usually caused by rupture of a cerebral aneurysm.**
2. Ischemic stroke in older adults, not a subarachnoid hemorrhage, often occurs during sleep when circulation and BP decrease.
3. **Irritation of the meninges from bleeding into the subarachnoid spaces causes a severe headache.**
4. Thrombolytic therapy with tPA lyses clots and is contraindicated in subarachnoid hemorrhage.
5. **Bleeding into the subarachnoid space will cause the CSF to be bloody.**

▸ *Test-taking Tip: You should select the statements that are correct when evaluating whether the new nurse understands information about subarachnoid hemorrhage.*

Content Area: Adult; **Concept:** Neurologic Regulation; **Integrated Processes:** Teaching/Learning; Nursing Process: Evaluation; **Client Needs:** Physiological Integrity: Physiological Adaptation; **Cognitive Level:** Evaluation [Evaluating]

## 1369. ANSWER: 2

1. A carotid endarterectomy involves removal of plaque from the carotid artery.
2. **NPH is treated with the placement of a permanent shunt in a lateral ventricle of the brain to the peritoneal cavity. The excess CSF drains into the peritoneal cavity.**

3. A lumbar drain can be used to remove CSF with disorders that increase CSF in the subarachnoid space in the lumbar area; this does not remain permanently.
4. Anticonvulsant medications are used to treat seizures.

▸ *Test-taking Tip: NPH is a reversible neurological condition in older adults resulting from excess production of CSF. The client's ventricles in the brain are dilated despite normal CSF pressure.*

Content Area: Adult; **Concept:** Neurologic Regulation; **Integrated Processes:** Nursing Process: Planning; **Client Needs:** Physiological Integrity: Reduction of Risk Potential; **Cognitive Level:** Comprehension [Understanding]

## 1370. ANSWER: 4

1. A normal temperature does not strengthen the immune system.
2. Although hypothermia may increase the client's chance for survival, the question is asking for the rationale for bringing the temperature to a normal level.
3. Hyperthermia, not a normal temperature, is associated with lower scores on the Glasgow Coma Scale.
4. **The nurse should initiate temperature reduction measures because a temperature elevation in the client poststroke can cause an increase in the infarct size. This may be due to the increased oxygen demand with hyperthermia and peripheral vasodilation that decreases cerebral perfusion.**

▸ *Test-taking Tip: Associate the word "deteriorating" in the stem with the only option that suggests a worsening status.*

Content Area: Adult; **Concept:** Thermo-regulation; Neurologic Regulation; **Integrated Processes:** Nursing Process: Analysis; **Client Needs:** Physiological Integrity: Reduction of Risk Potential; **Cognitive Level:** Application [Applying]

## 1371. CJ ANSWER:

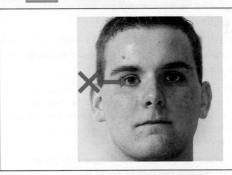

**The client should be looking straight ahead. Then, the penlight should be brought in from the right side and the light shown into the right eye to check its pupillary response.**

▸ *Test-taking Tip: Be sure to check the right eye and not the left.*

Content Area: Adult; **Concept:** Assessment; Neurologic Regulation; **Integrated Processes:** Nursing Process: Application; **Client Needs:** Physiological Integrity: Physiological Adaptation; **Cognitive Level:** Application [Applying]

**1372. ANSWER: 1, 2, 3, 4**

1. **Surgery, radiation therapy, and/or chemotherapy may be used to treat a slowly or rapidly growing tumor.**
2. **Surgery, radiation therapy, and/or chemotherapy may be used to treat a benign or malignant tumor.**
3. **Surgery, radiation therapy, and/or chemotherapy may be used to treat tumors of different cell types.**
4. **The tumor's location in the brain may affect whether surgery is an option or whether the surgical approach with radiation therapy and/or chemotherapy is used to treat the tumor.**
5. Comorbid conditions, not age, may be determining factors in treatment options. The type of insurance is irrelevant to treatment unless treatment is experimental.

▶ *Test-taking Tip: The client's ability to pay may influence choosing one treatment option over another; however, all treatment options would be made available if they are appropriate for the client's diagnosis.*

Content Area: Adult; Concept: Nursing Roles; Neurologic Regulation; Integrated Processes: Teaching/Learning; Client Needs: Physiological Integrity: Physiological Adaptation; Cognitive Level: Application [Applying]

**1373. ANSWER: 2**

1. The client with endocarditis has an infective process within the body's circulation and is at risk for septic emboli, which could progress to a brain abscess.
2. **The client who has idiopathic epilepsy has the lowest risk of developing a brain abscess because epilepsy from an unknown cause does not have the risk factors of an active infectious process or an impaired immune system.**
3. The client with the liver transplant is at risk for brain abscess because immunosuppressant medications depress the immune system.
4. The client with meningitis has an infective process in close proximity to the brain and should be monitored for a brain abscess.

▶ *Test-taking Tip: Brain abscess is a collection of pus in the brain that occurs from an infection. Risk factors for development of a brain abscess include an infectious process or an impaired immune system. The key word is "lowest." Select the client with the lowest risk.*

Content Area: Adult; Concept: Infection; Neurologic Regulation; Integrated Processes: Nursing Process: Assessment; Client Needs: Physiological Integrity: Reduction of Risk Potential; Cognitive Level: Application [Applying]

**1374. ANSWER: 2**

1. Cogwheel rigidity, a symptom of PD, is interrupted muscular movement and is not treated with the DBS.
2. **DBS is a treatment used for intractable tremors associated with PD. The electrical current interferes with the brain cells initiating the tremors.**

3. Severe facial pain is associated with trigeminal neuralgia, not PD. The DBS will not affect facial expression.
4. Auras are unusual sensations experienced before a seizure occurs and are not associated with PD.

▶ *Test-taking Tip: Identify that the question calls for improvement in the symptoms of PD. Consider the symptoms specific to PD: bradykinesia, tremors, and muscle rigidity. Then, evaluate each option for improvement of these symptoms. This should lead you to select Option 2.*

Content Area: Adult; Concept: Sensory Perception; Neurologic Regulation; Integrated Processes: Nursing Process: Evaluation; Client Needs: Physiological Integrity: Reduction of Risk Potential; Cognitive Level: Evaluation [Evaluating]

**1375.** **PHARM** **ANSWER: 1**

1. **When first taking levodopa/carbidopa (Sinemet), the client is likely to experience dizziness and orthostatic hypotension due to the dopamine agonist properties. The client and spouse must be alerted about the increased risk for falls.**
2. Levodopa/carbidopa can be taken with multiple vitamins.
3. Levodopa/carbidopa can be taken with food to decrease GI upset.
4. There are many, not few, adverse effects associated with levodopa/carbidopa, including involuntary movements, anxiety, memory loss, blurred vision, and mydriasis.

▶ *Test-taking Tip: Levodopa/carbidopa (Sinemet) is an antiparkinsonian agent. Levodopa is converted to dopamine in the CNS, where it serves as a neurotransmitter, and carbidopa, a decarboxylase inhibitor, prevents peripheral destruction of levodopa. You need to consider the side effects of levodopa/carbidopa to correctly answer the question.*

Content Area: Adult; Concept: Medication; Neurologic Regulation; Integrated Processes: Teaching/Learning; Client Needs: Physiological Integrity: Pharmacological and Parenteral Therapies; Health Promotion and Maintenance; Cognitive Level: Application [Applying]

**1376. ANSWER: 2**

1. There is no information that the client is working too much. Telling the client to avoid thinking the worst belittles the client's concern.
2. **This is the most appropriate response because it focuses on the client's concern, encourages verbalization, and solicits more information.**
3. ALS (Lou Gehrig's disease) is a degenerative disease that affects the motor system and does not have a dementia component; thus, a question about memory is inappropriate.
4. This response does not take the client seriously and does not address the client's concern.

▶ *Test-taking Tip: You should apply therapeutic communication principles. Only one option addresses the client's concern.*

Content Area: Adult; Concept: Communication; Neurologic Regulation; Integrated Processes: Communication and Documentation; Client Needs: Psychosocial Integrity; Cognitive Level: Application [Applying]

## 1377. ANSWER: 4

1. Ptosis (drooping eyelids) is a sign of muscle weakness often seen with MG.
2. If the muscles involved with speech are weak in the client with MG, the client may exhibit slurred speech.
3. Clients with MG may demonstrate weakness in the lower extremities.
4. **Numbness around the mouth is not associated with muscle weakness but could be indicative of a calcium deficiency or some other problem.**

▶ *Test-taking Tip:* MG is an autoimmune condition affecting the neuromuscular junction, causing muscle weakness. Only one option does not address muscle weakness.

Content Area: Adult; Concept: Mobility; Neurologic Regulation; Assessment; Integrated Processes: Nursing Process: Assessment; Client Needs: Physiological Integrity: Physiological Adaptation; Cognitive Level: Analysis [Analyzing]

## 1378. ANSWER: 1

1. **Stooping and avoiding bending and twisting motions when lifting objects lessen the likelihood of injury.**
2. The client should wear supportive shoes.
3. The client should include regular daily exercise as a program (not excessive walking over 2 days on the weekend).
4. Clients should avoid prolonged sitting or standing.

▶ *Test-taking Tip:* The key phrase is "positive lifestyle changes."

Content Area: Adult; Concept: Promoting Health; Neurologic Regulation; Mobility; Integrated Processes: Nursing Process: Evaluation; Client Needs: Health Promotion and Maintenance; Cognitive Level: Analysis [Analyzing]

## 1379. MoC PHARM CJ ANSWER: 1

1. **Exaggerated spasticity, muscle rigidity, and tinnitus are adverse effects of baclofen (Lioresal) that the nurse should discuss with the HCP.**
2. The prescribed medications for bowel elimination may be working for the client. There is inadequate information to warrant addressing these with the HCP.
3. The WBC and liver enzymes are WNL. The glucose, although elevated, is not as important as addressing the assessment findings with the HCP.
4. All prescribed medications are appropriate for the client who has a T12 SCI and can be safely given when the client has a penicillin allergy.

▶ *Test-taking Tip:* With a chart/exhibit type of question, it is often faster and easier to arrive at the answer by reviewing the options before analyzing the chart information.

Content Area: Adult; Concept: Collaboration; Neurologic Regulation; Medication; Diversity; Integrated Processes: Nursing Process: Implementation; Culture and Spirituality; Client Needs: Safe and Effective Care Environment: Management of Care; Physiological Integrity: Pharmacological and Parenteral Therapies; Cognitive Level: Analysis [Analyzing]

## Chapter Thirty-One

# Renal and Urinary Management

**1380.** The nurse is planning care for the client, who is scheduled for an IVP. Which intervention should the nurse plan to implement?

1. Teach that a warm, flushing sensation may occur as the dye is injected.
2. Prepare the client for urinary catheterization before the procedure.
3. Keep the client NPO after the procedure until test results are obtained.
4. Ambulate the client in the hall to promote excretion of the dye.

**1381.** MoC The nurse notes bright red blood and clots in the client's urine after a cystoscopy. Which is the most appropriate **initial** action by the nurse?

1. Irrigate the client's bladder.
2. Notify the HCP.
3. Apply heat over the client's bladder.
4. Give the prescribed antispasmodic agent.

**1382.** PHARM The client is concerned about having brown-colored urine after starting nitrofurantoin for treating a UTI. Which response by the nurse is **most** appropriate?

1. "Your urine is too concentrated. Take only one-half the dose of nitrofurantoin."
2. "Stop taking nitrofurantoin and make an appointment to have a urine culture."
3. "Nitrofurantoin normally does discolor urine; continue taking it as prescribed."
4. "Drink at least 500 mL of fluid every 3 hours to lighten the color of your urine."

**1383.** MoC The nurse is caring for the client experiencing a possible hospital-acquired bladder infection. Which nursing action should the nurse perform **first?**

1. Obtain an order for urine culture and sensitivity.
2. Administer the prescribed antibiotic medication.
3. Teach about wiping the perineum front to back.
4. Prepare the client for removal of the catheter.

**1384.** The nurse is caring for the female client experiencing recurrent UTIs. Which statement would **best** help the client reduce her risk for another UTI?

1. "Eliminate caffeine and tea from your diet."
2. "Take tub baths rather than showering."
3. "Wear good-quality synthetic underwear."
4. "Abstain from having sexual intercourse."

**1385.** The client with acute pyelonephritis of the left kidney is hospitalized. The nurse should monitor for which most frequently occurring symptom?

1. Low-grade fever
2. Bradycardia
3. Left-sided flank pain
4. Right quadrant rebound tenderness

**1386.** The nurse is caring for the client diagnosed with obstructing left ureterolithiasis. The nurse evaluates that the client may have passed the calculi in the urine when which outcome has been achieved?

1. Voiding clear amber urine greater than 30 mL per hour
2. No evidence of hematemesis or urinary tract infection
3. Absence of epigastric pain, nausea, and vomiting
4. Absence of colicky pain in the left lateral flank and groin

**1387.** During a teaching session, the nurse uses an illustration to show the client where inflammation occurs in left-sided pyelonephritis. Place an X to identify this area of inflammation.

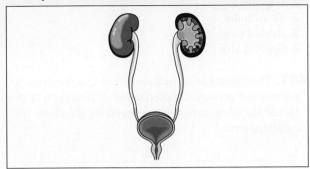

**1388.** The nurse is completing an admission assessment of the client with a possible obstructing struvite calculus of the right ureter. Which is the best question for the nurse to ask?

1. "Are you experiencing any pain in your left flank?"
2. "Do you like to drink cranberry, prune, or tomato juice?"
3. "Have you had a history of chronic urinary tract infections?"
4. "How often do you eat organ meats, poultry, fish, and sardines?"

**1389.** **MoC** The nurse is admitting the hospitalized client who has a renal calculus. Which should be the nurse's **priority?**

1. Encourage the client to increase the amount of oral fluids.
2. Obtain necessary supplies to measure and strain all urine.
3. Assess the location and the severity of the client's pain.
4. Obtain consent for extracorporeal shock wave lithotripsy (ESWL).

**1390.** The nurse is planning care for the client who is to undergo extracorporeal shock wave lithotripsy (ESWL). Which actions should the nurse include in the plan of care **immediately** following the procedure? **Select all that apply.**

1. Instruct about measuring and straining all urine.
2. Give no fluids or foods for 24 hours post-ESWL.
3. Check for flank ecchymosis on the affected side.
4. Assess the incision for clean, dry, and intactness.
5. Remove the stent that was placed during ESWL.

**1391.** **MoC** The client has new-onset urge urinary incontinence. Which prescribed interventions should the nurse verify with the HCP? **Select all that apply.**

1. Have the client taken to the bathroom q4h.
2. Give the daily prescribed diuretics at suppertime.
3. Turn on the water to assist the client to void.
4. Avoid caffeine and fluids that contain aspartame.
5. Instruct about vaginal weights for daytime use.

**1392.** **PHARM** The client has xerostomia secondary to oxybutynin use for treating urge incontinence. Which interventions should the nurse implement to relieve xerostomia?

1. Have the client bathe in tepid water.
2. Offer sugar-free candy or gumdrops.
3. Massage the client's skin with lotion.
4. Place a fan by the client at a low setting.

**1393.** The client, being treated for stress incontinence with vaginal cone therapy, calls a clinic to report burning when urinating, chills, and fever. Which is the nurse's **best** instruction?

1. "Take acetaminophen to relieve the pain and reduce your fever."
2. "Come to the clinic. We need to complete a urine culture and sensitivity."
3. "Discontinue the use of the vaginal weights to see if the symptoms subside."
4. "Drink cranberry juice and increase your fluid intake for the next 48 hours."

**1394.** **MoC** The HCP writes orders for the newly hospitalized client who has polycystic kidney disease (PKD) and dull flank pain, nocturia, and low urine specific gravity dilute urine. Which admission order should the nurse clarify with the HCP?

1. Fluid intake of at least 2000 mL daily
2. Restrict sodium intake to 500 mg daily
3. Initiate referral for genetic counseling
4. Metoprolol 12.5 mg (oral) bid

**1395.** The client has PKD. The nurse should consider that a cyst may have ruptured when collecting which information on assessment?

1. Reports a decrease in pain
2. Voids cola-colored urine
3. Passes stools that are bloody
4. Has a decreased serum creatinine level

**1396.** The client is scheduled for a cystectomy with an ileal conduit for urinary diversion. Which explanation should the nurse provide when the client asks about postsurgery urination?

1. "The normal urinary flow is maintained with this type of surgery."
2. "Doing Kegel exercises may help you achieve urinary continence."
3. "Bladder retraining will be taught later during your recovery."
4. "A urine collection bag is placed over the stoma that will be created."

**1397.** The client had continent urinary diversion surgery with creation of a Kock pouch. Which intervention should the nurse plan when caring for the client?

1. Insert a catheter in the pouch every 4 to 6 hours to drain the urine.
2. Cleanse the skin around the stoma with alcohol and water every day.
3. Encourage sleeping on the side of the stoma for good urine drainage.
4. Apply the stoma pouch so that it fits snugly to avoid urine leakage.

**1398.** **MoC** The female nurse is preparing to empty the urostomy bag of a female client. Which statement would be **most** respectful of the client?

1. "Do you want your spouse in the room when I empty the urine from this bag?"
2. "You need to increase your fluid intake. What beverages do you like to drink?"
3. "I need to move the covers to the side to empty the bag. Can I do this now?"
4. "You didn't eat lunch, and you need protein for healing. Don't you like the food?"

**1399.** **MoC** The client has had a kidney transplant from a live donor. The nurse should notify the HCP to report a possible complication of urine leakage when noting which findings on assessment?

1. Urine output 15 mL/hr; serum creatinine 3.4 mg/dL; lower abdominal discomfort
2. Urine output 200 mL/hr; serum creatinine 1.2 mg/dL; incisional discomfort
3. Urine output 20 mL/hr; elevated temperature; tenderness over the transplanted kidney
4. Urine output 0 mL for 1 hr, then 300 mL/hr; erratic output; incisional discomfort

**1400.** **PHARM** The client who had a kidney transplant has newly prescribed medications. Which prescribed medication should the nurse administer for BP control?

1. Digoxin
2. Tacrolimus
3. Amlodipine
4. Epoetin alfa

**1401.** The client has an Indiana pouch that requires intermittent urinary catheterization. Which type of stoma should the nurse expect when preparing the client for catheterization?

1.
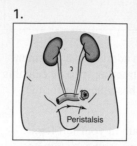

2.
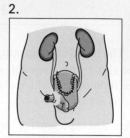

3.
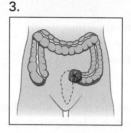

4.
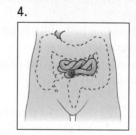

**1402.** **MoC** The NA reports to the nurse that urine in the client's urostomy bag is dark amber colored with a large amount of thick mucus. Which should be the nurse's instruction to the NA?

1. Obtain a urine specimen for culture.
2. Change the client's urostomy bag.
3. Offer the client fluids more often.
4. Ambulate the client in the hall.

**1403.** The client has a nephrostomy tube in place after a partial nephrectomy. Which actions should the nurse include when caring for a nephrostomy tube? **Select all that apply.**

1. Clamp and unclamp the tube every 4 hours.
2. Irrigate with 30 mL of sterile saline solution daily.
3. Observe for cloudy, foul-smelling urinary drainage.
4. Keep the nephrostomy tube below kidney level.
5. Record nephrostomy and urinary tube output separately.

**1404.** The nurse is caring for four clients. Which client requires further nursing assessment due to risk of prerenal failure?

1. The client diagnosed with renal calculi
2. The client undergoing an IV pyelogram
3. The client who has congestive heart failure
4. The client who had a transfusion reaction

**1405.** PHARM The nurse assesses that the client with ARF has a serum potassium level of 6.8 mEq/L. Which medications, if prescribed, should the nurse plan to administer **now**? **Select all that apply.**

1. Erythropoietin
2. Regular insulin
3. 0.45% saline bolus
4. Calcium gluconate
5. Sodium polystyrene sulfonate

**1406.** Three weeks after developing ARF following trauma, the hospitalized client has a significantly increased urinary output. Which assessment finding should the nurse report to the HCP immediately?

1. Absence of adventitious breath sounds
2. A drop in BP and an increase in pulse rate
3. A 3-pound weight loss over 24 hours
4. A serum potassium level of 3.7 mEq/L

**1407.** The client with CRF receives a hemodialysis treatment. The client's weight before dialysis was 83 kg and after dialysis is 80 kg. How many liters should the nurse estimate that the client lost during the hemodialysis treatment?

_____ L (Record your answer as a whole number.)

**1408.** The nurse is planning meals for the client on hemodialysis and fluid restriction secondary to ARF. Which afternoon snack should the nurse include?

1. Large banana
2. Glass of milk
3. Ham sandwich
4. A small apple

**1409.** The nurse is caring for the client who developed ARF. Which findings support the nurse's conclusion that the client is in the recovery phase of ARF? **Select all that apply.**

1. Increased urine specific gravity
2. Increased serum creatinine level
3. Decreased serum potassium level
4. Absence of nausea and vomiting
5. Absence of muscle twitching

**1410.** MoC The experienced nurse and new nurse are caring for clients with CRF. Which statement made by the new nurse should the experienced nurse correct?

1. "The client with CRF is starting on peritoneal dialysis and should have a high-protein diet."
2. "The amount of outflow from peritoneal dialysis should equal the amount that was instilled."
3. "I should hold the client's dose of lisinopril because the client is going for hemodialysis now."
4. "I will ensure that the client with CRF has more carbohydrates because protein is restricted."

**1411.** PHARM After a diagnosis of CRF, the client was started on epoetin alfa. Which finding indicates that the medication has been effective?

1. Decrease in serum creatinine levels
2. Increase in WBCs
3. Increase in serum hematocrit
4. Decrease in BP

**1412.** ABGs are prescribed for the client with CRF who has hypotension, cold and clammy skin, and dysrhythmias (see table). The nurse should notify the HCP to report that the client is experiencing which imbalance?

| ABG Laboratory Value | Client's Value | Normal Values |
|---|---|---|
| pH | 7.20 | 7.35–7.45 |
| $Paco_2$ | 32 | 35–45 mm Hg |
| $HCO_3$ | 14 | Bicarb 22–26 mEq/L |
| Base excess/ deficit | −3 | +2 mEq/L |
| $Pao_2$ | 80 | 80–100 mm Hg |

1. Respiratory acidosis
2. Respiratory alkalosis
3. Metabolic acidosis
4. Metabolic alkalosis

**1413.** The 75-year-old client is hospitalized with ESRD. Which finding in the client's medical record should the nurse associate with the diagnosis of ESRD?

1. A urinary output of less than 100 mL in 24 hours
2. A glomerular filtration rate less than 15 mL/min/ 1.73 m$^2$
3. A serum creatinine level greater than 12.0 mg/dL
4. A serum blood urea nitrogen greater than 100 mg/dL

**1414.** The nurse is caring for the client with CRF. Which statement should the nurse document as an appropriate outcome in the plan of care?

1. Eats three large meals daily without nausea
2. Daily weight gain of no more than 3 pounds
3. Reduced serum albumin levels within 1 week
4. No evidence of bleeding

**1415.** **MoC** The NA reports to the nurse that the client with CRF has "white crystals" and dry, itchy skin. On the basis of this information, which instruction should the nurse give to the NA?

1. Apply the prescribed antipruritic cream.
2. Offer the client a glass of warm milk.
3. Prepare a tepid-water bath for the client.
4. Assess the skin for areas of breakdown.

**1416.** The client has a newly placed left forearm internal arteriovenous (AV) fistula for hemodialysis. Which interventions should the nurse plan to implement? **Select all that apply.**

1. Tell the NA to take the BP on the right arm.
2. Palpate for a thrill over the left forearm fistula.
3. Aspirate blood from the fistula for lab tests.
4. Check left radial pulse, finger movement, and sensation.
5. Instruct about the hand exercises that start in about a week.

**1417.** **MoC** A nursing home resident returns to the facility after receiving a hemodialysis treatment. Which symptom observed by the nurse suggests that the client may have developed disequilibrium syndrome?

1. Shortness of breath with a nonproductive cough
2. Pitting edema in both of the hands and feet
3. Inability to palpate a thrill in the arteriovenous (AV) fistula
4. Headache with a decreased level of consciousness

**1418.** After determining that the client with CRF has no signs of an infection, the nurse initiates the first peritoneal dialysis treatment for the client. During the infusion of the dialysate, the client reports abdominal pain. How should the nurse **best** respond to the situation?

1. Raise the bed to a high Fowler's position.
2. Stop the infusion rate until the pain goes away.
3. Ask when the client last had a bowel movement.
4. Explain that the pain will subside after a few exchanges.

**1419.** The nurse is assessing the client who has a right forearm AV fistula. Place an X at the location where the nurse should palpate for a thrill.

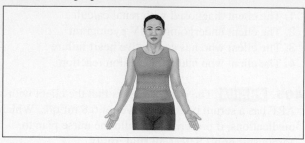

**1420.** The nurse is assessing the client receiving peritoneal dialysis. Which finding suggests that the client may be developing peritonitis?

1. Abdominal numbness
2. Cloudy dialysis output
3. Radiating sternal pain
4. Decreased WBC count

**1421.** The nurse is caring for four clients. For which client should the nurse anticipate treatment with continuous renal replacement therapy (CRRT)?

1. The client who has an increased serum creatinine level after receiving vancomycin IV to treat a wound infection
2. The client who is in stage 4 chronic kidney disease (CKD) as a complication of type 1 diabetes mellitus
3. The client who had an acute MI during coronary artery bypass graft (CABG) surgery and develops ARF
4. The client who can no longer have peritoneal dialysis (PD) due to thickening of the peritoneal membrane

**1422.** **MoC** The nurse is caring for a group of clients on a hospital unit with the assistance of the LPN. Which aspect of client care would be **most** appropriate for the nurse to delegate to the LPN?

1. Completing the admission for the client who has flank pain
2. Preparing the client for a newly prescribed renal biopsy
3. Administering sevelamer hydrochloride to the client with CRF
4. Observing the client self-catheterize a continent ileal reservoir

**1423.** **MoC** The nurse is admitting the client with possible renal trauma after an MVA. Prioritize the nurse's actions when caring for the client.

1. Teach the client signs of a UTI.
2. Palpate both flanks for asymmetry.
3. Assess for pain in the flank area.
4. Prepare the client for a CT scan.
5. Inspect the abdomen and the urethra for gross bleeding.

Answer: _____

# Answers and Rationales

**1380. ANSWER: 1**

1. **The nurse should teach that the client may experience a warm, flushing sensation up the arm or upper body and have a strange taste as the dye is injected.**
2. Urinary catheterization is needed only if the client is unable to void.
3. The client should increase intake of fluids after the IVP to promote clearance of the dye.
4. The client is usually allowed activity as tolerated, but fluids, not ambulation, promote dye excretion.

▶ *Test-taking Tip: You should focus on key words in the stem. Intravenous suggests that something is injected. Thus, narrow the Options to 1 and 4.*

Content Area: Adult; Concept: Nursing Roles; Urinary Elimination; Integrated Processes: Nursing Process: Planning; Client Needs: Physiological Integrity: Reduction of Risk Potential; Cognitive Level: Application [Applying]

**1381. MoC ANSWER: 2**

1. Although the HCP may prescribe a bladder irrigation, this should not be the nurse's initial action.
2. **Blood-tinged urine is expected after a cystoscopy, but bright red bleeding and clots are abnormal and should be reported to the HCP. Hemorrhage is a complication of cystoscopy.**
3. Heat may decrease the client's discomfort but may increase bleeding.
4. An antispasmodic medication will reduce the pain from spasms and contractions of the bladder and sphincter but will not control bleeding.

▶ *Test-taking Tip: Note the key word "initial." Clots suggest a potential complication of hemorrhage.*

Content Area: Adult; Concept: Critical Thinking; Urinary Elimination; Perfusion; Management; Integrated Processes: Nursing Process: Implementation; Client Needs: Safe and Effective Care Environment: Management of Care; Cognitive Level: Analysis [Analyzing]

**1382. PHARM ANSWER: 3**

1. Concentrated urine would be dark amber, not necessarily brown-colored. A medication dose should not be changed without first consulting the HCP.
2. A urine culture would have been completed before treatment was initiated. Another urine culture is not indicated at this time.
3. **The chemical makeup of the antibiotic nitrofurantoin (Furadantin) produces a harmless brown color to the urine. Nitrofurantoin should be discontinued only after the client's symptoms are alleviated or the prescribed dose is completed.**
4. Although increasing fluid intake will lighten the urine color, the urine will remain brown-colored from nitrofurantoin.

▶ *Test-taking Tip: You should recall that certain medications discolor the urine.*

Content Area: Adult; Concept: Medication; Infection; Urinary Elimination; Integrated Processes: Communication and Documentation; Client Needs: Physiological Integrity: Pharmacological and Parenteral Therapies; Cognitive Level: Application [Applying]

**1383. MoC ANSWER: 1**

1. **Urine should be obtained for culture and sensitivity (C&S) to identify the causative organism, the number of bacteria present, and the antibiotic that would be most effective. Urine should be collected before antibiotic treatment begins to avoid affecting results. The HCP must prescribe the C&S.**
2. The nurse should first obtain the urine for C&S. Once the results of the urine culture are obtained (24–48 hours), the antibiotic may need to be changed to one to which the causative organism is sensitive.
3. Although the client should be taught to wipe the perineum from front to back, this is not the first action.
4. If a urinary catheter is in place, it may need to be removed, but the C&S should be obtained first.

▶ *Test-taking Tip: Note the key word "first" in the stem.*

Content Area: Adult; Concept: Infection; Urinary Elimination; Integrated Processes: Nursing Process: Implementation; Client Needs: Safe and Effective Care Environment: Management of Care; Physiological Integrity: Physiological Adaptation; Cognitive Level: Application [Applying]

**1384. ANSWER: 1**

1. **Caffeine-containing beverages, such as coffee, tea, and cocoa, and alcoholic beverages irritate the bladder and should be eliminated from the diet.**
2. Showers, rather than tub baths, are recommended.
3. Synthetic underwear and constricting clothing, such as tight jeans, should be avoided.
4. Abstinence is unnecessary. The client should urinate after intercourse.

▶ *Test-taking Tip: Note the key words "reduce her risk." Look for key words in the options that make them incorrect: "tub baths," "synthetic," and "abstain."*

Content Area: Adult; Concept: Nursing Roles, Infection; Urinary Elimination; Integrated Processes: Teaching/Learning; Client Needs: Health Promotion and Maintenance; Cognitive Level: Application [Applying]

**1385. ANSWER: 3**

1. A high fever, rather than a low-grade fever, occurs with acute pyelonephritis.
2. Tachycardia, not bradycardia, occurs due to the elevated temperature.
3. **Flank pain on the affected side with costovertebral angle tenderness frequently occurs with acute pyelonephritis due to inflammation.**
4. Rebound tenderness in the right lower quadrant could indicate appendicitis.

▶ **Test-taking Tip:** *You should note that "-itis" means inflammation or infection.*

**Content Area:** Adult; **Concept:** Assessment; Infection; Urinary Elimination; **Integrated Processes:** Nursing Process: Assessment; **Client Needs:** Physiological Integrity: Physiological Adaptation; **Cognitive Level:** Application [Applying]

### 1386. ANSWER: 4

1. Voiding greater than 30 mL per hour does not indicate that the stone has passed. The kidneys will continue to produce urine, and the ureter will dilate, causing colicky pain.
2. Hematemesis occurs with GI problems. UTI may occur from the calculi's irritation to the ureter, but an absence of UTI does not mean the stone has passed.
3. Absence of epigastric pain, nausea, and vomiting is an outcome for the client with cholecystitis because it describes the pain characteristics of cholecystitis.
4. **Passage of a stone along the ureter produces flank pain and spasms of the ureter (colicky pain). The absence of the colicky pain indicates the stone may have been excreted.**

▶ **Test-taking Tip:** *Ureterolithiasis is a calculus (stone) in the ureter. The absence of symptoms from the presence of the stone would indicate that the stone has passed and the outcome is met.*

**Content Area:** Adult; **Concept:** Comfort; Urinary Elimination; **Integrated Processes:** Nursing Process: Evaluation; **Client Needs:** Physiological Integrity: Physiological Adaptation; **Cognitive Level:** Evaluation [Evaluating]

### 1387. ANSWER:

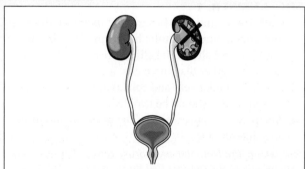

**Pyelonephritis is an inflammation, usually from an infection, that occurs in the renal parenchyma and collecting system, including the renal pelvis.**

▶ **Test-taking Tip:** *If pyelonephritis is unfamiliar, break the word down. "Pyelo" means pelvis, and "nephro" means kidney (pelvis of the kidney). The stem indicates that it is left-sided pyelonephritis, so focus on the client's left side.*

**Content Area:** Adult; **Concept:** Infection; Urinary Elimination; Nursing Roles; **Integrated Processes:** Teaching/Learning; **Client Needs:** Physiological Integrity: Physiological Adaptation; **Cognitive Level:** Application [Applying]

### 1388. ANSWER: 3

1. Although assessing pain is a priority, pain associated with a calculus in the right ureter would be in the right (not left) flank or costovertebral area.
2. Asking the client about juice preferences is irrelevant. The client with a UTI would be instructed to increase intake of cranberries, prunes, plums, and tomatoes because these acidify the urine. This is a good question to ask the client when planning teaching but is not the best question during the admission assessment.
3. **A frequent UTI is a predisposing factor for struvite stones. These stones are commonly referred to as "infection stones" because they form in alkaline urine that is rich in ammonia.**
4. Organ meats, poultry, fish, gravies, red wines, sardines, goose, and venison are high in purines. These can contribute to the development of uric acid, not struvite, stones.

▶ **Test-taking Tip:** *You should note that Options 2 and 4 are similar, and these would not be important to ask during an admission assessment; thus, these can be eliminated.*

**Content Area:** Adult; **Concept:** Infection, Assessment, Urinary Elimination; **Integrated Processes:** Nursing Process: Assessment; **Client Needs:** Physiological Integrity: Reduction of Risk Potential; **Cognitive Level:** Application [Applying]

### 1389. MoC ANSWER: 3

1. Increasing fluids will promote passage of the renal stone through the ureter and decrease pain, but it is not the priority.
2. Urine should be measured and strained, but this is not priority. Straining the urine is completed to determine if the stone has passed and was excreted in the urine.
3. **Assessment of the client's pain is priority. Severe colic pain, which is most severe in the first 24 to 36 hours, can cause a vasovagal reaction with syncope and hypotension. Pain can also interfere with the client's admission process.**
4. ESWL may be prescribed after other measures to assist the client to pass the stone are ineffective.

▶ **Test-taking Tip:** *Use the nursing process; assessment is the first step.*

**Content Area:** Adult; **Concept:** Assessment; Urinary Elimination: Management; **Integrated Processes:** Nursing Process: Implementation; **Client Needs:** Physiological Integrity: Physiological Adaptation; Safe and Effective Care Environment: Management of Care; **Cognitive Level:** Application [Applying]

### 1390. ANSWER: 1, 3

1. **Urine is strained to monitor the passage of stone fragments.**
2. Fluids and foods are given as soon as the client has recovered from the effects of the sedative. Drinking large amounts of fluid will assist with passage of the stone fragments.

3. **The flank should be checked for bruising. Some bruising may occur on the flank of the affected side after ESWL because sound, laser, or dry shock wave energies are used to break the stone into small fragments.**
4. There is no incision with ESWL. A small incision is made during percutaneous ultrasonic lithotripsy.
5. A stent is occasionally placed in the ureter before ESWL to dilate the ureter and ease passage of the stone fragments. Stent placement prevents the stone from coming in contact with the ureteral mucosa, thereby reducing pain. The stent is not removed until stone fragments have passed.

▶ *Test-taking Tip: ESWL uses laser and does not involve an incision.*

Content Area: Adult; Concept: Nursing Roles; Urinary Elimination; Integrated Processes: Nursing Process: Planning; Client Needs: Physiological Integrity: Reduction of Risk Potential; Cognitive Level: Synthesis [Creating]

### 1391. MoC ANSWER: 1, 2,

1. **An initial toileting schedule should be every 1 to 2 hours.**
2. **Diuretics should be given early in the day, preferably at breakfast time to avoid interrupting sleep.**
3. Turning on the water uses the power of suggestion to promote voiding. A type of urge urinary incontinence includes detrusor muscle hyperactivity with impaired contractility. The client is incontinent or voids a small volume of urine, is unable to void the remainder, and then has incontinence after leaving the bathroom.
4. Caffeine and aspartame are bladder irritants that increase detrusor muscle activity.
5. Vaginal weights (vaginal cone therapy) are helpful in strengthening the pelvic and bladder muscles. These can improve the ability to hold the urine until reaching a bathroom.

▶ *Test-taking Tip: The situation is urge urinary incontinence (overactive bladder). Focus on options that could result in a full bladder and increase incontinence.*

Content Area: Adult; Concept: Critical Thinking; Urinary Elimination; Integrated Processes: Nursing Process: Implementation; Client Needs: Safe and Effective Care Environment: Management of Care; Physiological Integrity: Physiological Adaptation; Cognitive Level: Application [Applying]

### 1392. PHARM ANSWER: 2

1. Bathing in tepid water will not relieve xerostomia (a dry mouth).
2. **The nurse should offer sugar-free candy or gumdrops; sucking on these will relieve xerostomia (a dry mouth).**
3. Using lotion will relieve itching but will not relieve xerostomia (a dry mouth).

4. Placing a fan by the client at a low setting may help with dyspnea or diaphoresis, but it will not relieve xerostomia (a dry mouth). It can increase the client's feeling of a dry mouth.

▶ *Test-taking Tip: Anticholinergics such as oxybutynin (Ditropan) block muscarinic receptors and can cause xerostomia or a dry mouth as a side effect.*

Content Area: Adult; Concept: Urinary Elimination; Sensory Perception; Integrated Processes: Nursing Process: Implementation; Client Needs: Physiological Integrity: Pharmacological and Parenteral Therapies; Cognitive Level: Analysis [Analyzing]

### 1393. ANSWER: 2

1. Although pain and temperature reduction are important, the client needs treatment for a possible infection.
2. **The client has symptoms of an infection, likely cystitis or a UTI, and should be seen in the clinic. The urine culture will establish the number and types of organisms present and help determine appropriate antibiotic therapy.**
3. The method of vaginal insertion of the weights may be the underlying cause of the infection, but discontinuing their use will not resolve the symptoms.
4. Drinking cranberry juice acidifies the urine and is thought to prevent the attachment of bacteria to the bladder wall. Fluids will help to "flush" the urinary tract; these measures do not treat the infection.

▶ *Test-taking Tip: The key word "best" indicates that more than one option may be appropriate, but that one option is better than another. Read the stem carefully and focus on the symptoms the client is experiencing, not the medical history.*

Content Area: Adult; Concept: Urinary Elimination; Nursing Roles; Communication; Integrated Processes: Nursing Process: Implementation; Client Needs: Safe and Effective Care Environment: Safety and Infection Control; Physiological Integrity: Physiological Adaptation; Cognitive Level: Application [Applying]

### 1394. MoC ANSWER: 2

1. When renal impairment results in decreased urine concentration with nocturia and low urine specific gravity, the client should drink at least 2 L of fluid daily to prevent dehydration.
2. **The client with PKD can have salt wasting and should not be on a sodium-restricted diet (500 mg). A low-sodium diet may be prescribed to control hypertension.**
3. Children of parents who have the autosomal dominant form of PKD (the most common form) have a 50% chance of inheriting the gene that causes the disease; a genetic counseling referral is appropriate.
4. BP control is necessary to slow the progression of the renal dysfunction and reduce cardiovascular complications.

▶ *Test-taking Tip: Salt wasting occurs with PKD.*

Content Area: Adult; Concept: Critical Thinking; Urinary Elimination; Management; Integrated Processes: Communication and Documentation; Client Needs: Safe and Effective Care Environment: Management of Care; Safe and Effective Care Environment: Safety and Infection Control; Cognitive Level: Analysis [Analyzing]

## 1395. ANSWER: 2

1. Sharp, intermittent pain (not decreased pain) occurs when a cyst ruptures.
2. **If a cyst ruptures, bleeding occurs, and the client could have bright red or cola-colored urine.**
3. Bloody stools would indicate a GI and not a renal problem.
4. Serum creatinine is a measure of renal function. As kidney function deteriorates, serum creatinine and BUN levels rise.

▶ *Test-taking Tip: You should think about the effects when bleeding occurs with a ruptured cyst.*

Content Area: Adult; Concept: Assessment; Urinary Elimination; Integrated Processes: Nursing Process: Analysis; Client Needs: Physiological Integrity: Reduction of Risk Potential; Cognitive Level: Application [Applying]

## 1396. ANSWER: 4

1. The normal urinary flow is not maintained. A stoma will be formed when the ileal conduit is created for the urinary diversion.
2. An ileal conduit creates a noncontinent stoma. Kegel exercises will have no effect on muscle strengthening because the bladder is removed during cystectomy.
3. Bladder retraining will have no effect on bladder control because the bladder is removed during cystectomy.
4. **An ileal conduit collects urine in a portion of the intestine that opens onto the skin surface as a stoma. After the creation of a stoma, the client must wear a pouch to collect urine.**

▶ *Test-taking Tip: The key word is "cystectomy," which is the removal of the bladder. You should also note that three options are similar and one is different; often the option that is different is the answer.*

Content Area: Adult; Concept: Nursing Roles; Urinary Elimination; Perioperative; Integrated Processes: Teaching/Learning; Client Needs: Physiological Integrity: Physiological Adaptation; Physiological Integrity: Basic Care and Comfort; Cognitive Level: Application [Applying]

## 1397. ANSWER: 1

1. **A Kock pouch is a continent internal ileal reservoir that should be catheterized every 4 to 6 hours to drain the urine.**
2. Alcohol is drying and can result in skin breakdown.
3. Sleeping on the side of the stoma is unnecessary. Urine will flow from the ureters into the reservoir regardless of the client's position.
4. A stoma pouch would not be required. The client may initially have a plastic catheter in the stoma until the incision heals.

▶ *Test-taking Tip: During the creation of the Kock pouch, the stoma is sutured to the abdominal wall. Fluid pressure closes the valve inside the pouch to prevent outflow of urine. Think about how this urine is removed.*

Content Area: Adult; Concept: Critical Thinking; Urinary Elimination; Integrated Processes: Nursing Process: Planning; Client Needs: Physiological Integrity: Basic Care and Comfort; Cognitive Level: Application [Applying]

## 1398. MoC ANSWER: 3

1. There is no indication in the stem that the client has a spouse.
2. The situation is about respect, not increasing the fluid intake.
3. **The nurse requesting permission before uncovering any part of the body is showing respect for the client.**
4. Although asking about food intake is important, the question will only elicit a yes or no response.

▶ *Test-taking Tip: The key word is "respect." Think about how you would want your care provided if you were hospitalized.*

Content Area: Adult; Concept: Critical Thinking; Urinary Elimination; Diversity; Integrated Processes: Culture and Spirituality; Caring; Client Needs: Safe and Effective Care Environment: Management of Care; Psychosocial Integrity; Cognitive Level: Application [Applying]

## 1399. MoC ANSWER: 1

1. **The complication of urine leaks manifests as diminished urine output, an increase in serum creatinine, and lower abdominal or suprapubic discomfort. It most commonly occurs at the site of the anastomosis.**
2. A normal, functioning kidney, from a live donor, produces large amounts of dilute urine. A reduction of serum creatinine and incisional discomfort are expected after renal transplant.
3. Oliguria, fever, and swelling or tenderness over the transplanted kidney could be a sign of kidney rejection.
4. A kidney from a cadaver donor may not function for 2 or 3 weeks, during which time anuria, oliguria, or polyuria may be present.

▶ *Test-taking Tip: Focus on the situation—complication of urine leakage. Eliminate Option 2 because there is a large amount of urine output. The key is the lower abdominal discomfort in Option 1 because urine is accumulating in the abdomen.*

Content Area: Adult; Concept: Critical Thinking; Urinary Elimination; Integrated Processes: Nursing Process: Analysis; Client Needs: Safe and Effective Care Environment: Management of Care; Physiological Integrity: Reduction of Risk Potential; Cognitive Level: Evaluation [Evaluating]

## 1400. PHARM ANSWER: 3

1. Digoxin (Lanoxin) is a cardiac glycoside used as an isotropic antidysrhythmic agent.
2. Tacrolimus (Prograf) is an immunosuppressant.

3. **Amlodipine (Norvasc) is a calcium channel blocking and antihypertensive agent. Antihypertensive agents are used to maintain optimal perfusion in the transplanted kidney and to control hypertension, an adverse effect associated with immunosuppressants.**
4. Epoetin alfa (Procrit) is given to treat anemia.

▶ *Test-taking Tip: A trade name for amlodipine is Norvasc. Use this as a clue that it is a vascular medication that will control hypertension.*

Content Area: Adult; Concept: Perfusion; Urinary Elimination; Medication; Integrated Processes: Nursing Process: Implementation; Client Needs: Physiological Integrity: Pharmacological and Parenteral Therapies; Cognitive Level: Knowledge [Remembering]

## 1401. ANSWER: 2

1. Option 1 is an ileal conduit. The urine is diverted by implanting the ureters into a loop of the ileum, and one end is brought out through the abdominal wall. A urostomy bag is used to collect the urine.
2. **In an Indiana pouch, the ureters are implanted into a segment of the ileum and cecum, and a pouch is created. Urine is drained intermittently by inserting a catheter into the stoma.**
3. Option 3 shows a sigmoid colostomy where a segment of the colon is brought outside the abdominal wall. It is a diversion for excreting feces when a lower portion of the large intestine has been removed.
4. Option 4 shows an ileostomy where a segment of the ileum is brought through the abdominal wall. It is a diversion for excreting feces when the large intestine, and at times a portion of the small bowel, has been removed.

▶ *Test-taking Tip: Note the key word "urinary." Eliminate options that illustrate bowel diversions. Of the remaining two options, select the option with the pouch.*

Content Area: Adult; Concept: Urinary Elimination; Integrated Processes: Nursing Process: Planning; Client Needs: Physiological Integrity: Physiological Adaptation; Cognitive Level: Comprehension [Understanding]

## 1402. MoC ANSWER: 3

1. Even though the urine is concentrated, there is no indication of an infection. A culture is unnecessary.
2. Changing the client's urostomy bag is unnecessary.
3. **An intestinal segment is used to create an ileal conduit. It continues to secrete mucus because of the irritating effect of the urine. Increasing the amount of fluids will flush the mucus from the client's ileal conduit.**
4. Ambulation may improve circulation, but increased amounts of fluids are needed.

▶ *Test-taking Tip: Dehydration can cause urine to become dark amber in color.*

Content Area: Adult; Concept: Urinary Elimination; Management; Regulations; Integrated Processes: Nursing Process: Implementation; Client Needs: Safe and Effective Care Environment: Management of Care; Cognitive Level: Application [Applying]

## 1403. ANSWER: 3, 4, 5

1. Clamping, compressing, or kinking the tube can cause renal damage.
2. Irrigation should be performed if prescribed, using no more than 5 mL of sterile solution. Irrigation may cause overdistention and renal damage.
3. **The output and surrounding tissue should be assessed for signs of infection.**
4. **The nephrostomy tube is draining urine from the kidney, so the tube must be kept below the flank level to prevent backflow of urine.**
5. **The nephrostomy tube drains urine from the affected kidney. The urinary drainage catheter drains urine from the bladder (collected from the other kidney). These should be recorded separately to evaluate kidney function, but the hourly urine output should be monitored by adding the two amounts together.**

▶ *Test-taking Tip: "Nephro" means kidney. Although Options 1 and 2 may sound plausible, but these are unsafe.*

Content Area: Adult; Concept: Urinary Elimination; Critical Thinking; Integrated Processes: Nursing Process: Implementation; Client Needs: Physiological Integrity: Physiological Adaptation; Cognitive Level: Application [Applying]

## 1404. ANSWER: 3

1. Renal calculi can cause postrenal failure.
2. An IV pyelogram can cause intra- or infrarenal renal failure (these are interchangeable terms) because the dye load can be toxic to the kidney.
3. **CHF can cause prerenal failure due to cardiac pump problems, volume depletion from fluid restriction or diuretics, or vasodilation from beta blocker medications. If the kidneys are not adequately perfused, the resulting hypoperfusion decreases GFR.**
4. A transfusion reaction can cause an intra- or infrarenal failure because of the hemoglobinuria produced by the breakdown of the wrong type of RBCs in the body.

▶ *Test-taking Tip: When determining the etiology of renal failure, you should think about the location in regard to the kidney itself. If the etiology is above the kidney, then it is prerenal.*

Content Area: Adult; Concept: Fluid and Electrolyte Balance; Urinary Elimination; Perfusion; Integrated Processes: Nursing Process: Assessment; Client Needs: Physiological Integrity: Physiological Adaptation; Cognitive Level: Analysis [Analyzing]

## 1405. PHARM ANSWER: 2, 4, 5

1. Erythropoietin triggers the production of RBCs by bone marrow. It is used to treat anemia, which is common in renal failure. It will not have an effect in treating hyperkalemia.
2. **Regular insulin forces the potassium into the cells, temporarily lowering serum potassium levels. It should be given now if prescribed.**

3. Five to 50% dextrose (not 0.45% saline bolus) is given along with regular insulin and calcium gluconate to force the potassium into the cells.

4. **Calcium gluconate raises the threshold for cardiac muscle excitation, thereby reducing the incidence of life-threatening dysrhythmias that can occur with hyperkalemia. It should be given now if prescribed.**

5. **Sodium polystyrene sulfonate (Kayexalate) is a cation-exchange resin that removes potassium by exchanging it with sodium ions in the large intestine. It should be given now if prescribed.**

▶ *Test-taking Tip: Note the key word "now." Eliminate options that may be used in ARF but do not need to be administered now and another that could be harmful.*

Content Area: Adult; Concept: Medication; Fluid and Electrolyte Balance; Urinary Elimination; Integrated Processes: Nursing Process: Planning; Client Needs: Physiological Integrity: Pharmacological and Parenteral Therapies; Cognitive Level: Application [Applying]

## 1406. ANSWER: 2

1. Adventitious breath sounds are abnormal breath sounds; absence of these is a normal finding.

2. **A decrease in BP and increase in pulse rate are physiological responses to a decrease in circulating blood volume that occurs in the diuretic phase of ARF. Uncorrected dehydration will complicate the client's recovery.**

3. Weight loss is an expected finding with diuresis.

4. A serum potassium level of 3.7 mEq/L is WNL of 3.5 to 5.0 mEq/L.

▶ *Test-taking Tip: With ARF, the onset is followed by three phases: oliguric, diuretic, and recovery. This client is now in the diuretic phase, which places the client at risk for dehydration and complications.*

Content Area: Adult; Concept: Fluid and Electrolyte Balance; Urinary Elimination; Perfusion; Integrated Processes: Nursing Process: Assessment; Client Needs: Physiological Integrity: Physiological Adaptation; Cognitive Level: Application [Applying]

## 1407. ANSWER: 3

**Because 1 kg of weight is equivalent to 1 L of fluid, a weight loss of 3 kg would be approximately 3 L of fluid loss.**

▶ *Test-taking Tip: Knowledge that 1 L of fluid is equivalent to 1 kg is needed to answer this question.*

Content Area: Adult; Concept: Fluid and Electrolyte Balance; Urinary Elimination; Integrated Processes: Nursing Process: Analysis; Client Needs: Physiological Integrity: Reduction of Risk Potential; Cognitive Level: Analysis [Analyzing]

## 1408. ANSWER: 4

1. Bananas are high in potassium. Potassium is restricted because clients with oliguria are unable to eliminate it.

2. Fluid is usually restricted to 500 mL plus the previous day's output to prevent fluid overload; a glass is 240 mL. Milk has a significant amount of potassium and phosphorus and should be avoided. Small amounts of rice milk or soy milk are alternatives.

3. Ham is high in sodium, which is restricted to minimize sodium and fluid retention.

4. **A small apple is low in potassium and an acceptable snack. Other snack options include grapes, celery, or 1 pita bread with 2 oz turkey (not processed meats). The amount of protein the client can have is increased when on hemodialysis.**

▶ *Test-taking Tip: You should eliminate options with foods high in potassium, phosphorus, sodium, and fluids because these are restricted in ARF.*

Content Area: Adult; Concept: Nutrition; Urinary Elimination; Integrated Processes: Nursing Process: Planning; Client Needs: Physiological Integrity: Basic Care and Comfort; Cognitive Level: Application [Applying]

## 1409. ANSWER: 1, 3, 4, 5

1. **During the recovery phase of ARF, urine specific gravity increases because of the kidneys' ability to concentrate urine and excrete electrolytes.**

2. The client should have a decreased, not increased, serum creatinine level in the recovery period.

3. **Potassium is decreased because of the kidneys' ability to excrete potassium.**

4. **Nausea, vomiting, and diarrhea are common in ARF because of accumulation of nitrogenous wastes. An absence of these indicates that the client is in the recovery phase of ARF.**

5. **Neurologically, the client in ARF may have muscle twitching, drowsiness, headache, and seizures because of the electrolyte imbalances and accumulation of metabolic wastes. In the recovery period, the client should not have muscle twitching.**

▶ *Test-taking Tip: Look for signs that show improvement, thus eliminating Option 2. Avoid reading into the question. You need to consider the effects of electrolyte alterations.*

Content Area: Adult; Concept: Urinary Elimination; Integrated Processes: Nursing Process: Evaluation; Client Needs: Physiological Integrity: Physiological Adaptation; Cognitive Level: Evaluation [Evaluating]

## 1410. MoC ANSWER: 2

1. During peritoneal dialysis (PD), protein moves out of the blood with the waste products and into the dialysate fluid, which is discarded. A high-protein diet is necessary to replace the losses.

2. **In PD, the amount of outflow should be more than what was instilled because fluid is being removed. This statement should be corrected by the experienced nurse.**

3. Antihypertensive medications, such as lisinopril (Prinivil), should be withheld before hemodialysis. Hypotension can occur when fluid is removed.

4. With CRF, kilocalories are supplied by carbohydrates and fat. Inadequate amounts of nonprotein kilocalories will lead to tissue breakdown and aggravate uremia.

▶ *Test-taking Tip: Three options pertain to client diet or medications, and one option is different (a procedure). Often the option that is different is the answer.*

Content Area: Adult; **Concept**: Critical Thinking; Urinary Elimination; **Integrated Processes**: Nursing Process: Evaluation; **Client Needs**: Safe and Effective Care Environment: Management of Care; Physiological Integrity: Physiological Adaptation; **Cognitive Level**: Evaluation [Evaluating]

## 1411. PHARM  ANSWER: 3

1. Epoetin alfa (Epogen) does not have a direct effect on serum creatinine levels.
2. Elevated WBCs could indicate that the client has an infection. Epoetin alfa does not affect WBCs.
3. **Epoetin alfa (Epogen) stimulates RBC production and increases Hct. Initial effects should be seen in 1 to 2 weeks, and normal Hct should be achieved within 2 to 3 months.**
4. As the Hct increases, there can be a transient increase in BP.

▶ *Test-taking Tip: Use the medication name as a cue to its effect on the bone marrow.*

Content Area: Adult; **Concept**: Medication; Hematologic Regulation; Urinary Elimination; **Integrated Processes**: Nursing Process: Evaluation; **Client Needs**: Physiological Integrity: Pharmacological and Parenteral Therapies; **Cognitive Level**: Evaluation [Evaluating]

## 1412. ANSWER: 3

1. Respiratory acidosis would result in a decreased pH, an increased $Paco_2$, and a normal or decreased $HCO_3$.
2. Respiratory alkalosis would result in an increased pH, a decreased $Paco_2$, and a normal or decreased $HCO_3$.
3. **In metabolic acidosis, the pH and $HCO_3$ are decreased, and the $Paco_2$ is normal (or decreased if compensation is occurring). In compensation, the client would be hyperventilating to decrease the $Paco_2$ and conserve the $HCO_3$. In CRF, metabolic acidosis occurs because the kidneys are unable to excrete the increased amounts of acids. The inability of the kidney tubules to excrete ammonia and to reabsorb sodium bicarbonate causes the decreased acid secretion. The decreased excretion of phosphates and other organic acids contributes to the accumulation of acids.**
4. Metabolic alkalosis would result in an increased pH, an increased $HCO_3$, and a normal or increased $Paco_2$.

▶ *Test-taking Tip: Recall that the $Paco_2$ is the respiratory component and that $HCO_3$ is the metabolic component of ABGs. For abnormal values, visualize the pH, $Paco_2$, and $HCO_3$ each separately on an acid-base scale to determine whether the client's value is acidic, basic, or within a normal pH range. Write this down. The value that matches the pH as being either acidic or basic is the system (respiratory or metabolic) that initiated the imbalance.*

Content Area: Adult; **Concept**: pH Regulation; Urinary Elimination; **Integrated Processes**: Nursing Process: Analysis; **Client Needs**: Physiological Integrity: Reduction of Risk Potential; Physiological Integrity: Physiological Adaptation; **Cognitive Level**: Analysis [Analyzing]

## 1413. ANSWER: 2

1. Anuria is defined as a urine output of less than 100 mL/24 hr and is not used to define ESRD.

2. **ESRD is defined as a GFR of less than 15. Creatinine clearance (based on urinary creatinine in a timed specimen and a serum creatinine level) is a calculated measure of GFR.**
3. Serum creatinine levels (normal 0.5–1.2 mg/dL) are elevated with renal failure but do not define ESRD.
4. Serum BUN is elevated in renal failure but is not used to define ESRD.

▶ *Test-taking Tip: The issue of the question is the definition of ESRD. Select the option that is more global and encompasses creatinine present in the serum and excreted in the urine.*

Content Area: Adult; **Concept**: Urinary Elimination; Communication; **Integrated Processes**: Nursing Process: Analysis; **Client Needs**: Physiological Integrity: Physiological Adaptation; **Cognitive Level**: Application [Applying]

## 1414. ANSWER: 4

1. The client with CRF has the potential for imbalanced nutrition due to anorexia, nausea, and stomatitis secondary to the effects of urea excess on the GI system. The client should consume small, frequent meals, not large meals.
2. The client with CRF is at risk for fluid volume excess because of the kidneys' inability to excrete water. A 3-lb weight gain in 1 day indicates fluid retention.
3. The client with CRF has the potential for imbalanced nutrition because of a protein-restricted diet. Serum albumin levels should be WNL.
4. **No evidence of bleeding is an appropriate client outcome. The client with CRF is at risk for bleeding because of impaired platelet function.**

▶ *Test-taking Tip: Use the ABC's to identify Option 4 as the correct answer to the question.*

Content Area: Adult; **Concept**: Critical Thinking; Urinary Elimination; Communication; **Integrated Processes**: Communication and Documentation; **Client Needs**: Physiological Integrity: Physiological Adaptation; **Cognitive Level**: Synthesis [Creating]

## 1415. MoC  ANSWER: 3

1. Although an antipruritic cream could be applied to relieve itching, applying the medication would not be within the scope of practice of the NA.
2. Fluid intake is usually restricted for the client with CRF.
3. **Bathing the client in cool water will remove crystals, decrease itching, and promote client comfort. The crystals (uremic frost) and itching are from irritating toxins and deposits of calcium-phosphate precipitates on the skin.**
4. Assessment is not within the scope of practice of the NA.

▶ *Test-taking Tip: Narrow the options by eliminating those that are not within the NA's scope of practice. Then, of the two remaining options, consider which would best relieve itching.*

Content Area: Adult; **Concept**: Nursing Roles; Urinary Elimination; Management; Regulations; **Integrated Processes**: Nursing Process: Implementation; **Client Needs**: Safe and Effective Care Environment: Management of Care; Physiological Integrity: Basic Care and Comfort; **Cognitive Level**: Analysis [Analyzing]

### 1416. ANSWER: 1, 2, 4, 5

1. **A BP should not be taken on the arm with the AV fistula because it could damage the fistula.**
2. **An AV fistula is created by the anastomosis of an artery to a vein. A thrill is the arterial blood rushing into the vein. Its presence indicates that the fistula is not occluded.**
3. Aspirating for blood can damage the fistula because it takes 4 to 6 weeks to mature.
4. **CMS is important to assess because complications of the fistula creation include impairment of circulation and nerve damage.**
5. **Hand exercises such as squeezing a rubber ball help the fistula to mature. These are not started until the incision heals. The fistula is not used until it matures in about 4 to 6 weeks.**

▸ *Test-taking Tip: You should eliminate an option that will cause damage to the newly created fistula.*

Content Area: Adult; Concept: Assessment; Urinary Elimination; Integrated Processes: Nursing Process: Planning; Client Needs: Physiological Integrity: Reduction of Risk Potential; Cognitive Level: Application [Applying]

### 1417. MoC ANSWER: 4

1. Shortness of breath is a symptom associated with fluid volume excess.
2. Pitting edema is associated with fluid volume excess.
3. Loss of a palpable thrill is associated with a thrombosed AV fistula.
4. **Rapid changes in fluid volume and BUN levels during hemodialysis can result in disequilibrium syndrome. Symptoms include headache and decreased level of consciousness from the associated cerebral edema and increased ICP.**

▸ *Test-taking Tip: The phrase disequilibrium suggests the loss of balance (equilibrium) involving the brain. This should direct you to the only option associated with neurological symptoms.*

Content Area: Adult; Concept: Fluid and Electrolyte Balance; Urinary Elimination; Integrated Processes: Nursing Process: Assessment; Client Needs: Safe and Effective Care Environment: Management of Care; Physiological Integrity: Physiological Adaptation; Cognitive Level: Application [Applying]

### 1418. ANSWER: 4

1. Positioning the client supine in a low Fowler's position reduces intra-abdominal pressure.
2. The infusion should not be stopped or slowed; the pain, due to initial peritoneal irritation, will subside only after a few exchanges.
3. A full bowel may cause slowing during inflow of the dialysate solution, and the client may feel pressure, but not pain. This is not the best response by the nurse.
4. **Peritoneal irritation, from the inflow of the dialysate, commonly causes pain during the first few exchanges and usually subsides within 1 to 2 weeks. The nurse should monitor for signs of peritonitis, such as cloudy effluent and abdominal pain.**

▸ *Test-taking Tip: The nurse is initiating peritoneal dialysis. Consider that pain may occur initially with the infusion of the dialysate.*

Content Area: Adult; Concept: Comfort; Urinary Elimination; Integrated Processes: Nursing Process: Implementation; Client Needs: Physiological Integrity: Reduction of Risk Potential; Cognitive Level: Application [Applying]

### 1419. ANSWER:

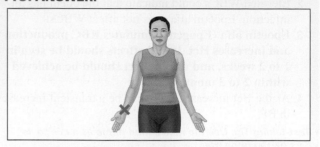

**An AV fistula is created by the anastomosis of an artery to a vein. A thrill is the arterial blood rushing into the vein. The thrill should be palpated at the site of the AV fistula.**

▸ *Test-taking Tip: Pay attention to the location identified in the stem of the question.*

Content Area: Adult; Concept: Assessment; Urinary Elimination; Integrated Processes: Nursing Process: Implementation; Client Needs: Physiological Integrity: Reduction of Risk Potential; Cognitive Level: Application [Applying]

### 1420. ANSWER: 2

1. The client would experience abdominal tenderness and pain with peritonitis, not numbness.
2. **Cloudy dialysate output suggests peritonitis.**
3. Abdominal pain rather than sternal pain occurs with peritonitis.
4. WBCs would increase (not decrease) in the presence of an infection.

▸ *Test-taking Tip: Normal peritoneal dialysis outflow is light yellow and clear.*

Content Area: Adult; Concept: Infection; Assessment; Urinary Elimination; Integrated Processes: Nursing Process: Assessment; Client Needs: Physiological Integrity: Physiological Adaptation; Cognitive Level: Application [Applying]

### 1421. ANSWER: 3

1. The client who develops reduced renal function after receiving vancomycin requires medical support and observation but does not necessarily require dialysis.
2. A diabetic client with CKD is a candidate for hemodialysis or peritoneal dialysis.
3. **CRRT is hemofiltration used to treat ARF in critically ill clients who have an unstable BP and cardiac output, such as the client who developed ARF post MI and CABG surgery. CRRT is performed continuously to avoid rapid shifts in fluids and electrolytes.**
4. The client who can no longer tolerate PD can be treated with hemodialysis.

▶ **Test-taking Tip:** *Read the question carefully and note the word "continuous" in CRRT. Select the client most acutely ill and most likely to benefit from continuous dialysis.*

**Content Area:** Adult; **Concept:** Fluid and Electrolyte Balance; Urinary Elimination; **Integrated Processes:** Nursing Process: Planning; **Client Needs:** Physiological Integrity: Physiological Adaptation; **Cognitive Level:** Application [Applying]

**1422.** MoC **ANSWER: 3**

1. The client being admitted with acute flank pain needs an admission and pain assessment that should be performed by the RN.
2. The client with a newly prescribed renal biopsy will need teaching that should be completed by the RN.
3. **Administering medications is within the scope of practice for the LPN. Sevelamer hydrochloride (Renagel) binds dietary phosphorus in the intestinal tract.**
4. Although "observing" would be within the scope of practice of the LPN, "evaluating" client performance is not.

▶ **Test-taking Tip:** *Note the key words "most appropriate." Read each situation carefully. Use delegation principles of right circumstances, right task, and right person to answer the question. Because it is not known if this is the first time the client is self-catheterizing, the most appropriate option to choose is Option 1.*

**Content Area:** Adult; **Concept:** Collaboration; Urinary Elimination; Regulations; **Integrated Processes:** Nursing Process: Implementation; **Client Needs:** Safe and Effective Care Environment: Management of Care; **Cognitive Level:** Application [Applying]

**1423.** MoC **ANSWER: 3, 5, 2, 4, 1**

3. **Assess for pain in the flank area. This is priority. Unrelieved pain can prolong the stress response.**
5. **Inspect the abdomen and the urethra for gross bleeding. If gross bleeding is present, the abdomen should not be palpated.**
2. **Palpate both flanks for asymmetry. Lack of symmetry may indicate renal damage.**
4. **Prepare the client for a CT scan. Preparation for tests should occur after the physical examination is completed.**
1. **Teach the client signs of a UTI. Physiological needs should be met before psychosocial needs such as teaching are met.**

▶ **Test-taking Tip:** *Use the nursing process and the physical assessment process to prioritize the nursing actions. Assessment is the first step in the nursing process. Look for the key word "assess." Inspection should occur before palpation because the findings could lead to deciding not to palpate because it could cause harm. Use the other steps of the nursing process to prioritize the remaining items.*

**Content Area:** Adult; **Concept:** Critical Thinking; Safety; Urinary Elimination; Trauma; Management; **Integrated Processes:** Nursing Process: Analysis; **Client Needs:** Safe and Effective Care Environment: Management of Care; Psychosocial Integrity; **Cognitive Level:** Synthesis [Creating]

## Chapter Thirty-Two

# Reproductive and Sexually Transmitted Infection Management

**1424.** The nurse is preparing a women's seminar. Which factors that increase the risk for breast cancer should the nurse plan to include? **Select all that apply.**

1. Fibrocystic breast disease
2. Onset of menarche occurring at a young age
3. Breastfeeding infants older than 6 months
4. Postmenopausal with a BMI less than 20
5. Sister diagnosed with breast cancer

**1425.** The nurse overhears the client talking with her husband about her new diagnosis of stage 1 breast cancer. Which statement by the client indicates that she does not fully understood the diagnosis?

1. "I won't be here to see our daughter graduate this spring."
2. "I understand that I will need either radiation or chemotherapy."
3. "I will need surgery to remove the cancerous breast tissue."
4. "The cancer was in an early stage, and it was contained."

**1426.** **PHARM** The client states, "My doctor suggested I take tamoxifen because of my risk for developing breast cancer. How does this drug reduce my risk?" Which information about tamoxifen should be the basis for the nurse's response?

1. Tamoxifen is an anti-inflammatory drug that reduces the body's response to the tumor.
2. Tamoxifen is a chemotherapy agent that has minimal side effects if taken prophylactically.
3. Tamoxifen will protect against the development of other cancers such as endometrial cancer.
4. Tamoxifen will block estrogen receptors on tumor cells and thus cause the tumor to regress.

**1427.** The client with newly diagnosed breast cancer asks the nurse to explain the advantages of a sentinel lymph node biopsy (SLNB). Which explanation should the nurse state to the client?

1. "This biopsy will improve the chances that all of the tumor will be removed."
2. "This biopsy can reduce the number of lymph nodes that must be removed."
3. "This biopsy makes breast reconstruction easier to perform."
4. "This biopsy, if performed, will make hormonal therapy unnecessary."

**1428.** The nurse plans care for the client who had a TRAM (transverse rectus abdominis myocutaneous) flap breast reconstruction. Which actions should the nurse plan?

1. Initiate passive ROM to the affected side immediately after surgery and q4h.
2. Assess capillary refill, color, and temperature of the flap hourly for 24 hours.
3. Maintain a pressure dressing on the reconstructed breast for the first 48 hours.
4. Keep the affected arm below the level of the reconstructed breast for 48 hours.

**1429.** The client has been having breast pain and has had several diagnostic procedures that all have been negative. Which suggestions should the nurse include when the client asks for advice on controlling this breast pain? **Select all that apply.**

1. Put a towel wet with primrose oil on the breasts.
2. Go without a bra for at least 4 hours every day.
3. Reduce the amount of caffeine in the diet.
4. Supplement the diet with B complex vitamins.
5. Apply hot packs to the breasts for 20 minutes.

**1430.** The client tells the nurse that she is considering breast reduction but wants to know if she could breast-feed in the future after this procedure. Which response by the nurse is correct?

1. "Breast reduction will not affect whether you choose to breastfeed."
2. "Breastfeeding is possible if the nipples are left connected to breast tissue."
3. "The amount of breast tissue removed will make breastfeeding impossible."
4. "Changes in the nipple structure from surgery will prevent milk production."

**1431.** **PHARM** A 15-year-old client's mother asks the nurse why the HCP prescribed oral contraceptives (OCPs) for treating her daughter's dysmenorrhea. Before responding to the mother, which fact about oral contraceptives should the nurse consider?

1. OCPs inhibit uterine inflammation, which indirectly causes the dysmenorrhea.
2. OCPs increase blood flow to the uterus during menstruation, thereby reducing pain.
3. OCPs inhibit the progesterone production that causes uterine contractions and pain.
4. OCPs suppress ovulation and thus prostaglandin production, which causes pain.

**1432.** The 17-year-old female client receives treatment for primary amenorrhea caused by hyperthyroidism. Which finding during a clinic visit should indicate to the nurse that treatment for amenorrhea was effective?

1. Weight increased by 10 pounds
2. Denies having menstrual cramps
3. Just started having her menses
4. No longer has a fine hand tremor

**1433.** The nurse is completing a health assessment of the female client with menorrhagia of unknown origin. Which serum laboratory result should the nurse carefully review?

1. Calcium level
2. Blood urea nitrogen
3. Hemoglobin level
4. White blood cell count

**1434.** The nurse is caring for the 30-year-old female client. Which concerns stated by the client should alert the nurse to the possibility of endometriosis? **Select all that apply.**

1. Vaginal dryness
2. Premenstrual tension headache
3. Pain during her menstrual period
4. Inability to conceive
5. Dyspareunia

**1435.** **MoC** The nurse is assessing the client who had a vaginal hysterectomy 8 hours ago. Which assessment finding should prompt the nurse to immediately notify the surgeon?

1. Three dime-size areas of serosanguineous drainage is noted on her perineal pad.
2. Urine output is 300 mL over the past 8 hours.
3. Hemoglobin dropped from presurgical 12 mg/dL to 10 mg/dL.
4. Urine is red in color and transparent.

**1436.** **PHARM** The HCP prescribed mifepristone for the 35-year-old female client to treat a leiomyoma. Before the client begins the medication, which information is **most** important for the nurse to obtain?

1. Baseline BP
2. Liver enzyme test results
3. Pregnancy test results
4. Baseline height and weight

**1437.** A female client has an abdominal hysterectomy to remove a uterine fibroid. Which action should the nurse include when caring for the client postoperatively?

1. Monitor the perineal pad for bleeding.
2. Administer hormone replacement therapy.
3. Maintain bedrest for the first 48 hours.
4. Start a regular diet 6 hours postsurgery.

**1438.** The 21-year-old who has been diagnosed with polycystic ovary syndrome (PCOS) asks about changes she could make to help control her disease. Which statement is the nurse's **best** response?

1. "Take ibuprofen to reduce your pain."
2. "Avoid oral contraceptives for birth control."
3. "Avoid having more than one sexual partner."
4. "Keep your BMI within the acceptable range."

**1439.** **MoC** The HCP writes orders for the client who is 24 hours postvulvectomy. Which order should the nurse verify with the HCP?

1. Cleanse perineal wound with warm saline daily.
2. Maintain high Fowler's position for 24 hours.
3. Begin low-residue diet when tolerating oral intake.
4. Apply antiembolic stockings; remove 20 minutes bid.

**1440.** The client asks the nurse how a woman can recognize when she is ovulating. Which should be the nurse's response?

1. "The mucus produced by the cervix during ovulation becomes abundant and stretchy."
2. "The body temperature drops and stays low for the remainder of the menstrual cycle."
3. "Do an over-the-counter urine test; with ovulation, luteinizing hormone is negative."
4. "You may notice a decrease in your desire for sexual activity when you are ovulating."

**1441.** The otherwise healthy menopausal client tells the nurse, "Over the past 2 years, I've been having vaginal itching, burning, and more vaginal infections. Which statement is the nurse's **best** response?

1. "The frequent vaginal infections could be a precursor to vulvar cancer."
2. "You could have a contact allergy that is causing your vaginal itching."
3. "The vagina becomes more acidic after menopause, causing your symptoms."
4. "The vaginal pH increases during menopause, predisposing you to these symptoms."

**1442.** The 54-year-old client who is postmenopausal reports increasing episodes of urinary leakage. Which lifestyle practice is **most** important for the nurse to discuss with the client?

1. Eliminate the consumption of caffeine.
2. Establish an hourly voiding schedule.
3. Decrease the intake of water and other fluids.
4. Strengthen pelvic muscles with Kegel exercises.

**1443.** The client, who is postmenopausal, reports pain with sexual intercourse. Which effective treatments should the nurse review with the client? **Select all that apply.**

1. Use estradiol vaginal tablets as prescribed by the HCP.
2. Have regular intercourse to enhance vaginal blood flow.
3. Soak in a bath with fragrant oil or bubble bath every day.
4. Use feminine cleansing cloths or a vaginal douche daily.
5. Insert a vaginal lubricant prior to having intercourse.

**1444.** **PHARM** The client, who had been prescribed sildenafil 2 weeks ago for erectile dysfunction, calls the clinic to report that nothing happens, despite taking sildenafil orally and waiting for his erection to develop. Which fact should the nurse consider before responding to the client?

1. In clinical trials, the sildenafil was effective only 20% of the time.
2. Sildenafil is not effective if taken orally and should be taken rectally.
3. In the absence of sexual stimuli, sildenafil will not cause an erection.
4. Sildenafil is ineffective if taken with foods high in saturated fats.

**1445.** **PHARM** The nurse teaches the client with erectile dysfunction about the use of alprostadil via subcutaneous penile injection. Which statement indicates the client needs further teaching?

1. "I need to keep the needle sterile before I inject my penis."
2. "The erection won't last long after alprostadil is injected."
3. "The injection will produce an erection within 30 minutes."
4. "I should report if I am feeling dizzy after an injection."

**1446.** **PHARM** The client, with known BPH, telephones the clinic with concerns of increased urinary frequency and urgency that started a few days ago after having a cold. Which question should the nurse immediately ask the client?

1. "Have you been drinking large amounts of water?"
2. "Have you been exercising more than usual?"
3. "Have you been taking any over-the-counter cold remedies?"
4. "Have you increased the amount of dairy products in your diet?"

**1447.** The client undergoes a TURP and CBI is started. When assessing the client, the nurse finds dark red urine containing several small clots. Which intervention should the nurse implement?

1. Increase the flow of the bladder irrigation fluid.
2. Immediately stop the bladder irrigation flow.
3. Irrigate the urinary catheter manually.
4. Deflate the balloon on the urinary catheter.

**1448.** The nurse is caring for the client following a TURP. At the end of an 8-hour shift, the nurse determines that the client received 3050 mL of CBI fluid and that 4030 mL of output was emptied from the urinary drainage bag. How many mL should the nurse document for the client's actual urine output for the 8 hours?

_____ mL (Record your answer as a whole number.)

**1449.** PHARM The client who is 24 hours post-TURP is having painful bladder spasms. Which intervention should the nurse plan to implement **first?**

1. Give the prn dose of morphine sulfate IV.
2. Give the prn suppository of belladonna/opium.
3. Assist the client out of bed to ambulate.
4. Apply a cold cloth to the client's abdomen.

**1450.** The nurse is obtaining a hospital admission history for the client. Which statement should prompt the nurse to consider that the client has chronic prostatitis?

1. "I am having difficulty sustaining an erection."
2. "I have pain with ejaculation during intercourse."
3. "I have been feeling pressure around my rectum."
4. "I don't think I am totally emptying my bladder."

**1451.** The nurse is reviewing hospital admission orders for the client who has acute prostatitis. Which order should the nurse verify with the HCP?

1. Give trimethoprim/sulfamethoxazole 1 g IV q6h.
2. Administer ibuprofen 600 mg orally q6h prn.
3. Increase fluid intake to 3 L daily; have client void often.
4. Insert an indwelling urinary drainage catheter now.

**1452.** The clinic nurse is reviewing the history of the client diagnosed with bacterial vaginosis (BV). Which identified disorder places the client at a higher risk for developing BV?

1. Gastroesophageal reflux
2. Hypothyroidism
3. Cardiovascular disease
4. Diabetes mellitus

**1453.** The nurse reviews the laboratory results exhibited of the client hospitalized with testicular cancer. Which conclusion by the nurse is **most** accurate?

| Lab Serum | Client Value | Normal Values |
|---|---|---|
| BUN | 20 | 5–25 mg |
| Creatinine | 1.0 | 0.5–1.5 mg/dL |
| Na | 137 | 135–145 mEq/L |
| K | 3.4 | 3.5–5.3 mEq/L |
| Cl | 99 | 95–105 mEq/L |
| $CO_2$ | 24 | 22–30 mEq/L |
| Glucose | 148 | 70–110 mg/dL |
| Hgb/Hct | 10%/33% | 13.5–17 g/dL, 40%–54% |
| WBC | 9000 | 4500–10,000/ microL or mm³ |
| Neutrophils | 65% | 50%–70% |
| AST | 200 | 8–38 unit/L |
| ALT | 150 | 10–35 units/L |

1. The client may have developed an infection.
2. The client's nutrient intake has been inadequate.
3. The client should be checked for type 2 DM.
4. The client's disease may have metastasized.

**1454.** The client is informed that he will require a right orchiectomy as part of his treatment of testicular cancer. The client asks the nurse if he will be infertile after this procedure. Which response by the nurse is **best?**

1. "You need to plan ahead; this procedure will make you infertile."
2. "Has your surgeon discussed cryopreservation of your sperm?"
3. "With the removal of only one testicle, your fertility will not be affected."
4. "I can't answer this; no one really knows whether fertility will be affected."

**1455.** The client, preparing to have a vasectomy, asks the nurse where the vasectomy incision will be made. Place an X within the circle on the illustration where the nurse should show the client the location of the vasectomy incision.

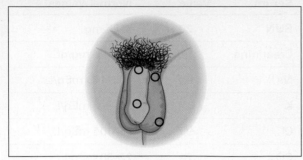

**1456.** The nurse is obtaining a health history on the Caucasian client with a possible left-sided varicocele. Which question is **most** important?

1. "Did your father have any testicular problems?"
2. "Does the left scrotum feel different from the right?"
3. "Do you have children or plan to have children?"
4. "Do you have any discomfort in your groin?"

**1457.** The nurse is discharging the client after an elective abortion by suction curettage. Which statement should the nurse include in the client's discharge instructions?

1. Sexual intercourse can be resumed once vaginal discharge has stopped.
2. Perform a vaginal douche with clean tap water twice daily for 48 hours.
3. Notify the HCP immediately if the vaginal discharge develops a foul odor.
4. Increase fluid intake, rest, and make plans to return to work in 1 week.

**1458.** The married couple tells the nurse they have been unsuccessful at achieving a pregnancy. What should be the nurse's **initial** question when they ask if they should begin infertility testing?

1. "Do either of you use tobacco products or drink alcohol?"
2. "What are your ages, and how long ago were you married?"
3. "Did either of you ever have an infection in your reproductive tract?"
4. "How long have you been having regular intercourse without contraception?"

**1459.** The nurse is providing information to the client who has genital herpes. What **priority** information should the nurse provide to the client?

1. Genital herpes simplex virus-2 (HSV-2) is more common in women than in men.
2. A herpes simplex virus-1 (HSV-1) genital infection can occur with oral–genital contact.
3. After a diagnosis of HSV-2, there are likely to be two to three outbreaks during the first year.
4. Transmission of genital herpes can occur from a partner who does not have a visible sore.

**1460.** The female client has been diagnosed with genital warts. Which assessment findings should the nurse associate with genital warts?

1. Painful vesicles on the labia, perineum, or anus
2. Painful ulcers on the vagina, labia, or perineum
3. Painless, cauliflower-appearing lesions near the vaginal opening or anus
4. Painless chancre or ulcers on the labia or perineum

**1461.** **PHARM** **MoC** The client is diagnosed with chlamydia and syphilis, and medication is prescribed. Which medication requires the nurse's immediate review with the HCP?

1. Doxycycline
2. Azithromycin
3. Metronidazole
4. Penicillin G

**1462.** **PHARM** The nurse is teaching the client about metronidazole, which has been prescribed for treating trichomoniasis. Which client comment indicates the need for additional education?

1. "I may have a bad metallic taste in my mouth."
2. "I'm glad I can still drink beer with these pills."
3. "My urine may look a little darker than usual."
4. "These pills may make me sick to my stomach."

**1463.** The client is angry about a new diagnosis of gonorrhea and informs the nurse, "I absolutely will not allow the release of this information to anyone." Which response by the nurse is **most** appropriate?

1. "I see you are upset. Tell me more about what you mean by this statement."
2. "I'm sorry, but I'm required by law to report this to the Health Department."
3. "Are you worried that your spouse wouldn't want the information released?"
4. "I can see you are angry, but there is no reason for you to be upset with me."

**1464.** After assessing the client, the nurse initiates the process for reporting the client's STI to the state health agency. Which client has the STI that the nurse is reporting?

1.

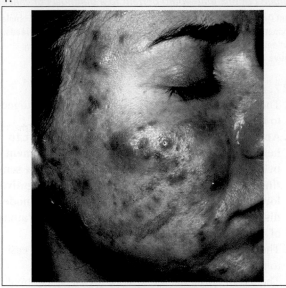

2.

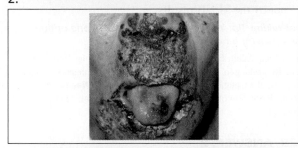

3.

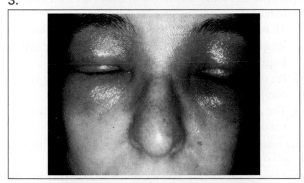

4.

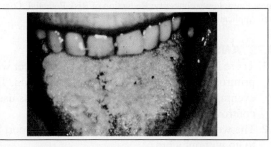

**1465.** MoC The female client diagnosed with AIDS is having vaginal itching and thick, white vaginal discharge. The nurse notifies the client's HCP concerned that the client may have which infection?

1. Herpes simplex
2. Candida albicans
3. Histoplasmosis
4. Kaposi's sarcoma

**1466.** The nurse is teaching the client and the family members about protection measures when the client, diagnosed with AIDS, returns home. Which instruction indicates that the nurse is unclear about the disease transmission?

1. "Disinfect items in your home using a bleach solution of 1 part bleach to 10 parts water."
2. "Place contaminated items, except sharps, in a plastic bag and then put them in the garbage."
3. "Use separate dishes and wash them with hot, soapy water or place them in the dishwasher."
4. "Wear gloves to clean body fluid spills with soap and water; then clean with bleach solution."

**1467.** MoC The nurse is planning care for the female client, who is newly diagnosed with herpes simplex virus type 2 (HSV-2, herpes genitalis). In which order should the nurse complete the planned actions? Place the nurse's planned actions in order of priority.

1. Teach abstinence from sexual intercourse during treatment and use of condoms.
2. Determine if the woman is pregnant.
3. Discuss the benefits of joining a support group such as HELP (Herpetics Engaged in Living Productively).
4. Administer an analgesic.
5. Administer the first dose of acyclovir.

Answer: _____

# Answers and Rationales

## 1424. ANSWER: 2, 5

1. Fibrocystic breast disease is not related to breast cancer development, but fibrocystic changes can make it more difficult to feel early cancerous lumps during breast examination.
2. **Early menarche and/or late menopause increase the risk of developing breast cancer.**
3. Childless women, not those who have breastfed, are at increased risk. It is thought that pregnancy and lactation interrupt ovulation and alter the hormonal environment, reducing breast cancer risk.
4. Postmenopausal women who are obese, not those with a lower BMI, are at increased risk.
5. **Women with first-degree relatives, such as a mother or sister, who had breast cancer are at risk.**

▶ *Test-taking Tip: Age, diet (overeating), and heredity are risk factors for breast cancer development.*

**Content Area:** Adult; **Concept:** Promoting Health, Cellular Regulation; Female Reproduction; **Integrated Processes:** Nursing Process: Planning; **Client Needs:** Health Promotion and Maintenance; **Cognitive Level:** Application [Applying]

## 1425. ANSWER: 1

1. **Ninety percent of women with localized tumors (stage 1 and 2) can be expected to achieve long-term disease-free survival. This statement indicates she did not understand the diagnosis of stage 1 breast cancer.**
2. Either chemotherapy or radiation is recommended for treatment of stage 1 breast cancer. This statement indicates understanding.
3. Surgery will be needed to treat the stage 1 breast cancer. This statement indicates understanding.
4. Stage 1 cancer means that it was contained in the area where the first abnormal cells began to develop or that only a tiny area of cancer has spread in the sentinel lymph node.

▶ *Test-taking Tip: The phrase "not fully understood" indicates a false-response item. Look for the incorrect statement.*

**Content Area:** Adult; **Concept:** Nursing Roles, Cellular Regulation; Female Reproduction; **Integrated Processes:** Nursing Process: Evaluation; **Client Needs:** Physiological Integrity: Physiological Adaptation; **Cognitive Level:** Evaluation [Evaluating]

## 1426. PHARM ANSWER: 4

1. Tamoxifen does not have anti-inflammatory properties.
2. Tamoxifen is a hormonal rather than a chemotherapeutic agent.
3. A major side effect of tamoxifen is that it increases the risk of developing endometrial cancer.
4. **Tamoxifen (Soltamox) blocks estrogen receptors on tumor cells, and thus the cell growth declines and the tumor regresses.**

▶ *Test-taking Tip: Focus on the information provided and note that the woman does not have cancer but is at high risk. Eliminate options that would pertain to a diagnosis of cancer.*

**Content Area:** Adult; **Concept:** Medication, Cellular Regulation; Female Reproduction; **Integrated Processes:** Teaching/Learning; **Client Needs:** Physiological Integrity: Pharmacological and Parenteral Therapies; **Cognitive Level:** Application [Applying]

## 1427. ANSWER: 2

1. The SLNB will not improve the ability of the surgeon to remove all of the tumor.
2. **An SLNB uses a radioactive substance or dye to help to identify axillary lymph node involvement before axillary dissection has occurred. If the sentinel node is identified and is found to be negative for tumor cells, then further axillary lymph node dissection is unnecessary. Thus the lymph drainage of the involved arm can be preserved.**
3. The SLNB will not make breast reconstruction easier to perform.
4. The use of hormonal therapy for breast cancer treatment is determined by the receptor status of the tumor, not by the SLNB results.

▶ *Test-taking Tip: You should note that only one option mentions lymph nodes.*

**Content Area:** Adult; **Concept:** Communication, Cellular Regulation; Female Reproduction; Nursing Roles; **Integrated Processes:** Nursing Process: Implementation; Teaching/Learning; **Client Needs:** Physiological Integrity: Reduction of Risk Potential; **Cognitive Level:** Application [Applying]

## 1428. ANSWER: 2

1. Upper-extremity exercise and ROM are restricted to reduce strain on the incision site.
2. **To monitor for viability and adequacy of blood supply to the TRAM flap, the flap must be assessed hourly for the first 24 hours.**
3. Pressure over the flap is avoided until healing is complete.
4. The affected arm should be elevated to promote venous return.

▶ *Test-taking Tip: Use the nursing process and ABC's to select the option that ensures that circulation is adequate.*

**Content Area:** Adult; **Concept:** Assessment; Female Reproduction; Cellular Regulation; **Integrated Processes:** Nursing Process: Planning; **Client Needs:** Physiological Integrity: Reduction of Risk Potential; **Cognitive Level:** Application [Applying]

## 1429. ANSWER: 3, 4, 5

1. There is no evidence that placing a towel wet with primrose oil over the breasts will reduce pain. Taking evening primrose oil orally may help, but its use is controversial.
2. The women should be taught to wear a support bra, not to go without a bra.

3. **Reducing caffeine has been shown by some to reduce breast pain.**
4. **B complex vitamins have been shown by some to reduce breast pain.**
5. **Applying hot packs to the breasts for 20 minutes has been shown by some to reduce breast pain.**

▶ *Test-taking Tip: Focus on the treatment for noncancerous breast pain. Eliminate any option that potentially could increase pain through gravitational pull.*

Content Area: Adult; Concept: Comfort; Nursing Roles; Female Reproduction; Integrated Processes: Teaching/Learning; Client Needs: Physiological Integrity: Basic Care and Comfort; Cognitive Level: Application [Applying]

## 1430. ANSWER: 2

1. Breast reduction has the potential to negatively affect lactation (breastfeeding) if large amounts of breast tissue are removed.
2. **Lactation can usually be accomplished if the nipples are left connected to breast tissue.**
3. The amount of breast tissue removed will determine whether lactation is possible.
4. The nipple structure is not changed with breast reduction; however, some surgeries may necessitate relocation of the nipple.

▶ *Test-taking Tip: Acini cells, which produce milk, are connected to ducts that eventually empty into lactiferous sinuses under the nipple. These connections must be maintained for lactation to occur.*

Content Area: Adult; Concept: Female Reproduction; Nursing Roles; Integrated Processes: Communication and Documentation; Teaching/Learning; Client Needs: Physiological Integrity: Reduction of Risk Potential; Cognitive Level: Application [Applying]

## 1431. PHARM ANSWER: 4

1. OCPs do not inhibit inflammation.
2. OCPs do not increase uterine blood flow; the amount of menstrual discharge may decrease with OCP usage as a result of decreased endometrial stimulation.
3. OCPs do inhibit progesterone production, but it is not progesterone that stimulates uterine contractions and pain; rather, it is prostaglandins.
4. **OCPs block ovulation by preventing the release of follicle stimulating hormone from the pituitary. The absence of ovulation decreases the sequential stimulation of the endometrium by estrogen and progesterone. This results in a decrease in the prostaglandin production by the endometrium and thus a decrease in pain.**

▶ *Test-taking Tip: Dysmenorrhea is caused by excessive endometrial prostaglandin production, which increases myometrial contraction and constriction of small endometrial blood vessels, resulting in ischemia and pain.*

Content Area: Adult; Concept: Promoting Health; Female Reproduction; Integrated Processes: Nursing Process: Planning; Client Needs: Physiological Integrity: Pharmacological and Parenteral Therapies; Cognitive Level: Comprehension [Understanding]

## 1432. ANSWER: 3

1. An increased weight may help with initiating a menstrual cycle if the cause is a body fat composition of less than 10%, but this does not indicate that the woman has started her menstrual cycle.
2. If the client is not menstruating (amenorrhea), she will not have menstrual cramps.
3. **Hyperthyroidism and a body fat composition of less than 10% can be contributing factors to amenorrhea (absence of menses). The start of a menstrual cycle indicates that treatment of the underlying cause of amenorrhea is effective.**
4. The absence of a fine hand tremor may indicate treatment is effective for the hyperthyroidism. It does not indicate that the primary amenorrhea is resolved.

▶ *Test-taking Tip: Amenorrhea is absence of menses. Only one option is directly related to menses. Avoid reading into the options.*

Content Area: Adult; Concept: Female Reproduction; Integrated Processes: Nursing Process: Evaluation; Client Needs: Physiological Integrity: Physiological Adaptation; Cognitive Level: Evaluation [Evaluating]

## 1433. ANSWER: 3

1. Calcium should not be affected by menorrhagia.
2. BUN should not be affected by menorrhagia.
3. **Persistent heavy bleeding can result in anemia, which would be reflected in the client's Hgb level.**
4. WBCs should not be affected by menorrhagia.

▶ *Test-taking Tip: Menorrhagia is excessive or prolonged bleeding at the time of the regular menstrual flow. Only one laboratory value is affected by bleeding.*

Content Area: Adult; Concept: Assessment; Female Reproduction; Integrated Processes: Nursing Process: Assessment; Client Needs: Physiological Integrity: Reduction of Risk Potential; Cognitive Level: Application [Applying]

## 1434. ANSWER: 3, 4, 5

1. Vaginal dryness is not a symptom of endometriosis.
2. Premenstrual tension headache is not a symptom of endometriosis.
3. **Endometriosis is the presence of normal endometrial tissue in sites outside the endometrial cavity. The tissue responds to hormonal influence, and therefore during menstruation, the tissue bleeds. This bleeding causes inflammation and pain at the time of menstruation.**
4. **Women with endometriosis are at increased risk for infertility, although the exact reason is unknown.**
5. **Depending on the location of the endometrial tissue, clients may experience pain with intercourse (dyspareunia).**

▶ *Test-taking Tip: Focus on symptoms that would arise when endometrial tissue appears in sites outside of the endometrial cavity.*

Content Area: Adult; Concept: Female Reproduction, Assessment; Integrated Processes: Nursing Process: Analysis; Client Needs: Physiological Integrity: Physiological Adaptation; Cognitive Level: Application [Applying]

**1435.** **MoC** **ANSWER: 4**

1. A moderate amount of serosanguineous vaginal drainage is expected after a vaginal hysterectomy.
2. The urine output is more than 30 mL/hour and thus not concerning at this time.
3. Decreased hemoglobin levels are expected after surgery as a result of blood loss or dilution of circulating blood volume by intravenous fluids.
4. **Red, transparent urine indicates blood in the urine. This should be reported to the surgeon. Injury to the bladder or ureters is a possible complication of a vaginal hysterectomy.**

▶ *Test-taking Tip: Focus on expected physiological changes after vaginal hysterectomy.*

Content Area: Adult; Concept: Collaboration; Female Reproduction; Integrated Processes: Nursing Process: Evaluation; Client Needs: Safe and Effective Care Environment: Management of Care; Cognitive Level: Evaluation [Evaluating]

**1436.** **PHARM** **ANSWER: 3**

1. Mifepristone does not cause changes in BP.
2. Mifepristone does not cause changes in liver enzymes.
3. **The pregnancy test results should be known because mifepristone is also used in conjunction with other medications for termination of early intrauterine pregnancy.**
4. Although weight can influence the dose, this information is not the most important. Mifepristone does not cause weight changes.

▶ *Test-taking Tip: Mifepristone (Mifeprex) is a synthetic steroid that blocks receptors for progesterone. Therefore it would decrease the hormonal supply to the leiomyoma and cause it to shrink. You should select the option most closely associated with female reproductive hormones.*

Content Area: Adult; Concept: Medication; Female Reproduction; Safety; Integrated Processes: Nursing Process: Planning; Client Needs: Safe and Effective Care Environment: Safety and Infection Control; Physiological Integrity: Pharmacological and Parenteral Therapies; Cognitive Level: Application [Applying]

**1437. ANSWER: 1**

1. **Monitoring the perineal pad will alert the nurse to any increase in vaginal bleeding. Infection and hemorrhage are the major risks following a hysterectomy.**
2. HRT is needed only if the ovaries have been removed (oophorectomy).
3. The client should be encouraged to ambulate in the early postoperative period, rather than remain on bedrest. Development of DVT is a concern after abdominal hysterectomy.
4. Peristalsis is typically suppressed after abdominal hysterectomy, and the client will be on restricted oral intake until physical signs indicate the return of peristalsis.

▶ *Test-taking Tip: You need to consider that the uterus and vagina are connected and that when an abdominal hysterectomy is performed, only the uterus is removed.*

Content Area: Adult; Concept: Female Reproduction; Clotting; Perioperative; Integrated Processes: Nursing Process: Assessment; Client Needs: Physiological Integrity: Physiological Adaptation; Cognitive Level: Application [Applying]

**1438. ANSWER: 4**

1. Although an anti-inflammatory medication such as ibuprofen (Advil) may help reduce pelvic pain, this is not a lifestyle change.
2. Oral contraceptives are useful in regulating the menstrual cycle for clients with PCOS and are used (not avoided) to treat this syndrome.
3. Maintaining a monogamous sexual relationship will not affect PCOS.
4. **Obesity exacerbates insulin resistance and hyperinsulinemia associated with PCOS.**

▶ *Test-taking Tip: Recall the relationship of weight to PCOS. Use the process of elimination to rule out incorrect options. The key word is "lifestyle." Eliminate options that are not related to lifestyle.*

Content Area: Adult; Concept: Female Reproduction; Promoting Health; Integrated Processes: Nursing Process: Implementation; Communication and Documentation; Client Needs: Health Promotion and Maintenance; Cognitive Level: Application [Applying]

**1439.** **MoC** **ANSWER: 2**

1. The perineal wound is cleansed with saline, or the client is given sitz baths for cleansing to promote healing and prevent infection.
2. **A high Fowler's position places pressure on the perineal area and will increase discomfort. The client should be placed in a low Fowler's position to decrease tension on the suture line and promote comfort.**
3. A low-residue diet prevents straining at stool and wound contamination.
4. Antiembolic stockings increase venous return to decrease the risk of DVT and to assist in the development of collateral pathways for lymph drainage.

▶ *Test-taking Tip: Focus on the client's safety. Select the option that could potentially cause perineal trauma.*

Content Area: Adult; Concept: Female Reproduction; Safety; Integrated Processes: Nursing Process: Implementation; Client Needs: Safe and Effective Care Environment: Management of Care; Cognitive Level: Application [Applying]

**1440. ANSWER: 1**

1. **At the time of ovulation, the mucus produced by the cervix becomes more abundant and stretchy. It looks and feels like egg whites. The ability of the mucus to be stretched indicates the time of maximum fertility.**
2. At the time of ovulation, the basal body temperature drops slightly and then, under the influence of progesterone, increases and stays elevated until 2 to 4 days before menstruation starts.

3. Home measurement of luteinizing hormone (LH) is possible with dipstick urine tests. A positive test (not negative) for LH indicates ovulation. LH causes the egg to be released from the ovary.

4. At the time of ovulation, most females note an increase (not decrease) in libido.

▶ *Test-taking Tip: Look for key words in the options. Three options address a decrease or negative finding, and one option is different (abundant). Often the option that is different is the answer.*

**Content Area:** Adult; **Concept:** Female Reproduction; Promoting Health; **Integrated Processes:** Nursing Process: Implementation; Teaching/Learning; **Client Needs:** Health Promotion and Maintenance; **Cognitive Level:** Application [Applying]

## 1441. ANSWER: 4

1. Vaginal infections do not predispose a female to vulvar cancer.

2. Although vaginal itching may be related to a contact allergy, it is not the best response.

3. Acidic secretions would have a low pH value; the pH increases during menopause.

4. **Decreased estrogen in menopausal women causes thinning of the vaginal mucosa and an increase in pH of vaginal secretions. As a result, the vagina is easily traumatized and more susceptible to infection.**

▶ *Test-taking Tip: You should eliminate options that suggest a medical diagnosis; diagnosing a medical problem is not within the nurse's scope of practice.*

**Content Area:** Adult; **Concept:** Female Reproduction; Nursing Roles; **Integrated Processes:** Teaching/Learning; **Client Needs:** Health Promotion and Maintenance; **Cognitive Level:** Application [Applying]

## 1442. ANSWER: 4

1. Caffeine can increase urinary frequency, but the loss of muscle tone contributes to urinary leakage.

2. A regular voiding schedule improves bladder control, but beginning with an hourly voiding schedule is unnecessary and inconvenient.

3. Decreasing intake of fluids can contribute to dehydration.

4. **Kegel exercises improve urinary incontinence by strengthening the pelvic floor muscles that support the bladder.**

▶ *Test-taking Tip: The key words are "most important," indicating that more than one option may be correct but that one is more important than the other. You need to consider that urinary leakage can increase over time with aging.*

**Content Area:** Adult; **Concept:** Female Reproduction; Urinary Elimination; **Integrated Processes:** Teaching/Learning; **Client Needs:** Health Promotion and Maintenance; **Cognitive Level:** Application [Applying]

## 1443. ANSWER: 1, 2, 5

1. **Estradiol vaginal tablets increase vaginal lubrication production and have been shown to be effective for vaginal dryness and pain with intercourse.**

2. **Increased blood flow to the vagina through regular intercourse effectively helps to prevent further tissue atrophy.**

3. Fragrant bath oil or bubble bath will cause further drying of vaginal tissues.

4. Feminine cleansing cloths or douches will cause further drying of vaginal tissues.

5. **Vaginal lubricants have been shown to be effective for vaginal dryness and pain with intercourse.**

▶ *Test-taking Tip: Fragrances and cleansers tend to be drying to the vagina.*

**Content Area:** Adult; **Concept:** Sexuality; Female Reproduction; **Integrated Processes:** Nursing Process: Planning; **Client Needs:** Physiological Integrity: Physiological Adaptation; **Cognitive Level:** Application [Applying]

## 1444. PHARM ANSWER: 3

1. In clinical trials, some improvement in erectile hardness and duration was reported by 70% of men taking sildenafil.

2. Sildenafil should be taken orally.

3. **Sildenafil (Viagra) enhances the normal erectile response to sexual stimuli by promoting relaxation of arterial and trabecular smooth muscle. The resultant arterial dilation causes engorgement of sinusoidal spaces in the corpus cavernosum. In the absence of sexual stimuli, however, nothing will happen.**

4. A fatty meal delays absorption, and, as a result, plasma levels peak in 2 hours instead of an hour; it does not cause sildenafil to be ineffective.

▶ *Test-taking Tip: "Waiting for an erection" is a key phrase in the stem.*

**Content Area:** Adult; **Concept:** Medication; Male Reproduction; **Integrated Processes:** Nursing Process: Planning; **Client Needs:** Physiological Integrity: Pharmacological and Parenteral Therapies; **Cognitive Level:** Application [Applying]

## 1445. PHARM ANSWER: 2

1. The client is correct in using sterile technique for the injection.

2. **The nurse should correct the statement about an erection not lasting long. Alprostadil (Caverject) injection therapy has the potential of producing a prolonged erection.**

3. Alprostadil will begin to produce the desired effect within 30 minutes.

4. Dizziness is a side effect of alprostadil and should be reported.

▶ *Test-taking Tip: The phrase "needs further instruction" is a false-response item. Look for the incorrect statement.*

**Content Area:** Adult; **Concept:** Medication, Male Reproduction, Promoting Health, Safety, Nursing Roles; **Integrated Processes:** Nursing Process: Evaluation; **Client Needs:** Physiological Integrity: Pharmacological and Parenteral Therapies; **Cognitive Level:** Evaluation [Evaluating]

**1446.** PHARM **ANSWER: 3**

1. Clients with BPH should maintain fluid intake at normal levels to prevent dehydration. Drinking large amounts of water, however, could lead to bladder distention, which would result in abdominal discomfort.
2. Increased exercise will not alter BPH symptoms.
3. **Compounds found in common cough and cold remedies, such as pseudoephedrine and phenylephrine, are alpha-adrenergic agonists that cause smooth muscle contraction. Because the bladder is a smooth muscle, these medications may increase symptoms of urinary urgency and frequency.**
4. Increased amounts of alcohol and caffeine can increase BPH symptoms, but dairy products should not affect BPH symptoms.

♦ *Test-taking Tip: The key information is that the client has a cold and that his symptoms increased with the onset of the cold symptoms. Option 3 directly mentions cold remedies.*

Content Area: Adult; Concept: Male Reproduction; Medication; Assessment; Integrated Processes: Nursing Process: Analysis; Client Needs: Physiological Integrity: Pharmacological and Parenteral Therapies; Cognitive Level: Application [Applying]

**1447. ANSWER: 1**

1. **If the urine is dark red, the flow rate of the CBI should be increased. The purpose of the CBI is to remove clots from the bladder and to ensure drainage of urine through the urinary catheter. The flow rate of the CBI fluid should be set so that the outflow remains free from clots and remains light red to pink.**
2. Stopping the CBI would increase the risk that the urinary catheter would become blocked and the flow of urine interrupted.
3. There is no need to manually irrigate a catheter if a CBI is flowing, unless the urinary catheter becomes obstructed.
4. Deflating the urinary catheter balloon would be contraindicated because this could result in dislodging the catheter.

♦ *Test-taking Tip: The purpose of a CBI is to maintain urinary catheter patency. Eliminate Option 2, as this would negate the functioning of the CBI.*

Content Area: Adult; Concept: Urinary Elimination; Male Reproduction; Integrated Processes: Nursing Process: Implementation; Client Needs: Physiological Integrity: Reduction of Risk Potential; Cognitive Level: Application [Applying]

**1448. ANSWER: 980**

**Subtract the amount of CBI solution from the total amount of fluid emptied from the urinary drainage device: 4030 mL – 3050 mL = 980 mL.**

♦ *Test-taking Tip: Be sure to subtract the amount of irrigation solution from the total amount in the urinary drainage bag to obtain the urine output.*

Content Area: Adult; Concept: Urinary Elimination; Male Reproduction; Perioperative; Integrated Processes: Nursing Process: Assessment; Client Needs: Physiological Integrity: Basic Care and Comfort; Cognitive Level: Application [Applying]

**1449.** PHARM **ANSWER: 2**

1. Opioid medications will decrease the pain sensations but will not decrease the muscle spasms.
2. **The belladonna and opium (B&O) suppository will inhibit smooth muscle contraction and decrease bladder spasms; thus, it will also reduce pain.**
3. Ambulation will not decrease the discomfort.
4. Heat, rather than cold, is the recommended nonpharmacological treatment for bladder spasms.

♦ *Test-taking Tip: Think about therapies to relieve muscle spasms. That should allow elimination of Options 1 and 3. Then consider the effects of applying cold versus warmth to the skin.*

Content Area: Adult; Concept: Medication; Male Reproduction; Perioperative; Integrated Processes: Nursing Process: Planning; Client Needs: Physiological Integrity: Pharmacological and Parenteral Therapies; Cognitive Level: Application [Applying]

**1450. ANSWER: 2**

1. Chronic prostatitis does not cause erectile dysfunction.
2. **Both chronic bacterial prostatitis and chronic prostatitis/pelvic pain syndrome manifest with ejaculatory pain.**
3. Chronic prostatitis does not cause rectal pain.
4. Obstructive bladder symptoms, such as incomplete bladder emptying, are uncommon unless the client also has BPH.

♦ *Test-taking Tip: You should think about the physiology of male sexual response: During ejaculation, the prostate gland contracts. Thus, disease in the prostate gland would predispose to ejaculation pain.*

Content Area: Adult; Concept: Inflammation, Male Reproduction; Integrated Processes: Nursing Process: Assessment; Client Needs: Physiological Integrity: Physiological Adaptation; Cognitive Level: Application [Applying]

**1451. ANSWER: 4**

1. Trimethoprim/sulfamethoxazole (Bactrim) is a common antibiotic used to treat acute prostatitis.
2. Analgesics, such as ibuprofen (Motrin), should be used for pain control, and rest should be encouraged.
3. Increasing fluid intake and voiding often help decrease irritation when emptying the bladder.
4. **Passage of a urinary catheter through an inflamed urethra is contraindicated in acute prostatitis. If urinary retention is a concern, a suprapubic catheter should be placed.**

♦ *Test-taking Tip: Select the option that is unsafe for the client with an inflamed prostate.*

Content Area: Adult; Concept: Inflammation; Male Reproduction; Integrated Processes: Nursing Process: Analysis; Client Needs: Safe and Effective Care Environment: Safety and Infection Control; Cognitive Level: Application [Applying]

**1452. ANSWER: 4**

1. Gastroesophageal reflux disorder is not a risk factor for BV.

2. Hypothyroidism does affect the reproductive system. However, it does not specifically alter the pH of the vagina, which could increase the incidence of BV.

3. Cardiovascular disease is not a risk factor for BV.

4. **Diabetes is a risk factor for a variety of vulvovaginal infections.**

▶ *Test-taking Tip: Diabetes affects the immune system, and clients may experience more frequent infections from a variety of sources.*

**Content Area:** Adult; **Concept:** Sexuality; Infection; **Integrated Processes:** Nursing Process: Analysis; **Client Needs:** Health Promotion and Maintenance; **Cognitive Level:** Application [Applying]

## 1453. ANSWER: 4

1. The WBCs are WNL; there is no indication of a developing infection.

2. There is no information in the stem about nutritional intake, and the serum albumin or prealbumin is not reported in the laboratory results to make a judgment about whether the client's nutrient intake is inadequate.

3. The elevated glucose level is likely related to the body's physiological response to stress.

4. **The decreased Hgb indicates anemia, and the liver enzymes are elevated (AST, ALT). These changes occur when testicular cancer has metastasized.**

▶ *Test-taking Tip: With question types that present a chart, it is often easier and quicker to review the options first and then analyze the chart to determine the answer.*

**Content Area:** Adult; **Concept:** Cellular Regulation; Male Reproduction; **Integrated Processes:** Nursing Process: Analysis; **Client Needs:** Physiological Integrity: Reduction of Risk Potential; **Cognitive Level:** Analysis [Analyzing]

## 1454. ANSWER: 2

1. The client's fertility can be affected to varying degrees, so it is inappropriate to say the client will be infertile.

2. **The impact of treatment for testicular cancer on fertility varies. The involvement of chemotherapy, lymph node removal, and/or radiation in the treatment plan may all influence the client's ability to procreate. Clients should be encouraged to consider cryopreservation of sperm in a sperm bank before beginning testicular cancer treatment.**

3. The client's fertility can be affected to varying degrees, so it is inappropriate to say the client will not be infertile.

4. Telling the client that the question can't be answered dismisses the client's concern and is not the best response. It may block further communication with the nurse about the client's concerns.

▶ *Test-taking Tip: Three options are similar, and one is different. Often the option that is different is the answer.*

**Content Area:** Adult; **Concept:** Communication; Male Reproduction; **Integrated Processes:** Communication and Documentation; Caring; **Client Needs:** Physiological Integrity: Physiological Adaptation; Psychosocial Integrity; **Cognitive Level:** Application [Applying]

## 1455. ANSWER:

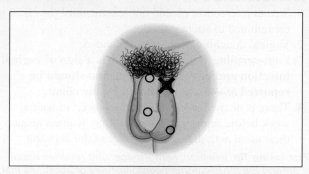

**The nurse should identify that the incision for the vasectomy will be made in the upper portion of the scrotum to expose the vas deferens. The vas deferens is then severed, and the severed ends are occluded with ligatures or by electrocautery. An incision in the upper or lower aspect of the penis or lower aspect of the scrotum would not expose the vas deferens.**

▶ *Test-taking Tip: A vasectomy is a resection of the vas deferens to prevent passage of sperm from the testes to the urethra during ejaculation. Because the vas deferens travels out of the scrotum and into the abdomen (gut cavity) through the inguinal canal, it cannot be seen from the outside of the body. Think about the location of the vas deferens and then where anatomically it would be most accessible.*

**Content Area:** Adult; **Concept:** Male Reproduction; Nursing Roles; **Integrated Processes:** Nursing Process: Implementation; Teaching/Learning; **Client Needs:** Physiological Integrity: Physiological Adaptation; **Cognitive Level:** Knowledge [Remembering]

## 1456. ANSWER: 3

1. Varicoceles are not inherited, and they are not related to ethnicity or race.

2. A varicocele does occur most frequently on the left side due to retrograde blood flow from the renal vein; however, a varicocele rarely produces symptoms.

3. **Asking about children is important because the most common cause of male infertility is a varicocele. Approximately 15% to 20% of the healthy, fertile male population is estimated to have varicoceles. However, 40% of infertile men may have them.**

4. A varicocele rarely produces any symptoms. It is usually diagnosed during physical examinations related to infertility. If symptoms do occur, pain and groin tenderness are the most common symptoms.

▶ *Test-taking Tip: A varicocele is abnormally dilated testicular vein. Infertility is a major concern.*

**Content Area:** Adult; **Concept:** Assessment; Male Reproduction; **Integrated Processes:** Nursing Process: Assessment; Culture and Spirituality; **Client Needs:** Physiological Integrity: Physiological Adaptation; **Cognitive Level:** Application [Applying]

## 1457. ANSWER: 3

1. Sexual intercourse should not resume until the client is reexamined in about 2 weeks.
2. Vaginal douching is not recommended.
3. **Foul-smelling vaginal discharge is a sign of vaginal infection and/or retained tissue and should be reported as soon as it is noted by the client.**
4. There is no evidence to support the need to wait a week before returning to work. Many women resume their usual activities the same day as the abortion.

♦ *Test-taking Tip:* Infection, hemorrhage, and retained tissue are among the more common complications of abortions that are performed via suction curettage.

**Content Area:** Adult; **Concept:** Infection; Female Reproduction; **Integrated Processes:** Teaching/Learning; **Client Needs:** Physiological Integrity: Reduction of Risk Potential; **Cognitive Level:** Application [Applying]

## 1458. ANSWER: 4

1. Using tobacco products and drinking alcohol are risk factors for infertility, but this is not the initial question.
2. Advancing age is a risk factor for infertility, but this is not the initial question.
3. A reproductive tract infection is a risk factor for infertility, but this is not the initial question.
4. **The definition of *infertility* is the inability to achieve a pregnancy after 1 year of regular intercourse without contraception. If the couple has not been attempting to achieve a pregnancy for that length of time, then there is no need for infertility testing. The other questions address risk factors for infertility, but those questions would be inconsequential if the criterion in Option 4 were not met.**

♦ *Test-taking Tip:* The key word is "initial." Eliminate the options that are risk factors for infertility.

**Content Area:** Adult; **Concept:** Promoting Health; Female Reproduction; Male Reproduction; **Integrated Processes:** Nursing Process: Assessment; **Client Needs:** Health Promotion and Maintenance; **Cognitive Level:** Application [Applying]

## 1459. ANSWER: 4

1. Information about females being infected more than males is important, and the client should be informed of this, but this is not the priority.
2. Information about the mode of transmission is important, and the client should be informed of this, but this is not the priority.
3. Typically in the first year after the diagnosis, the client will have four to five outbreaks, not two to three.
4. **The priority information to tell the client is that transmission can occur from a partner who does not have a visible sore.**

♦ *Test-taking Tip:* The key word is "priority." This indicates that more than one option is correct but that one is more important. Consider that genital herpes is caused by a virus that can be transmitted when no visible lesions are present.

**Content Area:** Adult; **Concept:** Sexuality; **Integrated Processes:** Nursing Process: Implementation; **Client Needs:** Safe and Effective Care Environment: Safety and Infection Control; **Cognitive Level:** Application [Applying]

## 1460. ANSWER: 3

1. Painful vesicles on the labia, perineum, or anus describe the lesions of genital herpes (herpes simplex virus 2).
2. Painful ulcerations of the vagina, labia, or perineum describe the lesions of genital herpes (herpes simplex virus 2).
3. **In females, genital warts appear as painless lesions near the vaginal opening, anus, vagina, or cervix. The lesions are textured, cauliflower appearing, and remain unchanged over time.**
4. A chancre is associated with syphilis, not genital warts.

♦ *Test-taking Tip:* Note the similarities in Options 1 and 2. Usually options that are similar are incorrect. Note the key word "chancre" in Option 4.

**Content Area:** Adult; **Concept:** Sexuality; Assessment; **Integrated Processes:** Nursing Process: Assessment; **Client Needs:** Physiological Integrity: Physiological Adaptation; **Cognitive Level:** Knowledge [Remembering]

## 1461. MoC PHARM ANSWER: 3

1. Doxycycline (Vibramycin), a tetracycline antibiotic, is an appropriate drug for treating chlamydia.
2. Azithromycin (Zithromax), a semisynthetic macrolide antibiotic, is an appropriate drug for treating chlamydia.
3. **Metronidazole (Flagyl) is an anti-infective against anaerobic organisms, an amoebicide, and an antiprotozoal agent. It is not indicated for either chlamydia or syphilis. Flagyl is used to treat bacterial vaginosis and trichomoniasis. Review with the HCP is necessary to discuss and clarify the order.**
4. Penicillin G (Bicillin) is an appropriate drug for treating syphilis.

♦ *Test-taking Tip:* The rights of medication administration include the right medication for the right reason. Chlamydia is an STI caused by bacteria that are usually spread through sexual contact. Narrow the options to the medication that would not be used for treating a bacterial infection.

**Content Area:** Adult; **Concept:** Sexuality; Infection; Medication; **Integrated Processes:** Nursing Process: Analysis; **Client Needs:** Safe and Effective Care Environment: Management of Care; Physiological Integrity: Pharmacological and Parenteral Therapies; **Cognitive Level:** Application [Applying]

## 1462. PHARM ANSWER: 2

1. Clients may experience a metallic taste while taking metronidazole.
2. **Drinking alcohol while on metronidazole (Flagyl) is contraindicated. It can cause a disulfiram-like reaction with nausea, vomiting, abdominal cramps, headache, and flushing.**
3. Metronidazole can turn urine dark. It is important to inform clients of this.
4. Nausea can occur when taking metronidazole. Taking it with food or milk may decrease GI irritation.

♦ *Test-taking Tip:* Examine all options and eliminate those that you know are anticipated side effects of metronidazole.

**Content Area:** Adult; **Concept:** Sexuality; Medication; **Integrated Processes:** Teaching/Learning; **Client Needs:** Physiological Integrity: Pharmacological and Parenteral Therapies; **Cognitive Level:** Application [Applying]

## 1463. ANSWER: 1

1. **Being diagnosed with an STI can cause emotional distress. This response acknowledges the client's reaction and provides the opportunity to clarify the statement's meaning.**
2. Although gonorrhea is reportable, this response is a closed statement and does not allow the opportunity for the client to express feelings.
3. The nurse is making an assumption about the client's spouse.
4. Although this response does acknowledge the client's reaction, the last portion becomes judgmental and places the emphasis on the nurse's feelings.

▸ **Test-taking Tip:** With a communication question, the correct response should be one that acknowledges the client's feelings and allows for a therapeutic interaction.

Content Area: Adult; Concept: Sexuality; Communication; Integrated Processes: Nursing Process: Implementation; Caring; Client Needs: Psychosocial Integrity; Cognitive Level: Application [Applying]

## 1464. ANSWER: 2

1. This illustrates acne vulgaris, which is not an STI.
2. **This illustrates herpes. Although herpes simplex may not necessarily be state reportable, it is an STI. By state law, the incidence of some STIs must be reported to the state.**
3. This illustrates a contact dermatitis; in this client, it was caused by nail polish.
4. This illustrates candidiasis or thrush. This is not reportable.

▸ **Test-taking Tip:** You should consider that only one of these options is an STI. If unsure, select the option that appears most severe. The nurse should consult agency requirements to determine which STIs are reportable in the practicing state.

Content Area: Adult; Concept: Sexuality; Infection; Integrated Processes: Communication and Documentation; Client Needs: Safe and Effective Care Environment: Safety and Infection Control; Cognitive Level: Application [Applying]

## 1465. MoC ANSWER: 2

1. Although herpes simplex can affect the genitalia, it is manifested by blister-like lesions that rupture and ulcerate, fever, pain, and bleeding.
2. **The nurse should consider possible *Candida albicans* infection. This is a fungal infection that can affect the mouth, esophagus, or the vaginal area. Perineal irritation, pruritus, and a thick, white vaginal discharge occur with vaginal candidiasis.**
3. Histoplasmosis, caused by *Histoplasma capsulatum*, begins as a respiratory infection and develops into a widespread infection. Dyspnea, fever, cough, weight loss, and an enlarged spleen, liver, and lymph nodes may be present.
4. Kaposi sarcoma is an AIDS-related malignancy that may begin with purplish-brown, raised lesions that are usually not painful or itchy.

▸ **Test-taking Tip:** Use knowledge of medical terminology to eliminate Option 3 because "-osis" is an abnormal increase and Option 4 because "-oma" means tumor. Herpes is associated with blisters, and blisters are not present. Therefore, eliminate Option 1.

Content Area: Adult; Concept: Sexuality; Infection; Immunity; Integrated Processes: Nursing Process: Implementation; Client Needs: Safe and Effective Care Environment: Management of Care; Physiological Integrity: Reduction of Risk Potential; Cognitive Level: Analysis [Analyzing]

## 1466. ANSWER: 3

1. This is the correct formula for mixing a bleach solution for disinfection.
2. Placing contaminated items in a plastic bag and then in the garbage is the correct method for disposing of contaminated articles. Sharps should first be placed in a rigid labeled container (such as a tin can), bleach solution added, the lid taped, and then placed in a bag for disposal in the garbage.
3. **Because sharing eating utensils does not transmit HIV, it is unnecessary to separately wash dishes and silverware used by the client. The client is prone to opportunistic and other infections.**
4. Cleaning with soap and water and then disinfecting with bleach solution is the correct method for cleaning body fluid spills.

▸ **Test-taking Tip:** Note the key word "unclear." Look for the incorrect instruction. Remember that HIV is not transmitted by kissing, hugging, shaking hands, or sharing eating utensils, towels, or bathroom fixtures with an HIV-positive person.

Content Area: Adult; Concept: Infection; Sexuality; Nursing Roles; Integrated Processes: Nursing Process: Evaluation; Client Needs: Safe and Effective Care Environment: Safety and Infection Control; Cognitive Level: Evaluation [Evaluating]

## 1467. MoC ANSWER: 2, 4, 5, 1, 3

2. **Determine if the woman is pregnant. This is priority because medications can be teratogenic, presenting a substantial risk to the developing fetus.**
4. **Administer an analgesic. Measures are needed to promote comfort. Itching, pain, macules, and papules occur initially with HSV-2. The infection can progress to vesicles and ulcers and can involve the labia, cervix, and vaginal and perianal areas.**
5. **Administer the first dose of acyclovir (Zovirax). An antiviral medication is needed to treat the infection.**
1. **Teach abstinence from sexual intercourse during treatment and use of condoms. The woman is unlikely to be receptive to teaching until some degree of comfort is achieved.**
3. **Discuss the benefits of joining a support group such as HELP (Herpetics Engaged in Living Productively). There is no cure for HSV-2 infection.**

▸ **Test-taking Tip:** Use the nursing process and Maslow's Hierarchy of Needs theory. Assessment should be completed before interventions.

Content Area: Adult; Concept: Sexuality; Infection; Integrated Processes: Nursing Process: Planning; Client Needs: Safe and Effective Care Environment: Management of Care; Cognitive Level: Synthesis [Creating]

## Chapter Thirty-Three

# Respiratory Management

**1468.** The client with asthma has obvious wheezing and signs of a possible impending asthma attack. Which intervention should the nurse implement **first?**

1. Have the client cough and deep breathe.
2. Prepare the client for possible intubation.
3. Give an inhaled beta-2 adrenergic agonist.
4. Notify the client's HCP.

**1469.** **PHARM** The client has recurrent asthma attacks. The HCP prescribes aminophylline 1000 mg in 250 mL of $D_5W$ to be infused at 30 mg/hr. The aminophylline ampule states 2000 mg/10 mL. How many mL of aminophylline should the nurse add to the IV fluid to obtain the prescribed concentration?

_____ mL (Record your answer as a whole number.)

**1470.** **PHARM** The nurse is teaching the client about using the illustrated attachment to the meter-dosed inhaler. The nurse should explain that this attachment is used for what purpose?

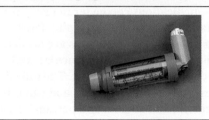

1. Allows for a greater amount of medication to be delivered
2. Permits visualization of the medication as it is delivered
3. Maintains the sterility of the mouthpiece and medication
4. Used for activating the medication canister by simply inhaling

**1471.** The client newly diagnosed with asthma is preparing for discharge. Which point should the nurse emphasize during the client's teaching?

1. Contact the HCP only if nighttime wheezing is a concern.
2. Avoid exposure to sources that might trigger an attack.
3. Use the peak flow meter only if symptoms are worsening.
4. Use the inhaled steroid medication as your rescue inhaler.

**1472.** The nurse is teaching the client newly diagnosed with asthma. Which instructions should the nurse include to reduce allergic triggers? **Select all that apply.**

1. Wash bedclothes and linens in cold water.
2. Use dust covers on mattresses and pillows.
3. Keep house fresh with a scented deodorizer.
4. Vacuum carpets daily in the bedrooms.
5. Clean the albuterol MDI daily under hot running water.

**1473.** The nurse and client are updating the client's asthma action plan. Which information should be updated on the action plan?

1. Drug adjustments for peak flows less than 50% of normal
2. Timeline for allergy skin testing to verify known triggers
3. The route the client may drive to the hospital during an attack
4. The best methods for performing chest physiotherapy (CPT)

**1474.** The nurse is assessing the client with chronic bronchitis. Which finding should the nurse expect?

1. Minimal sputum with cough
2. Copious pink, frothy sputum
3. Barrel chest appearance
4. Stridor on expiration

**1475.** The nurse is providing teaching to the client with COPD about the purpose of pursed-lip breathing. Which explanation is **most** appropriate?

1. It reduces upper airway inflammation.
2. It strengthens the respiratory muscles.
3. It improves inhaled drug effectiveness.
4. It reduces anxiety by slowing the HR.

**1476.** The nurse enters the room of the client with COPD and finds the client seated as illustrated. How should the nurse document the client's position?

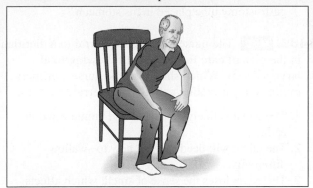

1. Orthopneic position
2. Abdominal breathing position
3. Pursed-lipped breathing position
4. Diaphragmatic breathing position

**1477.** The client with interstitial pulmonary disease has dyspnea and fatigue. Which recommendation by the nurse will be **most** helpful to this client?

1. Use energy conservation measures.
2. Use oxygen therapy while at home.
3. Remain in an upright position.
4. Use controlled coughing for airway clearance.

**1478.** The home health nurse is visiting the client whose chronic bronchitis has recently worsened due to not following previous instructions. Which instruction should the nurse reinforce?

1. Increase amount of bedrest.
2. Increase fluid intake to 3 liters.
3. Decrease carbohydrate intake.
4. Decrease use of home oxygen.

**1479.** **MoC** The client with COPD is in the third postoperative day following right-sided thoracotomy. At the change of the shift, the client's oxygen was increased to 10 L per mask to keep the $SaO_2$ greater than 88%. Which action should be taken by the oncoming shift nurse?

1. Work to wean oxygen down to 3 L by mask.
2. Call respiratory therapy for a nebulizer treatment.
3. Check the respiratory status and notify the HCP.
4. Administer a dose of the prescribed analgesic.

**1480.** The nurse enters the client's room after hearing the pulse oximeter alarming and sees the tracing illustrated on the screen. Which action should be immediately taken by the nurse?

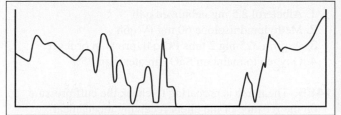

1. Call for the acute respiratory response team.
2. Remove the machine and call maintenance.
3. Give oxygen through a nasal cannula or mask.
4. Assess the client and the location of the probe.

**1481.** The nurse is helping the client newly diagnosed with obstructive sleep apnea to apply a CPAP mask at bedtime. When asked by the client about the purpose of CPAP, what should be the nurse's **best** response?

1. "The CPAP machine will breathe for you during sleep."
2. "Use of the CPAP will reduce intrathoracic pressure."
3. "The CPAP machine delivers higher levels of oxygen."
4. "Use of the CPAP prevents collapse of small air sacs."

**1482.** **MoC** The client is admitted with possible PE. In consulting with the HCP, the nurse learns that the V/Q scan shows a ventilation/perfusion quotient (V/Q) mismatch. Which intervention is appropriate?

1. Explain to the client that airborne precautions will be necessary.
2. Tell the client that the scan did not show a pulmonary embolus.
3. Explain to the client that further diagnostic testing will be needed.
4. Inform the client that the results of the V/Q scan were normal.

**1483.** The nurse is assessing the lung sounds of the client with pneumonia who is having pain during inspiration and expiration. Which information about lung sounds should the nurse document when hearing loud grating sounds over the lung fields?

1. Bronchial
2. Wheezing
3. Coarse crackles
4. Pleural friction rub

**1484.** **PHARM** The client, hospitalized with a lower respiratory tract infection, has a history of mild liver disease and asthma. Which prescription by an HCP should the nurse question?

1. Albuterol 2.5 mg nebulized q4h
2. Methylprednisolone 60 mg IV q6h
3. Aspirin 325 mg 2 tabs PO q4h prn pain or fever
4. Oxygen to maintain $SaO_2$ greater than 95%

**1485.** The nurse is preparing to check the cuff pressure on the ET tube of the client receiving mechanical ventilation. Place an X on the correct site where the nurse should check the cuff pressure.

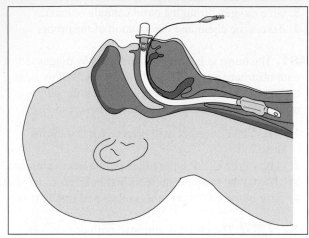

**1486.** The nurse is caring for the client requiring positive pressure mechanical ventilation. The client has been resisting the ventilator-assisted breaths, and the client's BP has been steadily decreasing. Which intervention should the nurse implement?

1. Place the client in the prone position to help aerate posterior alveoli.
2. Ask the respiratory therapist to adjust the machine's RRs.
3. Give the prescribed sedative-hypnotic medication if it is due now.
4. Prepare to administer an IV bronchodilator such as aminophylline.

**1487.** **MoC** The client had a total laryngectomy with tracheostomy placement. The nurse obtains two sets of postoperative VS that are WNL. Which is the nurse's **priority** now?

1. Check the stoma for the amount of mucus secretions.
2. Reposition so that the client is in a flat supine position.
3. Measure the amount of blood on the wound dressing.
4. Change the vital sign frequency to every 2 hours.

**1488.** On the third postoperative day following a total laryngectomy, the client's spouse asks when the client will be able to eat. Which response by the nurse is correct?

1. "He will be fed through a feeding tube, but eventually he will be able to eat normally."
2. "Before eating, he will need to learn a different way of swallowing to prevent aspiration."
3. "Because of his surgery, it will be several more days before his GI function begins again."
4. "He will likely always receive his food through a gastrostomy tube placed in his stomach."

**1489.** **MoC** The nurse includes a referral to a dietitian in the plan of care for the client following total laryngectomy. Which should be the nurse's primary rationale for initiating a dietician referral?

1. The client is likely depressed and uninterested in eating.
2. The client will need to learn how to swallow differently.
3. The client loses the sense of smell, which affects eating.
4. The client must learn strategies for preventing aspiration.

**1490.** The nurse is preparing to perform tracheostomy care for the client with a laryngectomy. Prioritize the steps that the nurse should take to correctly perform this client's tracheostomy care after assessing the client and explaining the procedure.

1. Apply clean gloves.
2. Wash hands and apply sterile gloves.
3. Wash hands and establish a sterile field.
4. Clean the inner cannula.
5. Reinsert the inner cannula.
6. Remove the inner cannula and place in the cleaning solution.
7. Clean the incision site and tracheostomy tube flange.

Answer: _____

**1491.** The nurse is evaluating discharge teaching that has been completed for the client following total laryngectomy. Which client statement should the nurse correct?

1. "I will be sure to carry an extra supply of facial tissue with me."
2. "I probably will not be able to go swimming at all anymore."
3. "I will plan for closure of my tracheostomy in about a month."
4. "I will check that our smoke detector batteries are working."

**1492.** The nurse is assessing the client post-hemilaryngectomy and radical neck dissection for treatment of cancer. Which finding should the nurse expect due to the surgical procedure?

1. A permanent loss of voice
2. Shoulder drop only on one side
3. Numbness of the mouth, lips, and face
4. An inability to cough to clear secretions

**1493.** The client with CF is visiting with the nurse in preparation for leaving home for college. Which client statement should the nurse clarify?

1. "I'll bring cough medicine to use at night so I don't wake up my roommate."
2. "I'll contact the college's health center and pass on my medical records."
3. "I'll check to make sure that the school has a facility for me to exercise."
4. "I'll carry and use a hand hygiene product and stay away from sick friends."

**1494.** The client telephones the clinic after having 3 days of symptoms that strongly suggest influenza. What should the nurse advise?

1. "Return to work after another day of rest."
2. "Rest and drink at least 3 liters of fluid daily."
3. "Obtain over-the-counter antihistamines."
4. "Come in to the clinic for a flu shot now."

**1495.** The nurse is developing a plan of care for the client admitted with a cough, fever, dyspnea, and a diagnosis of pneumonia. Which is the **best** intervention to include in the client's plan of care to prevent atelectasis?

1. Suction oral secretions every 2 to 4 hours.
2. Provide continuous use of oxygen at 2 L/NC.
3. Teach and reinforce coughing every 4 hours.
4. Encourage hourly use of an incentive spirometer.

**1496.** The nurse is preparing to admit the client who has been diagnosed with TB. Which interventions should the nurse plan to implement? **Select all that apply.**

1. Ensure that the room assigned is a positive-pressure airflow room.
2. Wear gown and gloves when handling the client's stool or urine.
3. Put on an N95 respirator mask before entering the client's room.
4. Keep the client in the room until antibiotics have been started.
5. Begin prescribed doses of isoniazid, rifampin, pyrazinamide, and ethambutol.

**1497.** **PHARM** The nurse is preparing to administer vancomycin 500 mg IV to the client with pneumonia. The vancomycin is supplied in a 100-mL piggyback that is to be given over 1 hour. At what rate in mL/hr should the nurse set the infusion pump?

_____ mL/hr (Record your answer as a whole number.)

**1498.** The nurse assesses the client brought to the ED via ambulance after a motorcycle crash. The client has paradoxical chest movement with respirations, multiple bruises across the chest and torso, crepitus, and tachypnea. What should the nurse do **next?**

1. Remove and reapply the cervical collar.
2. Prepare for the client's imminent intubation.
3. Insert another IV catheter to give medications.
4. Tape around the client's chest for rib protection.

**1499.** The client experienced a spontaneous pneumothorax. In explaining this to the client, which illustration should the nurse select?

1.
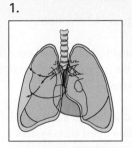
2.
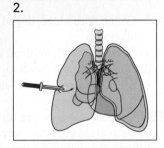
3.
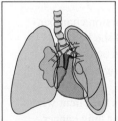
4.
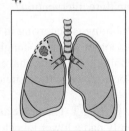

**1500.** **MoC** **PHARM** The nurse is caring for the client in an ED who has five fractured ribs from blunt chest trauma. The client is rating pain at 9 out of 10 on a 0 to 10 scale. When contacting the HCP, the nurse should advocate for which pain management option?

1. Oral nonsteroidal anti-inflammatory drugs
2. Oral narcotic analgesic and acetaminophen
3. Epidural analgesic or intercostal nerve block
4. Meperidine IV administered q1–2h prn

**1501.** The nurse is assessing the client who just arrived by ambulance following an MVA. Which assessment finding should the nurse associate with a possible pulmonary contusion?

1. Stridor
2. Bloody sputum
3. Unilateral rhonchi
4. Increased breath sounds

**1502.** **PHARM** **MoC** The nurse is caring for the client whose condition has progressed from an acute lung injury from near-drowning to ARDS. Which intervention should the nurse question with the HCP?

1. Place in prone position if tolerated
2. Normal saline 1000-mL bolus, then at 250 mL/hr
3. Ventilatory support with positive end-expiratory pressure (PEEP)
4. Methylprednisolone 175 mg IV now and q4h

**1503.** The nurse assesses the client being treated for smoke inhalation. Which early signs indicate the possible onset of ARDS in this client?

1. Cough with blood-tinged sputum and respiratory alkalosis
2. Decrease in white blood cell and red blood cell counts
3. Diaphoresis and low $SaO_2$ despite oxygen administration
4. Steadily increasing BP and elevated $PaO_2$

**1504.** The nurse is caring for the client with a left-sided chest tube attached to a wet suction chest tube system. Which observation by the nurse would require **immediate** intervention?

1. Bubbling is occurring in the suction chamber.
2. A loop of tubing is hanging off the bed.
3. Tubing connections have bands on them.
4. Chest tube insertion site dressing is occlusive.

**1505.** **PHARM** The nurse assesses the client who recently had a lower lobectomy for lung cancer. Findings include dyspnea with respirations at 45 bpm, hypotension, $SaO_2$ at 86% on 10 L close-fitting oxygen mask, trachea deviated slightly to the left, and the right side of the client's chest not expanding. Which action should be taken by the nurse **first**?

1. Notify the client's HCP.
2. Give the prn prescribed lorazepam.
3. Check the chest tube for obstruction.
4. Increase the oxygen flow to 15 liters.

**1506.** The nurse is assisting the client with arm and shoulder exercises on the client's first postoperative day following a right-sided thoracotomy. The client reports pain with the exercises and wants to know why they must be performed. Which explanation about the exercises is **best**?

1. "These will promote expanding the left lung."
2. "These increase blood flow back to your heart."
3. "These rebuild the muscle that was removed."
4. "These prevent stiffening and loss of function."

**1507.** Following a thoracotomy to remove a lung tumor, the nurse is preparing the client for discharge to home. Which information should the nurse include in discharge teaching? **Select all that apply.**

1. Avoid lifting greater than 20 pounds.
2. Gradually build up exercise endurance.
3. Continue to exercise even when dyspneic.
4. Expect normal strength in about 1 month.
5. Make time for frequent rest periods.

**1508.** **MoC** The NA is reporting to the nurse about the care given to assigned clients. After receiving this report, which client should the nurse attend to **first**?

1. The client with a PE who has not had a bowel movement in 2 days
2. The client after a thoracoscopy is on 4 L oxygen/NC and has $SaO_2$ of 88%
3. The client who had a right lobectomy and has a BP of 100/65 mm Hg
4. The client who has rib fractures and has not voided for 6 hr

**1509.** The client who had an open thoracotomy received fluid resuscitation during surgery due to extensive blood loss. Upon postoperative assessment, the nurse finds that the client is cyanotic, dyspneic, and drooling pink, frothy secretions. Which intervention should the nurse implement **now**?

1. Place the bed in high Fowler's position.
2. Administer a 500-mL NS fluid bolus.
3. Activate the respiratory code system.
4. Have the client cough and deep breathe.

**1510.** While performing tracheostomy care for the client who experienced facial trauma, the nurse discovers that more air is needed to inflate the cuff to maintain a seal. Which complication related to the tracheostomy should the nurse further explore?

1. Tracheal stenosis
2. Tracheomalacia
3. Tracheal sclerosis
4. Tracheal-innominate artery fistula

**INSTRUCTIONS:** Read the case study illustrated, noting the times and the nurse's assessment and intervention over time. Refer to the case study to answer Questions 1511 and 1512.

| Client: 52-year-old, African American | Allergies: Penicillin | Diagnosis: Lung Cancer; Right Lateral Thoracotomy and Pneumonectomy |
|---|---|---|
| **Time** | **Assessment** | **Interventions** |
| 1100 | Admitted from PACU; sleepy; BP 138/74, P. 110, RR 22. SaO₂ 89%. On 2L/NC. Chest tube (CT) in place to drainage system on waterseal. 50 mL bloody returns. Lung sounds absent on right. Ringer's Lactate at 100 mL/hr via pump. Epidural in place, CDI, with morphine sulfate infusing at 3 mg/hr (prescribed range 0-8 mg/hr). | Increased oxygen to 3L/NC. Attached CT drainage system to suction; dry suction control dial set at 20cm as prescribed. Positioned onto right side. Sequential compression stockings on; device started. |
| 1145 | BP 142/74, P. 112, RR 28. SaO₂ 92%. Rates pain right chest at 7 out of 10. Diaphoretic. | Increased epidural analgesic to 4 mg/hr. Tipped and tilted CT tubing towards suction container; bloody drainage now at 75 mL. Placed cool cloth on forehead. |
| 1200 | BP 118/70, P. 80, RR 18. SaO₂ 92%. Pain right chest at 5 out of 10. States feeling better but "hurts lying on incision." | Repositioned onto left side. Right incisional dressing CDI. |
| 1215 | BP 110/70, P. 88, RR 18. SaO₂ 89%. Bloody CT drainage at 100 mL. Left lung sounds diminished. | Increased oxygen to 4L/NC. Encouraged coughing and deep breathing. Gave prescribed dose of cefuroxime 1.5 gm IV. |
| 1230 | Diaphoretic. Chest pain 10 on 0-10 scale. BP: 88/38, P. 132, RR 30, SaO₂ 85%. CT returning bloody; drainage system at 140 mL. | |

**1511.** CJ MoC At which time did the nurse intervene incorrectly?

1. 1100
2. 1145
3. 1200
4. 1215

**1512.** CJ MoC The nurse intervened for this client at 1230. Based on the case study, which interventions are appropriate? **Select all that apply.**

1. Lowered the head of the client's bed
2. Asked LPN to place a call for the ART
3. Set CT drainage system suction dial to 30 cm
4. Telephoned the HCP regarding client status
5. Applied nonrebreather mask at 10L oxygen

# *Answers and Rationales*

**1468. ANSWER: 3**

1. Neither coughing nor deep breathing will stop the attack.
2. Intubation is not effective in treating the underlying cause of the attack, which is an inflammatory response, and would not be a first-line intervention.
3. **The client with asthma who is experiencing wheezing and an impending attack is best treated with inhaled beta-2 adrenergic agonist drugs such as albuterol (Ventolin). Oxygen and corticosteroids may also be used.**
4. The client should be given a rescue medication before the HCP is notified.

▶ *Test-taking Tip: You need to consider the intervention that will treat the narrowed airways.*

**Content Area:** Adult; **Concept:** Medication, Oxygenation; **Integrated Processes:** Nursing Process: Implementation; **Client Needs:** Physiological Integrity: Physiological Adaptation; **Cognitive Level:** Application [Applying]

**1469. PHARM ANSWER: 5**

**Using dimensional analysis, the formula would be:**

$$\underline{\quad} \text{mL} = \frac{X \text{ mL}}{X \text{ mg}} \left| X \text{ mg} = \frac{X}{X} ; \quad \underline{\quad} \text{mL} = \frac{10 \text{ mL}}{2,000 \text{ mg}} \right| 1,000 \text{ mg} = \frac{10,000}{2,000} = 5$$

▶ *Test-taking Tip: First identify the unit of measure being calculated (mL). Then identify the complete clinical ratio that contains that unit. Avoid being confused with the 250 mL of $D_5W$ and the rate of the infusion. Focus on what the question is asking.*

**Content Area:** Adult; **Concept:** Oxygenation; Nursing Roles; Medication; **Integrated Processes:** Nursing Process: Planning; **Client Needs:** Physiological Integrity: Pharmacological and Parenteral Therapies; **Cognitive Level:** Application [Applying]

**1470. PHARM ANSWER: 1**

1. **The attachment illustrated is a spacer or extender. This device holds the medication in suspension for a few moments longer, allowing improved medication delivery. These devices are recommended for children or older adults who might not have the dexterity or knowledge to time an inhalation with medication delivery.**
2. Visual confirmation of delivery is not the main reason that the spacer is attached.
3. The mouthpiece may be kept cleaner with a spacer but does not ensure sterility.
4. Although some inhalers allow for inhalation "trigger" delivery, this is not the purpose of the spacer/extender.

▶ *Test-taking Tip: If unfamiliar with the item pictured, think logically about the situation and link it to the aspects of the question that you do know.*

**Content Area:** Adult; **Concept:** Medication; Nursing Roles; Oxygenation; **Integrated Processes:** Nursing Process: Implementation; Teaching/ Learning; **Client Needs:** Physiological Integrity: Pharmacological and Parenteral Therapies; **Cognitive Level:** Analysis [Analyzing]

**1471. ANSWER: 2**

1. Symptoms such as worsening peak flow meter readings and nighttime wheezing are two of the many health changes that should signal the client to contact the HCP.
2. **The nurse should emphasize ways to prevent an attack, such as avoiding known triggers.**
3. A peak flow meter is generally used daily to document and identify worsening symptoms over time.
4. Generally, inhalers with steroid medications are not to be used as a rescue inhaler in the event of an asthma attack.

▶ *Test-taking Tip: Options with absolute words such as "only" are often incorrect.*

**Content Area:** Adult; **Concept:** Promoting Health; Nursing Roles; Oxygenation; **Integrated Processes:** Teaching/Learning; **Client Needs:** Health Promotion and Maintenance; **Cognitive Level:** Application [Applying]

**1472. ANSWER: 2, 4**

1. Bedclothes should be washed in hot water or cooler water with detergent and bleach to reduce allergen levels.
2. **The nurse should instruct the client to use dust covers on mattresses and pillows to reduce exposure to dust mites.**
3. Scented sprays should be avoided because they may trigger an asthmatic attack.
4. **Vacuuming the carpets in the bedrooms daily helps to remove dust mites and dust particles.**
5. Albuterol (Proventil, Ventolin) is a beta-2 adrenergic agonist. Only the plastic sleeve, and not the canister, should be placed under warm (not hot) running water.

▶ *Test-taking Tip: Remember that a frequent trigger for an asthma attack is dust mites. Use "dust" as a clue to narrow the options to Options 2 and 4, the only options that relate to dust in their descriptions.*

**Content Area:** Adult; **Concept:** Promoting Health; Oxygenation; **Integrated Processes:** Teaching/Learning; **Client Needs:** Health Promotion and Maintenance; Physiological Integrity: Reduction of Risk Potential; **Cognitive Level:** Application [Applying]

**1473. ANSWER: 1**

1. **A peak flow of less than 50% of normal indicates that the asthma action plan should be updated. If asthma worsens, adjustments are primarily made with the medication regimen.**
2. Allergy skin testing would be completed in the early phases of diagnosis.
3. The plan should identify the best ways to access and alert emergency personnel if an acute attack occurs, but the client should not be driving himself or herself to the hospital.
4. CPT is not usually a part of asthma therapy.

▶ **Test-taking Tip:** *Look for key words in the stem and options, such as "updates" in the stem and "adjustments" in the options.*

**Content Area:** Adult; **Concept:** Promoting Health; Oxygenation; **Integrated Processes:** Nursing Process: Implementation; **Client Needs:** Health Promotion and Maintenance; **Cognitive Level:** Synthesis [Creating]

## 1474. ANSWER: 3

1. Minimal sputum with cough is more indicative of emphysema than chronic bronchitis, which usually is characterized by copious secretions.
2. Pink, frothy sputum is indicative of pulmonary edema.
3. **Barrel chest is indicative of the client with chronic bronchitis because of lung hyperinflation.**
4. Stridor indicates some type of upper respiratory edema, which would not be expected with chronic bronchitis.

▶ **Test-taking Tip:** *Three options are similar, dealing with breathing, and one is different; often the option that is different is the answer.*

**Content Area:** Adult; **Concept:** Assessment; Oxygenation; **Integrated Processes:** Nursing Process: Assessment; **Client Needs:** Physiological Integrity: Physiological Adaptation; **Cognitive Level:** Comprehension [Understanding]

## 1475. ANSWER: 2

1. Pursed-lip breathing does not have an effect on upper airway inflammation.
2. **Pursed-lip breathing increases the strength of respiratory muscles and helps to keep alveoli open.**
3. Pursed-lip breathing is not a part of medication administration.
4. Pursed-lip breathing may reduce the client's anxiety, but this effect is usually due to improved breathing and not to slowing of the HR.

▶ **Test-taking Tip:** *Narrow the options to the two that pertain to the respiratory nature of the disease. The key phrase "most appropriate" indicates that one option is better than the other.*

**Content Area:** Adult; **Concept:** Nursing Roles; Oxygenation; **Integrated Processes:** Nursing Process: Implementation; Teaching/Learning; **Client Needs:** Physiological Integrity: Physiological Adaptation; **Cognitive Level:** Knowledge [Remembering]

## 1476. ANSWER: 1

1. **The client with chronic airflow issues, such as those with COPD, assumes an orthopneic position to ease the work of breathing. The illustration shows the Tripod position (leaning forward, hands on knees).**
2. Abdominal breathing is a breathing technique for chest and lung expansion; it is used to manage dyspneic episodes but does not require an upright position.
3. Pursed-lipped breathing can be done in any position and is not depicted in the exhibit.
4. Diaphragmatic breathing is a breathing technique for chest and lung expansion; it is used to manage dyspneic episodes but does not require an upright position.

▶ **Test-taking Tip:** *You need to understand that orthopnea is difficulty breathing while lying. You should be able to eliminate Options 2 and 4 because these can be performed in a lying position. Pursed-lipped breathing does not require a leaning-forward position; thus eliminate Option 3.*

**Content Area:** Adult; **Concept:** Oxygenation; Communication; **Integrated Processes:** Nursing Process: Analysis; Communication and Documentation; **Client Needs:** Physiological Integrity: Physiological Adaptation; **Cognitive Level:** Comprehension [Understanding]

## 1477. ANSWER: 1

1. **Energy conservation includes the use of rest periods and breathing techniques and is the only option that focuses on both the dyspnea and fatigue associated with interstitial pulmonary disease.**
2. Using oxygen focuses only on the symptom of dyspnea; there is no information about the client's oxygen saturation to indicate that oxygen is needed.
3. Although sitting upright will help expand the lungs, energy conservation will be more helpful to prevent dyspnea and fatigue.
4. There is no indication that this client has ineffective airway clearance.

▶ **Test-taking Tip:** *Focus on the key words "most helpful" and the client's symptoms of dyspnea and fatigue. The answer should be helpful to relieving both symptoms.*

**Content Area:** Adult; **Concept:** Oxygenation; Nursing Roles; **Integrated Processes:** Teaching/Learning; **Client Needs:** Psychosocial Integrity; Physiological Integrity: Physiological Adaptation; **Cognitive Level:** Application [Applying]

## 1478. ANSWER: 2

1. Imposing bedrest on the client with shortness of breath may worsen the situation. Physical activity interspersed with adequate rest can improve respiratory function.
2. **Increasing the fluid intake may help liquefy secretions for easier expectoration.**
3. A diet high in calories can compensate for this client's hypermetabolic state, dyspnea, and poor appetite.
4. Reducing home oxygen use in this situation would most likely exacerbate the client's symptoms.

▶ **Test-taking Tip:** *The key word is "reinforce." Think about which instruction would have been included in earlier teaching.*

**Content Area:** Adult; **Concept:** Nursing Roles; Oxygenation; **Integrated Processes:** Teaching/Learning; **Client Needs:** Physiological Integrity: Physiological Adaptation; **Cognitive Level:** Application [Applying]

## 1479. MoC ANSWER: 3

1. Working to wean oxygen by mask below 3 L will cause retention of $CO_2$; oxygen by mask generally should be set at 4 L or greater.
2. Although a nebulizer treatment may assist the client, the immediate need is to determine if the high flow oxygen is affecting the client's respiratory drive and to further determine the cause of the low oxygen saturations.

3. The oncoming shift nurse should check the client's RR and report these abnormal findings to the HCP. Although uncommon, clients with COPD on high flow oxygen can lose their respiratory drive, or the client may have developed a respiratory complication.

4. Analgesics may assist the client if he or she is in pain, but the immediate need is to determine if the high flow oxygen is affecting the client's respiratory drive and to further determine the cause of the low $SaO_2$.

▶ *Test-taking Tip: An option that includes an assessment is often the correct answer because the nursing process is driven by the data collected in an assessment.*

Content Area: Adult; Concept: Oxygenation, Critical Thinking; Management; Integrated Processes: Nursing Process: Implementation; Client Needs: Safe and Effective Care Environment: Management of Care; Physiological Integrity: Reduction of Risk Potential; Cognitive Level: Application [Applying]

## 1480. ANSWER: 4

1. A pulse oximeter or any other technology should never replace the direct assessment of the client by the nurse.

2. The nurse should always treat the client and not the monitor.

3. Applying oxygen would be a good choice if the nurse continued to be unable to determine the client's pulse oximetry reading within a few seconds, but oxygen may not be necessary or appropriate.

4. This pleth wave tracing is generally the result of an artifact from the client moving the area where the probe is placed. By immediately assessing the client and then the probe's location, the nurse can quickly determine whether the tracing constitutes an emergency or is just an artifact.

▶ *Test-taking Tip: Consider the steps of the nursing process in answering this question. An intervention is generally guided by the nurse's assessment findings. This should direct you to the correct option.*

Content Area: Adult; Concept: Assessment; Oxygenation; Safety; Integrated Processes: Nursing Process: Assessment; Client Needs: Safe and Effective Care Environment: Safety and Infection Control; Cognitive Level: Analysis [Analyzing]

## 1481. ANSWER: 4

1. A ventilator, and not a CPAP machine, can be used to breathe for the client who is unresponsive.

2. CPAP is not intended to reduce intrathoracic pressure.

3. Although oxygen can be administered with a CPAP device, it is not always necessary.

4. CPAP devices are intended for clients who can breathe on their own but need assistance in maintaining adequate oxygenation. The CPAP device keeps the alveoli open, allowing for maximal perfusion to occur.

▶ *Test-taking Tip: The client with sleep apnea is able to breathe but needs assistance in keeping the airway open to allow for maximal perfusion.*

Content Area: Adult; Concept: Oxygenation; Integrated Processes: Nursing Process: Implementation; Client Needs: Physiological Integrity: Reduction of Risk Potential; Cognitive Level: Application [Applying]

## 1482. MoC ANSWER: 3

1. A CXR, sputum culture, and Gram stain are used to diagnose TB; placement in airborne precautions is not indicated.

2. A V/Q mismatch is highly suspicious but not diagnostic of multiple lung diseases, including PE.

3. An imbalanced or mismatched V/Q scan indicates some type of problem with either ventilation or perfusion. Further testing is required, especially in the case of suspected PE.

4. A V/Q mismatch is not a normal finding.

▶ *Test-taking Tip: A mismatch should be a clue to you that the findings are not normal.*

Content Area: Adult; Concept: Oxygenation, Critical Thinking; Consultation; Integrated Processes: Nursing Process: Implementation; Client Needs: Safe and Effective Care Environment: Management of Care; Physiological Integrity: Physiological Adaptation; Cognitive Level: Application [Applying]

## 1483. ANSWER: 4

1. Bronchial sounds are normal tubular sounds auscultated over the trachea and bronchus.

2. Fine or coarse crackles will have a moist, bubbling, or Velcro-tearing sound.

3. Wheezing tends to have a high-pitched sound.

4. A pleural friction rub tends to be loud, grating, and heard easily over the lung fields upon auscultation. A pleural friction rub is often associated with painful breathing.

▶ *Test-taking Tip: The client with pneumonia may have crackles, rhonchi, and wheezes as well as a pleural friction rub, but the clue in the question is pain during inspiration and expiration.*

Content Area: Adult; Concept: Assessment; Oxygenation; Communication; Integrated Processes: Communication and Documentation; Client Needs: Health Promotion and Maintenance; Cognitive Level: Comprehension [Understanding]

## 1484. PHARM ANSWER: 3

1. The prescription of albuterol (Ventolin, Proventil), a bronchodilator, is appropriate for the client with a respiratory infection, asthma, and mild liver disease.

2. The prescription of methylprednisolone (Medrol), a glucocorticoid, is appropriate for the client with a respiratory infection, asthma, and mild liver disease.

3. Use of aspirin is avoided in clients with asthma because it is a known trigger for asthma attacks.

4. Oxygen is appropriate for the client with a respiratory infection, asthma, and mild liver disease.

▶ *Test-taking Tip: Use your knowledge of pharmacology and oxygen therapy to determine that all options include correct information. Next, consider the client's condition of a respiratory infection, mild liver disease, and asthma to identify that aspirin is the only drug that cannot be used in these conditions.*

Content Area: Adult; Concept: Oxygenation; Medication; Integrated Processes: Nursing Process: Analysis; Communication and Documentation; Client Needs: Physiological Integrity: Pharmacological and Parenteral Therapies; Safe and Effective Care Environment: Safety and Infection Control; Cognitive Level: Analysis [Analyzing]

## 1485. ANSWER:

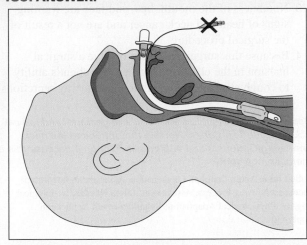

**The correct location to check cuff pressure is at the inflation assembly, which connects directly with the tube cuff. No other location allows cuff pressure to be assessed.**

▸ *Test-taking Tip: Closely inspect the illustrated tube to analyze its parts. Visualize the client with an ET tube and think about the purpose of the pilot tube attached to the ET tube.*

Content Area: Adult; Concept: Safety; Oxygenation; Integrated Processes: Nursing Process: Implementation; Client Needs: Safe and Effective Care Environment: Safety and Infection Control; Cognitive Level: Application [Applying]

## 1486. ANSWER: 3

1. Placing the client in the prone position will not correct the underlying issue and may increase resistance to the ventilator.
2. The respiratory therapist may help identify a possible cause for the client's response, but adjusting the RR may worsen the problem.
3. **Positive pressure ventilation can lead to decreased cardiac output and a drop in BP. Appropriate sedation promotes physical and mental relaxation and may improve cardiac output and BP.**
4. An IV-administered bronchodilator is not indicated and may further decrease the client's BP.

▸ *Test-taking Tip: Do not read into the question. Put the needs of the client first and consider the psychosocial and physiological responses to mechanical ventilation.*

Content Area: Adult; Concept: Oxygenation; Safety; Integrated Processes: Nursing Process: Implementation; Client Needs: Physiological Integrity: Physiological Adaptation; Cognitive Level: Analysis [Analyzing]

## 1487. MoC ANSWER: 1

1. **The nurse's priority action should be to check the amount of mucus secretions at the stoma because secretions are a potential cause of airway obstruction.**
2. The client should be positioned in an upright position (not flat supine) to prevent aspiration of secretions and to promote blood drainage.
3. Although monitoring the amount of bleeding at the wound site is important, it is not the priority.
4. The next set of VS should be taken in 15 minutes.

▸ *Test-taking Tip: Use the ABC's when selecting an option. Only Option 1 pertains to the client's airway.*

Content Area: Adult; Concept: Critical Thinking; Oxygenation; Integrated Processes: Nursing Process: Evaluation; Client Needs: Safe and Effective Care Environment: Management of Care; Cognitive Level: Evaluation [Evaluating]

## 1488. ANSWER: 1

1. **A feeding tube is generally placed during the surgical procedure and first used for stomach decompression and then for feeding until healing is near completion. Once healing occurs, the client can eat normally.**
2. The client should be able to swallow normally once healing is near completion.
3. Bowel function should be returning by the third postoperative day. However, when the GI function returns, the client will initially be fed by tube feeding and not orally.
4. Unless there are major complications, the client should be able to return to eating normally and should not need a permanent gastrostomy tube.

▸ *Test-taking Tip: Absolute words such as "always" usually indicate an incorrect option. If unsure, eliminate options that use complex medical terminology.*

Content Area: Adult; Concept: Nutrition; Oxygenation; Integrated Processes: Nursing Process: Implementation; Teaching/Learning; Client Needs: Physiological Integrity: Basic Care and Comfort; Cognitive Level: Analysis [Analyzing]

## 1489. MoC ANSWER: 3

1. Mental health concerns would not be handled by nutrition support staff.
2. Relearning how to swallow is more of a concern with a partial laryngectomy than with a total laryngectomy.
3. **The client's loss of the sense of smell and possibly the sense of taste after a total laryngectomy may reduce the desire to eat and may change the taste of certain foods. The dietician will plan a balanced diet of foods that the client likes and will eat to maximize healing.**
4. Aspiration is not a concern; there is no continuity between the lungs and the esophagus.

▸ *Test-taking Tip: The key term is "primary." You need to consider the role of the dietician in promoting the client's nutritional intake for wound healing.*

**Content Area:** Adult; **Concept:** Collaboration, Nutrition; Oxygenation; **Integrated Processes:** Nursing Process: Planning; **Client Needs:** Physiological Integrity: Basic Care and Comfort; Safe and Effective Care Environment: Management of Care; **Cognitive Level:** Synthesis [Creating]

## 1490. ANSWER: 3, 1, 6, 2, 4, 5, 7

3. **Wash hands and establish a sterile field; this does not require the use of gloves.**
1. **Apply clean gloves; clean gloves are used to avoid hand contamination.**
6. **Remove the inner cannula and place in the cleaning solution; the inner cannula should be removed before applying sterile gloves.**
2. **Wash hands and apply sterile gloves. Using sterile gloves reduces the incidence of introducing microorganisms.**
4. **Clean the inner cannula. The inner cannula needs to be cleaned before it is reinserted.**
5. **Reinsert the inner cannula. The inner cannula is only reinserted once it is cleaned.**
7. **Clean the incision site and tracheostomy tube flange; this performed last because movement during cleansing can cause increased secretions that can collect on the dressing and around the stoma.**

▶ *Test-taking Tip: First, visualize yourself performing tracheostomy care to the client. Recall the principles of asepsis, safety, and client teaching. With prioritization questions, it is easiest to select the first and last steps and then order the remaining options.*

**Content Area:** Adult; **Concept:** Oxygenation; **Integrated Processes:** Nursing Process: Implementation; **Client Needs:** Safe and Effective Care Environment: Safety and Infection Control; Physiological Integrity: Physiological Adaptation; **Cognitive Level:** Synthesis [Creating]

## 1491. ANSWER: 3

1. The client should carry extra tissue because usually nasal drip increases and there is the potential problem of managing oral secretions effectively after a total laryngectomy.
2. Swimming puts the client at risk for aspirating water and should be avoided.
3. **The nurse should correct this statement by the client. The tracheostomy is permanent after a total laryngectomy because the larynx and part of the trachea are removed.**
4. The client's loss of smell can be a safety concern in the home.

▶ *Test-taking Tip: You should narrow the options by eliminating the statements that would help keep the client free from harm and embarrassment.*

**Content Area:** Adult; **Concept:** Nursing Roles; Oxygenation; **Integrated Processes:** Nursing Process: Evaluation; **Client Needs:** Safe and Effective Care Environment: Safety and Infection Control; Physiological Integrity: Physiological Adaptation; **Cognitive Level:** Evaluation [Evaluating]

## 1492. ANSWER: 2

1. A hemilaryngectomy results in a hoarse voice rather than a loss of voice.
2. **During a radical neck dissection the 11th cranial nerve (spinal accessory muscle) is severed, resulting in shoulder drop on the side of the dissection.**
3. Numbness of the mouth, lips, and face are warning signs of head and neck cancer and are not a result of the surgical procedure.
4. Because this surgery does not involve a surgical incision in the chest or abdomen, the client's ability to cough effectively enough to clear airway secretions is intact.

▶ *Test-taking Tip: Visualize the hemilaryngectomy and radical neck dissection surgeries. Narrow the options to the neck, eliminating Options 3 and 4. Eliminate Option 1 because this is a hemilaryngectomy.*

**Content Area:** Adult; **Concept:** Oxygenation; Assessment; **Integrated Processes:** Nursing Process: Assessment; **Client Needs:** Physiological Integrity: Physiological Adaptation; **Cognitive Level:** Application [Applying]

## 1493. ANSWER: 1

1. **The nurse should clarify this statement. The client with CF should not be using cough suppressants because of the high importance of expectorating secretions.**
2. Contacting the college's health center will make them aware of any special care needs.
3. The client should exercise regularly to facilitate loosening and clearing secretions and to maintain physical strength.
4. Hand hygiene and avoiding sick friends will help to reduce the risk of respiratory illness.

▶ *Test-taking Tip: The health of the client with CF is dependent on his or her ability to have frequent productive coughing. This is a negative-response question. The key word "clarify" means you should select the option that is incorrect.*

**Content Area:** Adult; **Concept:** Nursing Roles; Promoting Health; Oxygenation; **Integrated Processes:** Nursing Process: Analysis; **Client Needs:** Physiological Integrity: Physiological Adaptation; Health Promotion and Maintenance; **Cognitive Level:** Application [Applying]

## 1494. ANSWER: 2

1. Influenza is highly contagious, so returning to work should not occur until the client is symptom-free.
2. **Rest to conserve energy and increased fluid intake to liquify secretions are essential when the client has influenza.**
3. Antihistamines are not the OTC medications of choice. Antitussives and antipyretics are usually used for symptom control.
4. The client who has influenza should not get the influenza vaccine.

▶ *Test-taking Tip: Influenza is generally a self-limiting condition but one that is also highly contagious.*

Content Area: Adult; Concept: Infection; Oxygenation; Medication;
Integrated Processes: Nursing Process: Implementation;
Client Needs: Physiological Integrity: Physiological Adaptation;
Cognitive Level: Application [Applying]

## 1495. ANSWER: 4

1. There is no indication that the client is unable to expectorate secretions.
2. Oxygen is used to treat hypoxia rather than to prevent atelectasis.
3. Clients should be encouraged to cough effectively at least every 2 hours while awake to promote airway clearance and expand the lungs.
4. **Incentive spirometry, also known as sustained maximal inspiration, is a type of bronchial hygiene used in pneumonia to prevent or reverse alveolar collapse (atelectasis).**

▸ *Test-taking Tip: Recall the pathophysiology of atelectasis (alveolar collapse). Associate each of the options with the prevention of atelectasis. This should lead you to select Option 4.*

Content Area: Adult; Concept: Oxygenation; Integrated
Processes: Nursing Process: Planning; Client Needs: Physiological
Integrity: Physiological Adaptation; Cognitive Level: Synthesis
[Creating]

## 1496. ANSWER: 3, 5

1. The client should be placed in a negative-airflow (not positive-pressure airflow) room, which pulls the air out of the room and vents it externally.
2. The appropriate PPE when handling stool or urine from the client with TB includes gloves and the N95 respirator mask.
3. **High-efficiency particulate masks (N95) should be worn by those entering the client's room to prevent inhalation of potentially infectious respiratory secretions.**
4. Although the client's movements around the hospital should be somewhat limited, the client can travel wearing a mask to reduce transmission risk and need not be confined to the room.
5. **The recommended initial treatment consists of a multiple-medication regimen of isoniazid (INH), rifampin (Rifadin), pyrazinamide (PZA), and ethambutol (Myambutol) given daily for 8 weeks. Vitamin B$_6$ 50 mg is also recommended.**

▸ *Test-taking Tip: Airborne precautions are used with clients who have TB, and clients receive an aggressive multiple-medication regimen.*

Content Area: Adult; Concept: Infection; Oxygenation; Integrated
Processes: Nursing Process: Planning; Client Needs: Safe and
Effective Care Environment: Safety and Infection Control;
Cognitive Level: Application [Applying]

## 1497. PHARM ANSWER: 100

Use the formula for calculating IV flow rates.
*Formula:*

$$\text{Infuse rate (in mL/hour)} = \frac{\text{Volume to be infused}}{\text{Infusion time}}$$

$$100 \text{ mL/hr} = \frac{100 \text{ mL}}{1 \text{ hr}} = 100 \text{ mL/hr}$$

▸ *Test-taking Tip: Identify the volume to be infused. The time over which it needs to be infused allows for quick and easy infusion rate calculations using the equation shown.*

Content Area: Adult; Concept: Medication; Infection; Oxygenation;
Integrated Processes: Nursing Process: Implementation;
Client Needs: Physiological Integrity: Pharmacological and
Parenteral Therapies; Cognitive Level: Application [Applying]

## 1498. ANSWER: 2

1. Although the position of the cervical collar should be checked, it does not need to be removed and reapplied unless it is incorrectly placed.
2. **Paradoxical chest movement suggests that the client has a flail chest, likely from broken ribs. The client's airway would be managed with intubation.**
3. There is no evidence to suggest that another IV catheter is needed for medication administration. EMS personnel should have placed an IV catheter already to give any needed emergency medications or IV fluids.
4. Taping the chest wall does not protect the ribs and can impair the client's breathing.

▸ *Test-taking Tip: Use the ABC's to determine the appropriate intervention.*

Content Area: Adult; Concept: Oxygenation; Critical Thinking; Integrated
Processes: Nursing Process: Planning; Client Needs: Physiological
Integrity: Physiological Adaptation; Cognitive Level: Analysis [Analyzing]

## 1499. ANSWER: 1

1. **This illustration shows a spontaneous pneumothorax from air entering the pleural space. This can occur from weakened lung tissue or a blister-like defect in the lung tissue (bullae or blebs).**
2. This illustration is a traumatic pneumothorax in which a penetrating trauma to the chest wall and parietal pleura allows air to enter the pleural space.
3. A tension pneumothorax occurs from an air leak in the lung or the chest wall on the affected side. The air that enters the pleural space does not exit during expiration and causes an increase in intrapleural pressure. This increased pressure pushes the heart and mediastinal structures to the contralateral side, compressing the contralateral lung.
4. This illustration shows a planned segmental resection of the lung to remove a tumor.

▸ *Test-taking Tip: With a spontaneous pneumothorax there is usually no external initiating event. Thus eliminate options that include external trauma. Of the two remaining, the one showing air in the pleural space is the answer.*

Content Area: Adult; Concept: Nursing Roles; Oxygenation; Integrated Processes: Teaching/Learning; Client Needs: Physiological Integrity: Physiological Adaptation; Cognitive Level: Application [Applying]

**1500. MoC PHARM ANSWER: 3**

1. Oral NSAIDs generally are not adequate to manage pain associated with rib fractures.
2. Oral analgesics generally are not adequate to manage pain associated with rib fractures.
3. **Epidural analgesics and intercostal nerve blocks are the most optimal modality for blunt chest trauma because they directly target the injury site.**
4. Meperidine (Demerol) is not the ideal narcotic for managing this type of pain because of its multiple adverse effects.

▶ *Test-taking Tip: Consider the physiological implications of the injury in selecting the best option that would give the highest level of pain control.*

Content Area: Adult; Concept: Medication; Oxygenation; Management; Integrated Processes: Nursing Process: Planning; Caring; Client Needs: Safe and Effective Care Environment: Management of Care; Physiological Integrity: Pharmacological and Parenteral Therapies; Cognitive Level: Application [Applying]

**1501. ANSWER: 2**

1. The alveoli are affected in pulmonary contusion; stridor involves the upper airway.
2. **The nurse should associate bloody sputum with a possible pulmonary contusion. In pulmonary contusion, hemorrhage occurs in and between the alveoli.**
3. Pulmonary contusion presents with crackles and wheezes (not unilateral rhonchi).
4. Pulmonary contusion presents with decreased (not increased) breath sounds.

▶ *Test-taking Tip: Contusion is bruising, which involves bleeding. Option 2 is the only option that pertains to bleeding.*

Content Area: Adult; Concept: Oxygenation; Trauma; Assessment; Integrated Processes: Nursing Process: Assessment; Client Needs: Physiological Integrity: Physiological Adaptation; Cognitive Level: Application [Applying]

**1502. MoC PHARM ANSWER: 2**

1. Prone positioning to promote gas exchange is appropriate in ARDS.
2. **Aggressive fluid therapy is inappropriate because it can result in pulmonary edema and worsening of ARDS.**
3. Ventilatory support with PEEP is appropriate in ARDS to prevent alveolar collapse.
4. Methylprednisolone (Solu-Medrol), a corticosteroid, decreases WBC movement and stabilizes the capillary membrane, possibly resulting in reduced fibrosis during late-phase ARDS.

▶ *Test-taking Tip: Clients who receive conservative fluid therapy (rather than aggressive) during ARDS have a significant increase in ventilator-free days during recovery.*

Content Area: Adult; Concept: Oxygenation; Medication; Integrated Processes: Nursing Process: Evaluation; Communication and Documentation; Client Needs: Safe and Effective Care Environment: Management of Care; Pharmacological and Parenteral Therapies; Cognitive Level: Evaluation [Evaluating]

**1503. ANSWER: 3**

1. Although blood-tinged sputum may occur due to lung damage, respiratory acidosis and not alkalosis is more likely initially.
2. The WBC and RBC counts could be affected in ARDS, but the WBC would increase if an infection is the causative factor of ARDS, and a low RBC count could be a contributing factor in ARDS if there are insufficient RBCs to carry oxygen.
3. **Due to lung damage and respiratory distress, early signs of ARDS include diaphoresis and low $SaO_2$ despite oxygen administration. Other signs of respiratory distress include tachypnea and use of accessory muscles.**
4. The BP could rise steadily if the client was in distress, but the $PaO_2$ would be low.

▶ *Test-taking Tip: ARDS is a respiratory problem. Narrow the options to those that the nurse can observe without invasive procedures.*

Content Area: Adult; Concept: Oxygenation; Critical Thinking; Integrated Processes: Nursing Process: Analysis; Client Needs: Physiological Integrity: Reduction of Risk Potential; Cognitive Level: Analysis [Analyzing]

**1504. ANSWER: 2**

1. Bubbling in a wet suction chest tube system indicates that the suction is working and is an expected finding.
2. **A dependent loop of the tubing creates pressure backup and prevents fluid from draining; this requires immediate intervention to prevent lung collapse.**
3. Banded connections between sections of tubing are expected. These are applied to prevent air leaks.
4. An occlusive dressing helps to prevent air from leaking into the subcutaneous space and maintains integrity of the closed drainage system.

▶ *Test-taking Tip: Visualize the different parts of a chest tube system and consider which of the options do not fit or seem negative.*

Content Area: Adult; Concept: Safety; Oxygenation; Integrated Processes: Nursing Process: Assessment; Client Needs: Safe and Effective Care Environment: Safety and Infection Control; Physiological Integrity: Reduction of Risk Potential; Cognitive Level: Application [Applying]

**1505. PHARM ANSWER: 3**

1. Although notifying the HCP is warranted, unkinking tubing if present would give some immediate relief and would be the best initial action.
2. Lorazepam (Ativan) is an antianxiety medication. Treating the client for anxiety would delay correcting the problem, and the client's lung could collapse.

3. **Tracheal deviation and the other signs and symptoms suggest a tension pneumothorax, which can occur from obstruction of the tubing. The chest tube tubing should be checked for kinks and the chest tube collection system for blockage.**
4. Turning up the oxygen flow would not correct this problem.

▸ *Test-taking Tip: Use the steps of the nursing process; assessment should be considered as the best answer.*

Content Area: Adult; Concept: Safety; Oxygenation; Critical Thinking; Integrated Processes: Nursing Process: Assessment; Client Needs: Physiological Integrity: Reduction of Risk Potential; Physiological Integrity: Pharmacological and Parenteral Therapies; Cognitive Level: Analysis [Analyzing]

## 1506. ANSWER: 4

1. Activity and deep breathing and coughing, not the arm and shoulder exercises, will promote lung expansion.
2. Activity will improve venous return, but this is not the reason for the exercises.
3. Although the girdle muscles are cut, they are generally not removed.
4. **Because of the location of the incision, disuse can cause contractures and loss of muscle tone. The exercises help to prevent stiffness and preserve function of the arm and shoulder.**

▸ *Test-taking Tip: You need to think about the location of the incision and the effects of scar tissue formation when you answer this question.*

Content Area: Adult; Concept: Mobility; Nursing Roles; Oxygenation; Perioperative; Integrated Processes: Teaching/Learning; Client Needs: Physiological Integrity: Basic Care and Comfort; Cognitive Level: Application [Applying]

## 1507. ANSWERS: 1, 2, 5

1. **To avoid injury to the incision, the client should be instructed to avoid lifting greater than 20 lb until healing is complete.**
2. **To avoid overuse, the client should gradually work up to an appropriate exercise level.**
3. The client should stop activity and rest if dyspnea occurs.
4. The client can expect to be weaker than normal for up to 3 to 6 months.
5. **The client should take rest periods before and after activity to maximize activity and conserve energy for healing.**

▸ *Test-taking Tip: During a thoracotomy for a lung tumor removal, an incision is made through the chest wall, and a segmental section of the lung is removed. You need to think about how long it will take for the client to resume normal activity and about indicators of possible exercise intolerance.*

Content Area: Adult; Concept: Nursing Roles; Oxygenation; Integrated Processes: Teaching/Learning; Client Needs: Physiological Integrity: Physiological Adaptation; Psychosocial Integrity; Cognitive Level: Application [Applying]

## 1508. MoC ANSWER: 2

1. The nurse can delay addressing this client's bowel needs until later.
2. **The nurse should attend to the client with the SaO$_2$ of 88% first; the client is not maintaining oxygen saturations despite receiving oxygen.**
3. Although this client's BP is low, it is only one data point. The nurse should delegate to the NA to obtain a repeat reading.
4. This client's urinary status should be addressed soon, but this client does not need to be attended to first.

▸ *Test-taking Tip: Use the ABC's to identify the priority client.*

Content Area: Adult; Concept: Oxygenation; Critical Thinking; Management; Integrated Processes: Nursing Process: Planning; Client Needs: Safe and Effective Care Environment: Management of Care; Cognitive Level: Analysis [Analyzing]

## 1509. ANSWER: 3

1. Placing the bed in high Fowler's position will not address the immediate problem of pulmonary edema.
2. Giving a fluid bolus would exacerbate the problem of pulmonary edema.
3. **The client's manifestations suggest pulmonary edema, likely from fluid overload. Emergency intervention is needed. Calling a respiratory code is essential so that intubation and appropriate interventions such as vasopressors and diuretics can be initiated.**
4. Having the client cough and deep breathe will not address the immediate problem of pulmonary edema.

▸ *Test-taking Tip: Pink, frothy secretions suggests pulmonary edema from fluid volume overload. This is a life-threatening situation.*

Content Area: Adult; Concept: Safety; Critical Thinking; Oxygenation; Integrated Processes: Nursing Process: Implementation; Client Needs: Physiological Integrity: Physiological Adaptation; Cognitive Level: Analysis [Analyzing]

## 1510. ANSWER: 2

1. Tracheal stenosis is a narrowed tracheal lumen due to scar formation from irritation of tracheal mucosa by the cuff. Stenosis is seen after the cuff is deflated or removed and does not present with the need to increase cuff pressure.
2. **Constant cuff pressure against the trachea can cause tracheomalacia (a dilation and erosion of the tracheal cartilage). This erosion results in a wider tracheal diameter and requires a larger, more inflated cuff to seal the diameter.**
3. Sclerosis is a hardening of tissues that is not caused by a tracheostomy tube.
4. A tracheal–innominate artery fistula is necrosis and erosion of the innominate artery from a malpositioned tube that causes its distal tip to push against the lateral wall of the tracheostomy. This is an emergency and presents with heavy bleeding from the stoma and a tube that pulses in synchrony with the heartbeat.

▶ **Test-taking Tip:** *Use your knowledge of medical terminology to define each of the options; this allows elimination of the option "Tracheal sclerosis." Visualize a cuffed tracheostomy tube and associate this scenario with a client from clinical practice, if possible. The need for increased cuff pressure is associated only with the correct option.*

**Content Area:** Adult; **Concept:** Oxygenation; **Integrated Processes:** Nursing Process: Analysis; **Client Needs:** Physiological Integrity: Reduction of Risk Potential; **Cognitive Level:** Application [Applying]

**1511.** CJ MoC **ANSWER: 3**

1. Interventions at 1100 are correct. Oxygen should be increased to maintain $SaO_2$ at 92% or above. The device for sequential compression stockings needs to be on for these to be effective in preventing a DVT.
2. Interventions at 1145 are correct. Epidural analgesia provides a continuous slow release of medication. An incremental increase in analgesic is appropriate when pain has not been relieved with the current dose. Due to intense pain after an open thoracotomy, pain management is needed to assist the client to participate in deep breathing and coughing to clear the airway and prevent postoperative complications.
3. **At 1200, the nurse positioned the client on the nonoperative side. After a pneumonectomy (complete removal of the lung), the client should be turned from the operative side to the back only. Positioning on the nonoperative side can result in a mediastinal shift.**
4. Interventions at 1215 are correct. Cefuroxime (Zinacef), a cephalosporin, should be used cautiously in clients with a penicillin allergy, but it is not contraindicated.

▶ **Test-taking Tip:** *You need to consider the positioning differences between a pneumonectomy and a lobectomy.*

**Content Area:** Adult; **Concept:** Management; Oxygenation; **Integrated Processes:** Nursing Process: Analysis; **Client Needs:** Safe and Effective Care Environment: Management of Care; Physiological Integrity: Physiological Adaptation; **Cognitive Level:** Analysis [Analyzing]

**1512.** CJ MoC **ANSWER: 2, 4, 5**

1. The client is still in the left side-lying position. Lowering the head of the bed can worsen mediastinal shift, further compromising the client's respiratory and cardiac status.
2. **In an emergency, the RN should delegate. Asking the LPN to place a call for the ART is appropriate delegation. Placing the ART call will ensure that adequate assistance is available.**
3. Increasing the suction dial on the chest drainage system to 30 cm can result in too much negativity, worsening the client's respiratory status.
4. **The HCP should be telephoned because there is a decline in client status, and new orders will be needed for treatment. The drop in BP with a MAP of 54.7 indicates inadequate perfusion (MAP = $[(88 + 38 + 38) \div 3] = 54.7$). The client is at risk for respiratory and cardiac arrest.**
5. **With a decrease in $SaO_2$ to 85%, a nonrebreather mask at 10L oxygen can deliver oxygen at 100%.**

▶ **Test-taking Tip:** *You need to consider the entire scenario before selecting your options. Consider that the client is African American. African Americans are more likely to die of lung cancer than Caucasians. Immediate intervention is required.*

**Content Area:** Adult; **Concept:** Management; Oxygenation; **Integrated Processes:** Nursing Process: Evaluation; Culture and Spirituality; **Client Needs:** Safe and Effective Care Environment: Management of Care; Physiological Integrity: Physiological Adaptation; **Cognitive Level:** Evaluation [Evaluating]

## Chapter Thirty-Four

# Sensory Management

**1513.** The nurse completes an assessment of the older adult client. Which disorder should the nurse associate with the finding illustrated?

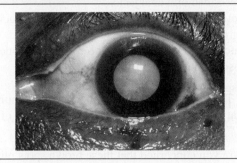

1. Glaucoma
2. Arcus senilis
3. Cataract
4. Mydriasis

**1514.** The 60-year-old client notices a gradual decline in visual acuity and asks if it could be from a cataract. Which question will help determine whether a cataract is developing?

1. "Has your ability to perceive colors changed?"
2. "Does your vision appear distorted or wavy?"
3. "Does the center of your visual field appear dark?"
4. "Do you see random flashes of bright light?"

**1515.** MoC The nurse telephones the client 1-day post–cataract surgery. Which client statement necessitates an evaluation by an ophthalmologist?

1. "My eye starts hurting about 4 hours after a pain pill."
2. "The redness in my eye is still there but less than yesterday."
3. "I'm ready to have my other cataract removed now."
4. "I can't see as well as I could yesterday after surgery."

**1516.** MoC The client is 1-day post–surgical repair of a retinal detachment. Which assessment finding is **most** important for the nurse to report immediately to the HCP?

1. Surgical eye pain rated 2 on a 10-point scale
2. Increased tearing from the surgical eye
3. Blurred vision and floaters in the surgical eye
4. Dryness and injection of the sclera in the surgical eye

**1517.** The client's eyes, tested with the use of a Snellen chart, show 20/40 vision in the right eye and 20/30 in the left eye. How should the nurse interpret these results?

1. The client has elevated intraocular pressure in both eyes.
2. The client needs testing for glaucoma with a tonometer.
3. The left eye is closer to normal vision than the right eye.
4. The client has errors of refraction indicating astigmatism.

**1518.** The client with severely diminished vision has difficulty with visual discrimination. Which interventions should the nurse recommend to improve the client's sight in the home environment? **Select all that apply.**

1. Ensure that all room walls are painted with colors that blend.
2. Use a white board and a black marker when writing out lists.
3. Place Velcro tabs on wall light switches to ease locating them.
4. Ensure that doorknobs on the doors are a bright contrasting color.
5. Match the color of dishes with the color of tablecloths or placemats.

**1519.** The client with diminished sight has problems with the glare from light. Which recommendation should the nurse make?

1. Install fluorescent lighting throughout the home.
2. Wear sunglasses and hats with brims when outdoors.
3. Avoid going outdoors on days that are sunny.
4. Use direct sunlight from windows rather than lights.

**1520.** The client tells the nurse, "My optometrist told me that cataracts are beginning to develop in both of my eyes." Which follow-up statement made by the client should the nurse correct?

1. "It is important that I schedule cataract surgery as soon as possible."
2. "Usually surgery is performed on each eye at different times."
3. "My own lens will be removed when I have cataract surgery."
4. "An intraocular lens may be inserted with the surgical procedure."

**1521.** A family member of the client undergoing cataract surgery asks the nurse if there are ways to prevent cataracts. Which recommendations should the nurse suggest? **Select all that apply.**

1. "Wear sunglasses that limit ultraviolet light penetration."
2. "Wear sunscreen with a high protection factor number."
3. "Wear eye protection if there is any risk for eye injury."
4. "Avoid activities and reading in dimly lit environments."
5. "Eat foods that are high in vitamin C, such as oranges."

**1522.** The nurse is reviewing the new nurse's discharge instructions for the client who had outpatient cataract surgery. Which statement should the experienced nurse remove from the discharge instructions?

1. Avoid lifting, pushing, or pulling objects heavier than 15 pounds.
2. Clean the eye with a clean tissue; wipe from the inner to outer eye.
3. Cough and deep breathe every 2 to 3 hours while you are awake.
4. Avoid lying on the side of the affected eye the night after surgery.

**1523.** The client asks the nurse about symptoms associated with retinal detachment. Which symptoms should the nurse identify? **Select all that apply.**

1. Seeing bright flashes of light
2. Shooting, throbbing eye pain
3. Severe frontal headache
4. Diminished visual acuity
5. Seeing floating dark spots in the vision field

**1524.** **MoC** The nurse is concerned that the client in a long-term care facility has a retinal detachment. Which intervention should the nurse plan to implement **first**?

1. Reassure that scleral buckling can be performed to repair retinal detachment.
2. Apply an eye shield to the affected eye and give a prescribed oral analgesic.
3. Notify the HCP; prepare for transport to a facility for ophthalmological care.
4. Patch both eyes and place the client in a prone position until blurring stops.

**1525.** The client who is dark-skinned asks the nurse, "What are the small brown spots in the whites of my eyes?" What is the nurse's **best** response?

1. "Are you concerned that these brown spots might be cancerous?"
2. "You don't need to worry about those spots; many people have them."
3. "These brown spots are a normal finding in a person with dark skin."
4. "I need to check your eyes so I can better inform your doctor about these."

**1526.** **PHARM** The client with glaucoma is prescribed pilocarpine hydrochloride 1% eye drops to both eyes four times per day. The nurse knows that this medication has which expected action?

1. Increases the outflow of aqueous humor
2. Improves vision in dimly lit environments
3. Increases production of aqueous humor
4. Increases ability of both pupils to dilate

**1527.** **PHARM** The client is receiving treatment with gentamicin ophthalmic solution for bacterial conjunctivitis. Which symptom, described by the client, indicates that the medication is **ineffective**?

1. Eyes feel strained
2. Yellowish eye drainage
3. Twitching of the eye
4. Unable to read small print

**1528.** MoC The nurse reviews the chart of the client diagnosed with closed-angle glaucoma. Which documented finding should the nurse question with the HCP?

1. Sudden onset of eye pain
2. Reduced central visual acuity
3. Normal intraocular pressure
4. Nausea and vomiting

**1529.** The client has open-angle glaucoma. Which instruction should the nurse include when teaching the client?

1. Limit oral fluid intake to 1000 mL daily.
2. Eat foods that are high in omega-3 fatty acids.
3. Have annual eye exams with an eye specialist.
4. Use timolol maleate eye drops when feeling eye pressure.

**1530.** PHARM The nurse is assessing the client receiving brimonidine eye drops. Which assessment findings will the nurse recognize as known side effects of brimonidine? **Select all that apply.**

1. Blurred vision
2. Ocular itching
3. Ocular stinging
4. Hearing loss
5. Conjunctivitis

**1531.** The nurse is reviewing home management strategies with the client who has dry macular degeneration. The nurse should review using which objects with the client? **Select all that apply.**

1. Protective goggles
2. Lighting that is bright
3. An Amsler grid
4. A soft eye patch
5. Magnification device

**1532.** The client with macular degeneration is told the condition is progressing to an advanced stage. Which findings should the nurse expect when completing the assessment? **Select all that apply.**

1. Curtain appearance over part of the visual field
2. Loss of peripheral vision in the affected eye
3. Difficulty seeing in dimly lit environments
4. Visual distortions in the central vision
5. Clouding of the lens in both eyes

**1533.** The nurse is caring for the client with macular degeneration. Which illustration should the nurse associate with the field disturbance seen by the client?

1.
2.

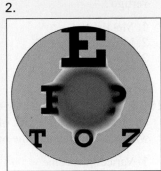

3.
4.

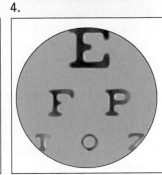

**1534.** The client has an hordeolum of the left eye, which is painful. Which intervention, if prescribed, should the nurse implement?

1. Apply an eye patch on the left eye.
2. Insert miotic eye drops twice daily.
3. Apply a warm compress four times daily.
4. Administer an antibiotic intravenously.

**1535.** The nurse completed teaching the client with a corneal abrasion about proper care of the injury. Which statements indicate that the client understood the teaching? **Select all that apply.**

1. "I should promptly report a sudden absence of pain."
2. "I should keep my affected eye uncovered when up."
3. "I should insert the eye drops 10 to 15 seconds apart."
4. "I should leave the eye patch in place for 24 hours."
5. "I will avoid rubbing my affected eye or the eye patch."

**1536.** MoC The nurse is planning care of the client with Ménière's disease. Which interdisciplinary team member should the nurse expect to consult regarding client care?

1. Rheumatologist
2. Otolaryngologist
3. Physical therapist
4. Oncologist

**1537.** **PHARM** The nurse is reviewing the medication list of the client with Ménière's disease. Which medication should the nurse give to treat the client's vertigo?

1. Meclizine
2. Megestrol
3. Meropenem
4. Metoprolol

**1538.** The nurse is teaching the client who has otitis media. To reduce the risk of recurrent otitis media, which vaccine should the nurse recommend?

1. Varicella vaccine
2. Pneumococcal vaccine
3. Typhoid vaccine
4. Zoster vaccine

**1539.** **PHARM** The client with severe otitis media and mastoiditis is prescribed levofloxacin IV, 250 mg every 12 hours. The medication is diluted in 100 mL of NS. To deliver the antibiotic in 30 minutes, how many mL/hr should the nurse set the infusion pump to deliver?

_____ mL/hr (Record your answer as a whole number.)

**1540.** The nurse is using a tuning fork to perform the Rinne test for air and bone conduction hearing. Place an X on the location where the nurse should place the stem of the tuning fork.

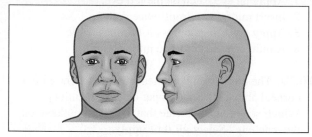

**1541.** The nurse is assessing the older adult client with otosclerosis. Which diagnostic characteristics should the nurse associate with otosclerosis?

1. Bone conduction is greater than air conduction.
2. Hearing aids are not effective in restoring hearing.
3. Surgical restoration of hearing is not possible.
4. The initial audiogram shows progressive hearing loss.

**1542.** **PHARM** The client, who has otosclerosis, is to take sodium fluoride tablets. The client asks the nurse, "What will this medication do for my ears?" Which response by the nurse is correct?

1. "Sodium fluoride prevents the breakdown of bone cells and hardens the bone in the ear."
2. "Sodium fluoride causes the breakdown of bone cells and softens the bone in the ear."
3. "Sodium fluoride blocks the effect of histamine and dries the fluid in the ear."
4. "Sodium fluoride causes the production of histamine and increases the fluid in the ear."

**1543.** The client recovering at home following a stapedectomy for otosclerosis reports having dizziness. To decrease symptoms, which interventions should the nurse recommend? **Select all that apply.**

1. Refrain from sudden movements.
2. Avoid chewing on the affected side.
3. Avoid lifting objects that are heavy.
4. Minimize bending over at the waist.
5. Restrict the intake of oral fluids.

**1544.** **MoC** The client, who underwent removal of a right-sided acoustic neuroma by a translabyrinthine approach, calls the nurse to report pain. The nurse finds that the client has new-onset right-sided facial drooping and numbness. Place the nurse's actions in priority order.

1. Close the client's right eye and place a patch over it.
2. Assess the operative incision site and assess the arms for drift.
3. Contact the stroke team and the HCP.
4. Medicate the client for pain unless contraindicated.

Answer: _____

**1545.** The client's daughter tells the nurse of frustration while communicating with her elderly mother who wears hearing aids. Which intervention should the nurse suggest to the client's daughter?

1. Minimize oral communication to essential matters.
2. Speak directly into her mother's better ear.
3. Use exaggerated mouth expressions while speaking.
4. Attract her mother's attention before speaking.

**1546.** A resident of a long-term care facility tells the nurse, "I'm having a hard time hearing people talk and can't understand the voices on TV." Which action is **most** appropriate?

1. Teach the client about eliminating background noises in the room.
2. Assess the client's hearing and use an otoscope for examination.
3. Schedule an appointment with the HCP for bilateral ear irrigations.
4. Instruct the client to look at the speaker's lips to decipher words.

**1547.** The nurse is examining the client's ear using an otoscope and sees the image illustrated. Which documentation by the nurse is **best**?

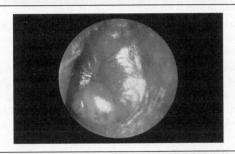

1. Tympanic membrane ruptured, no excessive cerumen
2. External ear canal showing no lesions or drainage
3. Tympanic membrane cone of light reflex distorted
4. Bony landmarks prominent on tympanic membrane

**1548.** The nurse is providing teaching on the home treatment of acute sinusitis. Which interventions should the nurse advise the client to implement? **Select all that apply.**

1. Take over-the-counter ranitidine.
2. Apply warm compresses to the face.
3. Use saline nasal spray as directed.
4. Take over-the-counter pseudoephedrine.
5. Spend time outdoors in the sunlight.

# Answers and Rationales

## 1513. ANSWER: 3

1. Glaucoma causes increased pressure within the eye and is not visible.
2. Arcus senilis is a bluish-white ring within the outer edge of the cornea, which is not present in this illustration.
3. **The illustration shows opacity of the lens of the eye. The nurse should associate this finding with a cataract.**
4. Mydriasis is dilation of the pupil, which is unable to be determined in this illustration due to opacity of the lens.

▶ *Test-taking Tip: The age of the client in the stem is often a clue to the correct option. You should associate the client's age with either Option 1 or 3. Realizing that glaucoma is not visible, you can eliminate Option 1.*

**Content Area:** Adult; **Concept:** Assessment; Sensory Perception; **Integrated Processes:** Nursing Process: Assessment; **Client Needs:** Physiological Integrity: Physiological Adaptation; **Cognitive Level:** Analysis [Analyzing]

## 1514. ANSWER: 1

1. **Asking about a change in the ability to perceive colors will help in determining cataract development. Cataract formation involves the lens of the eye becoming opaque, thus decreasing the vibrancy of colors.**
2. Distorted central vision is a sign of macular degeneration.
3. A darkened area in the center of the visual field is associated with macular degeneration.
4. Seeing flashes of bright lights is associated with retinal detachment.

▶ *Test-taking Tip: Cataracts appear as a cloudy white structure that light must pass through to get to the retina. Visualize the effect of an age-related cataract on vision. You can eliminate Options 2, 3, and 4 because they cannot be explained by a cloudy structure.*

**Content Area:** Adult; **Concept:** Sensory Perception; Assessment; **Integrated Processes:** Nursing Process: Assessment; **Client Needs:** Health Promotion and Maintenance; **Cognitive Level:** Analysis [Analyzing]

## 1515. MoC ANSWER: 4

1. Pain relieved by prescribed pain medication is within normal assessment parameters.
2. Decreasing redness is within normal assessment parameters.
3. The cataract of one eye is removed first. At least several weeks, preferably months, should separate the two procedures.
4. **A significant reduction in vision may indicate a complication such as infection or retinal detachment.**

▶ *Test-taking Tip: Only one option has abnormal findings.*

**Content Area:** Adult; **Concept:** Sensory Perception; Perioperative; **Integrated Processes:** Nursing Process: Evaluation; **Client Needs:** Safe and Effective Care Environment: Management of Care; Physiological Integrity: Reduction of Risk Potential; **Cognitive Level:** Evaluation [Evaluating]

## 1516. MoC ANSWER: 3

1. A low level of postoperative pain does not indicate a significant complication.
2. Watery drainage is not a specific sign for concern and is less serious than changes in visual acuity.
3. **Blurred vision and floaters in the surgical eye may occur with redetachment of the retina and would warrant additional surgery.**
4. Dryness and injection of the sclera may or may not resolve without treatment. However, a more important sign of complication that should be reported immediately is loss of visual acuity.

▶ *Test-taking Tip: The key phrase is "most important," indicating that more than one option may be correct, but only one option indicates a significant complication.*

**Content Area:** Adult; **Concept:** Sensory Perception; Management; **Integrated Processes:** Nursing Process: Implementation; Communication and Documentation; **Client Needs:** Safe and Effective Care Environment: Management of Care; **Cognitive Level:** Application [Applying]

## 1517. ANSWER: 3

1. The Snellen chart is not used to measure intraocular pressure.
2. There is no information suggesting that the client needs glaucoma testing.
3. **The Snellen chart is used to test distance vision. The numbers recorded indicate that at 20 feet (the first number) the client can read what a person with normal vision can read at another distance (second number). The left eye's vision recorded as 20/30 has better vision than the right eye with vision recorded as 20/40.**
4. The Snellen chart alone is not used to determine astigmatism, an abnormal curvature of the cornea. Testing for astigmatism includes examination of the eye with a slit lamp and taking measurements of the curvature of the corneas.

▶ *Test-taking Tip: The Snellen chart is used to test distance vision, so eliminate options that relate to other eye conditions.*

**Content Area:** Adult; **Concept:** Assessment; Sensory Perception; **Integrated Processes:** Nursing Process: Analysis; **Client Needs:** Physiological Integrity: Reduction of Risk Potential; **Cognitive Level:** Analysis [Analyzing]

## 1518. ANSWER: 2, 3, 4

1. When the client has limited vision, wall colors should contrast rather than blend so room openings can be easily identified.
2. **Using black on white can enhance the person's ability to read what has been written.**
3. **Placing Velcro tabs on light switches will make them easier to locate in dark environments or when vision is limited.**
4. **Using contrasting colors makes it easier to identify the doorknob and is a safety feature if the person needs to exit immediately.**
5. Similar colors will worsen the client's ability to discriminate visually.

▶ *Test-taking Tip: Clients who have difficulty with vision discrimination are helped by interventions that emphasize color contrast in the environment.*

**Content Area:** Adult; **Concept:** Sensory Perception; Nursing Roles; Safety; **Integrated Processes:** Nursing Process: Implementation; Teaching/Learning; **Client Needs:** Safe and Effective Care Environment: Safety and Infection Control; Physiological Integrity: Physiological Adaptation; **Cognitive Level:** Application [Applying]

## 1519. ANSWER: 2

1. Incandescent lighting produces less glare than fluorescent lighting.
2. **Wearing sunglasses and hats with brims while outdoors will block direct light from the client's eyes.**
3. The sun provides a source of vitamin D and should not be totally avoided; other measures can be taken to prevent glare.
4. Direct sunlight through windows can increase glare.

▶ *Test-taking Tip: Of the options, think about the action that would reduce strong light but not avoid it completely.*

**Content Area:** Adult; **Concept:** Sensory Perception; Nursing Roles; **Integrated Processes:** Nursing Process: Implementation; **Client Needs:** Physiological Integrity: Reduction of Risk Potential; **Cognitive Level:** Application [Applying]

## 1520. ANSWER: 1

1. **Although there is reduced vision with beginning cataract development, a person can wait until vision worsens before having surgery. When vision is reduced to the extent that ADLs are affected, surgery should be performed as soon as possible.**
2. If both eyes have cataracts, usually the eyes are treated in separate procedures.
3. Surgery for a cataract involves removal of the client's lens.
4. Although in most situations the client's lens is replaced with an intraocular lens at the time of surgery, other options include postoperative contact lenses or aphakic glasses.

▶ *Test-taking Tip: Cataract surgery is always elective and performed when the vision and lifestyle of the client are affected. The surgery is not urgent.*

**Content Area:** Adult; **Concept:** Nursing Roles; Sensory Perception; **Integrated Processes:** Nursing Process: Evaluation; **Client Needs:** Physiological Integrity: Physiological Adaptation; **Cognitive Level:** Evaluation [Evaluating]

## 1521. ANSWER: 1, 3

1. **Limiting eye exposure to UV light has been found to decrease the risk for cataracts.**
2. Sunscreen is applied to the skin, not the eyes.
3. **Avoiding trauma to the eye has been found to decrease the risk for cataracts.**
4. Straining the eyes to read does not lead to cataract formation.
5. There is no evidence that nutrition prevents or delays progression of cataracts.

▶ *Test-taking Tip: Cataracts are associated with aging, trauma, and exposure to toxic agents. Narrow the options to these factors.*

**Content Area:** Adult; **Concept:** Promoting Health; Sensory Perception; **Integrated Processes:** Teaching/Learning; **Client Needs:** Physiological Integrity: Reduction of Risk Potential; **Cognitive Level:** Application [Applying]

## 1522. ANSWER: 3

1. Lifting heavy objects increases pressure on the surgical eye.
2. The surgical eye should be cleaned with a clean tissue from the inner to outer canthus to prevent obstruction of the ducts with drainage.
3. **The client should not cough because this will increase the pressure within the eye and risk for complications.**
4. Lying on the side of the surgical eye can increase pressure on the surgical eye.

▶ *Test-taking Tip: This is a false-response item. You should select the option that would be an incorrect instruction and would increase the client's risk for complications.*

**Content Area:** Adult; **Concept:** Nursing Roles; Sensory Perception; **Integrated Processes:** Teaching/Learning; **Client Needs:** Health Promotion and Maintenance; Physiological Integrity: Reduction of Risk Potential; **Cognitive Level:** Analysis [Analyzing]

## 1523. ANSWER: 1, 4, 5

1. **As the choroid and retina partially separate, the client notices flashes of light.**
2. Pain is not associated with retinal detachment. There are few pain fibers in the retina.
3. Headache is not associated with retinal detachment.
4. **As the choroid and retina partially separate, the client notices decreased vision, often like "a curtain being drawn across."**
5. **As the choroid and retina partially separate, the client notices floating dark spots.**

▶ *Test-taking Tip: The retina is composed of cones and rods and transmits sensory impulses to the optic nerve. The retina is poorly innervated for pain. Eliminate the options that describe the physical appearance of the eye or pain.*

**Content Area:** Adult; **Concept:** Assessment; Sensory Perception; **Integrated Processes:** Nursing Process: Assessment; Teaching/Learning; **Client Needs:** Physiological Integrity: Reduction of Risk Potential; **Cognitive Level:** Knowledge [Remembering]

## 1524. MoC ANSWER: 3

1. Although providing support to the client is important, it is premature to discuss the surgical option of scleral buckling to repair the retinal detachment.
2. These actions will delay securing treatment. The nurse should follow the treatment prescribed by the HCP or ophthalmologist.
3. **The nurse should contact the HCP and secure an ophthalmological evaluation promptly.**
4. Blurred vision will not stop until the detachment is addressed.

▶ *Test-taking Tip: Early diagnosis and intervention for retinal detachment improve preservation of the client's vision. Three options are similar, and one is different; often the option that is different is the answer.*

**Content Area:** Adult; **Concept:** Communication; Assessment; Sensory Perception; Management; **Integrated Processes:** Nursing Process: Planning; **Client Needs:** Safe and Effective Care Environment: Management of Care; Physiological Integrity: Reduction of Risk Potential; **Cognitive Level:** Application [Applying]

## 1525. ANSWER: 3

1. Although asking about the client's concern may seem like an appropriate response, associating it with cancer can alarm the client unnecessarily.
2. Although many people have brown spots in the central sclera, they are usually only seen in dark-skinned individuals. This is an incomplete response. Telling the client not to worry is a block to therapeutic communication.
3. **The nurse's best response should be to inform that client that small brown spots in the central sclera is a normal finding in a person with dark skin.**
4. It is unnecessary to inform a HCP about a normal finding.

▶ *Test-taking Tip: Narrow the options by eliminating options that do not use therapeutic communication techniques and one that can alarm the client unnecessarily.*

**Content Area:** Adult; **Concept:** Development; Sensory; Diversity; **Integrated Processes:** Communication and Documentation; Nursing Process: Assessment; Culture and Spirituality; **Client Needs:** Health Promotion and Maintenance; Psychosocial Integrity; **Cognitive Level:** Analysis [Analyzing]

## 1526. PHARM ANSWER: 1

1. **Pilocarpine hydrochloride is a cholinergic agent used to treat glaucoma. It causes miosis (pupillary constriction), which then increases the angle of the channel in the anterior chamber of the eye. This improves the outflow of aqueous humor.**

2. Vision is limited in dimly lit environments, not improved due to the pupillary constriction from pilocarpine. When the pupil is constricted, less light reaches the retina to stimulate optic nerve function in sending impulses to the brain.

3. Pilocarpine does not increase production of aqueous humor.

4. Pilocarpine causes pupillary constriction, not dilation.

♦ *Test-taking Tip: In glaucoma, vision is slowly diminished due to increased intraocular pressure. Intraocular pressure will decrease if outflow of fluid is increased or production of fluid within the eyes is decreased. Constriction of the pupils improves the outflow of aqueous humor.*

Content Area: Adult; Concept: Medication; Sensory Perception; Integrated Processes: Nursing Process: Analysis; Client Needs: Physiological Integrity: Pharmacological and Parenteral Therapies; Cognitive Level: Knowledge [Remembering]

### 1527. PHARM ANSWER: 2

1. Eyestrain is not associated with an infectious process. Gentamicin is an antibiotic that would be administered to treat an infection.

2. **Mucopurulent eye drainage, especially yellowish or greenish, is associated with bacterial conjunctivitis; continuing with eye drainage indicates gentamicin is ineffective in treating the infection.**

3. Twitching is not associated with an infectious process. Gentamicin is an antibiotic that would be administered to treat an infection.

4. Inability to read small print is not associated with an infectious process. Gentamicin is an antibiotic that would be administered to treat an infection.

♦ *Test-taking Tip: The issue of the question is symptoms associated with bacterial conjunctivitis, an infectious process. Consider the symptom described in each option and determine whether it is consistent with an infectious process.*

Content Area: Adult; Concept: Infection; Sensory Perception; Integrated Processes: Nursing Process: Evaluation; Client Needs: Physiological Integrity: Pharmacological and Parenteral Therapies; Physiological Integrity: Reduction of Risk Potential; Cognitive Level: Evaluation [Evaluating]

### 1528. MoC ANSWER: 3

1. In closed-angle glaucoma, the flow of aqueous is blocked when the iris moves against the cornea (closed angle). The sudden rise in intraocular pressure causes eye pain.

2. Reduced central visual acuity is caused from the obstruction of aqueous outflow.

3. **Closed-angle glaucoma causes an increased, not normal, intraocular pressure. This documentation should be questioned.**

4. The sudden rise in intraocular pressure and vision changes contribute to nausea and vomiting.

♦ *Test-taking Tip: Note that three options are similar and that one is different. Often the option that is different is the answer.*

Content Area: Adult; Concept: Safety; Communication; Sensory Perception; Integrated Processes: Communication and Documentation; Client Needs: Safe and Effective Care Environment: Management of Care; Cognitive Level: Application [Applying]

### 1529. ANSWER: 3

1. Fluid restriction is not an effective treatment modality for open-angle glaucoma.

2. Consuming foods high in omega-3 fatty acids will not affect intraocular pressure.

3. **Glaucoma is a chronic progressive disease; annual eye examinations should be completed by an eye specialist physician.**

4. Elevated intraocular pressure cannot be felt; timolol maleate (Timoptic) is a nonselective beta-adrenergic receptor blocking agent and should be used as prescribed.

♦ *Test-taking Tip: Glaucoma is a chronic progressive disease that requires continued surveillance and treatment.*

Content Area: Adult; Concept: Promoting Health; Sensory Perception; Integrated Processes: Teaching/Learning; Client Needs: Physiological Integrity: Physiological Adaptation; Cognitive Level: Application [Applying]

### 1530. PHARM ANSWER: 1, 2, 3, 5

1. **Brimonidine (Alphagan) is an alpha-2 adrenergic agonist; the nurse should recognize blurred vision as a side effect of brimonidine.**

2. **Brimonidine (Alphagan) is an alpha-2 adrenergic agonist; the nurse should recognize ocular itching as a side effect of brimonidine.**

3. **Brimonidine (Alphagan) is an alpha-2 adrenergic agonist; the nurse should recognize ocular stinging as a side effect of brimonidine.**

4. Hearing loss is not a side effect of brimonidine (Alphagan).

5. **Brimonidine (Alphagan) is an alpha-2 adrenergic agonist; the nurse should recognize conjunctivitis as a side effect of brimonidine.**

♦ *Test-taking Tip: Alpha-2 adrenergic agonist ophthalmic drops are used in the treatment of glaucoma to decrease the production of aqueous humor and increase its outflow. Side effects will include those affecting the eye; ocular pertains to the eye.*

Content Area: Adult; Concept: Sensory Perception; Integrated Processes: Nursing Process: Assessment; Client Needs: Physiological Integrity: Pharmacological and Parenteral Therapies; Cognitive Level: Application [Applying]

### 1531. ANSWER: 2, 3, 5

1. Although the use of protective goggles does provide eye safety, their use is not specifically related to macular degeneration.

2. **The nurse should review using bright lighting because it improves vision and promotes safety.**

3. The nurse should review using an Amsler grid, a grid of horizontal and vertical lines used to monitor for a sudden onset or distortion of vision; its use may provide an early indication that macular degeneration is getting worse.
4. Eye patches are not used in macular degeneration.
5. The nurse should review using magnification devices to decrease eyestrain and promote safety.

▶ *Test-taking Tip:* An Amsler grid is a grid of horizontal and vertical lines used to monitor for a sudden onset of vision loss or distortion due to macular degeneration. Focus on options that prevent eyestrain with macular degeneration and client safety.

Content Area: Adult; Concept: Sensory Perception; Nursing Roles; Integrated Processes: Teaching/Learning; Client Needs: Health Promotion and Maintenance; Physiological Integrity: Reduction of Risk Potential; Cognitive Level: Application [Applying]

### 1532. ANSWER: 3, 4

1. A curtain appearance over the vision is associated with retinal detachment.
2. Peripheral vision deficits result from progressive glaucoma.
3. Difficulty seeing in dimly lit environments is from the slow breakdown of the outer layer of the retina and the formation of drusen within the macula.
4. The macula is the area of central vision. With macular degeneration there is the loss or distortion of central vision.
5. A cataract is the clouding of the lens.

▶ *Test-taking Tip:* The macula is the area near the fovea centralis, the area of most acute vision. Narrow the options to those visual defects associated with central vision.

Content Area: Adult; Concept: Assessment; Sensory Perception; Integrated Processes: Nursing Process: Analysis; Client Needs: Physiological Integrity: Physiological Adaptation; Cognitive Level: Application [Applying]

### 1533. ANSWER: 2

1. Limited peripheral vision is shown in Illustration 1. This is seen in glaucoma.
2. Distorted central vision as seen in Illustration 2 is characteristic of macular degeneration. The macula is the area of the fundus responsible for central vision. When the cells in the macula have been damaged, central vision is impaired.
3. Illustration 3 shows a normal visual field.
4. Illustration 4 shows a blurred visual field that can be found in many eye conditions, including cataracts, diabetic retinopathy, and refractory errors.

▶ *Test-taking Tip:* Visual field disturbances in clients with macular degeneration have distinct characteristics that affect central vision. Use the process of elimination to rule out Options 3 and 4. Apply knowledge of the anatomy and physiology and functions of the macula to rule out Option 1.

Content Area: Adult; Concept: Sensory Perception; Integrated Processes: Nursing Process: Analysis; Client Needs: Psychosocial Integrity; Cognitive Level: Application [Applying]

### 1534. ANSWER: 3

1. Patching the eye is not indicated because the infection is in the outer eye.
2. Miotic drops cause pupillary constriction and are commonly used to treat glaucoma.
3. Warm compresses are applied to promote drainage. A hordeolum, or stye, is an infected sweat gland in the eyelid at the base of the eyelashes.
4. An antibiotic ointment is used to treat the infection, often due to a *Staphylococcus* or *Streptococcus* organism. There is no need for IV-administered antibiotics.

▶ *Test-taking Tip:* A hordeolum occurs on the eyelid. Narrow the options to only those involving the eyelid.

Content Area: Adult; Concept: Infection; Sensory Perception; Integrated Processes: Nursing Process: Planning; Client Needs: Physiological Integrity: Basic Care and Comfort; Cognitive Level: Application [Applying]

### 1535. ANSWER: 4, 5

1. Some eye discomfort is expected with a corneal abrasion, but the client's pain should gradually diminish as the abrasion heals.
2. The eye is usually covered to protect it and reduce irritation from blinking.
3. It is recommended to allow more than 10 to 15 seconds between drops for more complete absorbance.
4. Patching the eye for the first 24 hours reduces irritation and promotes resting of the eye for optimal healing.
5. Rubbing the affected eye or eye patch may cause the healing abrasion to become reinjured.

▶ *Test-taking Tip:* Options 2 and 4 are opposites. Examine these options first and eliminate one of them. Then based on your selection, examine Option 5.

Content Area: Adult; Concept: Nursing Roles; Sensory Perception; Integrated Processes: Teaching/Learning; Nursing Process: Evaluation; Client Needs: Physiological Integrity: Reduction of Risk Potential; Cognitive Level: Evaluation [Evaluating]

### 1536. MoC ANSWER: 2

1. The rheumatologist treats arthritic and immune conditions.
2. Because Ménière's disease is a condition of the inner ear, the nurse would plan to include the otolaryngologist.
3. The physical therapist focuses on exercises and care for physical rehabilitation.
4. The oncologist treats clients with cancer.

▶ *Test-taking Tip:* Focus on the key term "Ménière's disease," a condition involving the inner ear that can lead to vertigo and hearing loss. "Oto-" refers to ear. Use knowledge of medical terminology to select the correct option.

Content Area: Adult; Concept: Communication; Collaboration; Sensory Perception; Integrated Processes: Nursing Process: Planning; Client Needs: Safe and Effective Care Environment: Management of Care; Cognitive Level: Comprehension [Understanding]

## 1537. PHARM ANSWER: 1

1. **The anticholinergic and antihistamine properties of meclizine (Antivert) treat the symptom of vertigo.**
2. Megestrol (Megace), an antineoplastic agent, is used to treat advanced breast cancer.
3. The antibiotic meropenem (Merrem) treats intra-abdominal infections.
4. The beta blocker metoprolol (Lopressor) is used in treatment of hypertension and heart disease.

▶ *Test-taking Tip: Narrow the options by using pharmacology cues; those ending in "-lol" are usually beta-adrenergic blockers; those ending in "-penem" often are penicillin derivatives. You need to select a medication that has anticholinergic and antihistamine properties.*

Content Area: Adult; Concept: Medication; Sensory Perception; Integrated Processes: Nursing Process: Implementation; Client Needs: Physiological Integrity: Pharmacological and Parenteral Therapies; Cognitive Level: Application [Applying]

## 1538. ANSWER: 2

1. Varicella vaccine is used to prevent chicken pox.
2. **Pneumococcal vaccine can reduce the risk of ear infections.**
3. Typhoid vaccine prevents typhoid fever.
4. Zoster vaccine is used to prevent the development of herpes zoster.

▶ *Test-taking Tip: Focus on the key term "otitis media" and think about the effect of each vaccine. Eliminate options with no association with ear infections.*

Content Area: Adult; Concept: Promoting Health; Immunity; Sensory Perception; Integrated Processes: Teaching/Learning; Client Needs: Health Promotion and Maintenance; Cognitive Level: Application [Applying]

## 1539. PHARM ANSWER: 200

**The rate of IV infusion uses a standard calculation formula. Start with what is known, the total fluid volume (100 mL) and the desired infusion time of 30 minutes. Form a ratio with the known values (100 mL in 30 min) and the unknown desired outcome ($X$ mL in 60 min). Thus 100 mL : 30 min :: $X$ mL : 60 min; $30X = 60 \times 100$; $30X = 6000$; $X = 6000 \div 30$; $X = 200$. The nurse should set the infusion at a rate of 200 mL/hr to deliver levofloxacin (Levaquin) over 30 min.**

▶ *Test-taking Tip: The information about the dosage of 250 mg levofloxacin (Levaquin) and the frequency every 12 hours is not relevant to the question. Use a standard formula for solving an unknown value, insert the known values, and double-check your calculations.*

Content Area: Adult; Concept: Infection; Sensory Perception; Integrated Processes: Nursing Process: Implementation; Client Needs: Physiological Integrity: Pharmacological and Parenteral Therapies; Cognitive Level: Application [Applying]

## 1540. ANSWER:

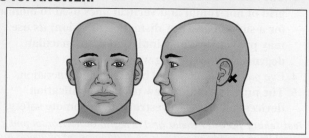

**For the Rinne test, the stem of the tuning fork is placed on the mastoid process, located posterior to the ear lobule.**

▶ *Test-taking Tip: Bone conduction can be tested by placing the tuning fork on the mastoid bone, which surrounds the ear canal.*

Content Area: Adult; Concept: Sensory Perception; Assessment; Integrated Processes: Nursing Process: Assessment; Client Needs: Health Promotion and Maintenance; Cognitive Level: Application [Applying]

## 1541. ANSWER: 1

1. **Otosclerosis impairs the air conduction of sound waves; therefore bone conduction is typically greater than air conduction.**
2. Amplification of sounds with a hearing aid may be helpful in otosclerosis.
3. Approximately 95% of clients experience resolution of conductive hearing loss after surgery on the stapes.
4. Otosclerosis develops gradually and therefore requires serial audiograms to detect the progressive loss of hearing.

▶ *Test-taking Tip: If unfamiliar with the term otosclerosis, dissect the parts of the words. "Oto" refers to the ear, and "sclerosis" implies stiffness and hardness. This may give you clues to the characteristics associated with the condition.*

Content Area: Adult; Concept: Sensory Perception; Integrated Processes: Nursing Process: Analysis; Client Needs: Physiological Integrity: Physiological Adaptation; Cognitive Level: Knowledge [Remembering]

## 1542. PHARM ANSWER: 1

1. **The medication, sodium fluoride, retards bone reabsorption (prevents the breakdown of bone cells) and promotes calcification (hardening) of the bony lesions in the ear.**
2. No drug action exists that causes the breakdown of bone cells and softens the bone in the ear.
3. Antihistamine drugs treat the symptoms of allergic reaction but do not affect the fluid in the ear.
4. No drug action exists that causes the production of histamine and increases the fluid in the ear.

▶ *Test-taking Tip: You should consider the action that fluoride has on protecting the teeth; then think about this in relation to the bones in the inner ear.*

Content Area: Adult; Concept: Medication; Nursing Roles; Sensory Perception; Integrated Processes: Teaching/Learning; Client Needs: Physiological Integrity: Pharmacological and Parenteral Therapies; Cognitive Level: Application [Applying]

**1543. ANSWER: 1, 3, 4**

1. **The occurrence of dizziness can be decreased by refraining from sudden movements. Sudden movements can stimulate the sensitive hairs inside the semicircular canal, causing dizziness.**
2. Dizziness is not associated with chewing.
3. **Avoiding heavy lifting may decrease the incidence of dizziness. The position changes associated with reaching down to lift a heavy object can cause fluid shifts in the inner ear and stimulation of the sensitive hairs inside the semicircular canal.**
4. **Avoiding bending may decrease the incidence of dizziness. Bending can cause fluid shifts in the inner ear and stimulation of the sensitive hairs inside the semicircular canal. Avoiding bending may decrease the incidence of dizziness.**
5. Restricting fluid intake has no effect on fluids in the inner ear and dizziness.

♦ **Test-taking Tip:** Three options pertain to movement, and two options are different. You should think about the relationship between movement and dizziness when answering this question.

**Content Area:** Adult; **Concept:** Nursing Roles; Safety; Sensory Perception; **Integrated Processes:** Nursing Process: Implementation; **Client Needs:** Physiological Integrity: Reduction of Risk Potential; **Cognitive Level:** Application [Applying]

**1544. MoC ANSWER: 2, 3, 4, 1**

2. **Assess the operative incision site and assess the arms for drift. Using the nursing process, assessment should occur before interventions.**
3. **Contact the stroke team and the HCP. This is next because facial drooping and numbness may indicate complications such as intracranial bleeding or nerve compression.**
4. **Medicate the client for pain unless contraindicated. The client is reporting pain.**
1. **Close the client's right eye and place a patch over it. The client will be unable to close the eye due to nerve compression or damage.**

♦ **Test-taking Tip:** Focus on the facial assessment. Visualize the process you would take in a real situation. Remember the urgent steps take priority (further assessment and contacting the HCP).

**Content Area:** Adult; **Concept:** Critical Thinking; Collaboration; Assessment; Sensory Perception; **Integrated Processes:** Nursing Process: Analysis; **Client Needs:** Safe and Effective Care Environment: Management of Care; **Cognitive Level:** Synthesis [Creating]

**1545. ANSWER: 4**

1. Normal conversation, including a variety of topics, helps the client avoid social isolation.
2. Speaking directly into the client's ear will amplify and perhaps distort the conversation. Additionally, the client will not be able to observe the speaker's mouth and receive visual cues.
3. Exaggerated mouth expressions distort the visual cues and hinder communication.
4. **Attracting the client's attention improves communication by including the client fully in the process from the start.**

♦ **Test-taking Tip:** Read the stem carefully and select the intervention that promotes communication and optimal functioning.

**Content Area:** Adult; **Concept:** Communication; Sensory Perception; **Integrated Processes:** Nursing Process: Implementation; Caring; **Client Needs:** Psychosocial Integrity; **Cognitive Level:** Application [Applying]

**1546. ANSWER: 2**

1. Eliminating background noise will help improve the client's ability to hear, but the most appropriate action is to further assess the client.
2. **The nurse should assess the client's hearing and perform an otoscopic examination to verify the client's symptoms and attempt to find the source of the problem.**
3. The nurse should obtain additional data before referring the client for medical evaluation.
4. Interventions to improve communication are useful to the client, but a new hearing loss must be investigated first.

♦ **Test-taking Tip:** Utilize the steps of the nursing process and select Option 2, which calls for the nurse to perform an assessment.

**Content Area:** Adult; **Concept:** Sensory Perception; Communication; Assessment; **Integrated Processes:** Nursing Process: Assessment; **Client Needs:** Psychosocial Integrity; **Cognitive Level:** Application [Applying]

## 1547. ANSWER: 3

1. The tympanic membrane is intact, and no excessive cerumen is visible; this documentation is incorrect.
2. The illustration does not show the external canal from this photo; this documentation is incorrect.
3. **This documentation is best. The tympanic membrane shown is reddened, and the cone of light is distorted. These findings indicate increased pressure behind the tympanic membrane.**
4. Bony landmarks of the ear are not prominent due to the bulging of the tympanic membrane.

▶ *Test-taking Tip:* In the normal ear, the tympanic membrane appears pearly gray, and the cone of light is at 7 o'clock in the left ear.

**Content Area:** Adult; **Concept:** Communication; Sensory Perception; **Integrated Processes:** Communication and Documentation; **Client Needs:** Physiological Integrity: Reduction of Risk Potential; **Cognitive Level:** Analysis [Analyzing]

## 1548. ANSWER: 2, 3, 4

1. Ranitidine (Zantac), an H2 blocker, will not treat sinusitis but will treat epigastric pain from dyspepsia.
2. **Applying warm compresses helps relieve nasal and sinus congestion.**
3. **Using a saline nasal spray loosens nasal and sinus secretions.**
4. **A decongestant, such as pseudoephedrine (Sudafed), helps relieve nasal and sinus congestion.**
5. Spending time in the sunlight will treat psoriasis but not sinusitis.

▶ *Test-taking Tip:* Note the key word "interventions" and use the process of elimination to exclude Options 1 and 5.

**Content Area:** Adult; **Concept:** Nursing Roles; Sensory Perception; **Integrated Processes:** Teaching/Learning; **Client Needs:** Physiological Integrity: Basic Care and Comfort; Health Promotion and Maintenance; **Cognitive Level:** Application [Applying]

# Chapter Thirty-Five

# Pharmacological and Parenteral Therapies for Adults

**1549.** **PHARM** The client who is to receive a scheduled dose of digoxin has an irregular apical pulse at 92 bpm and a serum potassium of 3.9 mEq/L. Which nursing documentation reflects the **most** appropriate action?

1. Serum potassium level WNL. Digoxin given for rapid apical pulse.
2. Digoxin withheld because the client's apical HR is irregular.
3. Digoxin withheld to prevent toxicity due to the low potassium level.
4. HCP informed of irregular HR and low serum potassium level.

**1550.** **PHARM** The client has been receiving clonidine 0.1 mg via transdermal patch once every 7 days. The NA removes the patch with morning cares. Eight hours later, the nurse discovers that the clonidine patch is no longer present. Which assessment finding should be **most** concerning to the nurse?

1. Skin tear is noted on the client's upper chest.
2. Client reports having an excruciating headache.
3. The current BP is noted to be 182/100 mm Hg.
4. The ECG monitor shows a HR of 120 bpm.

**1551.** **PHARM** The HCP prescribes a second antihypertensive medication for the client who has poorly controlled BP on one medication. If prescribed, which medication combination should the nurse question?

1. Atenolol and metoprolol
2. Metolazone and valsartan
3. Captopril and furosemide
4. Bumetanide and diltiazem

**1552.** **PHARM** The client with chronic, stable angina telephones the clinic nurse and reports a headache lasting for several days after taking isosorbide mononitrate as prescribed. The client also reports symptoms of orthostatic hypotension and palpitations. Which is the nurse's **best** recommendation?

1. "You need to come to the clinic to be seen."
2. "Retime the dose for later in the afternoon."
3. "Take two acetaminophen 325-mg tablets now."
4. "The headaches will subside with continued use."

**1553.** **PHARM** The client is taking metolazone and diltiazem for treatment of hypertension. Which statement made by the client indicates that the nurse should do further teaching?

1. "I eat foods high in potassium to prevent the development of hypokalemia."
2. "Metolazone makes me urinate more, so I take my last dose at suppertime."
3. "I took my medication at breakfast with eggs, toast, grapefruit juice, and milk."
4. "Ibuprofen affects my urine output, so I prefer to take acetaminophen for pain."

**1554.** **PHARM** The nurse is caring for the client taking atorvastatin. The nurse should assess for which adverse effects?

1. Constipation and hemorrhoids
2. Muscle pain and weakness
3. Fatigue and atrial fibrillation
4. Flushing and postural hypotension

**1555.** PHARM CJ The nurse is reviewing the chart illustrated of the client diagnosed with stage II HF. Which conclusion should the nurse make?

| Admitting History & Physical | Serum Laboratory Results |
|---|---|
| • Dyspnea on exertion<br>• Lung sounds: crackles in bilateral bases<br>• Reports seeing yellow halo around objects | • BNP: 886 ng/L*<br>• aPTT: 55 sec**<br>• K: 2.9 mEq/L |

| Diagnostic Results | Medications |
|---|---|
| • 12-lead ECG: Atrial fibrillation with frequent PVCs<br>• CXR: Pulmonary infiltrate bilateral bases<br>• Cardiomegaly | • Buffered aspirin 325 mg oral daily<br>• Digoxin 0.25 mg oral daily<br>• Furosemide 40 mg oral daily<br>• Atenolol 25 mg oral<br>• Heparin IV infusion per protocol |

\* BNP normal value 100 ng/L
\*\* aPTT normal range 24 to 33 seconds

1. The medications should be administered as prescribed.
2. The client may be experiencing toxicity from digoxin.
3. Hyperkalemia likely caused the client's cardiac dysrhythmias.
4. Seeing halos can result from the atrial fibrillation or anticoagulants.

**1556.** PHARM The client with CRF is receiving epoetin alfa. The nurse evaluates that the medication's action has been effective when noting which finding?

1. Urine output increased to 30 mL per hour
2. Hemoglobin 12 g/dL and hematocrit 36%
3. BP 110/70 mm Hg and HR 68 bpm
4. An increased energy level and less fatigue

**1557.** PHARM The client with CRF receives a sodium polystyrene sulfonate enema. Which finding indicates that the medication is achieving the desired therapeutic effect?

1. Returns of dark-colored stool
2. Able to retain solution for 1 hour
3. Verbalized relief of constipation
4. Serum potassium level at 4.0 mEq/L

**1558.** PHARM The nurse is educating the client receiving a thiazide diuretic. What information should the nurse plan to include? **Select all that apply.**

1. Take the radial pulse before setting up the medication.
2. Include fruits such as melons and bananas in the diet.
3. Report side effects such as muscle cramps, nausea, or a skin rash.
4. Take the last dose at bedtime when fluids are at the highest level.
5. Avoid high-fat foods; thiazide diuretics increase cholesterol levels.

**1559.** PHARM The nurse is reviewing the client's medication list, illustrated, prepared by the client's daughter. The nurse is **most** concerned about addressing which finding **first**?

| Client's Medication List | |
|---|---|
| Aspart insulin 1 unit per 1 carbohydrate choice (CHO) taken at meals | Captopril 25 mg three times daily |
| Aspirin 1 tab every a.m. | Glyburide 1 at breakfast |
| Atenolol 25 mg oral at breakfast | Hydrochlorothiazide 25 mg twice daily |
| Hydrochlorothiazide + captopril 1 daily | Simvastatin 10 mg daily in the evening |

1. Some medication doses are missing.
2. Some administration routes are missing.
3. Some medications are being duplicated.
4. Some medications have drug-drug interactions.

**1560.** PHARM Following a THR, the client asks the nurse, "Why am I receiving enoxaparin? With my last hip surgery, I was given a heparin injection." What is the nurse's **best** response?

1. "Enoxaparin is less expensive for you and much easier to administer than the heparin."
2. "There is less risk of bleeding with enoxaparin, and it doesn't affect your laboratory results."
3. "Enoxaparin is a low-molecular-weight heparin that lasts twice as long as regular heparin."
4. "Enoxaparin can be administered orally, whereas heparin is administered only by injection."

**1561. PHARM** The client with MS is prescribed baclofen. Which information is **most** important for the nurse to evaluate when caring for this client?

1. Serum baclofen levels
2. Muscle rigidity and pain
3. Intake and urine output
4. Daily weight pattern

**1562. PHARM** The client, hospitalized with an exacerbation of SLE, is to receive methylprednisolone 20 mg IV q8h. Which intervention should the nurse anticipate being included in the client's plan of care?

1. Take orthostatic BPs at least twice daily.
2. Administer a stool softener twice daily.
3. Premedicate with diphenhydramine.
4. Check blood glucose before meals and at bedtime.

**1563. PHARM** The client with tonsillar cancer is receiving filgrastim. Prior to administering the next dose of filgrastim, the nurse notes that the client's absolute neutrophil count is 11,000/mm³. What is the nurse's **best** action?

1. Administer filgrastim as prescribed.
2. Place the client on neutropenic precautions.
3. Notify the HCP to question giving filgrastim.
4. Apply gown, gloves, and mask to enter the room.

**1564. MoC PHARM** The HCP prescribes 5% albumin for four clients. The nurse should consult with the HCP if 5% albumin is prescribed for which client?

1. The client who is allergic to cephalosporins
2. The client experiencing hypovolemic shock
3. The client who refuses to receive blood or blood products
4. The client experiencing adult respiratory distress syndrome (ARDS)

**1565. PHARM** The nurse administered phenylephrine eye drops to the client before performing an ophthalmoscopic eye examination. Which assessment finding should the nurse expect?

1. Tremor
2. Hypotension
3. Pupil miosis
4. Pupil mydriasis

**1566. PHARM** The client using latanoprost eye drops for treatment of glaucoma calls the ophthalmology clinic after noting a brown pigmentation of the iris. Which nursing action is **most** appropriate?

1. Instruct the client to come to the clinic to have the eyes and medication evaluated.
2. Schedule an appointment for the client to see an internist for liver function studies.
3. Tell the client that the pigmentation is from the latanoprost but will eventually regress.
4. Recommend that the client wear sunglasses when outdoors to decrease iris pigmentation.

**1567. PHARM** The client has psoriasis vulgaris. Place an X on the illustration where the nurse should plan to apply a thin film of tazarotene topical medication.

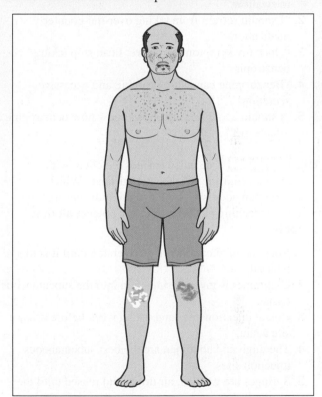

**1568. PHARM** The client is receiving multiple medications for treatment of PD. Which signs and symptoms should the nurse recognize as adverse effects of carbidopa-levodopa?

1. Dystonia and akinesia
2. Bradykinesia and agitation
3. Muscle rigidity and cardiac dysrhythmias
4. Orthostatic hypotension and dry mouth

**1569.** PHARM The client calls a clinic 2 weeks after taking oral carbidopa-levodopa, stating that the medication has been ineffective in controlling the symptoms of PD. What nursing action is **most** important?

1. Review how to correctly take the medication.
2. Contact the HCP to address a dosage change.
3. Reinforce that it takes 1 to 2 months to see effects.
4. Discuss eating a high protein diet with vitamin B$_6$.

**1570.** PHARM The nurse completes teaching the client who has PD about taking benztropine. Which statements made by the client indicate that teaching is effective? **Select all that apply.**

1. "I plan to crush the tablets so that they are easier to swallow."
2. "I should refrain from taking over-the-counter medications."
3. "Once my symptoms improve, I can stop taking benztropine."
4. "Benztropine can cause drooling and excessive secretions."
5. "I should avoid driving until I know how benztropine affects me."

**1571.** PHARM The nurse teaches the client with relapsing-remitting MS about glatiramer. Which information addressed by the client indicates that the nurse's teaching has been effective? **Select all that apply.**

1. Keep the medication vial refrigerated until it is to be used.
2. Glatiramer is given by injection into the subcutaneous tissue.
3. Rotate injection sites and wait a week before using a site again.
4. The thigh and abdomen are the best subcutaneous injection sites.
5. Syringes are washed, air dried, and reused until the needle is dull.

**1572.** PHARM The client taking carbamazepine XR for seizure control reports that pieces of the medication are being passed into the stool. Which action by the nurse is **most** important?

1. Report this to the HCP.
2. Reassure the client that this is normal.
3. Collect the stool for laboratory analysis.
4. Document the findings in the medical record.

**1573.** PHARM The nurse is caring for a group of clients all in need of pain medication. The nurse has determined the most appropriate pain medication for each client based on the client's level of pain. Prioritize the order that the nurse should plan to administer the pain medications, beginning with the most potent analgesic for the client with the most severe pain.

1. Ketorolac 10 mg oral
2. Fentanyl 0.1 mg IV bolus per patient-controlled analgesia (PCA)
3. Hydromorphone 5 mg oral
4. Morphine sulfate 4 mg IV
5. Propoxyphene 65 mg oral

Answer: _____

**1574.** PHARM The nurse applies a fentanyl transdermal patch to the client for the first time. Shortly after application, the client is experiencing pain. Which nursing action is **most** appropriate?

1. Remove the fentanyl patch and apply a new one.
2. Administer a short-acting opioid analgesic.
3. Vigorously rub the fentanyl transdermal patch.
4. Call the HCP to request a higher-dosed patch.

**1575.** PHARM The nurse is caring for the client who has received sumatriptan. The nurse evaluates that sumatriptan has been an effective treatment when the client reports which change?

1. Improvement in mood
2. Decrease in muscle spasms
3. Increase in ability to fall asleep
4. Relief of migraine headache attacks

**1576.** PHARM The nurse is caring for the client with OA receiving piroxicam. Which instruction is **most** important for the nurse to include in the medication teaching plan?

1. "Take piroxicam with food to decrease stomach irritation."
2. "If your pain is severe, you can take another piroxicam pill."
3. "Lie down until piroxicam is effective for controlling your pain."
4. "You can take ginkgo for an energy boost when taking piroxicam."

**1577.** PHARM The client experiencing an acute attack of gouty arthritis is prescribed colchicine 1 mg IV now and then 0.5 mg q6h. Colchicine 0.5 mg/mL in a 2-mL ampule is available. How many mL should the nurse administer for the **initial** dose?

_____ mL (Record your answer as a whole number.)

**1578.** PHARM The nurse is assessing the client. Which findings indicate that the client may be experiencing physical changes from long-term use of prednisone? **Select all that apply.**

1. Weight gain
2. Increased muscle mass
3. Fragile skin
4. Acne vulgaris
5. Alopecia

**1579.** PHARM Cyclosporine and methotrexate are prescribed for the client with severe rheumatoid arthritis. What information should the nurse address when teaching the client? **Select all that apply.**

1. Drink grapefruit juice to enhance the medication effects.
2. Drink plenty of fluids to prevent becoming dehydrated.
3. Avoid use of St. John's wort, echinacea, and melatonin.
4. These medications are administered weekly by injection.
5. Methotrexate and cyclosporine suppress the immune system.

**1580.** PHARM The client with CP is taking dantrolene. The nurse evaluates that the medication is effective when noting that the client has an increase in which findings? **Select all that apply.**

1. Muscle spasticity
2. Urinary frequency
3. Level of mobility
4. Ability to maintain balance
5. Level of alertness

**1581.** PHARM The nurse prepares to administer naloxone 0.4 mg IV to the client experiencing respiratory depression. Naloxone is supplied in a 1 mg/mL vial. How many mL should the nurse administer?

_____ mL (Round to the nearest tenth.)

**1582.** PHARM The client taking glyburide 5 mg orally once daily presents in the ED with headache, flushing, nausea, and abdominal cramps. The client's fingerstick blood sugar result is 56 mg/dL. Which question is **most** important for the nurse to ask the client?

1. "How many grams of protein do you normally eat?"
2. "What time did you eat your dinner last night?"
3. "How often do you check your blood sugar level?"
4. "What was your alcohol intake like this past week?"

**1583.** PHARM The 40-year-old client is receiving levothyroxine for treatment of hypothyroidism. Which serum laboratory results should lead the nurse to conclude that the client's dose is adequate?

| Serum Laboratory Value | Normal Value | Client Value |
| --- | --- | --- |
| WBC | 4500–11,100/mm$^3$ | 11,000/mm$^3$ |
| TSH | 0.4–4.2 micro units/mL | 0.5 micro units/mL |
| T$_3$ | 70–204 ng/dL | 80 ng/dL |
| Free T$_4$ | 0.8–2.3 ng/dL | 2.1 ng/dL |
| Cortisol | 5–25 mcg/dL | 10 mcg/dL |
| Glucose | 70–110 mg/dL | 80 mg/dL |
| Potassium | 3.5–5.0 mEq/L | 4.5 mEq/L |

1. Thyroid-stimulating hormone and cortisol
2. Thyroid-stimulating hormone and free thyroxine (T$_4$)
3. Triiodothyronine (T$_3$) and free T$_4$
4. White blood cells, glucose, and potassium

**1584.** PHARM The client with Addison's disease is taking fludrocortisone 100 mcg orally once daily. Which statement made by the client regarding the fludrocortisone therapy requires further teaching by the nurse?

1. "I should talk to my health care provider about getting a flu shot this year."
2. "I should stop taking fludrocortisone if my blood sugar levels are too high."
3. "I should check my weight, blood pressure, and pulse once every morning."
4. "I should eat foods higher in potassium like bananas, melons, and pears."

**1585. PHARM** The client is receiving fludrocortisone for treatment of adrenocortical insufficiency. The nurse is evaluating the client's serum laboratory values for adverse effects of the medication. Place an X on the laboratory tests that the nurse should specifically review to evaluate the adverse effects of fludrocortisone. **Select all that apply.**

| Serum Laboratory Test | Normal Value | Client Value |
|---|---|---|
| Glucose | 70–110 mg/dL | 180 mg/dL |
| Potassium | 3.5–5.0 mEq/L | 3.5 mEq/L |
| Calcium | 8.5–10.5 mg/dL | 8.0 mg/dL |
| Platelets | 179–450 K/mm³ | 165 K/mm³ |
| TSH | 0.4–4.2 micro units/mL | 9.4 micro units/mL |
| Free T$_4$ | 0.8–2.3 ng/dL | 0.1 ng/dL |

**1586. PHARM** Oral terbutaline is prescribed for the client with bronchitis. Which comorbidity **most** warrants the nurse's close monitoring of the client following administration of terbutaline?

1. Strabismus
2. Hypertension
3. Diabetes insipidus
4. Hypothyroidism

**1587. MoC PHARM** The client is admitted to the ED with tachypnea, tachycardia, and hypotension. The client has been taking theophylline for treatment of asthma and erythromycin for an upper respiratory tract infection. Which conclusions and actions taken by the nurse are correct? **Select all that apply.**

1. The client is having an asthma attack; the nurse requests an order for albuterol.
2. The client is experiencing septicemia; the nurse requests an order for blood cultures.
3. The client has theophylline toxicity; the nurse requests an order for a serum theophylline level.
4. The client is allergic to erythromycin; the nurse requests an order for diphenhydramine.
5. The client is having a drug-drug interaction; the nurse requests a change of medication.

**1588. PHARM** The client, admitted to the ED, is prescribed to receive 0.5 mg epinephrine subcutaneously for treatment of a severe asthma attack. The medication for injection is supplied in a vial that contains 5 mg/mL. How many mL of epinephrine should the nurse administer?

_____ mL (Round to the nearest tenth.)

**1589. PHARM** The hospitalized client is prescribed to receive ferrous fumarate 200 mg oral daily. When transcribing the medication onto the client's MAR, at which time in military time should the nurse schedule the daily dose for **best** absorption?

1. 0830
2. 1000
3. 1230
4. 1730

**1590. PHARM** Two hours after administering iron dextran, the nurse is drawing the client's blood sample for a laboratory test. Which intervention should the nurse implement when noting that the client's blood has a brownish hue?

1. Document the serum color.
2. Draw blood from another site.
3. Immediately notify the HCP.
4. Discard the sample of blood.

**1591. PHARM** The client has been successful at controlling gastroesophageal reflux symptoms without prescription medications. Which OTC medication should the nurse explore whether the client is taking for symptom control?

1. Aspirin once a day
2. Famotidine
3. Ibuprofen
4. Desloratadine

**1592. PHARM** The client with GERD is taking cimetidine. Which serum laboratory finding should the nurse determine is **most** concerning?

1. Increased liver enzymes
2. Increased platelet count
3. Decreased creatinine
4. Decreased prolactin

**1593.** **MoC** **PHARM** The client's medical record shows a contraindication for metoclopramide that was just prescribed. The nurse notifies the HCP. Which information in the client's medical record **most likely** prompted the nurse's notification of the HCP?

1. Use of nasogastric suctioning
2. History of diabetes mellitus
3. History of seizure disorders
4. Chemotherapy treatment for cancer

**1594.** **PHARM** The nurse is preparing to give medications at 1700 hours to multiple clients with GI problems. Which medication should be the nurse's **priority** when the meal trays are due to arrive at 1700?

1. Misoprostol
2. Famotidine
3. Cimetidine
4. Bisacodyl

**1595.** **PHARM** The client with ulcerative colitis is started on sulfasalazine. The nurse overhears the client talking with family members about sulfasalazine and recognizes the need for more teaching when the client makes which statement?

1. "I'll be taking sulfasalazine to help control my diarrhea."
2. "Sulfasalazine will decrease the inflammation in my colon."
3. "After a year of taking sulfasalazine, I'll be cured of the disease."
4. "Sulfasalazine will help to prevent exacerbations of my disease."

**1596.** **PHARM** The nurse evaluates that pancrelipase is having the optimal intended benefit for the client with CF. Which assessment finding prompted the nurse's conclusion?

1. The client lost 4 pounds in 1 month.
2. The client no longer has heartburn.
3. The client has increased steatorrhea.
4. The client has improved nutritional status.

**1597.** **PHARM** The nurse teaches the cli[...] lesions that have not healed and are recu[...] newly prescribed medication ganciclovir[...] should document that teaching about gan[...] completed for the client with which illustra[...]

1.

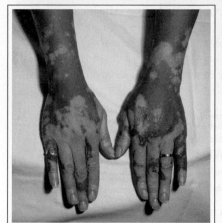

2.

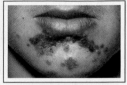

3.

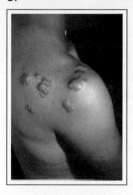

4.

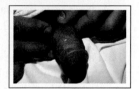

**1598.** **MoC** **PHARM** The client had a normal serum creatinine level on hospital admission. Four days later, the client's serum creatinine level is 3.7 mg/dL. The nurse should contact the HCP regarding a dosage change for which medications? **Select all that apply.**

1. Ceftriaxone
2. Insulin glargine
3. Diltiazem
4. Furosemide
5. Captopril

**599.** **PHARM** The nurse is to administer vancomycin to the client diagnosed with sepsis. The client is to have a peak and trough level completed on this dose of vancomycin. Which action should the nurse initiate **first?**

1. Determine if the trough level has already been drawn on the client.
2. Check drug compatibilities before infusing into an existing IV line.
3. Evaluate the client's culture and sensitivity (C&S) report results.
4. Calculate the rate at which the vancomycin should be infused.

**1600.** **MoC** **PHARM** The client is to receive the first dose of sulfamethoxazole 1g oral q12 h for treatment of recurrent UTIs. Which information about the client should prompt the nurse to consult the HCP before administration? **Select all that apply.**

1. History of gastric ulcer
2. Type 1 diabetes mellitus
3. Urine positive for *Escherichia coli*
4. Near-term pregnancy
5. Taking digoxin 0.25 mg daily

**1601.** **PHARM** The client with COPD is prescribed salmeterol diskus inhaler and fluticasone Rotadisk inhaler. Which instruction should the nurse include to prevent the client from developing oropharyngeal candidiasis?

1. "Drink a glass of water before taking your medications."
2. "Rinse your mouth after using your inhaler medications."
3. "Wait at least one minute before taking the next medication."
4. "Close your mouth tightly around the inhaler mouthpiece."

**1602.** **PHARM** The client calls a clinic to renew the prescription for insulin being administered subcutaneously via an insulin pump. Which insulin type, if prescribed by the HCP, should the nurse question?

1. Insulin lispro
2. Insulin aspart
3. Insulin glulisine
4. Insulin glargine

**1603.** **PHARM** The unresponsive client with DM is admitted to the ED with a serum glucose level of 35 mg/dL. Which medication should the nurse plan to administer?

1. Exenatide
2. Pramlintide
3. Miglitol
4. Glucagon

**1604.** **PHARM** The client taking rifampin brings an orange-colored urine sample to the clinic. Which interventions should the nurse implement? **Select all that apply.**

1. Send the urine to the lab for culture and sensitivity (C&S).
2. Reassure the client that this is normal and harmless.
3. Teach that the urine that is orange can stain clothing.
4. Question continuation of rifampin with the HCP.
5. Inform that sweat and tears can also turn orange-colored.

**1605.** **PHARM** Ciprofloxacin is prescribed for the client to treat a UTI. Which information should the nurse stress when teaching the client about the medication?

1. Avoid taking ciprofloxacin with dairy products such as milk or yogurt.
2. Treat diarrhea, a side effect of ciprofloxacin, with bismuth subsalicylate.
3. Avoid fennel because it will increase the absorption of the ciprofloxacin.
4. Take dietary calcium tablets 1 hour before or 2 hours after ciprofloxacin.

**1606.** **PHARM** The nurse is assessing the client with herpes zoster. The nurse determines that acyclovir is an effective treatment when which finding is noted?

1. Drying and crusting of genital lesions
2. Crusting and healing of vesicular skin lesions
3. Urticaria decreased and pruritus relieved
4. Decrease in intensity of chicken pox lesions

**1607.** PHARM The male client with known cardiac problem calls the clinic and informs the nurse that he is having extreme dizziness and feeling faint since taking his friend's sildenafil (Viagra) last night. Which question should be the nurse's **priority?**

1. "Do you take nitrates?"
2. "How old are you?"
3. "Do you have prostate hyperplasia?"
4. "How much sildenafil did you take?"

**1608.** PHARM The nurse receives the HCP order to start TPN for the client who has a PICC. Into which type of catheter illustrated should the nurse plan to administer the TPN?

1.

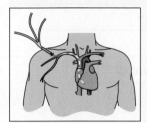

2.

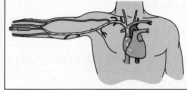

3.

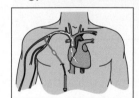

4.

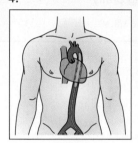

**1609.** PHARM The nurse completed teaching for the client who will be receiving TPN while at home. Which client statement indicates that further teaching is needed?

1. "My refrigerator is big enough to store several bags of parenteral solution."
2. "I will keep my cellular phone with me at all times to use in an emergency."
3. "I plan to use the main floor bedroom; it'll be best with the infusion pump."
4. "I'll sit at the table to remove the IV catheter cap to attach the IV tubing."

**1610.** PHARM The HCP prescribes 1200 mL of TPN solution to be administered over 24 hours for the homebound client. The home health nurse should instruct the client to set the infusion pump to deliver how many mL per hour?

_____ mL/hr (Record your answer as a whole number.)

**1611.** PHARM The nurse is initiating an IV infusion of lactated Ringer's (LR) for the client in shock. What is the purpose of LR for this client?

1. Increase fluid volume and urinary output.
2. Draw water from the cells into the blood vessels.
3. Provide dextrose and nutrients to prevent cellular death.
4. Replace potassium and magnesium for cardiac stabilization.

**INSTRUCTIONS:** Use the information provided in the table below to answer Question 1612.

| Client | 55-year old male |
|---|---|
| **Allergies** | Cefuroxime |
| **Admitting Diagnosis** | Left femoral neck fracture 72 hours ago |
| **Surgery** | Left total hip arthroplasty, anterior approach, 24 hours ago |
| **Medical History** | Hyperlipidemia, hypertension, depression |
| **Laboratory Test Results** | *Complete blood count:* Hemoglobin 16.6 g/dL (166 g/L), platelets 450 × 10³/microL (450,000/mm³), WBC 10.1 × 10³/microL (10,100/mm³) <br> *Serum Chemistry:* Sodium 143 mEq/L (143 mmol/L), potassium 4.8 mEq/L (4.8 mmol/L), creatinine 1.2 mg/dL (106.1 μmol/L), BUN 18 mg/dL (6.4 mmol/L) <br> *Coagulation:* PT 12 seconds, APTT 32 seconds |
| **Diet** | Low sodium, low saturated fat |
| **Scheduled Procedures** | Left hip x-ray in 30 minutes |
| **Current Vital Signs** | BP 146/92; pulse 46; respirations 20; oral temperature 99°F (37.2°C) |
| **Medications Due at This Time** | Cefazolin 500 mg IVPB <br> Enoxaparin 30 mg subcutaneously <br> Hydrocodone/acetaminophen 5 mg/325 mg 1 tab orally <br> Metoprolol succinate 100 mg orally <br> Pantoprazole 40 mg orally <br> Olanzapine 100 mg orally |

**1612.** `CJ` `MoC` `PHARM` The nurse is preparing to administer scheduled medications to the client. Which three medications would require clarification before administration? Complete the following statements by choosing the *number* for the medication from the left column that should be clarified with the HCP and the *letter* for the correct reason to clarify the medication with the HCP from the right column. Place the number and letter of the correct answer in the blank lines that follow.

| The nurse should <u>clarify</u> the: | because: |
|---|---|
| *1.* Cefazolin | A. The serum creatinine and BUN is elevated. |
| *2.* Enoxaparin | B. The client has an allergy to a cephalosporin antibiotic. |
| *3.* Hydrocodone/acetaminophen | C. The client has bradycardia. |
| *4.* Metoprolol succinate | D. The client has thrombocytopenia. |
| *5.* Pantoprazole | E. The dose is too high. |
| *6.* Olanzapine | F. The client has hyperkalemia. |

Answer:

Medication number _____ Reason letter _____
Medication number _____ Reason letter _____
Medication number _____ Reason letter _____

# Answers and Rationales

## 1549. PHARM ANSWER: 1

1. **A normal serum potassium level is 3.5 to 5.0 mEq/L. Digoxin (Lanoxin), a cardiac glycoside, slows and strengthens the heart. It is used for rate control in clients with atrial fibrillation, which often produces an irregular rhythm.**
2. Dysrhythmias can occur if digoxin is given when the serum potassium level is low, but the serum potassium level is WNL. Digoxin is used for rate control and would not be withheld due to an irregular HR.
3. Although it is important to monitor for digoxin toxicity, the serum potassium level is WNL.
4. Withholding digoxin and notifying the HCP are unnecessary; the serum potassium is WNL.

▶ *Test-taking Tip: The normal serum potassium level is 3.5 to 5.0 mEq/L.*

Content Area: Adult; Concept: Medication; Fluid and Electrolyte Balance; Integrated Processes: Communication and Documentation; Client Needs: Physiological Integrity: Pharmacological and Parenteral Therapies; Cognitive Level: Analysis [Analyzing]

## 1550. PHARM ANSWER: 3

1. Although a skin tear is concerning and may have occurred during removal, it is not the most concerning.
2. Headache can occur from the abrupt removal of clonidine but is not the most concerning.
3. **Clonidine (Catapres) is an antihypertensive medication. Rebound hypertension occurs from abrupt withdrawal. Immediate intervention is required to lower the BP.**
4. Tachycardia is an adverse effect of clonidine.

▶ *Test-taking Tip: The key words are "most concerning." Use the ABC's to determine the most concerning finding. Select Option 3 because it pertains to circulation.*

Content Area: Adult; Concept: Medication; Critical Thinking; Perfusion; Integrated Processes: Nursing Process: Assessment; Client Needs: Physiological Integrity: Pharmacological and Parenteral Therapies; Cognitive Level: Analysis [Analyzing]

## 1551. PHARM ANSWER: 1

1. **When two medications are used to treat hypertension, each should be from different drug classifications. Atenolol (Tenormin) and metoprolol (Lopressor) are both beta-adrenergic blockers and have the same general mechanism of action. The nurse should question this medication combination.**
2. Metolazone (Zaroxolyn) is a thiazide-like diuretic, and valsartan (Diovan) is an ARB.
3. Captopril (Capoten) is an ACE inhibitor, and furosemide (Lasix) is a loop diuretic.
4. Bumetanide (Bumex) is a loop diuretic, and diltiazem (Cardizem) is a calcium channel blocker.

▶ *Test-taking Tip: Beta blockers end in "-lol." Use this as a cue to identify the two medications that are within the same drug classification and would be inappropriately prescribed.*

Content Area: Adult; Concept: Medication; Perfusion; Integrated Processes: Nursing Process: Planning; Client Needs: Physiological Integrity: Pharmacological and Parenteral Therapies; Safe and Effective Care Environment: Safety and Infection Control; Cognitive Level: Application [Applying]

## 1552. PHARM ANSWER: 1

1. **Severe headaches, orthostatic hypotension, and palpitations may be a sign of isosorbide mononitrate (Imdur) toxicity; thus the client should be evaluated by an HCP. Other signs of toxicity include syncope, dizziness, blurred vision, and light-headedness.**
2. Isosorbide mononitrate should be taken in the morning to improve blood flow to the heart and prevent angina attacks that can occur due to increased oxygen demand from activity.
3. A headache (but not a severe headache) can be treated with or prevented by analgesics taken either before or at the same time as the isosorbide mononitrate.
4. Although the headaches will subside over time, the client may be experiencing symptoms of isosorbide mononitrate toxicity.

▶ *Test-taking Tip: The key words are "best action." Isosorbide mononitrate (Imdur) is a long-acting coronary vasodilator. Think about the toxic effects of isosorbide mononitrate.*

Content Area: Adult; Concept: Medication; Safety; Perfusion; Integrated Processes: Nursing Process: Implementation; Caring; Communication and Documentation; Client Needs: Physiological Integrity: Pharmacological and Parenteral Therapies; Cognitive Level: Application [Applying]

## 1553. PHARM ANSWER: 3

1. Consuming foods daily that are high in potassium is recommended. Thiazide diuretics such as metolazone (Zaroxolyn) can result in hypokalemia.
2. The diuretic metolazone (Zaroxolyn) should not be taken at bedtime to avoid nocturia and the subsequent loss of sleep.
3. **The client should not consume grapefruit juice because it inhibits the metabolism of diltiazem (Cardizem) and can cause toxicity. This client statement indicates the need for further teaching.**
4. NSAIDs such as ibuprofen (Advil, Motrin) can decrease the diuretic and antihypertensive effects of thiazide diuretics.

▶ *Test-taking Tip: The key words are "further teaching." Select the option that includes a contraindication when taking diltiazem.*

Content Area: Adult; Concept: Medication; Perfusion; Nutrition; Integrated Processes: Nursing Process: Evaluation; Client Needs: Physiological Integrity: Pharmacological and Parenteral Therapies; Cognitive Level: Evaluation [Evaluating]

**1554.** PHARM **ANSWER: 2**

1. Diarrhea, not constipation, has been found to be a side effect of statin medications. Bile acid sequestrants act by inhibiting bile acids from absorption by the small intestine. This results in fewer bile acids in the small intestine, which may lead to constipation and hemorrhoids.
2. **Atorvastatin (Lipitor) is a 3-hydroxy-3-methylglutaryl coenzyme A (HMG-CoA) reductase inhibitor (statin) used to lower lipid levels. Statins can cause muscle tissue injury manifested by muscle ache or weakness. Muscle injury can progress to myositis (muscle inflammation) or rhabdomyolysis (muscle disintegration).**
3. Research shows that atorvastatin decreased the risk of atrial fibrillation. Side effects of niacin, a lipid-lowering agent, include dysrhythmias.
4. Side effects of niacin, a lipid-lowering agent, include flushing and postural hypotension.

▶ *Test-taking Tip:* You need to know that the statin drugs can lead to muscle tissue injury.

Content Area: Adult; Concept: Medication; Assessment; Perfusion; Integrated Processes: Nursing Process: Assessment; Client Needs: Physiological Integrity: Pharmacological and Parenteral Therapies; Physiological Integrity: Reduction of Risk Potential; Cognitive Level: Comprehension [Understanding]

**1555.** PHARM CJ **ANSWER: 2**

1. The digoxin should be withheld and not given until a serum digoxin level is determined.
2. **Signs of digoxin (Lanoxin) toxicity include seeing yellow halos around objects and dysrhythmias. The furosemide (Lasix) diuretic increases urinary excretion of potassium and can cause hypokalemia. Hypokalemia can contribute to both cardiac dysrhythmias and digoxin toxicity.**
3. A serum potassium level of 2.9 mEq/L indicates hypokalemia, not hyperkalemia.
4. The yellow vision is a characteristic sign of digoxin toxicity and is not a sign of cerebral damage from an infarct due to atrial fibrillation or bleeding from the anticoagulants.

▶ *Test-taking Tip:* When charts are presented, it is often easier to review the options and then look at the information in the chart. Normal serum potassium level is 3.5 to 5.0 mEq/dL.

Content Area: Adult; Concept: Medication; Critical Thinking; Perfusion; Integrated Processes: Nursing Process: Analysis; Client Needs: Physiological Integrity: Pharmacological and Parenteral Therapies; Cognitive Level: Analysis [Analyzing]

**1556.** PHARM **ANSWER: 2**

1. Epoetin alfa does not have an effect on urine output.
2. **Epoetin alfa stimulates erythropoiesis, or the production of RBCs. It is used in treating anemias associated with decreased RBC production, such as in renal failure. Hgb and Hct are used to evaluate the medication's effectiveness. The target Hgb for the client with CRF is 12 g/dL.**

3. Epoetin alfa does not have an effect on BP or HR.
4. The client may report increased energy and less fatigue because of the increased Hgb levels, but these findings are not used to evaluate the medication's action.

▶ *Test-taking Tip:* Focus on the action of the medication in selecting an option. Epoetin alfa (Epogen, Procrit) affects the production of RBCs. This should lead you to select Option 2.

Content Area: Adult; Concept: Medication; Cellular Regulation; Urinary Elimination; Integrated Processes: Nursing Process: Evaluation; Client Needs: Physiological Integrity: Pharmacological and Parenteral Therapies; Cognitive Level: Evaluation [Evaluating]

**1557.** PHARM **ANSWER: 4**

1. Although sodium polystyrene sulfonate may be administered as an enema and stool may return, the purpose of the medication is to lower serum potassium levels and not to empty the bowel.
2. The client should be encouraged to retain the enema solution for as long as possible so that sodium ions can be exchanged for potassium ions in the intestine, but its retention for this length of time does not indicate its effectiveness in lowering the serum potassium level.
3. The client may be constipated prior to receiving the enema, but this is not the purpose of a sodium polystyrene sulfonate enema.
4. **Sodium polystyrene sulfonate exchanges sodium ions for potassium ions in the intestine and is administered when the client has hyperkalemia. A normal serum potassium level of 4.0 mEq/L indicates that the medication is achieving its desired therapeutic effect.**

▶ *Test-taking Tip:* If unsure of the medication polystyrene sulfonate, you should use the trade name, Kayexalate, as a clue to the action of the medication. The letter K represents potassium. Only Option 4 relates to potassium.

Content Area: Adult; Concept: Fluid and Electrolyte Balance; Medication; Urinary Elimination; Integrated Processes: Nursing Process: Evaluation; Client Needs: Physiological Integrity: Pharmacological and Parenteral Therapies; Cognitive Level: Evaluation [Evaluating]

**1558.** PHARM **ANSWER: 2, 3, 5**

1. It is unnecessary for the client to monitor the pulse prior to taking thiazide diuretics.
2. **Thiazide diuretics can cause hypokalemia, and potassium-rich foods, such as melons and bananas, can help maintain potassium levels.**
3. **Muscle cramps are a sign of possible medication side effects of hypokalemia and hypocalcemia. Nausea and rash are also medication side effects.**
4. A diuretic taken at bedtime can cause nocturia and loss of sleep. The usual timing of the last daily dose of a diuretic is at suppertime.
5. **Thiazide diuretics can increase serum cholesterol, LDL, and triglyceride levels, so teaching the client to avoid high-fat foods will help maintain cholesterol levels.**

▶ *Test-taking Tip: Thiazide diuretics lower BP through diuresis, which can result in hypokalemia. Focus on the common thiazide diuretic, hydrochlorothiazide (Microzide), and its effects and side effects when reading each of the options.*

Content Area: Adult; Concept: Medication; Fluid and Electrolyte Balance; Nursing Roles; Perfusion; Integrated Processes: Teaching/Learning; Client Needs: Physiological Integrity: Pharmacological and Parenteral Therapies; Health Promotion and Maintenance; Cognitive Level: Application [Applying]

## 1559. PHARM ANSWER: 3

1. Missing doses of medication is important to address; however, duplicate medications should be addressed first.
2. It is important to address the administration routes, but the duplication of medications is the priority to address.
3. **Hydrochlorothiazide + captopril (Capozide) is a combination product. The nurse should first determine if the client is taking the combination product along with the individual products due to the potential for overdosing. The client may be clear regarding the dose and the route but may not realize that two medications were replaced with one combination product.**
4. Drug-drug interactions are important to address and should be addressed, but the duplicate medications are the priority.

▶ *Test-taking Tip: The key words are "most concerned." The greatest safety risk for the client is medication overdosing.*

Content Area: Adult; Concept: Medication; Critical Thinking; Safety; Perfusion; Integrated Processes: Nursing Process: Evaluation; Caring; Client Needs: Physiological Integrity: Pharmacological and Parenteral Therapies; Safe and Effective Care Environment: Safety and Infection Control; Cognitive Level: Evaluation [Evaluating]

## 1560. PHARM ANSWER: 3

1. The cost of enoxaparin is more than twice the cost of the equivalent dose of heparin per injection. Both are available in prefilled syringes for subcutaneous injection.
2. Both enoxaparin and heparin increase aPTT, which affects clotting.
3. **Because enoxaparin is more specific in inhibiting active factor X, the response is more stable, and the effect is two to four times longer than that of heparin.**
4. Enoxaparin is only administered subcutaneously. Heparin can be administered both subcutaneously and intravenously.

▶ *Test-taking Tip: Focus on the issue: the difference between enoxaparin (Lovenox) and heparin. Note that Options 1, 2, and 4 are similar, addressing the supposed benefits of enoxaparin, whereas Option 3 is different, describing enoxaparin's action. The option that is different is usually the answer.*

Content Area: Adult; Concept: Medication; Nursing Roles; Clotting; Integrated Processes: Teaching/Learning; Client Needs: Physiological Integrity: Pharmacological and Parenteral Therapies; Safe and Effective Care Environment: Safety and Infection Control; Cognitive Level: Application [Applying]

## 1561. PHARM ANSWER: 2

1. There is no serum baclofen level.
2. **Baclofen (Lioresal) is used primarily to treat spasticity in MS and spinal cord injuries. The nurse should assess for muscle rigidity, movement, and pain to evaluate medication effectiveness.**
3. Although baclofen can cause urinary urgency, this is not the most important information.
4. Baclofen use is not associated with weight.

▶ *Test-taking Tip: Focus on the actions of baclofen, a medication commonly used in treating symptoms associated with MS.*

Content Area: Adult; Concept: Medication; Assessment; Mobility; Integrated Processes: Nursing Process: Assessment; Client Needs: Physiological Integrity: Pharmacological and Parenteral Therapies; Cognitive Level: Analysis [Analyzing]

## 1562. PHARM ANSWER: 4

1. Clients receiving systemic corticosteroids are at risk for hypertension, not orthostatic hypotension.
2. Constipation is not an adverse effect of corticosteroid therapy.
3. Antihistamine medications are not used before administration of corticosteroids.
4. **Methylprednisolone (Medrol, Solu-Medrol) is a corticosteroid. Therapy with corticosteroids causes hyperglycemia. The blood glucose level should be monitored.**

▶ *Test-taking Tip: Corticosteroids affect carbohydrate metabolism, leading to hyperglycemia.*

Content Area: Adult; Concept: Immunity; Medication; Integrated Processes: Nursing Process: Planning; Client Needs: Physiological Integrity: Pharmacological and Parenteral Therapies; Safe and Effective Care Environment: Safety and Infection Control; Cognitive Level: Synthesis [Creating]

## 1563. PHARM ANSWER: 3

1. Unnecessary doses can cause leukocytosis (WBCs above 100,000/mm$^3$), an adverse effect of filgrastim.
2. A normal neutrophil count is greater than 2000/mm$^3$. Neutropenic precautions and protective wear are unnecessary because the filgrastim has been effective in increasing the neutrophil count.
3. **Filgrastim (Neupogen) is a granulocyte colony-stimulating factor for treatment of neutropenia. Filgrastim is usually discontinued when the absolute neutrophil count reaches 10,000/mm$^3$.**
4. A high-efficiency particulate air (HEPA) or N95 mask rather than a regular mask should be worn if the client is severely neutropenic (less than 100/mm$^3$).

▶ **Test-taking Tip:** *Treatment for neutropenia in the stem is a cue to the correct option. A normal neutrophil count is greater than 2000/mm³.*

**Content Area:** Adult; **Concept:** Medication; Critical Thinking; Cellular Regulation; **Integrated Processes:** Nursing Process: Implementation; **Client Needs:** Physiological Integrity: Pharmacological and Parenteral Therapies; **Cognitive Level:** Application [Applying]

## 1564. MoC PHARM ANSWER: 3

1. A cephalosporin allergy is not a contraindication for receiving albumin.
2. Albumin is commonly given to clients in hypovolemic shock to increase vascular volume and increase the BP.
3. **Albumin is a blood derivative obtained by fractionating pooled venous and placental human plasma. Some people do not accept RBCs due to faith beliefs, and some do not accept blood products such as albumin or plasma.**
4. Albumin is commonly given to clients with ARDS to increase vascular volume when fluid has shifted from the vascular compartment into the cells.

▶ **Test-taking Tip:** *Albumin is used in the treatment of refractory edema, hypovolemic shock, cerebral edema, and ARDS. However, albumin is a blood derivative. Think about the religious group that does not accept blood or blood products.*

**Content Area:** Adult; **Concept:** Diversity; Medication; **Integrated Processes:** Nursing Process: Analysis; Culture and Spirituality; **Client Needs:** Physiological Integrity: Pharmacological and Parenteral Therapies; Safe and Effective Care Environment: Management of Care; **Cognitive Level:** Analysis [Analyzing]

## 1565. PHARM ANSWER: 4

1. Tremors are a side effect if phenylephrine is absorbed systemically.
2. Because phenylephrine absorbed systemically is a vasoconstrictor, hypertension (not hypotension) can occur as a side effect.
3. Miosis is pupil constriction, not an effect of phenylephrine.
4. **Phenylephrine (NeoSynephrine), an adrenergic agonist, produces pupil dilation (mydriasis) by activating alpha₁-adrenergic receptors on the dilator muscles of the iris.**

▶ **Test-taking Tip:** *If unsure of the action of phenylephrine, use the key words "ophthalmoscopic eye examination" to narrow the options. A memory aid to remember the difference between miosis and mydriasis is using the "o" in mi**o**sis to refer to c**o**nstriction and the "d" in my**d**riasis to refer to **d**ilation.*

**Content Area:** Adult; **Concept:** Medication; Assessment; Sensory Perception; **Integrated Processes:** Nursing Process: Assessment; **Client Needs:** Physiological Integrity: Pharmacological and Parenteral Therapies; **Cognitive Level:** Application [Applying]

## 1566. PHARM ANSWER: 1

1. **A side effect of latanoprost (Xalatan), a prostaglandin, includes a heightened brown pigmentation of the iris, which stops progressing when latanoprost is discontinued.**

2. Jaundiced sclera, and not brown iris pigmentation, would suggest the need to evaluate liver function.
3. The brown iris pigmentation from the latanoprost does not usually regress. The brown pigmentation stops progressing when latanoprost is discontinued.
4. Wearing sunglasses will have no effect on the iris pigmentation.

▶ **Test-taking Tip:** *Brown pigmentation of the iris is a side effect of latanoprost.*

**Content Area:** Adult; **Concept:** Medication; Critical Thinking; Sensory Perception; **Integrated Processes:** Nursing Process: Implementation; **Client Needs:** Physiological Integrity: Pharmacological and Parenteral Therapies; Physiological Integrity: Physiological Adaptation; **Cognitive Level:** Application [Applying]

## 1567. PHARM ANSWER:

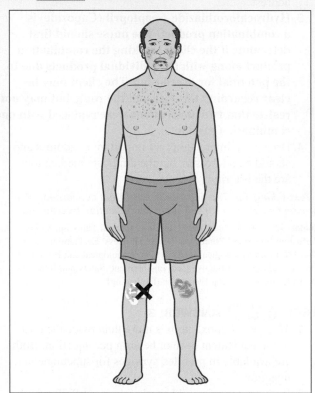

**Psoriasis, a noninfectious inflammatory disorder, is characterized by red, raised patches of skin covered with flaky, thick, silvery scales. Psoriasis vulgaris usually occurs on extensor surfaces of the knees, elbows, and scalp.**

▶ **Test-taking Tip:** *Psoriasis is characterized by flaky, thick, silvery scales. Use this information as a clue to direct you to the correct option.*

**Content Area:** Adult; **Concept:** Medication; Assessment; Skin Integrity; **Integrated Processes:** Nursing Process: Planning; **Client Needs:** Physiological Integrity: Pharmacological and Parenteral Therapies; Physiological Integrity: Physiological Adaptation; **Cognitive Level:** Application [Applying]

**1568. PHARM ANSWER: 4**
1. Although dystonia is an adverse effect of carbidopa-levodopa, akinesia is a symptom associated with PD.
2. Bradykinesia is a symptom associated with PD; agitation is an adverse effect of carbidopa-levodopa.
3. Muscle rigidity is a symptom associated with PD; cardiac dysrhythmia is an adverse effect of carbidopa-levodopa.
4. **Orthostatic hypotension and dry mouth are common adverse effects of carbidopa-levodopa (Sinemet). These can be minimized by slow position changes and sucking on sugarless candy or chewing gum.**

▶ *Test-taking Tip: You should first eliminate options that include a sign or symptom of PD; this will lead you to the answer.*

Content Area: Adult; Concept: Medication; Neurologic Regulation; Integrated Processes: Nursing Process: Analysis; Client Needs: Physiological Integrity: Pharmacological and Parenteral Therapies; Cognitive Level: Application [Applying]

**1569. PHARM ANSWER: 3**
1. Reviewing the method for taking carbidopa-levodopa, including foods to avoid, may be important, but Option 3 is most important. More information is needed to determine whether the client is taking it correctly.
2. A dosage change is unnecessary because it has been only 2 weeks since the client started carbidopa-levodopa.
3. **With oral administration of carbidopa-levodopa (Sinemet), it usually takes 1 to 2 months before an effect is noted, although in some cases it may require up to 6 months.**
4. A high-protein diet can slow or prevent absorption of carbidopa-levodopa. Vitamin $B_6$ increases the action of decarboxylases that destroy levodopa in the body's periphery, reducing the effects of carbidopa-levodopa. Foods high in pyridoxine should be avoided.

▶ *Test-taking Tip: Carbidopa-levodopa has a delayed onset of action.*

Content Area: Adult; Concept: Medication; Neurologic Regulation; Nursing Roles; Integrated Processes: Nursing Process: Implementation; Client Needs: Physiological Integrity: Pharmacological and Parenteral Therapies; Cognitive Level: Analysis [Analyzing]

**1570. PHARM ANSWER: 1, 2, 5**
1. **Benztropine (Cogentin) may be crushed; this statement indicates teaching is effective.**
2. **Many OTC medications contain alcohol. OTC medications containing alcohol should be avoided due to CNS depression and the addictive drowsiness that can occur. This statement indicates teaching is effective.**
3. Benztropine should not be abruptly discontinued; symptoms will recur, and it may precipitate parkinsonian crisis.

4. Benztropine is an anticholinergic that will cause a dry mouth, not drooling and increased secretions.
5. **Because benztropine (Cogentin) is a CNS depressant, driving should be avoided until the effects of the medication are known. This statement indicates teaching is effective.**

▶ *Test-taking Tip: The key words are "teaching is effective." You should select the options that are true statements.*

Content Area: Adult; Concept: Nursing Roles; Medication; Neurologic Regulation; Integrated Processes: Nursing Process: Evaluation; Client Needs: Physiological Integrity: Pharmacological and Parenteral Therapies; Health Promotion and Maintenance; Cognitive Level: Evaluation [Evaluating]

**1571. PHARM ANSWER: 1, 2, 3**
1. **Glatiramer is used to delay the progression of MS. To maximize the therapeutic effects of glatiramer, it should be refrigerated and reconstituted correctly.**
2. **Glatiramer is only administered subcutaneously; accidental IV administration must be avoided.**
3. **Injection sites are rotated to prevent skin breakdown or lumps at the injection sites.**
4. Appropriate subcutaneous injection sites for glatiramer include the thigh, back of the hip, abdomen, and upper arm.
5. Used syringes should be placed in a puncture-resistant container for proper disposal. Syringes and needles should not be reused.

▶ *Test-taking Tip: Focus on the fact that glatiramer (Copaxone) is only administered subcutaneously. Eliminate options that increase the risk for tissue trauma, infection, or injury.*

Content Area: Adult; Concept: Medication; Nursing Roles; Mobility; Integrated Processes: Teaching/Learning; Client Needs: Physiological Integrity: Pharmacological and Parenteral Therapies; Health Promotion and Maintenance; Cognitive Level: Analysis [Analyzing]

**1572. PHARM ANSWER: 2**
1. It is inappropriate to report an expected finding to the HCP.
2. **Carbamazepine XR (Tegretol XR) is a sustained-release medication with a coating that is not absorbed but is excreted in feces and may be visible in stool. The nurse should reassure the client that this is normal.**
3. Collecting the stool for laboratory analysis is not necessary because the coating is not absorbed but excreted in the stool.
4. The nurse should document the client teaching but usually would not document the presence of the coating in the client's stool.

▶ *Test-taking Tip: The abbreviation XR indicates that this is a controlled-release medication. Some controlled-release medications have a coating that is not absorbed in the GI tract.*

Content Area: Adult; Concept: Critical Thinking; Medication; Neurologic Regulation; Integrated Processes: Nursing Process: Implementation; Client Needs: Physiological Integrity: Pharmacological and Parenteral Therapies; Psychosocial Integrity; Cognitive Level: Application [Applying]

**1573.** PHARM **ANSWER: 2, 4, 3, 1, 5**

2. **Fentanyl 0.1 mg IV bolus per PCA. Fentanyl (Sublimaze), the most potent of the medications, is an opioid narcotic analgesic that binds to opiate receptors in the CNS, altering the response to and perception of pain. A dose of 0.1 to 0.2 mg is equivalent to 10 mg of morphine sulfate.**

4. **Morphine sulfate 4 mg IV. Morphine sulfate is also an opioid analgesic. This dose is IV and would be fast-acting.**

3. **Hydromorphone 5 mg oral. Hydromorphone (Dilaudid), another opioid analgesic, would be next in priority. The oral dosing of this medication would indicate that the client's pain is less severe than the client receiving fentanyl or morphine sulfate. Hydromorphone 7.5 mg oral is an equianalgesic dose to 30 mg of oral morphine or 10 mg parenteral morphine.**

1. **Ketorolac 10 mg oral. Ketorolac (Toradol) is an NSAID and nonopioid analgesic that inhibits prostaglandin synthesis, producing peripherally mediated analgesia.**

5. **Propoxyphene 65 mg oral. Propoxyphene (Darvon) should be given last. It binds to opiate receptors in the CNS but is used in treating mild to moderate pain. It has analgesic effects similar to acetaminophen.**

▶ *Test-taking Tip: Focus on ordering the medications starting with the most potent opioid analgesics and ending with the nonopioid analgesic.*

**Content Area:** Adult; **Concept:** Medication; Comfort; Critical Thinking; **Integrated Processes:** Nursing Process: Planning; **Client Needs:** Physiological Integrity: Pharmacological and Parenteral Therapies; **Cognitive Level:** Synthesis [Creating]

**1574.** PHARM **ANSWER: 2**

1. Removing the patch is unnecessary; effective analgesia may take 12 to 24 hours.

2. **The nurse should administer a short-acting opioid analgesic. When the first fentanyl (Duragesic) transdermal patch is applied, effective analgesia may take 12 to 24 hours because absorption is slow.**

3. Transdermal patches should not be rubbed to enhance absorption; it can cause the delivery of the medication to fluctuate.

4. It is premature to request a higher dose of fentanyl.

▶ *Test-taking Tip: Absorption from a fentanyl transdermal patch is slow.*

**Content Area:** Adult; **Concept:** Medication; Comfort; **Integrated Processes:** Nursing Process: Implementation; **Client Needs:** Physiological Integrity: Pharmacological and Parenteral Therapies; Physiological Integrity: Basic Care and Comfort; **Cognitive Level:** Application [Applying]

**1575.** PHARM **ANSWER: 4**

1. Sumatriptan is not used in the treatment of mood alterations.

2. Sumatriptan is not used in the treatment of muscle spasms.

3. Sumatriptan is not used in the treatment of insomnia.

4. **Sumatriptan (Imitrex) is a serotonin receptor agonist and a first-line medication for terminating a migraine or cluster headache attack.**

▶ *Test-taking Tip: The key words are "effective treatment." Sumatriptan is a serotonin receptor agonist. Narrow the options to those pertaining to the brain.*

**Content Area:** Adult; **Concept:** Medication; Comfort; **Integrated Processes:** Nursing Process: Evaluation; **Client Needs:** Physiological Integrity: Pharmacological and Parenteral Therapies; **Cognitive Level:** Evaluation [Evaluating]

**1576.** PHARM **ANSWER: 1**

1. **Piroxicam (Feldene) should be taken with food and a full glass of water to prevent gastric irritation and possible bleeding.**

2. Piroxicam is administered in a once-daily dose, and additional doses should not be taken.

3. Because of the gastric irritation and possible reflux, the client should sit upright after taking piroxicam.

4. Ginkgo interacts with piroxicam, increasing the risk for bleeding.

▶ *Test-taking Tip: You should focus on the gastric irritation that occurs with many anti-inflammatory medications.*

**Content Area:** Adult; **Concept:** Medication; Comfort; Nursing Roles; **Integrated Processes:** Communication and Documentation; **Client Needs:** Physiological Integrity: Pharmacological and Parenteral Therapies; **Cognitive Level:** Application [Applying]

**1577.** PHARM **ANSWER: 2**

**Use a proportion formula; multiply the extremes (outside values) and then the means (inside values), and solve for X.**

**0.5 mg : 1 mL :: 1 mg : X mL; 0.5X = 1; X = 1 ÷ 0.5; X = 2 mL**

**Colchicine (Colcrys) interferes with the function of WBCs in initiating and perpetuating the inflammatory response to monosodium urate crystals.**

▶ *Test-taking Tip: Read how colchicine is supplied. The question is asking for the milliliters to administer in the **first dose**. Double-check your answer, especially if it seems unusually large.*

**Content Area:** Adult; **Concept:** Medication; Comfort; **Integrated Processes:** Nursing Process: Implementation; **Client Needs:** Physiological Integrity: Pharmacological and Parenteral Therapies; **Cognitive Level:** Application [Applying]

**1578.** **PHARM** **ANSWER: 1, 3, 4**

1. **Weight gain and muscle atrophy are body changes that may occur with long-term glucocorticoid therapy.**
2. Muscle wasting (not increased muscle mass) is a side effect of prednisone.
3. **Fragile skin is a possible body change that may occur with long-term glucocorticoid therapy.**
4. **Acne vulgaris may occur with long-term glucocorticoid therapy.**
5. Hirsutism (not alopecia) is a side effect of prednisone.

▶ **Test-taking Tip:** Prednisone (Deltasone) is a glucocorticoid. Use the memory aid that glucocorticoids end in "-sone." Focus on the side effects of glucocorticoids to answer this question.

**Content Area:** Adult; **Concept:** Medication; **Integrated Processes:** Nursing Process: Analysis; **Client Needs:** Physiological Integrity: Pharmacological and Parenteral Therapies; **Cognitive Level:** Knowledge [Remembering]

**1579.** **PHARM** **ANSWER: 2, 3, 5**

1. Grapefruit juice should be avoided because it can increase the concentration of cyclosporine.
2. **Adequate hydration minimizes the risk of adverse effects.**
3. **St. John's wort decreases cyclosporine levels. Echinacea and melatonin interact with cyclosporine to alter immunosuppression.**
4. Methotrexate and cyclosporine can be taken orally instead of by injection. It is incorrect that both medications are taken weekly. Only methotrexate is taken weekly, whereas cyclosporine is usually taken twice daily.
5. **Methotrexate and cyclosporine both have immunosuppressive effects.**

▶ **Test-taking Tip:** Cyclosporine (Gengraf, Neoral, Sandimmune) and methotrexate are immunosuppressant medications. Focus on options related to the immune system.

**Content Area:** Adult; **Concept:** Medication; Nursing Roles; **Integrated Processes:** Teaching/Learning; **Client Needs:** Physiological Integrity: Pharmacological and Parenteral Therapies; Safe and Effective Care Environment: Safety and Infection Control; **Cognitive Level:** Analysis [Analyzing]

**1580.** **PHARM** **ANSWER: 3, 4**

1. Increased muscle spasticity indicates the medication is not effective.
2. Common adverse effects include urinary frequency.
3. **Dantrolene acts directly on skeletal muscles to inhibit muscle contraction, improving mobility.**
4. **Dantrolene acts directly on skeletal muscles to inhibit muscle contraction, improving the ability to maintain balance.**
5. Dantrolene does not increase alertness.

▶ **Test-taking Tip:** Dantrolene (Dantrium) is a direct-acting skeletal muscle relaxant. Consider the symptoms associated with CP.

**Content Area:** Adult; **Concept:** Medication; Assessment; Mobility; **Integrated Processes:** Nursing Process: Evaluation; **Client Needs:** Physiological Integrity: Pharmacological and Parenteral Therapies; **Cognitive Level:** Evaluation [Evaluating]

**1581.** **PHARM** **ANSWER: 0.4**

Use a proportion formula to calculate the correct amount. Multiply the extremes and then the means and solve for $X$.

1 mg : 1 mL :: 0.4 mg : $X$ mL; $X = 0.4$ mL

The nurse should administer 0.4 mL of naloxone (Narcan).

▶ **Test-taking Tip:** Use a medication formula to calculate the correct dosage. Double-check answers that seem unusually large.

**Content Area:** Adult; **Concept:** Medication; Oxygenation; **Integrated Processes:** Nursing Process: Implementation; **Client Needs:** Physiological Integrity: Pharmacological and Parenteral Therapies; **Cognitive Level:** Application [Applying]

**1582.** **PHARM** **ANSWER: 4**

1. Carbohydrate intake, not protein, is more important to consider in diabetic clients in relation to blood sugar levels.
2. Glyburide once daily dose is taken with breakfast, so asking the client about dinner is not consistent with drug administration.
3. Asking the client frequency of checking blood sugar levels will not help determine the possible causes of the client's symptoms.
4. **Alcohol use while taking sulfonylureas such as glyburide (DiaBeta, Micronase) can cause a disulfiram-like reaction, manifested by abdominal cramps, nausea, headache, flushing, and hypoglycemia.**

▶ **Test-taking Tip:** Focus on the key words "most important." Option 4 is the best option because alcohol is contraindicated with use of sulfonylureas due to drug-drug interactions that can lead to hypoglycemia and disulfiram-like symptoms.

**Content Area:** Adult; **Concept:** Medication; Metabolism; **Integrated Processes:** Nursing Process: Assessment; **Client Needs:** Physiological Integrity: Reduction of Risk Potential; Physiological Integrity: Pharmacological and Parenteral Therapies; **Cognitive Level:** Analysis [Analyzing]

**1583.** **PHARM** **ANSWER: 2**

1. Cortisol levels are used to evaluate adrenal and not thyroid function.
2. **Restoration of normal laboratory values for TSH and free $T_4$ indicates that the dose of levothyroxine (Synthroid) is therapeutic.**
3. $T_3$ is used to evaluate the effectiveness of liothyronine and propylthiouracil, used in the treatment of thyroid disorders.
4. The WBC count is used to determine if the client has an infection. Evaluation of serum glucose and potassium levels is unrelated to the use of levothyroxine.

▶ *Test-taking Tip: Levothyroxine is a synthetic preparation of T₄, a naturally occurring thyroid hormone. Thus eliminate Options 1 and 4 and focus on Options 2 and 3.*

**Content Area:** Adult; **Concept:** Medication; Metabolism; Critical Thinking; **Integrated Processes:** Nursing Process: Evaluation; **Client Needs:** Physiological Integrity: Reduction of Risk Potential; Physiological Integrity: Pharmacological and Parenteral Therapies; **Cognitive Level:** Evaluation [Evaluating]

### 1584. PHARM ANSWER: 2

1. The client should check with the HCP about getting vaccinations such as influenza; a chronic condition increases the client's risk for other illnesses and complications.
2. **Stopping mineralocorticoid replacement therapy abruptly may lead to Addisonian crisis. This statement indicates the need for further teaching.**
3. Common adverse effects of fludrocortisone include edema, arrhythmias, and hypertension; stating that he or she should monitor weight, BP, and pulse daily is appropriate.
4. Common adverse effects of fludrocortisone include hypokalemia; stating that he or she should consume potassium-rich foods is appropriate.

▶ *Test-taking Tip: The suffix "-sone" should help you determine that fludrocortisone is a mineralocorticoid that can increase blood glucose levels; however, as a general rule the client should first consult an HCP and not abruptly stop taking a medication.*

**Content Area:** Adult; **Concept:** Medication; Metabolism; **Integrated Processes:** Teaching/Learning; **Client Needs:** Physiological Integrity: Pharmacological and Parenteral Therapies; Health Promotion and Maintenance; **Cognitive Level:** Analysis [Analyzing]

### 1585. PHARM ANSWER:

| Serum Laboratory Test | Normal Value | Client Value |
|---|---|---|
| Glucose **X** | 70–110 mg/dL | 180 mg/dL |
| Potassium **X** | 3.5–5.0 mEq/L | 3.5 mEq/L |
| Calcium **X** | 8.5–10.5 mg/dL | 8.0 mg/dL |
| Platelets **X** | 179–450 K/mm³ | 165 K/mm³ |

**Adverse effects of fludrocortisone (Florinef) include hyperglycemia, hypokalemia, hypocalcemia, and thrombocytopenia. Thyroid hormones of TSH and free T4, although abnormal, are unaffected by fludrocortisone administration. The abnormal thyroid hormones suggest hypothyroidism.**

▶ *Test-taking Tip: The adverse effects of fludrocortisones include those related to the metabolic and hematological systems.*

**Content Area:** Adult; **Concept:** Medication; Assessment; Critical Thinking; **Integrated Processes:** Nursing Process: Evaluation; **Client Needs:** Physiological Integrity: Pharmacological and Parenteral Therapies; Physiological Integrity: Reduction of Risk Potential; **Cognitive Level:** Evaluation [Evaluating]

### 1586. PHARM ANSWER: 2

1. Terbutaline should be used with caution in clients with glaucoma (not strabismus).
2. **The client's history of hypertension warrants the nurse's close monitoring of the client when terbutaline (Brethine) is administered. It should be used with caution in clients with hypertension because it can precipitate a hypertensive episode.**
3. Terbutaline should be used with caution in clients with DM (not DI).
4. Terbutaline should be used with caution in clients with hyperthyroidism (not hypothyroidism).

▶ *Test-taking Tip: Terbutaline is a bronchodilator with relative selectivity for beta-2 adrenergic (pulmonary) receptor sites, with less effect on beta-1 adrenergic (cardiac) receptors. Think about the condition that could be exacerbated by its use.*

**Content Area:** Adult; **Concept:** Medication; Assessment; Critical Thinking; **Integrated Processes:** Nursing Process: Assessment; **Client Needs:** Physiological Integrity: Pharmacological and Parenteral Therapies; Physiological Integrity: Reduction of Risk Potential; **Cognitive Level:** Application [Applying]

### 1587. MoC PHARM ANSWER: 3, 5

1. Symptoms of an asthma attack would include wheezing and other signs of air hunger.
2. Additional signs would need to be present to suspect septicemia, such as an elevated temperature and skin flushing.
3. **Tachypnea, tachycardia, and hypotension are signs of theophylline (Theo-Dur) toxicity. These occur because macrolide antibiotics such as erythromycin inhibit the metabolism of theophylline. Obtaining an order for a theophylline level will expedite the client's treatment.**
4. Symptoms could suggest an allergic reaction, but epinephrine would be prescribed, not diphenhydramine.
5. **Macrolide antibiotics such as erythromycin (E-mycin) inhibit the metabolism of theophylline increasing the risk for theophylline toxicity. A request for a medication change is appropriate.**

▶ *Test-taking Tip: You should note that two options relate to the drugs and are different from the other options. Often the options that are different are the answers.*

**Content Area:** Adult; **Concept:** Medication; Safety; Critical Thinking; **Integrated Processes:** Nursing Process: Analysis; **Client Needs:** Safe and Effective Care Environment: Management of Care; Physiological Integrity: Pharmacological and Parenteral Therapies; **Cognitive Level:** Analysis [Analyzing]

**1588.** PHARM **ANSWER: 0.1**

Use a proportion to determine the amount in milliliters; then multiply the extremes (outside values) and the means (inside values) and solve for X.
5 mg : 1 mL :: 0.5 mg : X mL; 5X = 0.5 mL; X = 0.5 ÷ 5; X = 0.1 mL; the nurse should administer 0.1 mL of epinephrine (Adrenalin).

▶ *Test-taking Tip: Use the calculator provided and double-check the calculations. Remember a subcutaneous injection is likely to be less than 1 mL.*

Content Area: Adult; Concept: Medication; Integrated Processes: Nursing Process: Implementation; Client Needs: Physiological Integrity: Pharmacological and Parenteral Therapies; Cognitive Level: Analysis [Analyzing]

**1589.** PHARM **ANSWER: 2**

1. 0830 is near the time of breakfast in a health care facility. Food reduces the absorption of iron.
2. **For best absorption and therapeutic effectiveness, the nurse should schedule ferrous fumarate (Feosol) at 1000. Iron preparations should be administered 1 hour before or 2 hours after a meal because food diminishes iron absorption.**
3. 1230 is near lunchtime in a health care facility. Food reduces the absorption of iron.
4. 1730 is near the evening meal in a health care facility. Food reduces the absorption of iron.

▶ *Test-taking Tip: Look for the commonalities in options and for the option that is different. All except Option 2 are close to a meal; thus food consumption must affect the absorption of the medication.*

Content Area: Adult; Concept: Critical Thinking; Medication; Integrated Processes: Communication and Documentation; Client Needs: Physiological Integrity: Pharmacological and Parenteral Therapies; Cognitive Level: Application [Applying]

**1590.** PHARM **ANSWER: 1**

1. **The nurse should document the finding of the blood's brownish hue; iron dextran (DexFerrum) may impart a brownish hue to blood drawn within 4 hours after administration.**
2. Drawing blood from another site is unnecessary because iron dextran imparts the brown-colored serum, and the color will be unchanged even if blood is drawn at another site.
3. Notifying the HCP is unnecessary because the brown-colored serum is a normal finding after iron dextran administration.
4. The blood sample should not be discarded because the brown-colored serum is a normal finding after iron dextran administration and will not affect laboratory analysis.

▶ *Test-taking Tip: Iron dextran for administration is brown in color; the brownish hue to the blood is normal and harmless.*

Content Area: Adult; Concept: Critical Thinking; Cellular Regulation; Integrated Processes: Nursing Process: Implementation; Client Needs: Physiological Integrity: Pharmacological and Parenteral Therapies; Physiological Integrity: Reduction of Risk Potential; Cognitive Level: Application [Applying]

**1591.** PHARM **ANSWER: 2**

1. Aspirin increases gastric acid secretion and may worsen symptoms.
2. **The nurse should explore whether the client is taking famotidine (Pepcid) for symptom control. Famotidine blocks histamine-2 receptors on parietal cells, thus decreasing gastric acid production.**
3. NSAIDs, such as ibuprofen (Motrin), do not reduce gastric acid.
4. Desloratadine (Clarinex) blocks only histamine-1 receptors and is not effective against histamine-2 receptors.

▶ *Test-taking Tip: Focus on the classification of medications used to control gastroesophageal reflux, a histamine receptor blocker, to select the correct option.*

Content Area: Adult; Concept: Medication; Digestion; Nursing Roles; Integrated Processes: Teaching/Learning; Client Needs: Physiological Integrity: Pharmacological and Parenteral Therapies; Physiological Integrity: Basic Care and Comfort; Cognitive Level: Application [Applying]

**1592.** PHARM **ANSWER: 1**

1. **Elevation of liver enzymes should be most concerning because drug-induced hepatitis is an adverse effect of cimetidine (Tagamet HB) therapy.**
2. Histamine-2 receptor blockers can cause myelosuppression including thrombocytopenia. A decreased (not increased) platelet count would be concerning.
3. Renal adverse effects of the drug include elevated (not decreased) creatinine and BUN.
4. Cimetidine can increase (not decrease) secretion of prolactin from the anterior pituitary, inducing gynecomastia.

▶ *Test-taking Tip: Remember that many medications affect and are metabolized by the liver.*

Content Area: Adult; Concept: Medication; Digestion; Integrated Processes: Nursing Process: Evaluation; Client Needs: Physiological Integrity: Pharmacological and Parenteral Therapies; Physiological Integrity: Reduction of Risk Potential; Cognitive Level: Evaluation [Evaluating]

**1593.** MoC PHARM **ANSWER: 3**

1. The use of NG suctioning alone would not prevent metoclopramide use. Metoclopramide can be administered through the NG tube; the tube is then clamped for an hour after administration until absorption occurs.
2. Metoclopramide should be used with caution with DM, but it is not contraindicated.

3. The client's history of a seizure disorder would contraindicate the use of metoclopramide. Because metoclopramide (Reglan) blocks dopamine receptors in the chemoreceptor trigger zone of the CNS, it is contraindicated in seizure disorders.

4. Metoclopramide is used in the treatment of nausea and vomiting for clients receiving chemotherapy.

▶ **Test-taking Tip:** *Think about the CNS effects of metoclopramide. Select the only option that is related to the CNS.*

**Content Area:** Adult; **Concept:** Medication; Critical Thinking; Assessment; Digestion; **Integrated Processes:** Nursing Process: Analysis; Communication and Documentation; **Client Needs:** Safe and Effective Care Environment: Management of Care; Physiological Integrity: Pharmacological and Parenteral Therapies; **Cognitive Level:** Analysis [Analyzing]

### 1594. PHARM ANSWER: 1

1. **The nurse's priority should be to administer misoprostol (Cytotec), a gastric protectant, first because it should be taken with meals to minimize diarrhea.**

2. Famotidine (Pepcid), a histamine receptor agonist, should be taken after meals.

3. Cimetidine (Tagamet HB), a histamine receptor agonist, should be taken after meals.

4. Bisacodyl (Dulcolax), a laxative, should be taken at least 1 hour after meals.

▶ **Test-taking Tip:** *A gastric protectant that coats the stomach should be taken before meals. Because there are very few medications that should be taken at specific times, you should learn those medications.*

**Content Area:** Adult; **Concept:** Critical Thinking; Medication; Metabolism; **Integrated Processes:** Nursing Process: Analysis; **Client Needs:** Physiological Integrity: Pharmacological and Parenteral Therapies; **Cognitive Level:** Analysis [Analyzing]

### 1595. PHARM ANSWER: 3

1. Sulfasalazine reduces inflammation and thereby will reduce the number of diarrheal stools.

2. Sulfasalazine, commonly used to treat ulcerative colitis, decreases inflammation in the colon.

3. **This statement indicates the client needs additional teaching. Ulcerative colitis is a chronic illness. Sulfasalazine (Azulfidine) does not cure ulcerative colitis; the only cure is a total proctocolectomy.**

4. Sulfasalazine reduces inflammation and thereby will reduce the incidence of flare-ups from ulcerative colitis.

▶ **Test-taking Tip:** *"Needs further teaching" is a false-response item. Select the incorrect statement. Note that three options are similar and that one is different. Often the option that is different is the answer.*

**Content Area:** Adult; **Concept:** Medication; Nursing Roles; Bowel Elimination; **Integrated Processes:** Nursing Process: Evaluation; **Client Needs:** Physiological Integrity: Pharmacological and Parenteral Therapies; Psychosocial Integrity; **Cognitive Level:** Evaluation [Evaluating]

### 1596. PHARM ANSWER: 4

1. Weight gain, not weight loss, is an intended effect.

2. Pancrelipase is not used to treat abdominal heartburn.

3. Pancrelipase reduces the amount of fatty stools (steatorrhea).

4. **Pancrelipase (Pancreaze) is a pancreatic enzyme used in clients with deficient exocrine pancreatic secretions, CF, chronic pancreatitis, or steatorrhea from malabsorption syndrome. Because it aids digestion, the nutritional status should be improved.**

▶ **Test-taking Tip:** *The key words are "optimal intended benefit." Think about the role the pancreas plays in digestion when selecting the correct option.*

**Content Area:** Adult; **Concept:** Medication; Nutrition; Digestion; **Integrated Processes:** Nursing Process: Evaluation; **Client Needs:** Physiological Integrity: Pharmacological and Parenteral Therapies; Physiological Integrity: Physiological Adaptation; **Cognitive Level:** Evaluation [Evaluating]

### 1597. PHARM ANSWER: 4

1. Client A has vitiligo, a skin disorder characterized by the patchy loss of skin pigment. Vitiligo is treated with topical steroids.

2. Client B has dried herpes simplex, usually treated with the antiviral medication acyclovir.

3. Client C has keloids (hypertrophic scarring), which usually are not treated with medication.

4. **Ganciclovir (Cytovene) is an antiviral medication used in the treatment of recurrent genital herpes.**

▶ **Test-taking Tip:** *The key words are "not healing" and "recurring." Review each illustration and eliminate Options 1 and 3 because these are not recurring lesions. Of Options 2 and 4, determine which illustrates nonhealing lesions.*

**Content Area:** Adult; **Concept:** Medication; Communication; Infection; **Integrated Processes:** Communication and Documentation; **Client Needs:** Physiological Integrity: Pharmacological and Parenteral Therapies; **Cognitive Level:** Analysis [Analyzing]

### 1598. MoC PHARM ANSWER: 1, 5

1. **The nurse should contact the HCP regarding ceftriaxone (Rocephin). Ceftriaxone, a third-generation cephalosporin antibiotic, is 33% to 67% excreted in the urine unchanged. Dosage reduction or increased dosing interval is recommended in renal insufficiency because ceftriaxone is nephrotoxic and can further damage the kidneys.**

2. Insulin glargine (Lantus) is partially metabolized at the site of injection to active insulin metabolites and partially metabolized by the liver, the spleen, the kidney, and muscle tissue; no dose reduction is necessary unless serum glucose levels fluctuate.

3. Diltiazem (Cardizem) is mostly metabolized by the liver; no dose reduction is necessary.

4. Furosemide (Lasix) is 30% to 40% metabolized by the liver with some nonhepatic metabolism and renal excretion as unchanged medication; no dose reduction is necessary.

5. **Captopril (Capoten), an ace inhibitor that blocks the conversion of angiotensin I to angiotensin II, is 50% excreted in the urine unchanged. A 25% dosage reduction is recommended in renal insufficiency to prevent further damage to the kidneys.**

▶ *Test-taking Tip: Think about how medications are excreted from the body. Many antibiotics are nephrotoxic. If unsure, select the antibiotic.*

Content Area: Adult; Concept: Medication; Assessment; Critical Thinking; Urinary Elimination; Integrated Processes: Nursing Process: Implementation; Communication and Documentation; Client Needs: Safe and Effective Care Environment: Management of Care; Physiological Integrity: Pharmacological and Parenteral Therapies; Cognitive Level: Analysis [Analyzing]

## 1599. PHARM ANSWER: 1

1. **A trough level must be drawn before vancomycin (Vancocin) is administered. This is the first action because if the trough level has not been drawn, it will delay the vancomycin dose and could result in a medication error.**

2. Checking medication compatibilities is important, but this can be completed while the laboratory is obtaining the trough level.

3. Checking C&S report results is important, but this can be completed while the laboratory is obtaining the trough level.

4. Calculating the administration rate is important, but this can be completed while the laboratory is obtaining the trough level.

▶ *Test-taking Tip: Note the key word "first" and focus on the situation, "a peak and trough level." Eliminate options that do not pertain to obtaining a peak and trough level.*

Content Area: Adult; Concept: Medication; Critical Thinking; Integrated Processes: Nursing Process: Implementation; Client Needs: Physiological Integrity: Pharmacological and Parenteral Therapies; Cognitive Level: Application [Applying]

## 1600. MoC PHARM ANSWER: 4, 5

1. History of gastric ulcer is not a contraindication for the use of sulfamethoxazole.

2. Type 1 diabetes does not prevent the use of sulfamethoxazole.

3. A positive urine culture would be an indication for using sulfamethoxazole.

4. **Sulfamethoxazole (Bactrim, Septra), a sulfonamide antibiotic, is a category D medication for near-term pregnancy. This means there is positive evidence of human fetal risk, but the benefits from use in pregnant women may be acceptable despite the risk (e.g., for a life-threatening illness or a serious disease for which safer medications cannot be used or are ineffective).**

5. **Sulfamethoxazole will increase the effects of digoxin.**

▶ *Test-taking Tip: First review Option 3 because it is different from the other options. Eliminate this option knowing a positive urine culture would be an indication for antibiotic use. Of the remaining options, think about the conditions that would make the use of this medication most unsafe.*

Content Area: Adult; Concept: Medication; Pregnancy; Critical Thinking; Integrated Processes: Nursing Process: Analysis; Communication and Documentation; Client Needs: Safe and Effective Care Environment: Management of Care; Physiological Integrity: Pharmacological and Parenteral Therapies; Cognitive Level: Analysis [Analyzing]

## 1601. PHARM ANSWER: 2

1. Drinking fluids before inhaler use may moisten the mouth, but it does not prevent oropharyngeal candidiasis.

2. **Oropharyngeal candidiasis is a yeast infection that occurs in the mouth due to destruction of the normal flora with the use of a glucocorticoid inhaler (fluticasone [Advair]). The nurse should instruct the client to rinse the mouth after using the glucocorticoid inhaler to prevent its occurrence.**

3. For best effectiveness, the client should wait 5 minutes between medications, but this has no effect on prevention of oropharyngeal candidiasis.

4. This describes the correct technique for using an inhaler but does not reduce the risk of developing oropharyngeal candidiasis.

▶ *Test-taking Tip: Recall that glucocorticoid medications suppress inflammation and can destroy normal body flora. Think about the medication particles that remain in the mouth after inhaler use and how best to eliminate these.*

Content Area: Adult; Concept: Nursing Roles; Medication; Oxygenation; Integrated Processes: Teaching/Learning; Client Needs: Physiological Integrity: Pharmacological and Parenteral Therapies; Health Promotion and Maintenance; Cognitive Level: Application [Applying]

## 1602. PHARM ANSWER: 4

1. Lispro (Humalog) is a rapid-acting human insulin analog that can be delivered via an insulin pump.

2. Aspart (NovoLog) is a rapid-acting human insulin analog that can be delivered via an insulin pump.

3. Glulisine (Apidra) is a rapid-acting human insulin analog that can be delivered via an insulin pump.

4. **The nurse should question if glargine (Lantus) is prescribed. Glargine is long-duration insulin not suited for delivery by an infusion pump.**

▶ *Test-taking Tip: Only short-duration and short- or rapid-acting types of insulin can be administered through an insulin pump. These insulins can be administered as a slow continuous infusion (basal dose) or as a bolus dose that is triggered manually. Thus select the option with a long-duration insulin.*

Content Area: Adult; Concept: Medication; Metabolism; Critical Thinking; Integrated Processes: Nursing Process: Implementation; Communication and Documentation; Client Needs: Safe and Effective Care Environment: Safety and Infection Control; Physiological Integrity: Pharmacological and Parenteral Therapies; Cognitive Level: Application [Applying]

**1603.** PHARM **ANSWER: 4**

1. Exenatide (Byetta), a synthetic incretin mimetic, is used as an adjunct in type 2 diabetes to decrease blood glucose levels.
2. Pramlintide (Symlin) lowers postprandial glucose levels by slowing gastric emptying.
3. Miglitol (Glyset), an alpha-glucosidase inhibitor, lowers postprandial serum glucose levels.
4. **The nurse should plan to administer glucagon (GlucaGen). Glucagon, administered intramuscularly, intravenously, or subcutaneously, is used in unconscious clients with diabetes to reverse severe hypoglycemia from insulin overdose. Normal serum glucose is 70 to 110 mg/dL.**

▶ **Test-taking Tip:** Eliminate options that will lower the blood glucose level further. If unsure of the hypoglycemic agents, note that two options end in "-tide." Use this clue to eliminate these.

**Content Area:** Adult; **Concept:** Medication; Metabolism; **Integrated Processes:** Nursing Process: Planning; **Client Needs:** Physiological Integrity: Pharmacological and Parenteral Therapies; **Cognitive Level:** Analysis [Analyzing]

**1604.** PHARM **ANSWER: 2, 3, 5**

1. A C&S is unnecessary because orange-colored urine is a normal finding in the client taking rifampin.
2. **The nurse should reassure the client that orange-colored urine is a normal finding in the client taking rifampin (Rifadin).**
3. **The nurse should teach the client that the orange-colored urine and sweat can stain clothing and that the client should consider wearing nonwhite clothing or using undergarments if sweating is excessive.**
4. It is unnecessary to question continuation of rifampin if the urine is orange-colored because this is a normal finding.
5. **The nurse should inform the client that other body fluids, such as tears, sweat, and saliva, can also turn orange-colored with the use of rifampin (Rifadin).**

▶ **Test-taking Tip:** You should be able to narrow the options by noting that Options 1 and 4 suggest that orange-colored urine with rifampin use is an abnormal finding, and that Options 2, 3, and 5 suggest it is a normal finding and that other body fluids can also be affected.

**Content Area:** Adult; **Concept:** Critical Thinking; Medication; Oxygenation; **Integrated Processes:** Nursing Process: Implementation; **Client Needs:** Physiological Integrity: Pharmacological and Parenteral Therapies; Psychosocial Integrity; **Cognitive Level:** Analysis [Analyzing]

**1605.** PHARM **ANSWER: 1**

1. **Ciprofloxacin (Cipro) is a fluoroquinolone antibiotic. Milk or yogurt decreases its absorption and should be avoided.**
2. Bismuth subsalicylate decreases the absorption of ciprofloxacin and should be avoided.
3. Fennel will decrease, not increase, the absorption of the ciprofloxacin.

4. Dietary calcium can be taken at any time; it is unaffected by ciprofloxacin.

▶ **Test-taking Tip:** Select an option that will cause a decreased absorption of ciprofloxacin.

**Content Area:** Adult; **Concept:** Medication; Nursing Roles; Infection; **Integrated Processes:** Teaching/Learning; **Client Needs:** Physiological Integrity: Pharmacological and Parenteral Therapies; Health Promotion and Maintenance; **Cognitive Level:** Application [Applying]

**1606.** PHARM **ANSWER: 2**

1. Drying and crusting of genital lesions would indicate acyclovir's effectiveness for treating genital herpes, not herpes zoster.
2. **Herpes zoster produces painful vesicular skin eruptions along the course of a nerve. Crusting and healing of the vesicular skin lesions indicate that acyclovir (Zovirax) is effective.**
3. Urticaria (swollen, raised areas) and pruritus (itching) are not symptoms of herpes zoster.
4. The lesions of chicken pox are generalized, whereas herpes zoster lesions occur along the course of a nerve. Herpes zoster occurs when the chicken pox (varicella zoster) virus that has incorporated itself into nerve cells is reactivated years after the initial infection, but it is not chicken pox.

▶ **Test-taking Tip:** Apply knowledge of herpes zoster (shingles) to answer this question. Herpes zoster, herpes simplex, and genital herpes are all caused by a virus and develop vesicles, but these occur in different body locations.

**Content Area:** Adult; **Concept:** Medication; Infection; **Integrated Processes:** Nursing Process: Evaluation; **Client Needs:** Physiological Integrity: Pharmacological and Parenteral Therapies; **Cognitive Level:** Evaluation [Evaluating]

**1607.** PHARM **ANSWER: 1**

1. **Both nitrates (nitroglycerin and isosorbide) and sildenafil promote hypotension in the same way. Combining these drugs can cause life-threatening hypotension.**
2. Asking the age of the caller is important because as men age, the dosage of sildenafil should be reduced, but this question is not priority.
3. Clients who take alpha-adrenergic blockers for benign prostatic hyperplasia may also experience a synergistic hypotensive reaction when combining these drugs with sildenafil. This question is important but not the priority.
4. If the caller took more than the recommended dose of 50 mg, the side effects could be more intense. This question is important but not the priority.

▶ **Test-taking Tip:** Focus on the pharmacologic action of sildenafil. The most important question to ask would be a drug interaction that could have life-threatening consequences.

**Content Area:** Adult; **Concept:** Medication; **Integrated Processes:** Nursing Process: Planning; **Client Needs:** Physiological Integrity: Pharmacological and Parenteral Therapies; **Cognitive Level:** Application [Applying]

## 1608. PHARM ANSWER: 2

1. Illustration A is a central line that is percutaneously inserted into the jugular or subclavian vein and terminates in the central circulation. These are intended for short-term venous access.
2. **Illustration B is a PICC, which is inserted into the arm and terminates in the central circulation. A PICC is used when medications or solutions are too caustic to be peripherally administered or when therapy lasts more than 2 weeks.**
3. Illustration C is a tunneled catheter inserted into the upper chest wall and threaded through the cephalic vein; it terminates in the central circulation.
4. Illustration D is an intra-aortic balloon pump catheter that is inserted into the femoral artery and positioned in the descending aortic arch. The balloon on the end inflates during diastole. It is not used for medication or fluid administration.

▶ *Test-taking Tip: Focus on the illustrations. Note that only Options 2 and 4 are peripherally inserted catheters. Then note that only Option 2 is inserted into a vein, whereas the catheter in Option 4 is inserted into an artery.*

Content Area: Adult; Concept: Nutrition; Nursing Roles; Medication; Integrated Processes: Nursing Process: Planning; Client Needs: Physiological Integrity: Pharmacological and Parenteral Therapies; Safe and Effective Care Environment: Safety and Infection Control; Cognitive Level: Application [Applying]

## 1609. PHARM ANSWER: 4

1. Several total nutrient solution bags are kept on hand and require refrigeration.
2. A telephone is necessary for contacting home health personnel, arranging for supply deliveries, and calling emergency services.
3. The TPN is delivered through an infusion pump, which can limit the client's mobility.
4. **The central catheter lumen is capped with a needleless port. The IV infusion tubing is connected to the insertion site cap and not removed to administer the TPN solution. Caps are changed every 3 to 7 days during dressing changes, with the client in a flat position. An air embolus can occur if the cap is removed while the client is in a sitting position.**

▶ *Test-taking Tip: The key words are "further teaching is needed." This is a false-response item. Select the client's statement that is incorrect. Focus on which action could result in a complication.*

Content Area: Adult; Concept: Nursing Roles; Safety; Medication; Integrated Processes: Nursing Process: Evaluation; Client Needs: Physiological Integrity: Pharmacological and Parenteral Therapies; Safe and Effective Care Environment: Safety and Infection Control; Cognitive Level: Evaluation [Evaluating]

## 1610. PHARM ANSWER: 50

Use the formula:

$$\frac{\text{Total mL ordered}}{\text{Total hours ordered}} = \text{mL/hr}$$

$$\frac{1,200}{24} = 50 \text{ mL/hr}$$

▶ *Test-taking Tip: Use the formula for calculating IV flow rates for an infusion pump. Be sure to divide the milliliters per hour by the total hours to arrive at the answer.*

Content Area: Adult; Concept: Medication; Nutrition; Integrated Processes: Nursing Process: Implementation; Client Needs: Physiological Integrity: Pharmacological and Parenteral Therapies; Cognitive Level: Application [Applying]

## 1611. PHARM ANSWER: 1

1. **LR is an isotonic crystalloid solution containing multiple electrolytes in approximately the same concentration as plasma. It enters the cells from the blood, provides fluids, and increases urinary output.**
2. A hypertonic solution draws fluid from the cells into the vascular compartment; LR is isotonic.
3. LR alone does not contain dextrose. Formulations with dextrose are available.
4. Magnesium is not a component of LR.

▶ *Test-taking Tip: Apply knowledge of the components of LR and use the process of elimination. Eliminate Options 3 and 4 because neither dextrose nor magnesium is a component of LR.*

Content Area: Adult; Concept: Medication; Fluid and Electrolyte Balance; Integrated Processes: Nursing Process: Evaluation; Client Needs: Physiological Integrity: Pharmacological and Parenteral Therapies; Cognitive Level: Evaluation [Evaluating]

## 1612. CJ MoC PHARM ANSWER: 1B, 4C, 6E

1. **Cefazolin (Ancef) is a cephalosporin antibiotic. Because the client is allergic to cefuroxime, which is also a cephalosporin antibiotic, the medication should be clarified with the HCP (B). The client's laboratory values are all WNL. Thus options A, D, and F are incorrect reasons for contacting the HCP.**
2. Enoxaparin (Lovenox) is a low-molecular weight heparin. There are no reasons among the options to clarify it with the HCP.
3. Hydrocodone/acetaminophen (Vicodin, Lortab) is a narcotic analgesic. There are no reasons among the options to clarify it with the HCP.
4. **Metoprolol succinate (Toprol-XL) is a beta$_1$-selective (cardioselective) adrenoceptor blocking agent which will lower the HR. The client has a pulse of 50 bpm. The nurse should clarify the medication with the HCP because the client has bradycardia (C).**

5. Pantoprazole (Protonix) is a proton pump inhibitor. There are no reasons among the options to clarify it with the HCP.

6. **Olanzapine (Zyprexa) is an atypical antipsychotic which may be used in combination with other medications to treat depression. Olanzapine doses should not exceed 20 mg/day. The dose is too high and should be clarified with the HCP (E). Also, olanzapine is not indicated for monotherapy to treat depression.**

▶ **Test-taking Tip:** When there is an extensive scenario, it is best to read the questions first, then go to the information. Carefully, analyze the information in regards to the question.

**Content Area:** Adult; **Concept:** Medication; Collaboration; Management; Mobility; **Integrated Processes:** Nursing Process: Evaluation; **Client Needs:** Safe and Effective Care Environment: Management of Care; Physiological Integrity: Pharmacological and Parenteral Therapies; **Cognitive Level:** Evaluation [Evaluating]

# Growth and Development

**1613.** The nurse is preparing to assess a 3-week-old diagnosed with Epstein's pearls at birth. Which photograph illustrates the finding that the nurse should expect to observe if the Epstein's pearls are still present?

1.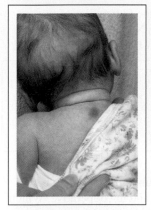

2.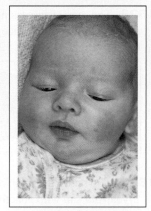

3.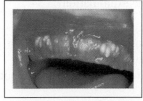

4.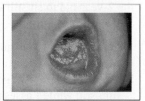

**1614.** The supervising nurse is instructing the student nurse on infant development. Which statements by the student nurse indicate understanding of the "oral phase" in Freud's theory of development? **Select all that apply.**

1. "An infant sucks for nourishment as well as pleasure."
2. "An infant may enjoy breastfeeding more than bottle feeding."
3. "An infant obtains little pleasure in the use of a pacifier."
4. "An infant explores the world through the mouth."
5. "An infant explores the genital area to learn sexual identity."

**1615.** The nurse is taking a BP on the 2-month-old. Which information reflects the nurse's critical thinking? **Select all that apply.**

1. Using too large of a cuff will result in a lower BP reading.
2. The cuff used should cover no more than two-thirds of the upper arm.
3. The normal range for infant and adult BP readings is the same.
4. The reading of the infant's upper arm should be higher than at the thigh.
5. A similar reading on the arm and the thigh could indicate coarctation of the aorta.

**1616.** The nurse is assessing the 3-month-old infant. Based on the infant's developmental age, which motor skill should the nurse expect?

1. Bangs objects held in hand
2. Begins to grab objects using a pincer grasp
3. Grabs objects using a palmar grasp
4. Looks and plays with own fingers

**1617.** The nurse is preparing the immunizations for a 6-month-old baby. The mother says, "My baby is afraid of strangers, including my mother-in-law, and afraid of separating from me. My mother-in-law is upset and thinks I am causing it." Which response by the nurse is **most** appropriate?

1. "Give your baby to strangers while you are present so your baby gets used to them."
2. "Your mother-in-law is correct; you need to include her more in your baby's needs."
3. "Separation anxiety is normal due to development and parent-infant attachment."
4. "Let your baby cry for a while; your baby will get used to being separated from you."

**1618.** The nurse is preparing to obtain the weight of the 6-month-old infant who weighed 7 lb 8 oz at birth. What should the nurse expect the child to weigh at 6 months of age?

_____ lb (Record your answer as a whole number.)

**1619.** The 8-month-old, who is developing appropriately, is hospitalized. The mother is holding the child, who is crying and trying to hide. Which of Erikson's Developmental Stages should the nurse identify as normal for this child?

1. Oral phase
2. Initiative versus guilt
3. Trust versus mistrust
4. Punishment versus obedience orientation

**1620.** The nurse is caring for the 10-month-old. Which nursing action is **most** appropriate for providing tactile stimulation for this child?

1. Caress the child while diaper changing.
2. Give the child a soft squeeze toy.
3. Swaddle the child at nap time.
4. Let the child squash food while sitting in a high chair.

**1621.** Various children are being seen in the clinic for well-baby checks. By what age should the nurse expect a child to begin to use simple words to communicate needs?

1. Age 1–2 years
2. Age 2–3 years
3. Age 6–9 months
4. Age 10–12 months

**1622.** The nurse is evaluating children's weights during a clinic visit. Which child should the nurse conclude has a weight that is normal for the child's age?

1. The child whose weight has tripled in the first 6 months of life
2. The child whose weight has doubled in the first year of life
3. The child whose weight doubled in the first 6 months of life and tripled in the first year
4. The child whose weight doubled in the first 6 months of life and quadrupled in the first year

**1623.** The nurse is teaching the mother regarding the nutritional needs of the 1-year-old. Which type of milk should the nurse recommend to the parent for this child?

1. 2% milk beginning at 1 year of age
2. 1% milk beginning at age 14 months
3. Whole milk until the age of 2 years
4. Skim milk beginning at age 18 months

**1624.** The nurse is assessing the 12-month-old. Which finding should the nurse document as a developmental delay?

1. Unable to lift own head to 90 degrees
2. Can smile and respond to own name
3. Says mama, dada, dog, eat, and milk
4. Unable to feed self with a spoon

**1625.** **PHARM** The nurse is scheduling immunizations for normally healthy children between ages 1 and 5 years who have been on schedule with previous immunizations. Which immunizations should the nurse plan to administer? **Select all that apply.**

1. Inactivated poliovirus
2. Diphtheria, tetanus, pertussis (DTaP)
3. Measles, mumps, rubella (MMR)
4. Hepatitis B (HepB)
5. Human papillomavirus HPV4 series

**1626.** The nurse is assessing the fontanelles of the 20-month-old child. Place an X on the fontanelle that should be closed at 12 to 18 months of age.

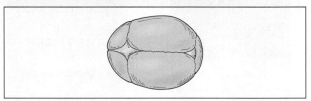

**1627.** The mother is in an examination room with her 2-year-old son who is active and uncooperative. Which statements by the nurse would be helpful in assisting the 2-year-old to sit still for the examination? **Select all that apply.**

1. To the child: "You can choose; do you want to sit in the chair or on the exam table?"
2. To the mother: "I'm going to get another nurse to hold him still while I assess him."
3. To the mother: "Can you hold your son in your lap while I examine him?"
4. To the child: "You can have a toy if you can be good and sit still for me."
5. To the mother: "Putting your son on the exam table will likely keep him still."

**1628.** The mother of the 2-year-old tells the clinic nurse that she is concerned that her child appears to be playing alongside other children but does not play with them. Which response by the nurse is correct?

1. "This type of play is representative of older children and shows your child's maturity."
2. "Some children just do not know how to play with others, but they will learn."
3. "Your child should be evaluated for developmental delays related to playing behaviors."
4. "During this age, children participate in parallel play, so this behavior is expected."

**1629.** During the examination of the 2-year-old, the parents ask the nurse when their toddler should be toilet trained. Which response by the nurse is **most** appropriate?

1. "Children should be placed on the potty chair often so they get used to the task."
2. "Sphincter control and an understanding of the task are needed for toilet training."
3. "Your 2-year-old should be ready to sit on a potty chair for toilet training now."
4. "First put training pants on your child so the child gets used to not wearing a diaper."

**1630.** The clinic nurse is meeting with a mother and her 3-year-old. The child is acting out, and the mother asks what a good form of discipline would be. The nurse recommends a "timeout" for the child. Which explanation regarding the timeout is **most** accurate?

1. "The child should sit still at a timeout for as many minutes as he misbehaved."
2. "The child should sit still at a timeout for as many minutes as the age in years."
3. "The child should sit still and be given a book to read during a 5-minute timeout."
4. "The child should sit for 3 minutes but not be expected to sit still until school age."

**1631.** The nurse reviewed the upper arm BP results for multiple children between the ages of 3 and 5 years. Which BP should the nurse evaluate as being an **abnormal** reading for this age group?

1. 86/42 mm Hg
2. 101/57 mm Hg
3. 112/66 mm Hg
4. 115/68 mm Hg

**1632.** MoC The nurse is assessing 3-year-olds in a clinic for well-child exams. Which observation would require further follow-up?

1. Has 26 respirations in 1 minute
2. Has 20 primary teeth
3. Builds a tower with four blocks
4. Is able to stand on one foot

**1633.** The visual acuity test results for a 4-year-old were 20/40 in both eyes using an Allen picture eye chart. Which nursing action is **most** appropriate?

1. Inform the parents that the child may need glasses.
2. Initiate a referral to an ophthalmologist.
3. Document the visual acuity test results.
4. Retest using the tumbling E eye chart.

**1634.** The nurse is preparing the 4-year-old child for surgery. Based on Erikson's developmental stages, which intervention is appropriate to include in preoperative teaching?

1. Allow the child to make a project related to surgery.
2. Have the child put a surgical mask on a doll.
3. Ask the child to describe feelings about the surgery.
4. Have the child listen to music without interruption.

**1635.** The mother of the hospitalized 4-year-old states, "I'm concerned because my son is sucking his thumb. He hasn't been doing this for 6 months." Which response by the nurse is **most** appropriate?

1. "I don't know why he is sucking his thumb; maybe he needs more attention while hospitalized."
2. "This regression is a normal response to hospitalization. Continue to love and support him."
3. "Is there anything else going on in your family right now that may be causing him to feel anxious?"
4. "Maybe the child wants his father. Are you able to contact him so that he comes for a visit?"

**1636.** The clinic nurse is reviewing the medical record of the 4-year-old. Which information would require further assessment by the nurse?

| Medical Record | | | |
| --- | --- | --- | --- |
| **Tab 1 Health and Physical** | **Tab 2 Growth and Development** | **Tab 3 Growth Chart** | **Tab 4 Vital Sign** |
| Child had chicken pox at 2 years of age | Can dress self without assistance | Weight 48 lb and in the 95th percentile | T 98.6°F (37°C), RR 20, BP 94/60, P 86 |

1. Vital signs
2. Growth chart
3. Health and physical
4. Growth and development

**1637.** The 7-year-old child lived in foster homes until adopted at the age of 1 year by an intact family that provided love and security. Which developmental task should the nurse identify that the child was **most likely** unable to complete as an infant?

1. Trust versus mistrust
2. Industry versus inferiority
3. Autonomy versus shame and doubt
4. Initiative versus guilt

**1638.** The nurse caring for the 9-year-old is planning ways to encourage normal growth and development during the child's hospitalization. Which option would **best** support the child's sense of industry?

1. Allow peers to visit the child in the hospital.
2. Allow the child to decide the time to go to bed.
3. Allow time for completing assigned schoolwork.
4. Allow for independent completion of hygiene.

**1639.** The clinic nurse is completing a school physical on the adolescent girl who is Caucasian. The girl is concerned because she is 13 years old and has not yet started menstruating. Which statement by the nurse would be **most** helpful in addressing the girl's concerns?

1. "The average age to start menstruating is $12^1/_2$ years; some girls are younger, and some are older."
2. "Don't worry; your period will come. You have not yet reached the average age for menstruation."
3. "I can see why you are concerned. Some girls have had their first period already at 10 years old."
4. "This is concerning; I can refer you to a specialist who can further explore this with you."

**1640.** The mother of the 14-year-old asks the nurse about the extended sleeping habits of her child. What is the nurse's **best** response?

1. "Due to the rapid growth during this period, adolescents need additional sleep."
2. "Your child needs to cut back on activities after school, as it is causing stress."
3. "Suggest a bedtime routine; this is important to allow for a good night's sleep."
4. "Have you observed any other behaviors that might suggest illicit drug use?"

**1641.** MoC The nurse is caring for the 14-year-old client hospitalized for dehydration from vomiting. The client is ready for discharge and says to the nurse, "I will tell you something, but you can't tell anyone." Which nursing action is **most** appropriate?

1. Promise the client that that the information will not be told to anyone due to HIPAA laws.
2. Inform the client that the information will remain confidential unless it is life-threatening or harmful.
3. Tell the client that only the physician will be told; otherwise, the information will remain confidential.
4. Ask the client to tell a social worker, who then can follow through with the information if it is concerning.

**1642.** MoC The nurse is triaging clients in a clinic. Prioritize the order in which the nurse should assess the four clients.

1. The 2-week-old healthy newborn being seen for a checkup
2. The 12-year-old male with gynecomastia
3. The 17-year-old with syncope and a BP of 86/62
4. The 6-month-old being seen for teething pain and fever of 99.9°F (37.7°C)

Answer: _____

# Answers and Rationales

**1613. ANSWER: 3**

1. In this illustration, the infant has a flat hemangioma, or "stork bite," at the back of the neck.
2. In this illustration, the infant has milia (white papules) on the face caused by immature sebaceous glands. They will disappear about 2–4 weeks after birth.
3. **This illustration shows that the infant has Epstein's pearls: small, white, pearl-like epithelial cysts on the palate that usually disappear within a few weeks after birth.**
4. This illustration shows *Candida albicans* (thrush), which is characterized by white patches on the tongue. It can be contracted during vaginal delivery.

♦ *Test-taking Tip: If unsure, use the word "pearls" to identify the correct illustration.*

Content Area: Child; Concept: Assessment; Promoting Health; Integrated Processes: Nursing Process: Assessment; Client Needs: Health Promotion and Maintenance; Physiological Integrity: Physiological Adaptation; Cognitive Level: Comprehension [Understanding]

**1614. ANSWER: 1, 2, 4**

1. **An infant has the desire to suck, which may actually build the ego and self-esteem of an infant.**
2. **Breastfeeding expends more energy and is more pleasurable for the infant than bottle feeding. It provides other comforting mechanisms, such as warmth.**

3. According to Freud, an infant finds pleasure in sucking on a pacifier.

4. **An infant explores the world through the mouth, especially the tongue.**

5. A preschooler, not an infant, learns sexual identity through awareness of the genital area.

▶ *Test-taking Tip: Eliminate options that include negative behaviors and one that is not age-appropriate.*

**Content Area:** Child; **Concept:** Promoting Health; Nursing Roles; **Integrated Processes:** Teaching/Learning; **Client Needs:** Health Promotion and Maintenance; **Cognitive Level:** Application [Applying]

## 1615. ANSWER: 1, 2

1. **An appropriately sized cuff should be used on the infant. A cuff that is too large results in a lower BP reading, and a cuff that is too small results in a higher BP reading.**

2. **The cuff should cover two-thirds or less of the arm for an accurate reading.**

3. The normal BP range for infants is much lower than the range for adults.

4. The readings of the upper arm and thigh should be equal or close to equal in an infant. If they are not equal, it could be a sign of coarctation of the aorta.

5. In coarctation of the aorta, the BP in the upper extremities is higher (more than 15 mm Hg) than in the lower extremities.

▶ *Test-taking Tip: Visualize taking a BP measurement on an infant prior to reading each of the options. Use the cue that the "l" in large results in a lower BP reading. This should prompt you to select Options 1 and 2.*

**Content Area:** Child; **Concept:** Assessment; Promoting Health; Nursing Roles; **Integrated Processes:** Nursing Process: Assessment; **Client Needs:** Safe and Effective Care Environment: Safety and Infection Control; Health Promotion and Maintenance; **Cognitive Level:** Application [Applying]

## 1616. ANSWER: 4

1. A 2-month-old infant will hold an object for a few minutes.

2. A 10-month-old infant uses a pincer grasp.

3. A 6-month-old infant uses a palmar grasp.

4. **Three-month-old infants can play with their own fingers. They can reach for objects in front of them, but they usually miss them due to their unpracticed grasp.**

▶ *Test-taking Tip: Awareness of the developmental stages of a 3-month-old will assist with answering this question correctly. Because Options 2 and 3 cannot both be correct, consider these options first and eliminate one or both of them.*

**Content Area:** Child; **Concept:** Promoting Health; Assessment; **Integrated Processes:** Nursing Process: Assessment; **Client Needs:** Health Promotion and Maintenance; **Cognitive Level:** Comprehension [Understanding]

## 1617. ANSWER: 3

1. It is not appropriate to force the baby to be with strangers.

2. The mother needs to be reassured, not told that the mother-in-law is correct. The baby will eventually pass through this stage of separation anxiety.

3. **This response is most appropriate. It is normal for the baby to exhibit separation anxiety at this developmental stage. Mothers are encouraged to have familiar people visit frequently so that babies can safely experience strangers.**

4. The baby doesn't need to cry to get used to strangers.

▶ *Test-taking Tip: Focus on the mother's comment and respond to her comment. The mother is not asking for advice.*

**Content Area:** Child; **Concept:** Promoting Health; Communication; **Integrated Processes:** Communication and Documentation; **Client Needs:** Psychosocial Integrity; **Cognitive Level:** Application [Applying]

## 1618. ANSWER: 15

**By 6 months of age, the child's birth weight should be doubled.**

▶ *Test-taking Tip: Growth is very rapid during the first year of life. Infants typically gain 5 to 7 oz per week. Use the equivalent; 1 pound equals 16 oz.*

**Content Area:** Child; **Concept:** Promoting Health; **Integrated Processes:** Nursing Process: Assessment; **Client Needs:** Health Promotion and Maintenance; **Cognitive Level:** Application [Applying]

## 1619. ANSWER: 3

1. The oral phase is based on Freud's, not Erikson's, theory of development.

2. Initiative versus guilt is a developmental task in the preschool stage.

3. **According to Erikson's developmental stages, trust versus mistrust is appropriate for a child under a year old. The child learns to love and be loved.**

4. Punishment-versus-obedience orientation is not a developmental stage.

▶ *Test-taking Tip: Erikson's developmental theory includes achievement of a task versus nonachievement of a task; thus eliminate Option 1, which does not include the term versus. Of the remaining options, think about the child's reaction of hiding.*

**Content Area:** Child; **Concept:** Promoting Health; Assessment; **Integrated Processes:** Nursing Process: Assessment; Caring; **Client Needs:** Health Promotion and Maintenance; **Cognitive Level:** Application [Applying]

## 1620. ANSWER: 4

1. Caressing during diaper change would be appropriate stimulation for a younger infant.

2. Providing a soft toy would be appropriate tactile stimulation for a younger baby.

3. Swaddling at nap time is an age-appropriate activity for providing tactile stimulation for a younger baby.

4. **The most appropriate action is to let the child squash and mash food. At this age, a child should be ready to touch and manipulate food and is capable of sitting up.**

▶ *Test-taking Tip: You should think about the physical activity of a 10-month-old.*

Content Area: Child; Concept: Sensory Perception; Promoting Health; Integrated Processes: Nursing Process: Implementation; Client Needs: Physiological Integrity: Basic Care and Comfort; Cognitive Level: Application [Applying]

## 1621. ANSWER: 4

1. By age 1 to 2 years, the child communicates in more than simple words, using about 50 words in two-word sentences.
2. At 2 to 3 years, the child's verbal language increases steadily; the child knows his or her full name, can name colors, and can hold up fingers to show age.
3. At 6 to 9 months, the child is learning to make sounds but does not yet communicate using words.
4. **By age 10 to 12 months, a child is able to communicate simple words, using four to six words by 15 months of age.**

▶ *Test-taking Tip: The key word is "begins"; thus eliminate the older age ranges in years.*

Content Area: Child; Concept: Promoting Health; Communication; Integrated Processes: Nursing Process: Assessment; Client Needs: Health Promotion and Maintenance; Cognitive Level: Knowledge [Remembering]

## 1622. ANSWER: 3

1. This child's weight is heavier than expected for the child's age; the weight should double (not triple) in the first 6 months of life.
2. This child's weight is less than expected for the child's age; the child's weight needs to double in the first 6 months, not the first year.
3. **This child's weight is normal for the child's age; the weight doubled in the first 6 months of life and tripled by the end of the first year.**
4. This child's weight is heavier than expected for the child's age; the child's weight should triple, not quadruple, in the first year.

▶ *Test-taking Tip: For their ages, two children are heavier than expected: One is lighter, and one is normal. If unsure of the answer, use this information to narrow the options.*

Content Area: Child; Concept: Promoting Health; Integrated Processes: Nursing Process: Evaluation; Client Needs: Physiological Integrity: Basic Care and Comfort; Cognitive Level: Evaluation [Evaluating]

## 1623. ANSWER: 3

1. Milk that is 2% has reduced amounts of fat and is not recommended for the 1-year-old.
2. Milk that is 1% has reduced amounts of fat and is not recommended for the 1-year-old.
3. **Whole milk until the age of 2 years should be recommended. The child should not have fat intake limited until the age of 2 years. Fats are necessary to ensure myelination of nerve fibers.**
4. Milk that is skim has reduced amounts of fat and is not recommended for the 1-year-old.

▶ *Test-taking Tip: You should select the option that has the highest amount of fat.*

Content Area: Child; Concept: Nutrition; Promoting Health; Integrated Processes: Nursing Process: Assessment; Client Needs: Physiological Integrity: Basic Care and Comfort; Cognitive Level: Application [Applying]

## 1624. ANSWER: 1

1. **Infants at 4 months of age should be able to lift their own head to 90 degrees. By 4 to 6 months, head control should be well established. The nurse should document the inability to lift own head to 90 degrees as a developmental delay.**
2. Smiling and responding to own name are expected achievements of the 6-month-old.
3. The ability to say up to five words is expected in language development at 12 months.
4. Feeding self with a spoon would not be expected until the child is 18 months old.

▶ *Test-taking Tip: You should examine options of what the child is unable to do to arrive at the answer.*

Content Area: Child; Concept: Development; Integrated Processes: Nursing Process: Analysis; Client Needs: Health Promotion and Maintenance; Cognitive Level: Analysis [Analyzing]

## 1625. PHARM ANSWER: 1, 2, 3

1. **Inactivated poliovirus dose three is given between ages 6 and 18 months; dose four between ages 4 and 6 years.**
2. **DTaP dose four is given between 15 and 18 months; dose five between ages 4 and 6 years.**
3. **MMR dose one is given between ages 12 and 15 months; dose two between ages 2 and 6 years.**
4. The hepatitis B vaccine is given to all infants in the United States at birth; a second dose at 1 to 2 months and a third dose at 6 or 18 months.
5. Human papillomavirus HPV4 series is given to males and females in the United States in a three-dose series between the ages of 11 and 12 years.

▶ *Test-taking Tip: If uncertain, recognize that there is a 5-year span of time in the question.*

Content Area: Child; Concept: Immunity; Promoting Health; Nursing Roles; Medication; Integrated Processes: Teaching/Learning; Client Needs: Health Promotion and Maintenance; Physiological Integrity: Pharmacological and Parenteral Therapies; Cognitive Level: Application [Applying]

## 1626. ANSWER:

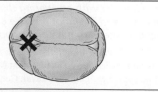

**The anterior fontanelle normally closes at 12 to 18 months of age. The posterior fontanelle closes by 6 to 8 weeks of life.**

♦ *Test-taking Tip: The anterior fontanelle is the soft spot located in the anterior aspect of the skull at the site where the frontal bones and the parietal bones meet.*

**Content Area:** Child; **Concept:** Promoting Health; Neurologic Regulation; Assessment; **Integrated Processes:** Nursing Process: Assessment; **Client Needs:** Health Promotion and Maintenance; **Cognitive Level:** Application [Applying]

## 1627. ANSWER: 1, 3

1. **Letting the child choose what is best allows the child to be a part of the decision.**
2. Holding any child down instead of talking the child through the process increases the child's anxiety and uncooperativeness.
3. **Letting the mother be involved in the process shows the child that he won't be separated from his mother.**
4. Bribing a child with a future reward does not help him to adjust to the present situation.
5. Placing the uncooperative child on the examining table increases the child's risk for injury from a fall.

♦ *Test-taking Tip: Distractions and presenting choices are age-appropriate interventions.*

**Content Area:** Child; **Concept:** Promoting Health; **Integrated Processes:** Communication and Documentation; Caring **Client Needs:** Health Promotion and Maintenance; **Cognitive Level:** Analysis [Analyzing]

## 1628. ANSWER: 4

1. Older children participate in associative play within groups of peers.
2. Children progress through stages of play beginning at infancy.
3. Play would be one area evaluated for developmental delays, but not a sole evaluation.
4. **This response is correct; based upon social development of children, parallel play is expected.**

♦ *Test-taking Tip: Playing with peers is achieved through developmental stages.*

**Content Area:** Child; **Concept:** Promoting Health; Communication; **Integrated Processes:** Nursing Process: Implementation; **Client Needs:** Health Promotion and Maintenance; **Cognitive Level:** Application [Applying]

## 1629. ANSWER: 2

1. A 2-year-old may not want to sit on a toilet when he or she does not feel it is necessary.
2. **This response is most appropriate. Sphincter control, an understanding of the task, and the ability to delay immediate gratification are needed for toilet training to occur. The child's development is cephalocaudal, and therefore the child's body may not be able to control the rectal and urethral sphincters if started too soon.**
3. There is no set age for potty training. Each child is different in his or her development.
4. Training pants will not help if the child is not physiologically ready for controlling his or her bladder.

♦ *Test-taking Tip: All options except one give advice. Often the option that is different is the answer.*

**Content Area:** Child; **Concept:** Promoting Health; Nursing Roles; **Integrated Processes:** Teaching/Learning; **Client Needs:** Physiological Integrity: Basic Care and Comfort; **Cognitive Level:** Analysis [Analyzing]

## 1630. ANSWER: 2

1. The child should not have his timeout related to his minutes of misbehaving because the timeout may be too long an expectation.
2. **Three minutes may not seem long to an adult, but to a toddler, 3 minutes is an excellent form of discipline because it seems like a long time to be restricted from activity.**
3. The timeout is a form of discipline, and reading a book should not be related to misbehaving. Reading a book should be a reward. A 5-minute timeout is too long for a 3-year-old.
4. A 3-year-old can be expected to sit still for short periods of time.

♦ *Test-taking Tip: Eliminate Options 3 and 4 because these are different from the other options. Of the two remaining options, use the child's age as a guide to selecting Option 2.*

**Content Area:** Child; **Concept:** Promoting Health; Nursing Roles; **Integrated Processes:** Teaching/Learning; **Client Needs:** Psychosocial Integrity; **Cognitive Level:** Application [Applying]

## 1631. ANSWER: 1

1. **A BP reading of 86/47 mm Hg has a MAP of 60, indicating insufficient perfusion to tissues.**
2. The mean BP for the child 2 to 5 years is 101/57 (MAP = 74).
3. The 90th percentile BP is 112/66 mm Hg (MAP = 82).
4. The 95th percentile is 115/68 mm Hg (MAP = 85).

♦ *Test-taking Tip: If unsure of the BP values for this age group, calculate the MAP = (SBP + 2DBP) ÷ 3, and then select the option with a low MAP.*

**Content Area:** Child; **Concept:** Assessment; Promoting Health; Development; **Integrated Processes:** Nursing Process: Analysis; **Client Needs:** Physiological Integrity: Reduction of Risk Potential; **Cognitive Level:** Evaluation [Evaluating]

## 1632. MoC ANSWER: 3

1. The RR range of a 3-year-old is 18–35 respirations per minute.
2. By age 3, approximately 20 primary teeth should be seen.
3. **At age 3, the child should be able to build a tower consisting of 9–10 blocks; building a tower of only four blocks may require further follow-up to identify a developmental delay.**
4. By age 3, a child has improved coordination and should be able to stand on one foot for at least 10 seconds.

♦ *Test-taking Tip: An abnormal finding would require further follow-up. You need to consider the development of a 3-year-old to identify an abnormal finding.*

Content Area: Child; **Concept:** Nursing Roles; Assessment; Integrated Process: Nursing Process: Evaluation; **Client Needs:** Safe and Effective Care Environment: Management of Care; **Cognitive Level:** Evaluation [Evaluating]

## 1633. ANSWER: 3

1. Informing the parents about the need for glasses is inappropriate at this time. If the results are greater than 20/20 by age 6, then glasses may be needed.
2. A referral would be initiated if the results were greater than 20/40.
3. **A visual acuity test result of 20/40 would be considered normal for a 4-year-old. The nurse should document the results.**
4. An Allen picture eye chart is a developmentally appropriate chart for eye testing; there is no need to retest using the tumbling E eye chart, which could be confusing for a 4-year-old.

▶ **Test-taking Tip:** Focus on the child's developmental age. The child's visual acuity is normally not fully developed at 4 years of age.

Content Area: Child; **Concept:** Sensory Perception; Promoting Health; Integrated Processes: Nursing Process: Implementation; **Client Needs:** Health Promotion and Maintenance; **Cognitive Level:** Evaluation [Evaluating]

## 1634. ANSWER: 2

1. The child is too young to do a project related to surgery.
2. **The child can practice putting a mask on the doll. This allows the child to feel the mask and know how it will fit on the doll and can reduce the child's anxiety.**
3. The child is not old enough to verbalize his feelings related to the surgery.
4. Music may help, but it cannot replace appropriate preoperative teaching based on the child's developmental stage.

▶ **Test-taking Tip:** Focus on the age of the child. Recall that a 4-year-old likes doing things and relieves tension through play. Eliminate all options except option 2, which is related to play.

Content Area: Child; **Concept:** Nursing Roles; Assessment; Promoting Health; Perioperative; **Integrated Processes:** Nursing Process: Implementation; **Client Needs:** Physiological Integrity: Basic Care and Comfort; **Cognitive Level:** Application [Applying]

## 1635. ANSWER: 2

1. Thumb-sucking does not indicate that the child is not getting enough attention.
2. **It is common for preschoolers to revert to a behavior they have outgrown to cope with difficult situations. Sucking a thumb is a comfort measure.**
3. This question is intrusive and unnecessary. Thumb-sucking does not mean there are other contributing factors.
4. The hospitalization is enough stress in a child's life. Having a father present may or may not be helpful to the child.

▶ **Test-taking Tip:** Consider the developmental stages of the 4-year-old and the information that the child is hospitalized.

Content Area: Child; **Concept:** Development; Stress; **Integrated Processes:** Communication and Documentation; **Client Needs:** Psychosocial Integrity; **Cognitive Level:** Application [Applying]

## 1636. ANSWER: 2

1. The vital signs are within expected ranges for a 4-year-old.
2. **The data from the growth chart should initiate further assessment by the nurse. Because childhood obesity is becoming more prevalent, it is important to monitor the growth of children. The nurse should further assess nutritional and exercise habits and provide teaching on health promotion.**
3. Past medical history is good to note but would not require additional assessment by the nurse.
4. The ability to dress independently is an expected milestone of growth and development at this age.

▶ **Test-taking Tip:** An abnormal finding would require further assessment.

Content Area: Child; **Concept:** Development; Assessment; **Integrated Processes:** Nursing Process: Analysis; **Client Needs:** Health Promotion and Maintenance; Physiological Integrity: Reduction of Risk Potential; **Cognitive Level:** Analysis [Analyzing]

## 1637. ANSWER: 1

1. **Because the child lived in multiple foster homes with many caregivers, the child may not have learned to love and be loved as an infant and may have had delayed development in trust.**
2. Industry versus inferiority occurs in the school-aged child. Children learn how to do things well, such as assembling and completing a short project.
3. Autonomy versus shame and doubt occurs in toddlers. Children begin to want to be independent and complete activities by themselves.
4. Initiative versus guilt takes place in the preschool-aged child. Children begin to initiate activities rather than solely responding to or mimicking the actions of others.

▶ **Test-taking Tip:** Focusing on the developmental stage of an infant and not that of a 7-year-old child should lead you to select Option 1.

Content Area: Child; **Concept:** Development; Critical Thinking; **Integrated Processes:** Nursing Process: Analysis; **Client Needs:** Psychosocial Integrity; **Cognitive Level:** Analysis [Analyzing]

## 1638. ANSWER: 3

1. Allowing peers to visit is much more important for children ages 12 to 20, who are gaining a sense of identity.
2. Choices in bedtime do not affect psychosocial development.
3. **Through acquiring skills in reading, writing, and mathematics, children gain a sense of industry.**

4. Completing hygiene routines independently supports autonomy versus shame and doubt and is not an example of industry.

▶ *Test-taking Tip:* You should narrow the options to those in which a task is completed and then decide which is most appropriate for the 9-year-old.

**Content Area:** Child; **Concept:** Promoting Health; Perioperative; **Integrated Processes:** Nursing Process: Implementation; **Client Needs:** Health Promotion and Maintenance; **Cognitive Level:** Application [Applying]

### 1639. ANSWER: 1

1. **This response most directly answers the girl's question and provides the average age of 12¹/₂ years to start menstruating. The onset of menstruating can vary by ethnicity and weight. African-American girls have been reported to have an earlier age at menarche than do European-American girls.**
2. It is demeaning to make comments such as "don't worry about it."
3. It is unnecessary to remind the client when some girls begin menstruating.
4. There is no need for a specialist; the girl is within the normal age range for the onset of menarche.

▶ *Test-taking Tip:* Use principles of therapeutic communication. Eliminate options that are nontherapeutic.

**Content Area:** Child; **Concept:** Development; Communication; Promoting Health; Diversity; **Integrated Processes:** Communication and Documentation; Caring; Culture and Spirituality; **Client Needs:** Psychosocial Integrity; **Cognitive Level:** Application [Applying]

### 1640. ANSWER: 1

1. **This statement is the nurse's best response. Adolescents experience a growth spurt, and the body requires additional sleep.**
2. Stress is not the cause of the additional sleep needs. Even though there is a change in social activities during the period that might affect the amount of sleep obtained on a nightly basis, cutting back on activities may not influence the amount of sleep needed.
3. A bedtime routine is not appropriate for this age. Adolescents tend to want to stay up late and sleep in.
4. The nurse is making an inappropriate conclusion and is not addressing the concerns regarding sleeping.

▶ *Test-taking Tip:* Focus on communication techniques that address the mother's concern of an adolescent needing additional sleep.

**Content Area:** Child; **Concept:** Promoting Health; Communication; **Integrated Processes:** Nursing Process: Assessment; Communication and Documentation; **Client Needs:** Physiological Integrity: Basic Care and Comfort; **Cognitive Level:** Application [Applying]

### 1641. MoC ANSWER: 2

1. The HIPAA law does not state that all information is to remain confidential.
2. **The information can remain confidential unless there is abuse involved or if there are other legal implications.**
3. The nurse should not tell the physician unless the information is life-threatening or could potentially result in harm to the client or others.
4. The client may not feel comfortable with the social worker. Nurses and social workers have the same obligation to report the information if it is life-threatening or harmful.

▶ *Test-taking Tip:* Thinking about the legal requirements for reporting information should direct you to select Option 2.

**Content Area:** Child; **Concept:** Safety; Communication; Legal; **Integrated Processes:** Communication and Documentation; Caring; **Client Needs:** Safe and Effective Care Environment: Management of Care; **Cognitive Level:** Application [Applying]

### 1642. MoC ANSWER: 3, 4, 1, 2

3. **A 17-year-old with syncope and a BP of 86/62 has priority because the teenager is symptomatic with a low BP.**
4. **A 6-month-old being seen for teething pain and fever of 99.9°F (37.7°C). Even though this is a normal occurrence, an assessment is needed to rule out other possible complications, and the caregiver may need reassurance.**
1. **The 2-week-old healthy newborn being seen for a checkup. The 2-week-old infant does not have a built-up immune system and therefore should be seen quickly to reduce exposure to infectious disease processes. The caregivers may also have several questions or concerns that would need to be addressed by the nurse.**
2. **The 12-year-old male with gynecomastia. Even though gynecomastia may be causing psychosocial distress, this is a benign process that is often self-limiting.**

▶ *Test-taking Tip:* First use your ABC's to answer this question and select Option 3 due to circulation. Then use the process of elimination to decide which client is ill or experiencing an acute episode and should be seen next. When deciding between the final two options, look at the ages and apply Maslow's Hierarchy of Needs.

**Content Area:** Child; **Concept:** Critical Thinking; Management; **Integrated Processes:** Nursing Process: Planning; **Client Needs:** Safe and Effective Care Environment: Management of Care; Physiological Integrity: Reduction of Risk Potential; **Cognitive Level:** Synthesis [Creating]

## Chapter Thirty-Seven

# Cardiovascular Management

**1643.** **MoC** The nurse completes an assessment of the 2-month-old infant during a well-child checkup. The nurse should report which finding to the HCP?

1. Split $S_2$ heart sound
2. Apical HR of 140 bpm
3. Oxygen saturation of 97%
4. Femoral pulse 3+, brachial pulse 2+

**1644.** The 6-month-old being seen in the clinic has an HR of 167 bpm, RR of 65 bpm, and $SpO_2$ of 98%. The mother states the infant gets very tired with feedings, eating approximately 2 ounces every 4 hours. Which action should be the nurse's **priority**?

1. Check peripheral capillary refill time.
2. Auscultate for bowel sounds.
3. Auscultate for a heart murmur.
4. Attempt to bottle-feed the infant.

**1645.** The nurse is using a picture to educate the parents of the child with a congenital murmur about the etiology of the condition. Which location should the nurse identify to the child's parents for a murmur occurring at the tricuspid valve?

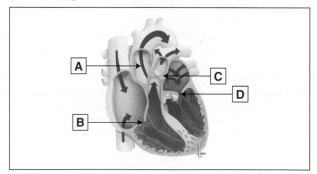

1. A
2. B
3. C
4. D

**1646.** The nurse is caring for the child who has liver enlargement secondary to infective endocarditis. The nurse should assess the child for which associated complication?

1. Pulmonary hypertension
2. Right-sided heart failure
3. Myocardial infarction
4. Tetralogy of Fallot

**1647.** **PHARM** The nurse is instructing the parents about the care of their infant with an unrepaired heart defect. Which information should the nurse include?

1. "Obtain monthly palivizumab injections during the RSV season."
2. "Restrict physical activity to avoid fatigue."
3. "Restrict caloric intake to minimize weight gain."
4. "Delay immunizations until the defect is repaired."

**1648.** The nurse is teaching the parents of the child with a history of hypoxemia. The nurse should instruct the parents to immediately notify the HCP if the child is experiencing which manifestation(s)?

1. Weight loss or gain
2. Excessive fussiness and crying
3. Dehydration and respiratory infection
4. Not achieving developmental milestones

**1649.** **PHARM** The 18-month-old, hospitalized with uncorrected cyanotic heart disease, experiences a hypercyanotic spell. Which actions should be taken by the nurse? **Select all that apply.**

1. Place the child in a knee-chest position.
2. Administer 2 L of oxygen via nasal cannula.
3. Administer intramuscular morphine sulfate.
4. Use a calm and comforting approach.
5. Administer oral propranolol if prescribed.

**1650.** The nurse is planning care for the infant with tetralogy of Fallot. Which intervention should the nurse include to **best** promote adequate nutrition?

1. Administer prostaglandin $E_1$ to keep fetal ducts open.
2. Provide rest periods to allow adequate digestion.
3. Administer fortified breast milk every 3 hours.
4. Encourage sips of water between feedings.

**1651.** The nurse is discussing the infant's diagnosis of hypoplastic left heart syndrome (HLHS) with the parents. The father states, "Shouldn't this get better when the heart grows in size with the baby?" How should the nurse respond to the father?

1. "The growth of the heart does not repair the problem of the small left ventricle."
2. "Surgery is needed; we are doing everything we can to save your baby's life."
3. "Your baby is very sick; many surgical procedures are needed for survival."
4. "The heart does not grow much in early childhood, so it still needs to be fixed."

**1652.** MoC The nurse is assessing the 3-month-old following the first surgery to repair hypoplastic left heart syndrome (HLHS). Which assessment findings require immediate intervention or notification of the HCP? **Select all that apply.**

1. HR of 120 bpm
2. Grade III heart murmur
3. Severe intercostal retractions
4. Oxygen saturation 80%
5. Hematocrit level 69%

**1653.** MoC The nurse is caring for the 12-kg child following cardiac surgery. The chest tube drainage totals 200 mL for the past hour. Which is the nurse's **best** action?

1. Check to be sure that the connections are secure.
2. Document the drainage and continue to monitor.
3. Tip and tilt the tube to promote adequate drainage.
4. Assess the child and notify the HCP immediately.

**1654.** The nurse is planning discharge teaching for parents of the child who had cardiac surgery. Which information should the nurse include in the discharge teaching? **Select all that apply.**

1. Taking the child's pulse before giving beta blocker medications
2. Contacting the HCP for a temperature greater than 100.3°F (37.9°C)
3. Preventing anyone from pulling the child up using the child's arms
4. Preparing an age-appropriate diet with vitamin C to promote wound healing
5. Taking prophylactic antibiotics before dental care to prevent pericarditis

**1655.** The 3-week-old is diagnosed with a patent ductus arteriosis (PDA). Which should the nurse include when teaching the parents about this condition? **Select all that apply.**

1. Prostaglandin $E_1$ ($PGE_1$) is prescribed to help close the PDA.
2. The infant has an increased risk of bacterial endocarditis.
3. There is increased pressure on the right side of the heart.
4. Blood is being shunted from the aorta back to the lungs.
5. Children with a PDA often have a heart murmur.

**1656.** MoC The nurse assesses the 6-kg infant following surgery to correct a VSD. In what order should the nurse address the assessment findings? Place the assessment findings in the order of priority.

1. Hemoglobin level of 25 g/dL
2. Chest tube drainage of 15 mL/kg in 1 hour
3. Pulse oximeter reading of 90%
4. Urine output of 20 mL over the past 2 hours

Answer: _____

**1657.** The nurse is questioning the 12-year-old who has frequent headaches and nosebleeds. Which focused assessments should the nurse include to **rule out** coarctation of the aorta? **Select all that apply.**

1. BP in all four extremities
2. Pulse quality of all four extremities
3. Deep palpation of the liver
4. Vision screening with a Snellen chart
5. Temperature and color of extremities

**1658.** The ED nurse is assessing the pediatric client with a tentative diagnosis of acute pericarditis. Which assessment finding should the nurse conclude supports acute pericarditis?

1. Bilateral lower-extremity pain
2. Pain on expiration
3. Pleural friction rub
4. Pericardial friction rub

**1659.** MoC The new nurse is preparing the pediatric client for a cardiac catheterization under the supervision of the experienced nurse. Which parameters, if identified by the new nurse, demonstrate understanding of the information that can be collected during cardiac catheterization? **Select all that apply.**

1. Oxygen saturation of blood within the heart chambers
2. Pressure of blood flow within the heart chambers
3. Cardiac output
4. Anatomical abnormalities
5. Ankle brachial index (ABI)
6. Ejection fraction

**1660.** The nurse is completing discharge teaching with the parents and their child who underwent a cardiac catheterization through the left femoral artery 8 hours ago. Which information should the nurse include? **Select all that apply.**

1. Check pulses on the affected leg hourly.
2. Call the HCP if the left foot is cooler than the right.
3. Encourage the child to drink fluids as tolerated.
4. Allow only quiet play activities until tomorrow.
5. Call the HCP if the child develops a fever.

**1661.** The nurse is caring for the 13-year-old client recently diagnosed with hypertension. Which diagnostic tests should the nurse anticipate being prescribed for this client? **Select all that apply.**

1. Complete blood count (CBC)
2. Serum chemistry
3. Renal ultrasound
4. Drug screen
5. Glucose tolerance test (GTT)

**1662.** PHARM The nurse is preparing to administer newly prescribed medications to the pediatric client with hypertension. Which medication classification, if prescribed, should the nurse question?

1. ACE inhibitor
2. Calcium channel blocker
3. Diuretic
4. Nitrate

**1663.** MoC The nurse is assessing the 1-month-old with HF. Which findings should alert the nurse to notify the HCP due to possible complications? **Select all that apply.**

1. HR of 145 bpm when asleep
2. Weight is the same as the birth weight
3. Breathing 70 times per minute at rest
4. BP of 90/60 mm Hg at rest
5. Absence of sweating when agitated and crying

**1664.** PHARM The nurse is managing the care of the pediatric client in CHF. Which medically delegated interventions should the nurse expect to include in the child's plan of care? **Select all that apply.**

1. Oral positive inotropic agents
2. Diuretic medications
3. ACE inhibitor medications
4. Hypolipidemic medications
5. Oral positive chronotropic agents
6. Beta blocker medications

**1665.** PHARM The nurse administers a calcium channel blocker to the 10-year-old who has fatigue and dependent edema from HF. The child's BP is 108/65 mm Hg. Which finding **best** indicates that the medication has had the desired therapeutic effect?

1. Voids 300 mL one hour after administration
2. BP decreases to 90/52 mm Hg
3. Able to do physical therapy without fatigue
4. Clubbing in the extremities begins to disappear

**1666.** The nurse is feeding the infant with HF. Which intervention should the nurse implement?

1. Hold the infant at a 45-degree angle for feeding.
2. Burp the infant only after completing the feeding.
3. Space feedings 6 hours apart to reduce fatigue.
4. Administer feedings only through a feeding tube.

**1667.** MoC PHARM The child with a cardiac defect is taking digoxin and captopril. The child is hospitalized with severe edema, and furosemide is prescribed. When reviewing the laboratory findings on day 3, which complication should be the nurse's concern and prompt notifying the HCP?

|  | Serum Lab Result Day 1 | Serum Lab Result Day 3 |
| --- | --- | --- |
| Digoxin | 0.9 ng/mL | 2.0 ng/mL |
| Potassium | 5.3 mEq/L | 3.4 mEq/L |
| Sodium | 150 mEq/L | 143 mEq/L |

1. Dehydration
2. Hyponatremia
3. Digoxin toxicity
4. Hyperkalemia

**1668.** The nurse assesses that the newly admitted pediatric client has tachycardia, edema, dyspnea, orthopnea, and crackles. The nurse should plan interventions to treat which possible condition?

1. Right-sided heart failure
2. Rheumatic fever
3. Kawasaki disease
4. Left-sided heart failure

**1669.** **PHARM** The nurse receives an order to administer digoxin 10 micrograms/kilogram (mcg/kg) orally to an 8-lb full-term infant. How many mcg should the nurse administer?

_____ mcg (Record your answer as a whole number.)

**1670.** **MoC** **PHARM** Prior to administering digoxin to the 6-year-old with HF, the nurse reviews the child's serum laboratory report. Which value should concern the nurse and be reported to the HCP?

1. Potassium 3.2 mEq/L
2. Hemoglobin 10 g/dL
3. Digoxin level 1.8 ng/mL
4. Creatinine 0.3 mg/dL

**1671.** **PHARM** Before administering oral digoxin to the pediatric client, the nurse assesses that the child has bradycardia and mild vomiting. Which is the nurse's **most** appropriate action?

1. Explain to the parent that bradycardia is an expected effect of the digoxin.
2. Give digoxin, document the observations, and reevaluate after the next dose.
3. Withhold digoxin and notify the HCP, as these signs indicate toxicity.
4. Give both the oral beta blocker that is prescribed now and the digoxin.

**1672.** **PHARM** The nurse is educating the adolescent client about simvastatin. Which information should the nurse include when teaching the client?

1. Contact the HCP if having new-onset muscle aches or dark urine.
2. Simvastatin is being prescribed to lower HDL cholesterol levels.
3. Take simvastatin in the morning when it is most effective.
4. Common side effects include sleepiness and altered taste.

**1673.** The nurse is educating the parents of the pediatric client in preparation for their child's home ECG monitoring. The nurse uses a picture to explain the different components of a normal ECG tracing. Place an X on the illustration where the nurse should be pointing when explaining repolarization of the ventricles.

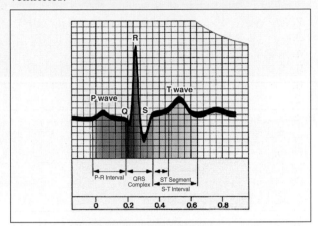

**1674.** The nurse is interpreting an ECG rhythm strip for the 2-year-old child with a congenital heart defect. The measurement for the PR interval is 0.26 seconds; the QRS is 0.08 seconds, and the QT is 0.28. The ventricular rate is 126 bpm. How should the nurse document the child's rhythm?

1. Sinus bradycardia
2. Sinus rhythm with a bundle branch block
3. Sinus rhythm with a first-degree AV block
4. Sinus tachycardia with a first-degree AV block

**1675.** The nurse is caring for multiple children with the rhythms illustrated. The nurse should activate the emergency response system when observing which ECG rhythm?

1.

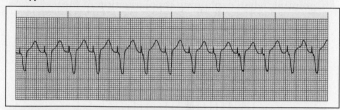

2.

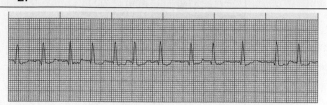

3.

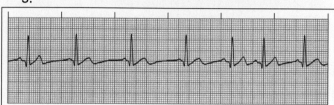

4.

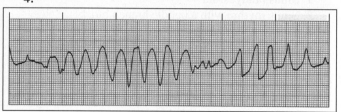

**1676.** The pediatric client receives treatment to convert a supraventricular tachycardia (SVT) rhythm to a sinus rhythm. The nurse instructs the child's parents on interventions to terminate the SVT rhythm should the rhythm recur. Which information stated by a parent indicates further teaching is needed?

1. Wrap the child's head with a cold, wet towel.
2. Massage both of the child's carotid arteries.
3. Have the child perform the Valsalva maneuver.
4. Insert a rectal thermometer for vagal stimulation.

**1677.** The nurse completed the health and social history of the adolescent client having palpitations and episodes of SVT. Which are possible contributing factors that the nurse should further explore? **Select all that apply.**

1. Uses alcohol
2. Is sexually active
3. Smokes cigarettes
4. Drinks coffee
5. Had recent chest injury

**1678.** MoC The nurse is caring for the pediatric client immediately following a permanent pacemaker placement. Which nursing intervention is **priority**?

1. Initiate continuous ECG monitoring.
2. Give a non-narcotic analgesic medication.
3. Transport to radiology for a chest x-ray.
4. Check whether an antibiotic has been prescribed.

**1679.** MoC The nurse is reviewing laboratory results for the Japanese child who has Kawasaki disease. Which result requires the nurse's immediate notification of the HCP?

1. White blood cells 14,000/mm$^3$
2. Slightly elevated liver enzymes
3. Platelets 569,000/mm$^3$
4. Elevated erythrocyte sedimentation rate (ESR)

**1680.** The nurse is caring for the child with Kawasaki disease. Which interventions should the nurse implement to provide comfort and reduce further skin breakdown? **Select all that apply.**

1. Provide warm baths twice daily.
2. Apply petroleum jelly to lips as needed.
3. Encourage loose-fitting cotton clothing.
4. Limit fluid intake to 500 mL.
5. Apply cool, moist cloths as desired.

## Answers and Rationales

**1643.** MoC **ANSWER: 1**

1. **A split S$_2$ sound may be abnormal if heard while respirations have paused. Because infants are unable to cooperate with the request to "hold a breath," the nurse should report the split S$_2$ sound to the HCP.**
2. An apical HR of 140 bpm is within the normal range for a 2-month-old infant.
3. Oxygen saturation of 97% is reassuring of oxygenation and perfusion status and a normal finding.
4. Femoral arteries are larger than brachial arteries and may have a higher pressure. A 3+ femoral pulse indicates that the pulse is bounding, whereas a 2+ brachial pulse indicates it is strong and normal.

♦ *Test-taking Tip: Look at the key words "report to the HCP." This tells you that you are looking for something abnormal in the assessment. Option 1 is the only option that falls outside of normal parameters.*

**Content Area:** Child; **Concept:** Perfusion; Management; **Integrated Processes:** Nursing Process: Analysis; **Client Needs:** Safe and Effective Care Environment: Management of Care; Physiological Integrity: Reduction of Risk Potential; **Cognitive Level:** Evaluation [Evaluating]

**1644. ANSWER: 3**

1. The SpO$_2$ is 98%, already suggesting that oxygenation and perfusion status is adequate; checking peripheral CRT does not have priority.
2. Assessment of bowel sounds does not have priority; fluid volume overload is of greater concern.
3. **Fatigue, tachycardia (HR of 167 bpm), and tachypnea (RR of 65 bpm) suggest fluid volume overload. Assessing for a heart murmur has priority to help identify the pathology of the underlying fluid overload.**
4. There is no need to attempt to feed the infant. The infant may not be hungry, thus giving inaccurate assessment data.

♦ *Test-taking Tip: Analyze the data that is already presented in the question. That should lead you to the need for a more focused cardiac assessment. After eliminating Options 2 and 4, eliminate Option 1 by understanding signs and symptoms of fluid volume overload.*

**Content Area:** Child; **Concept:** Perfusion; **Integrated Processes:** Nursing Process: Assessment; **Client Needs:** Physiological Integrity: Reduction of Risk Potential; **Cognitive Level:** Analysis [Analyzing]

**1645. ANSWER: 2**

1. Line A shows where blood is entering the aorta after flowing through the aortic valve.
2. **Blood is pumped from the right atrium to the right ventricle through the tricuspid valve shown at line B. Backflow (regurgitation) or stenosis may result in a murmur.**
3. Line C is the pulmonic valve.
4. Line D is the mitral valve.

♦ *Test-taking Tip: Apply basic knowledge of the anatomy and physiology of the heart to identify the tricuspid valve. A mnemonic for recalling the valves and the abnormal finding is APTM: **A**ll **P**oints **T**o **M**onitor. The letters signify the heart valves: A is for aortic, P for pulmonic, T for tricuspid, and M for mitral.*

**Content Area:** Child; **Concept:** Nursing Roles; Perfusion; **Integrated Processes:** Teaching/Learning; **Client Needs:** Physiological Integrity: Reduction in Risk Potential; **Cognitive Level:** Knowledge [Remembering]

**1646. ANSWER: 2**

1. Pulmonary hypertension is associated with left-sided, not right-sided, HF.
2. **The nurse should assess for the presence of right-sided HF. Back pressure in the portal circulation with resultant liver enlargement occurs in right-sided HF.**
3. Chest pain, dyspnea, and dysrhythmias, and not liver enlargement, would be initial signs of MI.
4. Tetralogy of Fallot occurs as a result of the malformation of the right ventricular infundibulum, which can lead to HF.

♦ *Test-taking Tip: The key words are "liver enlargement." Visualize each of the conditions presented to determine which is likely to result in back pressure and fluid accumulation in the liver.*

**Content Area:** Child; **Concept:** Assessment; Perfusion; **Integrated Processes:** Nursing Process: Assessment; **Client Needs:** Physiological Integrity: Physiological Adaptation; **Cognitive Level:** Application [Applying]

**1647.** PHARM **ANSWER: 1**

1. **Palivizumab (Synagis), a prophylaxis medication against RSV, is administered monthly during the RSV season to infants with unrepaired heart defects to decrease the risk of hospitalization with RSV.**
2. Activity is generally not restricted.
3. Infants with an unrepaired heart defect are often anorexic and require high-nutrient foods.
4. Infants should receive scheduled childhood immunizations according to current guidelines.

♦ *Test-taking Tip: When reviewing the options, think of the intervention that would prevent illness and hospitalization.*

**Content Area:** Child; **Concept:** Promoting Health; Perfusion; Medication; Nursing Roles; **Integrated Processes:** Communication and Documentation; **Client Needs:** Physiological Integrity: Pharmacological and Parenteral Therapies; Physiological Integrity: Physiological Adaptation; **Cognitive Level:** Analysis [Analyzing]

**1648. ANSWER: 3**

1. Weight change should be reported to the HCP but often is not an immediate concern.
2. Excessive crying should be reported to the HCP but often is not an immediate concern.

3. **Dehydration can increase the risk of stroke in hypoxemic children, and respiratory infection may compromise pulmonary function and increase the child's hypoxemia.**

4. Concerns over developmental milestones should be reported to the HCP but often are not immediate concerns.

▶ **Test-taking Tip:** *If unsure of the term "hypoxemic," break the word down. "Oxy-" means oxygen, and "-emia" pertains to blood. "Hypo-" refers to low. Of the options, only 2 and 3 potentially affect oxygenation. Select Option 3 because it is the most severe.*

**Content Area:** Child; **Concept:** Oxygenation; Perfusion; **Integrated Processes:** Communication and Documentation; **Client Needs:** Physiological Integrity: Physiological Adaptation; **Cognitive Level:** Application [Applying]

**1649. PHARM ANSWER: 1, 3, 4, 5**

1. **During a hypercyanotic episode, the child becomes dyspneic and hypoxic. The knee-chest position reduces cardiac output by decreasing blood return from the lower extremities and increasing the SVR.**

2. The child should receive 100% oxygen via facemask when having a hypercyanotic spell.

3. **Morphine sulfate should be administered to decrease preload and afterload.**

4. **A calm approach helps to settle the child and decrease oxygen demand.**

5. **Propranolol may be given to aid pulmonary artery dilation.**

▶ **Test-taking Tip:** *In a hypercyanotic episode, the partial pressure of oxygen ($PaO_2$) is lowered, and the partial pressure of carbon dioxide ($PaCO_2$) rises. As the respiratory center in the brain overreacts, hypoxemia progressively worsens. The increasing respiratory effort and cardiac output can cause a life-threatening decline unless rapid intervention is successful. You need to consider options that will decrease cardiac output, decrease preload and afterload, and promote pulmonary artery dilation.*

**Content Area:** Child; **Concept:** Perfusion; Critical Thinking; Safety; Medication; **Integrated Processes:** Nursing Process: Implementation; **Client Needs:** Physiological Integrity: Pharmacological and Parenteral Therapies; Physiological Integrity: Physiological Adaptation; **Cognitive Level:** Application [Applying]

**1650. ANSWER: 3**

1. Although prostaglandin $E_1$ (Cytotec) is given to dilate the ductus arteriosus, maintaining fetal duct patency does not address nutrition.

2. Providing rest periods helps decrease workload of the heart but does not directly affect nutritional status.

3. **Feeding the infant a higher-calorie food, such as fortified breast milk, directly increases caloric intake.**

4. Oral water is contraindicated, as it contains no calories and may cause electrolyte imbalances.

▶ **Test-taking Tip:** *The key words in the question are "adequate nutrition." Only one option will promote nutrition.*

**Content Area:** Child; **Concept:** Nutrition; Perfusion; **Integrated Processes:** Nursing Process: Planning; **Client Needs:** Physiological Integrity: Basic Care and Comfort; **Cognitive Level:** Application [Applying]

**1651. ANSWER: 1**

1. **This is a therapeutic response that answers the father's question.**

2. This is telling the father about the level of care but does not answer his question.

3. This is explaining medical care and does not answer his question.

4. This statement is incorrect; the heart continues to grow in early childhood.

▶ **Test-taking Tip:** *You should answer the patient's/family's question correctly and use therapeutic communication techniques to avoid increasing fear and anxiety.*

**Content Area:** Child; **Concept:** Perfusion; Communication; **Integrated Processes:** Communication and Documentation; Caring; **Client Needs:** Psychosocial Integrity; **Cognitive Level:** Application [Applying]

**1652. MoC ANSWER: 3, 5**

1. This HR of 120 bpm is WNL for a 3-month-old.

2. Murmurs are common following cardiac surgery.

3. **Severe intercostal retractions are a sign of severe respiratory distress. Without intervention, respiratory failure will occur.**

4. Decreased oxygen saturation levels are expected with HLHS. If oxygen saturations are normal, fetal ducts may close, thus worsening the problem.

5. **Extremely high Hct levels are associated with increased risk of stroke. The HCP should be notified to consider treatment.**

▶ **Test-taking Tip:** *Recognize what assessment findings are life-threatening to this child. Options 1 and 2 are normal findings. Option 4 is an expected finding for this child with HLSH and does not require intervention. Options 3 and 5 may lead to death without intervention.*

**Content Area:** Child; **Concept:** Perfusion; Management; **Integrated Processes:** Nursing Process: Analysis; **Client Needs:** Safe and Effective Care Environment: Management of Care; Physiological Integrity: Reduction of Risk Potential; **Cognitive Level:** Analysis [Analyzing]

**1653. MoC ANSWER: 4**

1. The tube is draining, so there is no reason to suspect an open connection.

2. Drainage of 200 mL requires further intervention, not just monitoring.

3. Although tipping and tilting the tubing will ensure drainage, the drainage of 200 mL is excessive; the best action is to notify the HCP.

4. **Because the drainage of 200 mL is excessive, the nurse's best action is to notify the HCP; this situation is emergent and can indicate hemorrhage.**

▶ **Test-taking Tip:** *Chest tube drainage greater than 5–10 mL/kg/hour, or >3 mL/kg for 3 consecutive hours, is indicative of hemorrhage.*

Content Area: Child; Concept: Perfusion; Critical Thinking; Integrated Processes: Nursing Process: Implementation; Client Needs: Safe and Effective Care Environment: Management of Care; Cognitive Level: Analysis [Analyzing]

## 1654. ANSWER: 1, 2, 3, 4

1. **Beta blocker medications lower the HR, and the HR should be known before administration.**
2. **A low-grade temperature could be a sign of an infection, and the HCP should be notified.**
3. **Pulling the child up by the child's arms can increase pain and cause sternal instability.**
4. **A diet high in vitamin C will promote wound healing.**
5. Although discharge instructions should include the importance of prophylactic antibiotic therapy prior to dental procedures, the purpose is to prevent bacterial endocarditis (not pericarditis).

▶ *Test-taking Tip: You should know the difference between pericarditis and endocarditis. Pericarditis is swelling and irritation of the thin saclike membrane surrounding the heart. Endocarditis is inflammation of the inner layer of the heart, which usually involves the heart valves.*

Content Area: Child; Concept: Nursing Roles; Perfusion; Integrated Processes: Teaching/Learning; Client Needs: Physiological Integrity: Physiological Adaptation; Health Promotion and Maintenance; Cognitive Level: Application [Applying]

## 1655. ANSWER: 2, 4, 5

1. Prostaglandin $E_1$ ($PGE_1$) is used to keep the ductus arteriosis open and indomethacin (Indocin) is used for closure.
2. **The infant does have a greater risk of bacterial endocarditis from increased pulmonary blood flow.**
3. With a PDA there is a greater pressure on the left side of the heart, not the right side.
4. **Blood is shunted from the aorta to the pulmonary artery and thus to the lungs.**
5. **A heart murmur may occur from the blood squirting through the small opening of the PDA.**

▶ *Test-taking Tip: Remember the pathophysiology of a PDA. This will allow Option 3 to be eliminated. Consideration of the effects of prostaglandin will eliminate Option 1.*

Content Area: Child; Concept: Perfusion; Nursing Roles; Integrated Processes: Teaching/Learning; Client Needs: Physiological Integrity: Physiological Adaptation; Cognitive Level: Application [Applying]

## 1656. MoC ANSWER: 3, 2, 4, 1

3. **Pulse oximeter reading of 90% has priority. It should be greater than 95%. The infant needs oxygen. The low level can be caused by the postoperative hemorrhage.**
2. **Chest tube drainage of 15 mL/kg in 1 hour should be addressed next. Any drainage greater than 5 to 10 mL/kg per hour is indicative of postoperative hemorrhage.**

4. **Urine output of 20 mL over the past 2 hours should be addressed third. Normal urine output for an infant is 2 to 3 mL/kg/hr.**
1. **Hgb level of 25 g/dL indicates polycythemia, which should correct itself over time as the oxygen levels are increased.**

▶ *Test-taking Tip: Use the ABC's to establish the order of priority.*

Content Area: Child; Concept: Critical Thinking; Perfusion; Management; Integrated Processes: Nursing Process: Planning; Client Needs: Safe and Effective Care Environment: Management of Care; Cognitive Level: Synthesis [Creating]

## 1657. ANSWER: 1, 2, 5

1. **The nurse should assess the BP in all four extremities. The BP may be higher in the right arm as compared to other extremities if coarctation of the aorta is present.**
2. **The nurse should assess the pulse quality in all four extremities. Pulses may be bounding in upper extremities as compared to weak in the lower extremities if coarctation of the aorta is present.**
3. Liver enlargement is related to HF, not an obstructive cardiac disorder.
4. Vision screening is not appropriate at this time to rule out coarctation of the aorta.
5. **Temperature and color may be less in the lower extremities if coarctation of the aorta is present.**

▶ *Test-taking Tip: Narrow the options to those related to the cardiovascular system.*

Content Area: Child; Concept: Perfusion; Assessment; Integrated Processes: Nursing Process: Assessment; Client Needs: Physiological Integrity: Reduction of Risk Potential; Cognitive Level: Application [Applying]

## 1658. ANSWER: 4

1. Decreased perfusion to the extremities can cause pain, but it does not occur with pericarditis.
2. Pain on inspiration, not expiration, is present with pericarditis.
3. The friction rub associated with pericarditis is pericardial, not pleural.
4. **Inflammation of the pericardial sac from acute pericarditis produces a pericardial friction rub.**

▶ *Test-taking Tip: Focus on the word "pericarditis." "Peri-" is around, "cardio-" pertains to the heart, and "-itis" is inflammation.*

Content Area: Child; Concept: Inflammation; Assessment; Perfusion; Integrated Processes: Nursing Process: Analysis; Client Needs: Physiological Integrity: Reduction of Risk Potential; Cognitive Level: Application [Applying]

## 1659. MoC ANSWER: 1, 2, 3, 4, 6

1. **Blood specimens can be obtained to determine oxygen saturation levels.**
2. **Pressure of blood flow in the heart chambers can be evaluated during cardiac catheterization.**

3. **Cardiac output and stroke volume can be evaluated during cardiac catheterization.**
4. **Contrast dye can be injected for angiography and for assessing anatomic abnormalities such as septal defects or obstruction of flow.**
5. ABI is a ratio of the ankle systolic pressure to the arm systolic pressure. It is an objective measurement of arterial disease quantifying the degree of stenosis and is not related to a cardiac catheterization procedure.
6. **Ejection fraction can be evaluated during cardiac catheterization.**

▶ **Test-taking Tip:** In cardiac catheterization, a radiopaque catheter is passed through a major vein in the arm, leg, or neck into the heart. Narrow the options to only those pertaining to the heart.

**Content Area:** Child; **Concept:** Safety; Critical Thinking; Nursing Roles; Perfusion; **Integrated Processes:** Nursing Process: Evaluation; **Client Needs:** Safe and Effective Care Environment: Management of Care; **Cognitive Level:** Evaluation [Evaluating]

### 1660. ANSWER: 2, 3, 4, 5
1. Hourly assessment is unnecessary at 8 hours postcatheterization.
2. **A cool foot is a sign of decreased perfusion that the parents can easily assess.**
3. **Oral liquids help to clear the dye from the body.**
4. **Activity should be limited for 24 hours after the procedure to prevent dislodgement of the clot.**
5. **Fever is a sign of infection, which can occur after an invasive procedure.**

▶ **Test-taking Tip:** Use the process of elimination. If unsure, think about whether parents would have the skill to adequately assess peripheral pulses.

**Content Area:** Child; **Concept:** Perfusion; Nursing Roles; **Integrated Processes:** Teaching/Learning; **Client Needs:** Physiological Integrity: Reduction of Risk Potential; **Cognitive Level:** Application [Applying]

### 1661. ANSWER: 1, 2, 3, 4
1. **The nurse should anticipate that a CBC may be prescribed to rule out anemia.**
2. **A serum chemistry may be prescribed to evaluate for altered BUN, creatinine, and electrolytes, which could indicate chronic renal disease or renal insufficiency secondary to hypertension.**
3. **A renal ultrasound may help identify a renal scar, congenital anomaly, or disparate renal size as a possible causative factor for the hypertension.**
4. **Drug screening is important to identify substances associated with hypertension.**
5. If a metabolic condition such as DM is suspected as a causative factor, a fasting serum glucose level should be drawn. Based on the test results, the need for a GTT would be determined.

▶ **Test-taking Tip:** Use the process of elimination to rule out the one test that requires a screening test be performed first.

**Content Area:** Child; **Concept:** Critical Thinking; Assessment; Perfusion; **Integrated Processes:** Nursing Process: Planning; **Client Needs:** Physiological Integrity: Reduction of Risk Potential; **Cognitive Level:** Comprehension [Understanding]

### 1662. PHARM ANSWER: 4
1. ACE inhibitors are used in treating hypertension in children.
2. Calcium channel blockers are used in treating hypertension in children.
3. Diuretics are used in treating hypertension in children.
4. **Nitrates are used to treat angina and are not prescribed to treat hypertension in children.**

▶ **Test-taking Tip:** Think about the action of each class of medications. Eliminate options that are classified as antihypertensive medications.

**Content Area:** Child; **Concept:** Medication; Critical Thinking; Perfusion; **Integrated Processes:** Nursing Process: Planning; **Client Needs:** Physiological Integrity: Pharmacological and Parenteral Therapies; **Cognitive Level:** Application [Applying]

### 1663. MoC ANSWER: 2, 3, 4
1. A HR of 145 bpm is within the normal rate of 100 to 160 bpm in a 1-month-old infant.
2. **Infants experiencing heart failure do not gain adequate weight due to their extremely high metabolic rate but do gain some weight.**
3. **The normal RR in a 1-month-old at rest is 50–60 respirations/minute; a rate of 70 is fast and could indicate complications.**
4. **A normal BP in a 1-month-old is a systolic BP of 65–85 and a diastolic BP of 45–55 mm Hg. A BP of 90/60 mm Hg at rest is elevated and could indicate possible complications.**
5. Although the infant may be agitated and crying, the 1-month-old infant would not sweat.

▶ **Test-taking Tip:** You should eliminate the options that are normal findings in a 1-month-old infant.

**Content Area:** Child; **Concept:** Perfusion; **Integrated Processes:** Nursing Process: Analysis; **Client Needs:** Safe and Effective Care Environment: Management of Care; Physiological Integrity: Reduction of Risk Potential; **Cognitive Level:** Analysis [Analyzing]

### 1664. PHARM ANSWER: 1, 2, 3, 6
1. **Positive inotropic agents increase the strength of muscular contractions.**
2. **Diuretics increase urine excretion and reduce volume overload.**
3. **ACE inhibitors (antihypertensive agents) relax arteries and promote renal excretion of salt and water by inhibiting the activity of an angiotensin-converting enzyme.**
4. Hypolipidemic agents are not standard management of CHF for pediatric clients. These agents are used to treat hyperlipidemia (elevated cholesterol and triglycerides). Hyperlipidemia contributes to the development of CAD.

5. Positive chronotropic agents will increase the HR, which can increase the heart's workload.
6. **Beta blockers decrease the workload of the heart by decreasing the amount of pressure against which it has to pump.**

▶ *Test-taking Tip: HF is inability of the heart to pump enough blood to meet the body's demand for energy. Select options that decrease the workload of the heart and improve cardiac output.*

Content Area: Child; Concept: Perfusion; Medication; Integrated Processes: Nursing Process: Planning; Client Needs: Physiological Integrity: Pharmacological and Parenteral Therapies; Physiological Integrity: Physiological Adaptation; Cognitive Level: Synthesis [Creating]

## 1665. PHARM ANSWER: 3

1. Calcium channel blockers do not have a diuretic effect.
2. The medication is not being given to lower the BP. This decrease in BP is not therapeutic, and results in a MAP of 52.
3. **A calcium channel blocker is being given to decrease the workload on the heart. An increase in activity tolerance should occur when cardiac workload is decreased.**
4. Clubbing is related to chronic hypoxia, not cardiac workload.

▶ *Test-taking Tip: Use the process of elimination. Eliminate Options 1 and 4, as they do not relate to any effect of a calcium channel blocker. Compare Options 2 and 3, reasoning that Option 2 is not a safe decrease in BP.*

Content Area: Child; Concept: Perfusion; Medication; Integrated Processes: Nursing Process: Evaluation; Client Needs: Physiological Integrity: Pharmacological and Parenteral Therapies; Cognitive Level: Evaluation [Evaluating]

## 1666. ANSWER: 1

1. **The infant with HF should be placed at a 45-degree angle during feedings. This angle decreases venous return of blood volume to the heart and eases the stress of feeding.**
2. The infant should be burped often and allowed a break during feedings to prevent undue fatigue.
3. Feedings should occur more frequently due to fatigue rather than be spaced farther apart.
4. A feeding tube is used only if the infant is unable to nipple feed or has tachypnea during feedings.

▶ *Test-taking Tip: Think about the action that would place the least amount of stress on the heart yet ensure adequate nutrition.*

Content Area: Child; Concept: Perfusion; Nutrition; Integrated Processes: Nursing Process: Implementation; Client Needs: Physiological Integrity: Reduction of Risk Potential; Cognitive Level: Application [Applying]

## 1667. MoC PHARM ANSWER: 3

1. The serum creatinine and BUN values are needed to determine whether or not the child is dehydrated from furosemide administration.

2. The child had a high sodium level on admission but is now within the normal range with the addition of the furosemide, which results in sodium excretion.
3. **A decrease in the potassium level can lead to an increased digoxin (Lanoxin) effect, resulting in digoxin toxicity. The great increase in the digoxin levels over 3 days is an indication that this may be occurring.**
4. The potassium levels were at the top of the normal range on admission and close to hyperkalemia. The potassium level is now WNL.

▶ *Test-taking Tip: Key information in the question is the large increase in the digoxin level over 3 days. Think about the effects of furosemide (Lasix) on potassium and then think about the effects this decrease in potassium can have on digoxin (Lanoxin). Captopril (Capoten) is an ACE inhibitor.*

Content Area: Child; Concept: Fluid and Electrolyte Balance; Medication; Perfusion; Integrated Processes: Nursing Process: Evaluation; Caring; Client Needs: Safe and Effective Care Environment: Management of Care; Physiological Integrity: Pharmacological and Parenteral Therapies; Cognitive Level: Evaluation [Evaluating]

## 1668. ANSWER: 4

1. In right-sided HF, the child would present with jugular venous distention, liver enlargement, splenomegaly, or ascites due to a reduced preload to the right side of the heart.
2. In RF, the child would present with an elevated temperature and a systolic murmur, mitral insufficiency, and a prolonged PR and QT interval.
3. In Kawasaki disease, the child would present with fever, rash, and lymph node enlargement.
4. **The child in left-sided HF will present with pulmonary symptoms of dyspnea, orthopnea, and crackles due to fluid accumulation in the lungs from ineffective pumping action of the heart.**

▶ *Test-taking Tip: Note that the child does not have an elevated temperature. Thus eliminate the conditions that would include temperature elevation. Then focus on Options 1 and 4, which are opposites. Only one of these is incorrect.*

Content Area: Child; Concept: Assessment; Perfusion; Integrated Processes: Nursing Process: Planning; Client Needs: Physiological Integrity: Reduction of Risk Potential; Cognitive Level: Analysis [Analyzing]

## 1669. PHARM ANSWER: 36

**First determine the weight. The infant weighs 8 lb or 3.6 kg (8 lb ÷ by 2.2 lb/kg = 3.6 kg). Next, determine the amount to administer: 3.6 kg × 10 mcg/kg = 36 mcg.**

▶ *Test-taking Tip: Recall that 2.2 lb equals 1 kg.*

Content Area: Child; Concept: Medication; Perfusion; Integrated Processes: Nursing Process: Implementation; Client Needs: Physiological Integrity: Pharmacological and Parenteral Therapies; Cognitive Level: Analysis [Analyzing]

**1670.** MoC PHARM **ANSWER: 1**

1. **The low serum potassium level should concern the nurse and be reported to the HCP. A low serum potassium level would increase the risk of digoxin toxicity.**
2. Although the Hgb level is a little low, this is not most concerning.
3. The digoxin level is on the high side of normal. Thus administering digoxin while the serum potassium level is low increases the risk further.
4. The serum creatinine level is a measure of renal function. It is WNL and not concerning.

♦ *Test-taking Tip: Focus on the abnormal values and eliminate Options 3 and 4 because these are normal values. Recall that potassium is involved in the conduction system of the heart, and digoxin (Lanoxin) will slow and strengthen the heart.*

**Content Area:** Child; **Concept:** Fluid and Electrolyte Balance; Medication; Perfusion; **Integrated Processes:** Nursing Process: Evaluation; **Client Needs:** Safe and Effective Care Environment: Management of Care; Physiological Integrity: Pharmacological and Parenteral Therapies; **Cognitive Level:** Evaluation [Evaluating]

**1671.** PHARM **ANSWER: 3**

1. Digoxin slows and strengthens the heart. Digoxin should not be given if the HR is too low.
2. Digoxin should be held if the HR is slow. Continuing to administer the medication would be unsafe.
3. **The nurse should withhold digoxin (Lanoxin) and immediately notify the HCP because bradycardia and mild vomiting are signs of digoxin toxicity. Digoxin slows and strengthens the heart.**
4. A beta-blocking agent should not be administered because it may further slow the rate.

♦ *Test-taking Tip: If unsure if these are signs of drug toxicity, recognize that the child is vomiting and would likely vomit the medication if administered.*

**Content Area:** Child; **Concept:** Medication; Perfusion; **Integrated Processes:** Nursing Process: Implementation; **Client Needs:** Physiological Integrity: Pharmacological and Parenteral Therapies; Safe and Effective Care Environment: Safety and Infection Control; **Cognitive Level:** Application [Applying]

**1672.** PHARM **ANSWER: 1**

1. **The nurse should instruct the client to contact the HCP if having muscle aches or dark urine when taking simvastatin (Zocor). These could be signs of a dangerous side effect of statins: rhabdomyolysis, the rapid breakdown of skeletal muscle tissue from the chemical effects of the medication.**
2. Simvastatin is an antilipidemic agent that lowers LDL and triglyceride levels; it will increase HDL cholesterol slightly (the good cholesterol).

3. The effectiveness of simvastatin is not affected by when it is taken; it can be taken in the morning or the evening.
4. A common side effect is insomnia, not sleepiness.

♦ *Test-taking Tip: Three options are similar, and one is different. Often the option that is different is the answer.*

**Content Area:** Child; **Concept:** Medication; Nursing Roles; Perfusion; **Integrated Processes:** Teaching/Learning; **Client Needs:** Physiological Integrity: Pharmacological and Parenteral Therapies; Health Promotion and Maintenance; **Cognitive Level:** Application [Applying]

**1673. ANSWER:**

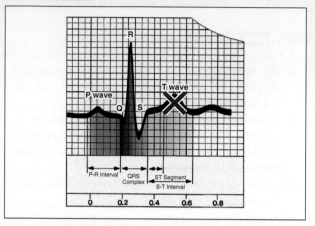

**The T wave represents repolarization of the ventricles—the process whereby the cell is polarized again with positive charges on the outer surface and negative charges on the inner surface.**

♦ *Test-taking Tip: The QRS represents ventricular depolarization. The next waveform would be repolarization.*

**Content Area:** Child; **Concept:** Perfusion; Nursing Roles; **Integrated Processes:** Teaching/Learning; **Client Needs:** Physiological Integrity: Physiological Adaptation; **Cognitive Level:** Analysis [Analyzing]

**1674. ANSWER: 3**

1. The ventricular rate in sinus bradycardia for a 2-year-old should be less than 80.
2. In a bundle branch block, the QRS interval should be greater than or equal to 0.12 seconds.
3. **A normal HR for a 2-year-old is 80 to 130 bpm. A normal PR interval measures 0.12 to 0.20 seconds. The PR interval is prolonged, indicating a first-degree AV block. The QRS is normal (0.6 to 0.10 seconds), and the QT is rate dependent. If the rate is fast, the QT will be shorter. The QT is within the normal range for the ventricular rate.**
4. In sinus tachycardia, the ventricular rate should be greater than 130 bpm for a 2-year-old; the rate is 126 bpm.

▶ *Test-taking Tip: To answer this question, knowledge of the normal ECG waveforms and the measurements is necessary. If this is unknown, then begin to eliminate options. The HR is normal for a 2-year-old. Eliminate Options 1 and 4. Next focus on the PR interval of 0.26 seconds. It is the time it takes the impulse to reach the AV node. Because it is prolonged, this should direct you to Option 3.*

**Content Area:** Child; **Concept:** Assessment; Perfusion; **Integrated Processes:** Communication and Documentation; **Client Needs:** Physiological Integrity: Physiological Adaptation; **Cognitive Level:** Analysis [Analyzing]

### 1675. ANSWER: 4

1. Option 1 is a ventricular paced rhythm with a pacemaker spike prior to the ventricular complex. This rhythm is expected with a pacemaker and would not require defibrillation.
2. Option 2 is atrial fibrillation and is not a rhythm that requires defibrillation.
3. This ECG shows a wandering atrial pacemaker with an irregular rhythm, variable PR interval, and multishaped P waves. Although abnormal, it would not require defibrillation.
4. **This ECG is a life-threatening torsades de pointes. The EMS should be activated.**

▶ *Test-taking Tip: If uncertain of life-threatening rhythms, you should select the most chaotic rhythm.*

**Content Area:** Child; **Concept:** Perfusion; **Integrated Processes:** Nursing Process: Implementation; **Client Needs:** Physiological Integrity: Physiological Adaptation; **Cognitive Level:** Analysis [Analyzing]

### 1676. ANSWER: 2

1. Wrapping the child's head with a cold, wet towel could potentially cause vagal stimulation. Vagal stimulation may convert the SVT rhythm to a sinus rhythm.
2. **Further teaching is needed when a parent states to massage both carotid arteries. Carotid artery massage is not recommended. Massaging both carotid arteries restricts blood flow.**
3. Having the child perform the Valsalva maneuver (bearing down) could potentially cause vagal stimulation. Vagal stimulation may convert the SVT rhythm to a sinus rhythm.
4. Inserting a rectal thermometer may initiate vagal stimulation.

▶ *Test-taking Tip: Narrow the options to the answer by eliminating options that can potentially cause vagal stimulation without restricting blood flow.*

**Content Area:** Child; **Concept:** Nursing Roles; Perfusion; Safety; **Integrated Processes:** Nursing Process: Evaluation; **Client Needs:** Physiological Integrity: Physiological Adaptation; Health Promotion and Maintenance; **Cognitive Level:** Evaluation [Evaluating]

### 1677. ANSWER: 1, 3, 4, 5

1. **Although alcohol is a depressant, it has been shown to be linked with SVT and heart palpitations because it irritates the cardiac muscle.**
2. Knowing sexual history is important for client care but is unlikely to contribute to the palpitations and SVT.
3. **Nicotine is a stimulant that increases the HR.**
4. **Caffeine is a stimulant that increases the HR.**
5. **Chest trauma can induce dysrhythmias.**

▶ *Test-taking Tip: Stimulants and irritants can affect the heart muscle, causing dysrhythmias.*

**Content Area:** Child; **Concept:** Assessment; Perfusion; **Integrated Processes:** Nursing Process: Assessment; **Client Needs:** Physiological Integrity: Reduction in Risk Potential; **Cognitive Level:** Application [Applying]

### 1678. MoC ANSWER: 1

1. **The nurse's priority should be to initiate continuous ECG monitoring. It is important in the recovery phase to assess pacemaker function immediately following placement.**
2. Analgesics, including narcotics, are administered as needed to control pain, but ensuring that the pacemaker is functioning properly has priority.
3. A CXR is performed within 24 hours for future comparison, but it does not have priority.
4. Although a prophylactic antibiotic may be prescribed, ensuring that the pacemaker is functioning correctly has priority.

▶ *Test-taking Tip: Use the ABC's to establish priority. Recall that the pacemaker initiates an impulse to stimulate the electrical conduction of a person's heart.*

**Content Area:** Child; **Concept:** Safety; Critical Thinking; Perfusion; **Integrated Processes:** Nursing Process: Implementation; **Client Needs:** Safe and Effective Care Environment: Management of Care; **Cognitive Level:** Analysis [Analyzing]

### 1679. MoC ANSWER: 3

1. This is a slight elevation in WBC count and is expected with the Kawasaki disease process.
2. Mild hepatic dysfunction is temporary for the child with Kawasaki disease. It requires no intervention.
3. **Extremely high platelets are associated with Kawasaki disease, but a platelet level of 569,000/mm³ requires treatment due to the increased risk of clots. This may be life-threatening.**
4. Increased ESR is expected with the underlying inflammatory process. This requires no intervention.

▶ **Test-taking Tip:** *Although all of the options are expected findings with Kawasaki disease, you need to identify the option that is potentially dangerous to the child. In Kawasaki disease there is vasculitis of medium-sized arteries, including the coronary arteries. Kawasaki disease also affects skin, mucous membranes, and lymph nodes. It is more common in Japanese children with an estimated 250/100,000 children < 5 years of age affected.*

**Content Area:** Child; **Concept:** Perfusion; Critical Thinking; Management; Diversity; **Integrated Processes:** Nursing Process: Analysis; Culture and Spirituality; **Client Needs:** Safe and Effective Care Environment: Management of Care; **Cognitive Level:** Analysis [Analyzing]

### 1680. ANSWER: 2, 3, 5

1. Warm baths may exacerbate the discomfort and skin breakdown associated with Kawasaki disease. Tepid or slightly cool baths are comforting.

2. Petroleum jelly is soothing and nonirritating and should be applied to the lips.
3. Breathable and loose-fitting cotton clothing will not irritate excoriated skin associated with Kawasaki disease.
4. Fluid intake should be increased (not limited) to maintain moist skin and mucous membranes.
5. Cool, moist cloths are similar to tepid baths and are comforting.

▶ **Test-taking Tip:** *Decide which interventions both provide comfort and reduce further skin breakdown. Options 1 and 4 should be eliminated because these may lead to further skin breakdown.*

**Content Area:** Child; **Concept:** Perfusion; Comfort; **Integrated Processes:** Nursing Process: Implementation; **Client Needs:** Physiological Integrity: Basic Care and Comfort; **Cognitive Level:** Application [Applying]

## Chapter Thirty-Eight

# Endocrine Management

**1681.** PHARM The medications for treating type 1 DM are changed for the Native American 12-year-old from NPH and rapid-acting insulin to a basal-bolus insulin regimen of glargine and insulin aspart. To achieve tight glucose control and for therapy to be effective, which instructions should the nurse provide to the child and parent? **Select all that apply.**

1. The long-acting insulin, glargine, is the basal insulin and administered once daily.
2. Insulin aspart, a rapid-acting insulin, is given as a bolus at mealtime and with snacks.
3. Extra rapid–acting insulin should be given when the child's daily exercise increases.
4. Consistently count the number of carbohydrates the child consumes during the day.
5. Obtain blood glucose four to eight times daily, and weekly at midnight and 3 a.m.
6. Obtain materials specific to Native Americans from the American Diabetes Association.

**1682.** PHARM The 9-year-old child with a history of type 1 DM for the past 6 years is diagnosed with diabetic ketoacidosis (DKA). Which intervention should the nurse plan to initiate?

1. Add sodium bicarbonate to the current IV fluids.
2. Add potassium chloride to the current IV fluids.
3. Give 0.9% or 0.45% NaCl for the maintenance IV fluid.
4. Administer regular insulin by subcutaneous injection.

**1683.** PHARM The parents of the 7-year-old child with type 1 DM are planning to drive 1200 miles for a vacation at the beach. They question the nurse about insulin storage for the trip. Which response by the nurse is **most** accurate?

1. "Because insulin must be refrigerated, you will need to obtain the medication from a pharmacy at your destination."
2. "Freeze the insulin before you leave home and take it in a cooler; it should be thawed by the time you get to the beach."
3. "Put the insulin in a cooler with an ice pack and store it out of the sun. Place unopened insulin in the refrigerator at your destination."
4. "It is illegal to transport needles and syringes across states; obtain a prescription now to buy the supplies at your destination."

**1684.** The 5-year-old has type 1 DM. The nurse is explaining the reason for counting the child's grams of carbohydrate intake to the mother. Which statement is **most** accurate?

1. "Carbohydrate counting helps to have lower blood glucose levels."
2. "Carbohydrate counting ensures sufficient energy for growth and development."
3. "Carbohydrate counting ensures consistent glucose levels to prevent hypoglycemia."
4. "Carbohydrate counting helps attain metabolic control of glucose and lipid levels."

**1685.** PHARM The adolescent with type 1 DM is taught how to use the device illustrated. Which client statement indicates the need for additional teaching?

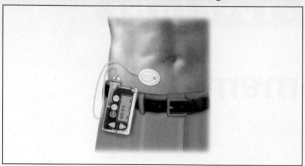

1. "I can put in the number of carbohydrates that I consume, and the insulin pump will calculate the bolus insulin dose that I will receive."
2. "I must check my blood glucose levels before meals and snacks and count the number of carbohydrates I eat so I get the correct bolus dose."
3. "With using the insulin pump, my blood glucose control should improve, and I should see a drop in the weight that I have gained."
4. "Every 2 to 4 days, I will need to change the cartridge, catheter, and site, moving away at least 1 inch from the last injection site."

**1686.** The 10-year-old child with a 6-year history of type 1 DM has had enuresis over the past 2 weeks. Which condition should the nurse consider as a cause of the enuresis?

1. Hemoglobin $A_{1c}$ levels lower than normal
2. Acquired adrenocortical hyperfunction
3. Sustained blood glucose levels higher than normal
4. Acquired SIADH

**1687.** The child with type 1 DM presents in the school nurse's office an hour before the lunch period reporting disorientation. Which information is **most** important for the nurse to obtain?

1. Blood glucose reading
2. Temperature reading
3. Morning insulin dose
4. Urine ketone amount

**1688.** The mother of the 12-year-old with type 1 DM asks the nurse whether changes in the daily routine are needed during her child's 4-week attendance at summer camp. Which is the **best** response by the nurse?

1. "The child will have an increased need for insulin due to the high carbohydrate content of camp food."
2. "The child's food intake should be decreased by 10%, while the insulin should be increased by 10%."
3. "Food intake should be increased as the child's activity increases; blood glucose levels need to be taken three to four times a day to evaluate results."
4. "The insulin injection should be given before every meal and snack to ensure that the food being eaten at camp can be utilized by the body."

**1689.** PHARM The 8-year-old child is to receive 1 unit of aspart insulin for every 15 g of carbohydrates consumed at mealtime and insulin per the sliding scale in the table presented. The child's fingerstick blood glucose before breakfast is 82 mg/dL, and the child ate 30 g of carbohydrates at breakfast. How many total units of insulin should the nurse administer?

_____ units (Record a whole number.)

| Mealtime Glucose Level (mg/dL) | Mealtime Units of Aspart Insulin for Glucose Level |
|---|---|
| 70–79 | –2 and call HCP |
| 80-89 | –1 |
| 90–180 | 0 |
| 181–200 | 1 |
| 201–250 | 2 |
| 251–300 | 3 |
| More than 300 | Call HCP |

**1690.** The nurse educates the parents and their 9-year-old child with type 1 DM about DM. Which statement, if made by the child, **best** indicates teaching was effective?

1. "If I get dizzy or lightheaded while in gym class, I should sit down and rest."
2. "It is okay for me to be barefoot if I am just walking around in the house."
3. "I should check my urine for ketones if my glucose is 240 mg/dL or more."
4. "If I get tearful and shaky, I should give myself a shot of glucagon in the thigh."

**1691.** **PHARM** The 4-year-old with type 1 DM consumed one-half cup of oatmeal, 60 mL of orange juice, and 60 mL of milk for breakfast. The child's blood glucose was 150 mg/dL before breakfast. No insulin was given before breakfast. Which conclusions by the nurse are correct? **Select all that apply.**

1. The total volume of fluid intake should be recorded as 120 mL.
2. Insulin will need to be administered to cover the carbohydrates eaten.
3. Insulin will not be needed, as the child's blood glucose was normal before breakfast.
4. A double-check of the amounts of carbohydrates eaten is needed before giving insulin.
5. Insulin should have been given before breakfast because the blood glucose was elevated.

**1692.** The 5-year-old, recently diagnosed with type 1 DM, is beyond the honeymoon phase of DM. In teaching the parents, which illustration should the nurse select to show the pathophysiology specific to type 1 DM at this stage?

1.

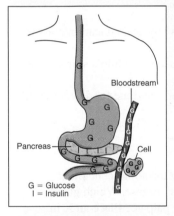

2.

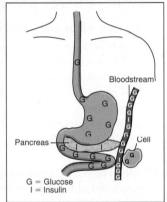

3.

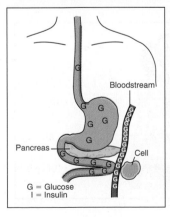

4.

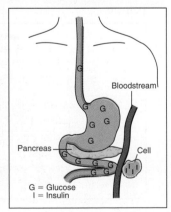

**1693.** The nurse completes teaching the parents of the child newly diagnosed with type 1 DM about sick day rules. What statements by a parent indicate that additional teaching is needed? **Select all that apply.**

1. "I will always give an extra dose of insulin when my child is ill."
2. "Even if unable to eat, my child should get the usual daily insulin dose."
3. "If urine ketones are high, I should notify my child's HCP."
4. "I should test my child's glucose level and urine ketones once a day."
5. "I should call the HCP if glucose levels are higher than 240 mg/dL."

**1694.** The child's parents inform the nurse about how they care for their 12-year-old child with type 1 DM, including sick day management, treating hyperglycemia, and managing ketosis. In which situation might the parents be able to safely manage the child's care at home?

1. Blood glucose 280 mg/dL; skin turgor very poor; lips and mouth parched
2. Blood glucose 250 mg/dL; vomiting and dizziness; having double vision
3. Blood glucose 240 mg/dL; polyuria; urine output 100 mL for past 8 hours
4. Blood glucose 300 mg/dL; urine positive for ketones; skin hot, flushed, and dry

**1695.** **MoC** The nurse is assessing the child with DM. Which findings support the nurse's immediate report to the HCP about the development of DKA? **Select all that apply.**

1. Kussmaul respirations
2. Slowing of the HR
3. Foul-smelling breath odor
4. Lethargic and unarousable
5. Blood glucose level 350 mg/dL

**1696.** The 5-year-old with type 1 DM develops hypoglycemia during a preschool class. Which simple carbohydrate should the nurse give now?

1. 1 slice of bread
2. 1 oz of peanuts
3. 120 mL of orange juice
4. 60 mL chocolate milk

**1697.** The hospitalized child is experiencing signs of a hypoglycemic episode. Place each nursing action in the order of priority.

1. Wait 15 minutes and check the blood glucose level a second time.
2. If the blood glucose level is 70 mg/dL or less, give 15 g of rapid-acting glucose, such as one-half cup fruit juice.
3. Recheck the blood glucose level for a third time in another 15 minutes.
4. Obtain a fingerstick blood glucose reading.
5. Assess for signs of pallor, sweating, tremors, irritability, or an altered mental status.
6. Repeat the rapid-acting glucose if the blood glucose level is 70 mg/dL or less.
7. Once the blood sugar has returned to at least 80 mg/dL, give a more substantial snack such as cheese and crackers.

Answer: _____

**1698.** The nurse is assessing recent Hgb $A_{1c}$ values for the 12-year-old. The most recent value is 8.9%, and the last three blood glucose results for the past 24 hours are 110 mg/dL, 138 mg/dL, and 130 mg/dL. What is the nurse's **best** interpretation of these values?

1. The client has good dietary control of his or her DM.
2. The client is under stress, causing these false high readings.
3. The client has had poor diet control except for the last 24 hours.
4. The client has had good long-term dietary control, but the recent diet is high in sugar.

**1699.** The nurse is interviewing the parents of the 3-year-old newly diagnosed with hypothyroidism. Which question is **most** important for the nurse to ask?

1. "Did your child's teeth come in earlier than usual?"
2. "Has your child's physical development been delayed?"
3. "Does your child seem to be hungry all of the time?"
4. "Does your child tell you about feeling too warm a lot?"

**1700. PHARM** The nurse is assessing the child with hypothyroidism. Which findings should indicate to the nurse that the child's levothyroxine dose is too high? **Select all that apply.**

1. Slow HR
2. Has lost a lot of weight
3. Puffy facial features
4. Has difficulty falling asleep
5. Elevated BP

**1701. PHARM** The infant, diagnosed with hypothyroidism, is prescribed levothyroxine sodium. Which assessments would assist the nurse in evaluating the effectiveness of levothyroxine sodium?

1. Monthly growth and development measurements
2. Monthly serum calcium and thyroxin levels
3. Bimonthly catecholamine level and ECG results
4. Weekly breast- or bottle-feeding intake measurements

**1702. MoC** The nurse observes the NA caring for the child newly diagnosed with hyperthyroidism. Which action by the NA requires the nurse to intervene?

1. Applies extra blankets over the child while the child is sleeping
2. Takes the child's BP with an automatic BP machine
3. Obtains a pudding snack that is requested by the child before bedtime
4. Rocks the child in a rocking chair when the child is unable to fall asleep

**1703.** The nurse is educating the parents of the school-aged child newly diagnosed with hyperthyroidism. Which instruction should be given as initial management until the disease is under control?

1. Discontinue your child's physical education classes at school.
2. Ask the teacher to increase your child's stimulation when at school.
3. Restrict calories from carbohydrate foods your child consumes.
4. Dress your child in cold weather clothing even in warm weather.

**1704.** The nurse is assessing the adolescent client suspected of having Graves' disease. Which gland illustrated should the nurse palpate? Place an X in the box pointing to the gland that the nurse should palpate.

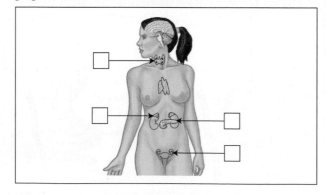

**1705.** The nurse is caring for the pediatric client with hyperthyroidism. Which intervention would the nurse plan to include in the child's plan of care?

1. Keep the temperature warm in the room.
2. Encourage increased food intake.
3. Increase physical activity.
4. Provide extra salt for meals.

**1706.** The nurse is providing teaching to the parents who have a child newly diagnosed with hypoparathyroidism. Which instruction should the nurse include?

1. Monitor for muscle spasms, tingling around the mouth, and muscle cramps.
2. Report side effects of medication excess, including dry, scaly, coarse skin.
3. Decrease the child's intake of foods high in calcium and phosphorus.
4. Increase environmental stimuli and encourage high-energy activities.

**1707.** **MoC** The 10-year-old is scheduled for a CT of the abdomen to identify a possible cause of acute adrenocortical insufficiency. Which HCP prescription should the nurse clarify before it is implemented?

1. Start D$_5$NS at 50 mL/hr per IV.
2. Pad bedside rails and ensure seizure precautions.
3. Place steroid medication on hold before CT.
4. Monitor VS q15 min pre- and post-CT.

**1708.** The adolescent is hospitalized with a tentative diagnosis of Addison's disease. Which nursing assessment findings would support the diagnosis of Addison's disease?

1. Long history of fatigue, weight loss, and muscle tetany
2. Sudden onset of skin hypopigmentation, polydipsia, and hyperactivity
3. Gradual onset of salt craving, decreased pubic and axillary hair, and irritability
4. Sudden onset of increasing weight gain, hirsutism, and skin hyperpigmentation

**1709.** The nurse teaches the parents of the child diagnosed with Addison's disease signs of Addisonian crisis. Which sign identified by the parents indicates that further teaching is needed?

1. Severe hypertension
2. Abdominal pain
3. Grand mal seizures
4. Dehydration

**1710.** **PHARM** The nurse instructs the parents of the child diagnosed with Addison's disease. Which instructions should be included by the nurse? **Select all that apply.**

1. Purchase and have the child wear a medical alert bracelet inscribed with Addison's disease.
2. Encourage the child to ingest adequate amounts of fluids, particularly on hot summer days.
3. Include emergency cortisone treatment for Addisonian crisis on the school medical care plan.
4. Repeat the cortisone dose if the child vomits the medication within 1 hour of administration.
5. Administer epinephrine subcutaneously immediately if an Addisonian crisis should occur.
6. Monitor your child for disturbed body image changes due to skin hyperpigmentation.

**1711.** The nurse is reviewing the plan of care for the child hospitalized with congenital adrenal hyperplasia. Which intervention is the nurse's **priority?**

1. Teach the parents about giving glucocorticoids.
2. Check chromosomal analysis for genetic sex.
3. Treat associated hyperkalemia and hyponatremia.
4. Place the child on a severe fluid restriction diet.

**1712.** **PHARM** Glucocorticoids are prescribed for the child diagnosed with congenital adrenal hyperplasia. Which nursing assessment finding indicates that therapy is successful?

1. Feminization if the child is a girl
2. Absence of symptoms of Cushing's syndrome
3. Penile enlargement if the child is a boy
4. Increased growth rate if either a boy or girl

**1713.** The nurse is caring for an infant hospitalized with congenital adrenal hypoplasia. Which problem is the nurse's **priority?**

1. Disproportionate growth
2. Excess fluid volume
3. Impaired parent-infant attachment
4. Knowledge deficit about lifelong medication use

**1714.** **MoC** The nurse is creating the plan of care for the child diagnosed with adrenal insufficiency. Which outcomes should the nurse include? **Select all that apply.**

1. The child demonstrates a positive body image.
2. The child demonstrates no complications related to inactivity.
3. The child responds to oxygen regimes to avoid hospitalization.
4. The child and family verbalize causes of the disease and treatments.
5. The child responds to activity restrictions to conserve energy.

**1715.** The 12-year-old being treated for GH deficiency is angry and refusing to go to school because everyone the same age is taller. The child is belligerent toward the mother, who gives the daily GH injection. Which **initial** intervention should the nurse attempt?

1. Teach the child about self-administration of the growth hormone.
2. Refer the family for counseling pertaining to anger management.
3. Assist the parents to contact the school to request home schooling.
4. Have the mother request an Individual Educational Plan (IEP) at school.

**1716.** The nurse is assessing the 3-year-old child. Which finding would alert the nurse to further explore for signs of hypopituitarism?

1. Lethargy
2. Hyperglycemia
3. Confusion
4. No growth since age 2

**1717.** **PHARM** The teenage client has been given education regarding goals of GH for treatment of hypopituitarism. The nurse determines that the client has adequate understanding of the treatment goals when making which statement?

1. "I need to record my growth on a growth chart."
2. "I will not need dentures to replace my soft teeth."
3. "I will start to grow at a normal rate and reach adult height."
4. "The hormone will allow me to build significant muscle mass."

**1718.** The nurse assesses the pediatric client who has DI. Which findings would require immediate investigation by the nurse? **Select all that apply.**

1. Blood glucose level of 126 mg/dL
2. Urine specific gravity of 1.000
3. Urine output of 2000 mL in 24 hours
4. Experiencing occasional upset stomach
5. Weight loss of 3 pounds in 24 hours

**1719.** The nurse is caring for the child newly diagnosed with DI. Which laboratory values should the nurse monitor? **Select all that apply.**

1. Serum calcium
2. Serum sodium
3. Serum glucose
4. Serum osmolality
5. Blood urea nitrogen

**1720.** The nurse caring for an infant with DI is documenting total output for a 12-hour shift. After reviewing the I&O flowsheet illustrated and subtracting the weight of 24 g for one dry diaper, how many mL of urine output should the nurse record?

_____ mL (Record your answer as a whole number.)

| Time | Wet Diaper Weight in Grams |
|------|----------------------------|
| 0800 | 340 |
| 1000 | 427 |
| 1130 | 75 |
| 1400 | 115 |
| 1545 | 235 |
| 1850 | 200 |

**1721.** The nurse is assessing the 4-year-old child diagnosed with precocious puberty. Which physical assessment findings should the nurse expect?

1. Short stature
2. Hypothalamic tumor
3. Advanced bone age
4. Pubic and axillary hair

**1722.** **PHARM** The nurse is caring for the older adolescent diagnosed with acromegaly. Which medication should the nurse plan to administer?

1. Somatropin
2. Desmopressin
3. Octreotide acetate
4. Clozapine

**1723.** **MoC** The 6-year-old child has pheochromocytoma. Which assessment finding should prompt the nurse to contact the HCP because this child is in crisis?

1. Systolic BP 120 mm Hg and bradycardia
2. Dark-colored urine and extreme muscle pain
3. Urine output 40 mL/hr and abdominal pain
4. Hyperexcitability and extreme agitation

# Answers and Rationales

## 1681. PHARM ANSWER: 1, 2, 4, 5

1. **With basal-bolus insulin therapy, basal insulin is administered once a day using a long-acting insulin such as glargine (Lantus).**
2. **A bolus of rapid-acting insulin, such as aspart (Novolog), is administered with each meal and snack based on the number of carbohydrates eaten and the child's blood glucose level.**
3. Exercise increases the need for carbohydrates, not insulin.
4. **It is important to count the carbohydrates to administer the appropriate amount of insulin.**
5. **Depending on the number of snacks eaten, blood glucose could be monitored up to eight times a day, and the child may get six to seven injections a day. Because of the potential for hypoglycemia at night, the child's blood glucose should be monitored at midnight and 3 a.m. once a week.**
6. **American Indians and Alaska Natives have the highest prevalence of DM among U.S. racial and ethnic groups. The American Diabetes Association has a specialized program and materials specific to the American Indian and Alaska Native population.**

♦ *Test-taking Tip: Eliminate the one option that is unsafe and will result in a hypoglycemic reaction.*

Content Area: Child; Concept: Metabolism; Nursing Roles; Medication; Diversity; Integrated Processes: Teaching/Learning; Culture and Spirituality; Client Needs: Physiological Integrity: Pharmacological and Parenteral Therapies; Cognitive Level: Analysis [Analyzing]

## 1682. PHARM ANSWER: 3

1. Research has shown no benefit to giving sodium bicarbonate to children with DKA to reverse metabolic acidosis.
2. Potassium is added only after laboratory studies have confirmed that the plasma potassium is low. Usually there is not a drop in plasma potassium.
3. **Both water and sodium are depleted in DKA; thus the child will require IV NaCl, either 0.9% or 0.45%.**
4. Regular insulin is given by IV in DKA for rapid effect and close monitoring. The onset by subcutaneous route is 15 to 30 minutes and can cause hypoglycemia if the dosage is excessive.

♦ *Test-taking Tip: DKA is a life-threatening condition, and the nurse needs to be ready to act when the child is admitted. High blood glucose levels cause osmotic diuresis and the loss of fluids. This information should direct you to Option 3.*

Content Area: Child; Concept: pH Regulation; Metabolism; Fluid and Electrolyte Balance; Medication; Integrated Processes: Nursing Process: Planning; Client Needs: Physiological Integrity: Pharmacological and Parenteral Therapies; Cognitive Level: Application [Applying]

## 1683. PHARM ANSWER: 3

1. It is unnecessary to refrigerate insulin when traveling. An ice cooler is sufficient.
2. Insulin is destroyed when frozen.
3. **Because insulin should be kept out of direct sunlight and extreme heat, it should be transported in a cooler with an ice pack. Unopened insulin should be refrigerated.**
4. It is not illegal to transport needles and syringes. However, the child/parent should have a prescription to identify the medication and justify the syringes. The prescription provides a means to obtain additional supplies if needed.

♦ *Test-taking Tip: Focus on what the question is asking, insulin storage. Eliminate Options 1 and 4 because these responses do not address insulin storage. Decide the best option, 2 or 3. Note that Option 3 is more complete, thus eliminate Option 2.*

Content Area: Child; Concept: Metabolism; Nursing Roles; Medication; Integrated Processes: Teaching/Learning; Client Needs: Physiological Integrity: Pharmacological and Parenteral Therapies; Health Promotion and Maintenance; Cognitive Level: Application [Applying]

## 1684. ANSWER: 4

1. This only partially correct; it also helps with lipid metabolism.
2. Children need energy for growth and development, but it is not the reason for counting carbohydrates.
3. This is only partially correct; it is important to control lipid levels as well.
4. **The overall goal of nutritional management by counting carbohydrates is to achieve and maintain control of glucose and lipid metabolism.**

♦ *Test-taking Tip: You should look for the most global response. Answers that are only partially complete should be eliminated.*

Content Area: Child; Concept: Metabolism; Promoting Health; Nursing Roles; Integrated Processes: Communication and Documentation; Client Needs: Physiological Integrity: Basic Care and Comfort; Cognitive Level: Application [Applying]

## 1685. PHARM ANSWER: 3

1. Insulin pumps can calculate the bolus insulin dose when the number of carbohydrates consumed is entered.
2. Monitoring blood glucose levels and calculating carbohydrates consumed are needed for correct dosing with an insulin pump.
3. **Weight gain, not weight loss, commonly occurs as blood glucose control improves because the glucose is being metabolized instead of excreted.**
4. About every 2 to 4 days when a cartridge is empty, a new cartridge and tubing are attached to the pump, along with a new skin setup. The injection site is also changed to prevent lipoatrophy.

▶ *Test-taking Tip:* The key phrase "need for additional teaching" indicates that this is a false-response question. Select the option that is incorrect. Note that Options 1, 2, and 4 relate to the pump operation, whereas Option 3 is different. Often the option that is different is the answer.

**Content Area:** Child; **Concept:** Metabolism; Medication; Nursing Roles; **Integrated Processes:** Nursing Process: Evaluation; **Client Needs:** Physiological Integrity: Pharmacological and Parenteral Therapies; **Cognitive Level:** Evaluation [Evaluating]

### 1686. ANSWER: 3

1. Children with type 1 DM who have higher (not lower) Hgb $A_{1c}$ levels are at risk for enuresis (bedwetting).
2. Adrenal hyperfunction will not cause enuresis.
3. **Children with type 1 DM who have higher Hgb $A_{1c}$ levels and higher fasting blood glucose levels, and who experience polydipsia and polyuria, are at risk for enuresis (bedwetting).**
4. Although SIADH will cause enuresis, the child with type 1 DM will more likely develop enuresis due to sustained, elevated blood glucose levels and not due to SIADH.

▶ *Test-taking Tip:* Note that Options 1 and 3 are opposites, so either one or both of these are incorrect. Think about the pathophysiology of type 1 DM to respond to this question.

**Content Area:** Child; **Concept:** Metabolism; Critical Thinking; **Integrated Processes:** Nursing Process: Evaluation; **Client Needs:** Physiological Integrity: Physiological Adaptation; **Cognitive Level:** Evaluation [Evaluating]

### 1687. ANSWER: 1

1. **Children who become disoriented or sleepy within an hour of a meal are most likely experiencing hypoglycemia. The nurse should obtain a blood glucose reading.**
2. The temperature will not provide the information needed to intervene.
3. The morning insulin dose would not provide the information needed to intervene.
4. Obtaining urine ketones is not indicated because ketones are not present in the urine at low plasma glucose levels.

▶ *Test-taking Tip:* Note the key words "most important." Look for the option that provides the information needed for the nurse to intervene immediately.

**Content Area:** Child; **Concept:** Assessment; Metabolism; Critical Thinking; **Integrated Processes:** Nursing Process: Assessment; **Client Needs:** Physiological Integrity: Reduction of Risk Potential; **Cognitive Level:** Application [Applying]

### 1688. ANSWER: 3

1. The nurse is making a generalization about the carbohydrate content of camp food that may not be true.
2. An increase of insulin with an increase in physical activity and/or a decrease in food consumption will result in profound hypoglycemia.

3. **Increases in muscle activity promote a more efficient utilization of glucose. School-aged children are more physically active during the summer months than during the school year.**
4. Giving regular insulin before every meal and snack is an option for older individuals who are usually engaged in regular, high-intensity physical activity and who consume the projected number of carbohydrates; it would not be recommended for the 12-year-old child attending 4 weeks of camp because food intake may be less than the projected amount of insulin.

▶ *Test Taking Tip:* You should eliminate options that can result in hypoglycemia.

**Content Area:** Child; **Concept:** Nursing Roles; Metabolism; Medication; **Integrated Processes:** Teaching/Learning; **Client Needs:** Physiological Integrity: Physiological Adaptation; **Cognitive Level:** Application [Applying]

### 1689. PHARM ANSWER: 1

**One unit of insulin aspart (Novolog) should be administered. The client should receive 2 units for the 30 g of carbohydrates (CHO) minus 1 unit for the blood glucose of 82 mg/dL, for a total of 1 unit.**

▶ *Test-taking Tip:* Carefully read what the question is asking. Be sure to note both the insulin "coverage dose" for the carbohydrate intake and the insulin "correction dose" for the blood sugar.

**Content Area:** Child; **Concept:** Metabolism; Medication; **Integrated Processes:** Nursing Process: Implementation; **Client Needs:** Physiological Integrity: Pharmacological and Parenteral Therapies; **Cognitive Level:** Analysis [Analyzing]

### 1690. ANSWER: 3

1. If the child with DM becomes dizzy or lightheaded, the child should check his or her blood glucose, not just sit down and rest.
2. Wearing shoes or slippers when indoors, rather than being barefoot, will prevent foot injuries. The risk for infection from injuries is increased in a person with DM.
3. **The child should check his or her urine for ketones if the blood glucose is ≥240 mg/dL. This statement indicates the child understood the teaching.**
4. Being tearful and shaky could indicate hypoglycemia. If conscious, the child should eat 10 to 15 g of simple carbohydrates, such as 8 oz of milk. If the child were unresponsive, glucagon would be administered.

▶ *Test-taking Tip:* The key word in the stem is "best," indicating that more than one option could be correct but that one statement is more complete than the others.

**Content Area:** Child; **Concept:** Metabolism; **Integrated Processes:** Nursing Process: Evaluation; Teaching/Learning; **Client Needs:** Physiological Integrity: Physiological Adaptation; **Cognitive Level:** Evaluation [Evaluating]

**1691. PHARM ANSWER: 1, 2, 4**

1. **The nurse should record the fluid intake of 120 mL for the child.**
2. **Insulin is not being produced in type 1 DM and should be given to transport the glucose into the cells.**
3. Although the blood glucose of 150 mg/dL is within the normal before-meal target range of 100 to 180 mg/dL for children under 6 years, insulin is still needed to transport the glucose into the cells.
4. **A double-check is completed for all medications that have a high potential for error. For insulin, this includes calculating the number of carbohydrates eaten and the insulin dose.**
5. A serum glucose of 150 mg/dL is within the normal before-meal range of 100 to 180 mg/dL for children under 6 years.

♦ **Test-taking Tip:** *Normal before-meal target range for blood glucose is 100 to 180 mg/dL for children less than 6 years of age. Note that Options 2 and 3 are opposites, so both cannot be correct.*

**Content Area:** Child; **Concept:** Metabolism; Medication; Assessment; **Integrated Processes:** Nursing Process: Analysis; **Client Needs:** Physiological Integrity: Pharmacological and Parenteral Therapies; **Cognitive Level:** Analysis [Analyzing]

**1692. ANSWER: 3**

1. Illustration 1 shows normal anatomy and physiology.
2. Illustration 2 shows type 2 DM in which a small amount of insulin is produced.
3. **The honeymoon phase is the period during new-onset diabetes when the child has some residual beta-cell function. In type 1 DM, after the honeymoon phase the pancreas is unable to produce insulin due to destruction of the beta cells in the islets of Langerhans. Without insulin, glucose is unable to enter the cells, thus causing hyperglycemia.**
4. Illustration 4 does not occur with DM. The cell does not enlarge and would not contain insulin because in type 1 DM after the honeymoon phase, no insulin is being produced.

♦ **Test-taking Tip:** *In type 1 DM there is a failure to produce insulin.*

**Content Area:** Child; **Concept:** Metabolism; Nursing Roles; **Integrated Processes:** Teaching/Learning; **Client Needs:** Physiological Integrity: Physiological Adaptation; **Cognitive Level:** Analysis [Analyzing]

**1693. ANSWER: 1, 2, 4**

1. **An extra dose of insulin is not always needed but is based on blood glucose levels. This statement indicates the parent needs additional teaching.**
2. **Although insulin should not be withheld during illness, the dosage requirements may increase, decrease, or remain unchanged, depending on the severity of the illness and blood glucose levels.**
3. Elevated urine ketones indicate that fat is being metabolized for energy; the HCP should be notified.
4. **Blood glucose levels and urine ketones should be tested more often than once daily. This statement indicates the parent needs additional teaching.**
5. The HCP should be notified when the blood glucose is higher than 240 mg/dL because this could indicate the development of DKA.

♦ **Test-taking Tip:** *The key phrase is "additional teaching is needed." You should be selecting options that are incorrect statements.*

**Content Area:** Child; **Concept:** Metabolism; Nursing Roles; **Integrated Processes:** Teaching/Learning; **Client Needs:** Physiological Integrity: Physiological Adaptation; **Cognitive Level:** Evaluation [Evaluating]

**1694. ANSWER: 4**

1. Poor skin turgor and parched mucous membranes are signs of severe dehydration. The child should be managed in the hospital.
2. Dizziness, double vision, and vomiting could be signs of cerebral involvement. The child should be managed in the hospital.
3. Urine output less than 30 mL per hour is a sign of severe dehydration. The child should be managed in the hospital.
4. **The child is experiencing DKA without vomiting and severe dehydration and can be managed at home if the parents are trained in sick day management and in hyperglycemia and ketoacidosis management. The parents should still notify the HCP.**

♦ **Test-taking Tip:** *Read each option carefully for the key words "hyperglycemia" and "ketosis," and look for like information within the options.*

**Content Area:** Child; **Concept:** Metabolism; Safety; Fluid and Electrolyte Balance; **Integrated Processes:** Nursing Process: Evaluation; **Client Needs:** Safe and Effective Care Environment: Safety and Infection Control; **Cognitive Level:** Evaluation [Evaluating]

**1695. MoC ANSWER: 1, 4, 5**

1. **Kussmaul respirations occur in DKA due to metabolic acidosis from the breakdown of fats into ketones and from the body attempting to compensate for the acidosis by increasing the RR and depth to eliminate the excess carbon dioxide.**
2. The HR would be increased in DKA, not decreased.
3. The breath odor would be sweet-smelling, not foul-smelling, in DKA.
4. **A change in consciousness occurs in DKA due to metabolic acidosis and the hyperglycemic state.**
5. **In DKA, blood glucose levels will be elevated (≥ 330 mg/dL).**

♦ **Test-taking Tip:** *This is an alternate-type question having more than one correct answer. Be sure to read all options to determine if each is associated with DKA.*

Content Area: Child; Concept: Metabolism; Assessment; Integrated Processes: Nursing Process: Assessment; Client Needs: Safe and Effective Care Environment: Management of Care; Physiological Integrity: Physiological Adaptation; Cognitive Level: Analysis [Analyzing]

## 1696. ANSWER: 3

1. Bread is considered a complex (not simple) carbohydrate.
2. Peanuts are a starch-protein snack that is considered a complex carbohydrate; caution is needed in giving peanuts to a 5-year-old.
3. **Fruit juices are considered a simple carbohydrate; 120 mL equals 15 g of carbohydrate.**
4. Although milk is a simple carbohydrate that also contains protein, 60 mL is an insufficient amount. The child would need 240 mL of milk to supply 15 g of carbohydrate.

♦ **Test-taking Tip:** Initial treatment for hypoglycemia includes ingesting 15 g of simple carbohydrate followed by a complex carbohydrate.

Content Area: Child; Concept: Critical Thinking; Metabolism; Nutrition; Integrated Processes: Nursing Process: Implementation; Client Needs: Physiological Integrity: Physiological Adaptation; Cognitive Level: Application [Applying]

## 1697. ANSWER: 5, 4, 2, 1, 6, 3, 7

5. **Assess for signs of pallor, sweating, tremors, irritability, or an altered mental status. Assessment is the first phase of the nursing process and should begin with observation.**
4. **Obtain a fingerstick blood glucose reading. Assessment continues with collecting additional information.**
2. **If the blood glucose level is 70 mg/dL or less, give 15 g of rapid-acting glucose, such as one-half cup fruit juice. The blood glucose needs to be known before interventions can be implemented.**
1. **Wait 15 minutes and check the blood glucose level a second time. Sufficient time needs to pass to evaluate whether treatment has been effective.**
6. **Repeat the rapid-acting glucose if the blood glucose level is 70 mg/dL or less. The brain needs glucose.**
3. **Recheck the blood glucose level for a third time in another 15 minutes. Blood glucose levels are reevaluated until the desired therapeutic effect with giving a carbohydrate choice (CHO) is observed.**
7. **Once the blood sugar has returned to at least 80 mg/dL, give a more substantial snack such as cheese and crackers. Giving a complex CHO should be last. The complex CHO will help maintain a normal blood glucose level.**

♦ **Test-taking Tip:** Use the nursing process. First select assessment options, then implementation, and then evaluation.

Content Area: Child; Concept: Critical Thinking; Metabolism; Integrated Processes: Nursing Process: Implementation; Client Needs: Physiological Integrity: Reduction of Risk Potential; Cognitive Level: Synthesis [Creating]

## 1698. ANSWER: 3

1. Hgb $A_{1c}$ registers the last 3 months of dietary control, with the targeted value less than 8%. The client has poor dietary control.
2. No information regarding the current health condition is available in the stem of the question.
3. **Hgb $A_{1c}$ values above 8% for the 12-year-old client indicate poor dietary control over the past 3 months.**
4. The client has poor long-term control and better short-term regulation of DM.

♦ **Test-taking Tip:** Hgb $A_{1c}$ values for the 12-year-old client should be less than or equal to 8%.

Content Area: Child; Concept: Metabolism; Critical Thinking; Integrated Processes: Nursing Process: Analysis; Client Needs: Physiological Integrity: Reduction of Risk Potential; Cognitive Level: Analysis [Analyzing]

## 1699. ANSWER: 2

1. In hypothyroidism, there is delayed (not early) eruption of teeth.
2. **Delayed physical development results from chronic deprivation of thyroid hormone in hypothyroidism. This question is most important for the nurse to ask the parents.**
3. Increased appetite is associated with hyperthyroidism, not hypothyroidism.
4. Heat intolerance is associated with hyperthyroidism, not hypothyroidism.

♦ **Test-taking Tip:** You should associate "hypo-," or "less than," with the symptoms listed to select the correct option and rule out those associated with "hyper-," or "increased."

Content Area: Child; Concept: Development; Metabolism; Integrated Processes: Nursing Process: Assessment; Client Needs: Physiological Integrity: Physiological Adaptation; Cognitive Level: Application [Applying]

## 1700. PHARM ANSWER: 2, 4, 5

1. A slow HR is associated with hypothyroidism and would indicate the thyroid medication dose is too low, not too high.
2. **Weight loss is associated with hyperthyroidism and could indicate that the thyroid medication dose is too high.**
3. Puffy facial features are associated with hypothyroidism and would indicate the thyroid medication dose is too low, not too high.
4. **Insomnia is associated with hyperthyroidism and could indicate that the thyroid medication dose is too high.**
5. **An elevated BP is associated with hyperthyroidism and could indicate that the thyroid medication dose is too high.**

♦ **Test-taking Tip:** Signs and symptoms of hyperthyroidism will appear if the dose is too high of levothyroxine (Synthroid, Levoxyl), the thyroid replacement hormone. Thus select the options associated with hyperthyroidism.

Content Area: Child; Concept: Medication; Metabolism; Integrated Processes: Nursing Process: Evaluation; Client Needs: Physiological Integrity: Pharmacological and Parenteral Therapies; Cognitive Level: Evaluation [Evaluating]

## 1701. PHARM ANSWER: 1

1. **The nurse should assess for normal growth and development. If the medication, levothyroxine sodium (Synthroid, Levoxyl), is effective, the child will grow and develop at a normal rate for age.**
2. Monthly serum calcium and thyroxin levels are insufficient to determine the effectiveness of levothyroxine sodium.
3. A bimonthly catecholamine level and ECG will not provide information about thyroid function and the effectiveness of levothyroxine sodium.
4. Determining the infant's intake may be helpful in evaluating the effectiveness of levothyroxine sodium, but assessment of the growth and development will give a more accurate indication of its effectiveness.

▶ *Test-taking Tip: Consider assessments that can be completed independently. Eliminate options that require collaboration with the HCP.*

Content Area: Child; Concept: Medication; Assessment; Integrated Processes: Nursing Process: Assessment; Client Needs: Physiological Integrity: Pharmacological and Parenteral Therapies; Psychosocial Integrity; Cognitive Level: Application [Applying]

## 1702. MoC ANSWER: 1

1. **The child with hyperthyroidism would have heat intolerance. Applying extra blankets could cause the child to overheat. The nurse should intervene by removing the extra blankets.**
2. Although the child with hyperthyroidism may have tachycardia and a high BP, taking the BP with an automatic BP machine is not contraindicated and may establish a more accurate BP.
3. The child with hyperthyroidism has an increased appetite. Providing a snack is appropriate.
4. The child with hyperthyroidism may have insomnia. Rocking the child to sleep is appropriate.

▶ *Test-taking Tip: When reviewing the options, consider the symptoms associated with hyperthyroidism and the action that will worsen the child's symptoms.*

Content Area: Child; Concept: Metabolism; Nursing Roles; Management; Integrated Processes: Nursing Process: Analysis; Client Needs: Safe and Effective Care Environment: Management of Care; Cognitive Level: Analysis [Analyzing]

## 1703. ANSWER: 1

1. **The child should avoid any vigorous activity and unnecessary external stimulation.**
2. The child should have decreased stimulation in school, not increased.
3. The child's appetite may increase, but the child will continue to lose weight until the problem is controlled. Food should not be restricted.

4. The child may experience heat intolerance and should be provided with warm weather clothing, even in winter.

▶ *Test-taking Tip: Knowledge of hyperthyroidism is needed to respond to this question. Note that Options 1 and 2 are somewhat opposite; Option 1 decreases stimulation, and Option 2 increases stimulation. Either one or both are incorrect.*

Content Area: Child; Concept: Metabolism; Nursing Roles; Promoting Health; Integrated Processes: Teaching/Learning; Client Needs: Physiological Integrity: Physiological Adaptation; Health Promotion and Maintenance; Cognitive Level: Application [Applying]

## 1704. ANSWER:

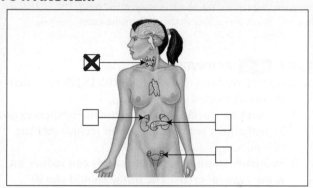

**The nurse should palpate the thyroid gland in Graves' disease.**

▶ *Test-taking Tip: If you are unfamiliar with Graves' disease, use the key word "palpate." Rule out glands that cannot be palpated.*

Content Area: Child; Concept: Metabolism; Promoting Health; Assessment; Integrated Processes: Nursing Process: Assessment; Client Needs: Health Promotion and Maintenance; Cognitive Level: Application [Applying]

## 1705. ANSWER: 2

1. With hyperthyroidism, the environment should be cool and calm due to increased metabolism.
2. **Metabolism is increased in hyperthyroidism; increased food intake is needed.**
3. The client should be encouraged to decrease physical activities due to increased metabolism.
4. Iodine salt increases thyroid hormone release and therefore should be limited.

▶ *Test-taking Tip: Distinguish between hyperthyroidism and hypothyroidism, remembering that in hyperthyroidism the metabolism is increased.*

Content Area: Child; Concept: Metabolism; Integrated Processes: Nursing Process: Planning; Client Needs: Physiological Integrity: Physiological Adaptation; Cognitive Level: Synthesis [Creating]

## 1706. ANSWER: 1

1. **In hypoparathyroidism, insufficient amounts of parathyroid hormone are produced. This affects serum calcium regulation. Muscle spasms, tingling around the mouth, and muscle cramps are signs of hypocalcemia. The nurse should include this instruction.**

2. Dry, scaly, and coarse skin is a sign of hypoparathyroidism, not medication overdose.

3. Phosphorus-rich foods (dairy products) are high in calcium and are usually not restricted unless serum phosphorus levels are exceptionally high. Calcium-rich foods, such as dark green vegetables, soybeans, and tofu, should be encouraged (not decreased in amounts).

4. During crisis episodes, environmental stimuli need to be decreased (not increased) and the child kept quiet.

▶ *Test-taking Tip: Focus on looking for key words in the options that are the opposite of the expected findings and treatment for hypoparathyroidism and eliminate those options.*

**Content Area:** Child; **Concept:** Metabolism; Nursing Roles; Safety; **Integrated Processes:** Teaching/Learning; **Client Needs:** Physiological Integrity: Reduction of Risk Potential; **Cognitive Level:** Analysis [Analyzing]

## 1707. MoC ANSWER: 3

1. Aggressive fluid resuscitation with $D_5NS$ is needed to correct electrolyte imbalances.

2. Seizures may occur due to electrolyte imbalances and hyperthermia; seizure precautions include padding side rails.

3. **Suddenly stopping corticosteroids can induce an acute adrenal crisis. The nurse should clarify this order.**

4. Taking vital signs frequently is necessary to evaluate for complications such as acute adrenal crisis or shock. Portable equipment is available for ongoing monitoring when the child leaves the unit.

▶ *Test-taking Tip: You should associate the key terms "adrenocortical insufficiency" in the stem with key terms "steroid medication" in the options when selecting the correct option.*

**Content Area:** Child; **Concept:** Safety; Metabolism; Management; **Integrated Processes:** Nursing Process: Implementation; **Client Needs:** Safe and Effective Care Environment: Management of Care; **Cognitive Level:** Analysis [Analyzing]

## 1708. ANSWER: 3

1. Weight loss and fatigue occur, but muscle tetany does not occur with Addison's disease.

2. Symptoms of Addison's disease are gradual, not sudden, and include hyperpigmentation and weakness.

3. **Signs and symptoms of Addison's disease do not usually appear until about 90% of the adrenal tissue is nonfunctional, so onset is very gradual. Irritability, decreased pubic hair, and craving for salt are symptoms.**

4. Onset is gradual, and symptoms include hyperpigmentation and weight loss, not gain.

▶ *Test-taking Tip: Narrow the options by first examining like options. Options 2 and 4 describe sudden onset, and 1 and 3 a gradual onset. Knowing that Addison's disease is gradual in onset, eliminate Options 2 and 4. Of the remaining options, consider that salt craving is associated with Addison's disease.*

**Content Area:** Child; **Concept:** Assessment; Critical Thinking; **Integrated Processes:** Nursing Process: Analysis; **Client Needs:** Physiological Integrity: Reduction of Risk Potential; **Cognitive Level:** Application [Applying]

## 1709. ANSWER: 1

1. **Addisonian crisis can lead to circulatory collapse with severe hypotension, not hypertension.**

2. Abdominal pain can be a symptom of Addisonian crisis.

3. Seizures can occur in Addisonian crisis due to electrolyte imbalances.

4. Dehydration can occur in Addisonian crisis due to fluid shifts and loss.

▶ *Test-taking Tip: The key words are "further teaching." Select the option that is not a sign of Addisonian crisis (Option 1).*

**Content Area:** Child; **Concept:** Nursing Roles; Safety; Fluid and Electrolyte Balance; **Integrated Processes:** Nursing Process: Evaluation; **Client Needs:** Physiological Integrity: Physiological Adaptation; **Cognitive Level:** Evaluation [Evaluating]

## 1710. PHARM ANSWER: 1, 2, 3, 4, 6

1. **Recommending that the child wear a medical bracelet will help to identify potential problems in emergency situations.**

2. **The child with Addison's disease is highly susceptible to dehydration and should be encouraged to drink adequate amounts of fluids.**

3. **The school medical plan should include emergency treatment for Addison's disease, and the school nurse should be instructed on appropriate emergency measures.**

4. **If the child vomits the dose of cortisone within 1 hour, the dose should be repeated.**

5. Epinephrine (EpiPen) is used for allergic reactions, such as food allergies or bee stings, and not for Addisonian crisis.

6. **In Addison's disease there is a dark pigmentation of the mucous membranes and the skin, especially of the knuckles, knees, and elbows. This hyperpigmentation may affect the child's body image.**

▶ *Test-taking Tip: Cortisone is administered in Addisonian crisis, and not epinephrine.*

**Content Area:** Child; **Concept:** Nursing Roles; Safety; Fluid and Electrolyte Balance; **Integrated Processes:** Teaching/Learning; **Client Needs:** Health Promotion and Maintenance; Physiological Integrity: Pharmacological and Parenteral Therapies; Psychosocial Integrity; **Cognitive Level:** Analysis [Analyzing]

## 1711. ANSWER: 3

1. Although glucocorticoids are given to treat congenital adrenal hyperplasia, teaching the parents about the medication is not priority among the options.

2. Determining genetic sex through chromosomal analysis may be an option provided to parents, and it may not have been performed.

3. **Symptoms associated with congenital adrenal hyperplasia include hyperkalemia and hyponatremia due to a deficiency in aldosterone. Treating these has priority.**
4. Fluids would not be restricted; children with congenital adrenal hyperplasia are prone to dehydration.

▶ *Test-taking Tip: Use Maslow's Hierarchy of Needs to determine the priority. Physiological problems have priority.*

Content Area: Child; Concept: Nursing Roles; Metabolism; Integrated Processes: Nursing Process: Planning; Client Needs: Physiological Integrity: Physiological Adaptation; Cognitive Level: Application [Applying]

**1712. PHARM ANSWER: 1**
1. **In congenital adrenal hyperplasia, the body lacks the enzyme to produce cortisol and aldosterone. The body produces more androgen, a male sex hormone. The goal of therapy is to reduce virilization (masculine characteristics) in girls.**
2. The presence of Cushing's syndrome is an adverse reaction and is not indicative of therapeutic success.
3. Precocious penile enlargement in males is not indicative of successful therapy.
4. Increased growth rate in both girls and boys indicates that medication therapy is not successful.

▶ *Test-taking Tip: Associate "hyper-" in hyperplasia with "more androgen." Recall that androgen is associated with the development of male characteristics. Select Option 1 because it emphasizes female characteristics.*

Content Area: Child; Concept: Critical Thinking; Medication; Development; Integrated Processes: Nursing Process: Evaluation; Client Needs: Physiological Integrity: Pharmacological and Parenteral Therapies; Cognitive Level: Evaluation [Evaluating]

**1713. ANSWER: 3**
1. There may be growth issues later as the child grows, but it has lesser priority.
2. Fluid volume excess is not a problem. Dehydration, hyponatremia, hyperkalemia, hypotension, and hypoglycemia are associated with adrenal hypoplasia from increased serum concentrations of ACTH.
3. **There is a high risk for impaired parental-infant attachment due to undetermined gender identity in an infant with congenital adrenal hypoplasia.**
4. The parents must be able to demonstrate understanding of the treatments and medications, including glucocorticoids and mineralocorticoids, to provide appropriate care, but it does not have priority.

▶ *Test-taking Tip: Note the key word, "priority." Look for an immediate concern and use the process of elimination. Physiological needs have priority, but because excess fluid volume is not a concern, eliminate Option 2. Note "growth" in Option 1 and "lifelong" in Option 4; eliminate these because they would be later concerns.*

Content Area: Child; Concept: Critical Thinking; Safety; Development; Integrated Processes: Caring; Client Needs: Physiological Integrity: Physiological Adaptation; Psychosocial Integrity; Cognitive Level: Application [Applying]

**1714. MoC ANSWER: 1, 4**
1. **The nurse should include the outcome of demonstrating a positive body image in the child's plan of care. Adrenal insufficiency is associated with stress, fluid volume regulation, and hyperpigmentation of the skin, which can affect body image.**
2. Problems related to activity usually do not occur with adrenal insufficiency.
3. Problems related to oxygenation usually do not occur with adrenal insufficiency.
4. **The nurse should include having the child and family verbalize causes and treatments. Verbalization of these is a measurable outcome.**
5. Problems related to activity usually do not occur with adrenal insufficiency.

▶ *Test-taking Tip: Knowledge of the outcomes of care for children with Addison's disease is needed to respond to this question.*

Content Area: Child; Concept: Nursing Roles; Promoting Health; Management; Integrated Processes: Nursing Process: Planning; Client Needs: Safe and Effective Care Environment: Management of Care; Physiological Integrity: Physiological Adaptation; Psychosocial Integrity; Cognitive Level: Synthesis [Creating]

**1715. ANSWER: 1**
1. **Allowing the child to participate in the care fosters a sense of control over the problem.**
2. The family may ultimately be referred to counseling, but the anger this child is displaying is a normal reaction to seeing him- or herself as different from other children the same age.
3. The child should not be removed from the school setting because that will just reinforce to the child that there is a difference.
4. There is no need for an IEP unless there are additional issues that could interfere with learning. No learning issues have been identified in the stem.

▶ *Test-taking Tip: Note the key word "initial." Only Option 1 addresses the immediate concern.*

Content Area: Child; Concept: Development; Promoting Health; Integrated Processes: Nursing Process: Implementation; Client Needs: Health Promotion and Maintenance; Psychosocial Integrity; Cognitive Level: Analysis [Analyzing]

**1716. ANSWER: 4**
1. Lethargy could be associated with many disease processes; however, it is not usually associated with hypopituitarism.
2. Increased levels of serum glucose are not an expected finding of hypopituitarism.
3. Confusion is usually associated with an injury or hypoglycemia.
4. **Children with hypopituitarism have normal growth patterns during the first year of life, then begins to have a slowing of the growth pattern or no growth growth during the second year of life.**

♦ **Test-taking Tip:** *You need to think about the hormones produced by the pituitary gland. Eliminate signs not associated with pituitary hormones.*

**Content Area:** Child; **Concept:** Development; **Integrated Processes:** Nursing Process: Analysis; **Client Needs:** Physiological Integrity: Reduction of Risk Potential; **Cognitive Level:** Application [Applying]

## 1717. PHARM ANSWER: 3

1. It is important to plot growth on a growth chart to monitor progress, but this is not a goal of treatment.
2. Hypopituitarism can cause soft teeth, but GH treatment will not affect the teeth.
3. **GH treatment should allow the child to grow at a normal rate and reach adult height. This statement indicates understanding of the treatment goals.**
4. Muscle mass may increase during treatment, but the goal is to increase linear growth.

♦ **Test-taking Tip:** *You should look for similar words between the stem and the options to narrow the options to the answer.*

**Content Area:** Child; **Concept:** Nursing Roles; Metabolism; **Integrated Processes:** Nursing Process: Evaluation; **Client Needs:** Physiological Integrity: Pharmacological and Parenteral Therapies; Physiological Integrity: Physiological Adaptation; **Cognitive Level:** Evaluation [Evaluating]

## 1718. ANSWER: 2, 3, 5

1. Blood glucose is only slightly elevated and not necessarily a concern with DI.
2. **A low urine specific gravity is a concern that treatment is not working, requiring further investigation.**
3. **Polyuria is one indication of DI and must be investigated further.**
4. An upset stomach is not a manifestation of DI, so it should just be noted.
5. **A significant weight loss in 24 hours' time is a sign of dehydration.**

♦ **Test-taking Tip:** *The key word is "immediate." If unsure, eliminate the options that are slightly abnormal.*

**Content Area:** Child; **Concept:** Fluid and Electrolyte Balance; **Integrated Processes:** Nursing Process: Analysis; **Client Needs:** Physiological Integrity: Reduction of Risk Potential; **Cognitive Level:** Analysis [Analyzing]

## 1719. ANSWER: 2, 4, 5

1. Serum calcium is not affected by DI.
2. **The nurse should monitor for an elevated serum sodium level. The deficiency in ADH causes massive amounts of water loss and the retention of sodium.**
3. Serum glucose would be monitored with DM, not DI.
4. **The nurse should monitor for an elevated serum osmolality. Polyuria and the sodium retention that occurs with DI increase serum osmolality.**
5. **The nurse should monitor for an elevated BUN, which indicates dehydration.**

♦ **Test-taking Tip:** *DI results from an insufficient production of ADH, resulting in uncontrolled diuresis. You need to consider laboratory value changes from both the condition and from the dehydration that occurs because of the diuresis.*

**Content Area:** Child; **Concept:** Fluid and Electrolyte Balance; **Integrated Processes:** Nursing Process: Assessment; Caring; **Client Needs:** Physiological Integrity: Reduction of Risk Potential; **Cognitive Level:** Application [Applying]

## 1720. ANSWER: 1248

**The total of the wet diapers is 1392 g. The dry weight of 6 diapers is 144 g (24 g × 6 = 144 g). The total urine output is 1392 g – 144 g = 1248 g. Convert grams to mL; 1 gram of urine is equal to 1 mL. Thus the urine output is 1248 mL.**

♦ **Test-taking Tip:** *You need to be sure to subtract the weight of a dry diaper. One gram of urine is equal to 1 milliliter.*

**Content Area:** Child; **Concept:** Fluid and Electrolyte Balance; **Integrated Processes:** Communication and Documentation; **Client Needs:** Physiological Integrity: Basic Care and Comfort; **Cognitive Level:** Application [Applying]

## 1721. ANSWER: 4

1. Children with precocious puberty do not have short stature but are tall for their age.
2. Children with precocious puberty may have a hypothalamic tumor, but it cannot be assessed on a physical exam.
3. Children with precocious puberty may have advanced bone age, but the nurse is unable to assess this on a physical exam.
4. **Secondary sex characteristics are present in children under 8 years of age and can be observed during a physical assessment.**

♦ **Test-taking Tip:** *The key phrase is "physical assessment." Narrow the options to physical findings that can be assessed during a physical examination.*

**Content Area:** Child; **Concept:** Assessment; Development; **Integrated Processes:** Nursing Process: Assessment; **Client Needs:** Physiological Integrity: Physiological Adaptation; **Cognitive Level:** Comprehension [Understanding]

## 1722. PHARM ANSWER: 3

1. Somatropin (Genotropin) is human GH and would not be given when acromegaly is present.
2. Desmopressin (DDAVP) is used to treat DI, not acromegaly.
3. **Octreotide (Sandostatin) suppresses GH release and would be given to treat acromegaly.**
4. Clozapine (Clozaril) is an antipsychotic medication used in the treatment of schizophrenia, not acromegaly.

♦ **Test-taking Tip:** *Acromegaly is a disorder caused by excess production of GH. Select the medication that suppresses the release of GH.*

**Content Area:** Child; **Concept:** Medication; Development; **Integrated Processes:** Nursing Process: Planning; **Client Needs:** Physiological Integrity: Pharmacological and Parenteral Therapies; **Cognitive Level:** Knowledge [Remembering]

**1723.** MoC **ANSWER: 2**

1. There is profound hypertension, up to 250 mm Hg, in a pheochromocytoma crisis and tachycardia (not bradycardia).

2. **Dark urine and extreme muscle pain may indicate skeletal muscle destruction (rhabdomyolysis) that occurs during a pheochromocytoma crisis.**

3. There is ARF with less than 30-mL/hr urine output in a crisis.

4. There is decreased level of consciousness (not hyperexcitability and agitation) in a crisis.

▶ *Test-taking Tip: Eliminate options that are within normal or near-normal parameters for the 6-year-old child.*

**Content Area:** Child; **Concept:** Assessment; Critical Thinking; Metabolism; **Integrated Processes:** Nursing Process: Analysis; Communication and Documentation; **Client Needs:** Safe and Effective Care Environment: Management of Care; Physiological Integrity: Physiological Adaptation; **Cognitive Level:** Analysis [Analyzing]

## Chapter Thirty-Nine

# Gastrointestinal Management

**1724.** MoC The new nurse is reviewing the lab results for the infant with diarrheal stools. Which statement indicates to the experienced nurse that the new nurse is correct in the analysis of the findings?

| Characteristic | Stool Sample |
|---|---|
| Color | Green |
| pH (less than 7 normal) | 6.8 |
| Odor | Sweet-smelling |
| Occult blood | Positive |

1. "The color is characteristic of diarrheal stools."
2. "The pH is abnormal, and the stool is alkaline."
3. "The odor is uncharacteristic for diarrhea."
4. "The stool is darker due to visible blood.

**1725.** PHARM The nurse is reviewing the HCP orders for the child weighing 40 lb who has infectious diarrhea caused by *Salmonella*. Which order should the nurse question?

1. Diphenoxylate/atropine 5 mg oral qid prn loose stools
2. Ibuprofen 65 mg oral q6h for fever >101°F (38.3°C)
3. Oral rehydration therapy per protocol if able to tolerate
4. Send stool sample to the lab for occult blood analysis

**1726.** The hospitalized 8-month-old child recovering from acute diarrhea has not had a loose stool for two hours. Which **initial** drink should the nurse give to the child hourly?

1. Half a glass of apple juice
2. Half a glass of Pedialyte®
3. Half a glass of clear soda
4. Half a glass of chocolate milk

**1727.** MoC An enema is prescribed for the 20-month-old who has had severe constipation. The experienced nurse observes the new nurse perform the procedure. Which action by the new nurse requires the experienced nurse to intervene?

1. Obtains the enema with 500 mL of solution from the unit supply
2. Places the infant on a bedpan for the duration of the procedure
3. Inserts a small soft catheter rectally for instilling the enema solution
4. Stops instillation when cramping is noted and resumes when it passes

**1728.** The nurse assesses that a neonate is passing meconium with urination. Which describes the nurse's **best** thinking about this assessment finding?

1. This is a normal finding immediately after birth.
2. The infant was not thoroughly cleaned after the first stool.
3. A fistula could exist between the colon and urinary tract.
4. If it appears again, then the HCP should be notified.

**1729.** The child is to have a breath hydrogen test to evaluate for malabsorption syndrome. Which instruction is **most** important for the nurse to include when teaching the parents about the preparation for the test?

1. "Be sure to administer the prescribed antibiotics an hour before the breath hydrogen test."
2. "Serve meat, rice, and water for the evening meal before the test; avoid other starchy foods."
3. "Give the child an enema for bowel cleansing the morning of the breath hydrogen test."
4. "Give fluids just before the test to moisten the child's mouth for blowing into the mouthpiece."

**1730.** The nurse is preparing to teach the parents of the child who is to have laparoscopic exploration for a possible Meckel's diverticulum. Which illustration should the nurse select when teaching the parents?

1.

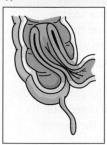

2.

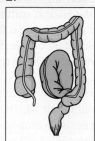

3.

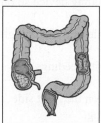

4.

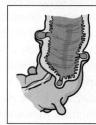

**1731.** The nurse is caring for the 2-month-old hospitalized for dehydration secondary to gastroenteritis. The nurse's assessment findings include irritability; pulse, 180 bpm; RR, 48 bpm; BP, 80/50 mm Hg; and dry mucous membranes. Which additional assessment finding supports moderate dehydration?

1. Capillary refill <2 seconds
2. Intense thirst
3. Sunken anterior fontanelle
4. Absence of tears

**1732.** MoC The infant is hospitalized with infectious gastroenteritis and dehydration. The nurse determines that the NA caring for the infant understands the necessary precautions when the NA makes which statements? **Select all that apply.**

1. "I should put on gloves when I am holding the infant."
2. "I should wear a gown and gloves to change the infant's diapers."
3. "I should keep the door to the infant's room closed most of the time."
4. "I should perform hand hygiene each time I change the infant's diaper."
5. "I should keep the infant in the room unless instructed otherwise."

**1733.** The nurse is developing a teaching plan for the parents of the 5-month-old diagnosed with gastroenteritis caused by a rotavirus. Which instructions should the nurse include to reduce the risk for transmission? **Select all that apply.**

1. Vacuum carpets and upholstery daily to rid the house of the infectious organism.
2. Wash the infant's clothing soiled with stool separately from other family clothing.
3. Perform frequent hand hygiene, especially after changing the infant's diaper.
4. When well, take the infant to the clinic to complete the rotavirus immunization series.
5. Use alcohol-based wipes to disinfect the infant's skin after each bowel movement.
6. Store toothbrushes, pacifiers, and personal items away from the diaper-changing area.

**1734.** The nurse is recording intake for the child hospitalized with diarrhea who has now begun to eat. How many mL should the nurse document for the 3 oz of ice pop that the child consumed?

_____ mL (Record a whole number.)

**1735.** PHARM The nurse admits the 22-lb 12-month-old with dehydration secondary to vomiting and diarrhea. The HCP prescribes $D_5\frac{1}{2}NS$ with 20 mEq KCL at 4 mL/kg/hr. How many mL/hr should the nurse set the infusion pump to deliver the IV infusion?

_____ mL/hr (Record your answer as a whole number.)

**1736.** The clinic nurse is teaching the parents of the 18-month-old who is experiencing acute diarrhea. The child weighs 12 kg. What information should the nurse emphasize? **Select all that apply.**

1. "Have your child drink plenty of fluids, including apple juice and other fruit juices."
2. "Feed your child bananas, rice, applesauce, tea, and toast until the diarrhea resolves."
3. "Avoid cow's milk or milk products; give small amounts of foods that your child eats."
4. "Avoid using commercial wipes that contain alcohol to cleanse your child's skin."
5. "Give one-half glass of a replacement fluid, such as Pedialyte®, for each diarrheal stool."

**1737.** MoC The experienced nurse is observing the new nurse caring for the 11-month-old child who is 12 hours postoperative from a cleft palate repair. Which action requires the experienced nurse to intervene?

1. Uses a suction catheter to remove oral secretions
2. Cautions the NA to not give toast or hard foods
3. Removes a restraint to check the skin and IV
4. Gives a prn prescribed analgesic via the IV route

**1738.** The nurse is developing a discharge plan for the parents of the 12-month-old who had a cleft palate repair. Which topics should the nurse address in the discharge plan? **Select all that apply.**

1. Checking the temperature of foods before feedings
2. Cleaning the suture line with water after each feeding
3. Demonstrating how to feed with a regular baby bottle
4. Using a bulb syringe to suction the baby's mouth
5. Addressing financial concerns for ongoing care
6. Monitoring for aspiration during and after bottle feeding

**1739.** The nurse is planning care for the infant newly diagnosed with esophageal atresia with tracheoesophageal fistula. Which nursing action has **priority** for preventing injury?

1. Assess lung sounds.
2. Withhold oral fluids.
3. Have suction accessible.
4. Monitor vital signs.

**1740.** MoC The nurse is caring for the infant who has respiratory distress and copious oral secretions. Which finding would prompt the nurse to notify the HCP with a concern about possible tracheoesophageal atresia (TEA)?

1. Respiratory distress decreases with oral suctioning.
2. NG tube gastric returns are greenish with some clots.
3. Abdomen is flat with hyperactive bowel sounds.
4. Meets resistance when trying to insert an orogastric tube.

**1741.** MoC The infant is postoperative day 1 after emergency surgery for tracheoesophageal atresia. Which unsafe nursing action would require the intervention of the more experienced nurse?

1. Provides a pacifier to help relax the infant
2. Performs oral and tracheal suctioning prn
3. Slightly elevates the head of the infant's bed
4. Has the gastrostomy tube to gravity drainage

**1742.** PHARM The nurse is developing the plan of care for the 2-month-old with GERD. Which interventions, if prescribed, should the nurse include? **Select all that apply.**

1. Provide feedings that have been thickened.
2. Notify the HCP if spitting up after a feeding.
3. Instruct the parents on the recommended surgery.
4. Keep the infant elevated 30 degrees after feedings.
5. Give oral ranitidine syrup 5 mg/kg q12 hr.

**1743.** The nurse completes teaching the parents of the 3-month-old infant who had surgical correction for pyloric stenosis. Which statement by the parents indicates teaching has been effective?

1. "We should use a special infant feeding device so our baby doesn't get so much air."
2. "We should handle our baby as little as possible right after giving the baby a bottle."
3. "Increasing the formula amount with feedings will help expand our baby's stomach."
4. "Our baby should be placed lying on the right side when put back to bed after a feeding."

**1744.** MoC The experienced nurse and the new nurse are caring for the infant newly diagnosed with pyloric stenosis. Using an illustration, the experienced nurse asks the new nurse to identify the area affected by pyloric stenosis. Place an X on the area that the new nurse should identify as the affected area.

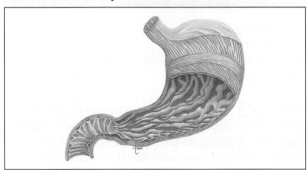

**1745.** The infant with prolonged vomiting secondary to pyloric stenosis has ABGs drawn. Which ABG results should the nurse expect with prolonged vomiting?

1. pH 7.49, PaCO$_2$, 38 mm Hg, HCO$_3$ 29 mEq/L
2. pH 7.26, PaCO$_2$ 40 mm Hg, HCO$_3$ 16 mEq/L
3. pH 7.52, PaCO$_2$, 48 mm Hg, HCO$_3$ 18 mEq/L
4. pH 7.30, PaCO$_2$, 32 mm Hg, HCO$_3$ 29 mEq/L

**1746.** The nurse is creating the plan of care for the infant newly diagnosed with pyloric stenosis. Which plans should the nurse include? **Select all that apply.**

1. Assess the amount and frequency of emesis.
2. Ensure that the infant is kept on NPO status.
3. Maintain patency of the nasogastric tube.
4. Monitor for signs of hyperkalemia.
5. Maintain patency of the rectal tube.

**1747.** The nurse is admitting the 5-week-old infant for a laparoscopic correction of pyloric stenosis. Which information should the nurse expect when asking the parents about the infant's symptoms? **Select all that apply.**

1. Projectile vomiting
2. Bile-colored emesis
3. Sweet-smelling vomitus
4. Weight loss
5. Absence of tears

**1748.** MoC Based on assessment findings, the nurse thinks the infant may have developed NEC. Place the nurse's planned interventions in order of priority.

1. Notify the HCP.
2. Stop feedings, especially any in progress.
3. Initiate prescribed antibiotics.
4. Prepare the infant for an abdominal x-ray.
5. Start prescribed intravenous fluids.

Answer: _____

**1749.** The nurse is admitting the infant with a tentative diagnosis of intussusception. Which question to the mother would be **most** helpful in obtaining additional information to confirm intussusception?

1. "Does your baby vomit after each feeding?"
2. "What does the infant do when experiencing pain?"
3. "Is your infant passing ribbonlike stools?"
4. "Have you felt a mass in your infant's abdomen?"

**1750.** The nurse is preparing the 4-month-old diagnosed with intussusception for surgery when the infant passes a normal brown stool. What is the nurse's **most** important action?

1. Palpate the infant's abdomen.
2. Notify the HCP.
3. Document the character of the stool.
4. Check the stool for the presence of blood.

**1751.** The nurse is taking the history from the parent of the infant with Hirschsprung's disease. Which statement is the parent **most** likely to make?

1. "My baby has ribbonlike stools that have a foul smell."
2. "My baby has projectile vomiting and swollen arms and legs."
3. "My baby has gained weight faster than my other children."
4. "My baby cries every evening and has leg and fist clenching."

**1752.** The nurse is caring for the infant with Hirschsprung's disease. Which statement by the parent indicates understanding of the treatment for Hirschsprung's disease?

1. "Our baby's symptoms can be controlled with a low-fiber diet."
2. "Our baby will need a permanent colostomy surgically placed."
3. "Our baby will be given enemas daily until the stools are normal."
4. "Our baby will need an operation to remove the diseased bowel."

**1753.** The nurse is assessing the neonate diagnosed with an anorectal malformation. Which abnormal assessment findings might the nurse observe? **Select all that apply.**

1. Vomiting
2. Stenosed anal opening
3. Abdominal distention
4. Dark green feces in the urine
5. Frequent meconium stools

**1754.** The nurse is planning care for children diagnosed with IBD. After collecting and analyzing the information about the clients, the nurse makes which statement that **best** reflects the conclusion about the information?

1. All of the clients diagnosed with Crohn's disease are adolescent females.
2. None of the clients have a family history of IBD or are of Jewish descent.
3. Most of those with either Crohn's disease or ulcerative colitis are adolescent males.
4. Of the clients, those with Crohn's disease have the most severe and bloody diarrhea.

**1755.** **MoC** The oncoming shift nurse is reviewing the medical record of the 16-year-old with ulcerative colitis. Which statement in the nurse's notes should the oncoming shift nurse **most** definitely clarify with the nurse from the previous shift?

1. Ate 75% of low-protein and low-carbohydrate breakfast meal of bran muffin, milk, and orange juice.
2. Antispasmodic given before breakfast effective. No abdominal pain or cramping after eating.
3. Client and parent instructed on azathioprine being used to wean the client off the steroids.
4. Four loose, bloody stools this shift. Taught on use and application of barrier cream for skin protection.

**1756.** The 4-year-old is diagnosed with celiac disease. In a follow-up visit, the parent is describing the number, consistency, appearance, and size of the child's stools. Which change in the child's stools should prompt the nurse to conclude that the child's ability to absorb nutrients is improving?

1. Disappearance of currant jelly-like stools
2. Reduction of ribbonlike stools
3. Absence of large, bulky, greasy stools
4. Absence of liquid green stools

**1757.** When counseling the parent of the child with celiac disease, the nurse uses a food list to address foods to be eliminated from the child's diet. Which foods should appear on the elimination food list?

1. Fruits and vegetables; meats, fish, poultry, and fresh eggs
2. Cereals and breads containing rice; cottage cheese
3. Cereal containing oat, wheat, or rye; certain frozen foods
4. Breads made with potato or corn; white whole or skim milk

**1758.** The child is diagnosed with early hypovolemic shock following surgical intervention for a ruptured appendix. Which nursing assessment findings **best** support early hypovolemic shock?

1. Irritability and anxiousness, capillary refill >2 seconds, and absent distal pulses
2. Bradycardia, hypotension, mottled skin coloring, cyanosis, and weak distal pulses
3. Tachycardia, capillary refill >2 seconds, cold extremities, and weak distal pulses
4. Lethargy, increased RR and urine output, and BP low for the child's age

**1759.** **MoC** The nurse is caring for the 10-year-old with peritonitis secondary to a ruptured appendix. Which prescribed intervention should the nurse question?

1. Wet-to-dry dressing change bid to open wound.
2. Empty and measure JP drain q8h or as needed.
3. NG to 180 mm Hg suction; call if NG output high.
4. Continue IV fluids; keep on NPO status for now.

**1760.** The 5-year-old diagnosed with peritonitis secondary to a ruptured appendix has abdominal pain and nausea, even though an NG tube is in place. When pulling back the covers, the nurse sees that the child's abdomen is distended. What should the nurse do **first?**

1. Report the findings to the HCP.
2. Look for fluid moving from the NG tube to the canister.
3. Check the child's VS.
4. Administer droperidol if prescribed.

**1761.** Before administering an enteral feeding to the 2-month-old infant, the nurse aspirates 5 mL of gastric contents. What should the nurse do **next?**

1. Return the aspirate and withhold the feeding.
2. Discard the aspirate and give the full feeding.
3. Return the aspirate before beginning the feeding.
4. Discard the aspirate and add 5 mL of saline to the feeding.

**1762.** The infant who is unable to suck effectively requires gavage feedings. Which statements **best** describe the proper protocol the nurse should follow when feeding the infant via gavage feedings? **Select all that apply.**

1. The gavage tube can be inserted in either the mouth or the nose.
2. The feedings should be similar in amount to the bottle feedings.
3. Continuous feedings rather than intermittent feedings are preferred.
4. Aspirate stomach contents before the feeding and discard the aspirates.
5. Warm the gavage formula to room temperature before starting the feeding.

**1763.** The nurse is caring for the 1-year-old who had a gastrostomy tube insertion. Which intervention should the nurse implement?

1. Place thick dressings under the gastrostomy tube area to keep it clean and dry.
2. Cleanse the gastrostomy site twice daily with saline solution and cotton applicators.
3. Apply tension on the gastrostomy tube to keep the balloon against the stomach wall.
4. Begin tube feedings as soon as the gastrostomy tube has been inserted.

**1764.** The clinic nurse completed teaching with the adolescent who recently started treatment for PUD caused by *Helicobacter pylori (H. pylori).* Which statement made by the client indicates the need for further teaching?

1. "I'll keep my antibiotic and antacid in my backpack so I can take these when at school."
2. "I should stop drinking caffeinated soda because it increases my abdominal pain and is irritating."
3. "Other members of my family could have *H. pylori*; our well should be checked for contamination."
4. "I was surprised that the breathing test I completed could determine whether or not I had *H. pylori.*"

**1765.** The nurse is analyzing laboratory data for an adolescent male who was attacked at a party. Which serum laboratory result should be **most** concerning to the nurse?

| Serum Laboratory Test | Client's Value | Normal Levels |
| --- | --- | --- |
| BUN | 32 | 5–25 mg/dL |
| Creatinine | 1.5 | 0.5–1.5 mg/dL |
| Potassium | 3.2 | 3.5–5.3 mEq/L |
| Amylase | 490 | <200 unit/L |

1. Blood urea nitrogen
2. Amylase
3. Potassium
4. Creatinine

**INSTRUCTIONS:** At 0800 hours, the nurse admits the client to the surgical unit from the ED and obtains the data illustrated in the table shown here. Use the information provided to answer Questions 1766 and 1767.

| | |
|---|---|
| **Client** | 16-year-old female |
| **Allergies** | Penicillin |
| **Admitting Diagnosis** | Appendicitis; type 1 DM |
| **Medical History** | Anorexia; depression; previous admission in adolescent psychiatric unit for suicidal verbalization without plan. |
| **0700 Laboratory Test Results** | *Complete blood count:* Hemoglobin 8.9 g/dL (89 g/L), platelets 450 × $10^3$/microL (450,000/mm³), WBC 14.1 × $10^3$/microL (14,100/mm³) <br> *Serum Chemistry:* Potassium 3.8 mEq/L (3.8 mmol/L), creatinine 1.2 mg/dL (106.1 μmol/L), BUN 40 mg/dL (14.3 mmol/L), glucose 140 mg/dL <br> *Coagulation:* PT 12 seconds |
| **Scheduled Procedures** | Appendectomy 1 hour |
| **Vital Signs** | **0730:** BP 92/58; pulse 90; respirations 22; oral temperature 100.8°F (39.1°C); weight 40 kg <br> **Current:** BP 78/41; pulse 128; respirations 32; oral temperature 102.8°F (39.1°C) |
| **Significant Assessment Data** | **0800** <br> *Neurologic:* Eyes glassy-appearance, reluctant to answer questions, arouses with stimulation <br> *Pain:* Rates 7 out of 10 on pain scale. Rebound tenderness right lower quadrant. Lying down, hips flexed, and knees bent up <br> *Skin:* Warm to touch; poor skin turgor <br> *Affect:* Does not smile, avoids eye contact, and cries easily <br> *Lines/Drains:* Right forearm, peripheral IV present and capped |
| **Medications on the MAR** | Acetaminophen 325 mg orally q4h; has not been given <br> Cefoxitin 1.5 gm I.V. due; not yet up from pharmacy <br> Morphine sulfate 2 mg IV q4h; last given at 0600 <br> 0.9% NaCl 500 mL fluid bolus IV STAT |
| **Diet** | NPO |

**1766.** CJ MoC Based on the case study, what should the nurse do **first?**

1. Insert an IV catheter into the left forearm.
2. Give morphine sulfate in the existing IV.
3. Start the 0.9% NaCl 500 mL fluid bolus IV.
4. Call pharmacy to deliver the cefoxitin now.

**1767.** CJ MoC The nurse is reviewing the client's data. Which statements are a correct analysis of the information? **Select all that apply.**

1. The client is showing signs and symptoms of severe dehydration.
2. The prescribed acetaminophen should be administered now.
3. The HCP should be contacted to prescribe insulin and glucose checks.
4. The data suggests sepsis and the HCP should be informed.
5. Potassium should be prescribed to treat the client's hypokalemia.

# Answers and Rationales

**1724.** MoC **ANSWER: 1**

1. **An infant's normal stool color is yellow. Diarrheal stools are green from lack of time for bile to be modified in the intestine.**
2. The pH is abnormal, but it is acidic rather than alkalotic because the pH is less than 7.
3. Diarrheal stools can be either sweet- or foul-smelling.
4. Only overt blood is visible in the stools, and a stool color change is dependent on the amount of blood and its source.

▶ *Test-taking Tip: Note that the client is an infant. Identify the normal finding for an infant's stool.*

**Content Area:** Child; **Concept:** Bowel Elimination; Assessment; Critical Thinking; **Integrated Processes:** Nursing Process: Analysis; **Client Needs:** Safe and Effective Care Environment: Management of Care; Physiological Integrity: Reduction of Risk Potential; **Cognitive Level:** Evaluation [Evaluating]

**1725.** PHARM **ANSWER: 1**

1. **Antidiarrheal medication such as diphenoxylate/ atropine (Lomotil) is generally not given to young children because it can mask a more serious illness. Children also are at risk for overdose with antidiarrheal agents.**
2. It is acceptable to treat temperature greater than 101°F with ibuprofen (Advil, Motrin).
3. Oral rehydration therapy provides the necessary fluid and electrolytes and is less invasive than IV replacement. Oral rehydration therapy is based on the child's weight and the amount of fluid and electrolyte losses.
4. Frequent diarrhea and some infectious organism can cause bleeding; sending a stool sample for occult blood analysis is an appropriate order.

▶ *Test-taking Tip: Of the options, consider which has the potential of causing the greatest harm to the child.*

**Content Area:** Child; **Concept:** Bowel Elimination; Nursing Roles; **Integrated Processes:** Nursing Process: Implementation; **Client Needs:** Safe and Effective Care Environment: Safety and Infection Control; Physiological Integrity: Pharmacological and Parenteral Therapies; **Cognitive Level:** Analysis [Analyzing]

**1726. ANSWER: 2**

1. Oral rehydration should not begin with juices high in sugar, such as apple juice, which could worsen the diarrhea.
2. **Oral rehydration should begin with an electrolyte replacement fluid such as Pedialyte®. This contains dextrose 25 g, sodium 45 mEq, potassium 20 mEq, chloride 35 mEq, and zinc 7.8 mg. It provides 100 kilocalories/L.**
3. Oral rehydration should not begin with sodas high in caffeine, which could irritate the bowel, or high in sugar, which increases GI motility.

4. Oral rehydration should not begin with chocolate milk, which contains caffeine and can irritate the bowel.

▶ *Test-taking Tip: When reviewing the options, consider the fluid that would provide the most electrolytes.*

**Content Area:** Child; **Concept:** Nutrition; Bowel Elimination; Fluid and Electrolyte Balance; **Integrated Processes:** Nursing Process: Implementation; **Client Needs:** Physiological Integrity: Physiological Adaptation; **Cognitive Level:** Application [Applying]

**1727.** MoC **ANSWER: 1**

1. **In infants, less than 250 mL of solution should be instilled when giving an enema; the amount should be stipulated by the HCP.**
2. Infants and children up to 3 or 4 years of age are unable to retain enema solution, so they must be on a bedpan during the procedure.
3. A soft catheter is used in place of an enema tip to prevent rectal trauma.
4. The amount of solution used in infants is usually so small that cramping is usually not a problem, but if it should occur, the flow should be stopped and resumed after the cramping sensation passes.

▶ *Test-taking Tip: You should think about the amount of enema solution that is appropriate for a 20-month-old.*

**Content Area:** Child; **Concept:** Bowel Elimination; **Integrated Processes:** Nursing Process: Evaluation; **Client Needs:** Safe and Effective Care Environment: Management of Care; Physiological Integrity: Basic Care and Comfort; **Cognitive Level:** Evaluation [Evaluating]

**1728. ANSWER: 3**

1. Meconium in the urine is an abnormal, not a normal, finding.
2. If the urethral opening is not cleansed well, meconium could appear in the urine, but this is unlikely and not the nurse's best thinking.
3. **A fistula could exist between the colon and urinary tract from an anorectal malformation.**
4. Anytime meconium appears in the urine of a neonate, it is concerning because of the potential for congenital anomalies. The HCP should be notified of this finding now, not with the next appearance.

▶ *Test-taking Tip: The key words are "best thinking," suggesting that more than one option could be correct but that one option is better than the other.*

**Content Area:** Child; **Concept:** Bowel Elimination; Critical Thinking; **Integrated Processes:** Nursing Process: Analysis; **Client Needs:** Physiological Integrity: Reduction of Risk Potential; **Cognitive Level:** Application [Applying]

**1729. ANSWER: 2**

1. Antibiotics should not be given because they may reduce hydrogen levels.
2. **The breath hydrogen test is used to detect a rise in expired hydrogen after oral loading with a specific carbohydrate. A meal high in starch can interfere with test results.**

3. Bowel cleansing is not required because the colon is not being examined.
4. The child should be NPO 12 hours before the test.

▶ *Test-taking Tip: If uncertain of a breath hydrogen test, focus on the words and eliminate any options not associated with the mouth. Of the three remaining options, note that two involve oral intake the morning of the test and that the other is different. Often the option that is different is the answer.*

**Content Area:** Child; **Concept:** Digestion; Nutrition; Nursing Roles; **Integrated Processes:** Teaching/Learning; **Client Needs:** Physiological Integrity: Reduction of Risk Potential; **Cognitive Level:** Analysis [Analyzing]

### 1730. ANSWER: 4

1. Illustration 1 shows intussusception where a distal segment of the bowel has invaginated into the cecum. Initial intense pain that passes when the peristaltic wave passes, vomiting, and "currant jelly" stools are characteristic symptoms of intussusception. It occurs more commonly in the second half of the first year of life.
2. Illustration 2 shows a volvulus, bowel twisting and dilated. The twist obstructs the passage of stools. Usually, a volvulus occurs during the first 6 months of life.
3. Illustration 3 shows tumors within different sections of the colon; tumors are rare in infants.
4. **Illustration 4 shows diverticula along the bowel segments. Meckel's diverticulum is the remains of a small pouch of a duct off the ileum. It is the most common congenital malformation of the GI tract, with most symptomatic cases seen in childhood. Tarry black or grossly bloody stools can occur with Meckel's diverticulum.**

▶ *Test-taking Tip: You should look for the illustration that has small bulging sacs pushing outward from the wall of the colon.*

**Content Area:** Child; **Concept:** Digestion; Nutrition; Nursing Roles; **Integrated Processes:** Teaching/Learning; **Client Needs:** Physiological Integrity: Physiological Adaptation; **Cognitive Level:** Application [Applying]

### 1731. ANSWER: 3

1. The moderately dehydrated infant will have slowed CRT of between 2 and 4 seconds.
2. Intense thirst is typical of severe, not moderate, dehydration.
3. **The anterior fontanelle closes between 16 and 18 months of age. In the infant with moderate dehydration, the fontanelle will be normal or sunken.**
4. Absence of tears is typical of severe, not moderate, dehydration.

▶ *Test-taking Tip: The key words are "moderate dehydration." Eliminate options pertaining to severe dehydration. Be aware of the age-appropriate VS, and if they are altered, the likely causes.*

**Content Area:** Child; **Concept:** Fluid and Electrolyte Balance; Assessment; **Integrated Processes:** Nursing Process: Analysis; **Client Needs:** Physiological Integrity: Physiological Adaptation; **Cognitive Level:** Application [Applying]

### 1732. MoC ANSWER: 2, 4, 5

1. If soiling or contact with infected surfaces or items is unlikely, neither a gown nor gloves are needed.
2. **Because the organisms causing gastroenteritis are eliminated in the feces, contact precautions should be used.**
3. The door is closed for airborne precautions; gastroenteritis is not airborne.
4. **Hand hygiene is included in standard precautions and should be performed before and after contact.**
5. **The infant's movement outside the room is limited to only what is necessary.**

▶ *Test-taking Tip: Narrow the options to only those that include contact precautions.*

**Content Area:** Child; **Concept:** Safety; Bowel Elimination; Nursing Roles; **Integrated Processes:** Nursing Process: Evaluation; **Client Needs:** Safe and Effective Care Environment: Management of Care; Safe and Effective Care Environment: Safety and Infection Control; **Cognitive Level:** Evaluation [Evaluating]

### 1733. ANSWER: 2, 3, 4, 6

1. Vacuuming and spraying the house are measures taken for other infectious diseases.
2. **Viral gastroenteritis is transmitted by the fecal-oral route. Washing soiled clothing separately can prevent transmission, especially if using hot water and soap and cleaning the washer with a bleach solution after use.**
3. **Proper hand washing is essential to prevent transmission.**
4. **Infants documented to have had rotavirus gastroenteritis before receiving the full course of rotavirus immunizations at 2, 4, and 6 months of age should still initiate or complete the 3-dose schedule because the initial infection frequently provides only partial immunity.**
5. Alcohol-based wipes, though disinfecting, can irritate the child's skin.
6. **Personal items should be stored away from soiled areas; contaminated items can cause reinfection or transmission to others.**

▶ *Test-taking Tip: "Viral" is the key word in the stem. Eliminate Option 1 because these measures are inappropriate for a viral infection and then Option 5 because alcohol has an irritating effect on the skin.*

**Content Area:** Child; **Concept:** Infection; Nursing Roles; Safety; Bowel Elimination; **Integrated Processes:** Nursing Process: Planning; **Client Needs:** Safe and Effective Care Environment: Safety and Infection Control; **Cognitive Level:** Analysis [Analyzing]

**1734. ANSWER: 90**

One ounce is equal to 30 mL. Use the proportion formula. Multiply extremes (outside values) and the means (inside values) to solve for *X*.

1 oz : 30 mL :: 3 oz : *X* mL; *X* = 90 mL.

♦ *Test-taking Tip: Recall that 1 oz is equal to 30 mL. Visualize a medicine cup, which is 1 oz or 30 mL.*

Content Area: Child; Concept: Fluid and Electrolyte Balance; Nutrition; Bowel Elimination; Integrated Processes: Communication and Documentation; Client Needs: Physiological Integrity: Basic Care and Comfort; Cognitive Level: Application [Applying]

**1735. PHARM ANSWER: 40**

Convert kilograms to pounds and then calculate the milliliters per kilogram per hour.

1 kg = 2.2 lb; 22 lb = 10 kg;
4 mL/kg/hr × 10 kg = 40 mL/hr

♦ *Test-taking Tip: Carefully read the question to ensure that the correct numbers are used in the calculation of the fluid to be administered. Remember 1 kg = 2.2 lb.*

Content Area: Child; Concept: Fluid and Electrolyte Balance; Bowel Elimination; Integrated Processes: Nursing Process: Implementation; Client Needs: Physiological Integrity: Pharmacological and Parenteral Therapies; Cognitive Level: Application [Applying]

**1736. ANSWER: 3, 4**

1. Fruit juices should be avoided because these contain a high amount of carbohydrates, pull circulating fluids into the gut, and can prolong diarrhea.
2. A diet of bananas, rice, applesauce, tea, and toast (BRATT diet) is low in energy and protein and, although recommended in the past, is no longer recommended.
3. **Cow's milk and milk products can be irritating to the GI tract and should be avoided. A normal diet and appropriate administration of fluids are advised.**
4. **Using alcohol-containing products can cause skin breakdown.**
5. Oral replacement solutions are used during maintenance fluid therapy to replace fluid losses from diarrheal stools. Rehydration is 50 mL/kg during the first 4 hours and 10 mL/kg for each diarrheal stool. The child's weight of 12 kg × 50 mL during the first 4 hours = 600 mL; there is no information about the size of the glass being recommended.

♦ *Test-taking Tip: You should be eliminating options that recommend low-energy foods, those that can prolong diarrhea, or the option that contains insufficient information to make a judgment as to whether the option is correct.*

Content Area: Child; Concept: Fluid and Electrolyte Balance; Nursing Roles; Bowel Elimination; Integrated Processes: Teaching/Learning; Client Needs: Physiological Integrity: Basic Care and Comfort; Health Promotion and Maintenance; Cognitive Level: Analysis [Analyzing]

**1737. MoC ANSWER: 1**

1. **Placing the suction catheter in the infant's mouth can disrupt the suture line and cause bleeding or injury.**
2. The infant will be fed blenderized food (no hard foods such as toast, hard cookies, crackers, or ice chips). The palate needs to heal, and hard foods may disrupt the sutures.
3. Restraints should be removed routinely to evaluate CMS and assess for skin breakdown. Elbow restraints are used to keep the hands away from the mouth.
4. Analgesics should be administered especially during the first 24 hours. Controlling pain helps to minimize crying and stress on the suture line.

♦ *Test-taking Tip: Note the key word "intervene." Select the option that could cause injury.*

Content Area: Child; Concept: Nutrition; Nursing Roles; Safety; Integrated Processes: Nursing Process: Evaluation; Client Needs: Safe and Effective Care Environment: Management of Care; Cognitive Level: Evaluation [Evaluating]

**1738. ANSWER: 1, 2, 5, 6**

1. **Checking the temperature of foods is important because the new palate has no nerve endings to sense when things are too hot; a burn can occur.**
2. **Cleaning the suture line with water after each feeding will avoid accumulation of food and promote healing.**
3. With cleft palate surgery, soft nipples or special feeding devices are recommended to maintain the approximation of the incision and intactness of the suture.
4. A bulb syringe has a hard tip and can damage the surgical repair.
5. **Financial stressors often exist because of the hospitalization and the need for ongoing care and speech therapy.**
6. **A special soft-sided bottle equipped with a soft nipple is used for feeding. This bottle allows the fluid to be introduced into the infant's mouth while the bottle is squeezed; this increases the risk for aspiration.**

♦ *Test-taking Tip: Eliminate any options that could damage the surgical incision.*

Content Area: Child; Concept: Safety; Nutrition; Nursing Roles; Integrated Processes: Nursing Process: Planning; Caring; Client Needs: Physiological Integrity: Physiological Adaptation; Psychosocial Integrity; Cognitive Level: Synthesis [Creating]

**1739. ANSWER: 2**

1. Assessing lung sounds is important to determine if aspiration has occurred but will not prevent respiratory distress.
2. **Withholding oral fluids has priority. The infant has a high risk for aspiration if feedings are not withheld and for aspirating secretions when there is a fistula connecting the esophagus and the trachea.**

3. Suction should be readily accessible to handle secretions but it does not have priority.

4. Monitoring VS is important for evaluating for complications but will not prevent respiratory distress.

♦ **Test-taking Tip:** *Use Maslow's Hierarchy of Needs theory to establish priority. A physiological need has priority; thus eliminate options pertaining to assessment.*

**Content Area:** Child; **Concept:** Nutrition; Safety; Oxygenation; **Integrated Processes:** Nursing Process: Planning; **Client Needs:** Physiological Integrity: Physiological Adaptation; **Cognitive Level:** Application [Applying]

## 1740. MoC ANSWER: 4

1. With TEA, respiratory distress is caused by aspiration and will not improve with oral suctioning.

2. In TEA, the NG tube cannot be advanced to the stomach; thus there would be no gastric returns.

3. In TEA, the stomach is usually distended due to air trapping; bowel sounds would be tympanic.

4. **There is a pouch at the end of the esophagus that does not connect to the stomach, so the tube will not advance past the pouch. Inability to pass the orogastric tube warrants further evaluation.**

♦ **Test-taking Tip:** *Atresia is the absence of a normal opening. Use this information to narrow the options to the answer.*

**Content Area:** Child; **Concept:** Safety; Oxygenation; Nutrition; **Integrated Processes:** Nursing Process: Analysis; **Client Needs:** Safe and Effective Care Environment: Management of Care; Physiological Integrity: Reduction of Risk Potential; **Cognitive Level:** Analysis [Analyzing]

## 1741. MoC ANSWER: 2

1. A pacifier can calm the infant and satisfy a sucking need.

2. **Tracheal suctioning should be avoided because it can disrupt the suture line from the repair. To remove secretions, shallow oral suctioning can be gently performed, but the catheter should be prevented from touching the suture line in the esophagus.**

3. Elevating the head of the bed minimizes aspiration of secretions into the trachea.

4. TPN is provided after surgery until gastrostomy or oral feedings are tolerated. If a gastrostomy tube is in place, it is attached to gravity drainage.

♦ **Test-taking Tip:** *The key word is "unsafe." This is a false-response item; select the action that should not be performed.*

**Content Area:** Child; **Concept:** Safety; Nursing Roles; **Integrated Processes:** Nursing Process: Evaluation; **Client Needs:** Safe and Effective Care Environment: Management of Care; Safe and Effective Care Environment: Safety and Infection Control; Psychosocial Integrity; **Cognitive Level:** Evaluation [Evaluating]

## 1742. PHARM ANSWER: 1, 4, 5

1. **Providing thickening feedings helps prevent reflux and improves pH scores.**

2. Spitting up is an expected symptom associated with GERD. The nurse should not notify the HCP.

3. GERD is usually self-limiting. As the esophageal sphincter matures and the child takes solid foods in a more upright position, GERD usually disappears.

4. **An infant should be placed with the head of the bed elevated 30 degrees or placed in an infant seat for at least 1 hour after feeding so gravity can help prevent reflux.**

5. **For infants older than 1 month of age, drug therapy in GERD includes H2 receptor antagonists such as ranitidine (Zantac), cimetidine (Tagamet), famotidine (Pepcid), or nizatidine (Axid).**

♦ **Test-taking Tip:** *Be careful when you read options. Sometimes options are the opposite of what is expected.*

**Content Area:** Child; **Concept:** Nutrition; Nursing Roles; Medication; **Integrated Processes:** Nursing Process: Implementation; **Client Needs:** Physiological Integrity: Physiological Adaptation; Physiological Integrity: Pharmacological and Parenteral Therapies; **Cognitive Level:** Synthesis [Creating]

## 1743. ANSWER: 4

1. A special infant feeding device is used in feeding children with cleft lip or palate and is unnecessary.

2. The infant should be bubbled well after a feeding so there is no pressure from air in the stomach.

3. Only the amounts prescribed should be given to preserve the integrity of the surgical repair site.

4. **Positioning side lying will prevent aspiration of vomitus; the right side aids stomach emptying through the pyloric valve by gravity.**

♦ **Test-taking Tip:** *The key word is "effective." Select the option that is a true statement.*

**Content Area:** Child; **Concept:** Nutrition; Safety; Nursing Roles; **Integrated Processes:** Teaching/Learning; **Client Needs:** Physiological Integrity: Basic Care and Comfort; **Cognitive Level:** Evaluation [Evaluating]

## 1744. MoC ANSWER:

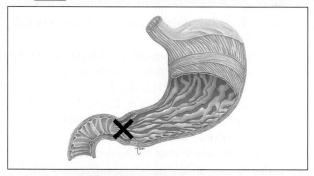

**In pyloric stenosis, fluid is unable to pass easily through the stenosed and hypertrophied pyloric valve (sphincter) at the lower portion of the stomach before the duodenum.**

♦ **Test-taking Tip:** *Carefully examine the illustration, noting the esophagus as the uppermost structure and the duodenum as the lowest structure on the illustration.*

**Content Area:** Child; **Concept:** Digestion; Nursing Roles; **Integrated Processes:** Teaching/Learning; **Client Needs:** Safe and Effective Care Environment: Management of Care; **Cognitive Level:** Knowledge [Remembering]

## 1745. ANSWER: 1

1. **An infant with pyloric stenosis often has been vomiting for 1 to 2 weeks, resulting in metabolic alkalosis as evidenced by an increase in both serum pH and bicarbonate.**
2. A decreased pH and bicarbonate are indicative of metabolic acidosis, which could result if overtreated for the acid-base imbalance or another complication.
3. An increased pH and decreased bicarbonate could be from respiratory alkalosis with compensation.
4. A decreased pH and increased bicarbonate could be from respiratory acidosis with compensation.

▸ *Test-taking Tip: To remember that acid is lost with vomiting and that base is lost with diarrheal stool (bowel movements), label the mouth with the letter "a" for acid and the bottom or bowel movements with "b" for base. A method to evaluate ABGs is to use the letters A for acidosis and B for alkalosis or base. Mark the pH as either acid (A) or alkaline (B). Next mark the $PaCO_2$ and then the $HCO_3$ value as either acid or base. The component that matches the pH is the system (respiratory or metabolic) initiating the acid-base imbalance. The other system is either normal or abnormal. If abnormal in the opposite direction of the initiating system, it is compensating. If both the systems match the pH as either acid or base, then it is both systems that initiate the imbalance.*

**Content Area:** Child; **Concept:** pH Regulation; Assessment; **Integrated Processes:** Nursing Process: Evaluation; **Client Needs:** Physiological Integrity: Reduction of Risk Potential; **Cognitive Level:** Evaluation [Evaluating]

## 1746. ANSWER: 1, 2, 3

1. **Infants dehydrate quickly; assessing the amount and frequency of vomiting should be included in the plan of care.**
2. **NPO status should be included in the plan of care. In pyloric stenosis, the frequent projectile vomiting from an overdistended stomach can be aspirated.**
3. **Maintaining patency of the NG tube should be included in the plan of care; the NG tube is needed for gastric decompression.**
4. Frequent vomiting causes a lack in adequate hydration and a loss of potassium, not hyperkalemia.
5. A rectal tube would not be placed. Stools will be minimal because of inadequate passage of food from the stomach to the duodenum due to constriction of the cardiac sphincter.

▸ *Test-taking Tip: If unsure, apply knowledge of medical terminology: pylorus is the opening from the stomach into the intestine, and stenosis is narrowing. Use this information to eliminate options not pertaining to the GI system from the end of the stomach and upward.*

**Content Area:** Child; **Concept:** Digestion; Nutrition; Fluid and Electrolyte Balance; **Integrated Processes:** Nursing Process: Implementation; **Client Needs:** Physiological Integrity: Physiological Adaptation; **Cognitive Level:** Synthesis [Creating]

## 1747. ANSWER: 1, 4

1. **Because the sphincter is stenosed and the muscle hypertrophied, preventing emptying of the stomach into the duodenum, the infant would begin to vomit immediately after each feeding.**
2. The emesis should not be bile colored because the feeding does not reach the duodenum to be mixed with bile.
3. The vomitus is sour- and not sweet-smelling because the feeding has reached the stomach, where it is in contact with stomach enzymes.
4. **Weight loss occurs due to lack of nourishment resulting from vomiting.**
5. Absence of tears could indicate dehydration in an older infant, but infants younger than age 6 weeks do not tear.

▸ *Test-taking Tip: Focus on the age of the infant when selecting options. You need to think about where the obstruction is occurring—before the duodenum—to be able to correctly identify the characteristics of the emesis.*

**Content Area:** Child; **Concept:** Assessment; Digestion; Nutrition; **Integrated Processes:** Nursing Process: Assessment; **Client Needs:** Physiological Integrity: Reduction of Risk Potential; **Cognitive Level:** Application [Applying]

## 1748. MoC ANSWER: 2, 1, 5, 3, 4

2. **Stop feedings, especially any in progress. The earlier the feedings are stopped in NEC, the better chance the infant has of bowel being preserved and not needing surgery.**
1. **Notify the HCP. The HCP will typically prescribe fluid replacement for the blood loss from bleeding from the bowel and prophylactic antibiotics.**
5. **Start prescribed intravenous fluids. Fluids should be initiated first to ensure that the IV access is patent before antibiotics are started.**
3. **Initiate prescribed antibiotics. Once the IV access is determined to be patent, antibiotics can be started.**
4. **Prepare the infant for an abdominal x-ray. This will determine whether perforation has occurred, as evidenced by air in the abdominal cavity. If a portion of the bowel is necrosed and perforated, the infant needs immediate surgical intervention. The abdomen should also be handled gently to prevent bowel perforation.**

▸ *Test-taking Tip: Use the ABC's to establish priority. The initial assessment requires an immediate intervention and then notifying the HCP. After notifying the HCP, focus on an intervention to preserve the circulation and then on interventions that prevent harm.*

**Content Area:** Child; **Concept:** Safety; Infection; Bowel Elimination; **Integrated Processes:** Nursing Process: Planning; **Client Needs:** Safe and Effective Care Environment: Management of Care; Physiological Integrity: Physiological Adaptation; **Cognitive Level:** Synthesis [Creating]

## 1749. ANSWER: 2

1. Vomiting can occur with the pain from the peristaltic wave; vomiting is unrelated to the time of feeding.
2. **Asking what the infant does when having pain may help establish the diagnosis. With intussusception, infants suddenly draw up their legs and cry as if in severe pain due to a peristaltic wave that occurs from the invagination of one portion of the intestine into another. When the peristaltic wave passes, the infant is symptom free.**
3. Ribbonlike stools occur in Hirschsprung's disease because stool passes through areas of impacted feces and narrowed aganglionic distal segments of the bowel. The stools of intussusception are red and currant jelly-like in appearance from the mix of blood and mucus.
4. A mass may exist and the baby's abdomen distended, but this is common to other GI conditions and too general to confirm the diagnosis.

▶ *Test-taking Tip: Focus on the key words "additional information." You should eliminate options that elicit a "yes/no" response.*

Content Area: Child; Concept: Comfort; Assessment; Bowel Elimination; Integrated Processes: Communication and Documentation; Client Needs: Physiological Integrity: Reduction of Risk Potential; Cognitive Level: Analysis [Analyzing]

## 1750. ANSWER: 2

1. Palpating the infant's abdomen may indicate a change in the presence of a palpable mass and is important before notifying the HCP but is not the most important action.
2. **The HCP should be notified because the passage of a normal brown stool may indicate reduction of the intussusception, and the course of treatment may be altered and surgery canceled.**
3. A change to a normal appearance indicates that the intussusception has been reduced. It is important to document the character of the stool, but this is not the most important action.
4. Checking for blood in the stool is important but is not the most important action.

▶ *Test-taking Tip: The stools of intussusception are currant jelly-like in appearance from the mixture of mucus and blood due to inflammation and mechanical rubbing with the intussusception. Notice that the stools are now normal. Select the option that is likely to alter the course of treatment.*

Content Area: Child; Concept: Communication; Bowel Elimination; Nursing Roles; Integrated Processes: Nursing Process: Implementation; Client Needs: Physiological Integrity: Physiological Adaptation; Cognitive Level: Analysis [Analyzing]

## 1751. ANSWER: 1

1. **Common features of Hirschsprung's disease are ribbonlike, foul-smelling stools, chronic constipation, and abdominal distention. These occur from the absence of ganglion cells in affected bowel segments and resulting lack of peristalsis and loss of internal sphincter relaxation.**

2. Projectile vomiting may occur from abdominal distention. Swollen arms and legs are not characteristics of Hirschsprung's disease, which affects the GI tract.
3. Weight loss and failure to thrive occur due to malabsorption of nutrients.
4. Recurrent evening crying with leg tensing and fist clenching is more typical of colic, which is associated with increased peristalsis.

▶ *Test-taking Tip: You should narrow the options to abnormal findings that affect the bowel.*

Content Area: Child; Concept: Assessment; Bowel Elimination; Integrated Processes: Nursing Process: Analysis; Client Needs: Physiological Integrity: Physiological Adaptation; Cognitive Level: Evaluation [Evaluating]

## 1752. ANSWER: 4

1. A low-fiber diet will not control symptoms; surgical intervention is necessary in Hirschsprung's disease.
2. A permanent colostomy is not always necessary; it depends on the location of the diseased colon. A two-stage surgery may be performed where a temporary colostomy is established, followed by a later repair at age 12 to 18 months.
3. Management of Hirschsprung's disease does not entail giving enemas daily until stools are normal because stools will not be normal in Hirschsprung's disease. Daily saline enemas may be given prior to surgery to achieve a bowel movement.
4. **Hirschsprung's disease treatment includes surgery to remove the unhealthy section of the bowel where the ganglions are absent. This statement indicates that the parent understands the treatment.**

▶ *Test-taking Tip: Hirschsprung's disease is absence of ganglionic innervation, usually in the lower portion of the bowel, causing chronic constipation, ribbonlike stools, and dilation of the colon proximal to the obstruction. When answering the question, you need to consider the treatment for bowel obstructions.*

Content Area: Child; Concept: Bowel Elimination; Nursing Roles; Integrated Processes: Teaching/Learning; Nursing Process: Evaluation; Client Needs: Physiological Integrity: Physiological Adaptation; Cognitive Level: Evaluation [Evaluating]

## 1753. ANSWER: 1, 2, 3, 4

1. **Vomiting can occur because stool has not passed due to the anorectal malformation.**
2. **The rectal opening can be narrowed, or stenosed, with an anorectal malformation.**
3. **Abdominal distention can occur because stool has not passed.**
4. **Meconium (dark green, first stools of the neonate) in the urine could indicate a fistula between the colon and urinary tract.**
5. Meconium stools are a normal finding. Stools are generally not passed in the infant with imperforate anus.

**Test-taking Tip:** The key term is "abnormal." You should eliminate normal findings. Anorectal malformation is a global term, so there may be many variations in findings ranging from simple imperforate anus to other associated complex anomalies of GU and pelvic organs.

**Content Area:** Child; **Concept:** Assessment; Bowel Elimination; **Integrated Processes:** Nursing Process: Assessment; **Client Needs:** Physiological Integrity: Reduction of Risk Potential; **Cognitive Level:** Application [Applying]

## 1754. ANSWER: 3

1. Because Crohn's disease is more common in males, it is unlikely that all clients will be females.
2. Both Crohn's disease and ulcerative colitis show familial tendencies. Crohn's disease can affect any ethnic group, but Caucasians and persons of Eastern European (Ashkenazi) Jewish descent have the highest risk.
3. **Both Crohn's disease and ulcerative colitis are more common in males, perhaps due to a familial or autoimmune tendency.**
4. The ileum is affected in Crohn's disease, whereas the colon and rectum are affected in ulcerative colitis. Because both diseases involve the development of ulcers of the mucosa or submucosal layers, both diseases manifest with diarrhea from irritation and unabsorbed fluids. However, because of the more severe ulcerations along the colon in ulcerative colitis, stools are more severe and bloody in ulcerative colitis (not Crohn's disease).

**Test-taking Tip:** Usually options with absolute words are incorrect. Thus you should eliminate the options with the absolute words "all" and "none" and then focus on the remaining two options.

**Content Area:** Child; **Concept:** Assessment; Bowel Elimination; Diversity; **Integrated Processes:** Nursing Process: Analysis; Culture and Spirituality; **Client Needs:** Physiological Integrity: Physiological Adaptation; **Cognitive Level:** Comprehension [Understanding]

## 1755. MoC ANSWER: 1

1. **The oncoming shift nurse should clarify an incorrect action. The diet used in the treatment of ulcerative colitis should be high in protein and carbohydrates (not low) with normal fat and decreased roughage. A bran muffin is high in roughage.**
2. Antispasmodic agents should be administered before meals.
3. Azathioprine (Imuran), an immunomodulatory agent, is used to wean the client off of steroids.
4. Ulcerative colitis is characterized by bloody diarrhea. The frequency of bloody stools can result in excoriation and skin breakdown. A barrier cream can help to protect the skin.

**Test-taking Tip:** The key phrase is "most definitely clarify," which suggests that either an action is incorrect or the documentation is incorrect. You need to consider if the interventions are appropriate for the client with ulcerative colitis.

**Content Area:** Child; **Concept:** Assessment; Bowel Elimination; Communication; **Integrated Processes:** Communication and Documentation; **Client Needs:** Safe and Effective Care Environment: Safety and Infection Control; Safe and Effective Care Environment: Management of Care; **Cognitive Level:** Analysis [Analyzing]

## 1756. ANSWER: 3

1. Currant jelly-like stools are characteristic of intussusception from the mixing of blood and mucus, and not celiac disease.
2. Ribbonlike stools occur in Hirschsprung's disease because stool passes through areas of impacted feces and narrowed aganglionic distal segments of the bowel.
3. **When gluten is ingested in celiac disease, changes occur in the intestinal mucosa or villi that prevent the absorption of foods into the bloodstream and affect the ability to absorb fat. Stools are large, bulky, and greasy, indicating steatorrhea. An absence of steatorrhea indicates that the child's ability to absorb nutrients is improving.**
4. Liquid green stools appear in diarrhea; nutrients are not being well absorbed.

**Test-taking Tip:** Carefully read what the question is asking. The key words are "absorb nutrients." Eliminate options that suggest bleeding or obstruction has improved.

**Content Area:** Child; **Concept:** Digestion; Nutrition; Bowel Elimination; **Integrated Processes:** Nursing Process: Evaluation; **Client Needs:** Physiological Integrity: Reduction of Risk Potential; **Cognitive Level:** Evaluation [Evaluating]

## 1757. ANSWER: 3

1. Foods in their natural form are usually gluten free.
2. Cereals and breads containing rice are acceptable foods, as is cottage cheese.
3. **Foods that contain gluten include wheat, rye, oats, and barley products. These should be included on the elimination list. Packaged and frozen foods typically contain gluten as fillers and should also be included.**
4. Potato bread or cornbread and whole, skim, or low-fat milk are acceptable. Chocolate milk and malt beverages contain gluten.

**Test-taking Tip:** Do not confuse celiac disease with lactose intolerance. Persons with celiac disease cannot have gluten-containing products. Those with lactose intolerance cannot have milk or milk products.

**Content Area:** Child; **Concept:** Nutrition; Digestion; Nursing Roles; **Integrated Processes:** Teaching/Learning; **Client Needs:** Physiological Integrity: Basic Care and Comfort; **Cognitive Level:** Application [Applying]

## 1758. ANSWER: 3

1. Absent distal pulses are associated with a later stage of hypovolemic shock.
2. Bradycardia is associated with a later stage of hypovolemic shock.

3. **Early hypovolemic shock is supported by these signs and symptoms due to blood or fluid loss: tachycardia, CRT >2 seconds, cold extremities, and weak distal pulses. Other findings are increased RR, pallor or mottled skin color, and decreased urine output. Usually the BP is normal for the child's age.**

4. A low BP is associated with a later stage of hypovolemic shock. Decreased (not increased) urine output (less than 1 to 2 mL/kg/hr in newborns and less than 0.5 to 1.0 mL/kg/hr in other age groups) is associated with a later stage of hypovolemic shock.

▶ **Test-taking Tip:** *The key phrase is "early hypovolemic shock." Narrow the options by first examining options that have opposite information, and eliminate one of these to arrive at the answer (bradycardia versus tachycardia; absent distal pulses versus weak distal pulses; irritability versus lethargy).*

**Content Area:** Child; **Concept:** Assessment; Fluid and Electrolyte Balance; Perfusion; **Integrated Processes:** Nursing Process: Analysis **Client Needs:** Physiological Integrity: Physiological Adaptation; **Cognitive Level:** Analysis [Analyzing]

---

**1759. MoC ANSWER: 3**

1. Due to the risk of peritonitis with a ruptured appendix, the HCP may leave the wound open to prevent infection and later close the wound. The wet-to-dry dressing changes will allow removal of infectious material through wicking and maintain tissue integrity.

2. The child with a ruptured appendix can be expected to have a JP drain. Emptying the JP drain q8h or as needed would be expected practice.

3. **The NG tube is used to decompress the bowel and remove gastric secretions until peristalsis returns. The NG tube on a child this age would be kept on low (40 mm Hg) intermittent suction to ensure that there would be no injury to the gastric lining.**

4. Continuing IV fluids and keeping the client NPO are needed because bowel peristalsis may not return for a few days.

▶ **Test-taking Tip:** *The key words are "should question." This is a negative-response item. You should choose the intervention that would be unsafe for the child.*

**Content Area:** Child; **Concept:** Collaboration; Inflammation; Safety; **Integrated Processes:** Nursing Process: Implementation; **Client Needs:** Safe and Effective Care Environment: Safety and Infection Control; **Cognitive Level:** Analysis [Analyzing]

---

**1760. ANSWER: 2**

1. Once the nurse determines that the NG is functioning correctly, the nurse should complete the assessment and contact the HCP. Nonmechanical paralytic ileus can develop in the immediate postoperative period.

2. **When the child has an NG tube in place and has abdominal pain, nausea, and abdominal distention, the first action is to check the functionality of the NG tube, including suction and correct placement. These findings can be due to a nonfunctioning NG tube.**

3. Further assessment of the abdomen and taking VS will delay determining whether the NG tube is functioning correctly.

4. An antiemetic such as droperidol (Inapsine) should be administered if prescribed, especially if reestablishment of a nonfunctioning NG tube does not relieve the nausea, but this is not the first action.

▶ **Test-taking Tip:** *The key word is "first." Focus on the client's symptoms. The NG tube, if functioning correctly, provides GI decompression.*

**Content Area:** Child; **Concept:** Inflammation; Bowel Elimination; **Integrated Processes:** Nursing Process: Implementation; **Client Needs:** Safe and Effective Care Environment: Safety and Infection Control; **Cognitive Level:** Application [Applying]

---

**1761. ANSWER: 3**

1. Five mL is equivalent to a teaspoon, which is a small amount for a 2-month-old infant. With a small amount of gastric aspirates, the feeding should not be withheld.

2. Discarding the aspirate with each feeding can result in acid-base and electrolyte imbalances.

3. **If the amount aspirated is small (a few mL), the aspirate should be returned at the beginning of the feeding to prevent the loss of electrolytes and gastric enzymes. If the amount is large as compared to the amount prescribed for the feeding, then the amount of the feeding should be reduced by the amount of the aspirate.**

4. Saline is not an electrolyte replacement for gastric contents.

▶ **Test-taking Tip:** *Examine options with duplicate words first. Determine whether the aspirate should be returned or discarded. After determining it should be returned, eliminate the discard options and then determine which of the two remaining options is best.*

**Content Area:** Child; **Concept:** Nutrition; Digestion; Fluid and Electrolyte Balance; **Integrated Processes:** Nursing Process: Planning; **Client Needs:** Physiological Integrity: Basic Care and Comfort; **Cognitive Level:** Application [Applying]

---

**1762. ANSWER: 1, 2, 5**

1. **Although orogastric insertion allows for easier breathing and less risk of vagal stimulation and is preferred, the tube may be inserted nasally if it is to stay in place.**

2. **The amount of gavage feeding should be similar to what the child normally would ingest at a feeding to prevent overdistention or undernourishment.**

3. Intermittent (not continuous) feedings are preferred to mimic the normal feeding pattern and allow the stomach to function more normally.

4. Unless the amount is excessive, aspirates should be measured and reinserted (not discarded) so electrolytes are retained.

5. **Warming to room temperature will prevent chilling of the infant.**

▶ ***Test-taking Tip:*** *Carefully read each option and look for key words in the options that are opposite of the actions in the protocol.*

**Content Area:** Child; **Concept:** Nutrition; Digestion; Fluid and Electrolyte Balance; **Integrated Processes:** Nursing Process: Implementation; **Client Needs:** Physiological Integrity: Basic Care and Comfort; **Cognitive Level:** Application [Applying]

### 1763. ANSWER: 2

1. Although there is the risk of infection at the gastrostomy site due to the area being moist and oozing fluid following insertion, a thick dressing puts tension on the tube. This tension could cause accidental removal or impaired tissue integrity from pressure.
2. **The nurse should cleanse the gastrostomy site with saline to prevent infection. An antibiotic ointment may be prescribed.**
3. Tension on the gastrostomy tube should be avoided to prevent tissue trauma or accidental removal.
4. Tube feedings are not begun until bowel function has returned.

▶ ***Test-taking Tip:*** *Identify the options that could cause harm and eliminate these.*

**Content Area:** Child; **Concept:** Digestion; Infection; Skin Integrity; **Integrated Processes:** Nursing Process: Implementation; **Client Needs:** Physiological Integrity: Basic Care and Comfort; **Cognitive Level:** Application [Applying]

### 1764. ANSWER: 1

1. **Keeping medications in a backpack and taking them as scheduled is unacceptable in a school setting. A permission form to take medications at school needs to be completed by the HCP, taken to school with the medications, and given to the appropriate school personnel (usually a school nurse). The medications are then placed in a safe location at school, usually the nurse's office.**
2. Beverages containing caffeine and alcohol can exacerbate the disease and should be stopped.
3. *H. pylori* is transmitted by the fecal-oral or oral-oral routes, and infections often occur in several members of a family. Water supplies can become contaminated with *H. pylori*.
4. A breathing test can be completed to measure urea in the breath and to diagnose *H. pylori* because the organism hydrolyzes urea.

▶ ***Test-taking Tip:*** *If uncertain of the answer, focus on selecting an option that is a safety concern. The key phrase "further teaching" indicates that you should select an incorrect statement made by the client.*

**Content Area:** Child; **Concept:** Digestion; Nursing Roles; **Integrated Processes:** Nursing Process: Evaluation; **Client Needs:** Safe and Effective Care Environment: Safety and Infection Control; Health Promotion and Maintenance; **Cognitive Level:** Evaluation [Evaluating]

### 1765. ANSWER: 2

1. The BUN is likely elevated due to tissue trauma. It is not life-threatening. If the serum creatinine were also elevated, that could indicate renal damage.
2. **An amylase level greater than 200 is indicative of acute pancreatitis. Abdominal trauma with injury to the pancreas can cause acute pancreatitis. Because the adolescent was attacked, there is the risk of other internal injuries. This value should be most concerning to the nurse.**
3. The serum potassium (K) does impact cardiac function, but typically a relatively healthy adolescent with no history of heart issues will tolerate a lower K level.
4. The serum creatinine level is WNL.

▶ ***Test-taking Tip:*** *When interpreting laboratory values, identify those that are abnormal and the systems affected. Then, determine which system or organ is more at risk. The key words are "most concerning."*

**Content Area:** Child; **Concept:** Nutrition; Safety; **Integrated Processes:** Nursing Process: Analysis; **Client Needs:** Physiological Integrity: Reduction of Risk Potential; **Cognitive Level:** Analysis [Analyzing]

### 1766. CJ MoC ANSWER: 3

1. Starting another IV line is important because the client is to receive multiple IV medications that need to be administered at different rates. But giving the fluid bolus IV should be first because the client is hypotensive and dehydrated.
2. It has only been two hours since the last dose of morphine sulphate; it is prescribed q4h. The nurse must first contact the HCP for a change of order before giving additional doses. The client is hypotensive; morphine sulphate may lower the BP further.
3. **The client is hypotensive with a current BP of 78/41 mm Hg. The BP has decreased since the ER admission and the client has inadequate perfusion. The nurse should first initiate the IV fluid bolus to increase circulating volume.**
4. Administering an antibiotic as soon as it arrives from pharmacy is important but giving the IV fluid bolus should be first. Although cefoxitin (Mefoxin) has been prescribed, the nurse should verify this with the HCP because the client has a penicillin allergy. Usually a carbapenem-type antibiotic, rather than a cephalosporin, is prescribed when a person has a penicillin allergy.

▶ ***Test-taking Tip:*** *With a scenario, it is best to read the questions before reviewing the scenario. Use the ABC's to determine the priority.*

**Content Area:** Child; **Concept:** Management; Nutrition; Perfusion; **Integrated Processes:** Nursing Process: Implementation; **Client Needs:** Safe and Effective Care Environment: Management of Care; Physiological Integrity: Physiological Adaptation; **Cognitive Level:** Analysis [Analyzing]

**1767.** `CJ` `MoC` **ANSWER: 1, 3, 4**

1. **Signs of dehydration include an elevated BUN, poor skin turgor, hypotension, and tachycardia.**

2. Although the client's elevated temperature should be treated with acetaminophen, the client is NPO and is sleepy. The nurse should contact the HCP to request an IV dose.

3. **The client's history includes DM type 1; the HCP should be contacted to prescribe insulin and glucose checks.**

4. **Signs of sepsis include hypotension, tachycardia, elevated temperature, and elevated WBC. The HCP should be informed of these symptoms.**

5. The serum potassium of 3.8 mEq/L (3.8 mmol/L) is within the normal range.

▶ *Test-taking Tip: You need to consider the entire scenario before selecting your options.*

**Content Area:** Child; **Concept:** Management; Nutrition; Perfusion; **Integrated Processes:** Nursing Process: Analysis; **Client Needs:** Safe and Effective Care Environment: Management of Care; Physiological Integrity: Physiological Adaptation; **Cognitive Level:** Analysis [Analyzing]

## Chapter Forty

# Hematological and Oncological Management

**1768.** The nurse is teaching the parents of the child who will have a bone marrow biopsy. Which location should the nurse identify as the site where bone marrow will be aspirated? Place an X on the site.

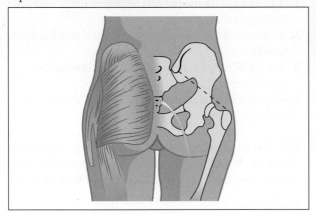

**1769.** The nurse teaches the 9-year-old who is to undergo bone marrow aspiration. Which statement by the child **best** indicates understanding of the teaching?

1. "I won't be able to go to the playroom again until tomorrow."
2. "I'll need to stay in bed for at least an hour after the procedure."
3. "I'll need to take a shower afterward to remove the cleansing dye."
4. "I'll have a dressing over the site, which will be removed later today."

**1770.** The nurse is planning care for the 18-month-old with iron-deficiency anemia. Which intervention should the nurse implement?

1. Review the lab findings for macrocytic RBCs.
2. Limit milk intake to no more than 1 liter per day.
3. Give prescribed iron with foods high in vitamin D.
4. Inform the HCP about hard, black-colored stools.

**1771.** **PHARM** After 7 days of iron therapy, the child with iron-deficiency anemia has serum laboratory tests completed. Which finding indicates that the iron therapy is beginning to correct the anemia?

1. Increased reticulocyte count
2. Increased granulocytes
3. Increased indirect bilirubin
4. Increased erythropoietin levels

**1772.** **MoC** The nurse is developing the plan of care for the child hospitalized in sickle cell crisis. Which nursing problem has **priority?**

1. Risk for deficient fluid volume related to inadequate fluid intake due to pain
2. Chronic pain related to chronic physical disability and clustering of sickled cells
3. Risk for infection related to ineffectively functioning spleen and poor health
4. Ineffective tissue perfusion related to pulmonary infiltrates of abnormal blood cells

**1773.** **PHARM** The parents' only child, who is 1-year-old, is hospitalized in sickle cell crisis. Which nursing intervention has **priority?**

1. Teach about keeping the child hydrated.
2. Ask if the parents would like to have genetic testing.
3. Obtain parental consent for a platelet transfusion.
4. Ensure that hydroxyurea is being prescribed.

**1774.** The parents of the child with sickle cell anemia are being taught pain control measures for their 4-year-old. Which measure is **most** important to teach the parents to prevent the onset of vaso-occlusive pain?

1. Apply ice packs to the child's joints.
2. Provide large amounts of fluids every day.
3. Give acetaminophen 650 mg orally twice daily.
4. Increase outdoor exercise in the afternoons.

**1775.** The child, recovering following ingestion of rat poison, develops aplastic anemia. Which findings associated with aplastic anemia should the nurse expect on assessment? **Select all that apply.**

1. Petechiae
2. Epistaxis
3. Easily fatigued
4. Watery, itching eyes
5. Mouth ulcerations

**1776.** The nurse is weighing gauze that was used to control bleeding for the child with hemophilia. A pack of 10 dry sponges weighs 75 g. The packs of 10 blood-soaked sponges weighed 188 g, 158 g, and 145 g, respectively. What amount in mL should the nurse document for the child's blood loss?

_____ mL (Record a whole number.)

**1777.** The child diagnosed with hemophilia has epistaxis. Which interventions should the school nurse implement? **Select all that apply.**

1. Have the child lie down and elevate the feet above heart level.
2. Apply pressure to the child's nose with the thumb and forefinger.
3. Keep pressure applied to the child's nose for at least 10 minutes.
4. Apply ice or a cold cloth to the bridge of the child's nose.
5. Ask whether the child is carrying medication to treat nosebleeds.

**1778.** The nurse is reviewing the laboratory results for the infant newly diagnosed with hemophilia A. Which finding should the nurse expect?

1. Prolonged prothrombin time (PT)
2. Decreased hemoglobin level (Hgb)
3. Decreased hematocrit level (Hct)
4. Prolonged activated partial thromboplastin time (aPTT)

**1779.** **PHARM** The child diagnosed with thrombocytopenia purpura (ITP) is being discharged from the hospital. Which nursing intervention is **most** important?

1. Teach parents to offer frozen juice pops to increase the child's fluid intake.
2. Inform the parents to keep flowers away from the child's living space.
3. Apply firm pressure to the IV site for 5 minutes following its removal.
4. Provide parental support because the child will have ITP for life.

**1780.** **MoC** The new nurse is telling the experienced nurse about treatments that the HCP discussed with the parents of the child who has thalassemia major. Which statement by the new nurse should the experienced nurse question?

1. "Plasmapheresis will be used to remove the toxins that are destroying the RBCs."
2. "Blood transfusions will need to be administered about every 2 to 4 weeks."
3. "A splenectomy may be necessary to reduce the child's abdominal discomfort."
4. "Bone marrow stem cell transplant might cure this child's thalassemia major."

**1781.** **PHARM** The African American child with thalassemia major has iron overload after receiving multiple blood transfusions. Which intervention should the nurse anticipate?

1. A meeting with the parents to determine if iron overload is hereditary
2. A change in the type of blood product that has been transfused
3. A reduction in the frequency of the transfusions administered
4. Initiation of chelation therapy to bind and excrete the excess iron

**1782.** The nurse is assessing the child newly diagnosed with ALL. Which assessment findings should the nurse relate to the child's diagnosis? **Select all that apply.**

1. Alopecia
2. Petechiae
3. Anorexia
4. Insomnia
5. Bleeding gums
6. Pallor

**1783.** The nurse is caring for the child with ALL. The nurse reviews the child's laboratory report after observing that the child has multiple bruises and a large amount of blood on bed linens and in tissues. Place an X on the specific laboratory value on the report illustrated that should be of greatest concern to the nurse.

| Laboratory Report | |
|---|---|
| **Hematology** | **Client Value** |
| Hgb (11.5–12.5 g/dL) | 9.0 g/dL |
| Hct (35%–50%) | 27% |
| WBC (5–15.5 K/mm³) | 22 K/mm³ |
| Platelets (Plt 150–300 K/mm³) | 20 K/mm³ |

**1784.** **PHARM** The child with leukemia is to receive a unit of platelets. The child weighs 33 lb, and the platelets are to be infused at 10 mL/kg/hr. The nurse should plan to transfuse the platelets at a rate of how many mL per hour?

_____ mL/hr (Record a whole number.)

**1785.** **PHARM** The child with leukemia is being discharged after an initial chemotherapy treatment. The nurse is teaching the parents about the allopurinol the child will continue to take at home. How should the nurse describe the **most** important purpose of allopurinol for this child?

1. Helps reduce the child's sleeplessness from chemotherapy
2. Treats joint pain and swelling caused by the child's gout
3. Prevents the child from development of gouty arthritis
4. Protects the child's kidneys by reducing uric acid formation

**1786.** The child with Hodgkin's disease is treated with irradiation to the cervical area in the neck. The child lacks energy and has malaise. What aspects should the nurse explore further? **Select all that apply.**

1. Thyroid function
2. Hemoglobin level
3. Nutritional status
4. Swallowing ability
5. Voiding patterns

**1787.** The hospitalized child is neutropenic due to chemotherapy treatments. Which instructions should the nurse plan to include when preparing the parents to take the child home? **Select all that apply.**

1. Ask those who were recently vaccinated not to come for a visit yet.
2. Keep the child's immediate surroundings free of plants and flowers.
3. Provide items such as goldfish, sanitized toys, or books for playtime.
4. Arrange for the child to sleep alone, preferably in his or her own room.
5. Take the child's temperature, respiratory rate, and pulse four times daily.

**1788.** The child receiving aggressive combination chemotherapy treatments has stomatitis. Which interventions should the nurse implement? **Select all that apply.**

1. Perform oral care with soft-sponged toothettes every 2 to 4 hours.
2. Use alcohol-based mouthwash diluted with water to lessen irritation.
3. Swab the child's mouth with viscous lidocaine before performing oral care.
4. Cleanse the child's gums using a piece of gauze soaked in saline or plain water.
5. Massage the back of the child's hands between the thumb and index finger with an ice cube for 5 to 7 minutes

**1789.** **MoC** Four parents call a clinic to have their children seen for unusual lumps or swelling. Which child should the nurse schedule to be seen by the HCP **first?**

1. The child with Down syndrome
2. The child who lives close to power lines
3. The child who has had chronic ear infections
4. The child whose sibling was treated for osteosarcoma

**1790.** **MoC** The nurse, concerned that the adolescent with NHL has superior vena cava syndrome, notifies the HCP. Which findings support this concern?

1. Thrombocytopenia and leukocytosis
2. Hyperuricemia, hypocalcemia, and hyperphosphatemia
3. Tingling and paresthesias of the lower extremities and pain on light touch
4. Upper chest, neck, and face cyanosis, upper-extremity edema, and distended neck veins

**1791.** The HCP explains the disease process and recommended treatment to the teenage client diagnosed with Hodgkin's lymphoma. Which statement to the nurse indicates that the client understands the diagnosis and treatment?

1. "I'm so relieved; I was worried that I had cancer and that nothing could be done to treat it."
2. "I have a good chance of being cured with radiation, chemotherapy, or both therapies."
3. "I'll need to have a laparotomy to stage the disease before I can start treatment."
4. "I'm so upset; I won't be able to go to college, marry, and raise a family."

**1792.** The nurse is completing a health history and an assessment for the male adolescent tentatively diagnosed with Hodgkin's lymphoma. Which findings should the nurse associate with Hodgkin's lymphoma? **Select all that apply.**

1. Firm, nontender, enlarged lymph node in the axillary area
2. Unexplained temperatures above 100.4°F (38°C) for 3 consecutive days
3. Unexplained weight loss of 10% or more in the previous 6 months
4. States consuming a diet consisting mostly of seafood and saturated fats
5. A brother who was diagnosed with Hodgkin's disease as an adolescent

**1793.** The nurse reviews the serum laboratory report of the 5-year-old hospitalized child. Based on the laboratory results, which intervention should be the nurse's **priority?**

| Serum Lab Report | Child's Result |
| --- | --- |
| Hgb | 12.9 g/dL |
| Hct | 39% |
| WBC | 2400/mm³ |
| Platelets | 215,000/mm³ |

1. Initiate neutropenic precautions.
2. Avoid administering any injections.
3. Use a favorite cup to increase fluid intake.
4. Call the HCP to request supplemental iron.

**1794.** PHARM The adolescent receiving chemotherapy for treatment of Hodgkin's lymphoma is to receive filgrastim. Which statement should reflect the nurse's thinking about filgrastim?

1. Filgrastim will increase the production of the RBCs by the bone marrow.
2. Filgrastim will increase the production of neutrophils by the bone marrow.
3. Filgrastim will destroy the cancer cells by inhibiting DNA synthesis.
4. Filgrastim will destroy the cancer cells by blocking DNA replication.

**1795.** MoC The experienced nurse and the new nurse are providing preoperative care for the 4-year-old with Wilms' tumor. Which action by the new nurse requires the experienced nurse to intervene?

1. Informs the child that water is not allowed now before the procedure.
2. Palpates the child's abdomen when completing the physical assessment.
3. Provides the child with a doll for play that has removable kidneys.
4. States, "You'll get medicine through this tubing to make you sleepy."

**1796.** The nurse is assessing a child who has a newly diagnosed retinoblastoma in one eye. If the child is experiencing the first sign of retinoblastoma, which assessment finding should the nurse expect when assessing the child's pupils with a flashlight?

1.
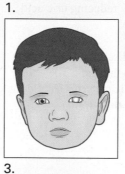

2.
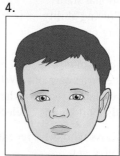

3.
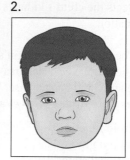

4.
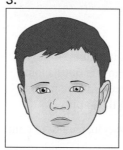

**1797.** The clinic nurse collects information from a parent and assesses the pediatric client one week after hospital discharge for removal of a brain tumor. Which finding **best** suggests the child may have developed a complication?

1. Reports having occasional headaches
2. Voids large amounts of dilute urine
3. Uses crutches to walk into the exam room
4. A tubing is palpable under the skin behind the ear

**1798.** The nurse is caring for the 17-year-old who is to have irradiation of the testes due to the presence of leukemic cells. The client asks the nurse if irradiation will make him sterile. What statements should be the basis for the nurse's response? **Select all that apply.**

1. The irradiation of the testes will lead to sterilization.
2. The irradiation of the testes will decrease sperm production but not cause sterilization.
3. This is a question that only the oncologist and radiologist would be able to answer.
4. A lead shield will be used to protect the pelvic area and preserve reproductive organs.
5. The 17-year-old is likely forming sperm; sperm banking may be an option before treatment.

**1799.** MoC PHARM Prior to administering asparaginase to the 12-year-old with ALL, the nurse reviews the child's laboratory report. Which result should prompt the nurse to notify the HCP before administering the asparaginase?

1. Hemoglobin 11.8 mg/dL
2. Blood glucose 252 mg/dL
3. Total bilirubin 1.2 mg/dL
4. Absolute neutrophil count 1078

**1800.** PHARM Prednisone is prescribed tid for a child receiving chemotherapy. Which is the **best** schedule for the nurse to suggest to a parent?

1. 6 a.m., 2 p.m., and 10 p.m.
2. 8 a.m., 1 p.m., and 6 p.m.
3. 10 a.m., 6 p.m., and 2 a.m.
4. 11 a.m., 4 p.m., and 9 p.m.

**1801.** The mother of the pediatric client consults the nurse because her daughter, who has hair loss from chemotherapy, refuses to wear the wig that she wants her to wear. The mother states she feels uncomfortable when people stare at her daughter. Which response is **most** appropriate?

1. "Is your daughter refusing to wear the wig because you are trying to make her wear it?"
2. "Does your daughter feel uncomfortable when others are looking at her hairless head?"
3. "You seem concerned about people staring. Tell me more about what you are feeling."
4. "Your daughter should cover her head when exposed to sunlight, wind, or the cold."

**1802.** The child is receiving radiation to the left thorax to treat metastases. Which interventions should the nurse include when planning care? **Select all that apply.**

1. Cleanse just with water on the irradiated area.
2. Apply lotion to the target skin area after bathing.
3. Leave the markings when providing skin care.
4. Wear a lead apron when in contact with the child.
5. Apply a dressing to the area after irradiation.

**1803.** PHARM The nurse is preparing a child for abdominal irradiation. Which medications should the nurse plan to administer to prevent nausea and vomiting?

1. Ondansetron and dexamethasone
2. Promethazine and cyclophosphamide
3. Metoclopramide and methotrexate
4. Marijuana and L-asparaginase

**1804.** MoC The nurse is planning the care of four assigned children. Place the children in the order of priority.

1. The 4-year-old receiving irradiation treatments who has a WBC of 3500/mm$^3$
2. The 3-year-old just diagnosed with ALL whose parents are crying at the bedside
3. The 6-year-old receiving chemotherapy treatments who has a platelet count of 40,000/mm$^3$
4. The child who had a CT scan to rule out a Wilms' tumor and needs discharge teaching

Answer: _____

**1805.** The adolescent is scheduled to have total body irradiation in preparation for a bone marrow transplant. The nurse has completed teaching about care following irradiation. Which statements by the adolescent indicate correct understanding of the information? **Select all that apply.**

1. "I should use a soft toothbrush to prevent bleeding and avoid getting myself injured."
2. "I will ensure that the raw fruits and vegetables I eat are well washed and not spoiled."
3. "To relieve my dry mouth, I can suck on lozenges or ice pops or drink cold liquids."
4. "I will need to take an antiemetic around the clock to help prevent nausea and vomiting."
5. "Once the irradiation is completed, I will no longer need to be in protective isolation."

# Answers and Rationales

## 1768. ANSWER:

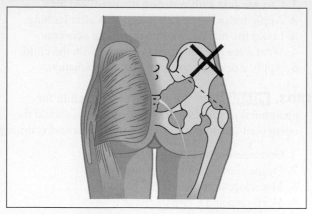

**A common site used for bone marrow aspiration in children is the posterior superior iliac crest.**

▶ *Test-taking Tip: Select an area in which the bone would be the largest and easily approached with a needle.*

Content Area: Child; Concept: Immunity; Hematologic Regulation; Nursing Roles; Integrated Processes: Teaching/Learning; Client Needs: Physiological Integrity: Reduction of Risk Potential; Cognitive Level: Application [Applying]

## 1769. ANSWER: 2

1. The child is on bedrest for an hour after the procedure. After this period of bedrest, activity is not restricted if the child can tolerate the activity.
2. **The child should be on bedrest for at least an hour after the bone marrow aspiration. Minimizing activity for an hour reduces the chance of bleeding from the aspiration site.**
3. Showering is contraindicated postprocedure; a dressing will be in place.
4. The dressing will need to remain intact for at least 24 hours postprocedure.

▶ *Test-taking Tip: Three options concern activity, and one is different. In this situation common sense should tell you that the dressing would not be removed the same day; thus eliminate Option 4. Of the three remaining options, eliminate the extremes in activity to arrive at the answer.*

Content Area: Child; Concept: Hematologic Regulation; Nursing Roles; Integrated Processes: Teaching/Learning; Client Needs: Physiological Integrity: Reduction of Risk Potential; Cognitive Level: Application [Applying]

## 1770. ANSWER: 2

1. Although the nurse should review the lab report, the RBCs in iron-deficiency anemia will be microcytic (small) and not macrocytic (large), and the RBC count will be reduced.
2. **Milk intake should be limited to promote intake of iron-rich food sources.**

3. Iron supplements should be given with foods or juices high in vitamin C, not D, which will enhance its absorption.
4. The HCP would not be notified for expected findings. Iron supplementation can cause constipation and black-colored stools.

▶ *Test-taking Tip: Treatment for iron-deficiency anemia includes iron supplementation and a diet high in iron. You need to consider whether milk is high in iron to answer this question correctly.*

Content Area: Child; Concept: Hematologic Regulation; Medication; Integrated Processes: Nursing Process: Planning; Client Needs: Physiological Integrity: Physiological Adaptation; Cognitive Level: Application [Applying]

## 1771. PHARM ANSWER: 1

1. **RBCs are small and pale because of the stunted Hgb in iron-deficiency anemia. Taking iron increases the production of RBCs. A reticulocyte count measures how fast the reticulocytes (slightly immature RBCs) are made by the bone marrow and released into the blood. An increased count indicates that the medication is beginning to correct the anemia.**
2. Granulocytes (neutrophils, basophils, and eosinophils) are a type of WBC filled with microscopic granules; granulocytes increase with infection or inflammation and are not associated with medication administration with iron-deficiency anemia.
3. Indirect bilirubin increases from the breakdown of the heme portion of RBCs. RBCs should not be breaking down.
4. Erythropoietin is a hormone produced by the kidneys that is stimulated whenever a child has tissue hypoxia. If anemia is correcting, hypoxia should not occur, and erythropoietin production should not be stimulated.

▶ *Test-taking Tip: Eliminate Options 2, 3, and 4 because these are not directly related to the development of RBCs.*

Content Area: Child; Concept: Hematologic Regulation; Medication; Integrated Processes: Nursing Process: Evaluation; Client Needs: Physiological Integrity: Pharmacological and Parenteral Therapies; Physiological Integrity: Reduction of Risk Potential; Cognitive Level: Evaluation [Evaluating]

## 1772. MoC ANSWER: 4

1. Risk for deficient fluid volume, although a concern, is not life-threatening.
2. Chronic pain, although a concern, is not life-threatening.
3. Risk for infection, although important, is not life-threatening.
4. **Although all are appropriate nursing problems, ineffective tissue perfusion is priority because it can be life-threatening. Acute chest syndrome is a common cause of hospitalization for sickle cell disease.**

◆ *Test-taking Tip: Use the ABC's to establish priority. Problems with any of the ABC's can be life-threatening.*

Content Area: Child; Concept: Hematologic Regulation; Comfort; Integrated Processes: Nursing Process: Analysis; Client Needs: Safe and Effective Care Environment: Management of Care; Cognitive Level: Synthesis [Creating]

## 1773. PHARM ANSWER: 4

1. Teaching about adequate hydration is important because inadequate hydration can precipitate a crisis episode, but this does not have priority.
2. Sickle cell anemia has an autosomal recessive characteristic. If both parents carry the sickle cell trait, there is a 25% chance that a child will be born with sickle cell disease. Sickle cell disease is more common in African Americans. Although the parents may want to be genetically tested, this does not have priority.
3. The RBC count would be reduced from destruction of RBCs during the sickling process. The child needs RBCs and not platelets.
4. **Hydroxyurea (Hydrea) is the only medication approved to reduce crisis episodes. Hydroxyurea promotes production of HbF and therefore reduces the concentration of HbS.**

◆ *Test-taking Tip: Use Maslow's Hierarchy of Needs to establish a physiology need as priority. Of the two physiological needs, you need to consider which cells are affected by sickle cell anemia.*

Content Area: Child; Concept: Hematologic Regulation; Diversity; Integrated Processes: Nursing Process: Implementation; Culture and Spirituality; Client Needs: Physiological Integrity: Physiological Adaptation; Physiological Integrity: Pharmacological and Parenteral Therapies; Psychosocial Integrity; Cognitive Level: Application [Applying]

## 1774. ANSWER: 2

1. Ice packs can cause vasoconstriction and decrease tissue perfusion, thereby increasing pain and sickling.
2. **Hydration promotes hemodilution, reduces blood viscosity, and prevents vessel occlusion. The information is most important to teach the parents.**
3. Acetaminophen (Tylenol) may be used for pain relief, but the dose is excessive for a child.
4. Exercise increases oxygen demand, decreases oxygen tension, and increases sickling. Sun exposure can lead to dehydration, which increases blood viscosity.

◆ *Test-taking Tip: The key phrase is "prevent the onset." Determine if each option would increase or decrease pooling of sickled cells and tissue hypoxia. This should prompt you to select Option 2.*

Content Area: Child; Concept: Comfort; Fluid and Electrolyte Balance; Nursing Roles; Integrated Processes: Teaching/Learning; Client Needs: Physiological Integrity: Basic Care and Comfort; Cognitive Level: Application [Applying]

## 1775. ANSWER: 1, 2, 3

1. **Reduced platelet production results in easy bruising and petechiae.**
2. **Reduced platelet production can result in bleeding such as nosebleeds (epistaxis).**

3. **The lower RBC count and resultant tissue hypoxia produce symptoms of fatigue.**
4. Watery, itching eyes are unrelated to aplastic anemia and could be from an allergic reaction.
5. Mouth ulcerations could be burns from the rat poison ingestion, and not aplastic anemia.

◆ *Test-taking Tip: Acquired aplastic anemia can result from chemicals, such as rat poisoning, that depress the hematopoietic activity in the bone marrow. Select only the signs and symptoms that would be associated with a decreased bone marrow function, eliminating options that may be related to ingestion of rat poison but that do not also indicate depressed hemolytic activity.*

Content Area: Child; Concept: Safety; Hematologic Regulation; Assessment; Integrated Processes: Nursing Process: Assessment; Client Needs: Physiological Integrity: Reduction of Risk Potential; Cognitive Level: Application [Applying]

## 1776. ANSWER: 266

**Determine the total weight of the dry sponges: Three packs would be 3 × 75 g = 225 g. Add the weight of the blood-soaked sponges: 188 g + 158 g + 145 g = 491 g or 491 mL. Recall that 1 g in weight is equivalent to 1 mL. Subtract the weight of the dry sponges from the blood-soaked sponge total: 491 mL − 225 mL = 266 mL.**

◆ *Test-taking Tip: Recall that 1 g in weight is equivalent to 1 mL of blood. Use this equivalent in calculating the child's blood loss.*

Content Area: Child; Concept: Hematologic Regulation; Integrated Processes: Communication and Documentation; Client Needs: Physiological Integrity: Physiological Adaptation; Cognitive Level: Application [Applying]

## 1777. ANSWER: 2, 3, 4

1. Lying down and elevating the feet can increase the blood flow to the head, increasing bleeding.
2. **Most of the bleeding occurs in the anterior part of the nasal septum; therefore compression helps stop the flow of blood.**
3. **Because of delayed clotting due to insufficient clotting factors in von Willebrand disease, pressure needs to be prolonged for at least 10 minutes.**
4. **The application of cold constricts blood vessels and reduces bleeding.**
5. The medication and supplies, if available at school, should be kept in a locked medication cupboard in the nurse's office and would not be carried by the student.

◆ *Test-taking Tip: Use principles from the ABC's to eliminate the options that compromise the child's airway, breathing, or circulation. While at school, medications are usually locked in the nurse's office.*

Content Area: Child; Concept: Hematologic Regulation; Safety; Integrated Processes: Nursing Process: Implementation; Client Needs: Physiological Integrity: Physiological Adaptation; Cognitive Level: Application [Applying]

## 1778. ANSWER: 4

1. The PT measures the action of prothrombin and will be prolonged with deficiencies of prothrombin and factors V, VII, and X. The deficient factor in hemophilia A is factor VIII.
2. The Hgb is not used to diagnose hemophilia A and should be normal unless the child is bleeding.
3. The Hct is not used to diagnose hemophilia A and should be normal unless the child is bleeding.
4. **Hemophilia A results from a deficiency of factor VIII. Because aPTT measures the activity of thromboplastin and factor VIII is deficient, the aPTT is prolonged.**

▶ *Test-taking Tip: Use a memory aid to remember that aPTT is prolonged in hemophilia A. Note the "A" in hemophilia A and the "a" in aPTT.*

**Content Area:** Child; **Concept:** Hematologic Regulation; Assessment; **Integrated Processes:** Nursing Process: Assessment; **Client Needs:** Physiological Integrity: Reduction of Risk Potential; **Cognitive Level:** Comprehension [Understanding]

## 1779. PHARM ANSWER: 3

1. Although enhancing the child's fluid intake is important, applying firm pressure during IV removal is more important.
2. The child is not at risk for infection; therefore there is no need to prevent contact with flowers.
3. **The nurse should plan to apply firm pressure to the site for at least 5 minutes after discontinuing the IV because the client is at increased risk for bleeding due to decreased platelets.**
4. Approximately 89% of children eventually recover from ITP; it may not be a life-long condition.

▶ *Test-taking Tip: Thrombocytopenia purpura is manifested by a decrease in platelet count, increasing the child's risk for bleeding.*

**Content Area:** Child; **Concept:** Hematologic Regulation; **Integrated Processes:** Nursing Process: Implementation; **Client Needs:** Physiological Integrity: Pharmacological and Parenteral Therapies; **Cognitive Level:** Application [Applying]

## 1780. MoC ANSWER: 1

1. **This statement is incorrect and should be questioned by the experienced nurse. Thalassemia major occurs from a deficiency in the synthesis of the beta-chain of the Hgb. This results in defective Hgb, destruction of RBCs, and anemia. Plasmapheresis, selective removal of the plasma, would be ineffective in treating thalassemia because the cells are not being destroyed by toxins in the plasma.**
2. Blood transfusions treat the anemia associated with thalassemia, providing sufficient RBCs to support growth and normal physical activity and to maintain the client's Hgb level at 9 to 10 g/dL. Blood transfusions also suppress endogenous erythropoiesis.
3. Spleen enlargement can occur due to the rapid destruction of RBCs; splenectomy may be necessary to increase the life span of supplemental RBCs and to minimize the disabling effects of the enlarged spleen.
4. Bone marrow stem cell transplantation can offer a cure. The diseased bone marrow is replaced by stem cells that develop into healthy bone marrow, which then produce normal cells.

▶ *Test-taking Tip: This is a false-response item. Select the statement that would be incorrect. Note the commonalities between Options 2, 3, and 4. Often the option that is different is the answer.*

**Content Area:** Child; **Concept:** Hematologic Regulation; Nursing Roles; **Integrated Processes:** Nursing Process: Evaluation; **Client Needs:** Safe and Effective Care Environment: Management of Care; Physiological Integrity: Physiological Adaptation; **Cognitive Level:** Evaluation [Evaluating]

## 1781. PHARM ANSWER: 4

1. Thalassemia major (not iron overload) is most often found in families of Chinese, South Asian, Middle Eastern, Mediterranean, or African origin.
2. Changing blood products does not treat iron overload.
3. Reducing the frequency of transfusions does not treat the iron overload.
4. **The nurse should anticipate chelation therapy. An iron-chelating drug, such as deferoxamine (Desferal), is administered to bind excess iron so it can be excreted by the kidneys.**

▶ *Test-taking Tip: Focus on treating the problem of iron overload from blood transfusions rather than on modifying the treatment plan for treating thalassemia major.*

**Content Area:** Child; **Concept:** Hematologic Regulation; Nursing Roles; Diversity; Medication; **Integrated Processes:** Nursing Process: Planning; Culture and Spirituality; **Client Needs:** Physiological Integrity: Pharmacological and Parenteral Therapies; **Cognitive Level:** Application [Applying]

## 1782. ANSWER: 2, 3, 5, 6

1. Alopecia (hair loss) may occur with chemotherapy but is not an expected sign with a new diagnosis of ALL.
2. **Petechiae, a sign of capillary bleeding, results from decreased platelet production and the ability of the blood to clot.**
3. **Anorexia occurs from enlarged lymph nodes and vague abdominal pain from inflammation within the intestinal tract.**
4. Because of the bone marrow, depression, fatigue, and increased time sleeping (not insomnia) are signs associated with ALL.
5. **Bleeding gums may be present related to decreased platelet production and decreased ability of the blood to clot.**
6. **Pallor occurs from decreased production of erythrocytes.**

▶ *Test-taking Tip: Recall that in leukemia, the proliferation of immature WBCs depresses bone marrow production, decreasing erythrocytes, platelets, and the formation of mature WBCs. Therefore select options that relate to the functions of these blood cells.*

Content Area: Child; **Concept:** Assessment; Hematologic Regulation; **Integrated Processes:** Nursing Process: Assessment; **Client Needs:** Physiological Integrity: Reduction of Risk Potential; **Cognitive Level:** Knowledge [Remembering]

## 1783. ANSWER:

| Laboratory Report | |
| --- | --- |
| **Hematology** | **Client Value** |
| Platelets (Plt 150–300 K/mm³) | 50 K/mm³ **X** |

**The low platelets are of greatest concern. The child is bleeding and platelets are needed for coagulation, but they are too low for effective coagulation. The low platelets are directly related to the leukemia, which causes a rapid proliferation of lymphocytes and a reduction in the production of platelets and RBCs. The Hgb and Hct are low and would be concerning if the bleeding continues, but these will not affect whether or not coagulation occurs. The WBC is elevated, which could indicate an infection, but this is not of greatest concern because WBCs will not affect coagulation.**

▶ *Test-taking Tip: The key words are "greatest concern." Focus on the child's diagnosis of leukemia and the function of each of the blood components listed in the hematology report. Eliminate Options 1, 2, and 3 because these are not related to blood clotting.*

Content Area: Child; **Concept:** Hematologic Regulation; Assessment; **Integrated Processes:** Nursing Process: Evaluation; **Client Needs:** Physiological Integrity: Reduction of Risk Potential; **Cognitive Level:** Evaluation [Evaluating]

## 1784. PHARM ANSWER: 150

**First convert pounds to kilograms using a proportion formula (2.2 lb = 1 kg).**
**2.2 lb : 1 kg :: 33 lb : X kg**
**Multiple the extremes and then the means and solve for X.**
**2.2X = 33; X = 33 ÷ 2.2; X = 15 . The child weighs 15 kg.**
**Next determine the rate: mL per hour at 10 mL/kg/hr.**
**10 mL : 1 kg :: X mL : 15 kg; X = 15 × 10;**
**X = 150 mL/hr.**

▶ *Test-taking Tip: Read the question carefully to determine what is being asked. Recall that 2.2 pounds equals 1 kilogram. The commonly accepted rate for transfusions in a child is 10 mL/kg/hr.*

Content Area: Child; **Concept:** Medication; Hematologic Regulation; **Integrated Processes:** Nursing Process: Planning; **Client Needs:** Physiological Integrity: Pharmacological and Parenteral Therapies; **Cognitive Level:** Application [Applying]

## 1785. PHARM ANSWER: 4

1. Although allopurinol can cause drowsiness, this is not the purpose for this child.
2. There is no indication that the child has gout or is likely to develop gout.
3. Although high levels of uric acid can lead to gouty arthritis, this is not the most important purpose for the child receiving chemotherapy.
4. **Rapid cell destruction from chemotherapy results in a high level of uric acid being excreted during treatment. This can plug the glomeruli and renal tubules, causing loss of kidney function. Allopurinol (Zyloprim) reduces the uric acid formation and protects the kidneys.**

▶ *Test-taking Tip: Three options are similar, and one is different in that it describes the action of allopurinol.*

Content Area: Child; **Concept:** Cellular Regulation; Medication; **Integrated Processes:** Teaching/Learning; **Client Needs:** Physiological Integrity: Pharmacological and Parenteral Therapies; **Cognitive Level:** Application [Applying]

## 1786. ANSWER: 1, 2, 3, 4

1. **Irradiation to the cervical area in the neck could result in damage to the thyroid gland and cause hypothyroidism.**
2. **Malaise and lack of energy can be signs of anemia from decreased RBC production.**
3. **Nutrition can be impaired with hypothyroidism, depression, or the effects of the radiation, which could influence the child's energy level.**
4. **The inflammation from a mild skin reaction with radiation to the neck area can cause difficulty swallowing and affect nutritional status.**
5. Lack of energy and malaise are not common symptoms associated with the renal system.

▶ *Test-taking Tip: Visualize the area that is being treated with radiation before reading each of the options.*

Content Area: Child; **Concept:** Assessment; Cellular Regulation; **Integrated Processes:** Nursing Process: Assessment; **Client Needs:** Physiological Integrity: Reduction of Risk Potential; **Cognitive Level:** Application [Applying]

## 1787. ANSWER: 1, 2, 4

1. **If exposed to a recently vaccinated person, especially those vaccinated with a live virus, the child would be unable to initiate an immune response and could develop an infection. Those recently vaccinated should not come for a visit.**
2. **Plants and flowers could harbor mold spores and should not be within the child's immediate surroundings.**
3. Goldfish in the home should be placed in an area that is off limits to the child because they harbor mold spores.
4. **Sleeping alone prevents exposure to those who may be developing an illness.**

5. Temperature, respiratory rate, and pulse should be taken daily; qid is unnecessary.

▶ *Test-taking Tip: Neutropenia is a reduction of circulating neutrophils, the most common type of granular WBC. With a reduction in WBCs, there is an increased risk of infection. Select options that will reduce the child's risk of infection and eliminate options that are harmful or excessive.*

**Content Area:** Child; **Concept:** Hematologic Regulation; Immunity; Cellular Regulation; **Integrated Processes:** Nursing Process: Planning; **Client Needs:** Safe and Effective Care Environment: Safety and Infection Control; **Cognitive Level:** Analysis [Analyzing]

### 1788. ANSWER: 1, 4, 5

1. **Soft toothbrushes or sponges are used to reduce trauma to the oral mucosa. Frequent oral care rids mucosal surfaces of debris, which is an excellent medium for bacterial and fungal growth.**
2. Alcohol-based mouthwash increases pain and tissue trauma because it has a drying effect.
3. Viscous lidocaine is not recommended for young children because it may depress the gag reflex, increasing the risk of aspiration.
4. **A moistened gauze is appropriate for cleaning the gums to remove debris that could be a medium for bacterial and fungal growth.**
5. **Massaging the area on the backs of both hands between the thumb and index finger with an ice cube for 5 to 7 minutes until numb is a reflexology strategy to reduce oral pain.**

▶ *Test-taking Tip: Focus on selecting options that will cleanse the mouth of debris, reduce pain, and decrease the risk of infection. Remember to consider complementary therapies.*

**Content Area:** Child; **Concept:** Cellular Regulation; Skin Integrity; Comfort; **Integrated Processes:** Nursing Process: Planning; **Client Needs:** Physiological Integrity: Basic Care and Comfort; **Cognitive Level:** Synthesis [Creating]

### 1789. MoC ANSWER: 1

1. **A correlation exists between some genetic disorders, such as Down syndrome (trisomy 21), and childhood cancer. In a child with Down syndrome, the probability of developing leukemia is about 20 times greater than that in other children. This child should be scheduled to be seen first.**
2. Studies have found marginally significant relationships between electromagnetic exposure and developing childhood cancer.
3. Chronic infections do not automatically increase the risk for cancer.
4. Studies suggest that in general there is not a strong constitutional genetic component for childhood cancers other than retinoblastoma.

▶ *Test-taking Tip: If unsure, think about the child who would most benefit by being seen first.*

**Content Area:** Child; **Concept:** Critical Thinking; Cellular Regulation; Safety; **Integrated Processes:** Nursing Process: Implementation; **Client Needs:** Safe and Effective Care Environment: Management of Care; **Cognitive Level:** Application [Applying]

### 1790. MoC ANSWER: 4

1. Thrombocytopenia and leukocytosis, although not signs of superior vena cava syndrome, increase the risk for vascular damage and life-threatening hemorrhage.
2. Hyperuricemia, hypocalcemia, and hyperphosphatemia are signs of tumor lysis syndrome (not superior vena cava syndrome).
3. A mass obstructing the spinal cord (not superior vena cava syndrome) can be manifested by symptoms of tingling and paresthesias of the lower extremities and pain on light touch.
4. **Mediastinal tumors, especially from NHL, may cause compression of the great vessel (superior vena cava syndrome). Signs of compression include upper chest, neck, and face cyanosis, upper-extremity edema, and distended neck veins.**

▶ *Test-taking Tip: You should think about the location of the superior vena cava when selecting the options. Only one option would be associated with the location.*

**Content Area:** Child; **Concept:** Cellular Regulation; Perfusion; Hematologic Regulation; **Integrated Processes:** Nursing Process: Analysis; **Client Needs:** Safe and Effective Care Environment: Management of Care; Physiological Integrity: Reduction of Risk Potential; **Cognitive Level:** Application [Applying]

### 1791. ANSWER: 2

1. Hodgkin's lymphoma is cancer that starts in WBCs and affects the reticuloendothelial and lymphatic systems.
2. **Hodgkin's lymphoma, which peaks at 20 years of age, is potentially curable with radiation therapy alone or with a combination of chemotherapeutic agents.**
3. A laparotomy is no longer performed for staging. A biopsy may be performed if lesions are suspicious and if the findings might alter the treatment regimen.
4. There is no indication that the client has an advanced stage of lymphoma.

▶ *Test-taking Tip: Select the statement that is a true statement. Eliminate options that include the client's emotional response to the diagnosis.*

**Content Area:** Child; **Concept:** Cellular Regulation; Nursing Roles; **Integrated Processes:** Nursing Process: Evaluation; Caring; **Client Needs:** Physiological Integrity: Physiological Adaptation; Psychosocial Integrity; **Cognitive Level:** Evaluation [Evaluating]

### 1792. ANSWER: 1, 2, 3, 5

1. **Hodgkin's disease is characterized by painless enlarged lymph nodes most commonly in the cervical area and less frequently in the axillary and inguinal areas.**
2. **An unexplained temperature above 100.4°F (38°C) for 3 consecutive days, along with lymph node enlargement and weight loss, has been recognized by the Ann Arbor Staging System as having prognostic significance in Hodgkin's disease.**

3. **Unexplained weight loss of 10% or more in the previous 6 months, along with lymph node enlargement and unexplained fever, has been recognized by the Ann Arbor Staging System as having prognostic significance in Hodgkin's disease.**
4. There is no conclusive association between dietary habits and the development of Hodgkin's disease.
5. **There is a genetic predisposition with an increased incidence among same-sex siblings.**

▶ **Test-taking Tip:** *If uncertain, you should select options that suggest an illness. Apply knowledge that Hodgkin's lymphoma begins in the lymphoid system.*

**Content Area:** Child; **Concept:** Cellular Regulation; Assessment; **Integrated Processes:** Nursing Process: Assessment; **Client Needs:** Physiological Integrity: Physiological Adaptation; **Cognitive Level:** Application [Applying]

## 1793. ANSWER: 1

1. **The nurse's priority should be to initiate neutropenic precautions because the child has an extremely low WBC count, which increases the risk for infection. The normal WBC count for a 5-year-old is 4500–13500/mm³.**
2. Injections would be avoided if the platelet count were low and the risk for bleeding were increased, but the platelet count is normal. Normal is 150,000 to 400,000/mm³.
3. Using a favorite cup may be helpful to promote the child's fluid intake. However, because the BUN is not reported and there is no indication that the child is dehydrated, this does not have priority.
4. The Hgb and Hct are normal; the HCP should not be notified for supplemental iron. Normal Hgb is 10.2–13.4 g/dL and normal Hct is 31.7%–39%.

▶ **Test-taking Tip:** *You would be expected to know normal laboratory ranges for common laboratory values on the NCLEX-RX® Examination.*

**Content Area:** Child; **Concept:** Infection; Hematologic Regulation; **Integrated Processes:** Nursing Process: Implementation; **Client Needs:** Physiological Integrity: Reduction of Risk Potential; **Cognitive Level:** Application [Applying]

## 1794. PHARM ANSWER: 2

1. Epoetin alfa (Epogen) is a glycoprotein that stimulates the bone marrow in RBC formation.
2. **Filgrastim (Neupogen) is a colony-stimulating factor that increases the production of neutrophils by the bone marrow.**
3. Antibiotic chemotherapeutic agents inhibit DNA synthesis.
4. Alkylating agents block DNA replication to destroy cancer cells.

▶ **Test-taking Tip:** *A trade name for filgrastim is Neupogen. Use this as a clue to selecting the correct option.*

**Content Area:** Child; **Concept:** Hematologic Regulation; Medication; **Integrated Processes:** Nursing Process: Analysis; **Client Needs:** Physiological Integrity: Pharmacological and Parenteral Therapies; **Cognitive Level:** Application [Applying]

## 1795. MoC ANSWER: 2

1. The child would typically be NPO for 2 hours prior to the procedure, though this time period can vary.
2. **Wilms' tumor (nephroblastoma) is an intrarenal abdominal tumor. Palpating the abdomen can potentially spread the cancerous cells.**
3. Play therapy is an appropriate means for teaching the child about the surgical procedure and assisting the child to cope.
4. When explaining the surgery and anesthesia, words that the child understands should be used.

▶ **Test-taking Tip:** *Consider both the age of the child and the type of tumor when reading the options.*

**Content Area:** Child; **Concept:** Cellular Regulation; Nursing Roles; Safety; **Integrated Processes:** Nursing Process: Evaluation; **Client Needs:** Safe and Effective Care Environment: Management of Care; **Cognitive Level:** Evaluation [Evaluating]

## 1796. ANSWER: 1

1. **The first sign of retinoblastoma is a white reflection in the affected pupil (leukokoria) due to the intraocular malignancy of the retina.**
2. The red reflex is absent, asymmetrical, or may be a different color in the eye affected by a retinoblastoma. This illustration shows that the red reflex is present in both eyes.
3. Unequal pupil size occurs from compression on the oculomotor nerve. The retinoblastoma affects the retina of the eye.
4. This illustration shows the child with normal pupil size and shape.

▶ **Test-taking Tip:** *You need to consider that in a retinoblastoma, the retina of the eye is affected. When a light is shined into the eyes, it may reflect off of the tumor, and a white reflex can be observed.*

**Content Area:** Child; **Concept:** Assessment; Cellular Regulation; **Integrated Processes:** Nursing Process: Evaluation; **Client Needs:** Physiological Integrity: Physiological Adaptation; **Cognitive Level:** Evaluation [Evaluating]

## 1797. ANSWER: 2

1. Headaches may be a symptom associated with a complication but also may occur due to the removal of the brain tumor.
2. **Voiding large amounts of dilute urine is a sign of DI caused by a deficiency in ADH secreted by the posterior pituitary gland. When ADH is inadequate, the renal tubules do not reabsorb water, leading to polyuria.**
3. Physical mobility may be impaired because of the location of the tumor. Being able to walk with crutches is an expected outcome if mobility was affected.
4. A ventriculoperitoneal shunt tubing is used to drain excess CSF. It is inserted into the ventricle, and a tract is made that travels behind the ear, along the neck and chest wall, and into the peritoneal cavity. The shunt may be felt under the skin behind the ear and along the neck.

▶ **Test-taking Tip:** *If unsure, select an option that is atypical for any person regardless of surgery.*

**Content Area:** Child; **Concept:** Assessment; Cellular Regulation; **Integrated Processes:** Nursing Process: Evaluation; **Client Needs:** Physiological Integrity: Reduction of Risk Potential; **Cognitive Level:** Evaluation [Evaluating]

## 1798. ANSWER: 1, 5

1. **Sperm will be destroyed during irradiation, and no sperm will be produced after irradiation of the testes.**
2. This statement is incorrect; no sperm will be produced after irradiation of the testes.
3. The nurse would be expected to answer the client's question and not defer the question. Deferring could cause distrust between the client and nurse or lead the client to suspect that there is more that is not being told to him.
4. The testes are reproductive organs of the male and would need to be exposed during irradiation. A lead shield may be used to cover other body organs.
5. **The 17-year-old is past puberty and is making sperm. Because irradiation of the testes leads to sterilization, sperm banking might be suggested before treatment.**

▶ **Test-taking Tip:** *Note that Options 1 and 2 are opposites. Eliminate one of these because both cannot be correct. Usually options with absolute words such as "only" are incorrect statements.*

**Content Area:** Child; **Concept:** Male Reproduction; Cellular Regulation; Nursing Roles; **Integrated Processes:** Communication and Documentation; **Client Needs:** Physiological Integrity: Physiological Adaptation; **Cognitive Level:** Comprehension [Understanding]

## 1799. MoC PHARM ANSWER: 2

1. The normal Hgb for ages 6 to 12 years is 11.5 to 15.5 g/dL.
2. **The normal fasting blood glucose level for a 12-year-old is 80–180 mg/dL; 252 mg/dL is high. An adverse effect of asparaginase (Elspar, Erwinaze) is hyperglycemia, which may need to be treated with insulin before administration of another dose.**
3. Total bilirubin is 0.3 to 1.2 mg/dL.
4. An ANC of 1078 is acceptable for asparaginase administration. An ANC of less than 1000 increases the child's risk of infection.

▶ **Test-taking Tip:** *Eliminate options that are known to be within normal ranges. Of the remaining two options, 2 and 4, determine which would require intervention.*

**Content Area:** Child; **Concept:** Medication; Safety; Communication; **Integrated Processes:** Nursing Process: Evaluation; **Client Needs:** Safe and Effective Care Environment: Management of Care; Physiological Integrity: Pharmacological and Parenteral Therapies; **Cognitive Level:** Evaluation [Evaluating]

## 1800. PHARM ANSWER: 2

1. Giving prednisone at 6 a.m., 2 p.m., and 10 p.m. spaces the medication over a 24-hour time period, but it is not given consistently in relation to meals.

2. **Prednisone (Deltasone) should be taken with meals or snacks to decrease or prevent GI upset. Giving prednisone at 8 a.m., 1 p.m., and 6 p.m. is the closest of the options to mealtime, yet it spaces the medication for effectiveness.**
3. Giving prednisone at 10 a.m., 6 p.m., and 2 a.m. spaces the medication over 24 hours, but it is not given consistently with meals.
4. Giving prednisone at 11 a.m., 4 p.m., and 9 p.m. would be administering prednisone before meals and at bedtime, rather than with meals.

▶ **Test-taking Tip:** *Prednisone should be taken with food. Note that only one option gives the medication closest to mealtime.*

**Content Area:** Child; **Concept:** Medication; Nursing Roles; **Integrated Processes:** Nursing Process: Implementation; **Client Needs:** Physiological Integrity: Pharmacological and Parenteral Therapies; **Cognitive Level:** Application [Applying]

## 1801. ANSWER: 3

1. This statement is challenging and can make the mother defensive. The mother already stated she would like her daughter to wear a wig.
2. This statement focuses on the daughter's feelings rather than the mother's feelings. Using the phrase "hairless head" may increase the mother's discomfort.
3. **Hair loss is often a greater problem for the parents than the child. The parent may be grieving the loss of a "normal" child. Acknowledging the parent's feelings and focusing the communication on the parent use the therapeutic communication technique of a broad opening statement.**
4. Although this statement is correct, it ignores the mother's concern of discomfort.

▶ **Test-taking Tip:** *The most appropriate response would be one that responds to the mother's feelings.*

**Content Area:** Child; **Concept:** Cellular Regulation; Self; Communication; **Integrated Processes:** Caring; Communication and Documentation **Client Needs:** Psychosocial Integrity; **Cognitive Level:** Application [Applying]

## 1802. ANSWER: 1, 3

1. **Only water should be used to gently cleanse the area. Soaps should not be applied to the irradiated area because they are irritating and can lead to skin breakdown. Radiation can cause burns to the skin.**
2. Lotions and rubbing to apply the lotion can cause skin breakdown if applied to traumatized skin.
3. **The markings outline the irradiation target area for precise positioning of the radiation and should remain until treatment is completed.**
4. A lead apron is unnecessary because radiation is not present in the client's body or in the room.
5. The irradiated area should be left open to air. A dressing can cause skin tearing when removed.

▶ **Test-taking Tip:** *There is the potential for impaired skin integrity following irradiation to an area. You need to focus on selecting options that protect the irradiated skin and the markings on the skin.*

Content Area: Child; Concept: Skin Integrity; Safety; Integrated Processes: Nursing Process: Planning; Client Needs: Physiological Integrity: Physiological Adaptation; Cognitive Level: Synthesis [Creating]

## 1803. PHARM ANSWER: 1

1. **Ondansetron (Zofran) is an antiemetic used to control nausea and vomiting. Dexamethasone (Decadron) is a corticosteroid anti-inflammatory agent used in the adjunctive management of nausea and vomiting from chemotherapy.**
2. Promethazine (Phenergan) is a phenothiazine-type antiemetic, but cyclophosphamide (Cytoxan) is a chemotherapeutic agent.
3. Metoclopramide (Reglan) is an antiemetic, but it causes extrapyramidal reactions in children. Methotrexate (Trexall) is a chemotherapeutic agent.
4. Synthetic cannabinoids are being used in children, but asparaginase (Elspar, Erwinaze) is a chemotherapeutic agent. Some states have legalized marijuana use, but it is not federally approved for use in the U.S. and thus not dispensed in health care agencies that are under federal regulations.

▶ *Test-taking Tip:* Eliminate options that include chemotherapeutic agents.

Content Area: Child; Concept: Medication; Cellular Regulation; Integrated Processes: Nursing Process: Planning; Client Needs: Physiological Integrity: Pharmacological and Parenteral Therapies; Cognitive Level: Application [Applying]

## 1804. MoC ANSWER: 3, 1, 4, 2

3. **The 6-year-old receiving chemotherapy treatments who has a platelet count of 40,000/mm³ should be assessed first. With a low platelet count, the child is at risk for bleeding.**
1. **The 4-year-old receiving irradiation treatments who has a WBC of 3500/mm³ should be assessed second. With a borderline low WBC, the child is at risk for an infection.**
4. **A child who had a CT scan to rule out a Wilms' tumor and needs discharge teaching should be assessed third. The nurse should provide the discharge teaching so that the child can go home.**
2. The 3-year-old just diagnosed with ALL whose parents are crying at the bedside should be assessed last. There is no indication that the child has immediate concerns, and attending to the child last would ensure that the nurse has adequate time to spend with the parents, answering questions, and providing support.

▶ *Test-taking Tip:* When prioritizing, use Maslow's Hierarchy of Needs. Clients with life-threatening issues should be assessed first, followed by those with physiological needs, and then those with psychosocial and learning needs.

Content Area: Child; Concept: Hematologic Regulation; Cellular Regulation; Critical Thinking; Integrated Processes: Nursing Process: Planning; Client Needs: Safe and Effective Care Environment: Management of Care; Psychosocial Integrity; Cognitive Level: Synthesis [Creating]

## 1805. ANSWER: 1, 2, 3, 4

1. **Irradiation results in bone marrow suppression and pancytopenia. Bleeding precautions are necessary. This statement indicates correct understanding.**
2. **Recent research has found that raw fruits and vegetables do not increase the risk of infection. These are allowable as long as they are well washed and not spoiled. Vegetable sprouts, such as alfalfa, should not be eaten.**
3. **Xerostomia (dry mouth) is a side effect that can be combated by lozenges, liquids, or oral hygiene.**
4. **Antiemetics are given around the clock to control nausea.**
5. Protective isolation continues until after the bone marrow transplant, not just during irradiation.

▶ *Test-taking Tip:* You need to consider that the adolescent will be in protective isolation until after the bone marrow transplant; thus eliminate options that can increase the client's risk for infection.

Content Area: Child; Concept: Cellular Regulation; Nursing Roles; Evidence-based Practice; Integrated Processes: Nursing Process: Evaluation; Client Needs: Physiological Integrity: Physiological Adaptation; Cognitive Level: Evaluation [Evaluating]

## Chapter Forty-One

# Infectious and Communicable Disease Management

**1806.** The nurse is caring for the 4-year-old hospitalized with complications from chicken pox. Which type of precautions should the nurse plan?

1. Airborne and droplet with negative-airflow room
2. Airborne and droplet with positive-airflow room
3. Contact and droplet with negative-airflow room
4. Standard and airborne with positive-airflow room

**1807.** **MoC** **PHARM** The medical resident admits the 4-year-old with complications related to chicken pox. Which prescribed medication is **most** important for the nurse to question with the HCP?

1. Acetaminophen
2. Ampicillin
3. Acyclovir
4. Acetylsalicylic acid

**1808.** **MoC** The nurse is reviewing the laboratory results for the 10-year-old diagnosed with chicken pox. Place an X next to the **most concerning** value that warrants the nurse notifying the HCP.

| Serum Laboratory Test | Client's Value | Normal Levels |
| --- | --- | --- |
| BUN | 32 | 5–25 mg/dL |
| Creatinine | 1.4 | 0.5–1.5 mg/ dL |
| Na | 130 | 135–145 mEq/L |
| K | 3.4 | 3.5–5.3 mEq/L |
| Cl | 110 | 95–105 mEq/L |
| SGOT | 75 | 0–42 units/L |
| Amylase | 190 | <200 units/L |

**1809.** **PHARM** The nurse is preparing acetaminophen for the 6-year-old who has chicken pox. The prescribed dose is 15 mg/kg. How many mg should the nurse give if the child weighs 55 lb?

_____ mg (Record a whole number.)

**1810.** The 1-year-old with a temperature of 103°F (39.4°C) is diagnosed with roseola. Which information should the nurse provide to the parent? **Select all that apply.**

1. Expect a rose-pink rash that usually appears once the fever subsides.
2. Administer aspirin every 4 hours as needed for an elevated temperature.
3. Bathe the child in oatmeal baths twice daily to reduce the child's itching.
4. Avoid contact with the child's secretions and perform hand hygiene often.
5. Isolate the child from other family members until after the rash subsides.

**1811.** The nurse in the ED plans to assess four children. Based on the type of infection, which child should the nurse plan to assess **first?**

1. The 2-year-old child with roseola
2. The 5-year-old child with rubeola
3. The 6-year-old child with rubella
4. The 8-month-old with blistering eczema

**1812.** The clinic nurse is teaching the parent of the 3-year-old with rubella. Which information should the nurse provide?

1. "The period of communicability is 7 days before and 5 days after the rash appears; many cases are asymptomatic, and complications are rare."
2. "You need to observe for pneumonia, a common complication; if pregnant, you do not need to worry about being exposed to rubella."
3. "The period of communicability is 5 days before and 14 days after the rash appears; there are no teratogenic effects from the virus on fetuses."
4. "The incubation period is 7 to 14 days; complications are rare, but those who are pregnant should not be exposed to rubella."

**1813.** The nurse is assessing the 18-year-old diagnosed with mumps. Which findings should be **most** concerning to the nurse?

1. Parotid swelling, fever, headache
2. Earache, anorexia, painful chewing
3. Headache, stiff neck, photophobia
4. Vomiting, swelling above the jawline

**1814.** The 17-year-old student visits the high school nurse's office experiencing a sore throat, headache, fever of 101°F (38.3°C), malaise, and abdominal pain. How should the nurse plan to proceed?

1. Call the HCP's office and send the student to be evaluated.
2. Give an antipyretic and have the student stay and rest for an hour.
3. Ask if the student would like to go see the HCP or be sent home.
4. Call the parent and have the student go home with recommendations to see the HCP.

**1815.** MoC The adolescent shows the school nurse the arm illustrated. The nurse recommends contacting the HCP immediately because this erythema pattern is characteristic of which condition?

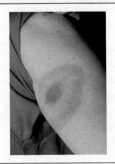

1. A bee sting
2. Cat scratch disease
3. A tick bite
4. Cellulitis

**1816.** PHARM The nurse completes teaching about Lyme disease and doxycycline use. The nurse recognizes the need for further education when the client makes which statement?

1. "I'm glad this isn't contagious so I can get back to tanning."
2. "I'll complete my entire dose of doxycycline even if I no longer have joint pain."
3. "I should abstain from sexual intercourse while on doxycycline."
4. "I'll notify my doctor if I get a fever, diarrhea, or my muscle or joint pain worsens."

**1817.** The adolescent, who has been sick for several days, is being seen in a clinic with a tentative diagnosis of mononucleosis. Which assessment findings should the nurse expect?

1. Weakness, loss of appetite, and extreme constipation
2. Fever, an enlarged spleen, and a rash similar to chicken pox
3. White coating on the throat and depressed lymphocyte levels
4. Extreme fatigue and enlarged lymph nodes in the neck and axilla

**1818.** The college health nurse is teaching the student athlete diagnosed with infectious mononucleosis. The student asks, "Can I play soccer after I rest up for a few days?" Which is the nurse's **best** response?

1. "You need to stay away from playing soccer for at least 3 months."
2. "You may be as active as you wish now if you are not feeling fatigued."
3. "There are no limitations on activity with infectious mononucleosis."
4. "You need to avoid soccer and activities that can injure your abdomen for a few weeks."

**1819.** PHARM The nurse is caring for the child who has a virulent infection. The HCP prescribes cefazolin sodium IV 50 mg q6hr. The *Pediatric Dosage Handbook* states the safe range of cefazolin is 6.25 to 25 mg per kg per day. The child weighs 18 lb. What is the **most** appropriate action by the nurse?

1. Notify the HCP because the dose is too high.
2. Request the pharmacy to send the correct dose.
3. Administer cefazolin sodium as prescribed.
4. Notify the HCP because the dose is too low.

**1820.** **PHARM** The nurse is caring for four pediatric clients who have the skin conditions illustrated. For which client should the nurse expect to administer acyclovir orally?

1.

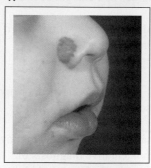

2.

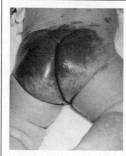

3.

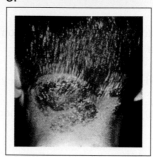

4.

**1821.** The 14-year-old client has impetigo on the hands and neck. When reviewing the client's history, which predisposing factors should the nurse associate with bacterial skin infections?

1. Diabetes insipidus, moisture, anorexia
2. Obesity, diabetes mellitus, eczema
3. Dry skin, acne, congenital heart defect
4. Systemic corticosteroids, strabismus

**1822.** The nurse is preparing to cleanse the skin of the hospitalized child with impetigo. Which nursing action is **most** important?

1. Apply clean gloves to prevent the spread of the infection to others.
2. Use sterile technique to prevent any further infection of the lesions.
3. Ensure that the water is cold to help reduce pain during cleansing.
4. Keep the child in contact precautions until the child is discharged.

**1823.** The clinic nurse is assessing the 17-year-old male and observes multiple lesions on both upper arms. Some of these lesions are covered with a honey-colored crust. Which skin condition should the nurse consider?

1. Herpes zoster
2. Impetigo
3. Cellulitis
4. Ringworm

**1824.** The nurse is teaching the parent skin care for the child diagnosed with impetigo. Which instruction is **best**?

1. Refrain from putting anything on the lesions.
2. Remove skin, crusts, and debris by debridement.
3. Avoid bathing the child until the scabs are gone.
4. Wash the crusts daily with soap and water.

**1825.** The nurse is caring for the 2-month-old newly hospitalized with pertussis (whooping cough). Which interventions, if prescribed, should the nurse implement? **Select all that apply.**

1. Administer erythromycin 15 mg/kg IV q6h.
2. Administer pertussis immune globulin.
3. Initiate airborne isolation precautions.
4. Place suction equipment at the child's bedside.
5. Report the pertussis to the state health department.

**1826.** The clinic nurse is teaching the mother of the child with head lice how to apply permethrin. Place the steps in the order that they should be performed.

1. Comb hair with fine-tooth or nit comb.
2. Thoroughly wet hair and scalp with permethrin lotion.
3. Ensure that the scalp and hair are dry.
4. Allow permethrin lotion to remain on hair for 10 minutes.
5. Massage permethrin into the hair one section at a time.

Answer: _____

**1827.** The school nurse is talking with the adolescent who is concerned about hair loss due to tinea capitis. Which response by the nurse is **most** appropriate?

1. "Others have gone through this. Would you like to talk with someone about this?"
2. "What did your doctor tell you about your hair growing back?"
3. "Your hair is styled nicely to cover the bald spot; why is this bothering you?"
4. "Don't worry. Your hair will grow back in about 6 to 12 months."

**1828.** The clinic nurse is assessing the 12-year-old who has multiple scaly-ringed lesions on the face, neck, and arms. Which is the **most** important question that the nurse should ask?

1. "Do others at home have similar lesions?"
2. "When did these lesions first appear?"
3. "Do you have an animal in your house?"
4. "Have you been picking at these sores?"

**1829.** The clinic nurse is advising the parent of the 8-year-old who has ringworm and now has an extensive, itchy rash. Which instruction should the nurse provide?

1. Use an over-the-counter topical steroid and an antihistamine to treat the reaction.
2. Bring the child immediately to the clinic for further assessment by a professional.
3. Observe for another 24 hours and call the clinic if the rash does not subside by then.
4. Stop all medication immediately because this could indicate an allergic reaction.

**1830.** While caring for the 2-year-old child who has a colostomy, the nurse observes small threadlike objects on and around the stoma. Which statement **best** reflects the nurse's thinking about these objects?

1. These are possible signs of a wound infection.
2. The objects may be indicative of hookworm.
3. The objects may be indicative of pinworms.
4. These are sutures left from the surgical procedure.

**1831.** The nurse is providing information to the parents about how to obtain a test tape specimen to determine if their child has pinworms. Place the nurse's instructions in the order that they should be completed for obtaining the specimen.

1. Place the tongue depressor in a glass jar or in a loose plastic bag.
2. Loop a piece of transparent tape, sticky side out, and place it on the end of a tongue depressor.
3. Repeat the procedure the following day.
4. Bathe the child.
5. As soon as the child wakes up in the morning and prior to the child having a bowel movement, place the tongue depressor firmly against the child's perianal area.

Answer: _____

**1832.** The nurse is assessing the adolescent involved in an MVA and sees the lesions illustrated. What should the nurse do? **Select all that apply.**

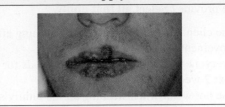

1. Ensure that this infection is reported to the CDC.
2. Prepare for possible testing of the lesions.
3. Prepare to give acyclovir as prescribed.
4. Tell the client to avoid touching his or her face.
5. Use standard precautions when providing care.

**1833.** The nurse is assessing an adolescent male diagnosed with gonorrhea. Which specific signs and symptoms should the nurse associate with the gonorrheal infection? **Select all that apply.**

1. Subnormal temperature
2. Purulent urethral discharge
3. Dysuria and frequency
4. Lesions on the penis
5. Generalized skin rash

**1834.** The nurse completes teaching the adolescent receiving treatment for an STI. Which statement indicates further teaching is needed?

1. "I should abstain from sexual intercourse while I am receiving treatment for chlamydia."
2. "If I use a latex rather than a nonlatex condom, there is less likelihood of it breaking."
3. "I'll apply podophyllin resin 10% solution to each wart and wash it off in 1 to 4 hours."
4. "There is no cure for genital herpes, but I'll be taking an analgesic and an antiviral drug."

**1835.** **PHARM** The school nurse is reviewing the immunization record of the 8-year-old incoming student. Which finding warrants further follow-up by the nurse?

1. The client has received two doses of hepatitis A.
2. The client has received two doses of hepatitis B.
3. The client has received five doses of DTaP.
4. The client has received two doses of MMR.

**1836.** **MoC** Ten adolescent factory workers developed symptoms of hepatitis within 2 days of each other. The source was contaminated cafeteria food. Which type of hepatitis should the nurse expect to be reported to the CDC?

1. Hepatitis A
2. Hepatitis B
3. Hepatitis C
4. Hepatitis D

**1837.** The adolescent is diagnosed with hepatitis A. The nurse is teaching the client and parents about preventing the spread of hepatitis A. Which information should the nurse provide? **Select all that apply.**

1. The client should use strict hand washing after bowel movements.
2. Everyone should avoid eating raw foods for the next 2 weeks.
3. Use hot water when washing all the family's laundry together.
4. Clean the common toilet seat with bleach after each use by the client.
5. The client should avoid kissing anyone until symptoms disappear.

**1838.** The nurse reviews the serology report of the hospitalized adolescent who has a history of ongoing IV drug use since age 13 years. After considering the serology report results, the nurse makes which correct conclusion?

| Laboratory Test | Client Values | Normal Values |
|---|---|---|
| HBsAg | Positive | Negative |
| Anti-HBc IgM | Positive | Negative |
| AST | 200 units/L | 8–38 units/L |
| ALT | 150 units/L | 10–35 units/L |

1. The client has acute hepatitis B, which can be transmitted by blood and body fluids.
2. The client had hepatitis B in the past, is currently immune, and cannot transmit it.
3. The client has acute hepatitis A, and contact precautions should be implemented.
4. The client is not currently infected with hepatitis, and no extra precautions are required.

**1839.** The nurse completes teaching with an adolescent newly diagnosed with acute hepatitis C. Which statement indicates the need for additional teaching?

1. "I know that my liver will be enlarged for several more weeks."
2. "Once my jaundice is gone, I will be cured of my hepatitis C."
3. "I understand that my loss of appetite is related to my disease."
4. "My liver function will need to be monitored closely in the future."

**1840.** The adolescent diagnosed with hepatitis is reporting pruritus. Which therapy should the nurse suggest?

1. Take a hot tub bath three times daily for a week.
2. Rub the skin well with a terry cloth bath towel.
3. Apply cool, moist washcloths on affected areas.
4. Use an exfoliating brush to scratch affected areas.

**1841.** The nurse is completing a follow-up visit at the home of the child recovering from a serious salmonella infection. The nurse should address a concern about reinfection with salmonella after noting that the family has which pets? **Select all that apply.**

1. The family has an indoor dog.
2. The family has a salamander.
3. The child has a large turtle.
4. The child's sister has a cat.
5. The family has baby chicks.

**1842.** The adolescent client with acute vomiting and diarrhea is diagnosed with a norovirus infection. Which instruction should the nurse include when teaching the client?

1. "Symptoms subside in 1 to 2 days; you can return to school and work and resume usual activities then."
2. "The virus can be present in the stool for 2 to 3 weeks after you feel better; strict hand washing is important."
3. "Wash soiled clothing in very hot water to destroy the virus; do this now and for 3 weeks after you feel better."
4. "The virus can be transmitted by respiratory droplets; be sure to wear a mask when in contact with others."

**1843.** The normally healthy adolescent client has a 5-mm skin induration 72 hours after receiving a tuberculin skin test. Which conclusions should the nurse make regarding the test results?

1. This 5-mm skin induration is negative for a normally healthy individual.
2. This finding indicates that active TB is present and treatment is needed.
3. This result is inconclusive, and a chest x-ray is needed to detect active TB.
4. The result is inaccurate; the site assessment occurred too long after the test.

**1844.** The nurse is caring for the pediatric client who was diagnosed with AIDS. Which assessment findings should alert the nurse to the development of *Pneumocystis carinii* pneumonia (PCP)?

1. Dyspnea, elevated temperature, nonproductive cough, and fatigue
2. Weight loss, night sweats, persistent diarrhea, and hypothermia
3. Dysphagia, yellow-white plaques in the mouth, and sore throat
4. Lung crackles, chest pain, and small, painless purple-blue skin lesions

**1845.** The adolescent client diagnosed with HIV has a CD4-positive T-lymphocyte count of 160 mcL. The nurse evaluates that interventions have been **most** effective when which outcome in the client's plan of care is achieved?

1. Soft, formed stools daily
2. Skin integrity nonintact
3. Free of opportunistic infections
4. Weight gain of 1 pound weekly

**1846.** The nurse is planning care for the adolescent client being admitted with newly diagnosed active TB secondary to AIDS. Which planned intervention is **most** important?

1. Monitor for signs of bleeding.
2. Teach strategies for skin care.
3. Institute airborne precautions.
4. Assess CD4 and T-lymphocyte counts.

**INSTRUCTIONS:** At 0800 hours after receiving shift report, the nurse assesses the child and documents the information in the record illustrated. Use the record illustrated to answer Questions 1847 and 1848.

| Client | 3-year-old | **Diagnosis:** Rubeola | **Allergies:** None |
|---|---|---|---|
| **Vital Signs** | **1600:** BP 108/64; P 100; RR 20; temp 100.2°F (37.9°C)<br>**2000:** BP 110/60; P 115; RR 24; temp 100.2°F (37.9°C)<br>**2400:** BP 100/60; P 120; RR 26; temp 101.6°F (38.7°C)<br>**0400:** BP 110/76; P 120; RR 30<br>**0800:** BP 120/80; P 130; RR 40; temp 103.6°F (39.8°C) | | |
| **Significant Assessment Data** | **0800:**<br>*Respiratory:* Crackles and rhonchi in bilateral bases; drooling copious secretions; nasal drainage<br>*Pain:* Crying, clenching eyes, rolling head, and grimacing<br>*Skin:* Warm to touch; generalized rash<br>*Behavior:* Restless, hard to calm | | |
| **Medications in Last 4 hours** | **0600:** Acetaminophen 320 mg oral suspension | | |

**1847.** `CJ` `MoC` After assessing the child, what should be the nurse's **priority**?

1. Recheck the vital signs again in one-half hour.
2. Give another dose of antipyretic medication.
3. Have the chart available and notify the HCP.
4. Implement airborne and standard precautions.

**1848.** `CJ` Which intervention would **best** ensure the child's comfort?

1. Have the lights dimmed and curtains drawn.
2. Provide baby oil baths to soothe the child.
3. Use a warm mist tent to loosen secretions.
4. Request a decongestant to reduce nasal drainage.

# Answers and Rationales

**1806. ANSWER: 1**

1. **Varicella zoster (chicken pox) is transmitted by direct mucous membrane contact, direct lesion contact, and airborne spread of secretions. In a hospital setting, strict airborne and droplet precautions and a negative-airflow room that prevents unfiltered air from leaving the room are used to prevent transmission to vulnerable and susceptible clients.**
2. Airborne and droplet precautions should be used, but the airflow should be negative and not positive.
3. Airborne precautions are also needed with this option.
4. A positive-airflow room is one that prevents unfiltered air from outside the room from entering the room.

▶ *Test-taking Tip:* Note that all options include airflow. First narrow the options by selecting the appropriate type of airflow, positive or negative, and then deciding which would be the most appropriate.

Content Area: Child; Concept: Infection; Critical Thinking; Integrated Processes: Nursing Process: Planning; Client Needs: Safe and Effective Care Environment: Safety and Infection Control; Cognitive Level: Application [Applying]

**1807. MoC PHARM ANSWER: 4**

1. Acetaminophen (Tylenol) is appropriate for a 4-year-old and can be administered for treating fever.
2. Ampicillin (Principen) is appropriate for a 4-year-old and may be used to treat a bacterial infection.
3. Acyclovir (Valtrex) is appropriate for a 4-year-old and may be used to treat a viral infection.
4. **There is a strong association with the use of acetylsalicylic acid (aspirin) for treating fever in children who have a viral illness and the onset of Reye's syndrome. Thus aspirin use is contraindicated for treating fever in children.**

▶ *Test-taking Tip:* Acetylsalicylic acid is aspirin; there is a strong association between Reye's syndrome and aspirin use.

Content Area: Child; Concept: Medication; Infection; Integrated Processes: Communication and Documentation; Client Needs: Safe and Effective Care Environment: Management of Care; Physiological Integrity: Pharmacological and Parenteral Therapies; Cognitive Level: Evaluation [Evaluating]

**1808. MoC ANSWER:**

| Serum Laboratory Test | Client's Value | Normal Levels |
| --- | --- | --- |
| SGOT | 75 **X** | 0–42 units/L |

**SGOT is an enzyme released by the liver when it is damaged. Hepatitis is a complication of varicella. Although the BUN and chloride values are elevated, indicating possible dehydration, and the potassium is marginally low, these are less concerning because these can be quickly treated with fluids and potassium replacement.**

▶ *Test-taking Tip:* Review the chart carefully and think of the laboratory alterations that could be indicative of complications from chicken pox and that would be more difficult to treat than other abnormal values.

Content Area: Child; Concept: Infection; Critical Thinking; Integrated Processes: Nursing Process: Analysis; Client Needs: Safe and Effective Care Environment: Management of Care; Physiological Integrity: Reduction of Risk Potential; Cognitive Level: Analysis [Analyzing]

**1809. PHARM ANSWER: 375**

**Step 1: First convert the child's weight of 55 lb to kilograms: 55 lb ÷ 2.2 lb/kg = 25 kg
Step 2: Multiply 25 kg by 15 mg/kg = 375 mg
The nurse should administer 375 mg of acetaminophen (Tylenol).**

▶ *Test-taking Tip:* Remember that 1 kg equals 2.2 lb.

Content Area: Child; Concept: Infection; Medication; Integrated Processes: Nursing Process: Implementation; Client Needs: Physiological Integrity: Pharmacological and Parenteral Therapies; Cognitive Level: Application [Applying]

**1810. ANSWER: 1, 4**

1. **A rose-pink rash appears once the fever drops to a normal temperature. It starts usually at the trunk and lasts 1 to 2 days.**
2. Aspirin should be avoided with viral illnesses because of its association with Reye's syndrome. Acetaminophen can be administered.
3. The rash of roseola does not itch; oatmeal baths are not necessary.
4. **Transmission is by person-to-infectious-person contact through oral secretions and is possible during the febrile and viremic phase of the illness. Avoiding contact with secretions and performing hand hygiene will help prevent transmission of roseola.**
5. Roseola is communicable during the febrile period; the rash appears after the fever subsides. Isolation is not necessary. Roseola is usually a self-limited illness with no long-term effects.

▶ *Test-taking Tip:* Three options have incorrect information for treating roseola, which is usually a mild illness that is characterized initially with a high fever.

Content Area: Child; Concept: Infection; Nursing Roles; Integrated Processes: Teaching/Learning; Client Needs: Physiological Integrity: Physiological Adaptation; Cognitive Level: Application [Applying]

**1811. ANSWER: 2**

1. Roseola is an acute benign disease characterized by a history of a febrile illness lasting approximately 3 days, followed by the appearance of a faint pink maculopapular rash once the fever subsides. It is not contagious.

2. **Rubeola (measles) has the most severe symptoms, the longest course for illness, and the most detrimental complications. The nurse should plan to assess this child first.**
3. Rubella infection in younger children is characterized by mild symptoms, rash, and suboccipital adenopathy.
4. Eczema is a common skin condition characterized by itchy and inflamed patches of skin. The skin areas can blister and bleed. It sometimes can be due to a reaction to an irritant. The blisters can become infected, but this child's condition will be less severe than the child with rubeola.

▶ *Test-taking Tip: You can narrow the options by using the infection name as a clue. Roseola rash is "rosy," whereas rubeola and rubella are "ruby." A ruby color would be stronger. Then think about Ebola as being very serious. Although not related, you can use this to remember that rubeola (measles) is the most severe infection of the options.*

Content Area: Child; Concept: Infection; Management; Integrated Processes: Nursing Process: Planning; Client Needs: Safe and Effective Care Environment: Safety and Infection Control; Cognitive Level: Application [Applying]

### 1812. ANSWER: 1

1. **The nurse should inform the parents that the period of communicability with rubella is 7 days before and 5 days after the rash appears, that many cases are asymptomatic, and that complications are rare. The greatest concern with this illness is the teratogenic effects on a fetus.**
2. Pneumonia is not a common complication, and exposure by a pregnant woman to rubella can have teratogenic effects.
3. The period of communicability is 5 days before and 14 days after the rash appears is incorrect, and there are teratogenic effects.
4. The incubation period is 14 to 21 days, not 7 to 14 days.

▶ *Test-taking Tip: Three options include effects on the fetus, and one option is different. Often the option that is different is the answer.*

Content Area: Child; Concept: Infection; Nursing Roles; Integrated Processes: Nursing Process: Implementation; Client Needs: Physiological Integrity: Physiological Adaptation; Cognitive Level: Application [Applying]

### 1813. ANSWER: 3

1. Parotid swelling, fever, and headache are associated with mumps and would be expected findings.
2. Earache, anorexia, and painful chewing are associated with mumps and would be expected findings.
3. **Headache, stiff neck, and photophobia are associated with aseptic meningitis and should be most concerning to the nurse. Around 15% of individuals diagnosed with mumps will develop this complication.**
4. Vomiting and swelling above the jawline are associated with mumps and would be expected findings.

▶ *Test-taking Tip: Narrow the options by eliminating the signs and symptoms associated with mumps. Think of the physiology of mumps and of a neurological complication that is potentially life-threatening.*

Content Area: Child; Concept: Infection; Assessment; Integrated Processes: Nursing Process: Analysis; Client Needs: Physiological Integrity: Reduction of Risk Potential; Cognitive Level: Application [Applying]

### 1814. ANSWER: 4

1. The parent, and not the nurse, should make the arrangements for a visit with the HCP.
2. Although the antipyretic may decrease the symptoms, these are not administered in a school setting without an HCP prescription. The responsibilities of the nurse include both providing care to the student and protecting others from possible transmission of an infectious disease.
3. Although the student is 17 years old, the parent will make the decision regarding seeing the HCP, and not the student.
4. **The student's signs and symptoms are consistent with strep throat. The nurse's responsibility is to provide care for this student and to prevent disease transmission. The parent should be notified, and the student should be sent home with a recommendation to be seen by an HCP.**

▶ *Test-taking Tip: You need to consider that the 17-year-old is still under parental guidance and may be under the parent's insurance unless the student is emancipated.*

Content Area: Child; Concept: Infection; Critical Thinking; Integrated Processes: Nursing Process: Planning; Client Needs: Safe and Effective Care Environment: Safety and Infection Control; Cognitive Level: Analysis [Analyzing]

### 1815. MoC ANSWER: 3

1. A bee sting will have an area of redness but will not have a bull's-eye pattern.
2. With cat scratch disease, a single papule or pustule first appears that lasts 1 to 3 weeks, followed by lymph node swelling 1 to 2 weeks after the scratch.
3. **A tick bite can transmit Lyme disease. A distinguishing characteristic of Lyme disease is the development of erythema migrans (a bull's-eye-type pattern) 3 to 31 days after a tick bite. The person should be seen by an HCP and treated immediately to prevent disease development.**
4. Cellulitis is a bacterial skin infection that appears as a swollen, red area of skin that feels hot and tender. It will not have a bull's-eye pattern.

▶ *Test-taking Tip: Focus on the pattern in the illustration. Lyme disease can present with the distinctive pattern of a "bull's eye."*

Content Area: Child; Concept: Infection; Promoting Health; Collaboration; Integrated Processes: Communication and Documentation; Client Needs: Safe and Effective Care Environment: Management of Care; Cognitive Level: Comprehension [Understanding]

**816.** **PHARM** **ANSWER: 1**

1. **The client needs further teaching about avoiding tanning when taking doxycycline (Vibramycin, Doryx). Doxycycline, a common medication used in the treatment of Lyme disease, can cause photosensitivity and requires the use of sunscreen and protective clothing to prevent skin reactions.**
2. It is appropriate for clients to complete their entire prescription of antibiotics. Lyme disease is accompanied by acute viral-like symptoms, including joint and muscle pain.
3. Doxycycline has a pregnancy classification of category D, which means that there is positive evidence of human fetal risk, and pregnancy should be avoided.
4. Diarrhea can be a side effect, but diarrhea and fever could indicate a more serious complication of pseudomembranous colitis. The HCP should be notified for these symptoms or if the disease worsens.

♦ **Test-taking Tip:** Three options are similar, indicating the actions the client will take, and one is different. Often the option that is different is the answer.

Content Area: Child; Concept: Infection; Medication; Nursing Roles; Integrated Processes: Teaching/Learning; Client Needs: Physiological Integrity: Pharmacological and Parenteral Therapies; Cognitive Level: Evaluation [Evaluating]

**1817. ANSWER: 4**

1. Weakness, loss of appetite, and diarrhea (not constipation) would be assessment findings with mononucleosis.
2. Although fever is associated with mononucleosis, the spleen enlarges only about 50% of the time. Occasionally a rash appears that is similar to measles, not chicken pox.
3. Although a white coating on the tongue and throat are present with mononucleosis, lymphocyte levels would be elevated, not depressed.
4. **The nurse can expect to assess extreme fatigue, loss of appetite, and chills that occur within the first 3 days of having mononucleosis. Then severe reddened sore throat and tonsils with a white coating, high fever, headache, diarrhea, and generalized lymphadenopathy occur.**

♦ **Test-taking Tip:** Narrow the options by first examining Options 3 and 4 because both address the lymph system with opposite information. Eliminate Option 3 because with a white coating on the throat, the lymphocyte level would increase.

Content Area: Child; Concept: Infection; Assessment; Integrated Processes: Nursing Process: Assessment; Client Needs: Physiological Integrity: Physiological Adaptation; Cognitive Level: Application [Applying]

**1818. ANSWER: 4**

1. It is unnecessary to refrain from playing soccer for 3 months. Contact sports such as soccer should be avoided while the spleen is enlarged.

2. The student cannot be active now. Bedrest is advised during the acute stage, usually 2 to 3 weeks, to prevent the spleen from rupturing.
3. Activity is limited. Bedrest is advised during the acute stage, usually 2 to 3 weeks, to prevent the spleen from rupturing.
4. **Hepatosplenomegaly is a potential complication of infectious mononucleosis. Because soccer is a contact sport, injury to the spleen can occur.**

♦ **Test-taking Tip:** Two options avoid activity, and two options limit activity. Look at the like options first and eliminate either one or both of these. You need to consider the splenomegaly that occurs with infectious mononucleosis and the length of the illness when selecting an option.

Content Area: Child; Concept: Infection; Nursing Roles; Integrated Processes: Communication and Documentation; Client Needs: Physiological Integrity: Physiological Adaptation; Cognitive Level: Analysis [Analyzing]

**1819. PHARM** **ANSWER: 3**

1. The dose is safe and appropriate.
2. Pharmacy can only dispense what is prescribed unless the HCP writes to have pharmacy calculate the dose.
3. **The daily dose of cefazolin (Ancef) falls within the safe range, so the dose is appropriate and should be administered. To determine the safe range, multiply the child's weight in kg (8.1 kg) by the low end of the medication range (8.1 kg × 6.25 mg = 50.6 mg/kg) and then multiply the child's weight by the high end of the medication range (8.1 kg × 25 mg = 202.5 mg/kg); the safe range is 50.6 mg to 202.5 mg per day. Next determine the daily dose, 50 mg × 4 = 200 mg. The dose of 200 mg falls within the safe range of 50.6–202.5 mg per day.**
4. The dose is safe and appropriate.

♦ **Test-taking Tip:** To determine the correct answer, you need to calculate the safe range and compare this to the amount prescribed to treat the infection.

Content Area: Child; Concept: Infection; Medication; Integrated Processes: Nursing Process: Planning; Client Needs: Physiological Integrity: Pharmacological and Parenteral Therapies; Cognitive Level: Analysis [Analyzing]

**1820. PHARM** **ANSWER: 2**

1. This child has a capillary hemangioma, a congenital disorder. There is no need to administer acyclovir.
2. **Acyclovir (Valtrex) is used to treat viral infections. The nurse can expect to administer acyclovir to this child who has herpes simplex, which is caused by a virus.**
3. This child has hair loss from tinea capitis, or head lice. A pesticide- or insecticide-free preparation is used to treat head lice and not acyclovir.
4. This child has a diaper rash. Topical applications would be used to treat a diaper rash and not acyclovir.

♦ **Test-taking Tip:** Use the medication name as a clue. Only one option shows a skin condition caused by a virus.

Content Area: Child; **Concept:** Infection; **Integrated Processes:** Nursing Process: Analysis; **Client Needs:** Physiological Integrity: Pharmacological and Parenteral Therapies; **Cognitive Level:** Application [Applying]

## 1821. ANSWER: 2

1. DI is not a predisposing factor for a bacterial skin infection.
2. **Predisposing factors placing the child at a greater risk for a bacterial skin infection include obesity, DM, and eczema. Others include excessive skin moisture and use of systemic corticosteroids or antibiotics.**
3. Excessive skin moisture, not dry skin, predisposes the child to a bacterial skin infection. A congenital heart defect does not predispose the child to a bacterial skin infection.
4. Strabismus does not predispose the child to a bacterial skin infection, although systemic corticosteroids do.

▶ **Test-taking Tip:** *Narrow the options by reviewing options with like terms first, Options 2 and 3, and decide if either of these could be the answer. Both cannot be correct. Then move to examining the other options for conditions that would not be associated with an increased risk for a skin infection.*

Content Area: Child; **Concept:** Infection; Assessment; **Integrated Processes:** Nursing Process: Analysis; **Client Needs:** Physiological Integrity: Reduction of Risk Potential; **Cognitive Level:** Analysis [Analyzing]

## 1822. ANSWER: 1

1. **Impetigo is transmitted by direct contact. Clean gloves are used to prevent the spread of infection to the nurse or others.**
2. Sterile technique is not needed because the infection is already present and the goal is to prevent spread of the infection to others.
3. The water temperature should be tepid or one that is comforting to the child.
4. Contact precautions can be discontinued 24 hours after initiation of therapy and do not need to continue during the entire hospitalization time period.

▶ **Test-taking Tip:** *The key phrase is "most important." Impetigo is transmissible from contact with the lesions.*

Content Area: Child; **Concept:** Skin Integrity; Infection; Safety; **Integrated Processes:** Nursing Process: Implementation; **Client Needs:** Safe and Effective Care Environment: Safety and Infection Control; **Cognitive Level:** Application [Applying]

## 1823. ANSWER: 2

1. Herpes zoster inflammation presents with vesicles and pain, and it is usually unilateral.
2. **Impetigo is a contagious, itchy skin lesion with honey-colored crusts.**
3. Cellulitis is a bacterial infection of the subcutaneous tissue that is usually associated with an injury or break in the skin. The client could have a fever, swelling, purulent drainage, redness of the area, and pain.
4. Ringworm is a fungal infection that can affect the scalp, skin, perineal area or inner thighs, feet, or the nails.

▶ **Test-taking Tip:** *The key phrase in the stem is "honey-colored crust." Narrow the options by eliminating those that do not have a crust.*

Content Area: Child; **Concept:** Infection; **Integrated Processes:** Nursing Process: Analysis; **Client Needs:** Physiological Integrity: Physiological Adaptation; **Cognitive Level:** Knowledge [Remembering]

## 1824. ANSWER: 4

1. Mupirocin (Bactroban) ointment for 7 to 10 days is often prescribed to treat the lesions.
2. Debridement (removal of undermined skin, crusts, and debris) occurs only after the skin is softened with wet compresses placed over the areas that are to be debrided.
3. The child should be bathed daily.
4. **Washing the crusts daily with soap and water promotes quick healing of the lesions.**

▶ **Test-taking Tip:** *Options 3 and 4 are opposites. Either one or both are incorrect.*

Content Area: Child; **Concept:** Infection; Nursing Roles; **Integrated Processes:** Teaching/Learning; Caring; **Client Needs:** Physiological Integrity: Basic Care and Comfort; Health Promotion and Maintenance; **Cognitive Level:** Application [Applying]

## 1825. ANSWER: 1, 2, 4

1. **Erythromycin, a macrolide antibiotic, is the preferred treatment for infants at least 1 month of age. The dose is within the recommended range.**
2. **Pertussis immune globulin is administered for passive immunization against pertussis.**
3. Droplet (not airborne) precautions are required. Transmission occurs through droplets, contact, and contaminated articles. Droplet precautions remain in place until the infant has had five days of effective antimicrobial therapy.
4. **Suction equipment may be needed if the infant is unable to cough up mucus to prevent airway obstruction.**
5. Although pertussis is a reportable communicable disease, a designated person in the facility does the reporting, not the nurse caring for the infant.

▶ **Test-taking Tip:** *Pertussis is a communicable disease spread by droplets. Use this information to eliminate incorrect options.*

Content Area: Child; **Concept:** Infection; **Integrated Processes:** Nursing Process: Implementation; **Client Needs:** Safe and Effective Care Environment: Safety and Infection Control; **Cognitive Level:** Analysis [Analyzing]

## 1826. ANSWER: 3, 2, 5, 4, 1

3. **Ensure that the scalp and hair are dry. Wet hair dilutes the permethrin (Elimite) and can contribute to product failure.**
2. **Thoroughly wet hair and scalp with permethrin lotion. A thorough application is necessary to reach the nits at the hair shafts.**

5. **Massage permethrin into the hair one section at a time. This will help to ensure that all of the hair and scalp are covered with permethrin.**

4. **Allow permethrin lotion to remain on hair for 10 minutes. This amount of time is necessary to kill the lice.**

1. **Comb hair with fine-tooth or nit comb. This step is last. The nits cling to the hair shaft and must be manually pulled down the hair with the comb. The hair should be combed one section at a time and pinned out of the way when the section is completed.**

▶ *Test-taking Tip: Finding the first and last step makes it easier to place the steps in the correct order.*

**Content Area:** Child; **Concept:** Infection; Nursing Roles; **Integrated Processes:** Teaching/Learning; **Client Needs:** Physiological Integrity: Physiological Adaptation; **Cognitive Level:** Synthesis [Creating]

## 1827. ANSWER: 2

1. Telling the student that others have experienced this is insensitive. Offering counseling is premature.

2. **Asking what information is known to the client allows the nurse to either supplement or clarify the information. Personal appearance is important to an adolescent.**

3. Asking a why question can block therapeutic communication and initiate defensiveness.

4. Telling the adolescent that the hair will grow back in 6 to 12 months is accurate information, but the client may need the nurse to provide further support rather than accurate, but challenging, information.

▶ *Test-taking Tip: Identify the most important issues for an adolescent and what statement would promote communication and allow the adolescent to discuss his or her feelings.*

**Content Area:** Child; **Concept:** Infection; Communication; **Integrated Processes:** Communication and Documentation; Caring; **Client Needs:** Psychosocial Integrity; **Cognitive Level:** Application [Applying]

## 1828. ANSWER: 3

1. Although it is important to know if others in the household have similar lesions, the most important question should focus on the causative agent to establish a diagnosis.

2. The location of the lesions and the adolescent's age should direct the questioning.

3. **Ringworm is a fungal infection that affects the skin, hair, and nails. Transmission can be human-to-human as well as animal-to-human. Because of the placement of these lesions, they would be consistent with cuddling an animal. Asking about an animal in the house would be the most important question.**

4. Unless there is evidence of picking at the sores, the question is irrelevant.

▶ *Test-taking Tip: Focus on the age of the adolescent and the location of the lesions in selecting the "most important" question. You should think about the transmission of ringworm.*

**Content Area:** Child; **Concept:** Infection; Assessment; **Integrated Processes:** Nursing Process: Assessment; **Client Needs:** Physiological Integrity: Physiological Adaptation; **Cognitive Level:** Analysis [Analyzing]

## 1829. ANSWER: 1

1. **The extensive, itchy rash is related to the development of a hypersensitivity to the fungal antigen. A topical steroid and an antihistamine should be used to treat the rash and help the child be more comfortable.**

2. Because an itchy rash is associated with ringworm, immediate treatment in the clinic is unnecessary. Both topical steroids and antihistamines can be purchased OTC.

3. Observation will not relieve the child's symptoms.

4. Stopping medications is unnecessary because it is unlikely to be an allergic reaction to medications. An itchy rash is associated with ringworm.

▶ *Test-taking Tip: To identify the answer, you should eliminate options that do not treat the child's symptoms. Often options that contain absolute words such as "all" are incorrect.*

**Content Area:** Child; **Concept:** Infection; **Integrated Processes:** Nursing Process: Implementation; **Client Needs:** Physiological Integrity: Physiological Adaptation; **Cognitive Level:** Application [Applying]

## 1830. ANSWER: 3

1. Threadlike objects are not a typical sign of an infection.

2. Although hookworm is a common soil-transmitted helminth infection, hookworm produces an intensely pruritic dermatitis at the entrance site (usually the feet), and as the infection migrates from the pulmonary to the intestinal system, eggs or evidence of the worms would be present in the feces.

3. **Pinworms (enterobiasis) look like tiny pieces of white thread and are about as long as a staple. It is the most common helminthic infection in the U.S. Infection begins when eggs are ingested or inhaled (eggs float in the air).**

4. Suture are not present on the stoma.

▶ *Test-taking Tip: It is important to consider that a surgical procedure has occurred, but it is also important to consider that the child may have been exposed to a variety of organisms prior to being hospitalized.*

**Content Area:** Child; **Concept:** Infection; **Integrated Processes:** Nursing Process: Analysis; **Client Needs:** Physiological Integrity: Physiological Adaptation; **Cognitive Level:** Application [Applying]

## 1831. ANSWER: 2, 5, 1, 4, 3

2. **Loop a piece of transparent tape, sticky side out, and place it on the end of a tongue depressor. The sticky tape is used for collection of the pinworms.**

5. As soon as the child wakes up in the morning and prior to the child having a bowel movement, place the tongue depressor firmly against the child's perianal area. The pinworms are best collected in the morning. At night, the female pinworm migrates within the intestinal tract to the anus to deposit eggs on the anus and skin.
1. Place the tongue depressor in a glass jar or in a loose plastic bag. This will preserve the collection until the pinworms can be inspected under a microscope.
4. Bathe the child. The movement of the worms causes itching, and some eggs can be carried in the fingernails and ingested.
3. Repeat the procedure the following day. It may take several collections to verify or rule out pinworm.

▸ **Test-taking Tip:** *Think about the supplies needed to collect the specimen. This should lead you to the first option. Then review the options and select the last option. Use cues within the options (e.g., following day) to identify the last step in the collection process.*

Content Area: Child; Concept: Infection; Nursing Roles; Integrated Processes: Teaching/Learning; Client Needs: Safe and Effective Care Environment: Safety and Infection Control; Cognitive Level: Synthesis [Creating]

### 1832. ANSWER: 2, 3, 4

1. Herpes simplex 1 (HSV-1) and 2 (HSV-2) are not reportable infections, even though they are highly contagious.
2. **Visualization of the lesion is often only needed to diagnose the HSV-1. However, a viral culture of an open area may be completed to determine if the lesions are the herpesvirus or a different virus, such as the varicella virus (chickenpox), that is similar in appearance.**
3. **Acyclovir (Avirix) is an antiviral medication used to treat viral infections.**
4. **HSV-1 is highly contagious. Keeping the hands away from the face will help prevent transmission to other areas.**
5. According to the CDC, standard and contact precautions are required until the lesions are dry and crusted.

▸ **Test-taking Tip:** *Use the process of elimination, eliminating options that would take minimal precautions. Select options that help to prevent the spread of HSV-1.*

Content Area: Child; Concept: Infection; Integrated Processes: Nursing Process: Analysis; Teaching/Learning; Client Needs: Safe and Effective Care Environment: Safety and Infection Control; Cognitive Level: Application [Applying]

### 1833. ANSWER: 2, 3

1. The temperature is elevated, not subnormal, with a gonorrheal infection.
2. **Urethral discharge, which appears after a 2- to 7-day incubation period, is associated with an infection caused by *Neisseria gonorrhoeae*.**

3. **Signs of urethritis with pain on urination and urinary frequency are associated with an infection caused by *Neisseria gonorrhoeae*.**
4. Lesions on the penis are associated with syphilis, not a gonorrheal infection.
5. A generalized skin rash is associated with syphilis, not a gonorrheal infection.

▸ **Test-taking Tip:** *You need to focus on a gonorrheal infection and eliminate options indicative of syphilis.*

Content Area: Child; Concept: Infection; Integrated Processes: Nursing Process: Assessment; Client Needs: Physiological Integrity: Physiological Adaptation; Cognitive Level: Application [Applying]

### 1834. ANSWER: 1

1. **This statement indicates the need for further teaching. Persons treated for chlamydia should abstain from sexual intercourse for 7 days after treatment is completed and until all sexual partners have completed a full course of treatment.**
2. Nonlatex condoms are more likely to break than latex condoms.
3. Podophyllin (Podoben) is a cytotoxic agent recommended for small external genital warts and should be carefully applied to just the wart, avoiding normal tissue, and washed off in 1 to 4 hours.
4. Genital herpes is caused by herpesvirus type 2. The virus remains in the body for life. The antiviral medication suppresses viral replication and shortens the course of illness, but it does not destroy the virus.

▸ **Test-taking Tip:** *The key phrase is "further teaching." Select the option that is an incorrect statement.*

Content Area: Child; Concept: Infection; Nursing Roles; Integrated Processes: Nursing Process: Evaluation; Teaching/Learning; Client Needs: Safe and Effective Care Environment: Safety and Infection Control; Physiological Integrity: Physiological Adaptation; Cognitive Level: Evaluation [Evaluating]

### 1835. PHARM ANSWER: 2

1. Two doses of hepatitis A is appropriate and would not require further evaluation.
2. **The 8-year-old should have completed the three-part series of hepatitis B. Having only two of the three doses is a reason for further follow-up. The reason for the missing vaccine may vary, but parental refusal of vaccines is a growing a concern. Parental refusal may be due to religious or personal beliefs, safety concerns, and a desire for more information from the HCP.**
3. The 8-year-old having five doses of DTaP is appropriate and would not require further evaluation.
4. The 8-year-old having two doses of MMR would be appropriate and would not require further evaluation.

▸ **Test-taking Tip:** *The key word in the stem is "follow-up." You need to select an option with incomplete immunizations for the 8-year-old.*

**Content Area:** Child; **Concept:** Immunity; Assessment; **Integrated Processes:** Nursing Process: Assessment; Culture and Spirituality; **Client Needs:** Health Promotion and Maintenance; Physiological Integrity: Pharmacological and Parenteral Therapies; **Cognitive Level:** Analysis [Analyzing]

### 1836. MoC ANSWER: 1

1. **Foodborne hepatitis A outbreaks are usually due to contamination of food during preparation by an infected food handler. Outbreaks of hepatitis within a group are consistently caused by hepatitis A virus.**
2. Hepatitis B is transmitted by exposure to blood or body fluids and therefore doesn't cause group outbreaks.
3. Hepatitis C is transmitted by exposure to blood or body fluids and therefore doesn't cause group outbreaks.
4. Hepatitis D virus requires the presence of hepatitis B virus to infect a host.

▶ *Test-taking Tip: Focus on the different methods of transmission of each type of hepatitis virus. Hepatitis A is the only one that can be transmitted through contaminated food.*

**Content Area:** Child; **Concept:** Infection; Nursing Roles; **Integrated Processes:** Nursing Process: Analysis; **Client Needs:** Safe and Effective Care Environment: Management of Care; Safe and Effective Care Environment: Safety and Infection Control; **Cognitive Level:** Comprehension [Understanding]

### 1837. ANSWER: 1, 4

1. **Hepatitis A virus is present in the client's feces for 2 weeks after symptoms appear. Careful hand washing after defecation will prevent the spread of the virus.**
2. The virus is not present on raw foods that have been cleansed; no one needs to abstain from eating these.
3. The client's laundry should be washed separately from the rest of the family's in hot, soapy water.
4. **Private toilet facilities are ideal; however, if there is a common family toilet, it should be wiped with bleach after each use by the infected individual. Bleach kills the virus.**
5. The virus is not present in saliva, so there is no reason to avoid kissing.

▶ *Test-taking Tip: Think about how hepatitis A is transmitted. A memory aid to remember the mode of transmission for hepatitis A would be the letter "A," which is for **a**nus. This should enable elimination of Options 2 and 5.*

**Content Area:** Child; **Concept:** Infection; Nursing Roles; **Integrated Processes:** Teaching/Learning; **Client Needs:** Safe and Effective Care Environment: Safety and Infection Control; **Cognitive Level:** Analysis [Analyzing]

### 1838. ANSWER: 1

1. **The client most likely has contracted hepatitis B. Immunoglobulin M (IgM) is responsible for the primary immune response. Thus the presence of IgM indicates an acute infection. In this case the positive anti-HBc IgM plus the positive HBsAg (hepatitis B surface antigen) indicates acute infection with hepatitis B. Elevated ALT and AST indicate liver cell injury and acute infection. Transmission of the hepatitis B virus occurs through contact with infectious blood or other body fluids. Standard precautions should be implemented.**
2. There is no indication of immunity to hepatitis B in the laboratory report, and transmission can occur through contact with infected blood or body fluids.
3. The laboratory tests for HBsAg and anti-HBc IgM indicate that the client is being tested for hepatitis B, not A.
4. Anti-HBc IgG subtype is indicative of chronic hepatitis infection. A positive anti-HBc IgM and HBsAg indicates acute infection with hepatitis B.

▶ *Test-taking Tip: The key laboratory values are the positive HBsAg and anti-HBc IgM. Recognizing that these indicate acute infection and are specific for hepatitis B allows elimination of Options 2, 3, and 4. Use the B in hepatitis B to remember that it is transmitted through blood and body fluids.*

**Content Area:** Child; **Concept:** Infection; **Integrated Processes:** Nursing Process: Analysis; **Client Needs:** Physiological Integrity: Reduction of Risk Potential; **Cognitive Level:** Analysis [Analyzing]

### 1839. ANSWER: 2

1. Liver enlargement remains for several weeks after the acute phase of hepatitis C has ended.
2. **The disappearance of jaundice does not mean that the client has totally recovered. Most hepatitis C infections result in chronic illness. When the client's jaundice begins fading, this is a sign that the convalescent phase of hepatitis C is beginning.**
3. The liver inflammation and accumulation of bilirubin that occurs with hepatitis C cause nausea and anorexia.
4. Hepatitis C carries a high risk of leading to chronic liver disease. The results of liver function tests will be closely monitored.

▶ *Test-taking Tip: "Need for more teaching" is a false-response item. Select the incorrect statement.*

**Content Area:** Child; **Concept:** Infection; Nursing Roles; **Integrated Processes:** Nursing Process: Evaluation; **Client Needs:** Physiological Integrity: Physiological Adaptation; **Cognitive Level:** Evaluation [Evaluating]

### 1840. ANSWER: 3

1. Hot water will increase blood flow to the area and thus increase the itching.
2. Rubbing affected skin areas increases skin irritation.
3. **Cool baths and cool, moist compresses will cause vasoconstriction and thus provide relief.**
4. Scratching affected skin areas increases skin irritation.

▸ **Test-taking Tip:** *Focus on the physiological action of heat and cold application. Knowing that heat and friction increase blood flow should allow elimination of Options 1 and 2.*

**Content Area:** Child; **Concept:** Infection; Nursing Roles; Comfort; **Integrated Processes:** Nursing Process: Implementation; Teaching/ Learning; **Client Needs:** Physiological Integrity: Basic Care and Comfort; **Cognitive Level:** Application [Applying]

## 1841. ANSWER: 2, 3, 5

1. Dogs are not a common source of salmonella infection.
2. **Reptiles, such as a salamander, are a common source of salmonella infection. Appropriate hand hygiene following contact is essential.**
3. **Turtles are common sources of salmonella infection. Appropriate hand hygiene following contact is essential.**
4. Cats are not a common source of salmonella infection.
5. **Chicks are common sources of salmonella infection. Appropriate hand hygiene following contact is essential.**

▸ **Test-taking Tip:** *Three options are less common pets in the home.*

**Content Area:** Child; **Concept:** Infection; Nursing Roles; **Integrated Processes:** Nursing Process: Assessment; **Client Needs:** Safe and Effective Care Environment: Safety and Infection Control; **Cognitive Level:** Application [Applying]

## 1842. ANSWER: 2

1. Vomiting and diarrhea usually last longer than 1 to 2 days. The CDC recommends not working and avoiding handling or preparing food for others until 2 or 3 days after the person recovers (not once the symptoms subside).
2. **Because the virus is highly contagious and continues to be present in the stool for as long as 2 to 3 weeks, strict hand washing must be performed to ensure that the person does not infect others. This is especially important after using the bathroom and before handling food.**
3. Washing soiled clothing immediately can reduce the transmission of the virus, but the virus can withstand environmental extremes of heat or cold and is resistant to chemical disinfection.
4. The virus is not transmitted by respiratory droplets. Droplets from a violent emesis can be transmitted to water, objects, or surfaces where others can pick up the virus when placing their hands in their mouths.

▸ **Test-taking Tip:** *Rule out Option 4 because the stem of the question addresses the GI and not the respiratory system.*

**Content Area:** Child; **Concept:** Infection; Nursing Roles; **Integrated Processes:** Teaching/Learning; **Client Needs:** Safe and Effective Care Environment: Safety and Infection Control; **Cognitive Level:** Analysis [Analyzing]

## 1843. ANSWER: 1

1. **An area of induration measuring 15 mm in diameter or greater in a person with no known risk factors for TB and read 48 to 72 hours after injection is a positive TB test. An induration of 5 mm or greater would be a positive result in HIV-infected persons but not for a normally health individual.**
2. A positive test indicates exposure to, and not active, TB.
3. The result is negative for TB rather than inconclusive.
4. Evidence-based practice guidelines indicate that a reading at 72 hours is more accurate than one at 48 hours; the time of assessment was not too long.

▸ **Test-taking Tip:** *Identify similar words in the stem and options. Note the key phrase "normally healthy" in both the stem and Option 1.*

**Content Area:** Child; **Concept:** Infection; Critical Thinking; **Integrated Processes:** Nursing Process: Analysis; **Client Needs:** Safe and Effective Care Environment: Safety and Infection Control; **Cognitive Level:** Evaluation [Evaluating]

## 1844. ANSWER: 1

1. **PCP is caused by a fungus that produces symptoms of dyspnea, elevated temperature, nonproductive cough, and fatigue. It is the most common opportunistic infection in HIV/AIDS.**
2. Weight loss, night sweats, and persistent diarrhea are symptoms of AIDS and not PCP; hypothermia is not associated with either AIDS or PCP.
3. Dysphagia, yellow-white plaques in the mouth, and sore throat are symptoms of *Candida albicans*.
4. Although PCP could cause lung crackles and chest pain, the skin lesions are found with Kaposi's sarcoma.

▸ **Test-taking Tip:** *Focus on symptoms of PCP, not AIDS. Narrow the options to 1 and 4 because only these options pertain to the respiratory system. Option 1 contains more respiratory symptoms than Option 4; thus eliminate Option 4.*

**Content Area:** Child; **Concept:** Infection; Assessment; **Integrated Processes:** Nursing Process: Assessment; **Client Needs:** Physiological Integrity: Physiological Adaptation; **Cognitive Level:** Application [Applying]

## 1845. ANSWER: 3

1. Soft, formed stools daily is an outcome for altered elimination.
2. Skin integrity nonintact is a problem and not a desired outcome.
3. **The CD4-positive T-lymphocyte count is low, increasing the client's risk for bacterial, fungal, and viral infections as well as for cancer. Interventions have been effective if the client does not develop an infection.**
4. Weight gain of 1 lb weekly is an outcome for altered nutrition: less than body requirements.

▸ **Test-taking Tip:** *The key phrase in the stem is "T-lymphocyte count." Knowing that T-lymphocytes are associated with an infection should direct you to Option 3.*

Content Area: Child; Concept: Infection; Integrated Processes: Nursing Process: Evaluation; Client Needs: Physiological Integrity: Physiological Adaptation; Cognitive Level: Evaluation [Evaluating]

## 1846. ANSWER: 3

1. The client may be at risk for bleeding due to the effects of antiretroviral therapy, but the situation does not note whether or not the client is receiving treatment.
2. Teaching is important but not the most important of the options.
3. **Active TB can be transmitted by airborne droplet nuclei smaller than 5 microns. The client should be in a private room with negative air pressure and 6 to 12 air exchanges per hour. Persons entering the room should wear an N95 respirator. The client should wear a surgical mask when transported out of the room.**
4. Although it is important to determine the level of immunodeficiency because the client is at risk for infection, initiating airborne precautions is the most important to prevent transmission of TB.

▶ *Test-taking Tip: The key term is "intervention." Eliminate Options 1 and 4 because these pertain to assessment. Of the two remaining options, determine which is most important.*

Content Area: Child; Concept: Infection; Integrated Processes: Nursing Process: Planning; Client Needs: Safe and Effective Care Environment: Safety and Infection Control; Cognitive Level: Application [Applying]

## 1847. CJ MoC ANSWER: 3

1. The VS pattern suggests a potential secondary infection; waiting to obtain another set of VS will delay the child's treatment.
2. Dosing of acetaminophen (Tylenol) is usually every 4 hours; it is too early for another dose.

3. **The nurse should contact the HCP because the child's rising fever and other signs and symptoms suggest a possible respiratory complication secondary to rubeola; pneumonia is a common complication.**
4. Airborne and standard infection precautions should have been implemented when the child was first hospitalized.

▶ *Test-taking Tip: The nurse is responsible for preventing harm. Negligence can occur when the nurse fails to recognize potential complications and fails to notify the HCP.*

Content Area: Child; Concept: Infection; Collaboration; Integrated Processes: Nursing Process: Planning; Client Needs: Safe and Effective Care Environment: Management of Care; Cognitive Level: Analysis [Analyzing]

## 1848. CJ ANSWER: 1

1. **Children with measles have photophobia. Keeping the lights dim and curtains drawn will reduce the pain caused from bright lighting.**
2. Skin should be kept clean and dry. Baby oil would not be used for the rash of measles.
3. Mist tents are no longer recommended in hospital settings because they disperse fungus and molds.
4. A decongestant does not reduce the nasal drainage associated with rubeola.

▶ *Test-taking Tip: Three options include rationale and one is different. Often the option that is different is the answer.*

Content Area: Child; Concept: Infection; Sensory Perception; Integrated Processes: Nursing Process: Implementation; Client Needs: Physiological Integrity: Physiological Adaptation; Cognitive Level: Application [Applying]

# Chapter Forty-Two

# Integumentary and Sensory Management

**1849.** The child is presenting with burn injuries. What should be the nurse's priority during the **initial** assessment?

1. The location, extent, and shape of burn injuries
2. The parent's concerns regarding the child's burn
3. Signs of smoke inhalation and airway patency
4. The child's history of other illnesses or infections

**1850.** MoC The nurse is assessing four 2- to 3-year-old children presenting with burn injuries. Which injuries would **least** likely trigger the need for further follow-up for potential child abuse and mandatory reporting?

1. Rough burns with edema that encircle the wrists
2. Round-shaped burns on the soles of the feet
3. Splash burns on the front torso, face, and neck
4. Scald burns appearing on the feet and legs

**1851.** The nurse is preparing to care for the 4-year-old hospitalized for moderate burns. Which response from the child should the nurse anticipate based on the child's developmental age?

1. Pushes boundaries to gain further autonomy
2. Wants clear details of the planned treatment
3. Shows hostility to try to not appear to be young
4. Believes it was his or her fault for the burns

**1852.** The child, being treated for second-degree burns over 40% of the body, has just been diagnosed with DIC. Which is the **current** priority problem that the nurse should add to the child's plan of care?

1. Ineffective tissue perfusion
2. Impaired urinary elimination
3. Risk for deficient fluid volume
4. Impaired physical mobility

**1853.** The nurse is developing an educational program about burn prevention for parents of toddlers. Which **most** common cause of burns in toddlers should the nurse be sure to address?

1. Pulling on cords or pan handles left within reach
2. Touching a hot iron that is left unattended
3. Touching flames such as from a burning candle
4. Playing with matches left within the child's reach

**1854.** The nurse is using the Rule of 9's to calculate the burn area of a child. What percent should the nurse document for the shaded area in the illustration that was burned?

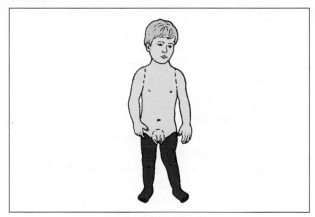

_____ % (Record your answer as a whole number.)

**1855.** MoC The nurse reviews HCP orders for the child with second- and third-degree burns over 10% of the total body surface area (TBSA). The child weighs 20 kg. Which order should the nurse clarify with the HCP?

1. Give Ringer's lactate IV at 50 mL/hr for 8 hrs.
2. Insert a urinary catheter to monitor hourly output.
3. Elevate extremities above the level of the heart.
4. Give morphine sulfate IV prn for pain control.

42 Integumentary and Sensory Management

**1856.** The ED nurse assessed the adolescent who has burns over 25% of the body. Which finding should be **most** concerning to the nurse?

1. Upper extremity burns are mottled.
2. Upper extremity burns are moist and red.
3. Lower extremity burns are waxy white.
4. Anterior lower extremity burns are red blistering.

**1857.** The nurse assessed the hospitalized child with severe burn injuries on the lower extremities. Findings include weak distal pulses in the right leg with capillary refill >3 seconds, and the child reports feeling numbness and tingling in the right leg. Which conclusion by the nurse is correct?

1. This is expected during initial burn healing.
2. This is an emergency; the HCP should be notified.
3. The extremity should be assessed again in 1 hour.
4. Fluid accumulation is decreasing blood flow.

**1858.** The parent of a toddler telephones the ED nurse and, sobbing hysterically, states, "My baby put an electrical cord in her mouth! What should I do?" Which statement by the nurse has **priority?**

1. "Call 911 to have your baby brought to the ED."
2. "Was the cord removed from the baby's mouth?"
3. "Is there bleeding inside the baby's mouth?"
4. "Describe the appearance of your baby's mouth."

**1859.** MoC The infant has burn injuries caused by the ingestion of a strong alkali. The parents, who have limited English, ask through an interpreter what will happen to their baby. Which intervention is **most** important for the nurse to address with the parents?

1. A chest x-ray will need to be performed to determine if there is lung injury.
2. Social services will be contacted due to this type of injury in an infant this age.
3. A barium swallow test will need to be performed to reveal the extent of injuries.
4. Surgery may be needed to correct esophageal strictures from the alkali ingestion.

**1860.** PHARM The nurse assesses the child's thermal burn from the scalding illustrated. Which interventions should the nurse plan? **Select all that apply.**

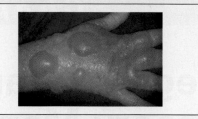

1. Give an analgesic prior to burn care.
2. Insert gauze between each of the fingers.
3. Pierce blisters prior to dressing the hand.
4. Secure any dressings applied with netting.
5. Apply vitamin E lotion to keep hand moist.
6. Apply silver sulfadiazine cream if prescribed.

**1861.** The child with a burn injury has had a skin graft. During the child's dressing change, the new nurse asks the experienced nurse why the skin appears lattice-like and is not smooth like the unburned areas. Which is the experienced nurse's **best** response?

1. "The skin is an allograft from a cadaver donor; the freezing of the skin causes this appearance."
2. "The skin is an autograft from an unburned area; it is meshed so it would stretch to cover more area."
3. "This is from indentations from the bulky dressing applied after the skin graft."
4. "Fluids seeping from tissues makes the new skin stretch; as it heals, the skin comes together."

**1862.** During the 2-year-old's skin grafting procedure to treat a severe burn injury, a bulky dressing is placed over 60% of the child's body. The parents are shocked when they see their child's appearance. Which is the nurse's **most** caring action?

1. Help the parents don the mask, gown, and gloves that are needed to enter the child's room.
2. Bring the parents to a quiet place to allow the parents to talk about immediate concerns.
3. When appropriately attired, accompany the parents to show them how to touch their child.
4. Arrange for a member of the clergy to come visit with the parents and child for support.

**1863.** The nurse is collecting information and preparing to assess the toddler with eczema. Which component is **most** important for the nurse to assess?

1. Child's emotional status
2. Child's fluid volume status
3. Infection control practices
4. Degree of lichenification

**1864.** **PHARM** The toddler with eczema is being seen in the clinic. What information should the nurse include when teaching the parent?

1. Bathe the child often to remove flaking skin.
2. Obtain mupirocin topical ointment.
3. Identify things that trigger eczema.
4. Remove the silvery scales from the child's skin.

**1865.** The adolescent has severe acne. Which information should the nurse teach about acne prevention measures and treatment? **Select all that apply.**

1. Squeeze comedones to express bacterial material.
2. Avoid eating chocolate and French fries.
3. If using makeup, only use oil-free makeup.
4. Use antibacterial soap to wash areas twice daily.
5. Apply benzoyl peroxide in the a.m. and before bed.

**1866.** **PHARM** The parent of the adolescent with acne telephones to clarify the prescription for minocycline 100 mg orally q6h for 3 doses, then 50 mg q6h. How many tablets should the nurse instruct the parent to give for the initial dose when 50-mg tablets were supplied?

_____ tablets (Record your answer as a whole number.)

**1867.** The mother calls the clinic due to the worsening of her 10-year-old's skin rash since the office visit. Which statement should alert the nurse that the parent may be using complementary therapies?

1. "My child plays outdoors in the woods."
2. "I've read about using alternative medicine."
3. "The cortisone cream doesn't seem to help."
4. "What do you think about using Echinacca?"

**1868.** The child has a tentative diagnosis of Albright's disease (neurofibromatosis). When caring for the child, what should the nurse expect to observe?

1. Pediculosis
2. Café-au-lait spots
3. Tick bites
4. Congenital nevi

**1869.** **PHARM** The 8-year-old is being seen in the clinic with contact dermatitis on the legs from poison ivy. Which instructions should the nurse include when teaching the child's parent? **Select all that apply.**

1. Apply an occlusive dressing and tape tightly.
2. Apply a thick paste made of baking soda.
3. Apply calamine lotion to promote drying.
4. Remove scabs from the lesions as they form.
5. Check the surrounding area for poison ivy plants.
6. Give OTC oral diphenhydramine as prescribed.

**1870.** The parents report that their child has been bumping into objects, seeing halos around objects, and sometimes has diplopia. A referral is made for a tonometry test. Which condition should the nurse discuss with the parents as the condition being evaluated for by the tonometry test?

1. Cataracts
2. Strabismus
3. Glaucoma
4. Lazy eye

**1871.** **PHARM** The child with a tentative diagnosis of otitis externa (OE) is to be evaluated in the clinic. The nurse should anticipate preparing the child for which procedures? **Select all that apply.**

1. A complete otoscopic examination
2. A complete blood count with differential
3. A culture of the external auditory canal
4. X-rays of the face, maxilla, and skull
5. Ear curettage to remove excess cerumen
6. Instillation of ear drops such as ciprofloxacin

**1872.** **MoC** The school nurse is meeting with the teacher of the child who has strabismus. Which suggestions should the school nurse make? **Select all that apply.**

1. Have the child select a desk for the best view.
2. Seat all the impaired children together.
3. Allow extra time for assignments and test taking.
4. Provide books and other materials in large print.
5. Speak louder than usual when the child is present.

**1873.** The child's mother tells the nurse, "My child's eyes are misaligned." The nurse observes that the child's eyes appear as illustrated. In reviewing the child's medical record, which condition should the nurse associate with the finding?

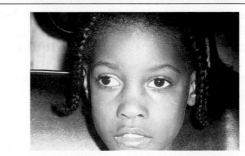

1. Strabismus
2. Diplopia
3. Hemianopsia
4. Pterygium

**1874.** The parent of a hospitalized child tells the nurse that the child's glasses for treating nearsightedness were damaged. Which observations should the nurse expect due to the child's nearsightedness? **Select all that apply.**

1. Has one eye that turns inward when focusing
2. Bends with head close to the table when coloring
3. Squints to see objects more clearly
4. Has a lens in one of the eyes that appears opaque
5. Reads holding a book at arm's length away from the eyes

**1875.** The nurse assesses that the 4-year-old child has difficulty with vision. The child's eyes do not adjust to focus on an object as it is brought toward the child's nose from a distance of 12 inches away. What is the nurse's correct documentation of this finding?

1. Altered reactivity
2. Impaired stereopsis
3. Presence of a red reflex
4. Inability to accommodate

**1876.** MoC The school nurse completed a second visual screen for preschool and school-aged children. Which child should the nurse plan to refer for follow-up evaluation of the child's vision?

1. The 4-year-old who has 20/40 vision in both eyes
2. The 6-year-old who has 20/30 vision in both eyes
3. The 7-year-old who has 20/40 vision in both eyes
4. The 9-year-old who has 20/15 vision in both eyes

**1877.** The nurse is presenting information about conjunctivitis to parents of preschool children. Which statement indicates that a parent understands the **most** important information about bacterial conjunctivitis?

1. "Conjunctivitis is almost always self-limiting without treatment."
2. "The most common cause of conjunctivitis is from a foreign body."
3. "Washcloths and towels should be used only by the infected person."
4. "Conjunctivitis can be transmitted to the newborn during the birth process."

**1878.** The mother tells the nurse that her 1-month-old infant does not react to light. Which response to the parent is **best?**

1. "You should have your infant's vision tested; I can help you with arranging an appointment."
2. "It's normal for your infant not to react to light; visual acuity improves as the infant grows."
3. "All babies react to light differently. See how your baby responds when in different lighting."
4. "This is nothing to worry about, but I'll inform the doctor so it can be evaluated."

**1879.** MoC The nurse is counseling the parents of the infant who was born blind. Which statement indicates that the parents need additional teaching?

1. "We will need to play with her so she will be stimulated and learn how to play."
2. "We'll teach her Braille and attach Braille clothing tags to help her learn to dress."
3. "She will need speech therapy because she will have difficulty learning verbal skills."
4. "We plan to obtain a seeing-eye dog so she can get used to the animal."

**1880.** The 6-year-old child is diagnosed with myopia. When teaching the child and parents about the reason for the visual problem, which illustration should the nurse select?

1.
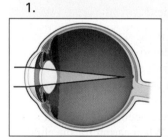

2.
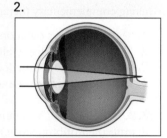

3.
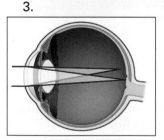

4.
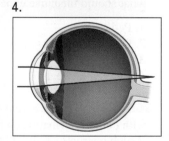

**1881.** [MoC] The 6-year-old is brought to the clinic after being hit in the eye by a baseball. The nurse assesses gross hyphema and a visible fluid meniscus across the iris. Which HCP order should the nurse anticipate?

1. Immediate referral to an ophthalmologist
2. Immediate transfer to the ED
3. Home treatment with ice application for 24 hours
4. Cortisone eye drops and an eye patch

**1882.** The nurse is assessing the toddler diagnosed with acute otitis media (AOM). Which signs and symptoms should the nurse expect? **Select all that apply.**

1. Fussy, restless
2. Irritable, crying
3. Pulling at the affected ear
4. Rhinitis, cough, and diarrhea
5. Rolls head from side to side

**1883.** The nurse is caring for the child who has drainage from the ears following insertion of tympanostomy tubes. Which interventions should the nurse implement? **Select all that apply.**

1. Insert earplugs to prevent infection.
2. Apply an ice compress over each ear.
3. Apply moisture barriers to each earlobe.
4. Administer analgesics for mild pain.
5. Clean the outer canal with sterile cotton swabs.

**1884.** The nurse is planning care for the toddler with otitis media who is returning from surgery following a tympanostomy. Prioritize the order in which the nurse should address the child's identified needs.

1. Interrupted family process related to illness and/or hospitalization of child and temporary hearing loss
2. Acute pain related to pressure caused by inflammatory process
3. Infection related to presence of infective organisms
4. Risk for delayed growth and development related to potential hearing loss

Answer: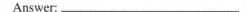

**1885.** [PHARM] The nurse is to instill ofloxacin 0.3% ear drops into the 18-month-old's left ear. Place an X at the location on the illustration where the nurse's fingers should be placed to straighten the child's ear canal.

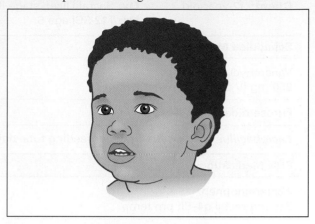

**1886.** The malnourished child has cheilosis of the lips, burning and itching eyes, and seborrheic dermatitis. The child is diagnosed with a vitamin $B_2$ (riboflavin) deficiency. Which additional assessment finding might the nurse expect based on the diagnosis?

1. Paresthesia
2. Irregular HR
3. Acanthosis nigricans
4. Cracks at the nasal angles

**INSTRUCTIONS:** Review the child's medical record illustrated, then answer Questions 1887 and 1888.

| Medication Administration Record (MAR) | | Date: Today | | |
|---|---|---|---|---|
| **Client:** 12-year-old | **Dx:** Sacral Ulcer, stage III; Sepsis  **Hx:** T12 SCI age 6 | **Allergies:** Cefdinir | **Weight:** 25 kg | |
| **Scheduled Medications** | | **2400–0759** | **0800–1559** | **1600–2359** |
| Vancomyci 250 mg IV q6h (give over 90 min) | | 0200 NSN | 0800 DSN  1300 DSN | |
| Furosemide 20 mg IV now | | | 1530 DSN | |
| *Lactobacillus acidophilus* 1 tab per feeding tube daily | | | 0800 DSN | |
| **PRN Medications** | | **2400–0759** | **0800–1559** | **1600–2359** |
| Acetaminophen 325 mg rectal q4–6h prn temp | | | | |
| Diphenhydramine 12.5–25 mg IV prn pruritus | | | | |
| Morphine Sulfate 0.5–0.1 mg q2h prn pain | | 0145 NSN (0.1 mg)  0630 NSN (0.1 mg) | 0945 DSN (0.1 mg)  1515 DSN (0.1 mg) | |
| Naloxone 12 mcg IV prn opioid reversal | | | | |
| **Sig: Night Shift Nurse, RN/NSN** | | **Day Shift Nurse, RN/DSN** | | |

**1887.** `CJ` `MoC` `PHARM` At 1600 hours, the nurse assesses that the child has a rash and pruritus. Based on the MAR, what should the nurse do now? **Select all that apply.**

1. Stop the IV pump with vancomycin infusing.
2. Notify the HCP of the rash and itching.
3. Give diphenhydramine 12.5 mg IV.
4. Administer naloxone 12 mcg IV.
5. Question about a possible furosemide allergy.

**1888.** `CJ` The nurse is preparing to provide wound care for the child's sacral ulcer. Which supplies should the nurse assemble? **Select all that apply.**

1. Soap and tap water
2. Half-strength hydrogen peroxide
3. Bottle of sterile sodium chloride
4. Hydrocolloid dressing
5. Tube of zinc oxide ointment

## Answers and Rationales

**1849. ANSWER: 3**

1. Although inspecting burn injuries is included in the initial assessment, it should not have priority.
2. The child's and parent's concerns should be addressed once the physiological status of the child is stabilized.
3. **Assessment of ABC's has priority. It is imperative to ensure that the airway has not been compromised by smoke or edema related to neck and facial burns.**
4. The child's history is important because it could influence the treatment, but it does not have priority.

♦ *Test-taking Tip: Use the ABC's to determine priority. Remember that smoke inhalation can compromise the airway.*

**Content Area:** Child; **Concept:** Skin Integrity; Assessment; **Integrated Processes:** Nursing Process: Assessment; **Client Needs:** Physiological Integrity: Physiological Adaptation; **Cognitive Level:** Application [Applying]

**1850. MoC ANSWER: 3**

1. Rope burns are often a result of child abuse and are not consistent with accidental burn injuries seen in a child. These types of burns should alert the nurse to further assess the situation.
2. Round-shaped burns are suspicious for cigarette burns and are not consistent with accidental burn injuries seen in a child. These types of burns should alert the nurse to further assess the situation.
3. **Splash burns on the front torso, face, and neck are consistent with a child pulling down a container of hot liquid.**
4. Scald burns are not consistent with accidental burn injuries seen in a child. These types of burns should alert the nurse to further assess the situation.

♦ *Test-taking Tip: Of the types of burn injuries presented, only one could occur by accident and is the answer.*

**Content Area:** Child; **Concept:** Violence; Safety; Skin Integrity; **Integrated Processes:** Nursing Process: Analysis; **Client Needs:** Safe and Effective Care Environment: Management of Care; **Cognitive Level:** Application [Applying]

**1851. ANSWER: 4**

1. Pushing boundaries would be a response by a toddler.
2. Wanting clear instructions would be characteristic of a school-aged child.
3. Anger and hostility is an adolescent response.
4. **The preschool child may experience feelings of guilt, anxiety, and fear when actions differ from perceived expected behavior. This may cause the child to believe that the injury was caused by a variation in expected behavior.**

♦ *Test-taking Tip: Think about the developmental stages outlined by Piaget, Erikson, and Freud and the responses expected by a toddler, a preschool-aged child, a school-aged child, and an adolescent when answering this question. Match options to the age groups and eliminate options not pertaining to a preschool-aged child.*

**Content Area:** Child; **Concept:** Promoting Health; Skin Integrity; Assessment; **Integrated Processes:** Nursing Process: Assessment; **Client Needs:** Health Promotion and Maintenance; Psychosocial Integrity; **Cognitive Level:** Application [Applying]

**1852. ANSWER: 1**

1. **The priority problem that should be added to the plan of care is inadequate tissue perfusion. DIC involves systemic activation of blood coagulation that leads to microvascular thrombi in various organs.**
2. Impaired urinary elimination is an important consideration and can occur secondary to DIC but is not the priority.
3. Risk for deficient fluid volume is a potential problem but is not the priority.
4. Impaired physical mobility is not the priority in the acute phase of DIC.

♦ *Test-taking Tip: Use the ABC's to determine priority. Note the vascular problem with DIC. This is a clue that there would be a perfusion problem; thus eliminate Options 2 and 4. Eliminate Option 3 because an actual problem (tissue perfusion) would have priority over a potential problem (risk).*

**Content Area:** Child; **Concept:** Perfusion; Skin Integrity; Critical Thinking; **Integrated Processes:** Nursing Process: Analysis; **Client Needs:** Physiological Integrity: Physiological Adaptation; **Cognitive Level:** Synthesis [Creating]

**1853. ANSWER: 1**

1. **The most common burn injury in toddlers occurs from the toddler pulling on pot and pan handles or cords within reach, resulting in a scalding burn.**
2. Burns from heat are usually more common in older children.
3. Burns from flames are typically seen in an older child.
4. Burns from flames are usually seen in older children.

♦ *Test-taking Tip: Think about the neuromuscular development of toddlers to identify the common type of burn injury. Note that Options 3 and 4 are similar in that these are flame injuries; thus eliminate these options. Options 1 and 2 are heat-related injuries. Think about whether a toddler is more likely to touch or to pull down an object.*

**Content Area:** Child; **Concept:** Promoting Health; Safety; Nursing Roles; **Integrated Processes:** Nursing Process: Planning; Teaching/Learning; **Client Needs:** Safe and Effective Care Environment: Safety and Infection Control; **Cognitive Level:** Application [Applying]

**1854. ANSWER: 27**

Using the Rule of 9's, each leg to the groin is 13.5% of the child's body surface area. Thus, both legs would equal 27% of the child's body surface area.

♦ *Test-taking Tip: The body surface area of both legs added together is a multiple of 9.*

**Content Area:** Child; **Concept:** Skin Integrity; Assessment; **Integrated Processes:** Communication and Documentation; **Client Needs:** Physiological Integrity: Reduction of Risk Potential; **Cognitive Level:** Analysis [Analyzing]

## 1855. MoC ANSWER: 4

1. In the first 24 hours, fluid resuscitation is 4 mL/kg body weight per percentage burn TBSA, with half over the first 8 hours and the remaining over the next 16 hours (4 mL/kg × 20 kg = 80 mL; 80 mL × 10 = 800 mL for 24 hours; half of this is 400 mL over 8 hours; 400 mL ÷ 8 = 50 mL).
2. A urinary catheter is inserted so that urine output can be closely monitored as a guide for volume status.
3. During the resuscitation phase, edema formation can decrease perfusion. Elevating the limbs above the heart level promotes gravity-dependent drainage.
4. **Because morphine sulfate does not state a dose, the order should be clarified with the HCP. If the HCP intended the dose to be based on the child's weight, then this should be included in the order.**

▶ *Test-taking Tip: Carefully read each option to determine if an option is missing information.*

Content Area: Child; Concept: Skin Integrity; Safety; Communication; Integrated Processes: Communication and Documentation; Client Needs: Safe and Effective Care Environment: Management of Care; Safe and Effective Care Environment: Safety and Infection Control; Cognitive Level: Analysis [Analyzing]

## 1856. ANSWER: 3

1. A mottled appearance is consistent with partial-thickness burns.
2. A moist-red appearance is consistent with partial-thickness burns.
3. **The waxy-white appearance should be most concerning because these areas indicate full-thickness or third-degree burns. These burns involve the entire epidermis and dermis and extend into the subcutaneous tissue. Hair follicles, nerve endings, and sweat glands are all destroyed. Full-thickness burns do not heal and will require some type of grafting.**
4. A blistering appearance is consistent with partial-thickness burns, which will heal spontaneously within about 14 days, but scarring will occur.

▶ *Test-taking Tip: Three options are consistent with partial-thickness burns, and one option is different. Often the option that is different is the answer.*

Content Area: Child; Concept: Skin Integrity; Perfusion; Assessment; Integrated Processes: Nursing Process: Analysis; Client Needs: Physiological Integrity: Physiological Adaptation; Cognitive Level: Analysis [Analyzing]

## 1857. ANSWER: 2

1. These are not expected findings during any phase of burn healing.
2. **The findings suggest inadequate circulation and impairment of nerve function, possibly from the tough, leathery scab (eschar). The eschar can form a tight constricting band, and an escharotomy may need to be performed by the HCP.**

3. Waiting an hour to do a comparative assessment will delay treatment.
4. This is not fluid accumulation but an emergency due to constriction from the eschar.

▶ *Test-taking Tip: Use the ABC's to reach the correct conclusion.*

Content Area: Child; Concept: Perfusion; Skin Integrity; Integrated Processes: Nursing Process: Analysis; Client Needs: Physiological Integrity: Physiological Adaptation; Cognitive Level: Analysis [Analyzing]

## 1858. ANSWER: 2

1. Telling the parent to call 911 is correct but not the priority because the baby may still have the cord in the mouth.
2. **The nurse should first ask whether the cord has been removed from the baby's mouth to prevent further injury. Electrical current is conducted from the plug to the underlying tissue. The actual amount of tissue damage is much larger than where the cord touched.**
3. Asking about bleeding inside and around the baby's mouth is important because this could compromise the airway, but it does not have priority.
4. Asking about the appearance of the baby's mouth is important due to airway compromise, but it does not have priority.

▶ *Test-taking Tip: Use Maslow's Hierarchy of Needs. The priority should be to protect from further harm.*

Content Area: Child; Concept: Safety; Nursing Roles; Skin Integrity; Integrated Processes: Nursing Process: Implementation; Communication and Documentation; Client Needs: Physiological Integrity: Physiological Adaptation; Cognitive Level: Application [Applying]

## 1859. MoC ANSWER: 1

1. **The most important information that the parents should know about is that a chest x-ray needs to be completed to determine whether there is any respiratory involvement from possible aspiration of the chemical.**
2. Contacting social services could be a possibility if the nurse or HCP suspects child neglect or abuse.
3. A barium swallow test would be done 2 weeks postburn; thus this is not information that the parents need at this moment.
4. Esophageal strictures may require surgery, but this will be determined later.

▶ *Test-taking Tip: You should prioritize the options to determine the intervention that would occur first. The priority intervention should be addressed with the parents at this time.*

Content Area: Child; Concept: Oxygenation; Management; Diversity; Integrated Processes: Caring; Communication and Documentation; Culture and Spirituality; Client Needs: Safe and Effective Care Environment: Management of Care; Cognitive Level: Application [Applying]

**1860.** **PHARM** **ANSWER: 1, 2, 4, 6**

1. **Analgesics help relieve pain and decrease anxiety for subsequent dressing changes.**
2. **Gauze should be inserted between fingers because burned surfaces should not touch. As healing takes place, webbing will form between burned surfaces that are touching.**
3. Some burn centers keep blisters intact, and others break them open. If blisters are broken, it is usually performed by the HCP and not the nurse. Tissue may be cut away to speed the healing process and prevent infection.
4. **Netting rather than tape should be used to hold dressings in place because it expands easily, and tape can be painful to remove and cause tissue injury.**
5. Antibiotic creams may be prescribed, but lotion should not be applied because it can increase the risk of infection to the burn area.
6. **Silver sulfadiazine (Silvadene) is a broad-spectrum antibacterial cream most commonly prescribed for treating burns.**

♦ *Test-taking Tip: Focus on the illustration and then determine whether each option applies.*

Content Area: Child; Concept: Skin Integrity; Comfort; Medication; Integrated Processes: Nursing Process: Planning; Client Needs: Physiological Integrity: Reduction of Risk Potential; Physiological Integrity: Pharmacological and Parenteral Therapies; Cognitive Level: Analysis [Analyzing]

**1861. ANSWER: 2**

1. An allograft can be from a cadaver or a donor and is sterilized and frozen until needed. However, unless it is meshed, it will not have a lattice-like appearance.
2. **The lattice-like appearance is from a mesh graft. In a meshed autograft, a partial thickness of skin is taken from another area of the body and is slit at intervals so that it can be stretched to cover a larger area.**
3. Although bulky dressings applied too tightly can leave indentations, it will not be a uniform lattice-like appearance.
4. Although fluid loss does occur with burn injuries, it does not cause the lattice-like appearance of a graft.

♦ *Test-taking Tip: To select the correct option, look for a word in the options that is closely related to the words "lattice-like appearance" in the stem.*

Content Area: Child; Concept: Skin Integrity; Communication; Integrated Processes: Communication and Documentation; Client Needs: Physiological Integrity: Reduction of Risk Potential; Cognitive Level: Application [Applying]

**1862. ANSWER: 3**

1. Although assisting the parents to dress in appropriate attire may be supportive to the parents, the most caring response is offering support to both the parents and child.

2. Bringing the parents to a quiet place may help the parents, but both the parents and child should be considered.
3. **The parents may not ask spontaneously to touch or hold their child because they are likely in a state of grief and may not react in a normal manner. Both the parents and the child are supported by the nurse's gesture of caring by accompanying the parents in the room and showing them how to touch their child.**
4. The presence of clergy may be supportive to the parent, but a 2-year-old is unlikely to recognize a member of the clergy as someone supportive.

♦ *Test-taking Tip: Two options pertain to just the parents, and two options pertain to both the parents and the child. The most supportive action would be one that pertains to both the parents and child; thus narrow the options to 3 and 4. Of Options 3 and 4, think about which would provide the most comfort to a 2-year-old.*

Content Area: Child; Concept: Nursing Roles; Skin Integrity; Grief and Loss; Integrated Processes: Caring; Client Needs: Psychosocial Integrity; Cognitive Level: Analysis [Analyzing]

**1863. ANSWER: 4**

1. There is no strong association between emotional upset and eczema exacerbation; toddlers can demonstrate emotional upset due to their developmental stage.
2. Skin hydration and turgor are important to assess, but fluid volume status is not typically a concern with eczema.
3. Although a secondary infection can occur from intense itching, eczema is not spread through touching a lesion.
4. **Lichenification, a thickening and hardening of the skin, occurs from chronic rubbing or scratching. Lichenification and hyperpigmentation can occur with childhood eczema.**

♦ *Test-taking Tip: The key word "eczema" in the stem is associated with the skin. You should look for a similar word in one of the options that pertain to the skin.*

Content Area: Child; Concept: Skin Integrity; Assessment; Integrated Processes: Nursing Process: Assessment; Client Needs: Physiological Integrity: Physiological Adaptation; Cognitive Level: Analysis [Analyzing]

**1864.** **PHARM** **ANSWER: 3**

1. Frequent bathing can cause skin dryness and trigger eczema.
2. Topical steroids such as OTC hydrocortisone cream (Corticaine) are used to treat inflammation. Mupirocin topical ointment (Bactroban) is an antibiotic. It may be prescribed by the HCP if excoriated skin becomes infected.

3. **Eczema is characterized by superficial skin inflammation of erythema and local edema followed by vesicle formations that can ooze, crust, and scale. The nurse should include information about things in the environment that can trigger eczema, such as dryness, temperature, and substances. Stress and infection can also trigger the inflammation, depending on the form of eczema.**

4. Silvery scaling is a characteristic of psoriasis and not eczema.

▶ *Test-taking Tip: Visualize the appearance of eczema and then use the process of elimination.*

**Content Area:** Child; **Concept:** Skin Integrity; Nursing Roles; **Integrated Processes:** Teaching/Learning; **Client Needs:** Physiological Integrity: Physiological Adaptation; Physiological Integrity: Pharmacological and Parenteral Therapies; **Cognitive Level:** Application [Applying]

### 1865. ANSWER: 3, 4, 5

1. Intentionally breaking comedones can increase the inflammation if the lesion ruptures below the skin surface; it can cause scarring and possibly a secondary infection.

2. No foods are known to cause acne. There is no evidence linking chocolate or greasy foods to acne.

3. **Oil-free products should be used on the face; products with a greasy base can worsen the acne.**

4. **Using an antibacterial soap will help prevent lesions from becoming infected.**

5. **Benzoyl peroxide applied topically has antimicrobial with bacteriocidal action and should be applied twice daily.**

▶ *Test-taking Tip: With multiple-response questions, options that are similar are often correct. Three options are related to skin care, and the other two options are different. These two options should be eliminated.*

**Content Area:** Child; **Concept:** Skin Integrity; Nursing Roles; **Integrated Processes:** Teaching/Learning; **Client Needs:** Physiological Integrity: Basic Care and Comfort; **Cognitive Level:** Application [Applying]

### 1866. PHARM ANSWER: 2

**Use a proportion formula to determine the number of tablets.**

**50 mg : 1 tablet :: 100 mg : $X$ tablet; $50X = 100$; $X = 100 \div 50$; $X = 2$**

▶ *Test-taking Tip: Be sure to carefully read the stem to know which dose you are calculating. The key words are "initial dose," which would be 100 mg of minocycline (Minocin).*

**Content Area:** Child; **Concept:** Medication; Skin Integrity; **Integrated Processes:** Communication and Documentation; **Client Needs:** Physiological Integrity: Pharmacological and Parenteral Therapies; **Cognitive Level:** Application [Applying]

### 1867. ANSWER: 4

1. Living in the woods and contact with vegetation could be the source of the skin rash, but this is not an intentional treatment.

2. Reading about alternative medicine may clue the nurse to further assess its use, but this is not the most alerting statement.

3. Cortisone is a medication and not a complementary therapy.

4. **Asking the nurse about a specific alternative modality is the most "nondisclosing" client remark without actually telling the nurse that an alternative treatment measure has been tried. Echinacea can reduce the effects of immunosuppressants; thus the skin rash may be worse with its use.**

▶ *Test-taking Tip: Focus on the fact that the skin rash has worsened, and that one option identifies a specific herb. Three options are statements, and one option is a question. Often the option that is different is the answer.*

**Content Area:** Child; **Concept:** Skin Integrity; Comfort; **Integrated Processes:** Nursing Process: Analysis; **Client Needs:** Physiological Integrity: Basic Care and Comfort; **Cognitive Level:** Analysis [Analyzing]

### 1868. ANSWER: 2

1. Pediculosis (lice infestations) is not a genetic disorder and has not been clinically shown to lead to neurofibromatosis.

2. **Neurofibromatosis or Albright's disease is a neurocutaneous autosomal dominant disorder that causes tumors to grow along nerves. The nurse should expect to see six café-au-lait spots or café-au-lait spots that are larger than 4 x 6 cm.**

3. Tick bites are not genetic and have not been shown to lead to neurofibromatosis.

4. Congenital nevi (moles) are present at birth and result from a proliferation of benign melanocytes in the dermis, epidermis, or both and may lead to melanoma. Congenital nevi differ in appearance from the café-au-lait spots of neurofibromatosis.

▶ *Test-taking Tip: Use the key word "disease" to eliminate options that are not associated with diseases (1, 3, and 4).*

**Content Area:** Child; **Concept:** Skin Integrity; Assessment; **Integrated Processes:** Nursing Process: Planning; **Client Needs:** Physiological Integrity: Physiological Adaptation; **Cognitive Level:** Application [Applying]

### 1869. PHARM ANSWER: 3, 5, 6

1. An occlusive dressing will increase itching and worsen the dermatitis.

2. A baking soda bath can relieve itching, but applying a thick paste can be harmful.

3. **Calamine lotion relieves itching and promotes drying of the lesions.**

4. Scabs should fall off naturally, not be removed, so that healing tissues are protected.

5. **The allergen should be identified and eliminated. The yard should be inspected, and poison ivy destroyed. Poison ivy is shiny with pointed oval leaflets. The color varies by season.**

6. **Diphenhydramine (Benadryl) is an antihistamine that will help relieve pruritus.**

▶ *Test-taking Tip: Read each option carefully, looking for key words such as "thick" that would make the option incorrect.*

Content Area: Child; Concept: Skin Integrity; Nursing Roles; Immunity; Integrated Processes: Teaching/Learning; Client Needs: Physiological Integrity: Reduction of Risk Potential; Physiological Integrity: Pharmacological and Parenteral Therapies; Cognitive Level: Application [Applying]

## 1870. ANSWER: 3

1. A characteristic of cataracts is lens opacity, which is not present.
2. Although symptoms of bumping into objects and diplopia can occur with strabismus (cross-eyes), it is not evaluated by tonometry.
3. **The child's symptoms suggest glaucoma. Tonometry is a method for measuring intraocular pressure (IOP) and detecting glaucoma.**
4. Tonometry is not used to detect lazy eye. Lazy eye results when one eye does not receive sufficient stimulation and poor vision results in the affected eye. A child may bump into objects because of the poor vision or exhibited diplopia.

▶ *Test-taking Tip: If unfamiliar with tonometry, focus on the child's symptom of seeing halos and eliminate options.*

Content Area: Child; Concept: Sensory Perception; Nursing Roles; Integrated Processes: Teaching/Learning; Client Needs: Physiological Integrity: Reduction of Risk Potential; Cognitive Level: Knowledge [Remembering]

## 1871. PHARM ANSWER: 1, 3, 5, 6

1. **OE is inflammation of the external ear canal. An otoscopic examination allows visualization of the tympanic membrane to ensure that there is no extension of the external otitis into the middle ear.**
2. A CBC is usually not indicated; the diagnosis is made based on the symptoms and physical examination.
3. **If there is any drainage in the ear, cultures are taken to identify the organism.**
4. X-rays are not beneficial in diagnosing otitis externa.
5. **Ear curettage to remove excess cerumen present in the ear canal may be necessary to visualize the tympanic membrane.**
6. **Most cases of OE are caused by superficial bacterial infections. Ciprofloxacin (Cetraxal), a fluoroquinolone antibiotic that inhibits bacterial synthesis and growth, may be used to treat OE.**

▶ *Test-taking Tip: You should eliminate options that are not directly related to the ear.*

Content Area: Child; Concept: Infection; Sensory Perception; Integrated Processes: Nursing Process: Planning; Client Needs: Physiological Integrity: Reduction of Risk Potential; Physiological Integrity: Pharmacological and Parenteral Therapies; Cognitive Level: Application [Applying]

## 1872. MoC ANSWER: 1, 3, 4

1. **Strabismus is unequally aligned eyes (cross-eyes) due to unbalanced muscle control. By law, this is a disability that allows for school accommodations. Preferential seating will enable the child to see assignments, class presentations, and the teacher.**

2. Seating or grouping impaired children violates federal Individual with Disabilities Education Act guidelines.
3. **Allowing for extra time to complete assignments ensures that the child has time to adjust and focus his or her vision to read the necessary documents.**
4. **Federal and state laws provide educational plans to ensure that individuals with disabilities have the materials and equipment needed to attain an education like any other student in the system.**
5. Speaking louder is unnecessary because this is a visual, not a hearing, problem.

▶ *Test-taking Tip: Think about the limitations from having "misaligned eyes," and then narrow the options to those that diminish these limitations.*

Content Area: Child; Concept: Sensory Perception; Nursing Roles; Promoting Health; Collaboration; Integrated Processes: Nursing Process: Implementation; Client Needs: Safe and Effective Care Environment: Management of Care; Cognitive Level: Analysis [Analyzing]

## 1873. ANSWER: 1

1. **Strabismus in children is noted when both eyes do not line up in the same direction, so they fail to focus on the same image.**
2. Diplopia is double vision and can occur because each eye transmits the images received, but this is not associated with the eyes being misaligned.
3. Hemianopia is seeing a portion of an object out of each eye.
4. Pterygium is a triangular growth of the bulbar conjunctiva from the nasal side of the eye toward the pupil and can obstruct the vision if the growth occludes the pupil.

▶ *Test-taking Tip: Narrow the options by eliminating options that are associated with symptoms from conditions, Options 2 and 3.*

Content Area: Child; Concept: Sensory Perception; Assessment; Integrated Processes: Nursing Process: Analysis; Client Needs: Physiological Integrity: Reduction of Risk Potential; Cognitive Level: Application [Applying]

## 1874. ANSWER: 2, 3

1. In esotropia strabismus (not nearsightedness), an eye turns inward.
2. **Nearsightedness is an inability to see objects clearly at a distance, so objects are brought closer to the eyes.**
3. **Because distant objects appear blurred with nearsightedness, squinting may occur to see objects more clearly.**
4. An opaque lens is seen with cataracts, and not nearsightedness.
5. Holding a book farther away is observed in farsightedness, not nearsightedness, because objects are better seen when farther away.

▶ *Test-taking Tip: Use the memory aid that in nearsightedness, objects need to be near to be seen. In farsightedness, objects are best seen if farther away.*

Content Area: Child; Concept: Sensory Perception; Assessment; Integrated Processes: Nursing Process: Assessment; Client Needs: Psychosocial Integrity; Cognitive Level: Analysis [Analyzing]

### 1875. ANSWER: 4

1. Reactivity refers to the pupil constricting in response to light.
2. Stereopsis is depth perception.
3. The red reflex suggests the corneas and retinas are intact.
4. **Accommodation occurs when the eye focuses on a close image.**

▶ *Test-taking Tip: You should look for related terms in the stem ("adjusting") and the options ("accommodate") to answer this question correctly.*

Content Area: Child; Concept: Sensory Perception; Assessment; Communication; Integrated Processes: Communication and Documentation; Client Needs: Health Promotion and Maintenance; Cognitive Level: Comprehension [Understanding]

### 1876. MoC ANSWER: 3

1. The 4-year-old with 20/40 vision is a normal finding for a preschool child.
2. The 6-year-old with 20/30 vision is a normal finding for a school-aged child.
3. **After a second screening, a child 6 years of age or older who has 20/40 vision or worse in one or both eyes should be referred to an eye doctor for corrective eye care.**
4. A result of 20/15 on visual acuity tests indicates vision that is better than normal.

▶ *Test-taking Tip: First, eliminate any options that are within normal or better-than-normal parameters. You need to consider that the sight of young children is still maturing.*

Content Area: Child; Concept: Sensory Perception; Promoting Health; Integrated Processes: Nursing Process: Planning; Client Needs: Safe and Effective Care Environment: Management of Care; Cognitive Level: Application [Applying]

### 1877. ANSWER: 3

1. Viral conjunctivitis is self-limiting. Ophthalmic antibiotics are used to treat bacterial conjunctivitis. These may include besifloxacin (Besivance), a broad-spectrum fluoroquinolone ophthalmic solution, or gentamicin (Garamycin, Gentak), an aminoglycoside antibiotic used for gram-negative bacterial coverage.
2. The most common cause of conjunctivitis is a bacterial infection, not from a foreign body.
3. **Washcloths and towels used by the infected person should be kept separate from others. Bacterial conjunctivitis can be easily transmitted to family members and others in direct contact with the child. Tissues used should be disposed of immediately, and good hand washing techniques should be followed by everyone.**

4. Conjunctivitis can occur after birth because of exposure to bacteria during the birthing process. This is not the most important point because the audience being addressed is parents of preschoolers.

▶ *Test-taking Tip: Options with absolute words such as "always" are usually not correct. The key word "most" indicates that more than one option is a correct statement but that one option is better than the others.*

Content Area: Child; Concept: Infection; Sensory Perception; Nursing Roles; Integrated Processes: Nursing Process: Evaluation; Client Needs: Safe and Effective Care Environment: Safety and Infection Control; Cognitive Level: Evaluation [Evaluating]

### 1878. ANSWER: 1

1. **Parent concerns should be taken seriously. If the infant does not respond to light, it could indicate blindness. This is an appropriate response.**
2. This statement is incorrect. A neonate can follow light or will cease body movement when a room is lighted.
3. Infants respond differently based on level of alertness and age. However, giving advice to try different lighting is inappropriate. The infant needs an eye examination and evaluation.
4. Telling the mother that there is nothing to worry about is providing false reassurance.

▶ *Test-taking Tip: Focus on therapeutic communication skills. Eliminate options that use barriers to effective communication or that do not address the parent's concern.*

Content Area: Child; Concept: Sensory Perception; Nursing Roles; Communication; Integrated Processes: Communication and Documentation; Client Needs: Physiological Integrity: Reduction of Risk Potential; Psychosocial Integrity; Cognitive Level: Application [Applying]

### 1879. MoC ANSWER: 3

1. Because blind children cannot imitate others or actively explore the environment, they rely much more on others to stimulate them and teach them to play.
2. Braille tags for clothing and other articles will help the child to distinguish items, colors, and prints.
3. **Verbalizing the need for speech therapy indicates that further teaching is needed. Blind children have little difficulty in learning verbal skills and can communicate with age-mates and participate in suitable activities.**
4. The use of a dog guide helps the child become independent in navigation.

▶ *Test-taking Tip: The key phrase "needs additional teaching" indicates that this is a false-response item; select the statement that is incorrect.*

Content Area: Child; Concept: Sensory Perception; Nursing Roles; Management; Integrated Processes: Teaching/Learning; Nursing Process: Evaluation; Client Needs: Safe and Effective Care Environment: Management of Care; Psychosocial Integrity; Cognitive Level: Evaluation [Evaluating]

## 1880. ANSWER: 1

1. **Myopia is nearsightedness and is caused by light rays focusing in front of the retina because the eyeball is elongated. Distance vision will be blurry, and the person holds the objects near the eyes to see them better.**
2. This option shows hyperopia and is caused by light rays focusing behind the retina because the eyeball is too short from front to back. The person can see images that are farther away more clearly than those up close.
3. This option shows astigmatism, in which corneal curvature is irregular and incoming light rays are bent unequally. The person will have blurred vision with distortion.
4. This option shows presbyopia, which is a loss of accommodation that occurs with aging. The person loses the ability to accommodate and focus on near objects and may compensate for blurred vision by holding objects farther away.

▶ *Test-taking Tip: Two images show the light rays beyond the retina. Because these are similar, they should be eliminated. With the two remaining images, consider which has the ray of light farthest away from the retina.*

Content Area: Child; Concept: Sensory Perception; Nursing Roles; Integrated Processes: Teaching/Learning; Client Needs: Physiological Integrity: Physiological Adaptation; Cognitive Level: Application [Applying]

## 1881. MoC ANSWER: 1

1. **An ophthalmologist referral is necessary to evaluate for further injury. Hyphmea is hemorrhage into the anterior chamber.**
2. Transfer to an ED will delay evaluation and treatment by an ophthalmologist.
3. If hyphema were not present, then ice would be applied for 24 hours to reduce swelling.
4. If eye contamination is suspected, antibiotic eye drops (not cortisone drops) may be prescribed. An eye patch is usually not necessary; the child should close and rest the affected eye.

▶ *Test-taking Tip: Use Maslow's Hierarchy of Needs theory to establish the priority action. Focus on preservation of eye function.*

Content Area: Child; Concept: Sensory Perception; Safety; Collaboration; Integrated Processes: Nursing Process: Planning; Client Needs: Safe and Effective Care Environment: Management of Care; Physiological Integrity: Physiological Adaptation; Cognitive Level: Application [Applying]

## 1882. ANSWER: 1, 2, 3, 5

1. **Fussiness and restlessness are common signs of acute otitis media due to the ear pain and pressure.**
2. **Irritability and crying are classic signs of acute otitis media due to the ear pain and pressure.**
3. **Pulling on the affected ear is often seen in acute otitis media due to the ear pain and pressure.**

4. Rhinitis, cough, and diarrhea are symptoms that occur with otitis media effusion and are not usually associated with AOM.
5. **Rolling the head from side to side is a classic sign of acute otitis media from the pain and pressure in the ear.**

▶ *Test-taking Tip: Read the question and think about the pathophysiology related to earaches; consider the age of the child and the limitations in speech.*

Content Area: Child; Concept: Sensory Perception; Assessment; Integrated Processes: Nursing Process: Assessment; Client Needs: Physiological Integrity: Physiological Adaptation; Cognitive Level: Knowledge [Remembering]

## 1883. ANSWER: 2, 3, 4, 5

1. Ear wicks, and not earplugs, should be inserted to facilitate drainage and should be kept clean and dry. These should be changed frequently to help prevent infection from spreading to the mastoid process.
2. **Ice compresses are used to decrease inflammation.**
3. **Moisture barriers such as petroleum jelly can be applied to earlobes to prevent excoriation from the exudate.**
4. **Analgesics, such as acetaminophen (Tylenol) and ibuprofen (Motrin), are used for minor pain, and codeine can be used for more severe episodes.**
5. **Keeping the outer ear canal clean and dry with sterile cotton swabs prevents excoriation.**

▶ *Test-taking Tip: Tympanostomy is an opening into the tympanic membrane and placement of tubes. Eliminate an option that does not facilitate drainage after the surgical procedure.*

Content Area: Child; Concept: Sensory Perception; Comfort; Nursing Roles; Integrated Processes: Nursing Process: Implementation; Client Needs: Physiological Integrity: Reduction of Risk Potential; Cognitive Level: Application [Applying]

## 1884. ANSWER: 2, 3, 1, 4

2. **Acute pain related to pressure caused by inflammatory process. Because the presence of pain influences both VS and the client's participation in measures needed for recovery, addressing pain should be first.**
3. **Infection related to presence of infective organisms. This is second because measures should be taken to eliminate the infection.**
1. **Interrupted family process related to illness and/or hospitalization of child and temporary hearing loss. This is third because physiological problems are priority over psychosocial problems.**
4. **Risk for delayed growth and development related to potential hearing loss can be addressed last. This is a potential and not actual problem.**

▶ *Test-taking Tip: Use Maslow's Hierarchy of Needs to place the child's needs in the correct sequence.*

Content Area: Child; Concept: Sensory Perception; Management; Integrated Processes: Nursing Process: Planning; Client Needs: Physiological Integrity: Reduction of Risk Potential; Cognitive Level: Synthesis [Creating]

**1885.** PHARM **ANSWER:**

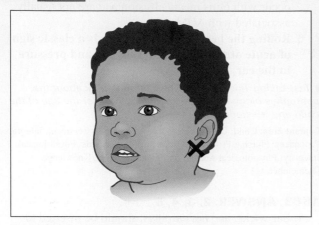

For a child younger than 3 years old, the nurse should place the fingers on the pinna of the earlobe and pull the pinna down and back to straighten the ear canal. Ofloxacin (Floxin), an antibiotic, has a broad-spectrum effect that inhibits bacterial growth.

♦ *Test-taking Tip: To remember the direction for straightening the ear canal for a child versus an adult, use the memory aid of age: Younger is down and older is up.*

**Content Area:** Child; **Concept:** Medication; **Integrated Processes:** Nursing Process: Implementation; **Client Needs:** Physiological Integrity: Pharmacological and Parenteral Therapies; **Cognitive Level:** Application [Applying]

**1886. ANSWER: 4**

1. Paresthesia, an abnormal sensation, is seen with vitamin B$_2$ excess.
2. Cardiac arrhythmias, which could present with an irregular HR, are seen in niacin excess.
3. Acanthosis nigricans—a brown to black, poorly defined, velvety hyperpigmentation in skin folds of the neck or under the arms—are seen with niacin excess.
4. **Irritation and cracks at the nasal angles of the nose are consistent with the diagnosis of a vitamin B$_2$ deficiency. Vitamin B$_2$ functions in maintaining healthy skin, especially around the mouth, nose, and eyes.**

♦ *Test-taking Tip: Eliminate the two options that do not pertain to skin changes. Of the two remaining options, determine which is most consistent with the skin changes in the situation.*

**Content Area:** Child; **Concept:** Nutrition; Assessment; **Integrated Processes:** Nursing Process: Assessment; **Client Needs:** Physiological Integrity: Physiological Adaptation; **Cognitive Level:** Application [Applying]

**1887.** CJ MoC PHARM **ANSWER: 2, 3, 5**

1. There is no need to turn off the IV pump for the vancomycin (Vancocin). The dose should be infused by 1430; it is now 1600. The IV needs to remain open to administer the diphenhydramine and other prescribed medications.
2. **The HCP should be notified to evaluate the child's symptoms and to review medications.**
3. **A rash and itching suggest an allergic reaction, and diphenhydramine (Benedryl) should be administered as the first action. The client already has one medication allergy to cefdinir (Omnicef). Antibiotics are well-known for causing allergic reactions.**
4. Naloxone (Narcan) is an opioid antagonist and is used for respiratory depression, not pruritus.
5. **All medications, including furosemide (Lasix) and morphine sulfate, should be reviewed to determine the cause.**

♦ *Test-taking Tip: After assessment, treat the client with medications already included on the client's MAR, examine the medications being administered, and then notify the HCP.*

**Content Area:** Child; **Concept:** Medication; Skin Integrity; Immunity; **Integrated Processes:** Nursing Process: Implementation; **Client Needs:** Safe and Effective Care Environment: Management of Care; Physiological Integrity: Pharmacological and Parenteral Therapies; **Cognitive Level:** Analysis [Analyzing]

**1888.** CJ **ANSWER: 3, 4**

1. Soap and tap water would be appropriate for a stage I ulcer but not stage III.
2. Hydrogen peroxide should not be used because it removes granulation tissue and has been found to be toxic to fibroblasts.
3. **Sodium chloride will be needed to cleanse the wound.**
4. **A hydrocolloid dressing forms an occlusive barrier over the ulcer to prevent bacterial contamination and keeps the wound environment moist for healing.**
5. Zinc oxide is appropriate for treating a diaper rash but not a stage 2 sacral ulcer.

♦ *Test-taking Tip: The pressure ulcer is stage III, which involves full thickness skin loss that extends to the subcutaneous fat but not the fascia. Eliminate options that will damage tissues.*

**Content Area:** Child; **Concept:** Medication; Skin Integrity; Immunity; **Integrated Processes:** Nursing Process: Planning; **Client Needs:** Safe and Effective Care Environment: Safety and Infection Control; **Cognitive Level:** Application [Applying]

## Chapter Forty-Three

# Neurological and Musculoskeletal Management

**1889.** The nurse is caring for the adolescent diagnosed with new-onset generalized tonic-clonic seizures of unknown etiology. Which nursing actions should be initiated by the nurse? **Select all that apply.**

1. Secure a tongue blade to the head of the bed.
2. Pad at least two of the side rails on the bed.
3. Ensure that an oropharyngeal airway is available.
4. Initiate and explain droplet isolation precautions.
5. Set up suction equipment near the head of the bed.

**1890.** The parent calls the clinic nurse voicing a concern that both she and her child's teacher are unable to "get the child's attention." The child stares for 10 to 30 seconds and does not seem to see or hear anything. Which type of seizure should the nurse recognize from the parent's report of her child's behavior?

1. Myoclonic seizure
2. Febrile seizure
3. Absence seizure
4. Atonic seizure

**1891.** The nurse is teaching the parent of the 8-year-old who was newly diagnosed with absence seizures. What information should the nurse emphasize?

1. For many, absence seizures usually cease during early adolescence.
2. They are likely to progress to a more serious type of seizure.
3. They are most likely to be diagnosed by the school nurse.
4. They usually occur as part of a larger neurological condition.

**1892.** PHARM The nurse is teaching parents about side effects of anticonvulsant medications. Which medication has the side effect of gingival hyperplasia?

1. Phenytoin
2. Valproic acid
3. Carbamazepine
4. Phenobarbital sodium

**1893.** MoC The nurse is assessing the child who had head trauma. Which **most** important assessment finding associated with ICP should the nurse report to the HCP?

1. Increasing temperature
2. Widening pulse pressure
3. Increasing HR
4. Decreasing systolic BP

**1894.** MoC The nurse is caring for the child who has a TBI. Which assessment finding should alert the nurse to question the HCP's order to place an NG tube?

1. Visible, penetrating scalp wound
2. Jerking movements of extremities for 1 minute
3. Leakage of clear fluid from the ears
4. Glasgow coma scale score of 10

**1895.** The pediatric client underwent a craniotomy. Which information should alert the nurse to further assess for the development of syndrome of inappropriate antidiuretic hormone secretion (SIADH)?

1. Hourly output of 300 mL of urine
2. Serum sodium level of 117/mEq/L
3. Dry oral mucous membranes
4. Nuchal rigidity

**1896.** The nurse is palpating the fontanelles of an infant hospitalized with a head injury. Which area should the nurse palpate to assess the posterior fontanelle? Place an X on the posterior fontanelle.

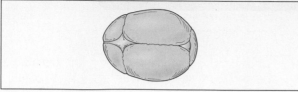

**1897.** MoC The nurse is planning care for the child who had spina bifida (myelodysplasia) at birth and has knee deformities, detrusor hyperreflexia, dyssynergia, and problems with constipation. Which is **most** important to include in the child's plan of care?

1. Avoid the child's exposure to latex.
2. Do intermittent urinary catheterization.
3. Provide dietary fiber supplements daily.
4. Complete a referral for physical therapy.

**1898.** The child had a myelomeningocele that was diagnosed at birth and surgically corrected. Which **most important** instruction should the nurse include when reinforcing teaching?

1. Place braces smoothly against the child's skin.
2. Shift the child's position at least every 3 hours.
3. Place a blanket on the child's wheelchair seat.
4. Check the child's skin daily for redness or irritation.

**1899.** The nurse is caring for multiple hospitalized children. In which conditions might the nurse assess for papilledema? **Select all that apply.**

1. Eczema
2. Craniosynostosis
3. Shaken baby syndrome
4. Hydrocephalus
5. Chest trauma

**1900.** The child just had a ventriculoperitoneal (VP) shunt placed for treatment of hydrocephalus. Which intervention should the nurse implement?

1. Keep the head of the bed elevated to 90 degrees.
2. Prevent movement of the child's extremities.
3. Check the pressure dressing at the insertion site.
4. Maintain a flat position and turn the child q2h.

**1901.** The 7-year-old child may have hydrocephalus secondary to a malignancy. Which assessment findings should the nurse associate with the development of hydrocephalus? **Select all that apply.**

1. Headache
2. Vomiting
3. Angioedema
4. Personality change
5. Increased head circumference

**1902.** The child is being screened for hydrocephalus. When teaching the parents, the nurse illustrates the location of the lateral ventricle. Place an X on the area that the nurse should show to the parents.

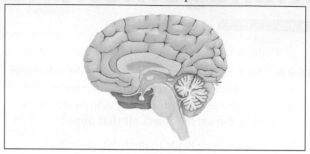

**1903.** The HCP's documentation states that the infant with meningitis is in an opisthotonus position. What should the nurse observe when performing an assessment?

1. Resistance with specific leg movement
2. Knee or hip flexion with head flexion
3. A high-pitched cry with neck flexion
4. Hyperextension of the head and neck

**1904.** The nurse is planning teaching about bacterial meningitis for a group of parents. Which statement should the nurse include when teaching the parents?

1. Symptoms of meningitis often develop over time, making it easier to diagnose than other infections.
2. Having a seizure associated with a high temperature usually indicates a problem other than meningitis.
3. High-risk children 2 to 10 years and other children 11 years and older should receive the meningococcal conjugate vaccine (MCV4).
4. Intravenous antibiotics are administered to family members who may have been in close contact with the child.

**1905.** The nurse is admitting the hospitalized child newly diagnosed with Reye's syndrome. Which action by the nurse would be **most** appropriate?

1. Determining if the child had a bacterial infection recently
2. Placing the child in a private room with droplet precautions
3. Taking the child to the unit's play area to interact with others
4. Assessing for signs of bleeding and prolonged bleeding time

**1906.** **MoC** The child with autism has been admitted to a four-bed ward on a pediatric unit. What should the nurse admitting the child do about the room assignment?

1. Request that the child be transferred to a private room.
2. Request that the child be transferred to a double room.
3. Admit the child to the room that has been preassigned.
4. Request that the child be assigned to an isolation room.

**1907.** The school nurse learns that the parents wish to enroll their 5-year-old child in school. Their child has autism. When preparing to meet with the parents and child, which behaviors should the nurse anticipate that the child might display? **Select all that apply.**

1. Polydactyly
2. Leukoderma
3. Poor eye contact
4. Restricted interests
5. Atypical language

**1908.** The nurse is preparing to care for the hospitalized child with autism. Which intervention should the nurse implement?

1. Massage the child while doing the assessment.
2. Play the radio or turn on the television.
3. Have the parent bring the child's favorite toy.
4. Offer choices of age-appropriate foods.

**1909.** The nurse is completing a health history and physical assessment for the 4-year-old who has spastic-type CP. Which statements made by a parent indicate that appropriate care is being provided? **Select all that apply.**

1. "I perform range of motion exercises every 4 hours to help prevent contractures."
2. "I give a therapeutic massage after the stretching exercises to help manage pain."
3. "I minimize the calories I provide because my child is more prone to obesity."
4. "I have my child wear a helmet because of chronic tonic-clonic seizures."
5. "Using silverware with large, padded handles makes it easier for my child to feed himself."

**1910.** While assessing the 18-month-old, the nurse observes genu varum. What should the nurse do?

1. Document the finding as normal.
2. Report this finding to the HCP.
3. Teach the parents about rickets.
4. Prepare the parent about using braces.

**1911.** The nurse is planning teaching for new mothers. The nurse should plan to include information about which common practice that can increase the risk for developmental dysplasia of the hip (DDH)?

1. Carrying a child in a backpack
2. Carrying a child in a frontpack
3. Swaddling of a child
4. Extended time in a car seat

**1912.** The nurse is preparing to teach the family of an infant with developmental dysplasia of the hip how to apply the Pavlik harness illustrated that has white Velcro straps. Place the steps for applying the harness in the correct sequence.

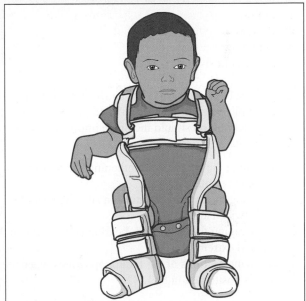

1. Connect the chest halter and leg straps in front.
2. Position the legs and feet in the stirrups.
3. Connect the chest halter and leg straps in back.
4. Position the chest halter at nipple line and fasten with Velcro.
5. Be sure the hips are flexed and abducted before fastening with Velcro.

Answer: _____

**1913.** The child has a newly applied fiberglass hip-spica cast. Which interventions should the nurse implement? **Select all that apply.**

1. Use a hair dryer on a low setting to dry the cast.
2. Check the weights on the Bradford frame.
3. Support the child's lower extremities on pillows.
4. Turn the child every 2 hours and check the CMS.
5. Petal the perineal area and edges of the cast.

**1914.** The nurse is teaching the adolescent who requires surgical treatment for scoliosis. Which is the nurse's **best** explanation regarding the goal of the surgery?

1. "The surgery will allow you to grow taller."
2. "The surgery will decrease the recurrence of pain."
3. "The surgery will prevent problems with breathing."
4. "The surgery will allow your clothes to fit you better."

**1915.** The nurse is completing a thorough assessment of the spine. The nurse is concerned about the spinal curve in the young child and documents the exaggerated lumbar curve. Which condition was likely documented?

1. Scoliosis
2. Lordosis
3. Kyphosis
4. Kyphoscoliosis

**1916.** The school-aged child has an Ilizarov external fixator applied to a lower extremity for bone lengthening. Which intervention should the nurse implement when providing care?

1. Loosening the bolts and lengthening the rods on the fixator every other day
2. Cleansing the external fixator pin sites with sterile saline twice daily
3. Discouraging the child from bearing any weight on the involved extremity
4. Removing sections of the fixator apparatus when the child is positioned in bed

**1917.** The school nurse is teaching high school sport trainers about the increased risk for sport-related deformities and injuries. The nurse should address that adolescent soccer players are **most** at risk for which deformity?

1. Varus knee
2. Valgus knee
3. Varus ankle
4. Valgus ankle

**1918.** The child with hip pain for several months was diagnosed with Legg-Calvé-Perthes disease. What should the nurse emphasize when preparing to teach the child and family about the treatment?

1. Once treatment starts, it likely will continue for about 6 months.
2. The treatment goal is a pain-free joint with full range of motion.
3. Activities requiring hip adduction are encouraged for joint alignment.
4. Most of the treatments will be completed while the child is hospitalized.

**1919.** The client tells the nurse that she is pregnant. The client is concerned that her unborn child may develop Duchenne muscular dystrophy (DMD) because her mother's brother and son have the condition. Which response by the nurse is **most** appropriate?

1. "You already have one child with muscular dystrophy; it's unlikely you'll have another."
2. "Your brother and son have DMD; it's unlikely that you'll have another child with the condition."
3. "As many as one-third of children born with DMD have no family history of the disease."
4. "If you deliver a female, she may carry the gene, but she will not develop DMD."

**1920.** The nurse is assessing the 4-year-old with DMD. Which observation indicates that the child has a Gowers sign?

1. Rises from the floor to stand by walking the hands up the legs
2. Is unable to initiate an effective cough or expectorate secretions
3. Has difficulty lifting the head and supporting it in an upright position
4. Tests at a high IQ and is advanced for the child's developmental age

**1921.** CJ PHARM The 10-year-old is scheduled to receive methotrexate to treat JRA. Which information in the child's medical record should prompt the nurse to withhold the dose and contact the HCP?

| History and Physical (H&P) | Laboratory Findings |
|---|---|
| • Age of onset 3 years<br>• Onset after severe illness<br>• Stiffness, swelling of hip joints with some loss of motion<br>• Stiffness worse upon rising after sleep<br>• No family history of JRA<br>• Chinese ethnicity<br>• Had last acupuncture treatment 9 days ago<br>• Indirect moxibustion by chiropractor 1 mo ago | • Urine pH 7.4<br>• Hgb 13 g/dL<br>• Serum creatinine 2.2 mg/dL<br>• ALT 38 international units/L |

| Vital Signs | Physical Assessment |
|---|---|
| • T: 100.1°F (37.8°C)<br>• BP: 124/69 mm Hg<br>• P: 102 bpm<br>• RR: 28 bpm | • Joint pain 10 out of 10<br>• Crying with movement<br>• Limited movement due to pain<br>• Respirations, deep and labored<br>• Had nausea after eating lunch of "hot" foods; no emesis |

1. H&P information
2. Laboratory findings
3. Vital sign abnormalities
4. Physical assessment findings

**1922.** The school nurse assesses the child who is crying and in pain after sustaining a twisting injury of the right arm. What interventions should the nurse implement? **Select all that apply.**

1. Elevate the arm and apply ice at the injured site.
2. Wrap the child's arm with an elastic bandage.
3. Contact the child's parent to discuss the injury.
4. Telephone the HCP identified by the child.
5. Schedule an x-ray of the child's arm.
6. Meet with the student who injured the child.

**1923.** The child is admitted to an ED with a dislocated kneecap that occurred while skiing. Which **most** immediate treatment by the HCP should the nurse anticipate?

1. Open surgical intervention to repair the kneecap
2. Arthroscopy to surgically repair the torn cartilage
3. Realignment of the kneecap by sliding it back into position
4. Application of a cast to the affected leg until the kneecap heals

**1924.** The child with myelodysplasia has a TEV (talipes equinovarus) repair that requires a cast application. In the postoperative period, the nurse notes serosanguineous drainage on the cast. What should the nurse do after making this observation?

1. Cut a window where the drainage is seeping through the cast.
2. Petal the cast to minimize skin irritation and decrease leakage.
3. Measure the area of drainage on the cast and document this.
4. Telephone the surgeon to report the serosanguineous drainage.

**1925.** The nurse is teaching the parents about how to care for their infant with osteogenesis imperfecta (OI). Which statement should the nurse include?

1. "Check the color of your infant's nailbeds and mucous membranes for signs of circulatory impairment."
2. "If you note signs of infection, bring your infant to the clinic; the infant has a significant immune dysfunction."
3. "Protect your infant from injury and handle your baby carefully; your infant's bones can break very easily."
4. "Notify your physician if your infant does not respond to sound; the infant's nervous system did not develop completely."

**1926.** MoC During an assessment of the 1-month-old, the nurse notes that the infant has blue sclerae. The nurse informs the HCP, recognizing that this may be a sign of which disorder?

1. Juvenile rheumatoid arthritis (JRA)
2. Tay-Sachs disease
3. Duchenne muscular dystrophy (DMD)
4. Osteogenesis imperfecta (OI)

**1927.** The nurse is preparing to assess the 9-year-old who has an intellectual disability with an IQ level of 45. Which level of participation should the nurse expect?

1. Able to communicate verbally but only with two-letter words
2. Able to read and comprehend simple written instructions
3. Able to walk independently and perform a simple skill
4. Able to perform tasks that require careful manual dexterity

**1928.** **PHARM** The teen is brought to an ED with a possible SCI. To minimize the extent of the damage to the spinal cord, which classification of medication should the nurse expect to administer?

1. An antibiotic
2. An analgesic
3. A steroid medication
4. An antihypertensive medication

**1929.** The nurse is teaching the adolescent who has a T12 SCI about the need to be diligent about skin protection. The nurse explains that the primary reason for the client's increased risk for altered skin integrity is due to which factor?

1. The inability to perceive extremes in temperature, leading to burns
2. The inability to feel skin irritation such as wrinkled linens or clothing
3. The increased likelihood of bowel and bladder dysfunction and skin irritation
4. The circulatory changes that cause vasoconstriction and decreased blood supply

**1930.** **PHARM** The child with an SCI is prescribed baclofen 5 mg TID orally to treat muscle spasticity. How many tablets should the nurse administer for one dose if 20 mg tablets are available?

_____ tablet (Round your answer to the nearest hundredth.)

**1931.** The nurse is caring for the 14-year-old who has a neurogenic bladder from an SCI with a lower motor neuron lesion occurring 2 years previously. Which intervention for bladder emptying should the nurse plan to implement?

1. Intermittent catheterization
2. Insertion of a retention catheter
3. Insertion of a suprapubic catheter
4. Giving an anticholinergic medication

**1932.** The nurse is teaching the parent of a 10-year-old who had an SCI about ROM exercises. Which illustration demonstrates abduction?

1.

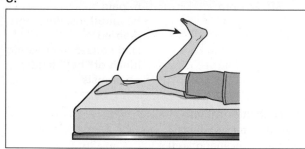

2.

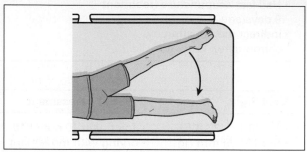

3.

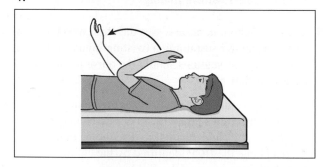

4.

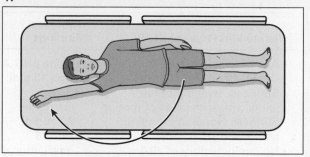

# Answers and Rationales

**1889. ANSWER: 2, 3, 5**

1. A tongue blade inserted into the adolescent's mouth during a seizure can cause injury.
2. **Padding protects the adolescent's limbs from injury against the hard side rails during a seizure.**
3. **Airway obstruction can occur during or after the seizure. An oropharyngeal airway should be available but should not be inserted during the seizure. If the seizure has commenced, nothing should be forced into the adolescent's mouth.**
4. The etiology is unknown. Only if an airborne or droplet infectious disease were suspected as the cause would droplet precautions be considered.
5. **Suctioning equipment may be needed to clear secretions after the seizure.**

▶ *Test-taking Tip: Generalized tonic-clonic seizures cause muscle rigidity and intense muscle jerking. You should select the options that will ensure the adolescent's safety during and following the seizure.*

Content Area: Child; Concept: Neurologic Regulation; Safety; Integrated Processes: Nursing Process: Implementation; Client Needs: Physiological Integrity: Reduction of Risk Potential; Cognitive Level: Application [Applying]

**1890. ANSWER: 3**

1. Myoclonic seizure involves muscle movement and not just loss of awareness.
2. Febrile seizures occur when the child's temperature is excessively elevated and usually includes tonic-clonic muscle movement.
3. **An absence seizure is a generalized seizure (involving loss of awareness) that might involve minor motor movements (e.g., eye blinking). The child appears to be staring.**
4. Atonic means absence of tone and would involve loss of muscle control and not eye blinking, which requires muscle control.

▶ *Test-taking Tip: Both myoclonic and atonic imply motor movements. Eliminate types of seizures related to motor movements because these are not described in this question.*

Content Area: Child; Concept: Neurologic Regulation; Safety; Integrated Processes: Nursing Process: Analysis; Client Needs: Physiological Integrity: Physiological Adaptation; Cognitive Level: Comprehension [Understanding]

**1891. ANSWER: 1**

1. **For most children, absence seizures stop during early teen years.**
2. Absence seizures rarely progress to other seizures.
3. Teachers often note signs of absence seizures, but seeing them is not adequate for diagnosis.
4. Absence seizures usually exist in isolation; usually the child has no other neurological condition.

▶ *Test-taking Tip: Read each option carefully. Think about what is appropriate information for a child.*

Content Area: Child; Concept: Neurologic Regulation; Nursing Roles; Integrated Processes: Nursing Process: Planning; Client Needs: Physiological Integrity: Physiological Adaptation; Cognitive Level: Application [Applying]

**1892. PHARM ANSWER: 1**

1. **Gingival hyperplasia (overgrowth of gum tissue) is unique to phenytoin (Dilantin) among antiepileptic medications. About 20% of people taking phenytoin have gingival hyperplasia. This can be minimized with thorough oral care.**
2. Valproic acid (Depakote) does not have a side effect of gingival hyperplasia.
3. Gingival hyperplasia is not a side effect of carbamazepine (Tegretol).
4. Gingival hyperplasia is not a side effect of phenobarbital (Luminal).

▶ *Test-taking Tip: Apply knowledge of medication side effects to answer this question.*

Content Area: Child; Concept: Medication; Neurologic Regulation; Nursing Roles; Integrated Processes: Teaching/Learning; Client Needs: Physiological Integrity: Pharmacological and Parenteral Therapies; Cognitive Level: Application [Applying]

**1893. MoC ANSWER: 2**

1. While an increasing temperature may be associated with ICP, it also may be due to an infection. It is more important for the nurse to report the widened pulse pressure as a sign of increased ICP.
2. **A widening pulse pressure (increased systolic BP and a decreased diastolic BP) is one of the signs of Cushing's triad and is indicative of ICP.**
3. Bradycardia (not tachycardia) is associated with ICP.
4. An increased systolic BP (not decreased systolic BP) is another sign of Cushing's triad.

▶ *Test-taking Tip: Three options typically are analyzed when evaluating the vital signs. One option is different and is unique to increasing ICP.*

Content Area: Child; Concept: Neurologic Regulation; Assessment; Collaboration; Integrated Processes: Nursing Process: Assessment; Client Needs: Safe and Effective Care Environment: Management of Care; Cognitive Level: Application [Applying]

**1894. MoC ANSWER: 3**

1. A visible, penetrating scalp wound is a sign of TBI but does not specifically indicate a basal skull fracture and is not a contraindication to the placement of an NG tube.
2. Jerking movements of extremities suggest seizure, which may be associated with TBI, but is not specific for basal skull fracture and is not a contraindication to the placement of an NG tube.

3. Clear fluid from the ears could be CSF, indicating a possible basal skull fracture. Suspected basal skull fracture is a contraindication to placement of an NG tube due to the concern that the tube may enter the brain through the fracture. The nurse should contact the HCP.

4. Loss of consciousness may be associated with TBI but is not specific for basal skull fracture and is not a contraindication for placement of an NG tube.

▸ **Test-taking Tip:** *Think about the disruption of the internal anatomical structures of the head and CSF leakage from the ears when selecting your answer.*

**Content Area:** Child; **Concept:** Neurologic Regulation; Management; **Integrated Processes:** Nursing Process: Implementation; **Client Needs:** Safe and Effective Care Environment: Management of Care; Physiological Integrity: Physiological Adaptation; **Cognitive Level:** Application [Applying]

## 1895. ANSWER: 2

1. An excessive urinary output such as 300 mL per hour is associated with DI (lack of antidiuretic hormone).

2. **The serum Na is low at 117 mEq/L (N = 135-145 mEq/L). The nurse should assess for other manifestations of SIADH such as low urinary output, fluid retention, and low plasma osmolarity. With SIADH, the body does not respond normally, and antidiuretic hormone (ADH) is released despite a low plasma osmolarity. The body retains fluid, thus lowering the plasma osmolarity and causing severe hyponatremia.**

3. Dry oral mucous membranes occur with dehydration.

4. Nuchal rigidity is a sign of meningeal irritation and not associated with SIADH.

▸ **Test-taking Tip:** *Recall the physiological action of ADH is conservation of fluid in response to high osmolarity.*

**Content Area:** Child; **Concept:** Fluid and Electrolyte Balance; Neurologic Regulation; **Integrated Processes:** Nursing Process: Assessment; **Client Needs:** Physiological Integrity: Physiological Adaptation; **Cognitive Level:** Application [Applying]

## 1896. ANSWER:

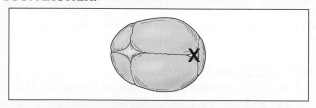

The posterior fontanelle is the smaller of the two fontanelles. Fullness of the fontanelles is a potential sign of increased ICP that can occur with head trauma.

▸ **Test-taking Tip:** *Focus on the size of the fontanelles and their location.*

**Content Area:** Child; **Concept:** Neurologic Regulation; Assessment; **Integrated Processes:** Nursing Process: Assessment; **Client Needs:** Physiological Integrity: Physiological Adaptation; **Cognitive Level:** Application [Applying]

## 1897. MoC ANSWER: 1

1. **About 50% of children with myelodysplasia develop a latex allergy. Because anaphylaxis can occur, exposure to latex should be avoided.**

2. Intermittent urinary catheterization may be needed to promote bladder emptying, especially if the child has detrusor hyperreflexia and dyssynergia, but this is not as life-threatening as the possible consequences of a latex allergy.

3. Dietary fiber supplements (recommended 10g/day), laxatives, suppositories, or enemas aid in producing regular evacuation to prevent constipation, but this is not as life-threatening as the possible consequences of a latex allergy.

4. Physical therapy (PT) is important to prevent contractures, but they are not as life-threatening as the possible consequences of a latex allergy. Common musculoskeletal problems with spina bifida include deformities of the knees, hips, feet, and spine.

▸ **Test-taking Tip:** *Three options are similar, and one is different. Often the option that is different is the answer.*

**Content Area:** Child; **Concept:** Neurologic Regulation; Safety; **Integrated Processes:** Nursing Process: Planning; **Client Needs:** Safe and Effective Care Environment: Safety and Infection Control; **Cognitive Level:** Synthesis [Creating]

## 1898. ANSWER: 4

1. Braces should never be directly against the skin; there always should be a cloth between the braces and the skin.

2. The child should shift position every hour (not every 3 hours).

3. The child should sit on a gel cushion because blanket folds can interrupt circulation.

4. **With a myelomeningocele, the spinal cord ended at the point where the spinal cord and the meninges protruded through the vertebrae. Thus, the child's motor and sensory functions are absent beyond this point. A daily thorough skin check is the best way to evaluate circulatory and skin alterations due to the child's immobility, altered sensation, or therapeutic treatments, such as braces.**

▸ **Test-taking Tip:** *Use the nursing process to identify the instruction. Only one option pertains to assessment.*

**Content Area:** Child; **Concept:** Safety; Skin Integrity; Neurologic Regulation; **Integrated Processes:** Teaching/Learning; **Client Needs:** Physiological Integrity: Basic Care and Comfort; **Cognitive Level:** [Applying]

## 1899. ANSWER: 2, 3, 4

1. Eczema does not cause increased ICP.

2. **Papilledema is edema and inflammation of the optic nerve caused by increased ICP. It can be assessed with the use of an ophthalmoscope.**

3. **Shaken baby syndrome can cause head trauma with bruising and bleeding in the brain, which can lead to ICP. This ICP can compress the optic nerve, resulting in papilledema.**

4. Hydrocephalus is excess CSF. This excess can increase ICP, which in turn can compress the optic nerve, resulting in papilledema.
5. Chest trauma does not cause increased ICP.

▶ **Test-taking Tip:** *Determine the commonality in some of the conditions (increased ICP) and then eliminate options that are not associated with ICP.*

**Content Area:** Child; **Concept:** Neurologic Regulation; Assessment; **Integrated Processes:** Nursing Process: Assessment; **Client Needs:** Physiological Integrity: Physiological Adaptation; **Cognitive Level:** Application [Applying]

## 1900. ANSWER: 4

1. An elevation of the head of the bed is contraindicated because it will increase the flow from the shunt.
2. Extremity movement is allowed and, as the child recovers, ROM of the extremities should be performed to maintain muscle strength.
3. A clear dressing (not a pressure dressing) is placed over the incision sites to allow observation.
4. **The child should be placed in a flat position following insertion of the shunt to prevent increasing the flow from the shunt. The skin should be protected by turning the child every 2 hours.**

▶ **Test-taking Tip:** *Narrow the options by first analyzing the items that are opposites (1 and 4) to determine if one of these is the correct answer.*

**Content Area:** Child; **Concept:** Neurologic Regulation; Nursing Roles; **Integrated Processes:** Nursing Process: Implementation; **Client Needs:** Physiological Integrity: Physiological Adaptation; **Cognitive Level:** Application [Applying]

## 1901. ANSWER: 1, 2, 4

1. **Headaches can result from fluid accumulation associated with hydrocephalus that is applying pressure on brain structures.**
2. **Vomiting can result from fluid accumulation associated with hydrocephalus that is applying pressure on brain structures.**
3. Angioedema is swelling and fluid accumulation under the skin and is not associated with hydrocephalus.
4. **Personality change can result from fluid accumulation associated with hydrocephalus that is applying pressure on brain structures.**
5. The fontanelles should be closed at 7 years of age. The head circumference will not increase in size.

▶ **Test-taking Tip:** *You should narrow the options to those associated only with neurological function.*

**Content Area:** Child; **Concept:** Neurologic Regulation; Assessment; Development; **Integrated Processes:** Nursing Process: Assessment; **Client Needs:** Physiological Integrity: Physiological Adaptation; **Cognitive Level:** Application [Applying]

## 1902. ANSWER:

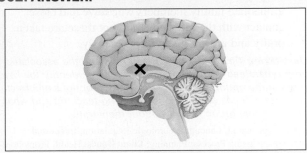

The two lateral ventricles, the largest of the four ventricles, are irregular in shape. Each consists of a central part with anterior, posterior, and inferior horns. Cerebral spinal fluid forms in the choroid plexus of the pia mater and flows through the two lateral ventricles, through the foramen of Monro into the third ventricle, and through the aqueduct of Sylvius to the fourth ventricle.

▶ **Test-taking Tip:** *Do not confuse the lateral ventricles with the corpus callosum, the band of nerve fibers that connects the left and right cerebral hemispheres, which is adjacent to the lateral ventricles.*

**Content Area:** Child; **Concept:** Neurologic Regulation; Nursing Roles; **Integrated Processes:** Teaching/Learning; **Client Needs:** Physiological Integrity: Physiological Adaptation; **Cognitive Level:** Knowledge [Remembering]

## 1903. ANSWER: 4

1. Resistance with particular leg movement is Kernig's sign.
2. Brudzinski's sign is knee or hip flexion with head flexion.
3. The specific quality of cry with neck flexion is not characteristic of opisthotonus.
4. **In an opisthotonus position, the child's neck and head are hyperextended to relieve discomfort.**

▶ **Test-taking Tip:** *Apply knowledge of medical terminology: "-tonus" is related to muscle tone. Select the option that would be caused by an extreme spasm of the muscles.*

**Content Area:** Child; **Concept:** Neurologic Regulation; Mobility; Assessment; **Integrated Processes:** Nursing Process: Assessment; **Client Needs:** Physiological Integrity: Physiological Adaptation; **Cognitive Level:** Application [Applying]

## 1904. ANSWER: 3

1. The symptoms of meningitis can occur insidiously, or suddenly.
2. A child with a febrile seizure is assumed to have meningitis until CSF findings prove otherwise.
3. **The MCV4 is recommended for certain high-risk children from ages 2 through 10 years and for all individuals 11 to 55 years. Those at high risk include children who travel to, and U.S. citizens who reside in, countries where meningitis is hyperendemic or epidemic; persons with terminal complement deficiency (an immune system disorder); and persons who have a damaged spleen or whose spleen has been removed.**

4. Prophylactic antibiotics may be prescribed for immediate family members who have had close contact with the infected child, but these are taken orally and are not given intravenously.

▶ **Test-taking Tip:** *Think about meningitis and the associated symptoms. Read each statement carefully to identify the key words in the option that make three of the options incorrect. If uncertain, focus on the group receiving teaching and what is best for that group to know about meningitis.*

**Content Area:** Child; **Concept:** Neurologic Regulation; **Integrated Processes:** Nursing Process: Planning; **Client Needs:** Health Promotion and Maintenance; Physiological Integrity: Reduction of Risk Potential; **Cognitive Level:** Application [Applying]

## 1905. ANSWER: 4

1. Although the cause is unknown, it usually occurs after a viral infection or influenza treated with a salicylate, and not after a bacterial infection.
2. Reye's syndrome is not infectious; droplet isolation is not necessary.
3. Treatment includes rest and decreasing environmental stimulation rather than play and interaction.
4. **Hypothrombinemia (abnormally low levels of thrombin in the blood leading to bleeding without clotting) occurs from fatty droplets invading the liver. The nurse should assess for signs of bleeding and prolonged bleeding time.**

▶ **Test-taking Tip:** *Use the nursing process to select an option that includes assessment.*

**Content Area:** Child; **Concept:** Neurologic Regulation; Assessment; **Integrated Processes:** Nursing Process: Assessment; **Client Needs:** Physiological Integrity: Physiological Adaptation; **Cognitive Level:** Application [Applying]

## 1906. MoC ANSWER: 1

1. **Because autistic children are unable to relate to other children or respond to emotional or social cues appropriately, the child should be in a private room. Autistic children may display a response to the environment, repetitive hand movement, rocking, and rhythmic body movements that can frighten other children. The private room also will decrease stimulation; it can precipitate a behavioral outburst.**
2. A double room is an inappropriate room assignment because the environment may be too stimulating and precipitate a behavioral outburst that may frighten other children.
3. The assigned room, a four-bed ward, is an inappropriate room assignment because the environment may be too stimulating and precipitate a behavioral outburst that may frighten other children.
4. Isolation is unnecessary because autism is not a communicable disease.

▶ **Test-taking Tip:** *Autism is a developmental disorder characterized by impairment of social and communication skills. Take this into consideration when selecting an option.*

**Content Area:** Child; **Concept:** Neurologic Regulation; Development; Safety; **Integrated Processes:** Nursing Process: Implementation; Caring; **Client Needs:** Safe and Effective Care Environment: Management of Care: Safe and Effective Care Environment: Safety and Infection Control; **Cognitive Level:** Analysis [Analyzing]

## 1907. ANSWER: 3, 4, 5

1. Polydactyly (having more than 10 fingers or toes) is not associated with autism.
2. Leukoderma (deficiency of skin pigmentation, usually in patches) is not associated with autism.
3. **The nurse should anticipate that the child may have poor eye contact from the social and communication impairments that occur with autism.**
4. **The nurse should anticipate that the child may have restricted interests (narrow range of interests) from the social and communication impairments that occur with autism.**
5. **The nurse should anticipate that the autistic child may have atypical language. It can include humming or grunting for extended periods, laughing inappropriately, or echolalia (echoing another's speech).**

▶ **Test-taking Tip:** *The key word in the stem is "behavior;" eliminate options pertaining to physical abnormalities.*

**Content Area:** Child; **Concept:** Neurologic Regulation; Development; Promoting Health; **Integrated Processes:** Nursing Process: Planning; **Client Needs:** Physiological Integrity: Physiological Adaptation; **Cognitive Level:** Application [Applying]

## 1908. ANSWER: 3

1. Physical contact often upsets a child with autism and can precipitate a behavioral outburst.
2. Auditory or visual stimulation can precipitate a behavioral outburst.
3. **Having a favorite toy may minimize the disruption of hospitalization and may help to control behavioral outbursts.**
4. An autistic child may have poor eating habits that can include throwing food or food refusal. Too many choices can precipitate a behavioral outburst.

▶ **Test-taking Tip:** *Think about the behavior of the child with autism and the intervention that would help most with any outbursts that may occur.*

**Content Area:** Child; **Concept:** Neurologic Regulation; Development; **Integrated Processes:** Nursing Process: Implementation; **Client Needs:** Psychosocial Integrity; **Cognitive Level:** Application [Applying]

## 1909. ANSWER: 1, 2, 4, 5

1. **A child with spastic CP has hypertonia and rigidity and is prone to contractures; ROM exercises every 4 hours are essential to maintain joint flexibility and prevent contractures.**
2. **Therapeutic massage can help control the pain associated with spasticity and stretching exercises.**

3. A child with CP requires high-calorie diets and sometimes supplements due to the feeding difficulties associated with spasticity.

4. **A child with chronic tonic-clonic seizures should wear a helmet to protect against head injury.**

5. **Utensils with large, padded handles are appropriate for a child with spasticity and can promote the child's independence in eating.**

▶ **Test-taking Tip:** *Eliminate the one option that is different from the other options.*

**Content Area:** Child; **Concept:** Neurologic Regulation; Development; **Integrated Processes:** Nursing Process: Evaluation; **Client Needs:** Physiological Integrity: Reduction of Risk Potential; **Cognitive Level:** Evaluation [Evaluating]

## 1910. ANSWER: 1

1. **Genu varum (bowlegs) is normal until 2 to 3 years of age. Bowlegs is a distance between the knees of greater than 2.5 cm. The nurse should document the observation.**

2. The persistence of bowlegs beyond the age of 3 years necessitates further evaluation; it is unnecessary to report a normal finding.

3. Rickets is a common pathological cause of bowed legs, but at age 18 months this is a normal finding.

4. Braces, worn usually at night, are used to correct bowlegs, but the child is too young for the nurse to determine if bowlegs will persist.

▶ **Test-taking Tip:** *Envisioning how a young toddler normally stands will help you answer this question.*

**Content Area:** Child; **Concept:** Mobility; Assessment; Development; **Integrated Processes:** Communication and Documentation; **Client Needs:** Physiological Integrity: Reduction of Risk Potential; **Cognitive Level:** Application [Applying]

## 1911. ANSWER: 3

1. The hip and leg are in abduction in a frontpack; this does not increase the risk of DDH.

2. The hip and leg are in abduction in a backpack; this does not increase the risk of DDH.

3. **The nurse should include information about the risks of swaddling. Although it has many benefits (e.g., neurological and musculoskeletal development, less physiological distress, better motor organization, more self-regulatory ability), swaddling can cause DDH because the legs are in extension and adduction.**

4. The leg and hip are in flexion and adduction in a car seat; this does not increase the risk for DDH.

▶ **Test-taking Tip:** *Look for the commonalities in leg and hip positions within the options. The option that is different is the answer.*

**Content Area:** Child; **Concept:** Mobility; Safety; Promoting Health; **Integrated Processes:** Nursing Process: Planning; Teaching/Learning; **Client Needs:** Physiological Integrity: Basic Care and Comfort; **Cognitive Level:** Application [Applying]

## 1912. ANSWER: 4, 2, 5, 1, 3

4. **Position the chest halter at nipple line and fasten with Velcro.** This first step needs to be applied before the legs can go into the stirrups; the leg straps are attached to the chest halter.

2. **Position the legs and feet in the stirrups.** Once the chest piece is in place, the infant's feet can be lifted into the stirrups.

5. **Be sure the hips are flexed and abducted before fastening with Velcro.** The legs need to be correctly positioned for hip reduction.

1. **Connect the chest halter and leg straps in front.** Once the legs are correctly positioned in the stirrups, then the leg straps can be connected to the chest halter.

3. **Connect the chest halter and leg straps in back.** This step is last because the legs need to be correctly positioned before the leg straps can be attached to the back of the halter.

▶ **Test-taking Tip:** *Often, finding the first and last steps makes it easier to place the items in the correct order.*

**Content Area:** Child; **Concept:** Mobility; Development; **Integrated Processes:** Nursing Process: Implementation; **Client Needs:** Safe and Effective Care Environment: Safety and Infection Control; Physiological Integrity: Basic Care and Comfort; **Cognitive Level:** Synthesis [Creating]

## 1913. ANSWER: 3, 4, 5

1. Hair dryers should never be used to promote drying because the heat can result in burn injuries.

2. A child with a plaster of Paris hip-spica cast is placed on a Bradford frame, which elevates the child off the bed and facilitates drying. Plaster of Paris casts take 10 to 72 hours to dry.

3. **A fiberglass cast dries within 30 minutes. Pillows are used to support the lower extremities to prevent pressure areas.**

4. **Turning every 2 hours prevents cast syndrome, and monitoring the CMS with turning will identify potential complications early.**

5. **Petaling (applying waterproof adhesive tape to the edges of the cast) protects it from soiling.**

▶ **Test-taking Tip:** *Recall that fiberglass casts dry more quickly than plaster of Paris casts. Eliminate options that would cause injury or that pertain to a plaster of Paris cast.*

**Content Area:** Child; **Concept:** Mobility; Critical Thinking; **Integrated Processes:** Nursing Process: Implementation; **Client Needs:** Safe and Effective Care Environment: Safety and Infection Control; Physiological Integrity: Basic Care and Comfort; **Cognitive Level:** Application [Applying]

## 1914. ANSWER: 3

1. Although the surgery may increase height, this is neither guaranteed nor a primary indication for the surgery.

2. Pain may decrease with surgery, but this is neither guaranteed nor a primary indication for surgery.

3. **A severe lateral spinal curvature can affect lung expansion. A goal for scoliosis surgery is to improve any current breathing problems and prevent future ones.**

4. The surgery may result in clothing fitting better, but this is neither guaranteed nor a primary indication for surgery.

▶ *Test-taking Tip:* Use the ABC's to determine which goal is priority.

**Content Area:** Child; **Concept:** Mobility; Promoting Health; Nursing Roles; **Integrated Processes:** Teaching/Learning; **Client Needs:** Physiological Integrity: Reduction of Risk Potential; **Cognitive Level:** Application [Applying]

## 1915. ANSWER: 2

1. Scoliosis is a lateral curve.

2. **Lordosis involves an exaggerated lumbar curve.**

3. Kyphosis is an exaggerated thoracic curve.

4. Kyphoscoliosis involves both curves in the same person.

▶ *Test-taking Tip:* The terms lordosis and lumbar start with the same letter, making it easier to remember this type of curvature.

**Content Area:** Child; **Concept:** Mobility; Communication; Assessment; **Integrated Processes:** Communication and Documentation; **Client Needs:** Physiological Integrity: Reduction of Risk Potential; **Cognitive Level:** Knowledge [Remembering]

## 1916. ANSWER: 2

1. Only the HCP should manipulate the rods to lengthen them.

2. **An Ilizarov external fixator is a device that uses wires, rings, and telescoping rods to permit limb lengthening to occur by manual manipulation of the rods. Pins secure the device in the bone. Pin site care is necessary to prevent infection and allow inspection for loosening of the pins.**

3. Partial weight bearing is allowed when a child has an Ilizarov external fixator to a lower extremity.

4. The fixation device must remain intact and should be supported on pillows when the child is in bed; sections should not be removed.

▶ *Test-taking Tip:* Two options involve complex procedures and should be eliminated. Of the two remaining options, select the one that involves care of the fixator.

**Content Area:** Child; **Concept:** Mobility; Safety; Infection; **Integrated Processes:** Nursing Process: Implementation; **Client Needs:** Physiological Integrity: Basic Care and Comfort; Safe and Effective Care Environment: Safety and Infection Control; **Cognitive Level:** Application [Applying]

## 1917. ANSWER: 1

1. **A varus deformity means that the structures are farther apart than expected. Soccer players are at risk for varus knee deformities because of the planting and forward-leaning actions that separate the knee joint when playing soccer.**

2. A valgus deformity means the structures are closer together than expected; when playing soccer, the knee structures are farther apart.

3. The ankle is less affected than the knee.

4. The ankle is less affected than the knee.

▶ *Test-taking Tip:* The letter "l" in a valgus deformity can be a reminder that the knees or ankles are together and should be eliminated.

**Content Area:** Child; **Concept:** Promoting Health; Mobility; Nursing Roles; **Integrated Processes:** Teaching/Learning; **Client Needs:** Physiological Integrity: Physiological Adaptation; **Cognitive Level:** Application [Applying]

## 1918. ANSWER: 2

1. Treatment for Legg-Calvé-Perthes disease likely will continue for as long as 2 years.

2. **Legg-Calvé-Perthes disease is avascular necrosis of the proximal femoral epiphysis occurring in association with incomplete clotting factors. The treatment goal is a pain-free joint with full ROM.**

3. Activities requiring abduction, not adduction, will promote proper joint alignment.

4. Most of the treatment will occur in community-based settings rather than during hospitalization.

▶ *Test-taking Tip:* The long time period to diagnose Legg-Calvé-Perthes disease should be a clue that the course of the disease is also likely to be longer. Thus, eliminate Options 1 and 4. Of the remaining options, think about which one would promote full joint motion.

**Content Area:** Child; **Concept:** Mobility; Management; **Integrated Processes:** Nursing Process: Planning; **Client Needs:** Physiological Integrity: Reduction of Risk Potential; **Cognitive Level:** Application [Applying]

## 1919. ANSWER: 4

1. Parents never can be assured they will not conceive another child with DMD.

2. Prevalence in the parents' generation does not predict incidence for DMD in the next generation.

3. Although as many as one-third of affected children have no family history of the disease, this statement does not address the woman's concern.

4. **Because DMD is usually X-linked recessive, a female can inherit the affected gene and be a carrier of DMD but not develop the condition because the expression of the disease is blocked. If the female has an affected gene on both X chromosomes, it is incompatible with life, and the female may die at or before birth.**

▶ *Test-taking Tip:* Focus on the question being asked by the woman and then eliminate any options that do not address the question. To select the correct option, consider that DMD is X-linked recessive.

**Content Area:** Child; **Concept:** Neurologic Regulation; Mobility; Development; Nursing Roles; **Integrated Processes:** Teaching/Learning; Caring; **Client Needs:** Physiological Integrity: Physiological Adaptation; Psychosocial Integrity; **Cognitive Level:** Evaluation [Evaluating]

**1920. ANSWER: 1**

1. **The progressive muscular weakness and wasting that occur with DMD make it difficult for the child to rise from the floor normally. The child will use the hands to walk up the legs.**
2. The inability to initiate an effective cough or expectorate secretions is due to respiratory musculature weakness associated with DMD but does not describe Gowers sign.
3. Difficulty lifting the head and supporting it in an upright position may be observed with juvenile dermatomyositis.
4. Mild to moderate mental retardation is associated with DMD, with the mean IQ approximately 20 points below normal.

▶ *Test-taking Tip: The age of the child in the stem of the question is important. Evidence of muscle weakness with DMD usually appears during the third to seventh year. Consider which observation would be an early sign of muscle weakness.*

Content Area: Child; Concept: Neurologic Regulation; Mobility; Assessment; Integrated Processes: Nursing Process: Assessment; Client Needs: Physiological Integrity: Physiological Adaptation; Cognitive Level: Evaluation [Evaluating]

**1921.** CJ PHARM **ANSWER: 2**

1. The documentation in the H&P includes the child's ethnicity, previous treatment, and information associated with JRA. Although the child is Chinese and has had acupuncture and moxibustion treatments (traditional Chinese medicine healing techniques), these do not influence the use of methotrexate.
2. **The serum creatinine of 2.2 mg/dL is elevated, indicating a concern for excreting methotrexate (Trexall). The nurse should withhold methotrexate and contact the HCP.**
3. The VS are within normal parameters for a child experiencing pain.
4. The physical assessment shows that the child is in pain; analgesics should be given, but this does not require notification of the HCP.

▶ *Test-taking Tip: Knowing how drugs are metabolized and excreted can give a clue as to which options should be considered.*

Content Area: Child; Concept: Mobility; Medication; Safety; Collaboration; Diversity; Integrated Processes: Nursing Process: Planning; Culture and Spirituality; Client Needs: Physiological Integrity: Reduction of Risk Potential; Physiological Integrity: Pharmacological and Parenteral Therapies; Cognitive Level: Analysis [Analyzing]

**1922. ANSWER: 1, 2, 3**

1. **Elevation and application of ice reduce edema at the site.**
2. **An elastic bandage will provide firm support and help control edema.**
3. **The parent should be notified to discuss the injury and should be advised to take the child to an HCP for examination.**

4. The parent, not the school nurse, should contact the child's HCP.
5. The school nurse's scope of practice does not include prescribing; the HCP needs to request an x-ray.
6. Appropriate channels should be used for reporting the incident rather than meeting with the offending student in the nurse's office.

▶ *Test-taking Tip: Consider that the child is describing a strain. Select options to treat a muscle strain. Remember the acronym RICE for rest, ice, compression, and elevation. The school nurse must function within the scope of nursing practice that does not include prescribing.*

Content Area: Child; Concept: Comfort; Assessment; Nursing Roles; Integrated Processes: Nursing Process: Implementation; Client Needs: Physiological Integrity: Physiological Adaptation; Cognitive Level: Analysis [Analyzing]

**1923. ANSWER: 3**

1. Open surgical intervention is unnecessary because the kneecap is movable.
2. A kneecap dislocation in itself does not cause torn cartilage.
3. **Dislocation of the kneecap causes it to move to the posterior surface of the knee. The kneecap is realigned by the HCP, sliding it back into position.**
4. After realignment, a leg immobilizer, not a cast, is applied and used for about a week.

▶ *Test-taking Tip: The key words are "most immediate." Select an option that can be accomplished quickly. Remember that the kneecap is movable.*

Content Area: Child; Concept: Mobility; Critical Thinking; Integrated Processes: Nursing Process: Planning; Client Needs: Physiological Integrity: Reduction of Risk Potential; Cognitive Level: Application [Applying]

**1924. ANSWER: 3**

1. It is not the nurse's responsibility to place a window in the cast. Windowing may be used to relieve pressure.
2. Petaling, or bending the edges of the cast away from the skin, may make it more comfortable for the child but will not help with drainage.
3. **The circumference of the drainage should be measured and the information documented for further comparison.**
4. Serosanguineous drainage on the cast is not an emergency situation that requires notification of the HCP unless it becomes bloody and copious.

▶ *Test-taking Tip: Focus on the color of the drainage on the cast to select the correct option. Recognize that this is not a medical emergency and that the nurse should not alter the cast.*

Content Area: Child; Concept: Hematologic Regulation; Mobility; Integrated Processes: Communication and Documentation; Client Needs: Physiological Integrity: Basic Care and Comfort; Safe and Effective Care Environment: Safety and Infection Control; Cognitive Level: Application [Applying]

## 1925. ANSWER: 3

1. OI is not a disease affecting circulation.
2. OI does not result in immune dysfunction.
3. **With OI, also known as brittle bone disease, the infant should be handled carefully and protected from injury. The nurse should include this statement when teaching the parents.**
4. OI is not a disease of the CNS.

▶ *Test-taking Tip:* Key words in the stem should be associated with words in an option. "Osteo-" refers to bone.

**Content Area:** Child; **Concept:** Mobility; Safety; Nursing Roles; **Integrated Processes:** Nursing Process: Analysis; **Client Needs:** Physiological Integrity: Physiological Adaptation; **Cognitive Level:** Evaluation [Evaluating]

## 1926. MoC ANSWER: 4

1. Blue sclerae are not associated with JRA, a chronic inflammation of the joints that can lead to damaged joint cartilage and bone, deformity, and impaired use of the joint. It is believed to be caused by a combination of genetic and environmental factors.
2. Blue sclerae are not associated with Tay-Sachs disease. This is a fatal genetic lipid storage disorder. The infant appears to develop normally for the first few months of life, then mental and physical abilities deteriorate as nerve cells become distended with fatty material.
3. Blue sclerae are not associated with DMD. This is a genetic disease causing progressive weakness and degeneration of skeletal muscles used in voluntary movement.
4. **Newborns may have sclerae that appear blue, but in children older than newborns, this is an indicator for osteogenesis imperfecta, a genetic disorder that causes fragile bones as well as other health problems. For a child who has not yet fractured a bone, blue sclerae may be the first sign that prompts further assessment and workup.**

▶ *Test-taking Tip:* If uncertain, select the condition that results in fragile bones. Remember that "osteo-" pertains to bones.

**Content Area:** Child; **Concept:** Assessment; Mobility; **Integrated Processes:** Nursing Process: Assessment; **Client Needs:** Safe and Effective Care Environment: Management of Care; Physiological Integrity: Physiological Adaptation; **Cognitive Level:** Application [Applying]

## 1927. ANSWER: 3

1. The child with an IQ level of 45 can use simple communication with more than two-letter words.
2. At an IQ level of 45, the child does not progress in functional reading or arithmetic and would be unable to read or comprehend written instructions.
3. **An IQ of 45 is considered to be a moderate intellectual disability. The IQ range for this is 36 to 49. At a 45 IQ, a 9-year-old should be able to walk independently and perform simple manual skills.**
4. While simple manual skills can be performed at an IQ level of 45, those requiring manual dexterity cannot.

▶ *Test-taking Tip:* An IQ level of 45 is considered moderate intellectual disability. Select an option that can be performed by a child younger than 9 years of age.

**Content Area:** Child; **Concept:** Neurologic Regulation; Development; Assessment; **Integrated Processes:** Nursing Process: Analysis; **Client Needs:** Physiological Integrity: Physiological Adaptation; **Cognitive Level:** Application [Applying]

## 1928. PHARM ANSWER: 3

1. An antibiotic may be unnecessary; there is no indication of impaired skin integrity or an associated risk of infection that could further damage the spinal cord.
2. Pain control is important but is not the most important medication for preventing swelling and compression of the spinal cord.
3. **Steroids administered shortly after injury help decrease inflammation and prevent further injury.**
4. While autonomic dysreflexia is a complication of SCI, and while the hypertensive crisis is treated with an antihypertensive medication, this will not protect the spinal cord from further injury.

▶ *Test-taking Tip:* The focus of the question is a medication that will minimize damage to the spinal cord. Eliminate options that do not have a direct effect on tissues surrounding the spinal cord.

**Content Area:** Child; **Concept:** Neurologic Regulation; Mobility; Medication; **Integrated Processes:** Nursing Process: Planning; **Client Needs:** Physiological Integrity: Pharmacological and Parenteral Therapies; Physiological Integrity: Physiological Adaptation; **Cognitive Level:** Application [Applying]

## 1929. ANSWER: 2

1. There are often sensation changes with an SCI, but burns are not the primary reason for an increased risk of altered skin integrity.
2. **The primary reason for an increased risk of altered skin integrity is the inability to perceive stimuli and the lack of sensation that would promote an uninjured person to take action. The person must be taught to plan movement, even in the lack of a physical prompt to move (e.g., discomfort).**
3. There is usually bowel and bladder dysfunction with SCI; however, good hygiene and a bowel and catheterization regimen minimize the likelihood of this as a cause of skin breakdown.
4. While there are circulatory changes with SCI, this is not the primary reason for an increased risk of altered skin integrity.

▶ *Test-taking Tip:* You should look for options that use the same or similar words as those used in the stem. Note "skin" in the stem and in Option 2.

**Content Area:** Child; **Concept:** Mobility; Safety; Skin Integrity; **Integrated Processes:** Teaching/Learning; **Client Needs:** Physiological Integrity: Basic Care and Comfort; **Cognitive Level:** Application [Applying]

**1930. PHARM ANSWER: 0.25**

Use a proportion formula to determine the number of tablets.

20 mg : 1 tablet :: 5 mg : $X$ tablet; $20X = 5$; $X = 5 \div 20$; $X = 0.25$

▶ **Test-taking Tip:** *Be sure to carefully read the stem to know which dose you are calculating for baclofen (Lioresal).*

**Content Area:** Child; **Concept:** Medication; Mobility; **Integrated Processes:** Communication and Documentation; **Client Needs:** Physiological Integrity: Pharmacological and Parenteral Therapies; **Cognitive Level:** Application [Applying]

**1931. ANSWER: 1**

1. **A lower motor neuron lesion produces a flaccid, neurogenic bladder that is unable to respond to changes in passive pressure, causing overdistention. Periodic emptying of the bladder with intermittent catheterization is necessary.**
2. A retention catheter is unnecessary and can increase the risk of infection.
3. There is no indication that a suprapubic catheter is needed.
4. An anticholinergic medication such as dicyclomine (Bentyl) relaxes the bladder musculature and promotes increased capacity and more adequate emptying, but it is used in persons with a spastic and not a flaccid bladder.

▶ **Test-taking Tip:** *Recognize that a lower motor neuron lesion of the spinal cord produces a flaccid bladder. Eliminate any options that pertain to just a spastic bladder. Of the remaining options, determine which is optimal.*

**Content Area:** Child; **Concept:** Mobility; Urinary Elimination; **Integrated Processes:** Nursing Process: Planning; **Client Needs:** Physiological Integrity: Basic Care and Comfort; **Cognitive Level:** Application [Applying]

**1932. ANSWER: 1**

1. **Abduction refers to increasing the angle between the extremity and the body's midline. This illustrates abduction of the shoulder.**
2. This illustrates leg adduction where the angle is decreased between the extremity and the body (bringing together).
3. This illustrates flexion of the knee; the knee is bent, and the heel is brought back toward the buttocks.
4. This illustrates elbow extension; the arm is straightened by bringing the lower arm forward and down.

▶ **Test-taking Tip:** *"Ad"-duction means decreasing the angle between the extremity and midline, or "adding."*

**Content Area:** Child; **Concept:** Mobility; Promoting Health; **Integrated Processes:** Nursing Process: Evaluation; **Client Needs:** Physiological Integrity: Basic Care and Comfort; **Cognitive Level:** Evaluation [Evaluating]

## Chapter Forty-Four

# Renal and Urinary Management

**1933.** The nurse reviews the child's laboratory report. Based on the findings, which order by the HCP should the nurse implement **now**?

| Serum Laboratory Test | Client's Value | Normal Values |
|---|---|---|
| BUN | 26 | 5–25 mg/dL |
| Creatinine | 2.0 | 0.5–1.5 mg/dL |
| Na | 140 | 135–145 mEq/L |
| K | 5.0 | 3.5–5.3 mEq/L |
| Cl | 100 | 95–105 mEq/L |
| CO | 28 | 22–30 mEq/L |
| Phosphate | 2.0 | 1.7–2.6 mEq/L |
| Calcium | 10 | 9–11 mg/dL |
| Hgb | 15 | 13.5–17 g/dL |
| Hct | 45 | 40%–54% |
| PTH | 30 | 11–54 pg/mL |

1. Obtain a urine culture.
2. Obtain a complete blood count (CBC).
3. Obtain a urinalysis (UA).
4. Obtain liver function tests.

**1934.** The nurse is calculating the 8-hour urine output for a hospitalized 18-month-old. The child had 6 wet diapers weighing 24 g, 24 g, 30 g, 31 g, 22 g, and 30 g. The weight of a dry diaper is 15 g. What amount in mL should the nurse document for the infant's total urine output for the 8 hours?

_____ mL (Record your answer as a whole number.)

**1935.** Parents bring their 1-year-old child to the ER of a large urban hospital. The child is lethargic and has bloody urine, and there is blood seeping through a diaper. The child's parents do not speak English. Which intervention should the nurse implement **first**?

1. Check the child's BP.
2. Arrange for an interpreter.
3. Inspect the child's genitalia.
4. Obtain urine and blood cultures.

**1936.** The nurse is collecting a 24-hour urine sample from the hospitalized adolescent. The client voids, and the nurse discards this. Each void for the next 24 hours is poured into a collection container that is placed on ice. At the end of hour 24, the client voids. What should the nurse do with this urine?

1. Discard the urine.
2. Add it to the urine container.
3. Measure and then discard it.
4. Pour it into a new container.

**1937.** The nurse is preparing to collect a urine specimen from the female infant. Prioritize the steps that the nurse should take to apply a urine-collection bag and collect the urine specimen from the female infant.

1. Check that the bag adheres firmly around the perineal area.
2. Explain the procedure to the parents, prepare supplies, and position the infant.
3. Check the bag frequently and remove it as soon as urine is available.
4. Carefully replace the diaper.
5. Cleanse and dry the perineum, and apply the adhesive portion of the collection bag.

Answer: _____

**1938.** The nurse is preparing the adolescent female for a renal/bladder ultrasound. Which explanation is **most** appropriate?

1. "Do not urinate before the procedure; a full bladder helps to identify important structures."
2. "Urinate immediately before the procedure; a full bladder impairs the viewing of important structures."
3. "You will be asked to urinate during the procedure to obtain the best results."
4. "A urinary catheter will be inserted to ensure that your bladder is empty during the test."

**1939.** MoC The nurse is taking a history of the 9-month-old. Which finding is **most** important for the nurse to report to the HCP for further follow-up?

1. The last diaper contained urine that was odorless.
2. The last diaper was stained with dark amber urine.
3. The child has not had a wet diaper in a 24-hour period.
4. Usual urinary output is about 250 mL per day.

**1940.** The nurse is caring for multiple clients preparing for placement of an external diversional urinary system. Which client has the greatest need for interventions to promote a positive body image?

1. The infant who has spina bifida
2. The toddler who is recently toilet trained
3. The school-aged child in foster care
4. The adolescent who is sexually active

**1941.** The nurse is caring for multiple clients. Which client would be **most** appropriate for the nurse to plan teaching about intermittent self-urinary catheterization?

1. The 15-year-old preparing to have a cesarean section
2. The 18-year-old newly diagnosed with MS
3. The 13-year-old with an SCI and no awareness of urge to void
4. The 16-year-old who is 8 months pregnant and reports dribbling

**1942.** The nurse is completing preoperative teaching with parents of the child who has hypospadias. Which principal objectives regarding surgical correction of hypospadias should be addressed? **Select all that apply.**

1. To preserve a sexually active organ
2. To correct an undescended testicle
3. To circumcise immediately after hypospadias is identified
4. To improve the physical appearance of the penis for psychological reasons
5. To enhance the child's ability to void a straight stream while in the standing position

**1943.** PHARM The nurse is educating the parent of the child with vesicoureteral reflux. The therapeutic use of which treatment is important to include in the teaching?

1. Steroidal therapy for at least 3 to 6 months
2. Acetaminophen three times daily for pelvic pain
3. Prophylactic antibiotics until the reflux resolves
4. Growth hormone injections to prevent ARF

**1944.** The nurse is teaching the parent of the male infant with phimosis. Which statement should the nurse include?

1. "Every day, retract the foreskin away from the glans penis to prevent urinary retention."
2. "Watch for and report enlargement of the testicles because fluid is likely to accumulate."
3. "Occasionally, the narrowing obstructs the flow of urine, resulting in a dribbling stream."
4. "Once the infant is older and begins toileting, urinating a straight stream will be impossible."

**1945.** MoC The nurse is assigned to care for the infant newly diagnosed with ambiguous genitalia. Which interventions should the nurse anticipate? **Select all that apply.**

1. Biochemical tests
2. Chromosome analysis
3. Radiographic contrast studies
4. Immediate surgical intervention
5. Referral to a pediatric urologist

**1946.** The nurse is caring for the child going home with an indwelling urinary catheter. Which important components should the nurse include in the discharge instructions? **Select all that apply.**

1. Keep the urine drainage bag below the level of the child's bladder.
2. Pull and tape the catheter securely down the length of the child's leg.
3. Have the child tub-bathe instead of showering to minimize standing time.
4. Reduce the child's fluid intake to limit the need for frequent bag emptying.
5. Ensure that the drainage bag does not rest on or touch the floor.

**1947.** The pediatric client requires clean intermittent catheterization while at home. Which early signs of infection should the nurse teach the parents to report **immediately?**

1. Tachypnea, tachycardia, hypertension
2. Mental confusion, diarrhea, dehydration
3. Increased appetite, anuria, sweet-smelling urine
4. Fever, pulse in the upper range of normal, foul-smelling urine

**1948.** The parent of the child with acute poststreptococcal glomerulonephritis is concerned about the child's ongoing care at home. What information should the nurse address? **Select all that apply.**

1. Recovery may take 2 years.
2. Return to pre-illness activities after discharge.
3. Avoid kissing to prevent spreading the infection.
4. The HCP will prescribe prophylactic antibiotics.
5. Weigh daily to check fluid retention or loss.
6. Give the prescribed BP-lowering drug if the diastolic BP exceeds 90 mm Hg.

**1949. MoC** The parent of the child recently diagnosed with acute poststreptococcal glomerulonephritis (APSGN) asks the new nurse about the usual prognosis. Which statement should the experienced nurse correct?

1. "All children with glomerulonephritis will develop chronic disease."
2. "Death from complications of APSGN may occur but fortunately are rare."
3. "Almost all children correctly diagnosed with APSGN recover completely."
4. "Specific immunity is conferred so that subsequent recurrences are uncommon."

**1950. MoC** The nurse caring for the hospitalized school-aged child writes a nursing problem of *altered urinary elimination* in the child's plan of care. Which outcome is **best** for the nurse to include?

1. Urinates six to eight times per day
2. Enuresis diminishes to every other day
3. Excretory function of the kidneys is improved
4. Ambulates to the bathroom independently

**1951. MoC** The 5-year-old with periorbital edema, anorexia, decreased urine output, and passage of cola-colored urine is brought to the ED by the parent. Which history information reported by the child's parent is **most** important to report to the HCP?

1. Fell from a skateboard the night before admission
2. Traveled from the U.S. to Europe a month ago
3. Had a "cold" 10 days prior to these symptoms
4. Ate new foods for the first time 2 days ago

**1952.** The nurse is reviewing the medical record of the school-aged child with acute glomerulonephritis (AGN) and finds that the child has proteinuria on UA and elevated serum BUN, creatinine, and uric acid levels. The child has had an elevated BP and low urine output for 24 hours. What should the nurse do **first**?

1. Contact the HCP.
2. Have the child drink more water.
3. Check the child's neurological status.
4. Document the findings in the medical record.

**1953. PHARM** The nurse is preparing to administer an analgesic for mild, short-term pain to the child who has a history of acute renal insufficiency. Which medication should the nurse select from the list of options in the HCP's symptom control protocol?

1. Ibuprofen
2. Meperidine
3. Acetaminophen
4. Morphine sulfate

**1954. PHARM** The nurse is evaluating whether treatment is effective for the 8-year-old with CRF who is receiving sevelamer hydrochloride. Place an X on each laboratory test result that indicates the medication is effective.

| Serum Laboratory Test | Client's Value | Normal Values |
|---|---|---|
| Potassium | 4.0 | 3.4–4.7 mEq/L |
| Calcium | 9.2 | 8.8–10.8 mg/dL |
| Phosphorus | 5.0 | 3.7–5.6 mg/dL |
| Albumin | 4.0 | 3.7–5.1 g/dL |
| RBCs | 4.9 | 3.89–4.96 m/mm³ |
| WBC | 15 | 4.5–11.1 K/microL or /mm3 |
| Hgb | 12 | 10.2–13.4 g/dL |
| Hct | 36% | 31.7%–39.3% |

**1955.** The pediatric client with chronic kidney disease (CKD) is hospitalized. The nurse should monitor for which associated complications? **Select all that apply.**

1. Anemia
2. Dehydration
3. Hypocalcemia
4. Osteodystrophy
5. Metabolic alkalosis

**1956.** The nurse is planning care for the child to be admitted for a hypospadias repair. Which illustration **best** reflects the nurse's critical thinking about the child's condition?

1.
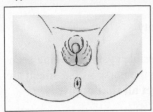

2.
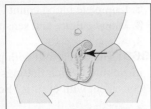

3.
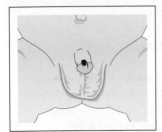

4.
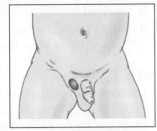

**1957.** MoC The nurse is assessing the genitalia of the 6-month-old male infant. Which documentation by the nurse is **most** accurate?

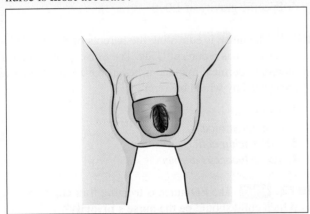

1. Hypospadias is noted on the upper area of the penis
2. Urethral opening is noted at the dorsum of the penis
3. Penis is normal in color, size, and appearance for a 6-month-old male
4. Ulcerations are present at tip of penis, extending almost to the foreskin

**1958.** PHARM The child is to receive 20 mcg intranasal desmopressin acetate (DDAVP) at bedtime for enuresis. DDAVP is supplied in a nasal spray pump of 10 mcg/spray in a 5-mL bottle (0.1 mg/mL), which contains 50 doses of DDAVP. How many nasal sprays should the nurse instruct the parent to deliver at bedtime?

_____ nasal sprays (Record your answer as a whole number.)

**1959.** The infant has an epispadias repair. Which interventions should the nurse include when noting that the infant has a urinary stent in place after the epispadias repair? **Select all that apply.**

1. Notifies the HCP if the penis becomes bluish-tinged
2. Notifies the HCP if the urine becomes blood-tinged
3. Sponge-bathes rather than immersing the infant in water
4. Places the distal end of the stent between a first and second applied diaper
5. Has the parent hold the infant by straddling on the parent's hip

**1960.** The pediatric client with CKD has elevations in serum creatinine and BUN. The nurse interprets this to mean that the child has a reduction in which component?

1. Growth hormone
2. Serum erythropoietin
3. Glomerular filtration rate
4. Blood flow to the kidneys

**1961.** MoC The ED nurse is triaging a group of pediatric clients. Which child should the nurse attend to **first**?

1. The child whose periorbital edema is worse in the morning
2. The previously well child who begins to gain weight insidiously over a few days
3. The child with a recent renal transplant who has hypertension and decreased urinary output
4. The child with fever, foul-smelling urine, dysuria, and frequency and urgency on urination

**1962.** The nurse is preparing peritoneal dialysis treatment for the 10-year-old. To promote a sense of control, what should the nurse allow the child to do?

1. Cleanse the abdomen before inserting the needle for the local anesthetic.
2. Select, from a list of options, liquids to drink during the dialysis procedure.
3. Play with a cloth doll that has a removable catheter inserted in the abdomen.
4. Play with a toy that is only allowed during the peritoneal dialysis procedure.

**1963.** The nurse is developing a teaching plan for the pediatric client and parents for home peritoneal dialysis. Which statement should the nurse **omit** from the teaching plan?

1. "The instilled solution remains for a variable length of time."
2. "A cooled solution is allowed to enter the peritoneal cavity by gravity."
3. "A sterile dialysis solution is instilled through a surgically implanted catheter."
4. "The solution is infused and the dialysate drained through a single catheter."

**1964.** The 9-year-old is to have a kidney transplant. What information should the nurse consider when preparing to teach the child and parents about the transplant? **Select all that apply.**

1. Eliminates dependence on dialysis
2. Restricted to blood relatives as donors
3. Eliminates the need for dietary restrictions
4. May result in rejection, hypertension, or infection
5. No activity restrictions once home

**1965.** **MoC** The nurse is assessing the 14-year-old who has a transplanted kidney. The nurse should notify the HCP when the child has which symptoms associated with organ rejection? **Select all that apply.**

1. Cloudy urine at 35 mL/hr
2. RR of 20 bpm
3. Serum creatinine of 0.9 mg/dL
4. BP of 142/92 mm Hg
5. Oral temperature of 101.8°F (38. 8°C)

**1966.** **PHARM** The 5-year-old who underwent a kidney transplant is receiving cyclosporine. Which laboratory finding should the nurse recognize as indicative that the treatment is having an adverse effect?

1. Hemoglobin of 9.0 g/dL
2. Total cholesterol of 220
3. Ammonia of 65 mg/dL
4. Random blood glucose of 60 mg/dL

**1967.** The nurse has completed teaching on strategies to prevent UTI recurrence with the female adolescent who is sexually active. Which statements made by the adolescent indicate that teaching was effective? **Select all that apply.**

1. "I should urinate after intercourse."
2. "I should be wearing silky underwear."
3. "I should drink 34 ounces of water daily."
4. "I should drink blueberry or cranberry juice."
5. "I should be sure that my partner uses a latex condom."

**1968.** The toilet-trained child presents with incontinence, strong-smelling urine, frequency, and urgency. What laboratory test should the nurse complete **first?**

1. Serum creatinine
2. Routine UA
3. Complete blood count
4. Blood culture and sensitivity

**1969.** The 6-year-old with possible cystitis is being seen in a clinic. Which findings in the nurse's assessment are consistent with cystitis? **Select all that apply.**

1. Enuresis
2. Hematuria
3. Suprapubic pain
4. Strong-smelling urine
5. Costovertebral angle tenderness

**1970.** **MoC** The 6-year-old with fever and painful urination is brought to the clinic by the parent. Which finding on a UA completed that morning is **most** important for the nurse to report to the HCP?

1. Hematuria
2. Urine pH of 6.5
3. Trace ketones
4. Specific gravity of 1.010

**1971.** The nurse is educating the parents of the pediatric client who has recurrent UTIs. The nurse's rationale for including perineal hygiene is because 80% of UTI cases are caused by which bacteria?

1. *Klebsiella*
2. *Candida albicans*
3. *Escherichia coli*
4. *Staphylococcus aureus*

**1972.** **MoC** The ED nurse is triaging four children. Which child should be the nurse's **priority?**

1. The child with vomiting and diarrhea for 24 hours
2. The child with a 3 cm facial laceration from a fall
3. The child with dyspnea and a palpable abdominal mass
4. The child with an oral temperature of 102.1°F (38.9°C)

**1973.** **PHARM** The child is hospitalized with nephrotic syndrome. Which medication should the nurse anticipate the HCP will prescribe to treat nephrotic syndrome?

1. Prednisone
2. Ibuprofen
3. Ampicillin
4. Hydrochlorothiazide

**1974.** The nurse is catheterizing the female adolescent. The nurse uses the nondominant hand to gently separate then pull up the labia minora to see the meatus. What should the nurse do next with the **nondominant hand?**

1. Pick up the sterile catheter 6 inches from the end.
2. Cleanse the urinary meatus with antiseptic swabs.
3. No longer use it during the procedure.
4. Continue separating the labia minora.

**1975.** MoC The child with ARF has not had a stool for a week. The resident physician prescribes a sodium biphosphate and sodium phosphate enema. What should the nurse do?

1. Administer the enema as prescribed by the resident physician.
2. Give the enema as prescribed after teaching is completed with the parent.
3. Give the enema as prescribed after consulting with another HCP.
4. Not give the enema and inform the resident physician of the enema's lethal risk.

**1976.** PHARM The 6-year-old with enuresis is to begin taking imipramine. The nurse should notify the HCP when the parent identifies that the child's history includes which problems? **Select all that apply.**

1. Asthma
2. Infantile seizures
3. Diabetes mellitus
4. Gastroesophageal reflux
5. Congenital heart disease

## Answers and Rationales

**1933. ANSWER: 3**

1. A urine culture will identify the presence of a UTI, is not specific to kidney function, and is not indicated at this time.
2. A CBC is not kidney function specific and is not indicated at this time.
3. **The elevated BUN and serum creatinine indicate abnormal kidney function; a UA is an additional study to further explore kidney function.**
4. Liver function tests are not indicated at this time because they are not specific to kidney function.

▶ *Test-taking Tip: Note that only the BUN and creatinine are abnormal. Thus, another kidney function test is needed next.*

Content Area: Child; Concept: Urinary Elimination; Critical Thinking; Integrated Processes: Nursing Process: Implementation; Client Needs: Physiological Integrity: Reduction of Risk Potential; Cognitive Level: Application [Applying]

**1934. ANSWER: 71**

**One mL of urine output equals 1 g of body weight. First, add the total weights of the diapers: 24 g + 24 g + 30 g + 31 g + 22 g + 30 g = 161 g. Next, determine the dry weight for 6 diapers: 15 g × 6 = 90 g. Finally, subtract the dry weight from the total weight of the diapers to determine the total urine output for 8 hours: 161 g − 90 g = 71 g. The 71 g of fluid loss equals 71 mL of urine output.**

▶ *Test-taking Tip: Use the equivalent of 1 mL of urine output equals 1 g of body weight to calculate the amount of urine output.*

Content Area: Child; Concept: Urinary Elimination; Assessment; Integrated Processes: Communication and Documentation; Client Needs: Physiological Integrity: Basic Care and Comfort; Cognitive Level: Application [Applying]

**1935. ANSWER: 2**

1. The BP is important to assess perfusion, but the parents may not allow the child to be touched without first communicating through an interpreter.
2. **The nurse first should request an interpreter because parental consent is needed for assessment and treatment of the child. Most major health care facilities have an on-site interpreter or on-demand remote video or telephone interpreting services.**
3. The genitalia may need to be inspected, but parental consent is needed first.
4. Blood and urine cultures may need to be obtained to determine if the child has a UTI or is septic or dehydrated, but an interpreter is needed first to explain the tests to the parents.

▶ *Test-taking Tip: Three options involve touching the child, and one is different. Often, the option that is different is the answer.*

Content Area: Child; Concept: Urinary Elimination; Diversity; Integrated Processes: Nursing Process: Implementation; Culture and Spirituality; Client Needs: Physiological Integrity: Reduction of Risk Potential; Cognitive Level: Application [Applying]

**1936. ANSWER: 2**

1. If the specimen is discarded, the test will need to be restarted.

2. At the end of the 24-hour period, the client is asked to void, and the urine is added to the container. This completes the 24-hour urine sample.

3. The final specimen should not be discarded.

4. It would be inappropriate to pour it into a new container unless the other container is full.

▶ *Test-taking Tip:* The key term is "24-hour."

**Content Area:** Child; **Concept:** Urinary Elimination; Nursing Roles; **Integrated Processes:** Nursing Process: Implementation; **Client Needs:** Physiological Integrity: Reduction of Risk Potential; **Cognitive Level:** Application [Applying]

### 1937. ANSWER: 2, 5, 1, 4, 3

2. **Explain the procedure to the parents, prepare supplies, and position the infant. Teaching and gathering supplies should be completed prior to the procedure to put the parent and infant at ease.**

5. **Cleanse and dry the perineum and apply the adhesive portion of the collection bag. The perineum must be cleansed and dried to ensure that the sample is not contaminated and that the adhesive sticks to the infant's skin.**

1. **Check that the bag adheres firmly around the perineal area. Adherence to skin is necessary to prevent urine leakage.**

4. **Carefully replace the diaper. It will help hold the collection bag in place.**

3. **Check the bag frequently and remove it as soon as urine is available. If a full bag is left in place, it will leak urine, which can irritate the skin.**

▶ *Test-taking Tip:* Visualize the steps prior to placing them in the correct order. Consider that the diaper should be replaced over the bag.

**Content Area:** Child; **Concept:** Urinary Elimination; Nursing Roles; **Integrated Processes:** Nursing Process: Planning; **Client Needs:** Physiological Integrity: Reduction of Risk Potential; **Cognitive Level:** Synthesis [Creating]

### 1938. ANSWER: 1

1. **During a renal ultrasound, a full bladder permits the best visualization of structures. The client should be informed to not urinate before the procedure.**

2. Voiding before the procedure is not recommended.

3. Voiding during the procedure is not recommended.

4. A urinary catheter would not be inserted because it would empty the bladder and structures would not be as visible.

▶ *Test-taking Tip:* Because three options involve an empty bladder and not all can be correct, the three should be eliminated.

**Content Area:** Child; **Concept:** Urinary Elimination; Nursing Roles; **Integrated Processes:** Teaching/Learning; **Client Needs:** Physiological Integrity: Reduction of Risk Potential; Psychosocial Integrity; **Cognitive Level:** Application [Applying]

### 1939. MoC ANSWER: 3

1. Infants often have odorless urine.

2. Dark amber urine may require more inquiry, although it is not the most important finding to report.

3. **Anuria, or lack of urine production, may be a sign of altered renal function.**

4. Output for a 9-month-old is usually between 250 and 500 mL daily.

▶ *Test-taking Tip:* The key phrase is "most important," indicating that more than one option may be correct but one is more critical than the others.

**Content Area:** Child; **Concept:** Urinary Elimination; Fluid and Electrolyte Balance; Management; **Integrated Processes:** Communication and Documentation; **Client Needs:** Safe and Effective Care Environment: Management of Care; **Cognitive Level:** Application [Applying]

### 1940. ANSWER: 4

1. An infant's developmental stage is trust versus mistrust. The infant is unaware of body alterations.

2. A toddler's developmental level is autonomy versus shame and doubt; the child could be at risk for altered body image, depending on the response of parents and others.

3. A school-aged child's developmental level is industry versus inferiority. The child would be at risk for body image disturbance if unable to develop competence with the device or if unable to achieve a sense of wholeness (one of Havighurst's developmental tasks).

4. **Because of the client's developmental stage and sexual activity status, an external urinary device places the adolescent at the greatest risk for body image disturbance, and thus this client has the greatest need for intervention. Developmentally, according to Havighurst, an adolescent's developmental task is to accept one's physique and use the body effectively; according to Erikson, the adolescent's task is to achieve a coherent sense of self.**

▶ *Test-taking Tip:* Think about the developmental stage of each individual before making a selection. The key phrase is "greatest need."

**Content Area:** Child; **Concept:** Self; Development; Promoting Health; **Integrated Processes:** Caring; Nursing Process: Evaluation; **Client Needs:** Health Promotion and Maintenance; **Cognitive Level:** Evaluation [Evaluating]

### 1941. ANSWER: 3

1. The 15-year-old would need only temporary indwelling urinary catheterization.

2. The 18-year-old newly diagnosed with MS likely would not have bladder involvement requiring intermittent catheterization. This may occur later in the disease process.

3. **The 13-year-old with SCI and no awareness of urge to void would require a means to empty the bladder.**

4. Dribbling is common in the third trimester of pregnancy. Catheterization should be avoided.

▶ **Test-taking Tip:** *The key word is "intermittent." You should find the commonalities in the options and eliminate these.*

**Content Area:** Child; **Concept:** Urinary Elimination; Mobility; Nursing Roles; **Integrated Processes:** Nursing Process: Planning; **Client Needs:** Physiological Integrity: Basic Care and Comfort; **Cognitive Level:** Analysis [Analyzing]

## 1942. ANSWER: 1, 4, 5

1. **Because the penis will be operated on during surgery, a surgical objective is to preserve its ability to be a sexually active organ.**
2. An undescended testicle is unrelated to hypospadias repair.
3. Circumcision may be delayed to save the foreskin for use in the hypospadias repair, if needed.
4. **The principal objectives of hypospadias repair include improving the physical appearance of the genitalia for psychological reasons.**
5. **In hypospadias, the urethra does not properly exit the penis at the tip. It can be a mild defect, with the urethral opening slightly out of place, or a severe defect, with the urethral opening closer to the scrotum. The objectives of the repair include voiding enhancement.**

▶ **Test-taking Tip:** *You should narrow the options by identifying the commonality involving the penis in the options.*

**Content Area:** Child; **Concept:** Male Reproduction; Sexuality; Urinary Elimination; **Integrated Processes:** Teaching/Learning; **Client Needs:** Physiological Integrity: Physiological Adaptation; **Cognitive Level:** Analysis [Analyzing]

## 1943. PHARM ANSWER: 3

1. Steroids are anti-inflammatory agents and are unnecessary.
2. High doses of acetaminophen can lead to renal impairment.
3. **Vesicoureteral reflux is the retrograde flow of urine from the bladder into the ureters due to an incompetent valve that does not prevent backflow. Because urine is retained in the ureters after voiding, stasis of this urine leads to infection. This is managed with prophylactic antibiotic therapy until the condition resolves.**
4. Growth hormone (GH) injections are used to treat a deficiency of GH, which is unrelated.

▶ **Test-taking Tip:** *Use knowledge of medical terminology. "Reflux" means backflow, and "ureteral" refers to ureters. Think about the effects of backflow on the ureters.*

**Content Area:** Child; **Concept:** Urinary Elimination; Infection; Nursing Roles; **Integrated Processes:** Teaching/Learning; **Client Needs:** Physiological Integrity: Pharmacological and Parenteral Therapies; Physiological Integrity: Reduction of Risk Potential; **Cognitive Level:** Application [Applying]

## 1944. ANSWER: 3

1. In phimosis, the foreskin already is retracted and causing the urinary problems.
2. Fluid does not accumulate in the testicles with phimosis; a hydrocele is the presence of fluid in the sac surrounding the testicles that causes an enlarged scrotum.
3. **Phimosis is a narrowing of the preputial opening that prevents retraction of the foreskin over the glans penis. Occasionally, the narrowing obstructs the flow of urine, resulting in a dribbling stream or the foreskin ballooning with accumulated urine during voiding.**
4. Hypospadias is a condition in which the urethral opening is located below the glans penis or anywhere along the ventral surface. If not corrected, a straight stream may not be possible. Hypospadias is unrelated to phimosis.

▶ **Test-taking Tip:** *The suffix "-osis" is the key in the stem. To identify the answer, relate it to something you already know such as "fibrosis," which causes a narrowing.*

**Content Area:** Child; **Concept:** Urinary Elimination; Nursing Roles; **Integrated Processes:** Teaching/Learning; **Client Needs:** Physiological Integrity: Physiological Adaptation; **Cognitive Level:** Application [Applying]

## 1945. MoC ANSWERS: 1, 2, 3, 5

1. **Biochemical tests help detect adrenocortical syndromes and are important components of the assessment to determine gender assignment.**
2. **Chromosome analysis will help determine chromosome abnormalities and precise genetic karyotype to help determine gender assignment.**
3. **Radiographic contrast studies are completed to identify the presence, absence, or nature of internal genital and urinary structures to help determine gender assignment.**
4. The assignment of a gender followed by immediate surgical intervention was the traditional treatment approach for ambiguous genitalia. A multidisciplinary team approach now is used to assign gender, and surgical reconstruction may be delayed to avoid irreversible surgical interventions.
5. **A referral to a specialist such as a pediatric urologist is necessary so the identification of appropriate gender is completed with precision and accuracy.**

▶ **Test-taking Tip:** *Consider ramifications of all options and delete the one that can have irreversible consequences.*

**Content Area:** Child; **Concept:** Male Reproduction; Female Reproduction; Sexuality; Management; **Integrated Processes:** Nursing Process: Planning; **Client Needs:** Safe and Effective Care Environment: Management of Care; Physiological Integrity: Physiological Adaptation; **Cognitive Level:** Application [Applying]

### 1946. ANSWER: 1, 5

1. **Keeping the drainage bag below the level of the bladder prevents reflux of urine into the bladder, which increases the risk of bladder infection.**
2. Placing tension on the catheter increases the risk of injury to the urinary meatus.
3. Showering rather than bathing minimizes the risk for contaminating the urinary drainage bag.
4. Fluid intake should be increased to reduce bacterial growth.
5. **The floor harbors many microorganisms. Allowing the bag to touch or rest on the floor increases the risk for a bladder infection.**

♦ **Test-taking Tip:** Focus on options that reduce the child's risk for infection.

**Content Area:** Child; **Concept:** Urinary Elimination; Promoting Health; Infection; **Integrated Processes:** Teaching/Learning; **Client Needs:** Safe and Effective Care Environment: Safety and Infection Control; Health Promotion and Maintenance; **Cognitive Level:** Application [Applying]

### 1947. ANSWER: 4

1. Elevated RR, pulse, and BP could be related to infection but would not likely be the early signs parents would be instructed to monitor.
2. Symptoms such as mental confusion, diarrhea, and dehydration would not be early signs of infection.
3. Changes in appetite and the odor of urine could be signs of infection or other conditions and need to be properly evaluated. Anuria, or the absence of urine production, requires immediate evaluation and intervention but is not an early sign of infection.
4. **Fever, increased pulse rate, and foul-smelling urine are early signs of infection that the parent should report to the HCP immediately.**

♦ **Test-taking Tip:** "Early signs of infection" are the key words in the stem. Avoid selecting options indicating later signs of infection.

**Content Area:** Child; **Concept:** Urinary Elimination; Infection; Promoting Health; **Integrated Processes:** Teaching/Learning; **Client Needs:** Safe and Effective Care Environment: Safety and Infection Control; **Cognitive Level:** Application [Applying]

### 1948. ANSWER: 1, 5, 6

1. **The recovery period may be as long as 2 years in AGN.**
2. Fatigue may restrict a return to the previous activity level. After 1 to 2 weeks, the child can attend school and engage in normal activities; however, competitive activities should be avoided because these stress the kidneys.
3. Acute poststreptococcal glomerulonephritis is not infectious; it is caused by an antigen-antibody inflammatory response to a past infection.
4. Antibiotics are usually ineffective because the disease is caused not by an active infection, but by an antigen-antibody inflammatory response to a past infection.
5. **The best indicator of fluid loss or retention is daily weight. Salt restriction may be needed to control edema, but most children do well on a normal diet with normal salt and protein content.**
6. **Antihypertensive therapy with calcium channel blockers is used to treat a diastolic BP >90 mm Hg.**

♦ **Test-taking Tip:** The word "poststreptococcal" is key to eliminating and narrowing the options.

**Content Area:** Child; **Concept:** Urinary Elimination; Inflammation; Nursing Roles; **Integrated Processes:** Teaching/Learning; **Client Needs:** Physiological Integrity: Physiological Adaptation; Health Promotion and Maintenance; **Cognitive Level:** Application [Applying]

### 1949. MoC ANSWER: 1

1. **A few children with APSGN will develop chronic disease, but many of these cases are believed to be different glomerular diseases misdiagnosed as poststreptococcal disease.**
2. Death from complications of APSGN may occur but fortunately are rare. This statement is correct.
3. Almost all children correctly diagnosed with APSGN recover completely. This statement is correct.
4. Specific immunity is conferred so that subsequent recurrences are uncommon in APSGN. This statement is correct.

♦ **Test-taking Tip:** When a definitive word such as "all" is used in an option, it is almost always an incorrect statement. This is a false-response item, so select the option that is an incorrect statement.

**Content Area:** Child; **Concept:** Urinary Elimination; Nursing Roles; **Integrated Processes:** Nursing Process: Evaluation; **Client Needs:** Safe and Effective Care Environment: Management of Care; Physiological Integrity: Reduction of Risk Potential; **Cognitive Level:** Evaluation [Evaluating]

### 1950. MoC ANSWER: 1

1. **The elimination system reaches maturity during school age, so the child should urinate six to eight times per day.**
2. Enuresis is no longer expected in this age group.
3. Improved excretory function is not measurable; thus, 1 is a better option.
4. Ambulating to the bathroom independently relates to mobility and not urinary elimination.

♦ **Test-taking Tip:** Use the nursing process step of evaluation to identify the option that is measurable and pertains to urinary elimination.

**Content Area:** Child; **Concept:** Urinary Elimination; Nursing Roles; **Integrated Processes:** Nursing Process: Evaluation; **Client Needs:** Physiological Integrity: Basic Care and Comfort; Safe and Effective Care Environment: Management of Care; **Cognitive Level:** Synthesis [Creating]

### 1951. MoC ANSWER: 3

1. A fall is not likely to cause kidney injury; if injury to the kidneys were to occur, the child also would have flank pain.

2. Exposure to an infectious disease could have occurred during travel a month ago, and the travel should be reported, but having a recent cold is most important to report.

3. **Periorbital edema, anorexia, and cola-colored urine (also tea-colored, reddish-brown, or smoky from hematuria) are the initial signs of nephrotic reaction in a child with AGN. Often, the child has been in good health with no history of infection except for symptoms described as a mild cold approximately 10 days before onset.**

4. The symptoms can be seen with an allergic reaction to food, but the onset would not be delayed by 2 days.

▶ *Test-taking Tip: The time periods in the options are significant in answering the question correctly.*

**Content Area:** Child; **Concept:** Urinary Elimination; Infection; **Integrated Processes:** Nursing Process: Analysis; **Client Needs:** Safe and Effective Care Environment: Management of Care; Physiological Integrity: Reduction of Risk Potential; **Cognitive Level:** Analysis [Analyzing]

### 1952. ANSWER: 3

1. The HCP should be contacted only after the child has been assessed by the nurse.

2. The increased BUN, serum creatinine and uric acid levels and proteinuria on UA are due to the accumulation of the by-products of metabolism from the failing renal function. Fluids usually would be limited.

3. **Hypertensive encephalopathy is a major complication that can occur during the acute phase of AGN. The child's neurological status should be assessed before notifying the HCP because the findings may affect the treatment plan.**

4. Documenting the findings is important, but the client is priority.

▶ *Test-taking Tip: Use the nursing process to determine the priority. Assessment is the first step.*

**Content Area:** Child; **Concept:** Urinary Elimination; Assessment; **Integrated Processes:** Nursing Process: Assessment; **Client Needs:** Physiological Integrity: Reduction of Risk Potential; **Cognitive Level:** Analysis [Analyzing]

### 1953. PHARM ANSWER: 3

1. Ibuprofen (Motrin) could contribute to renal impairment.

2. Meperidine (Demerol) is a narcotic analgesic and is best used for moderate to severe pain.

3. **Acetaminophen (Tylenol) is an appropriate analgesic for short-term, mild to moderate pain and will not contribute to the child's renal insufficiency.**

4. Morphine sulfate is a narcotic analgesic and is best used for moderate to severe pain.

▶ *Test-taking Tip: The key phrases are "short-term mild pain" and "renal insufficiency." Apply knowledge of pharmacology to eliminate all but Option 3.*

**Content Area:** Child; **Concept:** Medication; Comfort; Urinary Elimination; **Integrated Processes:** Nursing Process: Implementation; **Client Needs:** Physiological Integrity: Pharmacological and Parenteral Therapies; **Cognitive Level:** Application [Applying]

### 1954. PHARM ANSWER:

| Calcium | 9.2 **X** | 8.8–10.8 mg/dL |
|---|---|---|
| Phosphorus | 5.0 **X** | 3.7–5.6 mg/dL |

**Sevelamer hydrochloride (Renagel, Renvela) reduces absorption of phosphorus from the intestines. It will elevate the serum calcium level, thus decreasing the serum phosphorus level. Phosphorus is elevated in CRF because the kidneys are unable to excrete it.**

▶ *Test-taking Tip: If unsure, consider the kidney's role in excreting phosphorus and the inverse relationship between phosphorus and calcium.*

**Content Area:** Child; **Concept:** Urinary Elimination; **Integrated Processes:** Nursing Process: Evaluation; **Client Needs:** Physiological Integrity: Pharmacological and Parenteral Therapies; **Cognitive Level:** Evaluation [Evaluating]

### 1955. ANSWER: 1, 2, 3, 4

1. **Erythropoietin, which is formed by the kidneys, stimulates RBC production. Anemia develops with decreased erythropoietin and RBC production.**

2. **The few functioning nephrons cannot reabsorb enough sodium to maintain a functioning level of body fluid, so dehydration occurs.**

3. **Hypocalcemia and hyperphosphatemia occur due to the kidney's inability to excrete phosphate.**

4. **Osteodystrophy (bone disease) occurs as calcium is withdrawn from bones to compensate for hypocalcemia.**

5. Metabolic acidosis, not alkalosis, is caused by the kidney's inability to excrete hydrogen ion.

▶ *Test-taking Tip: Avoid reading options too quickly. Sometimes they state the opposite of what would be expected.*

**Content Area:** Child; **Concept:** Urinary Elimination; Fluid and Electrolyte Balance; Hematologic Regulation; **Integrated Processes:** Nursing Process: Planning; **Client Needs:** Physiological Integrity: Physiological Adaptation; **Cognitive Level:** Application [Applying]

### 1956. ANSWER: 2

1. Option 1 is ambiguous genitalia; the external reproductive organs cannot be easily identified as male or female. Note the urethra on the testicle.

2. **Hypospadias is a congenital anomaly involving the abnormal location of the urethral meatus on the ventral surface of the penis.**

3. In epispadias (Option 3), the urethral opening is on the dorsal surface of the penis.

4. Option 4 is undescended testicle and is unrelated to epispadias.

▶ *Test-taking Tip: Use the prefix "hypo-" as a cue to select the correct option.*

Content Area: Child; Concept: Male Reproduction; Assessment; Urinary Elimination; Integrated Processes: Nursing Process: Planning; Client Needs: Physiological Integrity: Physiological Adaptation; Cognitive Level: Application [Applying]

### 1957. MoC ANSWER: 2

1. The urethral opening in hypospadias is on the lower aspect or underside of the penis.
2. **The child is presenting with an epispadias. In epispadias the urethra ends in an opening on the upper aspect (the dorsum) of the penis. This documentation is accurate.**
3. The penis is malformed because of the presence of an epispadias, and not normal.
4. The reddened area is the urethral opening and not ulcerations.

▶ *Test-taking Tip: Recall that "dorsum" means upper. Carefully analyze the illustration to select the correct option.*

Content Area: Child; Concept: Male Reproduction; Assessment; Urinary Elimination; Integrated Processes: Communication and Documentation; Client Needs: Safe and Effective Care Environment: Management of Care; Cognitive Level: Analysis [Analyzing]

### 1958. PHARM ANSWER: 2

**Use a proportion formula:**
$$10 \text{ mcg} : 1 \text{ spray} :: 20 \text{ mcg} : X \text{ spray}; 10X = 20;$$
$$X = 20 \div 10; X = 2$$

▶ *Test-taking Tip: Carefully read the question and data provided to determine what is being asked. Sometimes more information is provided than is necessary for a drug calculation because the medication may contain all this information on the label.*

Content Area: Child; Concept: Medication; Safety; Urinary Elimination; Integrated Processes: Nursing Process: Implementation; Teaching/Learning; Client Needs: Physiological Integrity: Pharmacological and Parenteral Therapies; Cognitive Level: Application [Applying]

### 1959. ANSWER: 1, 3, 4

1. **A bluish-tinged discoloration of the penis could indicate impaired circulation.**
2. The urine will be blood-tinged for several days after surgery. The HCP should not be notified of an expected finding.
3. **Immersion in water when a stent is in place increases the risk for a UTI.**
4. **The stent should be placed between the first and second diaper placed on the infant. In double diapering, the inner diaper collects stool, and the outer diaper collects urine from the draining stent.**
5. Straddling the infant on the parent's hip can dislodge the stent.

▶ *Test-taking Tip: Eliminate any options that can increase the risk of dislodging the stent or that include normal findings.*

Content Area: Child; Concept: Urinary Elimination; Integrated Processes: Nursing Process: Implementation; Client Needs: Physiological Integrity: Reduction of Risk Potential; Cognitive Level: Application [Applying]

### 1960. ANSWER: 3

1. GH is an anabolic hormone that promotes protein application and mobilizes glucose and free fatty acids; it will not affect serum creatinine and BUN.
2. Serum erythropoietin is a measurement of the degree of hormonal stimulation to the bone marrow to release RBCs; it will not affect serum creatinine or BUN.
3. **A reduction in GFR results in an accumulation of nitrogenous wastes. This is reflected in an elevation of serum creatinine and BUN.**
4. Reduced blood flow to the kidneys is but one cause of CKD; other causes also can elevate serum creatinine and BUN.

▶ *Test-taking Tip: Think about the function of the kidneys in filtering urine. Then use the process of elimination to exclude all options but number 3. The other options do not relate to filtering urine.*

Content Area: Child; Concept: Urinary Elimination; Critical Thinking; Integrated Processes: Nursing Process: Analysis; Client Needs: Physiological Integrity: Reduction of Risk Potential; Cognitive Level: Application [Applying]

### 1961. MoC ANSWER: 3

1. This child likely has AGN. Almost all clients with this condition who are properly diagnosed and treated will recover completely.
2. This child likely has nephrotic syndrome, and the prognosis for ultimate recovery is good in most cases.
3. **The child with recent renal transplantation who has hypertension and decreased urinary output needs to be evaluated immediately for possible rejection.**
4. This child likely has a UTI. Adequate treatment at the time of diagnosis usually results in an excellent prognosis.

▶ *Test-taking Tip: Use the ABC's to determine the child who should be attended to first.*

Content Area: Child; Concept: Urinary Elimination; Safety; Critical Thinking; Integrated Processes: Nursing Process: Assessment; Client Needs: Safe and Effective Care Environment: Management of Care; Safe and Effective Care Environment: Safety and Infection Control; Cognitive Level: Analysis [Analyzing]

### 1962. ANSWER: 2

1. Allowing the 10-year-old to cleanse the abdomen is not the best option. The nurse needs to ensure sterility of supplies and prevent infection.
2. **Because the bulk of peritoneal fluid causes pressure on the stomach and causes a feeling of fullness, the child is provided with a liquid diet or small, frequent feedings. Allowing the child to choose the preferred, allowable liquid ensures a sense of control.**
3. Therapeutic play is used to enhance self-esteem and reduce anxiety.
4. Playing with a toy allowed only during dialysis helps to reduce boredom.

▶ **Test-taking Tip:** *The key words are "sense of control." Consider the safest action that allows the child a choice.*

**Content Area:** Child; **Concept:** Development; Urinary Elimination; Safety; **Integrated Processes:** Nursing Process: Implementation; Caring; **Client Needs:** Physiological Integrity: Physiological Adaptation; Psychosocial Integrity; **Cognitive Level:** Application [Applying]

## 1963. ANSWER: 2

1. The "dwell" time (time in the peritoneal cavity) varies by the type of PD.
2. **In PD, a warmed and not cooled solution enters by gravity. The solution is warmed to prevent a decrease in core body temperature. This incorrect statement should be omitted from the teaching plan.**
3. The sterile dialysis solution is instilled through a surgically implanted catheter into the peritoneal cavity. The catheter has an access device on the abdomen for attachment of the dialysis solution tubing.
4. A single catheter is used to infuse and drain the dialysis solution.

▶ **Test-taking Tip:** *The key word in the stem is "omit." An option that is incorrect would be excluded from the teaching plan.*

**Content Area:** Child; **Concept:** Urinary Elimination; Nursing Roles; **Integrated Processes:** Teaching/Learning; **Client Needs:** Safe and Effective Care Environment: Safety and Infection Control; **Cognitive Level:** Synthesis [Creating]

## 1964. ANSWER: 1, 3, 4

1. **Transplant does eliminate dependence on dialysis. However, dialysis may be used postoperatively, depending on the type of kidney donor.**
2. Kidney transplant donors are not restricted to blood relatives. The organs may come from living, asystolic, or deceased donors. Blood and tissue typing are completed to determine a match to prevent rejection.
3. **Kidney transplant eliminates the need to restrict the diet because the new organ should be able to remove nitrogenous wastes and assume the function lost by the diseased kidneys.**
4. **Kidney transplant may result in rejection, hypertension, or infection. The nurse needs to address signs and symptoms of these in postoperative teaching.**
5. Contact sports and other activities that could damage the kidney transplant will not be allowed.

▶ **Test-taking Tip:** *You should look for key words in the options when answering the question.*

**Content Area:** Child; **Concept:** Urinary Elimination; Nursing Roles; **Integrated Processes:** Nursing Process: Planning; **Client Needs:** Physiological Integrity: Reduction of Risk Potential; **Cognitive Level:** Application [Applying]

## 1965. MoC ANSWER: 4, 5

1. Cloudy urine may indicate a UTI, but not rejection.
2. The RR is WNL.
3. A serum creatinine of 0.9 mg/dL is normal for this age group.
4. **A BP of 142/92 mm Hg is high and may be associated with rejection.**
5. **An oral temperature of 101.8°F (38.8°C) represents fever, which is a sign of organ rejection.**

▶ **Test-taking Tip:** *Not all abnormal findings may be associated with a transplant rejection.*

**Content Area:** Child; **Concept:** Urinary Elimination; Collaboration; **Integrated Processes:** Nursing Process: Analysis; **Client Needs:** Safe and Effective Care Environment: Management of Care; **Cognitive Level:** Application [Applying]

## 1966. PHARM ANSWER: 1

1. **Hgb of 9.0 g/dL indicates anemia in a child this age and is an adverse effect related to the use of cyclosporine (Gengraf, Neoral, Sandimmune).**
2. Total cholesterol of 220 is normal for a 5-year-old.
3. An ammonia level of 65 mg/dL is normal for a 5-year-old.
4. A random blood glucose of 60 mg/dL is normal for a 5-year-old.

▶ **Test-taking Tip:** *Recall that clients with organ transplants are on long-term immunosuppression and that those medications generally have some amount of bone marrow depression associated with their use.*

**Content Area:** Child; **Concept:** Cellular Regulation; Medication; **Integrated Processes:** Nursing Process: Evaluation; **Client Needs:** Physiological Integrity: Pharmacological and Parenteral Therapies; **Cognitive Level:** Evaluation [Evaluating]

## 1967. ANSWER: 1, 4

1. **Voiding after intercourse helps to flush bacteria that may be present on the urethra.**
2. Cotton underwear is recommended rather than silk; silky underwear holds moisture and can promote bacterial growth.
3. Drinking 34 ounces of water daily is insufficient and amounts to a little over a liter. The adolescent should be consuming 2 to 3 liters of fluid daily.
4. **Blueberry and cranberry juice reduce bacterial adherence to the epithelial lining of the urinary tract.**
5. While condoms may prevent STIs, they do not prevent UTIs.

▶ **Test-taking Tip:** *Select options that are nonirritating and prevent bacterial growth.*

**Content Area:** Child; **Concept:** Urinary Elimination; Nursing Roles; **Integrated Processes:** Nursing Process: Evaluation; **Client Needs:** Health Promotion and Maintenance; **Cognitive Level:** Evaluation [Evaluating]

## 1968. ANSWER: 2

1. Serum creatinine evaluates kidney function. It may be part of the workup for this child but would not be the first test to be performed.
2. **Incontinence in a toilet-trained child, strong-smelling urine, frequency, and urgency are signs that should be evaluated for UTI. Routine UA is the first test to be performed. If the UA results suggest a UTI, then a urine specimen should be obtained through catheterization.**
3. A CBC is a test that may be used to evaluate for infection as it includes a WBC count, although it is unlikely it would be the first specimen collected by the nurse.
4. A urine culture and sensitivity may be obtained to evaluate for the presence of bacteria and determine appropriate antibiotic therapy, but a blood culture would not be necessary unless the child has an elevated temperature and other symptoms of sepsis.

♦ *Test-taking Tip: In a priority question, more than one option is correct, but one must be performed first. Options 1, 3, and 4 are all serum tests, whereas Option 2 pertains to the urine. The UA is also the least invasive, not requiring a blood draw.*

Content Area: Child; Concept: Urinary Elimination; Integrated Processes: Nursing Process: Planning; Client Needs: Physiological Integrity: Reduction of Risk Potential; Cognitive Level: Application [Applying]

## 1969. ANSWER: 1, 2, 3, 4

1. **Enuresis (bedwetting in a previously toilet-trained child) is due to inflammatory edema in the bladder wall that stimulates stretch receptors, producing urgency and frequency.**
2. **Hematuria (bloody urine) occurs due to bacterial infection and inflammation of the urethra and bladder wall.**
3. **Suprapubic pain is caused by inflammation and other effects of bacteria on the urethra and bladder wall.**
4. **Strong-smelling urine results from the accumulation of nitrates.**
5. Costovertebral angle tenderness is seen with an upper UTI such as pyelonephritis.

♦ *Test-taking Tip: Eliminate any option that pertains to an upper UTI.*

Content Area: Child; Concept: Urinary Elimination; Assessment; Integrated Processes: Nursing Process: Assessment; Client Needs: Physiological Integrity: Physiological Adaptation; Cognitive Level: Comprehension [Understanding]

## 1970. MoC ANSWER: 1

1. **Hematuria (RBCs in the urine) is an abnormal finding and should be reported, as it may be a sign of infection.**
2. Urine pH of 6.5 is within normal range (normal = 5–9). Urine is slightly acid in the morning (pH = 6.5–7.0) and more alkaline by evening (pH = 7.5–8.0).

3. Trace ketones may be abnormal but could be a result of mild dehydration.
4. Specific gravity of 1.010 is within normal range (normal = 1.001–1.029).

♦ *Test-taking Tip: Three options are similar, and one is different. Often the option that is different is the answer.*

Content Area: Child; Concept: Urinary Elimination; Integrated Processes: Nursing Process: Assessment; Client Needs: Safe and Effective Care Environment: Management of Care; Cognitive Level: Application [Applying]

## 1971. ANSWER: 3

1. *Klebsiella* is a gram-negative bacterium normally found in the mouth, skin, and intestinal tract, where it initially does not cause disease. It accounts for a small number of UTIs, generally in older women.
2. *Candida albicans* is not bacterial; it is fungal and can cause a yeast infection.
3. **The perineal area and urethra easily can become contaminated with *Escherichia coli* from fecal material. The bacterium is responsible for 80% of UTI cases.**
4. *Staphylococcus aureus*, present on the skin, accounts for a small number of UTIs.

♦ *Test-taking Tip: Use the memory aid of the "c" in each word to remember the bacteria commonly associated with UTIs:* <u>c</u>olon = E.<u>c</u>oli.

Content Area: Child; Concept: Urinary Elimination; Infection; Integrated Processes: Teaching/Learning; Client Needs: Safe and Effective Care Environment: Safety and Infection Control; Cognitive Level: Knowledge [Remembering]

## 1972. MoC ANSWER: 3

1. Vomiting and diarrhea are important to address, but this is not the priority.
2. Facial lacerations may require suturing, but this is not the priority.
3. **The nurse's priority should be the child who has dyspnea, which suggests respiratory compromise, and a palpable mass. The most common presenting sign of Wilms' tumor is a swelling or mass in the abdomen. Priority nursing care involves ensuring swift diagnosis and surgical intervention.**
4. Fever is important to address, but this is not the priority.

♦ *Test-taking Tip: Use the ABC's to determine priority. Option 3 is the only one that presents with oxygenation issues.*

Content Area: Child; Concept: Safety; Assessment; Critical Thinking; Integrated Processes: Nursing Process: Analysis; Client Needs: Safe and Effective Care Environment: Management of Care; Physiological Integrity: Reduction of Risk Potential; Cognitive Level: Evaluation [Evaluating]

## 1973. PHARM ANSWER: 1

1. **An immunological mechanism is involved in nephrotic syndrome. Corticosteroids such as prednisone (Deltasone) reduce inflammation and proteinuria. A corticosteroid is given until diuresis without protein loss is accomplished.**

2. Ibuprofen (Motrin) is an NSAID used to treat mild inflammation.

3. Ampicillin (Principen) is an antibiotic used to treat infection. Infection is not the cause of nephrotic syndrome.

4. Hydrochlorothiazide (Microzide, Oretic) is a thiazide diuretic used to treat hypertension or edema. It is not commonly used because it tends to decrease blood volume, which already is decreased in nephrotic syndrome.

▶ *Test-taking Tip: Two medications are similar in action, but one is more therapeutic than the other.*

Content Area: Child; Concept: Medication; Inflammation; Urinary Elimination; Integrated Processes: Nursing Process: Planning; Client Needs: Physiological Integrity: Pharmacological and Parenteral Therapies; Cognitive Level: Application [Applying]

## 1974. ANSWER: 4

1. The nondominant hand is no longer sterile after touching the skin and should not be used to pick up the sterile catheter.

2. Without visualization of the meatus because the hand has now moved to the swabs, it would be difficult to cleanse the urinary meatus adequately.

3. The hand needs to remain for the duration of the procedure to continue separating the labia. This hand cannot be used to pick up sterile materials.

4. **In catheterizing the female client, the nurse uses the nondominant hand to continue to gently separate and then pull up the labia minora. This visualizes the meatus for cleansing and then catheter insertion.**

▶ *Test-taking Tip: Visualize the steps in performing a sterile catheterization before making a selection. The key words in the stem are "nondominant hand" and not "next."*

Content Area: Child; Concept: Urinary Elimination; Nursing Roles; Integrated Processes: Nursing Process: Implementation; Client Needs: Safe and Effective Care Environment: Safety and Infection Control; Cognitive Level: Application [Applying]

## 1975. MoC ANSWER: 4

1. The enema should not be administered.

2. Teaching the parent is irrelevant when the enema should not be administered.

3. Consulting with another HCP does not prevent a lethal error.

4. **The use of a sodium biphosphate and sodium phosphate enema (Fleet) in a child with ARF is potentially lethal due to the kidneys' inability to excrete phosphate and the resulting hyperphosphatemia. The enema should not be given, and the resident should be informed of its lethal risk.**

▶ *Test-taking Tip: When three options are similar and one is different, the different option is likely the answer.*

Content Area: Child; Concept: Urinary Elimination; Critical Thinking; Safety; Integrated Processes: Nursing Process: Implementation; Client Needs: Safe and Effective Care Environment: Management of Care; Cognitive Level: Application [Applying]

## 1976. PHARM ANSWER: 2, 5

1. Imipramine is not contraindicated when the client has a history of asthma.

2. **Imipramine (Tofranil) is contraindicated in clients with seizure disorders. The nurse should clarify whether the medication is safe if the child had infantile seizures.**

3. Imipramine is not contraindicated when the client has a history of DM.

4. Imipramine is not contraindicated when the client has a history of GERD.

5. **TCAs such as imipramine may cause dysthymias and are contraindicated in heart disease unless their use has been cleared by a specialist who has noted that the child does not have a QTc prolongation. The nurse should notify the HCP.**

▶ *Test-taking Tip: TCAs are used in the treatment of enuresis in children but are contraindicated with certain neurological and cardiac conditions.*

Content Area: Child; Concept: Urinary Elimination; Medication; Integrated Processes: Nursing Process: Implementation; Client Needs: Physiological Integrity: Pharmacological and Parenteral Therapies; Cognitive Level: Application [Applying]

## Chapter Forty-Five

# Respiratory Management

**1977.** The child with a sore throat is hospitalized with a tentative diagnosis of epiglottitis. Which diagnostic test result should the nurse plan to review?

1. Blood culture
2. Throat culture
3. Lateral neck x-ray
4. Complete blood count

**1978.** **PHARM** The nurse completes teaching the parents of the 2-year-old hospitalized with epiglottitis about ciprofloxacin administration at home. The nurse should document that teaching was effective when the parent makes which statement?

1. "I'll taper ciprofloxacin to once daily when my child begins to 'feel better.'"
2. "I'll avoid giving ciprofloxacin with dairy products or calcium-fortified juices."
3. "I'll take my child outdoors; the sun exposure will help increase vitamin D levels."
4. "I should discontinue giving ciprofloxacin and contact the doctor if diarrhea occurs."

**1979.** The hospitalized child with severe asthma has ABGs of pH = 7.30, $Paco_2$ = 49 mm Hg, and $HCO_3$ = 24 mEq/L. Which findings should the nurse expect when performing an assessment?

1. Rapid and deep respirations, paresthesia, lightheadedness, twitching, anxiety, and fear
2. Rapid and deep respirations, fruity breath odor, drowsiness, vomiting, and abdominal pain
3. Slow, shallow breathing, hypertonic muscles, restlessness, twitching, confusion, and seizures
4. Diaphoresis, headache, tachycardia, confusion, restlessness, apprehension, and flushed face

**1980.** The triage nurse in the ED determines that the child is experiencing severe respiratory distress. Which assessment findings support the nurse's conclusion?

1. Agitation, vomiting, diarrhea, and tachycardia
2. Diaphoresis, restlessness, tachypnea, and anorexia
3. Pallor, coughing, expiratory wheeze, and confusion
4. Sternal retractions, grunting, cyanosis, and bradycardia

**1981.** The mother of the 2-year-old telephones the nurse to ask for advice. The child has a temperature of 104°F (40°C) and a sore throat and has been drooling for a few days. The child is now sleepy. Which advice is **best**?

1. "Take your child to the ED immediately."
2. "Bring your child to the clinic to be seen now."
3. "Give acetaminophen for the temperature and allow your child to sleep."
4. "Use a spoon to look inside your child's mouth and throat and tell me what you see."

**1982.** The new nurse places the infant diagnosed with tracheoesophageal fistula under a radiant warmer with the infant's head elevated at a 30-degree angle. Which statement to the infant's mother indicates that the new nurse understands the **most** important reason for this position?

1. "This position helps your baby to eat better and digest foods more easily."
2. "This position helps your baby breathe better by expanding her lungs."
3. "This position keeps your baby more comfortable and closer to the warmer."
4. "This position prevents gastric juices from going upward and into your baby's lungs."

**1983.** The child, admitted with a sudden onset of fever, lethargy, dyspnea, sore throat, and difficulty swallowing, is thought to have acute epiglottitis. What should the nurse do? **Select all that apply.**

1. Observe swallowing.
2. Review the vital signs.
3. Auscultate the lungs.
4. Obtain a throat culture.
5. Allay anxiety and fear.

**1984.** The nurse notes substernal retractions when assessing a child. Place an X in the box on the illustration that shows the area where the nurse made this observation.

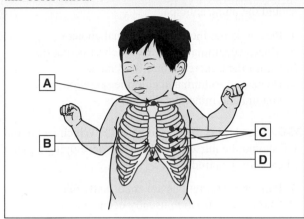

**1985.** The 6-month-old is diagnosed with LTB. Which findings should the nurse expect when completing the **initial** assessment? **Select all that apply.**

1. Dyspnea
2. Dysphagia
3. Hoarseness
4. Barking cough
5. Inspiratory stridor

**1986.** **PHARM** The 6-month-old hospitalized with LTB is given an albuterol nebulizer treatment. Which action should the nurse expect?

1. Relaxation of smooth muscles in the airways
2. Removal of excess fluid from the lungs
3. Loosening and thinning of pulmonary secretions
4. Reduction of inflammation and mucus from airways

**1987.** **PHARM** The 18-month-old is hospitalized with LTB. The child weighs 26 lb, is 33 inches tall, and has a body surface area (BSA) of 0.53. The HCP prescribes prednisolone 0.05 mg/kg oral daily, to be given with food or milk q6hr. How many mg should the nurse administer with each dose?

_____ mg (Round your answer to hundredths.)

**1988.** The infant with a history of streptococcus pneumonia is being admitted to the ED for bronchiolitis. The mother states the baby has been sneezing and wheezing and has had a runny nose for 2 days and has not eaten for 8 hours. The infant is placed in an ED room with droplet isolation precautions. Place the nurse's actions in priority order.

1. Initiate IV fluids.
2. Assess degree of respiratory distress.
3. Administer nebulized bronchodilator.
4. Initiate humidified oxygen therapy.
5. Provide family teaching.

Answer: _____

**1989.** **PHARM** The 8-year-old weighing 25 kg is prescribed azithromycin 250 mg oral tablet daily to treat bacterial pneumonia. Which intervention should the nurse implement?

1. Withhold azithromycin if the child has diarrhea or constipation.
2. Offer the child's preferred beverage after giving the medication.
3. Administer the tablets 1 hour before or 2 hours after a meal.
4. Verify the dose with the HCP; it exceeds the maximum dose for a child.

**1990.** The nurse is planning care for the child diagnosed with RSV. Which interventions should the nurse plan to implement? **Select all that apply.**

1. Promote rest by grouping care activities.
2. Encourage parents with young children to visit.
3. Question prescribed ceftriaxone 500 mg IV daily.
4. Assess skin turgor and mucous membranes q4h.
5. Give oxygen to maintain $SaO_2$ levels >95%.

**1991.** **PHARM** The infant is hospitalized after having a respiratory infection and severe diarrhea for 5 days. The child has poor skin turgor, respirations 30 bpm, T 101.3°F (39°C), and watery green stools. The HCP prescribes an antipyretic and IV fluid of $D_5NS$ with a potassium additive. What nursing action is **most** important?

1. Give the prescribed antipyretic medication.
2. Change the diaper that has watery green stool.
3. Apply oxygen to treat the infant's tachypnea.
4. Ensure adequate urine output before starting IV fluids.

**1992.** The nurse is caring for the infant with bronchiolitis. Which goal should the nurse identify as essential?

1. Promoting and maintaining adequate hydration
2. Setting up and facilitating the use of a mist tent
3. Ensuring that antibiotics are prescribed
4. Giving a cough suppressant when needed

**1993.** **PHARM** The child with asthma is prescribed albuterol MDI. Which statement should the nurse include when teaching the child how to take this medication?

1. "When using the MDI, avoid shaking the canister before discharging the medication."
2. "Press on the canister twice in succession to discharge two 'puffs' of the medication."
3. "Make a tight seal around the inhaler's mouthpiece before discharging the medication."
4. "Breathe out as much air as possible, put the mouthpiece in the mouth, press the canister, then slowly inhale."

**1994.** The nurse is triaging the child with asthma. The child is pale and has dry mucous membranes, cracked lips, and nasal flaring with inspiration. Which actions should the nurse perform while waiting for the HCP to assess the child? **Select all that apply.**

1. Assess lung sounds.
2. Obtain pulse oximetry.
3. Give a nebulizer treatment.
4. Elevate the head of the bed.
5. Offer the child's preferred oral fluid.

**1995.** The nurse completes teaching the parent of the child with asthma about the peak flow meter. Which statement indicates that the teaching was effective?

1. "I'll have my child do a meter reading each morning before getting out of bed while lying flat; the meter is set on the average peak flow."
2. "I'll have my child obtain the meter reading after doing morning exercises to get better airflow before testing the peak flow."
3. "I'll have my child set the meter at zero before testing and test peak flow every day; we'll record the best reading once a month."
4. "I'll set the meter gauge on zero; my child should stand and 'huff and cough' two times to clear the airway, then test the peak flow."

**1996.** Oxygen via simple face mask is prescribed for the hospitalized child diagnosed with mild intermittent asthma. Which items, brought by the parents from home, should the nurse remove from the room?

1. Plastic blocks and a handheld toy windmill
2. Electronic educational toy and electronic book
3. Washable cloth doll with cotton clothes
4. Synthetic stuffed animal and synthetic underwear

**1997.** The nurse is caring for the child with bronchial asthma. Which statement is **most** important for the nurse to make when teaching the parents?

1. "Bronchial asthma is also called hyperactive airway disease."
2. "Cold air and irritating odors can cause severe bronchoconstriction."
3. "Frequent occurrences of bronchiolitis before age 5 could indicate asthma."
4. "Severe respiratory alkalosis can result from respiratory failure in asthma."

**1998.** The nurse is planning care for the child with CF. What assessment finding and associated intervention should the nurse anticipate?

1. Pica appetite; increase nutritional choices
2. Mucus accumulation; perform chest percussion
3. Steatorrhea; increase oral fluid intake
4. Decreased sodium and chloride secretion; give vitamin and mineral supplements

**1999.** The child is diagnosed with CF. Which fact about CF should the nurse consider when developing a plan of care for the child?

1. Pulmonary secretions are abnormally thick.
2. Chronic constipation usually occurs in CF.
3. CF is an autosomal dominant hereditary disorder.
4. A child with CF also will have diabetes insipidus.

**2000.** The nurse is preparing to perform chest physiotherapy on the child with CF. When should the nurse plan to perform the treatment?

1. At least 1 hour before meals
2. Before performing postural drainage
3. Before a nebulized aerosol treatment
4. After suctioning the upper respiratory tract

**2001.** **MoC** The experienced nurse is observing the new nurse perform chest physiotherapy on the 8-month-old. The experienced nurse should intervene when observing the new nurse perform which action?

1. Laying the infant on the bed in a supine position
2. Setting the infant upright with the child's back toward the nurse
3. Laying the infant on the new nurse's lap with the child's head facing down
4. Setting the infant upright and facing the nurse with the child leaning forward

**2002.** MoC The nurse is preparing the child with CF for discharge to home. The nurse determines that the parent needs further education when the parent makes which statement?

1. "We will do chest therapy and postural drainage even if our child doesn't seem congested."
2. "Playing on the backyard swings and hanging upside down are exercises our child will enjoy."
3. "If a child at daycare has a cough, fever, or flu symptoms, we should keep our child home."
4. "We should withhold the pancreatic enzyme if our child has a good appetite and a stool daily."

**2003.** The nurse educates parents about the nutritional needs of their child with CF. Which response by a parent indicates an understanding of the child's nutritional needs?

1. "We will need to limit the amount of meat, carbohydrates, and fats in the diet plan."
2. "We will need to prepare a low-carbohydrate, high-fat diet plan with very little meat."
3. "We will need to prepare a lot of meat and carbohydrates and some fats in the diet plan."
4. "We will need to prepare moderate amounts of meats and low carbohydrates in the diet plan."

**2004.** MoC The nurse is developing a plan of care for the child with CF. Which outcomes would be **best** for the nurse to include?

1. Adequate hydration, absence of *Helicobacter pylori*, eating 75% of meals
2. Absence of pulmonary infection, weight normal for age, skin remains intact
3. Urine output 0.1 mL/kg/hr, absence of injury, normal growth and development
4. Absence of dehydration, maintains cleanliness, adheres to medication regimen

**2005.** The nurse is reviewing the lab report for the child hospitalized with hemoptysis. Based on the results, the nurse should plan to implement measures to treat the child for which condition?

| Laboratory Report | | |
|---|---|---|
| **Serum Laboratory Test** | **Client's Value** | **Normal Range** |
| Potassium | 4.0 | 3.5–5.0 mEq/L |
| Sodium | 128 | 135–145 mEq/L |
| Chloride | 88 | 94–106 mEq/L |
| Glucose | 110 | 60–100 mg/dL |
| SCr | 0.4 | 0.3–0.7 mg/dL |
| BUN | 25 | 5–20 mg/dL |
| Hgb | 10.8 | 11.5–13.5 g/dL |
| Hct | 34% | 35%–50% |
| WBCs | 11,500 | 4500–10,500/mm³ |
| **Other Laboratory Test** | **Client Value** | **Normal Range** |
| Sweat chloride levels | 66 | 23–47.5 mEq/L |

1. Renal failure
2. Cystic fibrosis (CF)
3. Cardiac dysrhythmias
4. Type 1 diabetes mellitus

**2006.** The child is scheduled to have a bronchoscopy to remove a foreign body. Which interventions should the nurse complete prior to the procedure? **Select all that apply.**

1. Provide pain medication to sedate the child.
2. Bring emergency equipment to the bedside.
3. Keep the child calm and environment quiet.
4. Have the child breathe deeply and try to cough.
5. Monitor for changes in the child's speech.

**2007.** The NA obtains the VS illustrated for a 15-year-old who just underwent a bronchoscopy. What should the nurse do **next?**

| Vital Sign | Results |
|---|---|
| Temperature | 100.4°F (38°C) |
| Pulse | 134 bpm |
| Respirations | 18 bpm |
| Blood Pressure | 122/76 mm Hg |
| Oxygen Saturation | 92% |

1. Complete a thorough respiratory assessment.
2. Ask the NA to recheck the VS in 15 minutes.
3. Continue to monitor the client's sedation level.
4. Ask if the adolescent had anything hot to drink.

**2008.** The nurse is auscultating posterior breath sounds of the infant who underwent a bronchoscopy to remove a foreign body. Which should the nurse expect to hear if the lung sounds are normal at the locations with Xs?

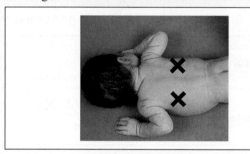

1. High-pitched sounds with a prolonged inspiration
2. Inspiration and expiration (I:E ratio) of equal length
3. Tracheal sounds with expiration longer than inspiration
4. Bronchovesicular sounds with inspiration longer than expiration

**2009.** The nurse is caring for the hospitalized adolescent who is being monitored by pulse oximetry. When the nurse enters the room, the pulse oximeter monitor shows an oxygen saturation of 84% and is alarming. What should the nurse do **next?**

1. Replace the pulse oximeter machine and probe.
2. Give oxygen at 2L via a nasal cannula or mask.
3. Assess the level of consciousness and skin color.
4. Call the HCP to obtain an order for ABGs.

**2010.** The nurse triages children involved in a school bus accident that resulted in the children being submerged in cold water. Which child has the greatest risk of a respiratory arrest and should be triaged as the **priority?**

1. The child who has hypoxia
2. The child who has asphyxia
3. The child who has aspiration
4. The child who has hypothermia

**2011.** The home health nurse is planning a follow-up visit to the parents after their first-born and only child died from SIDS. Which action is **most** important for the nurse to include in the **initial** visit?

1. Help the parents make plans for future children.
2. Complete a referral for genetic counseling.
3. Allow time to listen and explore their concerns.
4. Educate the family on the causes of SIDS.

**2012.** The nurse is evaluating the 16-year-old's tuberculin skin test (TST) result, which shows a 6 mm area of induration. During the evaluation, the client gives the nurse a personal history. Which details should be **most** concerning to the nurse?

1. Has a diagnosis of HIV infection
2. Recently had a chest x-ray to diagnose pneumonia
3. Is a recent immigrant from a country with high TB prevalence
4. Had recent contact with a person who has active TB

**2013.** **PHARM** The nurse is evaluating the laboratory report for the adolescent being treated with isoniazid for TB. After reviewing the report, the nurse should assess for signs and symptoms associated with which adverse effect of isoniazid?

| Serum Laboratory Test | Client's Value 1 Week Ago | Client's Value Today | Normal Ranges |
|---|---|---|---|
| BUN | 16 | 18 | 5–25 mg/dL |
| Creatinine | 0.8 | 0.9 | 0.4–1.2 mg/dL |
| Na | 135 | 139 | 135–145 mEq/L |
| K | 3.8 | 4.2 | 3.5–5.5 mEq/L |
| Cl | 99 | 99 | 98–105 mEq/L |
| $CO_2$ | 26 | 28 | 20–28 mEq/L |
| Hgb | 12 | 14 | 11–16 g/dL |
| Hct | 36 | 42 | 31%–43% |
| ALT/SGPT | 38 | 60 | 10–35 units/L |

1. Heart failure
2. Hepatotoxicity
3. Aplastic anemia
4. Renal insufficiency

**2014.** The child is diagnosed with TB after returning to the U.S. from a family trip out of the country. During the assessment, the nurse observes that the parents do not talk about the child's diagnosis as TB or use the term "TB" but rather use only the word "it." Which statement made by the nurse is **best**?

1. "Tell me how you feel about your child's diagnosis and illness."
2. "If your child takes the prescribed medications, 'it' can be cured."
3. "Why do you say 'it,' rather than referring to the diagnosis of tuberculosis?"
4. "How long has your child been having night sweats and a productive cough?"

**2015.** **MoC** The nurse is caring for the 22-month-old with LTB. Which symptoms should alert the nurse to notify the HCP due to impending respiratory failure?

1. Restlessness and irritability
2. Barking, rattling-sounding cough
3. Decreased inspiratory breath sounds
4. Voice hoarseness and weak-sounding cry

**2016.** The nurse is planning care for the infant diagnosed with esophageal atresia with lower tracheoesophageal fistula. Which illustration **best** shows the type of atresia that the nurse should visualize when thinking about the infant's diagnosis and care?

1.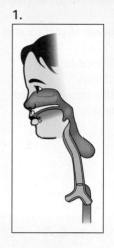
2.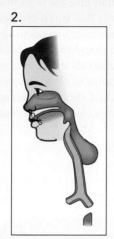
3.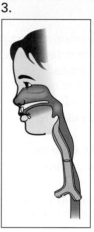
4.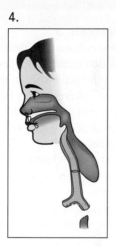

**2017.** The child who had a tonsillectomy and adenoidectomy (T&A) is brought to the postoperative recovery room. In which position should the nurse place the child?

1. Supine
2. Side-lying
3. Semi-Fowler's with the head turned to the side
4. High Fowler's, head slightly bent and to the side

**2018.** The nurse is caring for the child postoperatively following T&A surgery. Which assessment finding should alert the nurse to explore for hemorrhage?

1. Presence of "dark coffee ground" emesis
2. Frequent swallowing and clearing of the throat
3. Complaint of a sore throat and difficulty swallowing
4. Secretions and dried blood at the corners of the mouth

**2019.** The nurse completed teaching on home care to the mother of a child post-T&A surgery. The nurse determines that the mother understands the instructions when the mother makes which statement?

1. "I should give ice pops or cold drinks but avoid giving anything that is red-colored."
2. "Hemorrhage can occur up to a month after discharge due to sloughing from healing."
3. "My child should gargle and use a hard-bristled toothbrush to clean the mouth of debris."
4. "My child should cough and breathe deeply to keep the lungs clear and prevent pneumonia."

**2020.** The nurse determines that the 8-month-old aspirated a foreign body and is currently unresponsive. Place the steps in the order that the nurse should perform them.

1. Provide 2 rescue breaths for every 30 chest compressions.
2. Palpate the brachial artery.
3. Open the airway using the head-tilt, chin-lift or jaw-thrust maneuver.
4. Give 30 chest compressions at a depth of 1.5 inches at a rate of 100 per minute.
5. Place two or three fingers in the center of the chest just below the nipples.
6. Look for and remove object if seen.
7. Call for help.

Answer: _____

## Answers and Rationales

### 1977. ANSWER: 3

1. A blood culture will identify the organism and suggest antibiotic selection, but results will be delayed until the microorganism grows in the culture media.
2. A throat culture usually is not performed because gagging can cause complete airway obstruction.
3. **A lateral neck x-ray will show the enlarged epiglottis.**
4. The CBC will identify elevated WBCs and the presence of an infection but will not confirm the diagnosis.

▶ *Test-taking Tip: The key words are "confirm the diagnosis." Think about which results are available for each of the laboratory tests.*

**Content Area:** Child; **Concept:** Inflammation; Infection; Oxygenation; **Integrated Processes:** Nursing Process: Analysis; **Client Needs:** Physiological Integrity: Reduction of Risk Potential; **Cognitive Level:** Comprehension [Understanding]

### 1978. PHARM ANSWER: 2

1. All medication should be taken as directed; ciprofloxacin (Cipro) should not be tapered.
2. **Dairy products such as milk and yogurt, calcium-fortified juice, antacids, vitamins and mineral supplements negate the medication's effects and should be avoided.**
3. Although ciprofloxacin should not be taken with vitamin $D_3$ due to drug interactions, sun exposure as a source of vitamin D is not recommended because the skin is more sensitive and burns can occur.
4. Diarrhea is a common side effect of ciprofloxacin but usually is not severe enough to discontinue the medication; however, the parent should contact the HCP.

▶ *Test-taking Tip: Use the "c" in ciprofloxacin as a memory cue to avoid giving it with calcium-containing products, including dairy.*

**Content Area:** Child; **Concept:** Oxygenation; Medication; **Integrated Processes:** Communication and Documentation; **Client Needs:** Physiological Integrity: Pharmacological and Parenteral Therapies; **Cognitive Level:** Evaluation [Evaluating]

### 1979. ANSWER: 4

1. Rapid and deep respirations, paresthesia, light-headedness, twitching, anxiety, and fear are signs and symptoms of respiratory alkalosis. It may occur in asthma if excess artificial ventilation is used in treatment.
2. Rapid and deep breathing, fruity breath odor, fatigue, headache, lethargy, drowsiness, nausea, vomiting, and abdominal pain are signs and symptoms of metabolic acidosis.
3. Slow and shallow breathing, hypertonic muscles, restlessness, twitching, confusion, irritability, apathy, tetany, and seizures are signs and symptoms of metabolic alkalosis. Metabolic acidosis and alkalosis are not associated with asthma but may occur due to other complications.
4. **The decreased pH and increased $PaCO_2$ indicate respiratory acidosis. Diaphoresis, headache, tachycardia, confusion, restlessness, apprehension, and flushed face are manifestations of respiratory acidosis without compensation. These occur due to lack of oxygen and trapping of carbon dioxide in the lower airway from narrowed airway passages.**

▶ *Test-taking Tip: Analyze the ABG findings to determine if respiratory acidosis, respiratory alkalosis, metabolic acidosis, or metabolic alkalosis is present. Then think about how the bronchial constriction and bronchial spasms of asthma can cause these abnormal results. The assessment findings should be those noted in respiratory acidosis.*

Content Area: Child; **Concept:** pH Regulation; Oxygenation; Assessment; **Integrated Processes:** Nursing Process: Assessment; **Client Needs:** Physiological Integrity: Reduction of Risk Potential; **Cognitive Level:** Analysis [Analyzing]

## 1980. ANSWER: 4

1. Although agitation and tachycardia may be associated with respiratory problems, vomiting and diarrhea are more associated with GI problems.
2. Diaphoresis, restlessness, and tachypnea may indicate a possible electrolyte imbalance or mild respiratory distress.
3. Pallor, coughing, expiratory wheeze, and confusion may indicate moderate respiratory distress.
4. **Signs of severe respiratory distress include chest retractions, grunting, cyanosis, and bradycardia. Sternal retractions appear from the use of accessory muscles to breathe. Grunting is an involuntary response to end-stage respiratory effort. Cyanosis indicates that a state of hypoxia exists due to lack of circulating oxygen, and progression to bradycardia is an ominous sign that the body is so overtaxed that it is wearing out.**

▶ **Test-taking Tip:** *Narrow the choices by considering the number and severity of the respiratory distress symptoms noted in the options.*

Content Area: Child; **Concept:** Oxygenation; Assessment; **Integrated Processes:** Nursing Process: Assessment; **Client Needs:** Physiological Integrity: Physiological Adaptation; **Cognitive Level:** Application [Applying]

## 1981. ANSWER: 1

1. **An elevated temperature, sore throat, and drooling are symptoms of epiglottitis. The sleepiness could be from the effects of the elevated temperature or from respiratory depression. The child should be seen in an ED immediately because respiratory failure may develop.**
2. Bringing the child to the clinic could delay emergency treatment if needed.
3. Acetaminophen (Tylenol) may reduce temperature, but allowing the child to sleep without being assessed could be life-threatening.
4. If the epiglottis is swollen and inflamed, stimulating the gag reflex can cause complete obstruction of the glottis and respiratory failure and should never be performed when epiglottitis is suspected.

▶ **Test-taking Tip:** *A decreased level of consciousness can occur from impaired oxygenation. Use the ABC's to determine the best advice.*

Content Area: Child; **Concept:** Infection; Safety; Oxygenation; **Integrated Processes:** Communication and Documentation; **Client Needs:** Physiological Integrity: Physiological Adaptation; **Cognitive Level:** Analysis [Analyzing]

## 1982. ANSWER: 4

1. If the infant has not yet had a surgical repair, oral feedings should not be given. A gastrostomy tube may be inserted to drain the gastric secretions by gravity and prevent reflux into the lungs.
2. The infant will breathe better and be more comfortable with the head elevated, but that is not the most important reason.
3. Whether supine or with the head of the bed elevated, the infant should not be any closer to the warmer.
4. **Elevating the infant's head helps prevent gastric secretions from refluxing from the distal esophagus into the trachea, especially when intra-abdominal pressure is increased with crying.**

▶ **Test-taking Tip:** *The key phrase is "most important reason," indicating that more than one option is correct but that one is better than all the others. Focus on the infant's condition when answering this question.*

Content Area: Child; **Concept:** Oxygenation; Safety; **Integrated Processes:** Nursing Process: Evaluation; **Client Needs:** Physiological Integrity: Reduction of Risk Potential; **Cognitive Level:** Evaluation [Evaluating]

## 1983. ANSWER: 1, 2, 3, 5

1. **Swallowing should be observed to establish a baseline because the child may develop a greater risk of aspiration.**
2. **VS are needed to establish a baseline for further comparisons and determine deviations from normal.**
3. **Auscultating the lungs is important to determine if they sound diminished from airway impairment or if the sounds are rhonchi from oral secretions accumulating in the lungs.**
4. Obtaining a throat culture is contraindicated in the presence of epiglottitis because it may cause a complete airway obstruction.
5. **While assessing the child, the nurse should minimize anxiety and fear because they can increase oxygen requirements and cause dyspnea.**

▶ **Test-taking Tip:** *You should eliminate any options that are unsafe.*

Content Area: Child; **Concept:** Assessment; Infection; Inflammation; Safety; **Integrated Processes:** Nursing Process: Assessment; **Client Needs:** Physiological Integrity: Physiological Adaptation; **Cognitive Level:** Analysis [Analyzing]

## 1984. ANSWER:

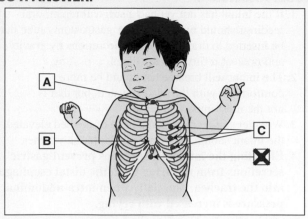

Line D indicates the substernal locations. Line A points to the suprasternal location. Line B points to the xiphoid process. Line C points to intercostal spaces.

▶ *Test-taking Tip: Remember anatomical locations and consider the prefix "sub-" in the word describing the location in the question, then visualize the area to be assessed.*

**Content Area:** Child; **Concept:** Oxygenation; Assessment; **Integrated Processes:** Nursing Process: Assessment; **Client Needs:** Physiological Integrity: Reduction of Risk Potential; **Cognitive Level:** Comprehension [Understanding]

## 1985. ANSWER: 1, 3, 4, 5

1. **Dyspnea occurs from impaired oxygenation due to inflammation, edema, mucus accumulation, or airway obstruction.**
2. Dysphagia (difficulty swallowing) occurs with epiglottitis because the obstruction is supraglottic, as opposed to the subglottic obstruction in LTB.
3. **Edema of the larynx causes hoarseness.**
4. **Inflammation in the larynx and trachea causes the characteristic barking cough.**
5. **Narrowing of the subglottic area of the trachea results in audible inspiratory stridor.**

▶ *Test-taking Tip: Read the options carefully; they may be the opposite of expected findings. These should be eliminated.*

**Content Area:** Child; **Concept:** Oxygenation; Inflammation; Assessment; **Integrated Processes:** Nursing Process: Assessment; **Client Needs:** Physiological Integrity: Reduction of Risk Potential; **Cognitive Level:** Knowledge [Remembering]

## 1986. **PHARM** ANSWER: 1

1. **Albuterol (Proventil, Ventolin) binds to beta-2 adrenergic receptors in the airway's smooth muscles, and cellular actions decrease intracellular calcium. Decreased intracellular calcium relaxes smooth muscle in the airways.**
2. Diuretics remove excess fluid through their actions on the kidneys. This affects circulating fluid volume and facilitates removal of excess fluid from the lungs.
3. Mucolytics reduce the thickness of pulmonary secretions by acting directly on the mucus plugs and dissolving them.

4. Expectorants reduce inflammation by liquefying mucus and stimulating natural lubricant fluids from the bronchial glands.

▶ *Test-taking Tip: Carefully read the options to determine which would have the most global effect in opening the airways.*

**Content Area:** Child; **Concept:** Medication; Oxygenation; **Integrated Processes:** Nursing Process: Analysis; **Client Needs:** Physiological Integrity: Pharmacological and Parenteral Therapies; **Cognitive Level:** Application [Applying]

## 1987. **PHARM** ANSWER: 0.15

**Calculate the child's weight in kilograms (pounds ÷ 2.2 lb/kg) = 26 lb ÷ 2.2 lb/kg = 11.818 kg. Weight in kilograms × daily mg/kg should be 11.818 kg × 0.05 mg/kg = 0.5909 mg. Determine the number of doses per day (ordered every 6 hours [24 ÷ 6 = 4]). Divide the daily dose by 4 (0.5909 mg ÷ 4 = 0.148 mg). Rounded to hundredths, the dose should be 0.15 mg.**

▶ *Test-taking Tip: Be sure to read the question carefully to determine what is being asked. You should be calculating one dose of prednisolone (Orapred) and not the daily dose.*

**Content Area:** Child; **Concept:** Medication; Inflammation; Safety; **Integrated Processes:** Nursing Process: Analysis; **Client Needs:** Physiological Integrity: Pharmacological and Parenteral Therapies; **Cognitive Level:** Analysis [Analyzing]

## 1988. ANSWER: 2, 4, 3, 1, 5

2. **Assess degree of respiratory distress. Assessment is the first step in the nursing process. Identifying respiratory status will help determine the type of oxygen delivery device that may need to be initiated.**
4. **Initiate humidified oxygen therapy. The oxygen delivery device will depend on the degree of respiratory distress. Oxygen is needed to counteract hypoxemia, and humidification keeps the respiratory membranes moist.**
3. **Administer nebulized bronchodilator. It will open the larger airways to promote oxygenation.**
1. **Initiate IV fluids. The infant has not eaten, and fluids are needed to prevent dehydration.**
5. **Provide family teaching. Meeting the physiological needs of the infant is priority; when that is completed, family teaching can occur. Explanations should be provided as the nurse performs each action.**

▶ *Test-taking Tip: Use the ABC's and nursing process to place items in the correct order.*

**Content Area:** Child; **Concept:** Inflammation; Infection; Oxygenation; **Integrated Processes:** Nursing Process: Implementation; **Client Needs:** Physiological Integrity: Physiological Adaptation; **Cognitive Level:** Synthesis [Creating]

## 1989. **PHARM** ANSWER: 2

1. Azithromycin has no significant adverse effects on GI function. It can be administered (not withheld) and the constipation or diarrhea treated.

2. **Offering a preferred beverage makes azithromycin (Zithromax) more palatable, and fluids should be encouraged to liquefy secretions in pneumonia.**
3. If given in capsule form, it should be given 1 hour before or 2 hours after a meal. Tablets may be taken without regard to food.
4. Verification with the HCP is unnecessary. The maximum dose of azithromycin for bacterial infections is 250 mg/day. It kills bacteria by inhibiting their protein synthesis.

▶ *Test-taking Tip: Azithromycin, a macrolide antibiotic, kills bacteria by inhibiting protein synthesis and is a recommended medication for bacterial pneumonia. Tablets may be given without regard to food. Thus, consider the option that will increase the child's fluid intake.*

Content Area: Child; Concept: Oxygenation; Medication; Integrated Processes: Nursing Process: Implementation; Client Needs: Physiological Integrity: Pharmacological and Parenteral Therapies; Cognitive Level: Application [Applying]

## 1990. ANSWER: 1, 3, 4, 5

1. **The child with RSV should have adequate rest to decrease the metabolic needs of the body. The nurse should plan to group care activities to promote this needed rest.**
2. RSV is extremely contagious; the child should be placed on droplet isolation precautions, and visits from other children should not be allowed.
3. **RSV is not a bacterial infection; therefore, administration of an antibiotic is not indicated. The nurse should question the HCP about giving ceftriaxone (Rocephin).**
4. **The child with RSV may experience impaired ability to consume food and fluids. The nurse should monitor hydration status to identify and prevent dehydration.**
5. **The nurse should plan to provide supplemental oxygen to maintain the child's oxygenation status.**

▶ *Test-taking Tip: RSV is a communicable viral infection. Use this information to delete options.*

Content Area: Child; Concept: Oxygenation; Critical Thinking; Integrated Processes: Nursing Process: Planning; Client Needs: Safe and Effective Care Environment: Safety and Infection Control; Cognitive Level: Application [Applying]

## 1991. PHARM ANSWER: 4

1. Giving an antipyretic is important because the temperature is elevated, but this is not the most life-threatening sign.
2. Changing the diaper to prevent skin breakdown is important, but this may not result in a life-threatening event.
3. A respiration rate of 20 to 40 breaths per minute is within the expected range for an infant; oxygen is not necessary.

4. **It is most important for the nurse to know if the infant's kidneys are functioning before giving fluid replacement with a potassium additive because potassium is excreted by the kidneys. A high serum potassium level can cause life-threatening events such as cardiac dysrhythmias.**

▶ *Test-taking Tip: You need to ask yourself if any of the options, if not performed, could result in a life-threatening event.*

Content Area: Child; Concept: Infection; Fluid and Electrolyte Balance; Oxygenation; Integrated Processes: Nursing Process: Implementation; Client Needs: Physiological Integrity: Pharmacological and Parenteral Therapies; Cognitive Level: Analysis [Analyzing]

## 1992. ANSWER: 1

1. **Hydration is an essential goal for a child with bronchiolitis (RSV) to loosen secretions, prevent shock, and maintain basic physiological needs.**
2. Studies have shown that mist tents offer no additional benefit in keeping secretions moist.
3. Antibiotics do not treat illnesses with viral etiologies; they may be used to treat secondary causes but are not primary for viral diseases.
4. Cough suppressants decrease a child's ability to effectively clear the airway.

▶ *Test-taking Tip: Note that three options are similar and one is different. The key word is "goal," which is usually a broad statement. Eliminate options that are interventions and thus more specific.*

Content Area: Child; Concept: Infection; Critical Thinking; Integrated Processes: Nursing Process: Evaluation; Client Needs: Physiological Integrity: Reduction of Risk Potential; Cognitive Level: Evaluation [Evaluating]

## 1993. PHARM ANSWER: 4

1. Shaking the MDI canister well before use supplies a better delivery of the aerosolized medication.
2. When taking two "puffs" of medication, waiting 1 minute between puffs allows for better absorption of the inhaled medication.
3. When taking inhaled medications via an MDI, wrapping the lips too tightly around the mouthpiece consolidates the medication in the buccal cavity and decreases its effectiveness.
4. **This statement should be included by the nurse. It is clear and in language that the child can understand.**

▶ *Test-taking Tip: Often, the most complete option is the answer.*

Content Area: Child; Concept: Medication; Oxygenation; Nursing Roles; Integrated Processes: Teaching/Learning; Client Needs: Physiological Integrity: Pharmacological and Parenteral Therapies; Physiological Integrity: Reduction of Risk Potential; Cognitive Level: Application [Applying]

## 1994. ANSWER: 1, 2, 4

1. **Assessing lung sounds provides important information about the child's respiratory status.**
2. **Pulse oximetry provides information about the child's oxygenation level.**
3. A nebulizer treatment needs to be prescribed by the HCP.
4. **Elevating the head of the bed promotes lung expansion.**
5. The nurse should wait until the HCP assesses the child and prescribes a diet before offering fluids.

♦ *Test-taking Tip: Use the nurse's scope of practice to identify the appropriate actions.*

Content Area: Child; Concept: Oxygenation; Assessment; Safety; Integrated Processes: Nursing Process: Assessment; Client Needs: Physiological Integrity: Physiological Adaptation; Cognitive Level: Application [Applying]

## 1995. ANSWER: 4

1. Lying flat would not allow for full lung expansion or provide an accurate peak flow rate.
2. Performing peak flow rates before (not after) exercise will help the parent and child determine if it would be safe to exercise.
3. Encouraging a child to test the peak flow meter every day and set the meter at zero before testing is an accurate statement; however, recording peak flow rating on a daily basis is essential.
4. **The meter gauge should be set at zero. Standing for the peak flow test allows full lung expansion; "huffing and coughing" clears the airways to allow for a complete full breath before testing a peak flow.**

♦ *Test-taking Tip: Visualize the actions in each option and eliminate any in which full lung expansion could not be achieved.*

Content Area: Child; Concept: Oxygenation; Nursing Roles; Promoting Health; Integrated Processes: Teaching/Learning; Nursing Process: Evaluation; Client Needs: Physiological Integrity: Reduction of Risk Potential; Cognitive Level: Evaluation [Evaluating]

## 1996. ANSWER: 4

1. Plastic blocks and handheld toys are safe and entertaining for the child receiving oxygen.
2. An electronic toy and electronic book are safe and entertaining for the child receiving oxygen.
3. Washable toys and clothing are safe and entertaining for the child receiving oxygen.
4. **Synthetic toys and clothing are restricted during oxygen use because these items can build up static electricity, create a spark, and start a fire. They should be removed from the room.**

♦ *Test-taking Tip: Narrow the options to those that can cause a spark through static electricity.*

Content Area: Child; Concept: Oxygenation; Safety; Integrated Processes: Nursing Process: Planning; Client Needs: Safe and Effective Care Environment: Safety and Infection Control; Cognitive Level: Analysis [Analyzing]

## 1997. ANSWER: 2

1. Although bronchial asthma is also called hyperactive airway disease, this is not the most important statement.
2. **It is most important for the nurse to teach the parents about asthma triggers such as exposure to cold air and irritating odors, which can cause severe bronchoconstriction, so that episodes can be avoided. Other triggers include inhalant antigens such as pollens, molds, house dust, food, and odors such as turpentine, smog, and cigarette smoke.**
3. Asthma tends to occur initially before 5 years of age, but in the early years it may be diagnosed as bronchiolitis instead. This information may be important if the child had frequent episodes of bronchiolitis, but it is not the most important of the options.
4. Severe respiratory acidosis, not alkalosis, can result from respiratory failure in asthma.

♦ *Test-taking Tip: The key words are "most important," indicating that more than one option is correct. Prioritize according to the ABC's to determine which statement is most important.*

Content Area: Child; Concept: Oxygenation; Promoting Health; Nursing Roles; Integrated Processes: Teaching/Learning; Communication and Documentation; Client Needs: Physiological Integrity: Physiological Adaptation; Health Promotion and Maintenance; Cognitive Level: Application [Applying]

## 1998. ANSWER: 2

1. Pica is an appetite for nonnutritive substances such as soil, chalk, coal, or paper. No research has linked pica directly with CF. Even though children with CF do manifest appetites for sweet or salty foods on occasion, that has not been termed "pica."
2. **CF is an autosomal recessive disorder of the exocrine gland. The thick, stagnant mucus secretions become a hospitable environment for bacteria, leading to infection. Chest percussion helps to loosen the mucus to prevent infection.**
3. Although steatorrhea may be present, the therapy does not include increasing oral fluids.
4. With CF there is increased (not decreased) sodium chloride secretion. Vitamin and mineral supplements are important, but pancreatic enzyme supplementation is more important.

♦ *Test-taking Tip: Think about the function of exocrine glands. Because they do not regulate appetite or fecal elimination, Options 1 and 3 can be eliminated.*

Content Area: Child; Concept: Digestion; Oxygenation; Integrated Processes: Nursing Process: Planning; Client Needs: Physiological Integrity: Physiological Adaptation; Cognitive Level: Application [Applying]

## 1999. ANSWER: 1

1. **Pulmonary secretions are abnormally thick, and the lungs are filled with mucus that the cilia cannot clear.**

2. The child with CF characteristically has large, bulky, frothy, foul-smelling stools from the inability to digest fats and protein.

3. CF is an autosomal recessive (not dominant) disorder. In CF, the acinar cells of the pancreas producing lipase, trypsin, and amylase are plugged, causing atrophy of the acinar cells and an inability to produce the enzymes.

4. DM (not DI) develops late in the disease. Thick secretions block the pancreatic ducts that later become fibrotic and reduce the number of islets of Langerhans in the pancreas.

♦ *Test-taking Tip: Read the question carefully. If uncertain, consider the priority physiological need based on Maslow's Hierarchy of Needs.*

Content Area: Child; Concept: Digestion; Oxygenation; Nursing Roles; Integrated Processes: Nursing Process: Planning; Client Needs: Physiological Integrity: Physiological Adaptation; Cognitive Level: Knowledge [Remembering]

## 2000. ANSWER: 1

1. **The nurse should perform chest physiotherapy between meals to prevent esophageal reflux and aspiration.**

2. Postural drainage is most effective after treatments and chest physiotherapy because secretions have been loosened.

3. Nebulizer treatments help to loosen secretions and are beneficial prior to chest physiotherapy.

4. Suction is used after treatments and therapy to help clear the airways.

♦ *Test-taking Tip: You should select the option that will prevent aspiration.*

Content Area: Child; Concept: Digestion, Oxygenation, Integrated Processes: Nursing Process: Planning; Client Needs: Physiological Integrity: Reduction of Risk Potential; Cognitive Level: Application [Applying]

## 2001. MoC ANSWER: 3

1. Laying the infant on the bed in a supine position allows for anterior and lateral lobes of the lungs to be percussed.

2. Setting the infant in an upright position with the infant's back toward the nurse exposes the posterior lobar areas to percussion.

3. **Laying an infant on the nurse's lap in a head-down position is contraindicated in infants because it increases gastroesophageal reflux.**

4. Sitting the infant upright and facing the nurse while leaning forward allows for anterior exposure to percussion.

♦ *Test-taking Tip: Three options are similar, and one is different. Often the option that is different is the answer.*

Content Area: Child; Concept: Oxygenation; Management; Integrated Processes: Nursing Process: Evaluation; Client Needs: Safe and Effective Care Environment: Management of Care; Cognitive Level: Evaluation [Evaluating]

## 2002. MoC ANSWER: 4

1. Performing chest therapy and postural drainage three to four times a day, even if the child is not congested, will help loosen and clear secretions and prevent future hospitalizations.

2. Backyard play including "hanging upside down" facilitates gravity drainage and can be considered if proper safety measures are enforced.

3. The child with CF should be kept away from areas of known communicable disease outbreaks because acquiring a respiratory disease can cause inflammation, tissue damage, and respiratory failure.

4. **In CF there is a lack of pancreatic enzyme production from clogged and atrophied cells. Pancreatic enzymes must be taken before all meals and snacks, even when nutritional intake and bowel movements are adequate.**

♦ *Test-taking Tip: The key phrase is "further education." This is a false-response option; select the option that is incorrect.*

Content Area: Child; Concept: Digestion; Nutrition; Nursing Roles; Integrated Processes: Nursing Process: Evaluation; Client Needs: Safe and Effective Care Environment: Management of Care; Physiological Integrity: Physiological Adaptation; Cognitive Level: Evaluation [Evaluating]

## 2003. ANSWER: 3

1. Limiting protein, carbohydrates, and fats is contraindicated in a child with CF due to the extra energy needs.

2. Low carbohydrates limit the amount of calories that the child with CF would need.

3. **A calorie-dense meal that includes high protein, high calories, and moderate fats will provide optimal nutrition and energy for a child with CF.**

4. Protein is essential for growth and development; carbohydrates are needed for energy and should not be limited.

♦ *Test-taking Tip: To narrow the options, examine those with duplicate words first and eliminate one or both. Beware of options that are opposite of what is expected.*

Content Area: Child; Concept: Oxygenation; Nutrition; Integrated Processes: Teaching/Learning; Client Needs: Physiological Integrity: Basic Care and Comfort; Cognitive Level: Evaluation [Evaluating]

## 2004. MoC ANSWER: 2

1. Although *Helicobacter pylori* infection can occur in a child with CF, it is not common.

2. **Thickened secretions in the bronchioles are a medium for infection. Plugging of pancreatic ducts results in enzymes for digesting fat, protein, and some sugars being unavailable, thus affecting nutrition. Stools can be bulky, foul-smelling, and irritating, or they can be diarrheal from pancreatic enzyme replacement, resulting in skin breakdown. These outcomes are best, and interventions would be implemented to achieve them.**

3. Urine output should be at least 0.5–1 mL/kg/hr.

4. Absence of dehydration, maintenance of cleanliness, and adherence to medication regimen are pertinent but are not the best outcomes among the options.

▶ *Test-taking Tip: The key word is "best," indicating that more than one option is correct, but one option is better. Focus on the pathophysiology of the child's diagnosis when selecting the best option.*

**Content Area:** Child; **Concept:** Digestion; Promoting Health; **Integrated Processes:** Nursing Process: Analysis; **Client Needs:** Safe and Effective Care Environment: Management of Care; Physiological Integrity: Physiological Adaptation; **Cognitive Level:** Synthesis [Creating]

## 2005. ANSWER: 2

1. Hypernatremia (not low serum sodium) and elevated serum creatinine (not normal) are present in renal failure.

2. **In CF, sodium and chloride are lost in the sweat, lowering serum levels. Chloride levels of more than 60 mEq/L in sweat are diagnostic of CF. Dehydration from loss of NaCl increases the BUN level. The Hgb is a little low due to hemoptysis, and the WBCs are elevated due to inflammation or infection.**

3. An elevated serum potassium level could result in dysrhythmias, but the potassium is normal.

4. Random glucose levels of 200 mg/dL or fasting glucose levels of 126 mg/dL are diagnostic for DM, but a level of 110 mg/dL, although elevated for a child, is not diagnostic for DM.

▶ *Test-taking Tip: Focus on the two laboratory values that relate to chloride first, and think about possible causative factors.*

**Content Area:** Child; **Concept:** Digestion; Assessment; Hematologic Regulation; **Integrated Processes:** Nursing Process: Analysis; **Client Needs:** Physiological Integrity: Reduction of Risk Potential; **Cognitive Level:** Analysis [Analyzing]

## 2006. ANSWERS: 2, 3, 5

1. Sedating the child can decrease respirations and further impair respiratory function.

2. **Emergency equipment should be at the bedside in case intubation is required.**

3. **When the airway is compromised, keeping the child calm reduces oxygen demand. Environmental noise and activity will increase the child's anxiety and oxygen demand.**

4. Deep breathing and coughing can cause further damage.

5. **Changes in speech can indicate airway edema that would require emergency intervention such as intubation.**

▶ *Test-taking Tip: Carefully read each option to determine if the intervention would promote or hinder oxygenation.*

**Content Area:** Child; **Concept:** Oxygenation; **Integrated Processes:** Nursing Process: Implementation; **Client Needs:** Physiological Integrity: Physiological Adaptation; **Cognitive Level:** Application [Applying]

## 2007. ANSWER: 1

1. **Increased HR (tachycardia) is an early sign of hypoxia. The nurse should perform a thorough respiratory assessment including RR and effort, lung sounds, color, recheck of oxygen saturation levels, and the adolescent's use of accessory muscles.**

2. The VS should be reassessed in 15 minutes for comparison; however, the nurse should perform an assessment after identifying an abnormal VS.

3. The nurse should assess the adolescent to determine the cause of the increased pulse rate and not just continue to monitor the sedation status.

4. Although the adolescent's temperature of 100.4°F (38°C) is elevated, it would not be affected by hot liquids. The client would have been sedated during the bronchoscopy and would have been NPO until the swallowing and gag reflexes were intact.

▶ *Test-taking Tip: Review the entire list of VS and identify any abnormal values. Use the nursing process to establish the initial action. Assessment should be the first action.*

**Content Area:** Child; **Concept:** Oxygenation; Assessment; **Integrated Processes:** Nursing Process: Analysis; **Client Needs:** Physiological Integrity: Reduction of Risk Potential; **Cognitive Level:** Analysis [Analyzing]

## 2008. ANSWER: 4

1. High-pitched sounds are an abnormal finding that could indicate wheezing.

2. The I:E ratio of equal length is an abnormal finding; normal I:E ratio is 3:1.

3. Tracheal breath sounds are usually heard only over the neck. Inspiration is longer than expiration; normal I:E ratio is 3:1.

4. **Vesicular sounds, which have an I:E ratio of 3:1, are heard in the peripheral parts (bases) of an infant's lung fields. Because infants have high body water content and water transmits sound, the upper airway bronchial sounds also may be transmitted.**

▶ *Test-taking Tip: Think about where the Xs are located on the illustration and the underlying anatomy. Then, narrow the options by eliminating those with abnormal sounds or an incorrect I:E ratio.*

**Content Area:** Child; **Concept:** Assessment; Oxygenation; **Integrated Processes:** Nursing Process: Assessment; **Client Needs:** Health Promotion and Maintenance; **Cognitive Level:** Application [Applying]

## 2009. ANSWER: 3

1. Replacing the machine or probe is only necessary if the machine is malfunctioning.

2. Applying oxygen may be necessary if the nurse is unable to determine the client's pulse oximetry reading within a few seconds.

3. **The nurse immediately should assess the client's mental status and skin color to quickly determine whether the signal tracing constitutes an emergency or whether it is an artifact. An artifact in the pulse oximeter monitoring system can be caused by altered skin temperature, movement of the client's finger, probe disconnection, or equipment malfunction.**
4. Calling the HCP is only necessary if the oxygen saturation reading of 84% is accurate.

▶ *Test-taking Tip: Use the steps of the nursing process in answering this question. An intervention generally is guided by the nurse's assessment findings. The significance of the reading can be determined by a more thorough assessment of the system affected.*

Content Area: Child; Concept: Oxygenation; Assessment; Integrated Processes: Nursing Process: Planning; Client Needs: Physiological Integrity: Physiological Adaptation; Cognitive Level: Application [Applying]

**2010. ANSWER: 2**

1. Hypoxia (oxygen deficiency in body tissues), although problematic, would not immediately cause respiratory arrest.
2. **Asphyxia (a condition caused by insufficient intake of oxygen) will cause respiratory arrest.**
3. Aspiration contributes to compromised respiratory function but will not immediately cause a respiratory arrest.
4. Hypothermia can contribute to compromised respiratory function but will not immediately cause a respiratory arrest.

▶ *Test-taking Tip: To narrow the options, associate the word "respiratory" in the stem with a related word in the options. Of the remaining options, consider the condition that is most life-threatening.*

Content Area: Child; Concept: Oxygenation; Integrated Processes: Nursing Process: Evaluation; Client Needs: Physiological Integrity: Physiological Adaptation; Cognitive Level: Evaluation [Evaluating]

**2011. ANSWER: 3**

1. Helping the parents make plans for future children is essential once the grieving process resolves.
2. There is no definitive etiology for SIDS, and making a referral for genetic counseling and education is not necessary.
3. **Many parents are unable to express their anger, grief, and loss openly. Making the focus of the first visit a time for listening may assist the parents in addressing their concerns, which may include grief, anger, and self-blame for the death of their child.**
4. Educating the family on causes of SIDS can help parents plan and use safety precautions for their future children, but this teaching is not appropriate for the first visit.

▶ *Test-taking Tip: Consider the stage of grief of the parents when selecting an option.*

Content Area: Child; Concept: Grief and Loss; Nursing Roles; Integrated Processes: Caring; Communication and Documentation; Client Needs: Psychosocial Integrity; Cognitive Level: Application [Applying]

**2012. ANSWER: 1**

1. **Usually a 10 mm induration in a nonimmunocompromised individual would not be a concern. However, an induration of greater than 5 mm in an HIV-positive individual requires follow-up and initiation of precautions.**
2. A chest x-ray to diagnose pneumonia should not affect the outcome of a TST.
3. A recent immigrant from a country with high TB prevalence is concerning as the client may have contracted TB while abroad; however, a 6 mm induration is inconclusive for the disease. Having another co-morbidity such as HIV that weakens the immune system increases the client's risk of actually having TB, and is more concerning.
4. Recent contact with a person who has active TB disease does ensure that a person will test positive for TB.

▶ *Test-taking Tip: If unsure, consider the effects of immunodeficiency on a TST.*

Content Area: Child; Concept: Oxygenation; Critical Thinking; Integrated Processes: Nursing Process: Evaluation; Client Needs: Physiological Integrity: Physiological Adaptation; Cognitive Level: Evaluation [Evaluating]

**2013. PHARM ANSWER: 2**

1. A BNP laboratory value would be needed to determine if HF was an adverse effect, but it is not reported.
2. **The adolescent should be assessed for signs of hepatotoxicity because the ALT or SGPT (serum glutamic pyruvic transaminase) is elevated. Isoniazid (Nydrazid) is metabolized by the liver.**
3. Aplastic anemia is an adverse effect of isoniazid, but the Hgb and Hct are normal.
4. The serum creatinine level would be elevated (not normal) with renal insufficiency.

▶ *Test-taking Tip: Eliminate all normal laboratory findings and focus on the abnormal values. Relate the abnormal laboratory values to the conditions listed in the options.*

Content Area: Child; Concept: Medication; Assessment; Oxygenation; Integrated Processes: Nursing Process: Analysis; Client Needs: Physiological Integrity: Pharmacological and Parenteral Therapies; Physiological Integrity: Reduction of Risk Potential; Cognitive Level: Analysis [Analyzing]

**2014. ANSWER: 1**

1. **An open-ended statement allows the parents time to express feelings and concerns, and they may provide the reason for referring to the TB as "it." In some cultures, people avoid calling the disease by name for fear that it may cause further harm.**
2. Telling the parents that the child will be cured by taking the prescribed medication is irrelevant during an assessment.

45 Respiratory Management Answers and Rationales

3. Asking a "why" question is a barrier to therapeutic communication and can result in defensiveness.

4. Although assessing the length of time the child may have had symptoms is important, this question ignores the parents' feelings.

▶ *Test-taking Tip: The key word is "best," indicating that more than one option is correct but one is better than the others. Remember to use therapeutic communication principles when answering questions.*

**Content Area:** Child; **Concept:** Infection; Stress; Assessment; Oxygenation; Diversity; **Integrated Processes:** Communication and Documentation; Culture and Spirituality; **Client Needs:** Psychosocial Integrity; **Cognitive Level:** Application [Applying]

## 2015. MoC ANSWER: 3

1. Restlessness and irritability are expected signs and symptoms of LTB.

2. The barking, rattling cough is due to fluid accumulation from inflammation and is an early, not impending, sign of respiratory failure.

3. **Decreased inspiratory breath sounds are a sign of physical exhaustion and may indicate impending respiratory failure.**

4. Hoarseness is usually associated with other disorders such as a sore throat or tonsillitis; a weak cry is associated with inflammation and pain.

▶ *Test-taking Tip: Another name for LTB is croup. Think about the effect of inflammation on the airways and the sounds heard if they are narrowed.*

**Content Area:** Child; **Concept:** Oxygenation; Assessment; **Integrated Processes:** Nursing Process: Evaluation; **Client Needs:** Safe and Effective Care Environment: Management of Care; Physiological Integrity: Reduction of Risk Potential; **Cognitive Level:** Evaluation [Evaluating]

## 2016. ANSWER: 1

1. **There are five classifications of esophageal atresia. In esophageal atresia with lower tracheoesophageal fistula, the proximal segment of the esophagus ends in a blind pouch and the distal segment connects with the trachea by way of a fistula. It is the most common type of esophageal atresia, occurring in 80%–90% of infants with this defect.**

2. This illustration shows both the upper and lower segments ending in blind pouches; there is no fistula.

3. This illustration shows both the upper and lower segments communicating with the trachea through a fistula.

4. This illustration shows the upper segment ending in a blind pouch and communicating with the trachea through a fistula.

▶ *Test-taking Tip: Use the term "esophageal atresia with lower tracheoesophageal fistula" to identify the blind pouch at the end of the esophagus.*

**Content Area:** Child; **Concept:** Digestion; Oxygenation; Assessment; **Integrated Processes:** Nursing Process: Analysis; **Client Needs:** Physiological Integrity: Physiological Adaptation; **Cognitive Level:** Comprehension [Understanding]

## 2017. ANSWER: 2

1. A supine position would allow secretions to pool at the back of the throat or in the buccal cavity.

2. **Following a T&A, the nurse should place the child in a side-lying position to facilitate drainage from the oropharynx.**

3. A semi-Fowler's position with the head turned to either side would hinder drainage and increase the risk for aspiration.

4. A high Fowler's position with the head slightly bent and to the side could hinder drainage and increase the risk for aspiration.

▶ *Test-taking Tip: Use the ABC's and visualization of what each position does to drainage to determine the best position to facilitate drainage from the oropharynx.*

**Content Area:** Child; **Concept:** Safety; Oxygenation; **Integrated Processes:** Nursing Process: Implementation; **Client Needs:** Physiological Integrity: Reduction of Risk Potential; **Cognitive Level:** Application [Applying]

## 2018. ANSWER: 2

1. "Coffee ground" emesis is an expected finding following a T&A.

2. **Frequent swallowing and clearing of the throat are signs and symptoms of hemorrhage, and they should be explored further by the nurse.**

3. Sore throat and difficulty swallowing are expected findings following a T&A.

4. Dried blood around the mouth is an expected finding following a T&A.

▶ *Test-taking Tip: Eliminate the options that would be expected following a T&A.*

**Content Area:** Child; **Concept:** Assessment; Oxygenation; Perfusion; **Integrated Processes:** Nursing Process: Assessment; **Client Needs:** Physiological Integrity: Reduction of Risk Potential; **Cognitive Level:** Analysis [Analyzing]

## 2019. ANSWER: 1

1. **Cold liquids will soothe the throat and decrease inflammation; red-colored food and beverages should be avoided because they can mask signs of bleeding.**

2. Hemorrhage may occur due to sloughing up to 10 days after surgery.

3. Gargling and toothbrushing are both recommended, but they should be performed gently with a soft toothbrush, and special care should be used to avoid traumatizing the surgical site.

4. Coughing should be avoided during the postoperative period because it can cause tissue disruption and hemorrhage.

▶ *Test-taking Tip: The key word is "understands." This is a positive-response item. Select the statement that is correct.*

**Content Area:** Child; **Concept:** Oxygenation; Nursing Roles; Comfort; **Integrated Processes:** Teaching/Learning; Caring; **Client Needs:** Physiological Integrity: Reduction of Risk Potential; Health Promotion and Maintenance; **Cognitive Level:** Evaluation [Evaluating]

**2020. ANSWER: 7, 2, 5, 4, 6, 3, 1**

7. Call for help. The emergency response system should be activated to ensure that others are available to perform CPR and get emergency supplies.

2. Palpate the brachial artery to determine if a pulse is present. Chest compressions should not be performed if an adequate pulse is present.

5. Place two or three fingers in the center of the chest just below the nipples. Correct placement is essential to avoid internal damage during chest compressions.

4. Give 30 chest compressions at a depth of 1.5 inches and a rate of 100 per minute. Sufficient depth and rate must be reached for adequate compression and perfusion.

6. Look for the object and remove it only if seen. A finger should not be placed in the mouth to search for the object because this could push the object deeper into the back of the throat.

3. Open the airway using the head-tilt, chin-lift or jaw-thrust maneuver. The method to open the airway will depend on whether the child has a neck injury.

1. Provide 2 rescue breaths for every 30 chest compressions. Rescue breaths and chest compressions are continued until the object is dislodged.

▶ *Test-taking Tip:* Use the acronym CAB (circulation, airway, and breathing) to place items in the correct order.

Content Area: Child; Concept: Oxygenation; Integrated Processes: Nursing Process: Implementation; Client Needs: Physiological Integrity: Physiological Adaptation; Cognitive Level: Synthesis [Creating]

# Chapter Forty-Six

# Pharmacological and Parenteral Therapies for Children

**2021.** **PHARM** The nurse is preparing an educational program on immunizations for parents of children 11 to 12 years of age. To ensure the information presented is accurate for this age group, which immunizations should the nurse plan to address?

1. Haemophilus influenza, varicella, and human papillomavirus (HPV)
2. Mumps, measles, and rubella (MMR); pneumococcal (PPSV); and hepatitis A
3. Diphtheria-tetanus-pertussis (DTaP), meningococcal, and haemophilus influenza
4. MMR; DTaP; and hepatitis B

**2022.** **MoC** **PHARM** The new nurse stored vaccines for future use. What observations by the supervisor indicate that they are properly stored? **Select all that apply.**

1. Placed all vaccines in a temperature-controlled refrigerator
2. Completed checks of the expiration date on the vaccines.
3. Placed bulk supplies of vaccines in a temperature-controlled freezer
4. Has no vaccines stored on the shelf in the door of the refrigerator
5. No food or beverage is stored in the same refrigerator or freezer as the vaccines
6. Protected light-sensitive vaccine vials with aluminum foil or aluminum packaging

**2023.** **MoC** **PHARM** The nurse observes a colleague about to administer an IM injection to the 12-month-old. Which intervention requires the nurse to intervene?

1. Prepares to give no more than 2 mL of fluid
2. Plans to give the injection using a 1-inch needle
3. Plans to inject into the dorsal gluteal site
4. Plans to apply lidocaine/prilocaine cream first

**2024.** **MoC** **PHARM** The nurse is preparing scheduled medications for hospitalized children. Which information should alert the nurse to withhold the medication and notify the HCP immediately?

1. Preparing oral hydrocodone with acetaminophen for the 10-year-old who has burn injuries and is feeling dizzy and light-headed
2. Preparing oral acetaminophen for the 6-month-old who has a fever of 102°F (38.9°C) from an infection and a new rash
3. Preparing clindamycin IV for the 16-year-old male who has aspiration pneumonia from near-drowning and has a BP of 92/56 mm Hg
4. Preparing phenobarbital IV for the 5-year-old who has intermittent seizures and is drowsy and states feeling tired

**2025.** **PHARM** The child, admitted to the ED, has nausea and vomiting, salivation, respiratory muscle weakness, and depressed reflexes an hour after exposure to pesticides. Which medications should the nurse anticipate administering to the child?

1. Atropine and flumazenil
2. Atropine and pralidoxime
3. Epinephrine and naloxone
4. Epinephrine and digoxin immune Fab

**2026.** PHARM The hospitalized child who has a blood lead level of 50 mcg/dL is to receive succimer 10 mg/kg oral capsule q8h for 5 days. The child weighs 20 kg. Which intervention by the student nurse should be corrected by the observing nurse?

1. Prepares to give the total dose of one 100-mg capsule with applesauce
2. Sprinkles the beads of two 100-mg capsules into pudding for administration
3. Offers fluids frequently during the shift to increase the child's urine output
4. Explains to the parent that chelation therapy removes the lead from the blood

**2027.** PHARM The 5-year-old is receiving an IV infusion of $D_5$ with 0.45 NaCl at 100 mL/hr. Which assessment findings suggest excessive parenteral fluid intake? **Select all that apply.**

1. Dyspnea
2. Lethargy
3. Gastric distention
4. Crackles in lung bases
5. Temperature of 102°F (38.9°C)

**2028.** PHARM The nurse has completed swaddling the 2-month-old infant, prepared supplies to cannulate the scalp vein for an IV infusion, and cleansed and shaved the hair at the site over the temporal bone. Place the remaining steps in the order that they should be performed by the nurse.

1. Return in 60 minutes and reswaddle the infant in a mummy restraint.
2. With an assistant holding the infant's head, insert a scalp vein needle and observe for blood return.
3. Apply lidocaine/prilocaine cream to the site selected and unswaddle the infant after the cream application.
4. Cleanse the shaved area with an antiseptic solution.
5. Remove the mummy restraint after initiating the infusion and comfort the infant.
6. Initiate the infusion and cover the infusion needle with a gauze dressing.

Answer: _____

**2029.** PHARM The child with CF is prescribed vitamin A supplements. Which finding by the clinic nurse indicates that the vitamin has been effective?

1. The skin is supple and healthy.
2. The viscosity of secretions is decreased.
3. The number of bleeding episodes is reduced.
4. The absorption of pancreatic enzyme is increased.

**2030.** MoC PHARM The new nurse is initiating TPN for four hospitalized pediatric clients. The experienced nurse should intervene when observing the new nurse attach the TPN infusion tubing into which IV catheter?

1. The catheter inserted in the right external jugular vein of the 2-year-old
2. The catheter inserted in the right subclavian vein of the 4-year-old
3. The peripherally inserted IV catheter in a hand vein of the 12-year-old
4. The PICC located in the right upper arm of the 6-year-old

**2031.** PHARM The child with CF is receiving albuterol. Which response should the nurse expect if albuterol is achieving the desired therapeutic effect?

1. Increased HR
2. Improved weight gain
3. Fewer hospitalizations
4. Fewer adventitious lung sounds

**2032.** PHARM The nurse is caring for the child from a non-English speaking country. The child is crying, and the interpreter is stating that the child has extreme pain. What should be the nurse's **priority?**

1. Administer morphine sulfate 1 mg IV as prescribed.
2. Have the child's mother, who knows limited English, ask the child what hurts.
3. Assess the child's pain level using an appropriate FACES pain rating scale.
4. Ask the HCP to change the analgesic dose due to inadequate pain control.

**2033.** PHARM The HCP prescribed acetaminophen according to weight recommendations for the child weighing 48 lb. The recommended dose is 15 mg/kg. How many mg should the nurse administer?

_____ mg (Record a whole number.)

**2034.** PHARM The adolescent, who is receiving morphine sulfate via PCA, has itching. Which medication listed on the client's MAR should the nurse plan to administer to relieve the itching?

1. Diazepam
2. Diphenhydramine
3. Naloxone hydrochloride
4. Butenafine hydrochloride

46 Pharmacological and Parenteral Therapies for Children

**2035.** PHARM The nurse is preparing to administer morphine sulfate IV to the child in severe pain. The child has an IV infusion of D₅W at 50 mL/hr through a PICC. Which intervention is **best** when administering the medication?

1. Disconnect the infusion, inject 3 mL of normal saline, and give the morphine sulfate undiluted.
2. Question the analgesic choice because morphine sulfate cannot be given through a PICC line.
3. Give the morphine sulfate undiluted into the existing IV tubing's medication port closest to the child.
4. Dilute the morphine sulfate with 5 mL of NS and give over 5 minutes into the IV tubing port closest to the child.

**2036.** MoC PHARM The HCP's progress notes state a plan to initiate an oral NSAID for the child's pain. Based on this information, the nurse should consult with the HCP when noting that which medication was the only analgesic prescribed?

1. Naproxen
2. Tolmetin
3. Ibuprofen
4. Hydromorphone

**2037.** PHARM A dose of albuterol 5 mg by nebulization is prescribed for the pediatric client experiencing wheezing from an asthma episode. The medication vial states 2.5 mg/3 mL. How many mL of medication should the nurse prepare for administration by nebulization?

_____ mL (Record your answer as a whole number.)

**2038.** MoC PHARM The home care nurse is observing the child with asthma self-administer a dose of albuterol via a metered-dose inhaler with a spacer. Within a short time, the child begins to wheeze loudly. What should the nurse do?

1. Reassure the parent that this usually only occurs with the initial dose.
2. Notify the HCP; wheezing may indicate paradoxical bronchospasms.
3. Consult with the HCP to have the child's medication dosage increased.
4. Reassess the technique; eye contact with albuterol can cause wheezing.

**2039.** PHARM The initial treatment regimen of isoniazid, rifampin, and ethambutol is prescribed for the adolescent who has a positive tuberculin skin test. The client confides that she thinks she may be pregnant and asks if she should be taking these medications. Which rationale should be the basis for the nurse's response?

1. These drugs cross the placental barrier, and treatment should be withheld until the postpartum period.
2. The medications should be taken, but the diagnosis is an indication for termination of the pregnancy.
3. The medications should be postponed because the risk for hepatitis is greatly increased in the intrapartum period.
4. The medications should be taken; untreated TB represents a far greater risk to the pregnant woman and her fetus.

**2040.** PHARM The 3-year-old with LTB is receiving aerosolized racemic epinephrine. Which assessment finding should alert the nurse that the treatment is having an adverse effect?

1. HR of 180 beats/min
2. BP of 60/40 mm Hg
3. RR of 25 breaths/min
4. Pulse oximetry of 90% on room air

**2041.** PHARM The HCP prescribes amoxicillin for the 8-month-old with acute otitis media that has not resolved. Which statement to the parents is correct regarding the primary purpose of amoxicillin?

1. "It will reduce the child's fever."
2. "It will reduce the child's severe ear pain."
3. "It will shrink swollen tissue in the Eustachian tube."
4. "It will treat the probable causative organism, *Haemophilus influenzae.*"

**2042.** MoC PHARM While the nurse is completing the assessment of the child with Reye's syndrome, the parent states that multiple OTC medications were given before hospitalization to treat the child's influenza symptoms. Which medication stated by the parent is **most** important for the nurse to report to the HCP?

1. Acetaminophen
2. Bismuth subsalicylate
3. Pseudoephedrine
4. Diphenhydramine

**2043.** **PHARM** The nurse is assessing the child's ear with an otoscope prior to administering medications to treat persistent otitis media. Which assessment finding should the nurse expect?

1.

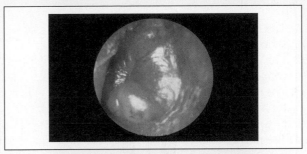

2.

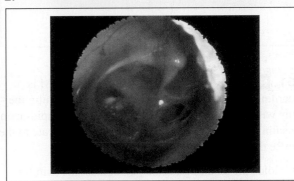

3.

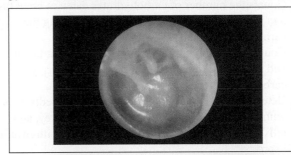

4.

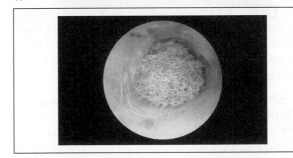

**2044.** **PHARM** The child weighing 20 kg is to receive ceftriaxone 2 g IVPB q12h and dexamethasone 3 mg IV-push q6h for 4 days to treat *Haemophilus influenzae* type b meningitis. The usual dose of ceftriaxone for a child is 100 mg/kg/dose with a maximum daily dose of 4 g. The recommended dose of dexamethasone for treating *H. influenzae* type b meningitis is 0.15 mg/kg q6h for 2 to 4 days. Based on the medications prescribed and these findings, which conclusion by the nurse is correct?

1. The dose of ceftriaxone is too high.
2. The dose of dexamethasone is too low.
3. Both medications are safe to administer as prescribed.
4. The ceftriaxone should be given before the dexamethasone.

**2045.** **PHARM** The nurse is reviewing the hospitalized child's medical record and serum laboratory report as illustrated. Based on the findings, which HCP order is **most** important for the nurse to question?

| Client: 12-year-old | Allergies: Penicillin, azithromycin, and cefazolin sodium |
|---|---|
| Diagnosis: Bacterial pneumonia and an upper respiratory tract infection | Weight: 50 kg |

| Serum Laboratory Test | Client's Value | Normal Values |
|---|---|---|
| BUN | 36 | 7–18 mg/dL |
| Creatinine | 1.2 | 0.3–0.7 mg/dL |
| Na | 136 | 138–145 mEq/L |
| K | 3.4 | 3.5–5.0 mEq/L |
| Cl | 96 | 98–106 mEq/L |
| Hgb | 11.5 | 11.5–15.5 g/dL |
| Hct | 34.5% | 35%–45% |
| WBC | 16.2 | 4.5–13.5 K/microL or mm$^3$ |
| Osmolality | 298 | 275–295 mOsm/kg H$_2$O |

1. Amikacin sulfate 375 mg IVPB q12h
2. Guaifenesin 50–100 mg q4h prn for cough
3. Dextrose 5% in 0.25 NaCl with 20 mEq/L KCL at 88 mL/hr
4. Acetaminophen 325–650 mg q4–6h prn, not to exceed 3000 mg/24 hr

**2046.** PHARM The nurse is teaching the 14-year-old who is being given captopril for the first time. Which explanation would be **most** appropriate?

1. "Captopril will help to control your asthma."
2. "Captopril will help to control your heart rate."
3. "Captopril will help to control your blood sugar."
4. "Captopril will help to control your blood pressure."

**2047.** PHARM The HCP orders a digitalizing dose of digoxin 225 mcg IV now to be given to a 3-year-old. The pharmacy sends a solution of 500 mcg in 50 mL of D₅W. How many mL should the nurse administer?

_____ mL (Round your answer to the nearest tenth.)

**2048.** PHARM The nurse is discharging the child with sickle cell disease who has undergone a splenectomy. The child has an allergy to penicillin. The nurse should anticipate teaching about which prophylactic medication?

1. Epoetin
2. Amoxicillin
3. Morphine sulfate
4. Erythromycin ethylsuccinate

**2049.** PHARM The 16-year-old, hospitalized for barbiturate overdose, is receiving low-dose dopamine at 1 mcg/kg/min. Which finding in the client's medical record illustrated should prompt the nurse to conclude that dopamine is effective?

| Time | Vital Signs | Cardiac Rhythm | Urine Output |
|------|-------------|----------------|--------------|
| 0800 | BP is 88/48 mm Hg HR 112 bpm | Sinus tachycardia with premature atrial contractions (PACs) | 20 mL |
| 1000 | BP is 94/64 mm Hg HR 116 bpm | Sinus tachycardia with rare PAC | 100 mL |

1. Decrease in PACs
2. Increase in urine output
3. Decrease in pulse pressure
4. Increase in the diastolic BP

**2050.** PHARM The nurse is showing the parents the preferred site for their child's insulin administration via an insulin pump. Place an X within the oval for the preferred site.

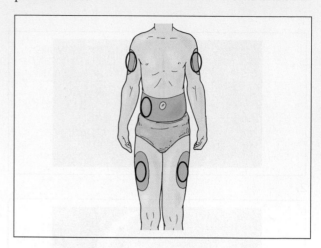

**2051.** PHARM The 12-year-old with type 1 DM is learning to use insulin pens for basal-bolus insulin therapy with both a very long-acting insulin and rapid-acting insulin. Which action by the child should indicate to the nurse that additional teaching is needed?

1. Holds the insulin glargine pen against the skin for 10 seconds after giving the correct amount of insulin
2. Counts the number of carbohydrates eaten at breakfast and selects the insulin lispro pen for covering the carbohydrates eaten
3. Counts the number of carbohydrates eaten at lunch and selects the insulin glargine pen for covering the carbohydrates eaten
4. Determines that the blood glucose level at bedtime is within the normal range, eats a piece of turkey, and tells the nurse that coverage is not needed with insulin lispro.

**2052.** PHARM The nurse completes teaching insulin administration to the parent of the toddler newly diagnosed with type 1 DM. The nurse concludes that the teaching was successful when the parent makes which statement?

1. "NPH insulin is only given at night immediately before the bedtime snack."
2. "I should use only the buttocks for the insulin injections until the child is older."
3. "Insulin lispro acts within 15 minutes and peaks 30 to 90 minutes after injection."
4. "Insulin detemir can be added to the insulin lispro pen to reduce the number of injections."

**2053.** **PHARM** The nurse is evaluating the effectiveness of lispro and glargine insulins being administered to the 2-year-old with type 1 DM. Which findings on the serum laboratory report indicate that treatment is effective? Place an X next to each laboratory result that reflects that treatment is effective.

| Laboratory Report | |
|---|---|
| **Serum Laboratory Test** | **Client Result** |
| Creatinine | 0.9 mg/dL |
| WBCs | 4000/mm³ |
| Hgb | 11 g/dL |
| Hgb A₁c | 4.5% |
| Potassium | 3.9 mEq/L |
| Glucose | 70 mg/dL |

**2054.** **MoC** **PHARM** The parent of the child brought to the ED states to the nurse, "My child is sweaty and shaky; I think some of my medication is gone." The parent hands the nurse the medication bottle as illustrated. Which action should the nurse take **first**?

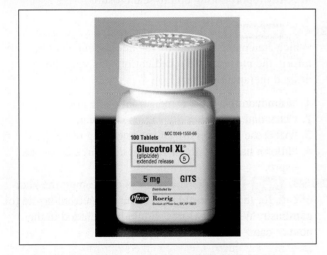

1. Start an infusion of D₅W at 40 mL/hr.
2. Give glucagon 1 mg subcutaneously.
3. Check the child's blood glucose level.
4. Determine how many tablets were taken.

**2055.** **PHARM** Trimethoprim-sulfamethoxazole is prescribed for the child who develops a UTI. What information should the nurse address when teaching the parents about administering the medication? **Select all that apply.**

1. Weigh the child daily in the morning.
2. Take the child's temperature once daily.
3. Encourage the child to drink plenty of fluids.
4. Give the medication at the prescribed times.
5. If a rash occurs, contact the HCP immediately.

**2056.** **MoC** **PHARM** The 9-year-old with SLE is receiving large doses of prednisolone. Which lab finding should be reported to the HCP as an untoward effect of prednisolone?

1. Total bilirubin of 4 mg/dL
2. WBC count of 18,000/mm³
3. Serum sodium of 130 mEq/L
4. Random glucose of 130 mg/dL

**2057.** **PHARM** Methylphenidate hydrochloride is prescribed for the child with ADHD. The nurse should teach the parents to administer the medication in which way?

1. Whenever the child exhibits inattention behaviors
2. Whenever the child exhibits hyperactive behaviors
3. With a snack before bed to calm the child for sleep
4. During or after meals to prevent a decreased intake of food

**2058.** **PHARM** Oral ranitidine 2 mg/kg twice daily is prescribed for the infant weighing 16 lb 8 oz. The medication is supplied as 15 mg/mL. How many mL should the nurse instruct the parent to withdraw in the syringe provided with the ranitidine for one dose?

_____ mL (Record a whole number.)

**2059.** **PHARM** The nurse is reviewing information for the 6-month-old who is being given ranitidine. Which finding should the nurse identify as an adverse effect of ranitidine?

1. A HR of 110 bpm
2. Oral temperature of 102.7°F (39.3°C)
3. Spitting up some formula after each feeding
4. A hard, pebble-like stool every 2 days

**2060.** **PHARM** The 14-year-old who has GERD is receiving lansoprazole. Which response should the nurse expect if lansoprazole is achieving the desired therapeutic effect?

1. Increased appetite
2. Increased GI motility
3. Decreased epigastric pain
4. Decreased rectal flatulence

**2061.** **PHARM** The nurse is preparing to care for the 14-month-old newly hospitalized toddler with bacterial gastroenteritis and severe dehydration. Which initial collaborative interventions should the nurse expect to implement? **Select all that apply.**

1. IV antibiotic to treat infection
2. Oral fluids for fluid rehydration
3. IV fluid therapy for rehydration
4. Analgesics for pain and discomfort
5. An antidiarrheal to control diarrhea
6. Antipyretic for elevated temperature

**2062.** **PHARM** The nurse is preparing to administer IV fluids to the 13-kg child who has dehydration. The daily IV fluid requirement is to administer 1000 mL + 50 mL/kg weight over 10 kg. How many mL/hr should the nurse calculate to administer the IV therapy correctly?

_____ mL/hr (Record a whole number.)

**2063.** **PHARM** The nurse is developing the plan of care for the 7-year-old with encopresis who has been started on lactulose. Which outcome would be **most** appropriate for the nurse to establish?

1. 2-pound weight gain
2. Nighttime continence
3. Blood glucose 70–110 mg/dL
4. Normal bowel movement daily

**2064.** **PHARM** The nurse is to administer phenobarbital 300 mg IV to the child weighing 18 kg who is in status epilepticus. Which actions should the nurse take to safely administer phenobarbital? **Select all that apply.**

1. Give the phenobarbital over 30 minutes via IV piggyback.
2. Monitor the IV site for signs of extravasation.
3. Dilute the phenobarbital dose in 10 mL D$_5$W.
4. Identify incompatible medications or solutions being infused.
5. Inject the phenobarbital over 10 minutes in the port closest to the child.

**2065.** **PHARM** The 4-year-old who has meningitis is to receive ceftriaxone 750 mg IVPB over 30 minutes. The pharmacy provided 750 mg in 50 mL D$_5$W to be infused IVPB through a microdrip infusion system (tubing drop factor 60 gtt/mL). At what rate, in gtt per min, should the nurse program the IVPB pump?

_____ gtt/min (Record a whole number.)

**2066.** **PHARM** The 17-year-old female is about to have a drug screen test for employment. The adolescent tells the nurse of a recent UTI that was treated with antibiotics. Which antibiotic, if identified by the client, could produce a false-positive urine screening test for opioids?

1. Cephalexin
2. Ceftazidime
3. Amoxicillin
4. Ciprofloxacin

**2067.** **MoC** **PHARM** The nurse is assessing the 13-year-old who has been taking somatropin recombinant. Which findings associated with the medication use should the nurse report to the HCP?

1. Erythematous palmar rash
2. BP of 122/74 mm Hg
3. Random blood glucose of 158 mg/dL
4. X-ray report noting epiphyseal closure

**2068.** **PHARM** The 16-year-old is taking valacyclovir. Which statement, if made by the adolescent, should inform the nurse that the medication is having the desired therapeutic effect?

1. "I am having a regular menstrual cycle now."
2. "That bad odor from my vagina is now gone."
3. "All those sores on my labia are getting better."
4. "I don't have that green vaginal discharge anymore."

**2069.** **MoC** **PHARM** The nurse is developing the plan of care for the 4-year-old who is taking metronidazole for giardiasis. Which measures should be included in the plan of care? **Select all that apply.**

1. Assess cardiac status.
2. Assess for signs of infection.
3. Reinforce strict hand washing.
4. Give metronidazole with food.
5. Monitor results of stool samples.

**2070.** **PHARM** The nurse is concerned that the adolescent with RA may be developing a side effect of methotrexate. Which test should the nurse review prior to administration?

1. Folic acid level
2. Serum electrolytes
3. Complete blood count
4. Activated partial prothrombin time

**2071.** **PHARM** Prior to administering filgrastim, the nurse reviews the laboratory results for the 3-year-old who completed the second round of chemotherapy three weeks ago. Which finding indicates a therapeutic response to filgrastim?

1. Hematocrit of 31%
2. Eosinophil count of 6%
3. WBC count of 6800/mm³
4. Platelet count of 150,000/mm³

**2072.** **PHARM** The nurse is teaching the parent of the 3-year-old being treated with vincristine sulfate for Wilms' tumor. The nurse should inform the parents to immediately notify the HCP of which **most** significant adverse effect?

1. The child develops diarrhea.
2. The child's hair begins to fall out.
3. The child develops dysphagia and paresthesia.
4. The child has signs or symptoms of depression.

**INSTRUCTIONS:** Refer to the information provided in the client's MAR illustrated to answer Questions 2073 and 2074.

### Medication Administration Record

| Client: 10-year-old | Allergies: Cefdinir | Weight: 66 lbs | Dx: New-Onset Seizure Disorder; Gastroenteritis | | |
|---|---|---|---|---|---|
| **Scheduled Medications** | | 0001–0759 | 0800–1559 | 1600–2400 | |
| Lamotrigine 18 mg orally bid | | | 0800_____ | 2000____ | |
| Metronidazole oral 225 mg q6h | | 0200_____ | 0800_____ 1400_____ | 2000____ | |
| NaCl 500 mL IV bolus now (20 mL/kg) | | | 0800_____ | | |

**2073.** **CJ** **PHARM** The nurse reads from the MAR illustrated that the child is to receive the first dose of lamotrigine at 0800 hours. The drug reference book recommends an initial pediatric dose of lamotrigine of 0.6 mg/kg/day in two divided doses for the first 2 weeks. Which action by the nurse is **most** appropriate?

1. Administer lamotrigine as written on the MAR.
2. Telephone the HCP to question the dose.
4. Withhold lamotrigine; it interacts with metronidazole.
3. Consult the pharmacist about the correct dose.

**2074.** **CJ** **PHARM** The nurse determines that the child's NaCl 500 mL IV bolus dose is incorrect. What should be the correct amount in mL for the bolus dose?

_____ mL (Record a whole number.)

# Answers and Rationales

**2021.** PHARM **ANSWER: 3**

1. Varicella vaccines are administered at 12 to 15 months, with the second dose at 4 to 6 years.
2. The first dose of hepatitis A vaccine is administered before 1 year of age, with the second dose 6 months after the first dose.
3. **The recommended immunization schedule for children 11 to 12 years old includes a DTaP booster and meningococcal and haemophilus influenza vaccines. Others include HPV, PPSV, and hepatitis A series.**
4. MMR vaccines are administered at 12 to 15 months, with the second dose at 4 to 6 years. A hepatitis B vaccine is administered to all newborns prior to hospital discharge, with the second dose at 1 to 2 months and the third dose at 6 to 18 months.

▶ **Test-taking Tip:** *Identify those diseases that younger children are more likely to have exposure to and that require early immunizations, a series for the immunization, or a later booster. Eliminate these options.*

**Content Area:** Child; **Concept:** Medication; Immunity; Promoting Health; **Integrated Processes:** Nursing Process: Planning; **Client Needs:** Health Promotion and Maintenance; Physiological Integrity: Pharmacological and Parenteral Therapies; **Cognitive Level:** Analysis [Analyzing]

**2022.** PHARM MoC **ANSWER: 2, 4, 5, 6**

1. Not all vaccines are refrigerated; some vaccines will be inactivated by refrigeration and freezing.
2. **Periodic checking for expiration dates is necessary to ensure that outdated vaccines are not administered.**
3. Not all bulk supplies should be placed in a freezer; some vaccines are inactivated by freezing.
4. **When refrigeration is required, a main shelf inside the refrigerator is best because a shelf in the door will have frequent temperature changes that will alter the potency of the vaccine.**
5. **Storing food and beverage in the same unit may "result in frequent opening of the unit, leading to greater chance of temperature instability and light exposure. Contamination may also result.**
6. **Aluminum foil or packaging can be used to protect light-sensitive vaccines.**

▶ **Test-taking Tip:** *Options that contain absolute words such as "all" are usually not correct and should be eliminated.*

**Content Area:** Child; **Concept:** Immunity; Medication; **Integrated Processes:** Nursing Process: Implementation; **Client Needs:** Safe and Effective Care Environment: Management of Care; Physiological Integrity: Pharmacological and Parenteral Therapies; Safe and Effective Care Environment: Safety and Infection Control; **Cognitive Level:** Application [Applying]

**2023.** PHARM MoC **ANSWER: 3**

1. No more than 2 mL of fluid should be injected into a muscle.
2. The appropriate needle length for an IM injection for children ages 2 to 12 months is 1 inch and 1¼ inch for toddlers.
3. **Use of the dorsal gluteal site is not recommended due to a high risk of nerve damage.**
4. Use of lidocaine/prilocaine cream (EMLA) to numb the area is suggested when time allows but is not required.

▶ **Test-taking Tip:** *The vastus lateralis muscle is the largest muscle in the infant, thus providing the safest IM injection site.*

**Content Area:** Child; **Concept:** Medication; Management; Safety; **Integrated Processes:** Nursing Process: Implementation; **Client Needs:** Safe and Effective Care Environment: Management of Care; Physiological Integrity: Pharmacological and Parenteral Therapies; **Cognitive Level:** Application [Applying]

**2024.** PHARM MoC **ANSWER: 3**

1. Dizziness and light-headedness are side effects of hydrocodone with acetaminophen (Vicodin), and the nurse may choose to withhold a scheduled dose. These are not potentially life-threatening or warranting an immediate call to the HCP.
2. A rash is a side effect of acetaminophen (Tylenol). However, the rash is not potentially life-threatening or warranting an immediate call to the HCP.
3. **An adverse effect of clindamycin (Cleocin) is hypotension. A BP of 92/56 mm Hg is low for a 16-year-old. Normal BP for a 16-year-old male is 111/63 mm Hg to 136/90 mm Hg, depending on height percentile. The nurse should compare the previous BP readings with the current one to determine the degree of BP variation and then immediately notify the HCP because the BP can decrease further.**
4. Tiredness and drowsiness are side effects of phenobarbital (Luminal). However, these are expected. The nurse would not withhold phenobarbital unless there were additional neurological alterations that would warrant contacting the HCP.

▶ **Test-taking Tip:** *The key word in the stem is "immediately." Use the ABC's to establish priority.*

**Content Area:** Child; **Concept:** Medication; Assessment; Safety; **Integrated Processes:** Nursing Process: Evaluation; Communication and Documentation; **Client Needs:** Safe and Effective Care Environment: Management of Care; Physiological Integrity: Pharmacological and Parenteral Therapies; **Cognitive Level:** Evaluation [Evaluating]

**2025. PHARM ANSWER: 2**

1. Although the nurse should anticipate administering atropine, flumazenil would not be used to treat organophosphate poisoning. Flumazenil (Romazicon) antagonizes the effects of benzodiazepines on the CNS, such as sedation, impaired recall, and psychomotor impairment.
2. **An organophosphate base in pesticides causes acetylcholine to accumulate at neuromuscular junctions. Atropine (Atropine), an anticholinergic medication, and pralidoxime chloride (Protopam), a cholinesterase reactivator, are effective antidotes to reverse the symptoms.**
3. Epinephrine (EpiPen) is an alpha- and beta-adrenergic agonist and cardiac stimulant that strengthens myocardial contractions, increases systolic BP, increases cardiac rate and output, and constricts bronchial arterioles, inhibiting histamine release. Naloxone (Narcan) is a narcotic antagonist that reverses the effects of opiates.
4. Although the nurse should anticipate administering epinephrine, digoxin immune Fab would not be used to treat organophosphate poisoning. Digoxin immune Fab (Digibind) is the antidote for digoxin and digitoxin, which acts by complexing with circulating digoxin or digitoxin, preventing the drug from binding at receptor sites.

▶ **Test-taking Tip:** The focus of the question is an antidote for organophosphates in pesticides. Examine options with duplicate information first. Use the drug names as cues for identifying the antidote and eliminate the antidotes for benzodiazepines, opiates, and digoxin.

Content Area: Child; **Concept:** Medication; Critical Thinking; Safety; **Integrated Processes:** Nursing Process: Planning; **Client Needs:** Physiological Integrity: Pharmacological and Parenteral Therapies; **Cognitive Level:** Analysis [Analyzing]

**2026. PHARM ANSWER: 1**

1. **The 20-kg child should receive two capsules of succimer (Chemet), not one.**
   **Dose (mg) = 20 kg × 10 mg/kg = 200 mg.**
2. Succimer capsules can be opened and sprinkled on a small amount of food or in liquid to be swallowed; two 100-mg capsules = 200 mg, which is the correct dose.
3. Fluids should be increased to prevent renal damage because succimer is excreted by the kidneys.
4. Succimer forms a water-soluble compound with lead, allowing urinary elimination of excessive amounts of lead. Lead is removed from the blood, and theoretically some lead is removed from tissues and organs.

▶ **Test-taking Tip:** The dose the child is to receive is stated in the options and not the stem. Carefully calculate the dosage based on information in the options.

Content Area: Child; **Concept:** Medication; Safety; **Integrated Processes:** Nursing Process: Evaluation; **Client Needs:** Physiological Integrity: Pharmacological and Parenteral Therapies; **Cognitive Level:** Evaluation [Evaluating]

**2027. PHARM ANSWER: 1, 2, 4**

1. **Dyspnea occurs in fluid volume overload from fluid rapidly shifting between the intracellular and extracellular compartments.**
2. **Lethargy and change in level of consciousness can occur from fluid shifting in brain cells.**
3. Gastric distention can occur from excessive oral (not IV) fluid intake or infection.
4. **Crackles indicate fluid volume overload and occur from fluid rapidly shifting into the alveoli.**
5. An elevated temperature is a sign of fluid volume deficit, not excess.

▶ **Test-taking Tip:** The key words in the stem are "excessive parenteral." Eliminate options that pertain to oral fluid intake or fluid volume deficit.

Content Area: Child; **Concept:** Fluid and Electrolyte Balance; Oxygenation; Medication; **Integrated Processes:** Nursing Process: Assessment; **Client Needs:** Physiological Integrity: Pharmacological and Parenteral Therapies; **Cognitive Level:** Application [Applying]

**2028. PHARM ANSWER: 3, 1, 4, 2, 6, 5**

3. **Apply lidocaine/prilocaine (EMLA) cream to the site selected and unswaddle the infant after the cream application. An anesthetic cream will numb the site and help reduce the infant's pain during insertion. The infant does not need to remain swaddled while the cream reaches its therapeutic effectiveness in about an hour.**
1. **Return in 60 minutes and reswaddle the infant in a mummy restraint. It takes about an hour for the lidocaine/prilocaine cream to reach its therapeutic effectiveness. The infant should be reswaddled to minimize movement during insertion.**
4. **Cleanse the shaved area with an antiseptic solution. Cleansing the area with an antiseptic solution will help prevent inadvertent introduction of microorganisms into the vascular system.**
2. **With an assistant holding the infant's head, insert a scalp vein needle and observe for blood return. Movement of the infant's head can result in loss of the vein access or a needle-stick injury to the infant or nurse.**
6. **Initiate the infusion and cover the infusion needle with a gauze dressing. Once the vein has been successfully cannulated, the site can be dressed and IV fluids started.**
5. **Remove the mummy restraint after initiating the infusion and comfort the infant. The mummy restraint is no longer needed after the IV catheter has been successfully inserted into a scalp vein.**

▶ **Test-taking Tip:** Visualize the procedure prior to placing the steps in the correct order. Look for key words in the options to determine if the step is an early or a later step.

Content Area: Child; **Concept:** Medication; Fluid and Electrolyte Balance; Safety; **Integrated Processes:** Nursing Process: Implementation; **Client Needs:** Physiological Integrity: Pharmacological and Parenteral Therapies; **Cognitive Level:** Synthesis [Creating]

**2029.** PHARM **ANSWER: 1**

1. **A water-miscible form of vitamin A is given in children diagnosed with CF because the uptake of the fat-soluble vitamins is decreased. One of the functions of vitamin A is to keep epithelial tissue healthy by aiding the differentiation of specialty cells.**
2. Other treatments for CF, such as bronchodilators and recombinant human deoxyribonuclease [dornase alfa (Pulmozyme)], decrease the viscosity of secretions.
3. Vitamin K, another fat-soluble vitamin administered in CF, increases coagulation.
4. Vitamin A has no effect on pancreatic enzyme absorption.

♦ **Test-taking Tip:** *Eliminate options that pertain to outcomes of the treatments for CF. Of the two remaining options, determine which pertains to vitamin A and which to vitamin K.*

**Content Area:** Child; **Concept:** Skin Integrity; Digestion; **Integrated Processes:** Nursing Process: Evaluation; **Client Needs:** Physiological Integrity: Pharmacological and Parenteral Therapies; **Cognitive Level:** Evaluation [Evaluating]

**2030.** PHARM MoC **ANSWER: 3**

1. The external jugular vein is a central IV access site.
2. The subclavian vein is a central IV access site.
3. **TPN is a concentrated hypertonic solution containing glucose, vitamins, electrolytes, trace minerals, and protein. Because it is hypertonic, it should be administered through a central IV access site or a PICC. A major vein is used to avoid inflammatory reactions and venous thrombosis from the high-caloric and high-osmotic fluid.**
4. A PICC is located in a central IV access site.

♦ **Test-taking Tip:** *Look for similarities in options. Identify the three central IV access sites and eliminate these.*

**Content Area:** Child; **Concept:** Medication; Safety; Nursing Roles; Nutrition; **Integrated Processes:** Nursing Process: Implementation; **Client Needs:** Physiological Integrity: Pharmacological and Parenteral Therapies; Safe and Effective Care Environment: Management of Care; **Cognitive Level:** Analysis [Analyzing]

**2031.** PHARM **ANSWER: 4**

1. Albuterol may increase HR, but this is not the desired therapeutic effect.
2. Weight should not be affected by albuterol.
3. The use of a bronchodilator has not been demonstrated to decrease hospitalization frequency.
4. **The desired therapeutic effect of a bronchodilator such as albuterol (Proventil) is a reduction in adventitious (abnormal) breath sounds.**

♦ **Test-taking Tip:** *Think about the nutritional and pulmonary effects that CF has in the body and narrow the options to nutrition and pulmonary. Also note that the question involves a pulmonary medication, and so you can eliminate options that are not related to pulmonary effects.*

**Content Area:** Child; **Concept:** Oxygenation; Medication; **Integrated Processes:** Nursing Process: Evaluation; **Client Needs:** Physiological Integrity: Pharmacological and Parenteral Therapies; **Cognitive Level:** Evaluation [Evaluating]

**2032.** PHARM **ANSWER: 3**

1. The nurse's judgment regarding the choice of pain medication and dose should be based on the reported level of pain.
2. The nurse should do an independent assessment because sometimes information can be misinterpreted if there is limited knowledge of the language.
3. **Assessment should be completed prior to a pain intervention. The FACES pain-rating scale has been translated into a variety of languages.**
4. There is no information indicating the need for the pain medication dose to be changed.

♦ **Test-taking Tip:** *Note the key word "priority." Use the nursing process. Assessment is the first step.*

**Content Area:** Child; **Concept:** Medication; Communication; Comfort; Assessment; Diversity; **Integrated Processes:** Nursing Process: Assessment; Caring; Culture and Spirituality; **Client Needs:** Physiological Integrity: Pharmacological and Parenteral Therapies; Psychosocial Integrity; **Cognitive Level:** Application [Applying]

**2033.** PHARM **ANSWER: 327**

**First change 48 lb into kilograms (48 lb ÷ 2.2 lb/kg = 21.8 kg). Next determine the dose (21.8 kg × 15 mg/kg = 327 mg). The child should receive 327 mg of acetaminophen (Tylenol).**

♦ **Test-taking Tip:** *Recall that 1 kg = 2.2 lb.*

**Content Area:** Child; **Concept:** Medication; Safety; **Integrated Processes:** Nursing Process: Implementation; **Client Needs:** Physiological Integrity: Pharmacological and Parenteral Therapies; **Cognitive Level:** Analysis [Analyzing]

**2034.** PHARM **ANSWER: 2**

1. Diazepam (Valium) acts on the CNS to produce sedation, hypnosis, skeletal muscle relaxation, and anticonvulsant activity.
2. **Diphenhydramine (Benadryl) is an antihistamine that blocks histamine release by competing for the histamine receptors.**
3. Naloxone (Narcan) is a narcotic antagonist that reverses the effects of opiates.
4. Butenafine (Mentax) is an antifungal antibiotic used to treat tinea pedis, tinea corporis, and tinea cruris.

♦ **Test-taking Tip:** *A medication that is an antihistamine can be used to treat itching.*

**Content Area:** Child; **Concept:** Medication; Comfort; **Integrated Processes:** Nursing Process: Planning; **Client Needs:** Physiological Integrity: Pharmacological and Parenteral Therapies; Physiological Integrity: Basic Care and Comfort; **Cognitive Level:** Application [Applying]

**2035.** PHARM **ANSWER: 4**

1. Unnecessary IV disconnections increase the risk for infection. Morphine sulfate is compatible with $D_5W$.
2. Morphine sulfate can be administered into a PICC access device.
3. Administering undiluted morphine sulfate to the child increases the risk of adverse effects.

4. **The nurse should dilute the morphine sulfate before administration to prevent too-rapid administration and adverse effects. A single dose should be given over 4 to 5 minutes.**

▶ *Test-taking Tip: Often the option that is most complete is the answer.*

Content Area: Child; **Concept:** Comfort; Medication; **Integrated Processes:** Nursing Process: Implementation; **Client Needs:** Physiological Integrity: Pharmacological and Parenteral Therapies; **Cognitive Level:** Analysis [Analyzing]

## 2036. PHARM MoC ANSWER: 4

1. Naproxen (Aleve) is an NSAID.
2. Tolmetin (Tolectin) is an NSAID.
3. Ibuprofen (Advil, Motrin) is an NSAID.
4. **Hydromorphone (Dilaudid) is an opioid analgesic, not an NSAID.**

▶ *Test-taking Tip: This is a false-response item; select the medication that is not an NSAID. If uncertain, use the generic name of the medication as a cue to determine the answer.*

Content Area: Child; **Concept:** Comfort; Medication; Management; **Integrated Processes:** Communication and Documentation; **Client Needs:** Safe and Effective Care Environment: Management of Care; Physiological Integrity: Pharmacological and Parenteral Therapies; **Cognitive Level:** Application [Applying]

## 2037. PHARM ANSWER: 6

**Use a proportion formula:**
**2.5 mg : 3 mL :: 5 mg : $X$ mL; multiply the outside values and then the inside values and solve for $X$;**
**$2.5X = 15$; $X = 15 \div 2.5$; $X = 6$ mL**

▶ *Test-taking Tip: The dose may seem unusually large, but albuterol (Proventil) is being administered by nebulization.*

Content Area: Child; **Concept:** Medication; Safety; Oxygenation; **Integrated Processes:** Nursing Process: Implementation; **Client Needs:** Physiological Integrity: Pharmacological and Parenteral Therapies; **Cognitive Level:** Application [Applying]

## 2038. PHARM MoC ANSWER: 2

1. Reassuring the parent is an inappropriate action; the wheezing is not a normal reaction. There is no indication that this is an initial dose.
2. **The client's wheezing suggests paradoxical bronchospasms, which can occur with excessive use of adrenergic bronchodilators such as albuterol (Proventil). The medication should be withheld and the HCP notified.**
3. A paradoxical bronchospasm can occur from excessive use, so the dosage should not be increased.
4. Contact with the eyes can cause eye irritation, not wheezing.

▶ *Test-taking Tip: Examine options with duplicate words first and eliminate one of these options. Then review the remaining options. Use the ABC's to determine that wheezing requires an immediate intervention.*

Content Area: Child; **Concept:** Medication; Oxygenation; **Integrated Processes:** Nursing Process: Implementation; **Client Needs:** Safe and Effective Care Environment: Management of Care; Physiological Integrity: Pharmacological and Parenteral Therapies; **Cognitive Level:** Analysis [Analyzing]

## 2039. PHARM ANSWER: 4

1. The medications do not cross the placental barrier, so treatment should not be withheld.
2. Administering antituberculosis medications would not be an indication for termination of pregnancy because the medications are safe during pregnancy.
3. The risk of hepatitis is slightly increased with the use of antituberculosis medications in pregnant women; however, the benefits of treatment strongly outweigh postponement of treatment.
4. **Infants born to women with untreated TB may be of lower birth weight, but rarely would the infant acquire congenital TB. Isoniazid (Nydrazid), rifampin (Rifadin), and ethambutol (Myambutol) are all considered safe for use in pregnancy.**

▶ *Test-taking Tip: Evaluate similar options first (not giving the medication) and eliminate one or both of these. Then examine the two remaining options. Think about the risk to others if the client is not treated.*

Content Area: Child; **Concept:** Medication; Pregnancy; Safety; **Integrated Processes:** Nursing Process: Analysis; **Client Needs:** Physiological Integrity: Pharmacological and Parenteral Therapies; **Cognitive Level:** Analysis [Analyzing]

## 2040. PHARM ANSWER: 1

1. **Tachycardia is an adverse effect of racemic epinephrine (AsthmaNefrin).**
2. Hypertension, not hypotension, is an adverse effect of racemic epinephrine; a BP of 60/40 mm Hg in a 3-year-old indicates hypotension.
3. A RR of 25 breaths/min is normal for a 3-year-old.
4. A pulse oximetry reading of 90% is concerning and may indicate the need for supplemental oxygen, but it is not an adverse effect from the medication.

▶ *Test-taking Tip: Epinephrine is an adrenergic medication, and response to the drug should mimic a sympathetic response (fight or flight). Adverse effects often exaggerate the expected action.*

Content Area: Child; **Concept:** Oxygenation; Medication; **Integrated Processes:** Nursing Process: Analysis; **Client Needs:** Physiological Integrity: Pharmacological and Parenteral Therapies; **Cognitive Level:** Application [Applying]

## 2041. PHARM ANSWER: 4

1. As the infection is treated, the fever will be reduced, but this is not the primary reason for treatment with amoxicillin.
2. Treating the ear infection will reduce the pain, but that is not the primary purpose for treatment with amoxicillin.
3. Reducing inflammation of the Eustachian tube will occur, but this is not the primary purpose for treatment with amoxicillin.
4. **Acute otitis media is frequently caused by the *Haemophilus influenzae* and *Streptococcus pneumoniae* bacteria. The primary purpose of amoxicillin (Amoxil) is to treat the infection caused by these two organisms.**

▶ *Test-taking Tip: The key words are "primary purpose." Focus on the main action of amoxicillin.*

**Content Area:** Child; **Concept:** Infection; Medication; Nursing Roles; **Integrated Processes:** Teaching/Learning; **Client Needs:** Physiological Integrity: Pharmacological and Parenteral Therapies; **Cognitive Level:** Application [Applying]

## 2042. PHARM MoC ANSWER: 2

1. Acetaminophen (Tylenol) is an aspirin-free analgesic and antipyretic.
2. **Although the etiology of Reye's syndrome is unknown, the condition typically occurs after a viral illness, such as influenza, and is associated with aspirin (acetylsalicylic acid) use during the illness. Bismuth subsalicylate (Pepto-Bismol) contains aspirin.**
3. Pseudoephedrine (Sudafed) is an allergy and/or cold remedy used for nasal drying and decongestion. This does not contain aspirin.
4. Diphenhydramine (Benadryl) is an antihistamine. This does not contain aspirin.

▶ *Test-taking Tip: Use the generic name as a cue to select the correct option. Reye's syndrome is thought to be associated with aspirin use during a viral illness.*

**Content Area:** Child; **Concept:** Medication; Safety; Communication; Collaboration; **Integrated Processes:** Communication and Documentation; **Client Needs:** Safe and Effective Care Environment: Management of Care; Physiological Integrity: Pharmacological and Parenteral Therapies; **Cognitive Level:** Analysis [Analyzing]

## 2043. PHARM ANSWER: 1

1. **This illustration shows otitis media characterized by a bulging contour to the tympanic membrane, unclear ossicular landmarks, and yellowish middle ear effusion.**
2. This illustration shows a perforated tympanic membrane, not otitis media.
3. This illustration shows a normal left ear tympanic membrane. The ossicular landmarks can be identified through the tympanic membrane. The nurse would not expect to see a normal tympanic membrane when the child has persistent otitis media.
4. This illustration shows the presence of a foreign body in the ear canal.

▶ *Test-taking Tip: The suffix "-itis" refers to inflammation. Narrow the options to those that look inflamed.*

**Content Area:** Child; **Concept:** Infection; Medication; **Integrated Processes:** Nursing Process: Assessment; **Client Needs:** Physiological Integrity: Pharmacological and Parenteral Therapies; Physiological Integrity: Physiological Adaptation; **Cognitive Level:** Comprehension [Understanding]

## 2044. PHARM ANSWER: 3

1. The dose for ceftriaxone is correct (100 mg/kg × 20 kg = 2000 mg; 1000 mg = 1 gm; 2000 mg = 2 gm).
2. The dose of dexamethasone is correct (0.15 mg/kg × 20 kg = 3 mg).
3. The doses of ceftriaxone (Rocephin) and dexamethasone (Decadron) are at the recommended doses. The dose for ceftriaxone is correct (100 mg/kg × 20 kg = 2000 mg; 1000 mg = 1 g; 2000 mg = 2 g). The dose of dexamethasone is correct (0.15 mg/kg × 20 kg = 3 mg).
4. An IV-push medication takes less time to administer than an IV piggyback (IVPB) medication. The dexamethasone should be administered first.

▶ *Test-taking Tip: Use a medication calculation formula and calculate the doses and the options; then select an answer.*

**Content Area:** Child; **Concept:** Medication; Safety; Infection; **Integrated Processes:** Nursing Process: Analysis; **Client Needs:** Physiological Integrity: Pharmacological and Parenteral Therapies; **Cognitive Level:** Analysis [Analyzing]

## 2045. PHARM ANSWER: 1

1. **Amikacin (Amikin) is an aminoglycoside, which is nephrotoxic and should be questioned. The serum creatinine and BUN levels are elevated, suggesting decreased renal function.**
2. Guaifenesin (Robitussin) is used for cough. The dose is within the range for a child of 12 years.
3. The serum osmolality is high, suggesting dehydration, and the potassium is low. $D_5$ in 0.25 NaCl with 20 mEq/L at 88 mL/hr will treat the dehydration and hypokalemia. The rate is appropriate; the child weighs 50 kg [1500 mL/day, plus 20 mL/kg/day for each kg over 20 kg = 1500 mL + (20 mL/kg × 30 kg) = 2100 mL; 2100 mL ÷ 24 hr = 87.5 mL/hr].
4. The acetaminophen (Tylenol) dose is within parameters (10–15 mg/kg/dose q4–6h prn, not to exceed five doses/24 hr), but it is concerning with the decreased renal function. Because acetaminophen is prn and amikacin is timed, the amikacin is more important to question.

▶ *Test-taking Tip: Carefully examine each laboratory value for abnormalities. Narrow the medications to those that are nephrotoxic.*

**Content Area:** Child; **Concept:** Infection; Medication; Safety; Management; **Integrated Processes:** Communication and Documentation; **Client Needs:** Physiological Integrity: Pharmacological and Parenteral Therapies; **Cognitive Level:** Analysis [Analyzing]

## 2046. PHARM ANSWER: 4

1. Captopril does not have any effect on asthma.
2. Although HR may slow in response to lowered BP, this is not the desired effect for which captopril is given.
3. Captopril does not have any effect on blood sugar.
4. **Captopril (Capoten) is an ACE inhibitor and is indicated for the treatment of hypertension in children.**

▶ *Test-taking Tip: Use the memory cue that ACE inhibitors end in the suffix "-pril" and that beta blockers end in the suffix "-lol." Narrow the options by identifying the one common effect for both of these medications.*

Content Area: Child; **Concept:** Perfusion; Medication; **Integrated Processes:** Teaching/Learning; **Client Needs:** Physiological Integrity: Pharmacological and Parenteral Therapies; **Cognitive Level:** Knowledge [Remembering]

## 2047. PHARM ANSWER: 22.5

**Using dimensional analysis:**

$$X \text{ mL} = \frac{50 \text{ mL}}{500 \text{ mcg}} \times \frac{225 \text{ mcg}}{1}$$

$$X \text{ mL} = \frac{50 \text{ mL}}{500 \text{ mcg}} \times \frac{225 \text{ mcg}}{1} \quad \text{Cancel the units and solve}$$

$$X = \frac{11{,}250}{500}$$

$$X = 22.5 \text{ mL}$$

**Using a ratio-proportion calculation:**
**500 mcg: 50 mL :: 225 mcg: $X$ mL**
**Multiple the outside values, then the inside values and solve for $X$.**
**$500X = 50 \times 225$; $500X = 11250$; $X = 11250 \div 500$;**
**$X = 22.5$ mL**

▶ *Test-taking Tip: Use either the ratio-proportion or dimensional analysis method for calculations. Use a calculator and be sure the answer is logical for digoxin (Lanoxin).*

Content Area: Child; **Concept:** Perfusion; Medication; **Integrated Processes:** Nursing Process: Planning; **Client Needs:** Physiological Integrity: Pharmacological and Parenteral Therapies; **Cognitive Level:** Application [Applying]

## 2048. PHARM ANSWER: 4

1. Epoetin (Epogen) stimulates the bone marrow to produce RBCs (erythropoiesis). In sickle cell disease, the RBCs "sickle," increasing the levels of hemoglobin S (HbS). Increasing the production of sickled RBCs can worsen the condition.
2. Amoxicillin (Amoxil) is an aminopenicillin and is contraindicated when allergies to penicillin are present; the nurse should question this medication if prescribed.
3. Opioids such as morphine sulfate are administered in sickle cell crises or for severe pain; its use depends on pain severity. It is usually not given prophylactically.
4. **The ability to fight infection is decreased following a splenectomy. Daily prophylactic antibiotics are given. Erythromycin ethylsuccinate (E.E.S.) is a macrolide antibiotic and safe to administer when a penicillin allergy exists.**

▶ *Test-taking Tip: Eliminate options that are contraindicated with a penicillin allergy. Consider the disease and surgery when reviewing the remaining options. The key word is "prophylactic."*

Content Area: Child; **Concept:** Hematologic Regulation; Medication; Infection; **Integrated Processes:** Nursing Process: Planning; **Client Needs:** Physiological Integrity: Pharmacological and Parenteral Therapies; **Cognitive Level:** Application [Applying]

## 2049. PHARM ANSWER: 2

1. Dopamine (Intropin) will have no effect on decreasing the incidence of PACs.
2. **Low-dose dopamine, 0.5–2.0 mcg/kg/min, acts on dopaminergic receptor sites along afferent arterioles in the glomerulus, dilates the renal vasculature, and improves urine output.**
3. Positive inotropic effects of dopamine include an increase in systolic BP with an increase (not decrease) in pulse pressure. Pulse pressure is the difference between the systolic BP and diastolic BP. The pulse pressure at 0800 hours is 40; at 1000 hours it is 30.
4. Positive inotropic effects of dopamine include an increase in systolic BP with little or no effect on DBP.

▶ *Test-taking Tip: The usual dose of dopamine for treating shock is 2–5 mcg/kg/min, increased gradually to 20–50 mcg/kg/min. Think about the effect of this low-dose dopamine. Note that three options involve the cardiovascular system, and one is different. Often the option that is different is the answer.*

Content Area: Child; **Concept:** Medication; Perfusion; **Integrated Processes:** Nursing Process: Evaluation; **Client Needs:** Physiological Integrity: Pharmacological and Parenteral Therapies; Physiological Integrity: Physiological Adaptation; **Cognitive Level:** Evaluation [Evaluating]

## 2050. PHARM ANSWER:

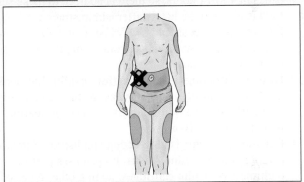

**The abdomen allows for a more consistent rate of absorption of insulin and is the preferred site for insulin administration via an insulin pump; it can be placed on either side of the umbilicus. The site is rotated within the abdominal area (green shaded area of the abdomen). More rapid absorption of insulin can occur when administered into the arms or legs.**

▶ *Test-taking Tip: You need to consider which area would have the most consistent absorption of insulin and be affected the least by muscle activity.*

Content Area: Child; **Concept:** Metabolism; Medication; Nursing Roles; **Integrated Processes:** Teaching/Learning; Caring; **Client Needs:** Physiological Integrity: Pharmacological and Parenteral Therapies; **Cognitive Level:** Application [Applying]

**2051.** **PHARM** **ANSWER: 3**

1. To ensure that the medication is administered with the insulin pens, the pen is held in place for 10 seconds after delivery of the medication. This action is correct.
2. Insulin lispro (Humalog) is rapid-acting insulin with an onset of 5 to 10 minutes. This action is correct.
3. **Insulin glargine (Lantus) is very long-acting insulin administered once daily and is not used for covering the number of carbohydrates eaten. This action indicates that the child needs additional teaching.**
4. The rapid-acting insulin lispro (Humalog) is not needed if the glucose level is WNL. Turkey does not contain carbohydrates; insulin is administered to cover only the carbohydrates eaten. This action is correct.

▶ *Test-taking Tip: Carefully read the situation. Examine the options that have duplicate information first and then eliminate either one or both of these.*

**Content Area:** Child; **Concept:** Metabolism; Medication; Nursing Roles; **Integrated Processes:** Nursing Process: Evaluation; **Client Needs:** Physiological Integrity: Pharmacological and Parenteral Therapies; **Cognitive Level:** Evaluation [Evaluating]

**2052.** **PHARM** **ANSWER: 3**

1. NPH (Humulin N) insulin can be given in the morning, but there is better glucose control if given at night. NPH peaks in 4 to 14 hours, so there is no need to make sure food is given immediately after administration.
2. Insulin injections should always be rotated to prevent subcutaneous tissue damage from giving the injections in the same location.
3. **Lispro (Humalog) is rapid-acting insulin that peaks in 30 to 90 minutes and may last as long as 5 hours in the blood. This statement is correct, indicating teaching is effective.**
4. Detemir (Levemir) is long-acting and lispro (Humalog) is rapid-acting insulin. An insulin pen uses prefilled, multiple-use insulin cartridges; adding other types of insulins should not be attempted.

▶ *Test-taking Tip: Eliminate options with absolute words such as "only." Focus on the type of insulin a newly diagnosed child with type 1 DM is most likely to receive.*

**Content Area:** Child; **Concept:** Metabolism; Medication; Nursing Roles; **Integrated Processes:** Teaching/Learning; **Client Needs:** Physiological Integrity: Pharmacological and Parenteral Therapies; **Cognitive Level:** Evaluation [Evaluating]

**2053.** **PHARM** **ANSWER:**

| Laboratory Report | |
| --- | --- |
| **Serum Laboratory Test** | **Client Result** |
| Hgb A$_{1c}$ | 4.5% **X** |
| Glucose | 70 mg/dL **X** |

**The treatment goal for children with type 1 DM is blood glucose levels within the normal range (60–105 mg/dL for a 2-year-old). Hgb A$_{1c}$ levels are indicative of the average blood glucose levels over the past 2 to 3 months; normal A$_{1c}$ is 3.9% to 7.7%. Although the other laboratory values are normal, these do not indicate the effectiveness of insulin therapy.**

▶ *Test-taking Tip: Hgb A$_{1c}$ is glycosylated hemoglobin. Lispro (Humalog) and glargine (Lantus) insulins lower glucose levels. Narrow options to only those pertaining to glucose levels.*

**Content Area:** Child; **Concept:** Metabolism; Medication; Management; **Integrated Processes:** Nursing Process: Evaluation; **Client Needs:** Physiological Integrity: Pharmacological and Parenteral Therapies; **Cognitive Level:** Evaluation [Evaluating]

**2054.** **PHARM** **MoC** **ANSWER: 3**

1. Initiating an IV access for glucose administration is more time-consuming than giving glucose by the oral route or glucagon (GlucaGen) subcutaneously to a child who is still responsive.
2. An oral form of glucose should be administered if the child is responsive and glucagon given only if the child is unresponsive or too uncooperative or upset to take oral glucose. Glucagon stimulates the release of liver glycogen and releases glucose into the circulation.
3. **The child may have ingested the glipizide (Glucotrol XL), a sustained-released hypoglycemic agent. The child's blood glucose level should be checked first to determine the appropriate treatment.**
4. Determining the number of tablets taken may delay the child's treatment.

▶ *Test-taking Tip: Use the steps of the nursing process. Assessment should be completed to determine an appropriate intervention.*

**Content Area:** Child; **Concept:** Metabolism; Medication; Assessment; **Integrated Processes:** Nursing Process: Assessment; **Client Needs:** Safe and Effective Care Environment: Management of Care; Physiological Integrity: Pharmacological and Parenteral Therapies; **Cognitive Level:** Analysis [Analyzing]

**2055.** PHARM **ANSWER: 3, 4, 5**
1. Weighing is unnecessary; it is important with medications that affect fluid balance but not with an antibiotic.
2. Monitoring temperature would be important to evaluate the effectiveness of antipyretic medications.
3. **Fluids should be increased to dilute bacterial toxins and increase urinary output.**
4. **The medication should be given in the exact amount at the times directed to maintain a therapeutic blood level. If the therapeutic blood level falls, organisms can build a resistance to the medication.**
5. **Trimethoprim-sulfamethoxazole (Bactrim) is a sulfonamide antibiotic. A rash can indicate an allergy to sulfonamides.**

♦ *Test-taking Tip: Eliminate options that are assessments and do not pertain to treatment with an antibiotic.*

Content Area: Child; Concept: Infection; Medication; Nursing Roles; Integrated Processes: Teaching/Learning; Client Needs: Physiological Integrity: Pharmacological and Parenteral Therapies; Cognitive Level: Analysis [Analyzing]

**2056.** PHARM MoC **ANSWER: 2**
1. The liver is not affected by prednisolone use, so an increased total bilirubin of 4 mg/dL is not related to the use of the drug. Normal total bilirubin in a 9-year-old should be less than 2 mg/dL.
2. **A WBC count of 18,000/mm³ may indicate an infection, an untoward effect of prednisolone (Omnipred). Prednisolone, a corticosteroid used to reduce inflammation, may increase the risk of infection. The normal WBC in a 9-year-old is 4500–11,100/mm³.**
3. Prednisolone has been associated with the adverse effect of hypokalemia but not hyponatremia (serum sodium of 130 mEq/L). Normal serum sodium is 135–145 mEq/L.
4. Although corticosteroids may have the effect of increasing blood glucose, a random glucose of 130 mg/dL is not abnormal.

♦ *Test-taking Tip: Prednisolone is a corticosteroid; consider expected adverse or untoward effects of this class of drugs, such as infection and hyperglycemia, to narrow the options.*

Content Area: Child; Concept: Inflammation; Medication; Integrated Processes: Nursing Process: Evaluation; Client Needs: Safe and Effective Care Environment: Management of Care; Physiological Integrity: Pharmacological and Parenteral Therapies; Physiological Integrity: Reduction of Risk Potential; Cognitive Level: Evaluation [Evaluating]

**2057.** PHARM **ANSWER: 4**
1. Methylphenidate is usually given twice daily at or before breakfast and at noon, not whenever inattention behaviors occur.
2. Methylphenidate is usually given twice daily at or before breakfast and at noon, not whenever hyperactive behaviors occur.

3. The last dose of the medication should be given before 6 p.m. to prevent insomnia.
4. **A side effect of methylphenidate hydrochloride (Ritalin) is anorexia. It should be given during or immediately after breakfast and lunch to prevent a decreased intake.**

♦ *Test-taking Tip: Options with absolute words such as "whenever" are usually incorrect. Think about the effect of psychostimulants on sleep.*

Content Area: Child; Concept: Medication; Development; Integrated Processes: Teaching/Learning; Client Needs: Physiological Integrity: Pharmacological and Parenteral Therapies; Cognitive Level: Application [Applying]

**2058.** PHARM **ANSWER: 1**
**First determine the dose for the child's weight:**
**16 lb 8 ounces = 16.5 lb ÷ 2.2 lb/kg = 7.5 kg**
**Next determine the prescribed dose. 7.5 kg ×**
**2 mg/kg = 15 mg.**
**The medication is supplied in 15 mg per 1 mL. The dose to administer is 1 mL of ranitidine (Zantac).**

♦ *Test-taking Tip: You need to convert pounds and ounces to kilograms to obtain the answer: 1 lb = 16 oz; 1 kg = 2.2 lb. The question is asking for mL and not mg.*

Content Area: Child; Concept: Medication; Safety; Integrated Processes: Nursing Process: Implementation; Client Needs: Physiological Integrity: Pharmacological and Parenteral Therapies; Cognitive Level: Application [Applying]

**2059.** PHARM **ANSWER: 4**
1. An HR of 110 bpm is normal for a 6-month-old; the range is 80–170 bpm.
2. Fever (temperature of 102.7°F or 39.3°C) is not an adverse effect of ranitidine.
3. Ranitidine is indicated for GERD; spitting up after feedings should improve. If not, then the medication dose may be too low or the medication itself ineffective. Spitting up is not a side effect.
4. **The nurse should identify that a hard, pebble-like bowel movement every 2 days demonstrates constipation; constipation is an adverse effect of ranitidine (Zantac).**

♦ *Test-taking Tip: Narrow the options to abnormal findings related to the GI tract.*

Content Area: Child; Concept: Bowel Elimination; Digestion; Medication; Integrated Processes: Nursing Process: Analysis; Client Needs: Physiological Integrity: Pharmacological and Parenteral Therapies; Cognitive Level: Application [Applying]

**2060.** PHARM **ANSWER: 3**
1. Lansoprazole would not be expected to change appetite.
2. Lansoprazole is not a gastric motility agent.
3. **Lansoprazole (Prevacid) is a PPI of stomach acid secretion. Decreasing the overall pH allows the gastric mucosa to heal.**
4. Flatulence is not affected.

▶ **Test-taking Tip:** *Use gastroesophageal in the stem and relate it to a similar word in an option.*

**Content Area:** Child; **Concept:** Digestion; Medication; **Integrated Processes:** Nursing Process: Evaluation; **Client Needs:** Physiological Integrity: Pharmacological and Parenteral Therapies; **Cognitive Level:** Evaluation [Evaluating]

## 2061. PHARM ANSWER: 1, 3, 6

1. **Antibiotics may be prescribed to treat bacterial gastroenteritis to ensure complete recovery.**
2. Oral fluid rehydration will be initiated later, but not initially, when the toddler presents with severe dehydration.
3. **The child who presents with severe dehydration needs IV therapy to stabilize the balance of fluids and electrolytes.**
4. The pain and discomfort the toddler will have are due to fever and cramping from the GI illness; thus analgesics are usually not prescribed.
5. An antidiarrheal medication is contraindicated.
6. **Fever is often a symptom of gastroenteritis. Ensuring that the fever is controlled with an antipyretic will provide some comfort.**

▶ **Test-taking Tip:** *The key phrase is "severe dehydration." You need to consider whether oral or IV fluids would be used for rehydration.*

**Content Area:** Child; **Concept:** Medication; Fluid and Electrolyte Balance; Infection; **Integrated Processes:** Nursing Process: Implementation; **Client Needs:** Physiological Integrity: Pharmacological and Parenteral Therapies; Physiological Integrity: Physiological Adaptation; **Cognitive Level:** Analysis [Analyzing]

## 2062. PHARM ANSWER: 48

**This child weighs 13 kg; the daily requirement is 1000 mL + (50 mL × 3) = 1150 mL over 24 hr. The hourly rate is 1150 mL ÷ 24 hr = 47.92; rounded to a whole number the rate is 48 mL/hr.**

▶ **Test-taking Tip:** *The daily fluid requirement is a cue that the total amount should be divided by 24 hours. Avoid multiplying the additional mL/kg by either 10 or 13 kg.*

**Content Area:** Child; **Concept:** Fluid and Electrolyte Balance; Medication; **Integrated Processes:** Nursing Process: Planning; **Client Needs:** Physiological Integrity: Pharmacological and Parenteral Therapies; **Cognitive Level:** Application [Applying]

## 2063. PHARM ANSWER: 4

1. Weight gain is not expected with an osmotic laxative.
2. Nighttime continence is not expected to be altered by an osmotic laxative.
3. Blood glucose is not expected to be altered by an osmotic laxative.
4. **Lactulose (Constulose) is an osmotic laxative used in treating encopresis to prevent constipation; the nurse should establish an outcome of a normal daily bowel movement.**

▶ **Test-taking Tip:** *Use the "lac-" in lactulose to remember that it is a laxative. With encopresis, the child holds the stool and resists having a bowel movement.*

**Content Area:** Child; **Concept:** Bowel Elimination; Medication; **Integrated Processes:** Nursing Process: Planning; **Client Needs:** Physiological Integrity: Pharmacological and Parenteral Therapies; Physiological Integrity: Basic Care and Comfort; **Cognitive Level:** Synthesis [Creating]

## 2064. PHARM ANSWER: 2, 4, 5

1. This dose of phenobarbital should be administered over 10 minutes; administering it over 30 minutes will delay the medication's effects to treat status epilepticus.
2. **Whenever IV medications are being administered by any route, the site should be evaluated for irritation and extravasation. An extravasation of phenobarbital (Luminal) may cause necrotic tissue changes that necessitate skin grafting.**
3. Phenobarbital, if diluted, should be mixed with sterile water for injection and not $D_5W$.
4. **When administering IV medications, identification of medications or solutions that would be incompatible with that medication must occur so that the tubing can be flushed to ensure that crystallization does not occur in the IV tubing.**
5. **For treating status epilepticus in infants and children the phenobarbital dose is 15–20 mg/kg IV infused at a rate no faster than 2 mg/kg/min, with a maximum of 30 mg over 1 minute. Giving the maximum of 30 mg over 1 minute, the child would receive the full dose of 300 mg over 10 minutes.**

▶ **Test-taking Tip:** *Quick termination of the seizure is desired; consider the actions that will best ensure that phenobarbital reaches the vascular system quickly and safely.*

**Content Area:** Child; **Concept:** Medication; Safety; **Integrated Processes:** Nursing Process: Planning; **Client Needs:** Physiological Integrity: Pharmacological and Parenteral Therapies; **Cognitive Level:** Analysis [Analyzing]

## 2065. PHARM ANSWER: 100

**Using dimensional analysis:**

$$X \text{ gtt/min} = \frac{60 \text{ gtt}}{1 \text{ mL}} \times \frac{50 \text{ mL}}{30 \text{ min}}$$

$$X \text{ gtt/min} = \frac{60 \text{ gtt}}{1 \text{ mL}} \times \frac{50 \text{ mL}}{30 \text{ min}} \quad \text{Cancel the units}$$

$$X \text{ gtt/min} = \frac{60}{1} \times \frac{50}{30}$$

$$X \text{ gtt/min} = \frac{3,000}{30} \quad \text{Solve the equation}$$

$$X \text{ gtt/min} = 100$$

▶ **Test-taking Tip:** *Learn the dimensional analysis method for medication and fluid administration. Use a calculator and be sure the answer is logical. Remember that drops should be rounded to the nearest whole number.*

**Content Area:** Child; **Concept:** Management; Medication; **Integrated Processes:** Nursing Process: Planning; **Client Needs:** Physiological Integrity: Pharmacological and Parenteral Therapies; **Cognitive Level:** Application [Applying]

**2066.** PHARM **ANSWER: 4**

1. Cephalexin (Keflex) is a first-generation cephalosporin that does not interfere with urine testing for opioids.
2. Ceftazidime (Fortaz) is a third-generation cephalosporin that does not interfere with urine testing for opioids.
3. Amoxicillin (Amoxil), an aminopenicillin, does not interfere with urine testing for opioids.
4. **Fluoroquinolones, such as ciprofloxacin (Cipro), can cause false-positive urine opiate screens.**

▶ *Test-taking Tip: Eliminate options from the same drug classification and then determine which of the two remaining medications is likely to cause false-positive opioid results.*

Content Area: Child; Concept: Medication; Infection; Promoting Health; Integrated Processes: Nursing Process: Analysis; Client Needs: Physiological Integrity: Pharmacological and Parenteral Therapies; Cognitive Level: Application [Applying]

**2067.** PHARM MoC **ANSWER: 4**

1. Erythematous palmar rash is not associated with the use of GH.
2. BP of 132/84 in a 13-year-old is considered normal.
3. Although GH use may be associated with blood glucose changes, a random blood glucose of 158 mg/dL is normal.
4. **Somatropin (Genotropin) recombinant is an injectable GH indicated for children with a deficiency of the hormone. It cannot be given once the epiphyses have closed. The nurse should notify the HCP.**

▶ *Test-taking Tip: If the drug is unfamiliar, think about the drug name, somatropin recombinant. "Soma-" refers to the body, and "-tropin" should be associated with growth, resulting in "body growth." Only one option relates to body growth.*

Content Area: Child; Concept: Development; Medication; Management; Integrated Processes: Nursing Process: Analysis; Communication and Documentation; Client Needs: Safe and Effective Care Environment: Management of Care; Physiological Integrity: Pharmacological and Parenteral Therapies; Physiological Integrity: Physiological Adaptation; Cognitive Level: Application [Applying]

**2068.** PHARM **ANSWER: 3**

1. A side effect of valacyclovir is a change in the menstrual cycle; however, having a regular menstrual cycle is not the desired therapeutic effect.
2. A bad odor from the vagina is a symptom of bacterial vaginosis or trichomoniasis vaginalis, and usually not a symptom of genital herpes simplex.
3. **Valacyclovir (Valtrex), an antiviral medication, is indicated for the treatment of genital herpes simplex virus, shingles (herpes zoster), or chicken pox. Labial sores are associated with genital herpes simplex. Improvement of labial sores indicates that valacyclovir is having the desired therapeutic effect.**
4. A green vaginal discharge may be a symptom of *Trichomonas*, which is treated with metronidazole (Flagyl), an amebicide.

▶ *Test-taking Tip: Drugs with the suffix "-vir" are generally antiviral or antiretroviral medications. Think about the symptoms of STIs and those treated with an antiviral medication.*

Content Area: Child; Concept: Infection; Medication; Sexuality; Integrated Processes: Communication and Documentation; Client Needs: Physiological Integrity: Pharmacological and Parenteral Therapies; Safe and Effective Care Environment: Safety and Infection Control; Cognitive Level: Analysis [Analyzing]

**2069.** MoC PHARM **ANSWER: 2, 3, 5**

1. Metronidazole is not associated with any cardiac changes or adverse events.
2. **Giardiasis is an infectious diarrheal disease; the plan of care should include assessing for infection. Infection should subside when treated with metronidazole (Flagyl).**
3. **Giardiasis is an infectious diarrheal disease; the plan of care should include reinforcing strict hand washing.**
4. Metronidazole should be given on an empty stomach.
5. **Giardiasis is an infectious diarrheal disease; the plan of care should include monitoring the results of stool samples.**

▶ *Test-taking Tip: The plan of care should include assessments and interventions for the child's problems as well as specifics regarding collaborative interventions.*

Content Area: Child; Concept: Critical Thinking; Medication; Sexuality; Management; Integrated Processes: Nursing Process: Planning; Client Needs: Safe and Effective Care Environment: Management of Care; Physiological Integrity: Pharmacological and Parenteral Therapies; Cognitive Level: Synthesis [Creating]

**2070.** PHARM **ANSWER: 3**

1. Although methotrexate is a folic acid antagonist, it does not alter serum levels.
2. Methotrexate has no effect on electrolytes.
3. **An adverse effect of methotrexate (Trexall) is aplastic anemia; thus the nurse should review the CBC results before administration.**
4. Methotrexate has no effect on coagulation.

▶ *Test-taking Tip: Methotrexate is an antineoplastic and antirheumatoid medication that has direct effects on bone marrow and rapidly dividing cells. The risk of infection during antineoplastic and antirheumatic therapy is increased. The CBC will provide information about both RBCs and WBCs.*

Content Area: Child; Concept: Cellular Regulation; Medication; Integrated Processes: Nursing Process: Assessment; Client Needs: Physiological Integrity: Pharmacological and Parenteral Therapies; Cognitive Level: Application [Applying]

**2071.** PHARM **ANSWER: 3**

1. The Hct of 31% is normal but is unaffected by filgrastim, a colony-stimulating factor.
2. The eosinophil count of 6 is elevated (0 to 2% is normal) but is not related to filgrastim use.

3. **Filgrastim (Neupogen) is a colony-stimulating factor used to increase the production of WBCs in persons who have bone marrow depression from chemotherapy.**

4. The platelet count of 150,000/mm$^3$ is normal but is not used to evaluate the therapeutic effectiveness of filgrastim.

▸ *Test-taking Tip: A trade name for filgrastim is Neupogen. Use the "Neu-" as a memory cue for neutrophils to help identify the answer.*

**Content Area:** Child; **Concept:** Cellular Regulation; Medication; **Integrated Processes:** Nursing Process: Analysis; **Client Needs:** Physiological Integrity: Pharmacological and Parenteral Therapies; **Cognitive Level:** Application [Applying]

## 2072. PHARM ANSWER: 3

1. Both diarrhea and severe constipation are adverse effects of vincristine, and prophylactic treatment is implemented at the beginning of therapy to decrease the potential of these occurring.

2. Hair loss is a common adverse reaction to the medication and is reversible.

3. **Dysphagia and paresthesia are CNS adverse effects from vincristine sulfate (Oncovin). The nurse should teach the parent to notify the HCP immediately if these occur.**

4. Three-year-old children may not show signs or symptoms of depression. If present, these should be distinguished as being associated with the neoplastic disease itself or as side effects of the medication.

▸ *Test-taking Tip: The key words are "most significant." Use Maslow's Hierarchy of Needs to identify a problem that has the potential for causing injury. Dysphagia is difficulty swallowing.*

**Content Area:** Child; **Concept:** Medication; Safety; Nursing Roles; **Integrated Processes:** Teaching/Learning; **Client Needs:** Physiological Integrity: Pharmacological and Parenteral Therapies; **Cognitive Level:** Evaluation [Evaluating]

## 2073. CJ PHARM ANSWER: 2

1. Although the medication is written on the MAR, an error still exists in the dose, and the medication should not be administered.

2. **The nurse should notify the HCP. The child weighs 30 kg; the recommended initial daily dose of the anticonvulsant lamotrigine (Lamictal) for this child would be 18 mg (0.6 mg/kg/day × 30 kg = 18 mg/day). If given 18 mg bid, the child would receive a daily dose of 36 mg, twice the recommended initial pediatric dose.**

3. There are no known drug interactions between lamotrigine (Lamictal), an anticonvulsant, and metronidazole (Flagyl), an antibiotic.

4. Consulting the pharmacist is unnecessary; the nurse still needs to seek clarification from the HCP.

▸ *Test-taking Tip: Carefully read the MAR to identify the child's weight and diagnosis. Note that three options address the dose. Use this information to eliminate options.*

**Content Area:** Child; **Concept:** Management; Medication; Neurologic Regulation; **Integrated Processes:** Communication and Documentation; **Client Needs:** Physiological Integrity: Pharmacological and Parenteral Therapies; Safe and Effective Care Environment: Safety and Infection Control; **Cognitive Level:** Analysis [Analyzing]

## 2074. PHARM CJ ANSWER: 600

**First convert lbs to kg: 66 lbs ÷ 2.2 lbs/kg = 30 kg**
**Next, determine the rate: 20 mL/kg × 30 kg = 600 mL**

▸ *Test-taking Tip: Recall that 1 kg = 2.2 lbs.*

**Content Area:** Child; **Concept:** Medication; Fluid and Electrolyte Balance; Infection; **Integrated Processes:** Nursing Process: Implementation; **Client Needs:** Physiological Integrity: Pharmacological and Parenteral Therapies; Safe and Effective Care Environment: Safety and Infection Control; **Cognitive Level:** Application [Applying]

# Crisis and Violence

**2075.** The nurse is caring for the client who was violently raped 3 months ago and has a diagnosis of rape-trauma syndrome. Which assessment findings, associated with rape-trauma syndrome, should the nurse anticipate? **Select all that apply.**

1. Anorexia
2. Nightmares
3. Hypertension
4. Fears and phobias
5. Sexual promiscuity

**2076.** **MoC** The client is being admitted to the ICU with drug overdose that resulted in extreme hypertension and an unstable cardiac rhythm. The client suddenly becomes physically combative and abusive. The nurse calls a behavioral situation code, and four-point restraints are applied by the team. Which **most** important intervention should be **next?**

1. Have staff who were harmed complete an incident report.
2. Contact the HCP to obtain an order for restraint use.
3. Document the client's behavior and action taken.
4. Check that the wrist restraints are tightly secured to the HOB.

**2077.** The nurse is delayed in changing the dressing on the client's leg. The client reacts by becoming verbally aggressive and telling the nurse, "None of you can be trusted. You all just make promises you never intend to keep." Which should the nurse do **now?**

1. Alert other staff to the client's apparent escalation.
2. Ask why the client is overreacting.
3. Leave the room until the client regains control.
4. Apologize to the client for being late with the treatment.

**2078.** The client is admitted to the ED with multiple lacerations and broken bones after being assaulted. The client's spouse barges into the client's ED room with a gun and states, "I'm going to kill you and anyone else who gets in my way." Which action should be taken by the nurse **initially?**

1. Yell for help to distract the person's attention away from the client.
2. Firmly state, "You don't want to hurt anyone else. Let's talk about it."
3. Use gestures to alert another nurse to clear others who may be nearby.
4. Use a nonaggressive posture and tone to state, "Put the gun on the floor."

**2079.** **MoC** The nurse observes that the client diagnosed with intermittent explosive disorder is becoming aggressive and that lorazepam was prescribed. The client is now exhibiting a tense posture, a clenched fist, and a defiant affect. Prioritize the nurse's actions to de-escalate the client's aggression.

1. Call other staff for assistance.
2. Attempt to talk the client down.
3. Apply wrist restraints.
4. Offer the client the choice of taking the medication voluntarily.
5. Provide an alternate use of physical energy, such as suggesting punching a pillow.

Answer: _____

**2080.** [PHARM] The nurse is to administer haloperidol 2 mg IV now to the hospitalized client. A vial of haloperidol 5 mg/mL is available. How many mL of medication should the nurse administer?

_____ mL (Round to the nearest tenth.)

**2081.** [MoC] Staff are debriefing following the client's violent episode. What information should be included in the debriefing session? **Select all that apply.**

1. The client's coping mechanisms postevent
2. The client's history of violent behavior
3. Adherence to instructional policies and procedures
4. The staff's feelings regarding the effectiveness of the team
5. The staff's ability to respond to the client therapeutically postevent

**2082.** The client has been placed in restraints for violent behavior. Which statement **best** indicates the nurse's understanding of the risk for client injury while being restrained?

1. "Can you arrange to order the client's favorite sandwich for his lunch?"
2. "I need to make sure the restraints' release mechanisms are working properly."
3. "I need someone to continuously monitor the client and relieve me for a few minutes."
4. "The client's feet feel a little cool, but they have a good pulse. I'll get a pair of socks."

**2083.** [MoC] The nurse is preparing to document the client's violent episode. Which statements should be included specifically about the violent episode? **Select all that apply.**

1. The client's wife called during the escalation cycle.
2. The client refused to voluntarily enter into seclusion.
3. The client stated, "All of you are just evil people."
4. Attempts to identify the cause of the client's agitation failed.
5. Five staff members responded to "Emergency Code."
6. The client asked to leave the seclusion room after 30 minutes.

**2084.** The client with Alzheimer's disease becomes increasingly agitated and states, "I must go and clean out the barn!" Which nursing response is **most** therapeutic?

1. "What makes you think that the barn needs to be cleaned?"
2. "So you've cleaned a barn. Tell me, did you live on a farm?"
3. "It's awfully hot today; maybe you should wait until tomorrow."
4. "There are no barns around here. Would you like something to eat?"

**2085.** The experienced nurse determines that the new nurse's actions are therapeutic when managing the cognitively impaired client whose agitated behavior is escalating. Which nursing actions should have occurred? **Select all that apply.**

1. Saying, "Mr. Smith, will you look at me, please?"
2. Saying, "You seem upset. How can I help you?"
3. Presenting the client with detailed expectations
4. Turning off the TV in the room to reduce noise
5. Saying, "Getting angry will not help you get what you want."
6. Speaking loudly to ensure that the client hears what is being said

**2086.** [MoC] The new nurse is working with the cognitively impaired client who has a history of violent behavior. Which statement, made by the new nurse, reflects an immediate need for follow-up by the mentor?

1. "My first concern is the safety of all those on the unit."
2. "I know to turn off the TV when the client starts pacing."
3. "When the client got aggressive, I tried talking the client down."
4. "I'm going to assign the same staff to work with the client each shift."

**2087.** The nurse is developing the plan of care for the client who has schizophrenia and is having an alcohol-induced crisis. Which specific outcome **best** reflects the primary goal of crisis intervention for this client?

1. The client will be successfully detoxified within 20 days.
2. The client will return to his or her part-time job within 20 days.
3. The client will state two effective coping mechanisms.
4. The client will self-administer medications before discharge.

**2088.** [MoC] Staff members have expressed fear of the client who has a history of violent behavior. Which response made by the lead nurse would be **most** beneficial in addressing the staff's expressed concerns?

1. "Let's not prejudge him. His medication should help him control his behavior."
2. "I will be very attentive to his behavior, monitoring it for any signs of escalation."
3. "It may be hard, but we need to appear calm and nonthreatening but alert to his behavior."
4. "As staff we are all trained to manage violent clients, and we can handle any crisis behavior."

**2089.** The newly admitted client is expressing anger with increasing intensity. Which therapeutic site should the nurse recommend to the client for gaining control over the increasing anger?

1. The client's own private room down the hall
2. The unit's common television dayroom
3. An outdoor sheltered client smoking area
4. An out-of-the-way corner near the nursing station

**2090.** The client with a history of aggressive behavior toward staff and peers states to the nurse, "Everyone is just so touchy; I don't see where I'm being too aggressive." Which nursing action should be included in the therapeutic plan of care to **best** effect a difference in perceptions?

1. Refamiliarize the client with the rules of the unit.
2. Introduce nonaggressive interpersonal behaviors.
3. Promote dialogue between the staff and client to discuss the staff's perceptions of aggressive behavior.
4. Encourage the staff to show patience because the client may have poor aggression control.

**2091.** The client is placed in seclusion for exhibiting violent behavior. Which should be the nurse's primary goal of this seclusion?

1. Assist the client in regaining self-control.
2. Ensure the safety of the client and others.
3. Regain control over the unit's environment.
4. Provide a consequence for the client's behavior.

**2092.** The client is experiencing withdrawal symptoms leading to sleep deprivation. The nurse should recognize that the client is at **greatest** risk for violent behavior due to which assessment finding?

1. Poor coping mechanisms
2. Physical pain from withdrawal
3. A sense of guilt/shame regarding family
4. Anxiety over lack of access to the substance of choice

**2093.** The 28-year-old is being seen in the ED with injuries after being assaulted by her live-in boyfriend. The client acknowledges that this is not the first time that she has been assaulted and that she is afraid. Which client action indicates that an outcome for the client has been achieved?

1. Elects to return to her boyfriend to make amends
2. Accepts arrangements made with a women's shelter
3. Verbalizes plans for staying at the hospital overnight
4. Asks the nurse to report the assault to Adult Health Protective Services

**2094.** The client on the mental health unit is becoming increasingly short-tempered with others; the client approaches the nurse's desk and, pounding on the counter, yells, "I want out of here now!" Document the client's violent behaviors on the flow sheet by placing an X in the column for each behavior exhibited.

| Violent Behaviors | Client's Violent Behaviors |
|---|---|
| Confusion | |
| Irritability | |
| Boisterousness | |
| Verbal threats | |
| Attacks on objects | |

**2095.** MoC During orientation to the behavioral care unit, the new nurse asks, "How will I know which clients are potentially violent?" Which response by the nurse educator is **best?**

1. "Just be alert and aware of your client's behavioral clues."
2. "The client prone to violence will usually tell you they are angry about something."
3. "As you plan care, review the clients' charts to determine who has a history of violence."
4. "Your orientation will include an in-service on violent clients and how to identify them."

**2096.** MoC The client who recently emigrated from another country to the U.S. has been placed in seclusion. The nurse assesses that the client is now calm and ready to be assimilated back into the mental health milieu. Which action by the nurse demonstrates cultural insensitivity?

1. Gives the client a thumbs-up gesture
2. Avoids looking at the clock or a watch
3. Has the NA bring the client a cup of tea
4. Offers to get a book that the client chooses

**2097.** The nurse manager, concerned about the potential for staff harm on a behavioral health unit, is assessing the unit's milieu. Which milieu situation should the nurse manager address because it is a predictive factor for violence?

1. Two clients have a history of spousal abuse.
2. Several clients have lost smoking privileges.
3. The unit is at less than full client capacity.
4. The nurse from a medical unit is assigned to work on the unit.

**2098.** Multiple clients are being cared for on the behavioral health unit. In which circumstances should the nurse plan the therapeutic use of seclusion and/or restraints? **Select all that apply.**

1. The client asks to be placed in seclusion.
2. The client expresses the likelihood of self-injury.
3. The staff feels the client is likely to harm others.
4. The legally detained client is threatening to "escape."
5. The staff identifies seclusion as a consequence of the client's behavior.
6. The client's threatening behavior is negatively affecting the therapeutic milieu.

**2099.** The client has been violent toward other clients on a mental health unit, and interventions have failed. During the application of restraints, which action by the team leader will gain the **greatest** cooperation from the client?

1. Showing sympathy by apologizing for the need to restrain the client
2. Dispassionately explaining why and how the restraints will be applied
3. Affording the client one last opportunity to avoid restraints by "behaving"
4. Offering to remove the restraints as soon as the client can "control the anger"

**2100.** The client who sustained a brain injury from a motor vehicle accident is now experiencing aggression, impulsivity, and poor judgment. In teaching the family, which area of the brain illustrated should the nurse identify as being affected?

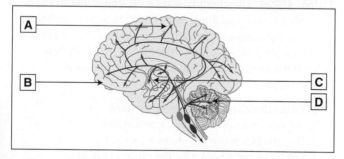

1. Line A
2. Line B
3. Line C
4. Line D

**2101.** The client has been placed in involuntary seclusion. Which information **best** indicates to the nurse that the client is ready to leave involuntary seclusion?

1. The client calmly stating, "I have control over my anger now."
2. BP is 110/64 mm Hg; P is 82 bpm and regular; RR is 16 bpm and regular.
3. The client is sitting in the seclusion room doorway asking staff for a drink.
4. Medical record states, "Seclusion of 45 minutes resulted in improved control."

**2102.** The client is visibly upset, pounding on the desk at the nurses' station, and shouting, "You're the nurse, so you have to fix this now." What should be the nurse's primary rationale for recognizing that the client is a danger to staff and other clients?

1. The client is verbally threatening the nurse to fix the situation now.
2. The client does not acknowledge his or her role in solving problems.
3. The client does not recognize that he or she is acting inappropriately.
4. The client uses intimidation and anger for meeting personal needs and wants.

**2103.** **PHARM** The client on a medical nursing unit is acutely agitated, getting out of bed unassisted despite having a high risk for falling, and is now hitting and biting staff. Which medication prescribed prn should the nurse administer to help calm the client?

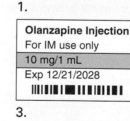

1.

| Olanzapine Injection |
| --- |
| For IM use only |
| 10 mg/1 mL |
| Exp 12/21/2028 |

2.

| Bupropion Oral |
| --- |
| 100 mg tablet |
| Exp 10/21/2028 |

3.

| Zolpidem Oral |
| --- |
| 5 mg tablet |
| Exp 11/16/2028 |

4.

| Ondansetron Injection |
| --- |
| For IV or IM use only |
| 4 mg/vial (2 mg/mL) |
| Exp 12/28/2028 |

**2104.** When debriefing the unit's staff after the client's catastrophic reaction, the nurse stresses the need for staff to remain calm during the event. Which statement should be the basis for the nurse's comment?

1. The client's safety is at jeopardy if the staff is feeling threatened.
2. An agitated staff will not be able to manage the situation as effectively.
3. The client will sense the staff's agitation, and aggressive behavior will escalate.
4. An agitated staff response is indicative of a need for additional crisis-control training.

**2105.** The client who is indigent and has emotional and physical diagnoses is attending a discharge planning session with the nurse. Which client behavior shows the greatest commitment to self-management?

1. Correctly stating the medications prescribed and the administration schedule
2. Asking to stay with a relative until an affordable place to live can be found
3. Researching the names of and calling contact people at local support centers
4. Promising the nurse to keep the scheduled follow-up appointments at the clinic

**2106.** The client is admitted to an ED with facial bruises, a broken arm, and rib fractures. The client states, "I fell down the stairs." During assessment, the nurse sees bruises and lacerations in various stages of healing. Which questions by the nurse are appropriate? **Select all that apply.**

1. "Has anyone hurt you?"
2. "Are you afraid of anyone at home?"
3. "Have you been falling down a lot lately?"
4. "Have you had any fainting spells or times that you have been weak?"
5. "I noticed you have more bruises. Can you tell me how they happened?"
6. "You look abused. Why haven't you reported that you have been abused?"

**2107.** MoC The nurse is caring for the unresponsive toddler in a PICU. The child's parent was arrested for alleged child abuse but released on bail. The parent is pounding at the door, belligerent, and demanding to visit the child. Which plan is **most** appropriate?

1. Allow the parent to enter the room and see the child.
2. Tell the parent that the HCP wants to speak with the parent first.
3. Contact Social Services to report the parent's abusive behavior.
4. Initiate the emergency response system for behavioral situations.

**2108.** MoC The toddler is hospitalized for observation after having apnea spells that led to cardiac arrest at home three times in the past 6 months. The nurse suspects Munchausen Syndrome by Proxy (MSP) and contacts the HCP. The HCP does not believe that this is a correct assessment of the child or of the family dynamics. What should the nurse do?

1. Contact the head of the department of pediatrics to report the incident.
2. Consult with the clinical charge nurse as to what action should be taken.
3. Call a case conference involving physicians, nurses, and social workers.
4. File a variance report indicating the HCP was notified but took no action.

**2109.** MoC The NA is helping the ED nurse admit a woman who is the victim of spousal abuse and marital rape. The NA asks the nurse what should be done with the woman's torn and soiled clothing. What is the nurse's **best** response?

1. "Place items in a plastic bag and avoid blood and body fluid contact."
2. "Ask the woman what she wants done with her clothing; she may want them discarded."
3. "These may be needed by the police. I will remove them and place each item in separate paper bags."
4. "Fold each article of clothing and leave them with her; she can decide later about disposal."

**2110.** The older, disheveled client is admitted to the ED with hypertension, severe dehydration, and malnourishment. During the admission interview, the daughter notes that she and her husband, who is temporarily out of work, have been living with the client. Which nursing action is **most** important?

1. Report the suspected elder abuse to Adult Health Protective Services.
2. Ask additional questions of the client in private without the family present.
3. Ask the daughter whether her father has been eating and taking his medication.
4. Call the resource hotline to ask whether abuse and neglect should be considered.

# Answers and Rationales

## 2075. ANSWER: 1, 2, 4

1. **Rape-trauma syndrome symptoms include physiological symptoms such as loss of appetite.**
2. **Rape-trauma syndrome symptoms may include nightmares of the attack occurring again.**
3. Although hypertension may be a result of long-term stress, it is not recognized as a symptom of rape-trauma syndrome.
4. **Rape-trauma syndrome symptoms include fears and phobias; these usually arise due to the victim's feelings of being unable to protect him- or herself from the assault. Fears may include the fear that the assailant might try to find the victim again.**
5. Fear of sexual encounters rather than sexual promiscuity is a recognized symptom of rape-trauma syndrome.

▶ *Test-taking Tip: Rape-trauma syndrome is a form of post-traumatic stress syndrome. You need to think about the emotional, cognitive, behavioral, and interpersonal reactions to a traumatic event.*

Content Area: Mental Health; Concept: Violence; Sleep, Rest, and Activity; Stress; Integrated Processes: Nursing Process: Assessment; Client Needs: Psychosocial Integrity; Cognitive Level: Analysis [Analyzing]

## 2076. MoC ANSWER: 2

1. Staff members who are injured should be seen by the employee health service and an incident report completed, but this is not the next intervention.
2. **If physical restraints are initiated, a HCP or licensed independent practitioner must prescribe the restraints, assess the client, and evaluate the need for restraints within 1 hour of the restraints being placed. The restraints could be placed immediately for client self-protection and protection of others.**
3. It is more important to contact the HCP first. Although documentation is important, the nurse would also include information about contacting the HCP.
4. The client should be restrained in the supine position with arms restrained so that one arm is flexed up and the other is extended at the side of the bed. The HOB should be elevated 30 degrees to decrease the risk of aspiration. Extending both arms overhead can impair circulation.

▶ *Test-taking Tip: To select the correct option, consider the legal implications for the use of four-point restraints.*

Content Area: Mental Health; Concept: Addiction; Safety; Violence; Integrated Processes: Nursing Process: Implementation; Client Needs: Safe and Effective Care Environment: Management of Care; Safe and Effective Care Environment: Safety and Infection Control; Cognitive Level: Application [Applying]

## 2077. ANSWER: 4

1. If the client does not de-escalate with an apology and the nurse's presence, then the nurse should alert the staff.

2. Asking a why question is challenging the client and can cause the client to become defensive or increase the client's distress.
3. The nurse should not leave but first validate the client's distress and then attempt to communicate with the client.
4. **By apologizing for being late with the treatment, the nurse is validating the client's distress and acknowledging his or her role in creating the situation.**

▶ *Test-taking Tip: Note the key word "initial" and then use the process of elimination. The initial approach should be the least drastic action.*

Content Area: Mental Health; Concept: Communication; Safety; Integrated Processes: Caring; Communication and Documentation; Client Needs: Safe and Effective Care Environment: Safety and Infection Control; Cognitive Level: Analysis [Analyzing]

## 2078. ANSWER: 4

1. A technique for de-escalating is to redirect and/or divert the person's emotions. Yelling does not redirect emotions; it may startle the person, and the nurse or the client could be shot.
2. The nurse is assuming that the client's spouse is the person who assaulted the client, which may be incorrect. Telling the client what to do is a block to therapeutic communication.
3. Gesturing that could be observed by the person holding the gun may escalate the situation. If the person barged into the room, others may already be aware of the situation, clearing the area and notifying security.
4. **The nurse should initially talk to the client's spouse who is holding the gun using a nonaggressive posture and tone of voice to diffuse the situation.**

▶ *Test-taking Tip: Note the key word "initially." Think about which action would help to diffuse the situation.*

Content Area: Mental Health; Concept: Addiction; Safety; Violence; Integrated Processes: Nursing Process: Analysis; Client Needs: Safe and Effective Care Environment: Safety and Infection Control; Psychosocial Integrity; Cognitive Level: Application [Applying]

## 2079. MoC ANSWER: 2, 5, 4, 1, 3

2. **Attempt to talk the client down. Talking the client down may promote a trusting relationship and help to diffuse the client's anger and determine the underlying cause.**
5. **Provide an alternate use of physical energy, such as suggesting punching a pillow. This activity provides an effective means for the client to release tension associated with high levels of anger.**
4. **Offer the client the choice of taking the medication voluntarily. Lorazepam (Ativan) or another tranquilizing medication may calm the client and prevent violence from escalating.**

1. **Call other staff for assistance. Client and staff safety are of primary concern if the behavior continues to escalate. Sufficient staff to indicate a show of strength may be enough to de-escalate the situation, and the client may agree to take the medication.**
3. **Apply wrist restraints. The client who does not have internal control over his or her own behavior may require external controls, such as mechanical restraints, to prevent harm to self or others.**

▶ *Test-taking Tip: Think about approaching the client who is angry and aggressive. The approach should be least restrictive to most restrictive.*

Content Area: Mental Health; Concept: Safety; Self; Violence; Integrated Processes: Nursing Process: Implementation; Client Needs: Safe and Effective Care Environment: Management of Care; Cognitive Level: Synthesis [Creating]

### 2080. PHARM ANSWER: 0.4

**Use a proportion formulation to calculate the dose. Then multiply the extremes (outside values) and means (inside values) to solve for $X$.**
**5 mg : 1 mL :: 2 mg : $X$ mL; $5X = 2$; $X = 2 \div 5$; $X = 0.4$**
**The nurse should administer 0.4 mL haloperidol (Haldol).**

▶ *Test-taking Tip: If the dose obtained is 1 or more mL, check your calculations.*

Content Area: Mental Health; Concept: Medication; Violence; Safety; Integrated Processes: Nursing Process: Implementation; Client Needs: Physiological Integrity: Pharmacological and Parenteral Therapies; Cognitive Level: Application [Applying]

### 2081. MoC ANSWER: 3, 4, 5

1. The client's coping mechanisms are not generally pertinent to the postevent debriefing.
2. A history of violence is not generally pertinent to the postevent debriefing.
3. **The staff debriefing should include whether everyone adhered to facility policies and procedures; this will help to identify the need for additional/remedial staff training.**
4. **The staff debriefing should include team effectiveness; this will help to identify readiness to respond and manage the event and the need for additional/remedial staff training.**
5. **The staff debriefing should include the staff's ability to respond to the client therapeutically postevent. This will help to identify the need for additional/remedial staff training.**

▶ *Test-taking Tip: Three options pertain to the staff, and two options pertain to the client. You need to consider that the purpose of debriefing is for quality improvement when selecting your options.*

Content Area: Mental Health; Concept: Violence; Safety; Management; Integrated Processes: Nursing Process: Analysis; Client Needs: Safe and Effective Care Environment: Management of Care; Cognitive Level: Application [Applying]

### 2082. ANSWER: 3

1. Although nutrition is an important consideration, the most important action regarding client safety while in restraints is monitoring.
2. Although the proper working of the restraints is important, it cannot be achieved without appropriate client monitoring.
3. **The client must be constantly monitored when in restraints to assess for and prevent any type of client injury.**
4. Assessing for adequate circulation is important, but it cannot be monitored effectively if the client is not being observed constantly.

▶ *Test-taking Tip: Note the key word "best." Three options are more specific, and one is more global. Often the more global option is the answer.*

Content Area: Mental Health; Concept: Safety; Management; Violence; Integrated Processes: Nursing Process: Evaluation; Client Needs: Safe and Effective Care Environment: Safety and Infection Control; Physiological Integrity: Basic Care and Comfort; Cognitive Level: Evaluation [Evaluating]

### 2083. MoC ANSWER: 2, 3, 4, 6

1. The fact that the client's wife telephones during the event does not reflect on the circumstances of the event, and so it does not need to be documented.
2. **Documentation of the client's violent cycle must include observations of client behavior during the entire cycle.**
3. **Documentation of the client's violent cycle must include observations of client behavior, including client statements, during the entire cycle.**
4. **Documentation of the client's violent cycle must include all nursing interventions used and the client's response to the interventions.**
5. The number of individuals responding to the emergency need not be documented.
6. **Documentation of the client's violent cycle must include how the client was reintegrated into the unit's milieu.**

▶ *Test-taking Tip: Note the key word "specifically." Eliminate options that do not pertain specifically to the violent episode.*

Content Area: Mental Health; Concept: Violence; Communication; Integrated Processes: Communication and Documentation; Client Needs: Safe and Effective Care Environment: Management of Care; Cognitive Level: Synthesis [Creating]

### 2084. ANSWER: 2

1. Although redirecting the client's attention is appropriate, asking the client this question may be interpreted as argumentative or challenging and may escalate the client's agitation.
2. **Rather than attempting to reorient the agitated, cognitively impaired client, asking the client to describe feelings or memories related to the situation may effectively divert the client's attention to a less problematic focus.**

3. Explaining that it is hot to the client may be seen as an obstacle to therapeutic communication.

4. Stating there are no barns here and attempting to redirect the client's attention may be viewed as merely putting an obstacle in the client's way.

▶ *Test-taking Tip: The key phrase is "most therapeutic." Consider which option would best promote reminiscence.*

Content Area: Mental Health; **Concept:** Cognition; Communication; **Integrated Processes:** Communication and Documentation; **Client Needs:** Psychosocial Integrity; **Cognitive Level:** Analysis [Analyzing]

## 2085. ANSWER: 1, 2, 4

1. **Calling the client by name and achieving eye contact may have a calming effect for a cognitively impaired, agitated client.**

2. **Acknowledging the client's agitation may help the client regain control.**

3. Complex explanations and extensive conversation are likely to be interpreted as more sensory stimuli to the agitated client.

4. **Decreasing the stimuli in the area may have a calming effect on the client.**

5. The client is not capable of rational thought; telling the client that being angry will not get the client what the client wants may be interpreted as a challenge to the client.

6. Speaking in a loud tone may escalate the client's agitation.

▶ *Test-taking Tip: Note the key word "therapeutic." Use understanding of the techniques for crisis intervention and managing catastrophic reactions, and eliminate Options 3 and 6 because these increase sensory stimuli and Option 5 because it can be interpreted as challenging.*

Content Area: Mental Health; **Concept:** Cognition; Communication; Stress; **Integrated Processes:** Nursing Process: Evaluation; **Client Needs:** Psychosocial Integrity; Physiological Integrity: Reduction of Risk Potential; **Cognitive Level:** Evaluation [Evaluating]

## 2086. MoC ANSWER: 3

1. Safety of all on the unit is a major concern and does not require follow-up.

2. Minimizing external stimuli and the use of sound judgment are important in providing a therapeutic milieu for an agitated client and do not require follow-up.

3. **The mentor should follow up when the new nurse attempts to talk to the agitated client. Until the client regains control, talking will be interpreted as external stimulation. As the client becomes calmer and more secure, attempts can then be made to redirect the client's attention and behavior.**

4. Surrounding the client with the same staff every day will be beneficial for the client and does not require follow-up.

▶ *Test-taking Tip: Note the key word "immediate." You need to consider which option can result in an escalation of the client's violent behavior.*

Content Area: Mental Health; **Concept:** Cognition; Safety; Violence; Stress; Management; **Integrated Processes:** Nursing Process: Evaluation; **Client Needs:** Safe and Effective Care Environment: Management of Care; Safe and Effective Care Environment: Safety and Infection Control; **Cognitive Level:** Evaluation [Evaluating]

## 2087. ANSWER: 2

1. Detoxification is directed toward treatment of the underlying condition, alcohol abuse, and is not focused on the goal of crisis intervention.

2. **The primary goal of crisis intervention is to return the client to his or her pre-crisis level of functioning. Returning to work is the most appropriate outcome directed toward that goal.**

3. The client should be demonstrating the use of effective coping mechanisms before discharge, not just stating them.

4. The client's ability to self-administer medication is necessary for treating schizophrenia but is not a goal specific to the crisis situation.

▶ *Test-taking Tip: The key phrase is "crisis intervention." Use the process of elimination to select the only option directly related to the client's crisis behavior.*

Content Area: Mental Health; **Concept:** Cognition; Addiction; Violence; Stress; **Integrated Processes:** Nursing Process: Planning; **Client Needs:** Psychosocial Integrity; **Cognitive Level:** Synthesis [Creating]

## 2088. MoC ANSWER: 3

1. This response focuses on the client and fails to address the concerns expressed by the staff members.

2. The concerns expressed by the staff are not taken into consideration. The lead nurse's response does not appear to value the staff's opinions.

3. **When dealing with potentially violent clients, although it may be very difficult, it is imperative to present a calm, relaxed, nonthreatening demeanor. This option both addresses the staff concerns and offers direction regarding client management.**

4. This response fails to address the concerns expressed and a means of controlling the feared behavior.

▶ *Test-taking Tip: Note the key phrase "most beneficial." The most beneficial response should focus on the staff's concerns.*

Content Area: Mental Health; **Concept:** Violence; Safety; Stress; Communication; Management; **Integrated Processes:** Caring; Communication and Documentation; **Client Needs:** Safe and Effective Care Environment: Management of Care; **Cognitive Level:** Analysis [Analyzing]

## 2089. ANSWER: 4

1. The client's room is not visible to the staff; the safety of everyone on the unit would be a concern.

2. The dayroom (lounge) is not quiet; stimulation can increase the agitation and anger.

3. An outside area is not visible to the staff; the safety of the client and others using the smoking area would be a concern.

4. **A quiet location that is visible to the staff is best. A quiet environment is critical for client de-escalation.**

▶ *Test-taking Tip:* Select the only option that is visible to the staff and quiet.

**Content Area:** Mental Health; **Concept:** Violence; Safety; Stress; **Integrated Processes:** Nursing Process: Implementation; **Client Needs:** Safe and Effective Care Environment: Safety and Infection Control; **Cognitive Level:** Application [Applying]

## 2090. ANSWER: 3

1. Refamiliarizing the client with unit rules may have little impact on the client's aggressive behavior.
2. Providing alternate behaviors is an appropriate option but is not the most therapeutic because the various perceptions need to be addressed first.
3. **Research has shown that staff and clients often have different perceptions of aggressive behaviors and of how to control or reduce aggression. Promoting a dialogue between the client and the staff can clarify the different perceptions.**
4. Suggesting "patience" is not appropriate because the client's aggressive behavior is a risk for injury to others in the environment.

▶ *Test-taking Tip:* Note the key word "best" and use the process of elimination. The focus of the question is clarifying misperceptions.

**Content Area:** Mental Health; **Concept:** Communication; Safety; Violence; Stress; Evidence-based Practice; **Integrated Processes:** Nursing Process: Planning; **Client Needs:** Psychosocial Integrity; **Cognitive Level:** Synthesis [Creating]

## 2091. ANSWER: 2

1. Regaining self-control is an outcome rather than the goal of seclusion.
2. **The primary goal of seclusion is always safety of the client and others by decreasing environmental stimuli.**
3. Unit control is an outcome rather than the goal of seclusion.
4. Seclusion should never be used as punishment for behavior.

▶ *Test-taking Tip:* Note the key word "primary." Eliminate options that are outcomes of seclusion.

**Content Area:** Mental Health; **Concept:** Violence; Safety; Stress; **Integrated Processes:** Nursing Process: Analysis; **Client Needs:** Safe and Effective Care Environment: Safety and Infection Control; **Cognitive Level:** Application [Applying]

## 2092. ANSWER: 4

1. Although the lack of coping skills may result in violent behavior, the primary cause is likely no access to drug/alcohol.
2. Although inadequately managed physical pain resulting from withdrawal may result in violent behavior, the primary cause is likely no access to drug/alcohol.
3. Although a sense of guilt or shame regarding family may result in violent behavior, the primary cause is likely no access to drug/alcohol.

4. **The client hospitalized for chemical dependency is at risk for developing violent behavior due to anxiety from the loss of access to the drug of choice.**

▶ *Test-taking Tip:* Note the key word "greatest" and use the process of elimination to determine the primary factor affecting violence in the client who abuses substances.

**Content Area:** Mental Health; **Concept:** Addiction; Sleep, Rest, and Activity; Violence; Stress; **Integrated Processes:** Nursing Process: Assessment; **Client Needs:** Psychosocial Integrity; **Cognitive Level:** Application [Applying]

## 2093. ANSWER: 2

1. Electing to return to the boyfriend poses a threat to client safety.
2. **Accepting an arrangement at a women's shelter is a positive outcome for this client.**
3. The woman's injuries are not such that she requires hospitalization. If the woman has insurance, third-party payers may not approve hospitalization that is based solely on abuse.
4. The nurse has a legal obligation to report the abuse whether or not the client requested this.

▶ *Test-taking Tip:* Focus on the client action that promotes the client's personal safety.

**Content Area:** Mental Health; **Concept:** Safety; Stress; Violence; **Integrated Processes:** Nursing Process: Evaluation; **Client Needs:** Safe and Effective Care Environment: Safety and Infection Control; **Cognitive Level:** Evaluation [Evaluating]

## 2094. ANSWER:

| Violent Behaviors | Client's Violent Behaviors |
|---|---|
| Confusion | |
| Irritability | X |
| Boisterousness | X |
| Verbal threats | |
| Attacks on objects | X |

**Violent behaviors displayed by the client include short-tempered (irritability), yelling (boisterousness), and pounding on the desk (attacks on objects). There is no evidence of confusion or making verbal threats.**

▶ *Test-taking Tip:* Avoid reading into the question; you should be looking for related words between the stem of the question and the options within the table.

**Content Area:** Mental Health; **Concept:** Violence; Stress; **Integrated Processes:** Communication and Documentation; Nursing Process: Assessment; **Client Needs:** Safe and Effective Care Environment: Safety and Infection Control; **Cognitive Level:** Application [Applying]

**2095.** MoC **ANSWER: 3**

1. Suggesting that the staff be alert and aware does not effectively address the staff's concerns about identifying potential violent clients.
2. The staff needs to be aware of potential violence well before the client verbally expresses the anger.
3. **The two most significant predictors of violence are a history of violence and impulsivity. Thus reviewing the client's chart for this information is best.**
4. Telling the nurse that the information will be provided during in-service education does not answer the nurse's question.

▶ **Test-taking Tip:** Note the key word "best." Eliminate any options that do not answer the client's question. Select the option that is most proactive.

**Content Area:** Mental Health; **Concept:** Violence; Safety; Nursing Roles; Stress; **Integrated Processes:** Teaching/Learning; Communication and Documentation; **Client Needs:** Safe and Effective Care Environment: Management of Care; **Cognitive Level:** Analysis [Analyzing]

**2096.** MoC **ANSWER: 1**

1. **Although a thumbs-up gesture may mean "good job" in the U.S., it is considered an offensive gesture by persons from some other cultures. It is comparable to a raised middle finger in the U.S.**
2. If it appears that the nurse is fixated on time, the nurse may not be trusted.
3. Tea is a common beverage consumed by people in many countries.
4. Although the client may want a book that is not available, the offer does not indicate cultural insensitivity.

▶ **Test-taking Tip:** Gestures are culturally learned and may not mean the same thing to everyone. Thus focus on the options that use gestures to select the answer.

**Content Area:** Mental Health; **Concept:** Violence; Communication; Diversity; **Integrated Processes:** Nursing Process: Implementation; Culture and Spirituality; **Client Needs:** Safe and Effective Care Environment: Management of Care; Psychosocial Integrity; **Cognitive Level:** Application [Applying]

**2097. ANSWER: 4**

1. A history of violent behavior is considered a predictor of potential violence, but it is a client-oriented and not a milieu-oriented factor.
2. Although revocation of privileges may contribute to the potential for violence, it is a client-oriented and not a milieu-oriented factor.
3. Unit overcrowding, and not less than capacity, is considered an environmental predictor of violence.
4. **Staff inexperience is a significant environmental predictor of violent behavior of clients. The nurse manager should address this situation.**

▶ **Test-taking Tip:** Note the key word "milieu." You should focus on the options that pertain only to the environment, not to the client.

**Content Area:** Mental Health; **Concept:** Violence; Safety; Management; Stress; **Integrated Processes:** Nursing Process: Assessment; **Client Needs:** Safe and Effective Care Environment: Safety and Infection Control; **Cognitive Level:** Application [Applying]

**2098. ANSWER: 1, 2, 3, 4**

1. **The client requesting to be placed in seclusion is a reason to therapeutically employ seclusion.**
2. **The likelihood of harming self or others is one of the reasons to therapeutically employ seclusion and/or restraints.**
3. **If the staff feels as though the client is likely to harm others, a plan of therapeutic use of seclusion and/or restraints should be utilized to protect others.**
4. **Therapeutic use of seclusion and/or restraints is appropriate for the involuntarily detained client who threatens to escape. The client is being legally detained.**
5. Neither seclusion nor restraints should ever be used as punishment for the client's behavior.
6. Although the client's behavior may result in disruption to the milieu, seclusion and restraints are therapeutic only after all alternative interventions have been tried.

▶ **Test-taking Tip:** Look for similarities in options and select only the options that can result in self-injury or injury to others.

**Content Area:** Mental Health; **Concept:** Safety; Management; Violence; Stress; **Integrated Processes:** Nursing Process: Planning; **Client Needs:** Safe and Effective Care Environment: Safety and Infection Control; **Cognitive Level:** Analysis [Analyzing]

**2099. ANSWER: 2**

1. To apologize would give the client the impression that the client is being mistreated. The nurse should not view the application of restraints as something to be sorry for; it is in the client's best interest to be assisted in the process of regaining control.
2. **By providing an explanation of what is to happen and why, the client may resist less or, in some instances, decide to alter the behavior, especially once an understanding of the intervention is achieved. A dispassionate explanation avoids the nurse's emotions being misinterpreted by the client.**
3. Once the decision is made that restraints are the appropriate intervention, the client is not given an opportunity to negotiate out of their application.
4. Offering a situation when the restraints can be removed will not have much impact on securing the client's cooperation when applying the restraints.

▶ **Test-taking Tip:** Options 1, 3, and 4 are similar, and Option 2 is different. Often the option that is different is the answer.

**Content Area:** Mental Health; **Concept:** Violence; Safety; Stress; **Integrated Processes:** Nursing Process: Implementation; **Client Needs:** Safe and Effective Care Environment: Safety and Infection Control; **Cognitive Level:** Analysis [Analyzing]

## 2100. ANSWER: 2

1. The cortex (line A) controls motor functions.
2. **An inability to modulate judgment, aggression, and impulsivity results from a failure of control systems in the prefrontal cortex (line B) and limbic systems.**
3. The hypothalamus (line C) controls temperature and fluid regulation.
4. The cerebellum (line D) controls balance.

♦ *Test-taking Tip: Think about the functions of the brain. Select an area of the brain that controls behavior and emotions.*

Content Area: Mental Health; Concept: Cognition; Safety; Violence; Stress; Integrated Processes: Teaching/Learning; Client Needs: Physiological Integrity: Physiological Adaptation; Cognitive Level: Application [Applying]

## 2101. ANSWER: 3

1. Although the client's statement is a positive indicator of regained control, it is not as definitive as observed behavior regarding exposure to increased stimulation.
2. VS may indicate physical calmness, but they are not as definitive as observed behavior regarding exposure to increased stimulation.
3. **The client is showing the ability to tolerate the stimulation provided by being in the doorway and still appropriately asking for needs to be met. The reintegration of the client into the milieu should be completed gradually so as to monitor the client's ability to handle increased stimulation.**
4. Although past behavior may indicate a pattern, it is not as definitive as observed behavior regarding exposure to increased stimulation.

♦ *Test-taking Tip: Note the key word "best." Select the option of an observed behavior showing tolerance of increased stimulation.*

Content Area: Mental Health; Concept: Assessment; Self; Violence; Stress; Integrated Processes: Nursing Process: Evaluation; Client Needs: Safe and Effective Care Environment: Safety and Infection Control; Cognitive Level: Evaluation [Evaluating]

## 2102. ANSWER: 4

1. Hitting the desk is a threatening gesture, but the client has not verbally threatened the nurse.
2. There is no information to assume that the client does not acknowledge his or her role in the problem-solving process.
3. There is no information to assume that the client does not recognize that he or she is acting inappropriately.
4. **For some, intimidation and anger are the primary strategies for obtaining needs and goals and for achieving feelings of mastery and control. The nurse should recognize that the client is a danger to staff and others when using intimidation and anger.**

♦ *Test-taking Tip: Avoid reading into the situation and making inappropriate assumptions. Use only the information provided in the question stem and focus on the client's behavior.*

Content Area: Mental Health; Concept: Violence; Safety; Assessment; Stress; Integrated Processes: Nursing Process: Analysis; Client Needs: Safe and Effective Care Environment: Safety and Infection Control; Cognitive Level: Analysis [Analyzing]

## 2103. PHARM ANSWER: 1

1. **Olanzapine (Zyprexa) is an antipsychotic and mood stabilizer. It antagonizes dopamine and serotonin type 2 in the CNS. It is useful in helping to control acute agitation. The initial dose would be 0.5 mg, and the dose should be increased cautiously because it produces hypotension.**
2. Bupropion (Wellbutrin, Zyban) is an antidepressant that decreases neuronal reuptake of dopamine in the CNS; it is also used for smoking cessation.
3. Zolpidem (Ambien) is a sedative/hypnotic that produces CNS depression and is used for sleep.
4. Ondansetron (Zofran) is an antiemetic that blocks serotonin at vagal nerve terminals and in the CNS; it would not be useful in controlling agitation.

♦ *Test-taking Tip: Use the suffix "-zapine" to identify a medication that can be used to control anxiety.*

Content Area: Mental Health; Concept: Cognition; Safety; Violence; Stress; Medication; Integrated Processes: Nursing Process: Implementation; Client Needs: Physiological Integrity: Pharmacological and Parenteral Therapies; Cognitive Level: Analysis [Analyzing]

## 2104. ANSWER: 3

1. Although an agitated staff member may find it more difficult to keep the client's safety in mind, it is not the primary reason to remain calm.
2. Although an agitated staff member may not be as in control of the situation, it is not the primary reason to remain calm.
3. **The presence of other agitated people leads to increased client agitation.**
4. A staff member's ineffective behavior would require additional training, but it is not the primary reason to remain calm.

♦ *Test-taking Tip: Note that two options pertain to the client and two to the staff. Eliminate options pertaining to the staff's behavior and focus on the client's response to the behavior.*

Content Area: Mental Health; Concept: Safety; Stress; Violence; Integrated Processes: Teaching/Learning; Client Needs: Safe and Effective Care Environment: Safety and Infection Control; Cognitive Level: Application [Applying]

## 2105. ANSWER: 3

1. Stating the medications prescribed and the administration schedule does not demonstrate that the client can actually carry out the correct administration schedule.
2. Asking to stay with a relative does not show as much commitment to self-improvement as does the correct option.

3. Telephoning contacts at support services shows both an understanding of and a willingness to utilize the services. Research has shown that beginning client linkage to services prior to discharge has a positive effect on client outcomes.

4. Making promises does not necessarily indicate that the client will follow through with these.

▶ **Test-taking Tip:** You should focus on the only option in which the client's behavior demonstrates an action, not just verbalizing a commitment to self-management.

**Content Area:** Mental Health; **Concept:** Self; Assessment; Promoting Health; Stress; Evidence-based Practice; **Integrated Processes:** Nursing Process: Evaluation; **Client Needs:** Health Promotion and Maintenance; **Cognitive Level:** Evaluation [Evaluating]

**2106. ANSWER: 1, 2, 3, 4, 5**

1. Asking if anyone hurt the client is exploring the possibility of abuse and an appropriate question.

2. Asking if the client is afraid of anyone at home is exploring the possibility of abuse and an appropriate question.

3. Neurological or cardiovascular alterations, such as TIAs or low BP or pulse rate, can also result in falls. Asking about the frequency of falls is appropriate.

4. Neurological or cardiovascular alterations, such as TIAs or low BP or pulse rate, can also result in falls. Asking about fainting spells and weakness is appropriate.

5. Whenever a person presents with multiple injuries in various stages of healing, the possibility of abuse should be explored. Having the client explain how these happened may help determine the source.

6. Asking why the client has not reported abuse is insensitive and presumptuous.

▶ **Test-taking Tip:** The key phrase is "various stages of healing." Focus on assessment questions that will help determine the cause of the injuries.

**Content Area:** Mental Health; **Concept:** Communication; Violence; Stress; **Integrated Processes:** Communication and Documentation; **Client Needs:** Physiological Integrity: Physiological Adaptation; **Cognitive Level:** Application [Applying]

**2107.** MoC **ANSWER: 4**

1. Without clear orders, the nurse must not allow contact between the parent and child.

2. There is no indication that the HCP wishes to speak with the parent. The HCP does not decide who has access to the child.

3. A report to Social Services should have already been filed because the parent had previously been arrested for alleged child abuse.

4. The nurse's primary responsibility is the safety of the child and others. The nurse would initiate the hospital's emergency response system for behavioral situations to a secure a supervisor, security staff, and others.

▶ **Test-taking Tip:** The key phrase is "most appropriate." Think about the action that would maintain the safety of the child and others.

**Content Area:** Mental Health; **Concept:** Safety; Violence; Stress; **Integrated Processes:** Caring; Nursing Process: Planning; **Client Needs:** Safe and Effective Care Environment: Management of Care; Safe and Effective Care Environment: Safety and Infection Control; **Cognitive Level:** Analysis [Analyzing]

**2108.** MoC **ANSWER: 2**

1. The chain of command should be used first. Contacting the pediatric department head may be necessary if the nurse and charge nurse are unable to identify a policy or method by which to proceed.

2. Nurses are mandated reporters of any suspected child abuse. This form of child abuse is one of the most difficult to confirm, and court-ordered video surveillance may be necessary. Therefore to talk with the charge nurse would be most appropriate. Typically, with MSP, there are covert pieces of evidence that would point to such a diagnosis, but hard evidence is difficult to identify.

3. Calling a case conference may be the method by which health care professionals share information about this family, but the charge nurse should be notified first.

4. Filing a variance report is inappropriate. There is no indication that the HCP took no action, only that the HCP disagrees with the nurse's diagnosis of MSP; the suspected abuse should be further investigated.

▶ **Test-taking Tip:** MSP is a pattern of behavior in which caretakers deliberately exaggerate, fabricate, or induce physical or mental health problems in others. Nurses are mandated reporters of any suspected child abuse. Use the chain of command to determine the nurse's next action.

**Content Area:** Mental Health; **Concept:** Management; Stress; Violence; **Integrated Processes:** Nursing Process: Implementation; **Client Needs:** Safe and Effective Care Environment: Management of Care; **Cognitive Level:** Analysis [Analyzing]

**2109.** MoC **ANSWER: 3**

1. Moisture in a plastic bag will cause mold and mildew and destroy the evidence.

2. Asking the woman what she wants done with her clothing is inappropriate. Assault is a criminal offense, and evidence should be preserved.

3. To preserve the evidence, items are placed in separate paper bags, labeled, and released with appropriate documentation to the requesting police officer. The nurse specially trained to deal with possible criminal offenses should handle the clothing.

4. The nurse specially trained to deal with possible criminal offenses should handle the clothing. The items should not be returned to the woman or discarded.

▶ *Test-taking Tip: Select the option that would preserve the evidence.*

**Content Area:** Mental Health; **Concept:** Management; Violence; **Integrated Processes:** Communication and Documentation; Caring; **Client Needs:** Safe and Effective Care Environment: Management of Care; Physiological Integrity: Physiological Adaptation; **Cognitive Level:** Application [Applying]

## 2110. ANSWER: 2

1. A careful history is crucial to elicit accurate information. Insufficient information has been obtained to report suspected abuse.
2. **Additional questions should be asked of the client in private to elicit information about abuse, maltreatment, or neglect.**

3. Questioning the daughter may be appropriate, but it is most important to collect information from the client.
4. The resource hotline can be used by health care workers to seek answers to questions about abuse and neglect, but obtaining additional information from the client is most important.

▶ *Test-taking Tip: Avoid reading into the question. Use the nursing process. Assessment is the first step and should be completed before implementing interventions.*

**Content Area:** Mental Health; **Concept:** Critical Thinking; Safety; Stress; Assessment; **Integrated Processes:** Nursing Process: Assessment; **Client Needs:** Safe and Effective Care Environment: Safety and Infection Control; **Cognitive Level:** Analysis [Analyzing]

## Chapter Forty-Eight

# Substance Abuse

**2111.** The client states, "I go out just about every weekend and drink pretty heavily with my friends. Does that mean I'm dependent on alcohol?" Which is the **best** response by the nurse?

1. "You're not dependent on alcohol if you never drink to the point of intoxication."
2. "It sounds like you feel guilty about how much you drink. Tell me more about this."
3. "With dependence, you have a strong need to drink and feel uncomfortable if you don't."
4. "You could be dependent. Consuming alcohol pretty heavily every weekend is excessive."

**2112.** MoC The nurse is teaching home health aides about monitoring for alcohol abuse in older adults. Which response by an aide indicates a need for further teaching?

1. "Alcohol abuse is the largest category of substance abuse problems in older adults."
2. "I should monitor more closely for alcohol abuse in single male clients who smoke."
3. "Retirement and freedom from work and family pressures tend to decrease alcohol use."
4. "Confusion, malnutrition, and self-neglect may be signs of alcohol abuse in the elderly."

**2113.** MoC The nurse is assigned four clients at a substance abuse crisis clinic. Place the clients in the order of priority for care by the nurse.

1. The client with cannabis use who has a P of 145, dry mouth, and states having an increased appetite.
2. The client with opioid abuse who has pinpoint pupils, BP of 84/46, and temperature of 103.6°F (39.8°C).
3. The client with a flushed face, unsteady gait, and incoordination from alcohol intoxication.
4. The client with opioid abuse who has dilated pupils, diaphoresis, RR of 44, BP of 205/100, and now is having radiating chest pain.

Answer: _____

**2114.** Based on client statements, the nurse determines that the client has enormous guilt about drinking and is using excessive rationalization and denial of drinking. Place an X on the current phase of the client's alcoholic drinking progression.

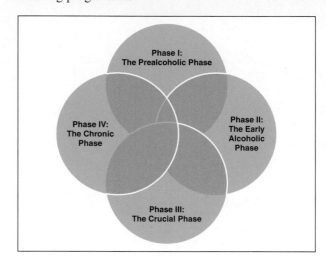

**2115.** PHARM The newly hospitalized client has Korsakoff's psychosis from alcohol abuse. Which intervention should the nurse plan?

1. Administer thiamine intravenously.
2. Give octreotide acetate intravenously.
3. Apply soft wrist restraints for safety.
4. Start oxygen at 2 L/min per nasal cannula.

**2116.** PHARM The client taking disulfiram has a throbbing headache, diaphoresis, and sudden vomiting. Which conclusions should the nurse explore **first?**

1. The client may have developed influenza.
2. The client may have recently consumed alcohol.
3. The client may have taken a cough suppressant.
4. The client may have eaten foods that interact with disulfiram.

**2117.** The nurse is preparing to lead a group therapy session with clients recovering from alcohol and other substances. Which seating arrangement would be **most** effective to facilitate group participation and discussion?

1.

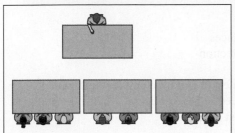

2.

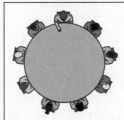

3.

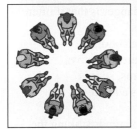

4.

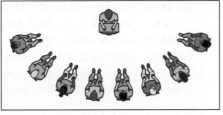

**2118.** The client, admitted 2 days ago to a medical unit, has a long history of heavy alcohol abuse. The nurse should monitor for which acute complications related to alcohol abuse? **Select all that apply.**

1. Seizures
2. Pancreatitis
3. GI bleeding
4. Exophthalmos
5. Delirium tremens (DTs)

**2119.** The hospitalized client has a history of weekly moderate alcohol use. Which symptoms assessed by the nurse indicate that the client may be experiencing alcohol withdrawal? **Select all that apply.**

1. Agitation
2. Hypotension
3. Tachycardia
4. Hallucinations
5. Tongue tremor

**2120.** **PHARM** The client experiencing severe withdrawal symptoms due to alcohol dependence is prescribed chlordiazepoxide 100 mg oral × 1, then 50 mg q2hrs until symptoms are controlled. The medication is supplied in 50-mg tablets. The nurse administered the initial dose 2 hours ago, and the client is still agitated and tremulous. How many tablets should the nurse prepare to give at this time?

_____ tablet(s) (Record a whole number.)

**2121.** The client brought to an ED is thought to have recent drug ingestion with possible overdose. Based on the table information illustrated, if the drug was ingested 6 hours ago, which are some of the drugs that the nurse should be able to detect in a urine specimen?

| Suspected Drug Duration for Witnessed Urine Sample | |
| --- | --- |
| **Drug** | **Detection Duration** |
| Amphetamines | 4 hours |
| Barbiturates | 24 hours to 7 days |
| Benzodiazepines | 3 days |
| Cannabinoids | 21 hours to 3 days |
| Cocaine | 2 to 3 days |
| Codeine | 4 hours |
| Methadone | 3 days |
| Methaqualone | 7 days |
| Morphine | 4 hours |
| Phencyclidine | 7 days |

1. Barbiturates, cocaine, and codeine
2. Amphetamines, codeine, and morphine
3. Phencyclidine, methaqualone, and morphine
4. Benzodiazepines, cocaine, and methaqualone

48 Substance Abuse

**2122.** The client receiving treatment for substance dependence has not been attending group therapy. Which statement by the nurse to confront this behavior is **best?**

1. "Why don't you want to go to group therapy? Other users are there waiting for you to attend."
2. "Talking about personal issues with others can be difficult. Try talking to the therapist alone."
3. "Therapy is important to your treatment. You need to attend therapy if you want to get better."
4. "You say you want to get better, but you are not actively participating in your treatment plan."

**2123.** MoC The nurse suspects that a coworker is working while impaired. Which **initial** action should be taken by the nurse?

1. Contact the Drug Enforcement Agency (DEA).
2. Contact the nurse manager to report the incident.
3. Confront the nurse and suggest to "get help."
4. File an anonymous report with the state's board of nursing.

**2124.** The spouse of the client who is currently in inpatient treatment for substance abuse tells the nurse, "We've done this so many times. I don't think my spouse is ever going to change. Do you think it's time for me to get a divorce?" Which response by the nurse is **most** helpful?

1. "You don't think your spouse is ever going to change?"
2. "It sounds like you're feeling discouraged in your marriage."
3. "Your spouse will likely continue to use and need treatment again."
4. "That's your decision; I can't tell you whether you should get a divorce."

**2125.** The nurse is in the working phase of a relationship with the client being treated for substance abuse. Which plan would be appropriate during this phase of treatment?

1. Assess the client's readiness to change substance-abusing behavior.
2. Evaluate the effectiveness of the client's newly adapted coping skills.
3. Confront the client's denial that substances have negatively impacted daily life.
4. Determine the extent to which substances have impaired the client's functioning.

**2126.** The nurse is assessing the client who presents with generalized fatigue, dry mouth, tachycardia, and an increased appetite. Which additional finding from the client's history and physical exam should alert the nurse to explore possible marijuana abuse?

1. Paranoia
2. Flashbacks
3. Gastric disturbances
4. Conjunctival infection

**2127.** The client states, "I don't see any problem with smoking a little weed. It isn't addictive." Which response by the nurse is **most** accurate?

1. "Marijuana is a natural chemical that has many therapeutic uses, but it is still illegal to use."
2. "Marijuana is not addictive. The danger is that it often leads to abuse of more illicit drugs."
3. "Marijuana has effects similar to alcohol, hallucinogens, and sedatives that are addictive."
4. "There are no withdrawal symptoms, so it is controversial whether marijuana is addictive."

**2128.** The client who abuses marijuana reports liking the drug for its perceived effects. Which experiences, if reported by the client, should the nurse attribute to marijuana use? **Select all that apply.**

1. Euphoria
2. Increased energy
3. Sexual enhancement
4. Appetite suppression
5. Improved fine-muscle coordination

**2129.** MoC The nurse educator is presenting a program on drug abuse to new nurses on the mental health unit. When explaining cocaine abuse, which street names for cocaine should the nurse include in the discussion?

1. Weed, chaw, fags
2. Toot, snow, crack
3. Uppers, dexies, crystal
4. Blue silk, cloud 9, white knight

**2130.** The nurse is discharging the client from an inpatient treatment program for cocaine abuse. Which statement by the client indicates an accurate understanding about the disease process of addiction?

1. "I'm really going to try to stay off cocaine. I'm not worried about alcohol. I've never had any problem with a glass or two of wine with dinner."
2. "Once my cravings go away, I won't need to go to Narcotics Anonymous (NA) anymore. I'll be recovered and will be able to stay away from using cocaine."
3. "I feel much better after talking to my therapist. I didn't realize that I was hurting so much emotionally. I must have been using to deal with my emotional problems."
4. "I didn't realize that staying off drugs meant changing my thoughts and emotions. I thought I could just learn to stop using cocaine. NA will help me make these changes."

**2131.** The client often avoids talking about cocaine use by refocusing on other problems such as losing a job and family discord. Which is the **most** helpful response by the nurse when the client avoids discussing using cocaine?

1. "Has your cocaine use helped you to cope with these problems in the past?"
2. "You need to consider that all these problems are related to your cocaine use."
3. "How do you think these problems will change once you no longer use cocaine?"
4. "You can't do anything about these while here. Just focus on getting off cocaine."

**2132.** The nurse completed an admission interview and assessment of the client who is under the influence of cocaine. Which findings should the nurse attribute to the client abusing cocaine? **Select all that apply.**

1. Decreased BP and HR
2. Lack of attention to the interview process
3. Hypersensitivity in response to personal questions
4. Underreporting the amount of cocaine used on a regular basis
5. Wheezing, coughing, red nose, and runny nose

**2133.** The client who is addicted to cocaine states, "I don't really need treatment. Things just got a little out of hand, causing some problems. I can handle things on my own. I really need to get back to my business." Which response by the nurse **best** assists the client to break through denial and get insight into the severity of the addiction?

1. "Tell me more about the business you feel you must return to at this time."
2. "You don't really need to be here? Tell me more about what you are thinking."
3. "You don't feel you need treatment. How often have you been using cocaine?"
4. "You say you can handle things, but you found yourself with a lot of problems."

**2134.** The parent expresses concern that her son, newly admitted to the mental health unit, may be using methamphetamine. Which nursing assessment findings are consistent with methamphetamine abuse?

1. Hypotension and bradycardia
2. Constricted pupils and fatigue
3. Anorexia and recent weight loss
4. Bruises and scrapes on extremities

**2135.** MoC The nursing is counseling the client who uses methamphetamine regularly. Which statements demonstrate the client using pathological projection as a coping mechanism?

1. "I'm here to get help. Everything will be all right again if I can just stop using drugs."
2. "My dad and I don't get along. He thinks that I'm a failure and can't do anything right."
3. "I'm not giving up alcohol, just the methamphetamine. I never had a problem with alcohol."
4. "I can't go back to work. I'd be so embarrassed if anyone found out I've been in treatment."

**2136.** The nurse is interacting with the client who abuses methamphetamine. The client states, "I don't plan to quit meth. I can work for days when I'm high." Which is the **best** response by the nurse?

1. "You'll exhaust yourself working days when you're high."
2. "You can't see the real problem yet because you're in denial."
3. "You say you don't plan to quit. Do you think using drugs helps you?"
4. "Good point. You probably do work long hours while you are on meth."

**2137.** The nurse is caring for the client who has methamphetamine toxicity. Which interventions, if prescribed, should the nurse include in the client's plan of care? **Select all that apply.**

1. Give olanzapine 10 mg IM q2h prn to treat agitation.
2. Allow the client to sleep and eat as much as desired.
3. Administer labetalol 20 mg IV to control hallucinations.
4. Monitor 1:1 to protect client from harm to self and others.
5. Encourage involvement in the therapeutic treatment milieu.

**2138.** The client has developed paranoia as a result of regular methamphetamine use. The nurse uses cognitive reappraisal to confront the client's persecutory thoughts. Which question should the nurse ask the client?

1. "How can you look at this differently?"
2. "Why would they want to cause you harm?"
3. "What did you do that makes others not like you?"
4. "How do you feel when others create problems for you?"

**2139.** **MoC** The 19-year-old is given a court order to enter treatment for cocaine abuse. The client threatens to leave the treatment facility AMA. Which statement by the nurse demonstrates an accurate understanding of the client's options?

1. "The client is of legal age and can leave if he wants; we can't stop him from leaving."
2. "Due to the court order, the client is not allowed to leave and will be placed in seclusion."
3. "The client is allowed to leave as long as the court is informed; I'll prepare the documents."
4. "The client cannot leave and will be returned to treatment, or another option, by court order."

**2140.** **PHARM** The nurse is educating the client on the methadone prescribed for replacement therapy while in an outpatient treatment program for heroin addiction. The client asks, "How is taking a pill going to help me stay substance-free?" Which statement is the nurse's **best** reply?

1. "The methadone will give you the same high, so you won't want heroin anymore."
2. "The methadone will cause you to become very sick if you take heroin at the same time."
3. "The methadone 'replaces' heroin in your body, so you will have fewer cravings for heroin."
4. "The methadone causes sedation; you'll sleep better, so you can participate in your treatment."

**2141.** The client is being discharged from treatment for addiction to alprazolam and will be attending an addiction self-help group. Which statement indicates that the client has an accurate understanding of maintaining sobriety according to 12-step self-help principles?

1. "I cannot take any mood-altering drugs, or I run the risk of relapsing."
2. "I will have to stay away from situations that I find anxiety-producing."
3. "I've learned how to safely use my nerve pills to avoid overusing them."
4. "Instead of these pills, I'll drink a small glass of wine when I feel anxious."

**2142.** **PHARM** The client is started on buprenorphine with naloxone sublingual for opiate addiction. Which statements indicate that the client understood the nurse's instructions about the medication? **Select all that apply.**

1. "The medication can slow or stop my breathing. I should only take what is prescribed."
2. "I'm taking this non–habit-forming medication to help stop my craving for opiate drugs."
3. "If I suddenly stop taking buprenorphine and naloxone, I could experience withdrawal."
4. "I can take the tablet whole or crush it and take it with food to make it more palatable."
5. "This drug is highly abused; I should not share this or keep it where it can be stolen."

**2143.** The nurse is counseling the client with a substance abuse disorder. Which defense mechanism is the nurse **most** likely to observe the client using in response to a stressful event?

1. Repression
2. Regression
3. Sublimation
4. Reaction formation

**2144.** **PHARM** The client is receiving clonidine to relieve selected symptoms of opioid withdrawal. Which assessment is **most** important for the nurse to complete before administering clonidine?

1. Check for presence of dilated pupils.
2. Investigate recent nausea or vomiting.
3. Test for abnormally heightened reflexes.
4. Verify that the BP is not low.

**2145.** **PHARM** The client in group therapy states, "I've enjoyed using methylphenidate because of how it makes me feel." The nurse should identify which additional statement with methylphenidate use?

1. "I love how it gave me energy to stay up all night."
2. "It really helped me sleep when I wasn't very tired."
3. "The bad part was that I gained weight when using it."
4. "I could really focus. I liked not worrying about anything."

**2146.** The mother of the 14-year-old tells the clinic nurse that she is concerned that her child may be "doing some sort of drug." The adolescent is confused and has difficulty answering questions clearly but admits to sniffing solvents in the family's garage. Which statement by the nurse is correct?

1. "Most inhalants can cause serious nervous system and respiratory system damage."
2. "There is little risk for physical harm; the effects will wear off within a few hours."
3. "By seeking help early you can discourage your child from future drug use."
4. "Your child will sleep for long periods after the drug effects are gone."

**2147.** **MoC** The nurse is planning care for the client receiving treatment for benzodiazepine abuse. Place the interventions in the order that they should be implemented during the client's course of treatment.

1. Review lifestyle changes that will need to be made.
2. Take vital signs.
3. Administer lorazepam as prescribed.
4. Emphasize personal responsibility for abstaining from substance abuse.
5. Provide information about the symptoms of withdrawal.
6. Encourage oral fluids.

Answer: _____

**2148.** **PHARM** The nurse is preparing to administer chlordiazepoxide 75 mg orally for the client experiencing severe withdrawal symptoms due to alprazolam dependency. The medication is supplied in 25-mg capsules. How many capsules should the nurse prepare to administer?

_____ capsule(s) (Record a whole number.)

**2149.** The client with a history of poly substance abuse is being medically detoxified in an acute care hospital. The client reported recently using alcohol, oxycodone, crack cocaine, and marijuana. In planning for detoxification, which substance for detoxification should be the nurse's **priority?**

1. Alcohol
2. Marijuana
3. Oxycodone
4. Crack cocaine

**2150.** **PHARM** The 19-year-old client regularly abuses dextromethorphan (DXM). Which activity, if performed under the influence of dextromethorphan, places the client at the greatest risk for complications related to DXM abuse?

1. Dancing at a nightclub
2. Competing in a swim meet
3. Snow-skiing on spring break
4. Fishing from a shaded shoreline

**2151.** **PHARM** The student participating in college sports is suspected of abusing anabolic steroids and is referred to the college's health service. Which nursing assessment findings are consistent with anabolic steroid abuse? **Select all that apply.**

1. Acne vulgaris
2. Aggressive behavior
3. Heavy menstruation
4. Urinary tract infection
5. Thickening of the hair
6. Edema of the hands and feet

**2152.** The client expresses ambivalence about quitting smoking and the fear of "getting fat" and "looking like a cow." The client wonders if that is worse than smoking. Which response by the nurse is **most** helpful?

1. "We could set up a diet for you to start at the same time to prevent you from gaining any weight."
2. "Don't you think it would be much better to breathe more easily, even if you gain a little weight?"
3. "You don't want to quit smoking because you think you might gain weight. Do you see yourself as overweight?"
4. "It sounds like you are afraid of weight gain. Tell me about both the good and bad things that might happen if you give up smoking."

# Answers and Rationales

## 2111. ANSWER: 3

1. Intoxication is not necessarily an indication of dependence. A person can be dependent without becoming intoxicated, or vice versa.
2. Dependence on alcohol is not defined by guilt or other feelings surrounding the drinking behavior.
3. **Dependence involves a compulsive or chronic requirement for a chemical. The need is so strong as to generate physical or psychological distress if left unfilled. More than 3 drinks per day or more than 7 drinks per week in women, more than 4 drinks per day or more than 14 drinks per week in men, or more than 1 drink per day if over age 65 is high-risk alcohol consumption.**
4. Dependency is not defined by frequency.

♦ *Test-taking Tip: Use the process of elimination. The key word is "dependent." Eliminate options that are definitive, and then select the most descriptive option for dependence.*

**Content Area:** Mental Health; **Concept:** Addiction; Communication; **Integrated Processes:** Communication and Documentation; **Client Needs:** Health Promotion and Maintenance; **Cognitive Level:** Application [Applying]

## 2112. MoC ANSWER: 3

1. The use of alcohol is the largest category of substance abuse in the elderly; this is a correct statement.
2. Being male and single, having less than a high school education, low income, and smoking are risk factors for heavy drinking in older adults; this statement is correct.
3. **This statement indicates more teaching is needed. Past work and family responsibilities may have kept a potential abuser from drinking too much, whereas isolation due to retirement and lack of family nearby can trigger alcohol abuse.**
4. Older clients abusing alcohol display vague geriatric signs or syndromes such as confusion, malnutrition, and self-neglect.

♦ *Test-taking Tip: The question asks you to identify an incorrect response. Be careful with words in an option such as "increase" or "decrease" that are opposite of what would make a statement correct.*

**Content Area:** Mental Health; **Concept:** Addiction; Nursing Roles; Management; **Integrated Processes:** Nursing Process: Evaluation; **Client Needs:** Safe and Effective Care Environment: Management of Care; **Cognitive Level:** Evaluation [Evaluating]

## 2113. MoC ANSWER: 4, 2, 3, 1

4. **The client with opioid abuse who has dilated pupils, diaphoresis, RR of 44, BP of 205/100, and now is having radiating chest pain is priority. Using ABC's, this client should be first. The client needs lifesaving intervention.**

2. **The client with opioid abuse who has pinpoint pupils, BP of 84/46, and temperature of 103.6°F (39.8°C) should be seen second. The client has inadequate perfusion with the low BP, and the high temperature could indicate sepsis.**
3. **The client with a flushed face, unsteady gait, and incoordination from alcohol intoxication can be attended to third. The client is walking, although with an unsteady gait and is not in any imminent danger.**
1. **The client with cannabis use who has a P of 145, dry mouth, and states having an increased appetite is not experiencing any unexpected effects. The client can be attended to last.**

♦ *Test-taking Tip: Use the ABC's to establish priority. Clients with life-threatening problems should be attended to first.*

**Content Area:** Mental Health; **Concept:** Addiction; Critical Thinking; Management; **Integrated Processes:** Nursing Process: Assessment; **Client Needs:** Safe and Effective Care Environment: Management of Care; Psychosocial Integrity; **Cognitive Level:** Synthesis [Creating]

## 2114. ANSWER:

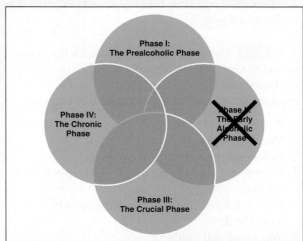

Jellinek (1952) outlined four phases through which the alcoholic's pattern of drinking progresses. During the early alcoholic phase (Phase II), the individual feels guilt and becomes defensive. Excessive use of denial and rationalization becomes evident. Phase I involves using alcohol to relieve everyday stress. In Phase III, control over alcohol is lost, and physiological dependence is evident. Drinking has become the total focus. Phase IV involves emotional and physical disintegration.

♦ *Test-taking Tip: Think about the progression of substance abuse. Recall that denial occurs early in the alcoholic process.*

**Content Area:** Mental Health; **Concept:** Addiction; Assessment; **Integrated Processes:** Nursing Process: Analysis; **Client Needs:** Psychosocial Integrity; **Cognitive Level:** Application [Applying]

**2115.** PHARM **ANSWER: 1**

1. **Confusion, loss of recent memory, and the use of confabulation occurs in Korsakoff's psychosis in alcoholics due to a deficiency in thiamine. Thiamine (vitamin B$_1$) deficiency occurs from insufficient intake and malabsorption of nutrients from the toxic effects of alcohol. Thiamine use may reduce confusion and prevent further impairment.**
2. Octreotide acetate (Sandostatin) is a vasoconstrictor given to lower portal BP and can prevent rebleeding from esophageal varices that can occur as a complication of alcohol abuse.
3. Least restrictive measures, such as a 1:1 sitter or family presence, should be used before applying restraints on a confused client.
4. Confusion due to Korsakoff's psychosis is treated with thiamine, not oxygen.

▶ **Test-taking Tip:** You need to consider the symptoms associated with Korsakoff's psychosis to determine the correct intervention.

**Content Area:** Mental Health; **Concept:** Addiction; Medication; **Integrated Processes:** Nursing Process: Planning; **Client Needs:** Physiological Integrity: Pharmacological and Parenteral Therapies; **Cognitive Level:** Application [Applying]

**2116.** PHARM **ANSWER: 2**

1. Throbbing headache, diaphoresis, and vomiting are symptoms associated with both influenza and alcohol ingestion, and should be explored if the client has not consumed alcohol recently.
2. **Throbbing headache, diaphoresis, and vomiting are symptoms associated with recent alcohol ingestion while taking disulfiram (Antabuse). Recent alcohol consumption should be explored first.**
3. Alcohol-containing cough suppressants can cause a disulfiram-alcohol reaction. This should be explored if the client has not consumed alcohol recently.
4. Foods cooked in wine or alcohol-containing preparations can cause a disulfiram-alcohol reaction. This should be explored if the client has not consumed alcohol recently.

▶ **Test-taking Tip:** The key word is "first," suggesting that all options are correct but that one option is more important than the others. A brand name for disulfiram is Antabuse.

**Content Area:** Mental Health; **Concept:** Addiction; Medication; **Integrated Processes:** Nursing Process: Analysis; **Client Needs:** Physiological Integrity: Pharmacological and Parenteral Therapies; **Cognitive Level:** Application [Applying]

**2117. ANSWER: 3**

1. Clients facing forward with the nurse at the front of the room establishes a communication barrier.
2. When the clients and nurse are seated in a circle around a conference table, the conference table poses a physical barrier.

3. **Clients and the nurse seated in chairs arranged in a circle is most effective for promoting communication. The room is arranged so that there are no barriers between members.**
4. The teacher standing in front of the group establishes a power position and poses a barrier to effective communication.

▶ **Test-taking Tip:** When selecting the option, you need to eliminate options that pose a barrier to effective communication.

**Content Area:** Mental Health; **Concept:** Addiction; Communication; **Integrated Processes:** Nursing Process: Planning; **Client Needs:** Psychosocial Integrity; **Cognitive Level:** Application [Applying]

**2118. ANSWER: 1, 2, 3, 5**

1. **Seizures can occur due to the electrolyte alterations and encephalopathy that occur with chronic alcohol abuse.**
2. **Acute pancreatitis can occur as an acute complication of heavy alcohol abuse. Alcohol abuse is the second most common cause of acute pancreatitis, after gallstones.**
3. **GI bleeding may be an acute complication due to cirrhosis or esophageal varices. Alcohol abuse is the second most common cause of cirrhosis in the United States.**
4. Exophthalmos is abnormal bulging of the eyeballs; it is not an acute complication associated with heavy alcohol abuse. Exophthalmos may be seen in thyrotoxicosis.
5. **DTs (tremors, hallucinations, anxiety, and disorientation) can occur 24 to 72 hours after the client last consumed alcohol. DTs is a complication due to alcohol withdrawal from chronic alcohol abuse.**

▶ **Test-taking Tip:** Use the ABC's to identify complications associated with chronic alcohol abuse.

**Content Area:** Mental Health; **Concept:** Addiction; Assessment; **Integrated Processes:** Nursing Process: Assessment; **Client Needs:** Physiological Integrity: Physiological Adaptation; **Cognitive Level:** Application [Applying]

**2119. ANSWER: 1, 3, 4, 5**

1. **Alcohol withdrawal leads to increased activity of postsynaptic $N$-methyl-D-aspartate (NMDA) receptors in the brain, resulting in agitation.**
2. Hypertension, not hypotension, is associated with alcohol withdrawal.
3. **Alcohol withdrawal leads to increased activity of NMDA receptors in the brain, resulting in tachycardia.**
4. **Alcohol withdrawal leads to increased activity of NMDA receptors in the brain, resulting in hallucinations.**
5. **Alcohol withdrawal leads to increased activity of NMDA receptors in the brain, resulting in tongue tremor.**

▶ **Test-taking Tip:** *Think about how all options except one might be related through increased brain activity.*

**Content Area:** Mental Health; **Concept:** Addiction; Assessment; **Integrated Processes:** Nursing Process: Assessment; **Client Needs:** Physiological Integrity: Physiological Adaptation; **Cognitive Level:** Application [Applying]

### 2120. PHARM ANSWER: 1

Use a proportion formula. Multiply the extremes (outside values) and then the means (inside values) and solve for *X*.

50 mg : 1 tablet :: 50 mg : *X* tablets; 50*X* = 50;
*X* = 50 ÷ 50; *X* = 1

The nurse should administer 1 chlordiazepoxide (Librium) tablet.

▶ **Test-taking Tip:** *Focus on the information in the question. Realize that it is 2 hours later, so a smaller amount is required.*

**Content Area:** Mental Health; **Concept:** Addiction; Medication; **Integrated Processes:** Nursing Process: Implementation; **Client Needs:** Physiological Integrity: Pharmacological and Parenteral Therapies; **Cognitive Level:** Application [Applying]

### 2121. ANSWER: 4

1. Although barbiturates and cocaine would be present in the urine, codeine can be detected in the urine for only up to 4 hours, not 6 hours.
2. Amphetamines, codeine, and morphine can be detected in the urine for only up to 4 hours, not 6 hours.
3. Although phencyclidine and methaqualone would be present in the urine for up to 7 days, morphine can be detected in the urine for only up to 4 hours, not 6 hours.
4. **According to the table, benzodiazepines can be detected for up to 3 days, cocaine for up to 2 to 3 days, and methaqualone for up to 7 days. If benzodiazepines, cocaine, and methaqualone were ingested 6 hours ago, these drugs could be detected in the urine.**

▶ **Test-taking Tip:** *Focus on what the question is asking: presence of the drug if the adolescent ingested these within the past 6 hours. First read the options, and then check the information in the table to eliminate options.*

**Content Area:** Mental Health; **Concept:** Medication; Addiction; Assessment; **Integrated Processes:** Nursing Process: Analysis; **Client Needs:** Physiological Integrity: Reduction of Risk Potential; **Cognitive Level:** Application [Applying]

### 2122. ANSWER: 4

1. A "why" question is a barrier to therapeutic communication and can initiate a defensive response.
2. Although this statement may seem to acknowledge the client's concerns, the client has not provided a reason for not attending group therapy.
3. Telling the client of the need to attend therapy to get better can be a threatening statement that can initiate a defensive response.

4. **The nurse should address the behavior in a matter-of-fact, nonjudgmental manner by using confrontation with a caring approach. Confrontation interferes with the client's ability to use denial. A caring attitude avoids putting the client on the defensive.**

▶ **Test-taking Tip:** *Use therapeutic communication principles. The key word in the stem is "confront."*

**Content Area:** Mental Health; **Concept:** Addiction; Communication; **Integrated Processes:** Caring; Communication and Documentation; **Client Needs:** Psychosocial Integrity; **Cognitive Level:** Application [Applying]

### 2123. MoC ANSWER: 2

1. The DEA may become involved if there has been diversion of controlled substances, but it is the nurse manager's responsibility to carry out the agency's policy for reporting to the DEA.
2. **The nurse suspecting a coworker of working while impaired should contact the nurse manager, who will investigate the allegation and initiate the appropriate action.**
3. Confronting an impaired nurse may result in denial or retaliation.
4. Many state boards of nursing have adopted mandatory reporting of suspected impairment, but the nurse should first report the impaired nurse's behavior to the nurse manager. It is the nurse manager's responsibility to take further action; reporting laws vary by state.

▶ **Test-taking Tip:** *The primary concern of the nurse should be ensuring client safety. Only one option allows for internal investigation, which should be carried out before further action is taken.*

**Content Area:** Mental Health; **Concept:** Legal; Addiction; Collaboration; **Integrated Processes:** Communication and Documentation; **Client Needs:** Safe and Effective Care Environment: Management of Care; **Cognitive Level:** Application [Applying]

### 2124. ANSWER: 2

1. Restatement is a therapeutic technique but is not the best option to encourage facilitation of feelings.
2. **Using validation assists the spouse in examining his or her feelings and facilitates further exploration of how that person is being affected by the substance abuse behavior.**
3. This response may or may not be true. The nurse should refrain from giving a personal opinion.
4. A direct answer, although refraining from opinion giving, closes the communication.

▶ **Test-taking Tip:** *Using a therapeutic communication technique that focuses on the client's or spouse's feelings is usually the most therapeutic option.*

**Content Area:** Mental Health; **Concept:** Addiction; Family; **Integrated Processes:** Caring; Communication and Documentation; **Client Needs:** Psychosocial Integrity; **Cognitive Level:** Application [Applying]

**2125. ANSWER: 3**

1. Assessing readiness to change occurs in the first phase and not the working phase of the nurse-client relationship.
2. Evaluating the extent of behavioral change occurs during the final, not working, phase of the nurse-client relationship.
3. **In the working phase, the nurse should determine the strength of the client's denial system and assist the client to accept the fact that substances are causing problems.**
4. Determining the extent of drug or alcohol's impact occurs during the assessment phase of the nurse-client relationship, where factual data is collected.

▶ **Test-taking Tip:** Key words are "working phase" and "intervention." Use the nursing process and eliminate options that represent different phases of the nursing process. Only one option is an intervention.

**Content Area:** Mental Health; **Concept:** Addiction; **Integrated Processes:** Nursing Process: Planning; **Client Needs:** Psychosocial Integrity; **Cognitive Level:** Application [Applying]

**2126. ANSWER: 4**

1. Methamphetamine abuse may present with paranoia, compulsive and aggressive behavior, and hallucinations.
2. Flashbacks are attributed to the use of hallucinogens.
3. Gastric disturbances are common in chronic alcohol abuse.
4. **Physical symptoms of cannabis intoxication include conjunctival infection, generalized fatigue, dry mouth, tachycardia, and an increased appetite.**

▶ **Test-taking Tip:** Focus on the client's initial symptoms and think about what may be missing and the methods for marijuana use.

**Content Area:** Mental Health; **Concept:** Addiction; Assessment; **Integrated Processes:** Nursing Process: Assessment; **Client Needs:** Psychosocial Integrity; **Cognitive Level:** Knowledge [Remembering]

**2127. ANSWER: 3**

1. Marijuana is believed to have some therapeutic use. Some states, but not all, have legalized its use.
2. Marijuana still remains a drug with addictive potential.
3. **Even at moderate doses, marijuana produces effects similar to those of CNS depressants, hallucinogens, and sedative-hypnotics. Psychological addiction has been shown to occur with marijuana.**
4. There is an identified withdrawal syndrome (insomnia and restlessness), so marijuana is considered an addictive substance.

▶ **Test-taking Tip:** The key word in the stem is "addictive." Narrow the options to those that address addiction.

**Content Area:** Mental Health; **Concept:** Addiction; Promoting Health; Nursing Roles; **Integrated Processes:** Teaching/Learning; Communication and Documentation; **Client Needs:** Psychosocial Integrity; **Cognitive Level:** Application [Applying]

**2128. ANSWER: 1, 3**

1. **Marijuana induces a sense of euphoria through its effects on the CNS.**
2. Cannabis induces amotivational syndrome, including lethargy and lack of motivation (not increased energy).
3. **It is thought that marijuana enhances the sexual experience in both men and women through the intensified sensory awareness and the subjective slowness of time perception. Its use also enhances the sexual functioning by releasing inhibitions for certain activities that would normally be restrained.**
4. CNS effects include increased appetite, not appetite suppression.
5. Muscle tremor, not increased fine-muscle coordination, is associated with marijuana use.

▶ **Test-taking Tip:** You need to carefully analyze options for information that is opposite of the findings associated with marijuana use.

**Content Area:** Mental Health; **Concept:** Addiction; Neurologic Regulation; **Integrated Processes:** Nursing Process: Analysis; **Client Needs:** Psychosocial Integrity; **Cognitive Level:** Comprehension [Understanding]

**2129.** MoC **ANSWER: 2**

1. Weed, chaw, and fags are common street names for nicotine products including cigarettes, cigars, pipe tobacco, and snuff.
2. **Street names for cocaine include toot, snow, and crack. Other street names are coke, blow, lady, and flake.**
3. Uppers, dexies, and crystal refer to amphetamines.
4. Blue silk, cloud 9, and white knight 3 are street names for synthetic stimulants.

▶ **Test-taking Tip:** Use the appearance of the drug and how it is used as cues to the street names. Narrow the options by using clues such as "dexies" within the options.

**Content Area:** Mental Health; **Concept:** Addiction, Nursing Roles; **Integrated Processes:** Teaching/Learning; **Client Needs:** Safe and Effective Care Environment: Management of Care; Psychosocial Integrity; **Cognitive Level:** Application [Applying]

**2130. ANSWER: 4**

1. Persons addicted to one substance appear to be susceptible to dependency on other substances.
2. Recovery is a lifelong process. There is no cure for addiction.
3. Substance dependence disorders are primary in nature; they are not secondary to other emotional problems.
4. **An emphasis on the requirement for a total lifestyle change is necessary for preventing relapse. Through NA people learn to change negative attitudes and behaviors into positive ones.**

▶ **Test-taking Tip:** Focus on the concept of total abstinence associated with recovery when answering this question.

**Content Area:** Mental Health; **Concept:** Addiction; Nursing Roles; **Integrated Processes:** Nursing Process: Evaluation; Teaching/Learning; **Client Needs:** Health Promotion and Maintenance; **Cognitive Level:** Evaluation [Evaluating]

## 2131. ANSWER: 3

1. This response is not helpful. Cocaine has likely contributed to other problems, not assisted in coping with or resolving them.
2. Giving an opinion may cause defensiveness in the client with little insight.
3. **Other problems encountered by the client are often related to drug use. Using a therapeutic communication technique of helping the client see relationships between drug use and other problems helps provide insight into the severity of the substance abuse.**
4. Significant problems should be addressed concurrently in treatment for substance abuse, not avoided.

▶ *Test-taking Tip: Apply principles of therapeutic communication as well as knowledge of thought processes commonly associated with substance abuse.*

Content Area: Mental Health; Concept: Addiction; Communication; Integrated Processes: Communication and Documentation; Client Needs: Psychosocial Integrity; Cognitive Level: Application [Applying]

## 2132. ANSWER: 3, 5

1. Physical effects include tachycardia (not decreased HR) and either elevated or lowered BP.
2. Hypervigilance and not lack of attention occurs with cocaine intoxication.
3. **Cocaine intoxication usually causes interpersonal sensitivity, changes in sociability, hypervigilance, and anxiety.**
4. Underreporting is common in all substance abusers and is not specific to cocaine intoxication.
5. **If snorting cocaine, wheezing, red nose, coughing, and runny nose can develop and persist.**

▶ *Test-taking Tip: Think "hyper" when considering the options and how cocaine is ingested.*

Content Area: Mental Health; Concept: Addiction; Stress; Integrated Processes: Nursing Process: Analysis; Client Needs: Physiological Integrity: Physiological Adaptation; Cognitive Level: Analysis [Analyzing]

## 2133. ANSWER: 4

1. Addressing the client's business changes the focus of the conversation.
2. Voicing doubt or parroting the client without presenting reality may cause defensiveness.
3. Addressing the pattern of cocaine use changes the focus.
4. **This statement assists the client to work on accepting the fact that using substances has caused problems in significant life areas.**

▶ *Test-taking Tip: Confrontation should be used as a therapeutic communication technique when the client uses denial.*

Content Area: Mental Health; Concept: Addiction; Communication; Integrated Processes: Communication and Documentation; Client Needs: Psychosocial Integrity; Cognitive Level: Application [Applying]

## 2134. ANSWER: 3

1. The nurse should expect to find an increase in BP and HR, not hypotension and bradycardia.
2. The nurse should expect to find dilated (not constricted) pupils. Constricted pupils may indicate opiate abuse. Fatigue can be associated with any drug use.
3. **Weight loss is associated with methamphetamine and other stimulant abuse due to their ability to cause a rise in metabolic rate and varying degrees of anorexia.**
4. Bruises and scrapes can be associated with gait impairments from intoxication. Bruises may be seen with methamphetamine use due to alterations in the immune system from nutritional deficiencies.

▶ *Test-taking Tip: Methamphetamine is a stimulant that increases metabolic rate. Narrow the options to only those pertaining to metabolism.*

Content Area: Mental Health; Concept: Addiction; Assessment; Integrated Processes: Nursing Process: Assessment; Client Needs: Physiological Integrity: Reduction of Risk Potential; Cognitive Level: Comprehension [Understanding]

## 2135. MoC ANSWER: 2

1. Believing that all problems will be solved if drugs are absent is a fallacy of ignoring.
2. **Projecting (blaming) involves placing the responsibility for one's behavior on someone or something else besides the person. The client is blaming the drug use and lack of behavior change on what the client believes about his or her dad. This is negative self-talk and is self-deprecating.**
3. Denial is evidenced in the statement that the client has no problem or intention to alter alcohol use.
4. Feeling embarrassed displays a fallacy of perfectionism rather than projection.

▶ *Test-taking Tip: The key word is "projection." Three options focus on the client, and one option is different. Often the option that is different is the answer.*

Content Area: Mental Health; Concept: Addiction; Stress; Communication; Integrated Processes: Communication and Documentation; Client Needs: Safe and Effective Care Environment: Management of Care; Psychosocial Integrity; Cognitive Level: Analysis [Analyzing]

## 2136. ANSWER: 3

1. Directive statements do not facilitate the client's thinking and disclosure.
2. Informing the client of denial before he or she indicates readiness does not facilitate the therapeutic relationship.
3. **The focus is on current reality, and the nurse must be nonjudgmental. Restatement is a neutral response that assists the client in reexamining the thought process.**
4. Agreeing with the client's irrational statement reinforces the denial process.

▶ *Test-taking Tip: Apply principles of therapeutic communication and eliminate options that use barriers to therapeutic communication.*

Content Area: Mental Health; Concept: Addiction; Communication; Integrated Processes: Communication and Documentation; Client Needs: Psychosocial Integrity; Cognitive Level: Application [Applying]

## 2137. ANSWER: 1, 2, 4

1. **Olanzapine (Zyprexa) is an atypical antipsychotic that binds to alpha-1, dopamine, histamine H1, muscarinic, and serotonin type 2 (5-HT2) receptors, and reduces agitation associated with methamphetamine withdrawal.**
2. **Treatment of CNS stimulant toxicity involves keeping the client in a quiet atmosphere and allowing the client to eat and sleep as much as needed.**
3. Labetalol (Normodyne, Trandate) when given IV acts primarily as a beta-receptor antagonist. It is used to lower BP, not control hallucinations.
4. **Agitation and violence are CNS manifestations of methamphetamine toxicity; 1:1 monitoring is needed for client and staff safety.**
5. Stimulation should be kept to a minimum during the acute phase of methamphetamine toxicity. Due to the severity of the condition, the client would not be on a mental health unit yet.

♦ *Test-taking Tip: Options 2 and 5 are opposites; evaluate these options first because usually one of these would be incorrect. Consider the severity of the condition and likely manifestations and treatment when examining the options.*

Content Area: Mental Health; Concept: Addiction; Medication; Sleep, Rest, and Activity; Integrated Processes: Nursing Process: Planning; Caring; Client Needs: Safe and Effective Care Environment: Safety and Infection Control; Cognitive Level: Synthesis [Creating]

## 2138. ANSWER: 1

1. **Cognitive restructuring involves stopping maladaptive thoughts and replacing them with more realistic ones. Reappraisal can be achieved by examining different perspectives.**
2. Asking a "why" question gives the client opportunity to reinforce the distorted belief.
3. Asking what the client did reinforces the irrational thought and places blame on the client.
4. Asking how one feels is not a cognitive restructuring technique.

♦ *Test-taking Tip: Note the key phrase "uses cognitive reappraisal" to consider the correct response. Eliminate options that focus on others and not on the client.*

Content Area: Mental Health; Concept: Addiction; Nursing Roles; Communication; Integrated Processes: Communication and Documentation; Nursing Process: Assessment; Client Needs: Psychosocial Integrity; Cognitive Level: Application [Applying]

## 2139. MoC ANSWER: 4

1. Persons committed to treatment by the court cannot leave voluntarily.
2. Placing the client in seclusion violates the law providing treatment in the least restrictive setting and can be considered false imprisonment.
3. The court is informed if the committed client leaves, but the court would determine the consequential action rather than the client being allowed to leave.
4. **With involuntary commitments, state standards require a specific impact or consequence. Court hearings determine commitment and length of stay, and a person is not allowed to leave and would be returned for treatment if attempting AMA.**

♦ *Test-taking Tip: The key phrase is "court order." Review options for similar words between the stem of the question and the options.*

Content Area: Mental Health; Concept: Addiction; Legal; Management; Integrated Processes: Nursing Process: Evaluation; Client Needs: Safe and Effective Care Environment: Management of Care; Cognitive Level: Evaluation [Evaluating]

## 2140. PHARM ANSWER: 3

1. Methadone does not exert the severe high of other abused opiates.
2. Methadone does not have a role in aversion therapy.
3. **Methadone (Methadose) is one of the more common medications for opioid detoxification. Methadone is a long-acting agonist that, in effect, displaces heroin (or other abused opioids) and restabilizes the receptor site, thereby lessening the cravings for heroin and reversing opioid withdrawal symptoms.**
4. Methadone does not cause sedation.

♦ *Test-taking Tip: Three options are similar, and one is different; often the option that is different is the answer.*

Content Area: Mental Health; Concept: Addiction; Medication; Integrated Processes: Teaching/Learning; Client Needs: Physiological Integrity: Pharmacological and Parenteral Therapies; Cognitive Level: Application [Applying]

## 2141. ANSWER: 1

1. **Alcoholics Anonymous and other 12-step self-help groups promote total abstinence as the only cure. Persons addicted to drugs cannot safely use any mood-altering chemicals.**
2. Avoiding anxiety-producing situations is not realistic.
3. Sobriety involves abstaining from the use of all substances, including anxiety medications.
4. Sobriety involves abstaining from alcohol to maintain optimal wellness.

♦ *Test-taking Tip: Alprazolam (Xanax) is a benzodiazepine anxiolytic drug. Narrow the options to those focusing on the use of addictive medications. Options 1 and 3 are opposites. Often when two options are opposite, one is the answer.*

Content Area: Mental Health; Concept: Addiction; Medication; Integrated Processes: Nursing Process: Evaluation; Client Needs: Psychosocial Integrity; Cognitive Level: Evaluation [Evaluating]

**2142. PHARM ANSWER: 1, 3, 5**

1. Buprenorphine with naloxone (Suboxone) is a combination drug. Buprenorphine is an opioid medication that, when taken in excessive doses, can cause respiratory depression. These should be taken as prescribed.
2. Buprenorphine and naloxone are habit-forming.
3. The buprenorphine contained in Suboxone is an opioid medication; withdrawal symptoms can occur if stopped abruptly.
4. Sublingual medication should not be crushed or chewed but should be placed under the tongue. No food or beverages should be consumed until the tablet is dissolved.
5. Buprenorphine with naloxone is widely prescribed as a detoxifying drug, but it is greatly abused. It has addictive effects when taken with alcohol and other CNS depressants. It should not be shared with others.

▸ *Test-taking Tip:* Buprenorphine is an opioid medication. Relate this information to the options to narrow the choices to the correct options.

Content Area: Mental Health; Concept: Medication; Addiction; Integrated Processes: Nursing Process: Evaluation; Client Needs: Physiological Integrity: Pharmacological and Parenteral Therapies; Cognitive Level: Evaluation [Evaluating]

**2143. ANSWER: 2**

1. Repression is involuntary exclusion of an event from consciousness.
2. Defense mechanisms utilized by persons who abuse substances include denial, regression, rationalization, and projection. Regression is the retreat to an earlier level of development and the comfort measures associated with that level of functioning; it may include behaviors such as crying, helplessness, rocking, or childlike behavior.
3. Sublimation involves channeling unacceptable desires into acceptable forms.
4. Reaction formation is acting opposite from one's desires.

▸ *Test-taking Tip:* Apply knowledge of medical terminology related to defense mechanisms.

Content Area: Mental Health; Concept: Addiction; Stress; Integrated Processes: Nursing Process: Assessment; Client Needs: Psychosocial Integrity; Cognitive Level: Application [Applying]

**2144. PHARM ANSWER: 4**

1. Dilated pupils are expected with opioid withdrawal but do not contraindicate the administration of clonidine.
2. Nausea and vomiting may occur with opioid withdrawal; although this is important to know before administering clonidine orally, verifying that the BP is not low is more important.
3. Heightened reflexes are associated with opioid withdrawal but do not contraindicate the administration of clonidine.

4. The nurse should verify the client's BP prior to administration and should withhold clonidine (Catapres) if the systolic BP is lower than 90 mm Hg or the diastolic BP is below 60 mm Hg.

▸ *Test-taking Tip:* Use the ABC's to identify the most important assessment.

Content Area: Mental Health; Concept: Addiction; Medication; Integrated Processes: Nursing Process: Assessment; Client Needs: Physiological Integrity: Pharmacological and Parenteral Therapies; Cognitive Level: Application [Applying]

**2145. PHARM ANSWER: 4**

1. Excessive energy is associated with amphetamine stimulants.
2. Methylphenidate increases alertness so it will not act as a sleep aid.
3. Weight loss, not weight gain, is a side effect of methylphenidate use.
4. Methylphenidate (Ritalin, Concerta) is a nonamphetamine stimulant that increases mental alertness, decreases distractibility, and aids in concentration and focus, but it can produce a false sense of euphoria and well-being.

▸ *Test-taking Tip:* Focus on the key word "enjoyed" and look for related words in the options.

Content Area: Mental Health; Concept: Addiction; Self; Integrated Processes: Nursing Process: Analysis; Client Needs: Physiological Integrity: Pharmacological and Parenteral Therapies; Cognitive Level: Analysis [Analyzing]

**2146. ANSWER: 1**

1. This statement is correct. Most inhalants produce some neurotoxicity with cognitive, motor, and sensory involvement. Respiratory effects range from coughing and wheezing to dyspnea, emphysema, and pneumonia.
2. There is physical harm including damage to the brain and internal organs, including the heart, lungs, kidneys, liver, pancreas, and bone marrow.
3. Even though the adolescent is 14 years old, there is no indication regarding the length of time the child has been sniffing solvents or whether help has been sought early.
4. A period of postdetoxification insomnia is expected and can be treated with good sleep practices such as avoiding caffeine, daytime napping, and overstimulation in the evening.

▸ *Test-taking Tip:* Options 1 and 2 are opposites, so one of these must be wrong.

Content Area: Mental Health; Concept: Addiction; Nursing Roles; Communication; Neurologic Regulation; Integrated Processes: Communication and Documentation; Client Needs: Health Promotion and Maintenance; Physiological Integrity: Reduction of Risk Potential; Cognitive Level: Application [Applying]

**2147.** **MoC** **ANSWER: 2, 3, 6, 5, 4, 1**

2. **Take VS; these are assessed to identify abnormalities associated with benzodiazepine withdrawal.**

3. **Administer lorazepam as prescribed. Lorazepam should be administered to reduce the potentially fatal withdrawal symptoms of the benzodiazepines.**

6. **Encourage oral fluids to maintain adequate hydration.**

5. **Provide information about the symptoms of withdrawal. Education on expected symptoms helps to ease the client's fear of the unknown. Education is accomplished once the client is physically stable.**

4. **Emphasize personal responsibility for abstaining from substance abuse. The client should be involved in the treatment plan once physically stable.**

1. **Review lifestyle changes that will need to be made. This step is last; the client needs to first acknowledge the need to change. Specific changes should be explored to help promote the client's drug-free lifestyle.**

▶ *Test-taking Tip: Use the nursing process and Maslow's Hierarchy of Needs theory. Recall that assessment and then analysis are priority in the nursing process. Physiological needs are addressed before psychosocial and teaching needs.*

Content Area: Mental Health; Concept: Medication; Addiction; Integrated Processes: Nursing Process: Implementation; Client Needs: Safe and Effective Care Environment: Management of Care; Physiological Integrity: Basic Care and Comfort; Cognitive Level: Synthesis [Creating]

**2148.** **PHARM** **ANSWER: 3**

**Use a proportion formula to calculate the dose of chlordiazepoxide (Librium). Multiply the extremes (outside values) and then the means (inside values) and solve for X.**

**25 mg : 1 capsule :: 75 mg : X capsules; 25X = 75; X = 75 ÷ 25; X = 3**

▶ *Test-taking Tip: Focus on the information in the question and use the on-screen calculator. Verify your answer, especially if it seems like an unusual amount.*

Content Area: Mental Health; Concept: Medication; Addiction; Integrated Processes: Nursing Process: Implementation; Client Needs: Psychosocial Integrity; Physiological Integrity: Pharmacological and Parenteral Therapies; Cognitive Level: Application [Applying]

**2149. ANSWER: 1**

1. **Alcohol should have priority when detoxifying because it produces the most serious withdrawal syndrome, which can be fatal. Withdrawal symptoms include tremors, nausea/vomiting, malaise, weakness, tachycardia, sweating, elevated BP, anxiety, depressed mood, irritability, hallucinations, headache, insomnia, and seizures. Safety issues during alcohol withdrawal are a concern.**

2. Withdrawal symptoms from marijuana include restlessness, irritability, insomnia, loss of appetite, depressed mood, tremors, fever, chills, headache, and stomach pain. These are less life-threatening than alcohol withdrawal symptoms.

3. Withdrawal symptoms from oxycodone include craving for the drug, nausea and vomiting, muscle aches, lacrimation or rhinorrhea, pupillary dilation, piloerection or sweating, diarrhea, yawning, fever, and insomnia. These are less life-threatening than alcohol withdrawal symptoms.

4. Withdrawal symptoms from crack cocaine include depression, anxiety, irritability, fatigue, insomnia or hypersomnia, psychomotor agitation, paranoid or suicidal ideation, apathy, and social withdrawal. These are less life-threatening than alcohol withdrawal symptoms. Safety issues are a concern with both alcohol and crack cocaine withdrawal.

▶ *Test-taking Tip: Think about the abused substances that produce the most serious withdrawal syndromes before answering this question.*

Content Area: Mental Health; Concept: Addiction; Management; Integrated Processes: Nursing Process: Planning; Caring; Client Needs: Psychosocial Integrity Safe and Effective Care Environment: Safety and Infection Control; Cognitive Level: Application [Applying]

**2150.** **PHARM** **ANSWER: 1**

1. **When consumed in large quantities, dextromethorphan (Delsym, Robitussin DM) can cause hyperthermia. Hyperthermia is a concern for clients who take DXM while exerting themselves and becoming hot, such as while dancing.**

2. When under the influence of DXM, swimming is a lower-risk activity for inducing complications due to the cooler environment.

3. When under the influence of DXM, snow-skiing is a lower-risk activity for inducing complications due to the cooler environment.

4. When under the influence of DXM, fishing is a lower-risk activity for inducing complications due to the cooler environment.

▶ *Test-taking Tip: Focus on the actions of the client and on the environments. Three environments are likely to be cooler than the other environment. Select the option that is different.*

Content Area: Mental Health; Concept: Addiction; Thermo-regulation; Sleep, Rest, and Activity; Integrated Processes: Nursing Process: Analysis; Client Needs: Physiological Integrity: Pharmacological and Parenteral Therapies; Cognitive Level: Analysis [Analyzing]

**2151.** **PHARM** **ANSWER: 1, 2, 4, 6**

1. **Acne vulgaris is a side effect of anabolic steroid usage.**

2. **Behavioral disturbances such as severe aggressiveness can occur with anabolic steroid usage.**

3. Females experience cessation of menses (not heavy menstruation) with the use of anabolic steroids.

4. **UTIs can result because of anabolic steroid usage.**

5. Hair usually thins (not thickens) with anabolic steroid usage.

6. **Edema of the extremities may be a result of anabolic steroid use.**

▶ *Test-taking Tip: Anabolic steroids are synthetic variations of testosterone. Think about the effects of testosterone as you review the options.*

**Content Area:** Mental Health; **Concept:** Addiction; Medication; Assessment; **Integrated Processes:** Nursing Process: Assessment; **Client Needs:** Physiological Integrity: Pharmacological and Parenteral Therapies; **Cognitive Level:** Knowledge [Remembering]

## 2152. ANSWER: 4

1. Dieting during smoking cessation is not recommended in general and has been shown to increase the likelihood of smoking relapse.
2. Pointing out the health gains of stopping smoking does little to assuage the client's fear of weight gain.

3. A closed-ended question has limited effectiveness in helping the client discuss fears.
4. **Fear of weight gain is a barrier for many who want to quit smoking. Acknowledging fears develops empathy. Exploring fears as well as benefits helps the client in decision-making. Cognitive reappraisal helps the client face fears more realistically. This is the most helpful response by the nurse.**

▶ *Test-taking Tip: Select the therapeutic communication technique that focuses on the client's fears.*

**Content Area:** Mental Health; **Concept:** Addiction; Nutrition; Promoting Health; **Integrated Processes:** Caring; Communication and Documentation; **Client Needs:** Health Promotion and Maintenance; Psychosocial Integrity; **Cognitive Level:** Application [Applying]

## Chapter Forty-Nine

# Mental Health Disorders

## ANXIETY AND MOOD DISORDERS

**2153.** The parents, whose child died after being accidently shot, tell the nurse about their involvement in gun safety legislation. The parents are using which defense mechanism?

1. Denial
2. Sublimation
3. Identification
4. Intellectualization

**2154.** The client states, "For 5 years, I have been physically ill and have had frequent crying episodes, feelings of worthlessness, and loss of appetite on the anniversary of when my spouse died." What should be the nurse's focus when counseling the client?

1. Anticipatory grief
2. Uncomplicated grief
3. Delayed grief reaction
4. Distorted grief reaction

**2155.** The client is being discharged after hospitalization for a suicide attempt. Which question asked by the nurse assesses the learned prevention and future coping strategies of the client?

1. "How did you try to kill yourself?"
2. "Why did you think life wasn't worth living?"
3. "What skills can you utilize if you experience problems again?"
4. "Do you have the phone number of the suicide prevention center?"

**2156.** The nurse is caring for the client with a major depressive disorder. Which client problem should be the nurse's **priority?**

1. Powerlessness
2. Attempted suicide
3. Anticipatory grieving
4. Disturbed sleep pattern

**2157.** MoC The nurse is interviewing the client at a mental health clinic who recently attempted suicide and continues to report active suicidal ideation. Which care setting is **most** appropriate for this client?

1. An acute care hospital unit
2. An inpatient mental health unit
3. An outpatient mental health clinic
4. A community detoxification center

**2158.** MoC The nurse is discharging the client who was hospitalized for suicidal ideation. The nurse advises the client to seek help from a mental health professional or the National Suicide Prevention Lifeline if experiencing which warning signs for suicide? **Select all that apply.**

1. Feelings of sadness
2. Feelings of hopelessness
3. Feelings of being trapped
4. Severe anxiety and agitation
5. Increasing alcohol or drug use

**2159.** PHARM The client is diagnosed with acute mania. What should the nurse ensure happens prior to initiating the prescribed lithium carbonate?

1. The client has been fasting for the past 12 hours.
2. Kidney function has been evaluated as WNL.
3. The client has not been in room seclusion.
4. Benzodiazepine therapy has been discontinued.

**2160.** PHARM The client is newly prescribed tramadol hydrochloride for chronic pain. The client is also taking fluoxetine 40 mg daily for depression. Which nursing action is **most** important?

1. Instruct the client to drink plenty of fluids daily.
2. Ask the HCP about increasing the fluoxetine dose.
3. Monitor for signs of serotonin syndrome.
4. Administer both medications with food.

**2161.** PHARM The client with a bipolar disorder presents to the ED with impaired consciousness, nystagmus, and seizures. The nurse determines that which result(s) on the client's serum lab report illustrated explains the client's symptoms?

| Serum Laboratory Test | Client's Value |
| --- | --- |
| Creatinine | 2.2 mg/dL |
| BUN | 44 mg/dL |
| Sodium | 140 mEq/L |
| WBC | 3500/mm³ |
| Lithium | 3.8 mEq/L |
| Dilantin | 15 mcg/dL |

1. Dilantin level
2. Lithium level
3. Sodium and WBC values
4. Creatinine and BUN values

**2162.** PHARM The nurse is educating the client about prescription antidepressant medications and the appropriate expectations when taking these medications. Which statement by the nurse is accurate?

1. "It is important to continue taking antidepressant medication even after you feel better."
2. "Your symptoms will subside about 72 hours after starting the antidepressant medication."
3. "You will be taking fluoxetine, which is the most potent SSRI antidepressant medication."
4. "Some common side effects of SSRIs are dry mouth, blurred vision, and urinary retention."

**2163.** PHARM The nurse is reviewing diet restrictions with the client taking an MAOI. The nurse should inform the client of which symptom that can occur when the client is nonadherent to diet restrictions?

1. Akathisia
2. Agranulocytosis
3. Severe hypotension
4. Explosive occipital headache

**2164.** The experienced nurse is orienting a new nurse on a mental health unit. Which intervention should the nurse suggest when attempting to establish a therapeutic relationship with the newly admitted client diagnosed with major depressive disorder?

1. Sit with the client in silence.
2. Invite the client to attend an exercise class.
3. Ask the client to join others to watch a 2-hour movie.
4. Ask the client how his or her day should be scheduled.

**2165.** PHARM The client who is taking amitriptyline 150 mg daily is scheduled for elective surgery. Which statement reflects accurate understanding of safety concerns in this situation?

1. The client could be switched to doxepin instead of amitriptyline prior to surgery.
2. Amitriptyline should be continued, as the stress of surgery will worsen depression.
3. Amitriptyline should be gradually discontinued prior to the client having surgery.
4. Oral medications should be taken 4 hours before surgery with only a sip of water.

**2166.** PHARM The HCP prescribes citalopram 20 mg daily. After 6 months, the HCP increases the dose to 30 mg daily. The client wants to use the fifteen 20-mg tablets remaining from the previous prescription but wants to know how many days these will last. How many days should the nurse state if the client takes the newly prescribed dose of 30 mg daily?

_____ days (Record your answer as a whole number.)

**2167.** The client recently diagnosed with depression tells the nurse that she is 2 months pregnant and is reluctant to take an antidepressant. Which type of therapy should the nurse discuss when the client asks about an alternate treatment for depression?

1. Gestalt therapy
2. Client-centered therapy
3. Therapeutic touch therapy
4. Cognitive behavioral therapy

**2168.** The nurse is assessing the client with possible major depressive disorder. Which symptoms, if identified by the client as occurring nearly daily for at least 2 weeks, should the nurse associate with major depressive disorder? **Select all that apply.**

1. Impaired concentration
2. Feelings of worthlessness
3. Having a depressed mood
4. Loss of interest or pleasure
5. Presence of psychomotor retardation
6. Talking rapidly with pressured speech

**2169.** During the client education class, the nurse is asked, "What is an effective treatment for seasonal affective disorder?" Which intervention should the nurse recommend as an evidenced-based practice for the first-line treatment of seasonal affective disorder?

1. Light therapy
2. Prescribing quetiapine
3. A 2-week trial of lithium carbonate
4. Individual therapy with a psychologist

**2170.** The nurse is assessing the client with dysthymia who reports symptoms of depressed mood. Which assessment finding should the nurse associate **most** with the essential feature of dysthymia?

1. Feelings of sadness and emptiness for the past 2 weeks
2. Decreased ability to think or concentrate daily for the past 2 weeks
3. Chronically depressed mood for most of the day for at least 2 years
4. Attempted suicide and had recurrent thoughts of death in the past week

**2171.** MoC The newly admitted client who is depressed tells the nurse, "Nothing gives me joy. Things seem hopeless." Prioritize the nurse's immediate care for this client by placing interventions in the order that they should be performed.

1. Initiate prescribed psychosocial treatment plans.
2. Determine the client's risk for suicide by direct questioning (asking about suicide intent and plan).
3. Assist the client in maintaining nutritional needs, hygiene, and grooming and in meeting other physical needs.
4. Contact the client's support system in collaboration with case manager and/or social services.
5. Initiate suicide precautions, as needed, according to policy and standards of care.

Answer: _____

**2172.** The nurse is assessing the client, attempting to differentiate the client's symptoms between delirium and depression. Which client symptoms are unique to depression? **Select all that apply.**

1. Sadness
2. Labile affect
3. Lack of motivation
4. Presence of hallucinations
5. Disturbance in sleep patterns

**2173.** The client who was recently divorced and has a court appearance the following week for DUI is seeing the nurse for possible depression. Which statement by the nurse is **most** therapeutic?

1. "You seem concerned. Were you surprised that your spouse left after you got a DUI?"
2. "Getting a DUI can be depressing. You aren't thinking about hurting yourself, are you?"
3. "I think you should have a substance abuse evaluation before we treat your depression."
4. "I'm concerned about your drinking. I'd like you to talk with our chemical dependency staff."

**2174.** MoC The nurse is teaching a class to assistive personnel on depression. Which statements by the nurse provide accurate information about depression? **Select all that apply.**

1. Behaviors can fluctuate between low mood and euphoria.
2. Children within all age groups can experience depression.
3. The rate of depression among adolescents increases with age.
4. Women are about twice as likely as men to develop depression.
5. Perfectionism and rigid thought patterns are signs of depression.

**2175.** The client diagnosed with mania tells the nurse, "I think you're nice looking. Maybe we could go to my room?" Which response by the nurse is **most** therapeutic?

1. "Let's walk down to the seclusion room."
2. "That's not appropriate, and I feel offended."
3. "I don't have that kind of relationship with clients."
4. "Let's focus on recovery; it's time for group therapy."

**2176.** MoC The NA comments to the nurse about the recently admitted client with bipolar disorder. "I think the new admit is faking being ill. Yesterday the client didn't say a word, and today it's nonstop talking." Which response by the nurse is **most** helpful?

1. "Thanks for letting me know. I think the client may be looking for attention."
2. "It is more appropriate to refer to the client by name and not as the new admit."
3. "The client has rapid-cycle bipolar disorder; this includes quickly changing moods."
4. "Some people are quiet; the client has the right to decide when and when not to talk."

**2177.** The nurse is planning care for the recently admitted client who is exhibiting agitation associated with acute mania. Which intervention should the nurse plan to implement?

1. Involve the client in group activities to provide structure.
2. Maintain a low level of stimuli in the client's environment.
3. Take the client to his or her room and leave the client alone.
4. Apply restraints to prevent the client from harming self or others.

**2178.** The nurse assesses the client who reports feeling full of energy despite having been awake for the past 48 hours. Which diagnosis is the nurse likely to find documented in the client's medical record?

1. Korsakoff's psychosis
2. Bipolar disorder/mixed type
3. Bipolar disorder/manic type
4. Obsessive-compulsive disorder

**2179.** The client is diagnosed with major depressive disorder and was started on an antidepressant 2 days ago. The nurse observes that 2 days ago the client appeared sad and remained in bed. Now the client is awake at 4 a.m. and planning a unit party. Which conclusion should the nurse make regarding the client's change in behavior?

1. The client is responding positively to the antidepressant medication.
2. Treatment was effective, and the client plans on being discharged soon.
3. The client is more familiar with the unit and is able to be self-expressive.
4. The client may have been misdiagnosed and may have a bipolar disorder.

**2180.** The client recently admitted to a psychiatric unit is experiencing acute mania. Which intervention should the nurse include when developing a plan of care for the client?

1. Initiate prolonged conversations to improve the client's concentration.
2. Provide finger foods that the client can eat while moving around the unit.
3. Teach the client and family about community resources that are available.
4. Instruct the family to confront the client's angry behavior, or it will escalate.

**2181.** **PHARM** The nurse assesses that the client with acute mania has coarse hand tremors, and the serum lithium level is 1.8 mEq/L. What should the nurse do?

1. Advise the client to limit the intake of fluids.
2. Continue to administer lithium as prescribed.
3. Withhold the lithium dose and notify the HCP.
4. Request a medication to treat the hand tremors.

**2182.** The nurse is planning a class for clients with mild to moderate anxiety. Which strategies should the nurse use when teaching the clients? **Select all that apply.**

1. Maintain a calm, nonthreatening manner.
2. Create an atmosphere of low stimulation.
3. Reinforce reality by focusing on the "here and now."
4. Limit the class time and the amount of information.
5. Remove objects that the client could use to cause harm.

**2183.** The newly admitted client is diagnosed with generalized anxiety disorder. Which nursing assessment findings would be consistent with the diagnosis? **Select all that apply.**

1. Irritability
2. Muscle tension
3. Expansive mood with pressured speech
4. Restlessness or feeling keyed up or on edge
5. Difficulty controlling the anxiety

**2184.** The client tells the nurse, "I have an intense fear of dogs. I can't visit others unless I know that there are no dogs around. This fear seems unreasonable, but it continues to be a problem." Which conclusion by the nurse is accurate?

1. The client has a recognized fear, but there is no evidence of psychopathology.
2. Phobias begin in childhood and are diagnosed more often in men than women.
3. A fear that is recognized as excessive and unreasonable is a criterion for phobias.
4. True phobias are rare in the general population, but common with anxiety disorders.

**2185.** **MoC** The nurse manager is planning an in-service that focuses on staff management of potential suicidal ideation among clients. Which activity has the **greatest** likelihood for improving the effectiveness of the staff?

1. Have staff review the policies pertaining to the suicide assessment protocol.
2. Ask clients who have experienced a suicidal ideation to participate in a discussion.
3. Have staff role-play communication techniques for assessing and managing suicidal ideation.
4. Have mental health experts present a roundtable discussion on suicidal ideation.

**2186.** **MoC** The client with an anxiety disorder tells the nurse that being in crowds creates thoughts of losing control and the need to quickly leave. Which therapy should the nurse recommend for this client?

1. Family systems therapy
2. Psychoanalytical therapy
3. Electroconvulsive therapy (ECT)
4. Cognitive behavioral therapy (CBT)

**2187.** The client has been seeking treatment for insomnia secondary to situational depression. Which statement made by the client requires follow-up by the nurse?

1. "I'm going to be tested for sleep apnea; this could be causing my sleep problems."
2. "Replacing my morning shower with an evening bath will take some adjustment."
3. "It's possible that once I'm no longer depressed, I'll be able to sleep better again."
4. "I will be including black tea and a snack as part of my nightly bedtime ritual."

# TRAUMA- AND STRESSOR-RELATED DISORDERS

**2188.** The recently discharged veteran who served in active combat reports having recurring intrusive thoughts, insomnia, and hypervigilance. Which question would be **most** helpful in establishing a diagnosis?

1. "Do you find yourself falling asleep while working?"
2. "Are you also having nightmares when you do sleep?"
3. "Your hair seems thin. Are you also pulling at your hair?"
4. "Have you ever been diagnosed with obsessive-compulsive disorder?"

**2189.** The nurse is caring for a victim of sexual assault brought to the ED by a roommate. How should the nurse respond when the client begins to angrily insist upon reporting the details of the assault?

1. Ask the roommate to sit with the client until the examination can be resumed.
2. Redirect the client to the physical tasks related to securing any existing evidence.
3. Encourage the client to use deep breathing techniques to regain emotional control.
4. Listen quietly as the client expresses the anger and rage currently being experienced.

**2190.** The young adult who was robbed is attending counseling sessions to address anxiety issues. What is the nurse's **best** response when the client asks, "When will things get better for me?"

1. "These types of crises are self-limiting, and usually things are better in 4 to 6 weeks."
2. "Try not to worry; it is best for you to think about the future and not focus on the past."
3. "Being assaulted is traumatic; in time the anxiety will lessen, and you'll feel more in control."
4. "By using the skills you're learning, the goal for you is to feel better or be back to normal in about 6 weeks."

**2191.** [MoC] The client who does not speak or understand English was assaulted and an agency interpreter is present at the time of assessment. Which action is most appropriate for the nurse while utilizing the interpreter?

1. Asking the questions directly to the client
2. Asking the questions directly to the interpreter
3. Asking the interpreter to step out of the room while completing the physical assessment
4. Allowing the interpreter to rephrase questions and responses instead of interpreting each word

**2192.** The 10-year-old who was sexually abused by a relative experiences flashbacks of a disagreement with that adult and the resulting sexual assault. Which suggestion by the nurse to the child's parents would help minimize this reaction?

1. "Have your child avoid arguments with adults until this reaction is unlearned."
2. "I will ask the HCP to prescribe a medication to minimize your child's aggressiveness."
3. "Adults in your family should learn to recognize and diffuse arguments effectively."
4. "You and your child should regularly discuss bad memories to decrease their effect."

**2193.** The child who was physically abused has begun pulling out hair. The behavior appears to be a result of the child's repressed anger. To facilitate the child's recovery, the nurse encourages the parent to **initially** implement which response?

1. Accept the hair pulling until therapy can substitute this behavior by addressing the anger.
2. Ignore the hair pulling and focus on reassuring the child that the abuse will never recur.
3. Distract the child from the hair pulling by introducing a pleasurable experience in its place.
4. Explain that hair pulling is unacceptable and must stop so that the therapy can be successful.

**2194.** The client's home was destroyed by a major flood. The client is attending a support group and says, "I will rebuild my home as good as new and be living in it in a few months." What should be the nurse's **initial** response?

1. "That's a very ambitious plan to undertake at this time."
2. "I'm proud of your resiliency and willingness to start over."
3. "Have you given thought to what may happen if it floods again?"
4. "Can you tell me how many months you think rebuilding will take?"

**2195.** The client is being treated after surviving a major hurricane that took the lives of many neighbors. Which statement by the client provides the nurse with the **best** evidence that therapy has been successful?

1. "Therapy has been a very helpful for me because the hurricane ruined everything."
2. "I'm ready and able to move on with my life in spite of all that has happened."
3. "Nothing can happen to me that is worse than what I have been through already."
4. "I have learned a lot about myself since agreeing to attend crisis therapy sessions."

## PERSONALITY DISORDERS

**2196.** The nurse is assessing the client with paranoid personality disorder. Which behavior should the nurse expect?

1. Able to trust only those who are fair and treat the client well
2. Sees the goodwill of another when that behavior does not exist
3. Acts the opposite of what the client may be thinking or feeling
4. Analyzes the behavior of others to find hidden and threatening meanings

**2197.** The nurse is working with the client with paranoid personality disorder. The nurse considers that the client likely experienced what in the past?

1. Little affection or approval during the childhood years
2. Lack of empathy and lack of nurturing during upbringing
3. Indifference and lack of affection during early upbringing
4. Recognition for accomplishments only in early childhood

**2198.** The nurse identifies that an individual with antisocial personality disorder exhibits poor judgment, emotional distance, aggression, and impulsivity. Place an X on the step of the nursing process illustrated being completed by the nurse.

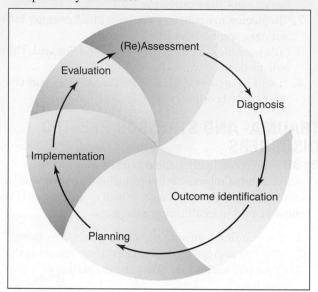

**2199.** The nurse is caring for the client with paranoid personality disorder. Which approach should the nurse use when working with the client?

1. Use a businesslike manner using clear, concrete, and specific words.
2. Use social conversation initially to work on developing social relationships.
3. Include jokes when conversing to work on reducing the client's serious behavior.
4. Confront when stating suspicious ideas to aid the client in seeing reality.

**2200.** The nurse reads in the medical record that the client with BPD has "splitting." What is the nurse's interpretation of "splitting"?

1. The client is having an intense psychotic episode and has become catatonic.
2. The client has an identity disturbance with an unstable self-image or sense of self.
3. The client is using a defense mechanism in which all objects are seen as good or bad.
4. The client's behavior shows a pattern of unstable and intense interpersonal relationships.

**2201.** The nurse is working with the client with histrionic personality disorder. Which behaviors should the nurse expect? **Select all that apply.**

1. Uses physical appearance to gain attention
2. Shows apathy in conversations until trust is established
3. Lacks close friends or companions other than first-degree relatives
4. Harbors recurrent suspicions about the fidelity of his or her marital partner
5. Discomfort in situations in which the client is not the center of attention

**2202.** The client with bipolar personality is taking lithium 300 mg tid. Fluoxetine 20 mg bid is prescribed. Before giving the medication, the nurse reviews the client's chart illustrated. What should the nurse do? **Select all that apply.**

| Client Chart | | | |
|---|---|---|---|
| Lab Test | 4 Months Ago | 2 Months Ago | Today |
| Lithium Level | 1.0 mEq/L | 1.2 mEq/L | 1.5 mEq/L |

1. Question the dose of lithium.
2. Question the dose of fluoxetine.
3. Notify the HCP of the lab results.
4. Administer the dose of fluoxetine.
5. Question the addition of fluoxetine.

**2203.** The client with BPD often attempts to manipulate staff to promote self needs. Which behavior indicates that the client can overcome manipulation?

1. The client insists on joining other clients in the dayroom because of feeling lonely.
2. The client asks for a cigarette 30 minutes after being told that cigarettes are allowed once an hour.
3. The client states to the nurse, "You are the best nurse; only you are allowed to care for me."
4. The client self-mutilates by cutting after the HCP discussed possible discharge with the client.

**2204.** The client with BPD states to the nurse, "Hey, you know what! You are my favorite nurse. That night nurse sure doesn't understand me the way you do." Which response by the nurse is **most** therapeutic?

1. "Hang in there. I won't enjoy coming to work as much after you are discharged."
2. "I'm glad you're comfortable with me. Which night nurse doesn't understand you?"
3. "I like you. Tomorrow you'll be discharged; I'm glad you will be able to return home."
4. "You are my favorite patient; I'll really miss caring for you when you are discharged."

**2205.** MoC PHARM The client diagnosed with BPD is prescribed phenelzine 15 mg tid. Based on the client's MAR illustrated, which should be the nurse's reasoning for questioning the medication order?

| Client: A | Diagnosis: Borderline Personality Disorder | Allergies: None | |
|---|---|---|---|
| Medication | 0001–0759 | 0800–1559 | 1600–2400 |
| Fluoxetine 20 mg daily | | 0900 | |
| Carbamazepine 400 mg bid | | 0900 | 2100 |
| Alprazolam 0.5 mg bid | | 0900 | 2100 |

1. The combination phenelzine and fluoxetine will drastically lower the BP.
2. Tension headaches may result when carbamazepine and alprazolam are combined.
3. MAOIs are not used to treat BPD due to the risk of suicide.
4. Phenelzine and fluoxetine should not be taken together due to excessive serotonin release.

**2206.** The client who has no psychiatric history is in the ED after physically assaulting his wife. The client is frightened by his loss of control, which he states was precipitated by his wife's complaining and lack of support. The client states, "I'm self-employed, expanded my company nationally, and have many well-known friends." The client's wife states, "The business is losing money, yet he continues his lavish lifestyle; what's important to him is who he knows and how it looks!" The nurse determines that the client's behavior is typical of which disorder?

1. Paraphilia
2. Psychogenic amnesia
3. Borderline personality disorder
4. Narcissistic personality disorder

**2207.** During an initial home visit, the nurse discovers cluttered possessions taking up 75% of the client's living space and obstructing access into the home and all rooms except the bathroom. How should the nurse interpret the client's behavior?

1. Inability to focus related to possible passive-aggressive personality disorder
2. An attention-seeking behavior related to possible histrionic personality disorder
3. Hoarding behavior related to possible obsessive-compulsive personality disorder
4. Inattentiveness to surroundings related to possible BPD

**2208.** MoC The nurse is developing the plan of care for the client with schizoid personality disorder. Which **primary** outcome should the nurse include?

1. Recognizes limits
2. Able to cope and control emotions
3. Validates ideas before taking action
4. Able to function independently in the community

**2209.** The nurse is planning care for the client with avoidant personality disorder. Which interventions should the nurse plan? **Select all that apply.**

1. Use reframing technique.
2. Explore positive self-aspects.
3. Practice social skills with client.
4. Use decatastrophizing technique.
5. Identify negative responses from others.

**2210.** The nurse is working with the individual with obsessive-compulsive personality disorder. Which approach should the nurse use?

1. Inflexible and autocratic
2. Calm and nonconfrontational
3. Direct, hurried, and organized
4. Uninterrupted and confrontational

**2211.** MoC The client with OCD is refusing treatment for hand and face wounds caused by excessive washing and treatment for the OCD diagnosis. Which nursing actions are appropriate? **Select all that apply.**

1. Do not treat the client; the client is competent.
2. Treat the client's injuries; the client is incompetent.
3. Notify the client's family; the client is incompetent.
4. Notify the HCP of the refusal; the client is competent.
5. Notify the HCP of the refusal; the client is incompetent.

**2212.** The nurse observes that the client diagnosed with obsessive-compulsive personality disorder is exhibiting reaction formation. The nurse should plan to assess for which other defense mechanisms commonly associated with this disorder? **Select all that apply.**

1. Isolation
2. Undoing
3. Projection
4. Introjection
5. Rationalization
6. Intellectualization

**2213.** The nurse is planning a counseling session with the client who has antisocial personality disorder. The nurse should anticipate that the client would use which primary ego defense mechanism?

1. Projection
2. Sublimation
3. Compensation
4. Rationalization

**2214.** PHARM The HCP writes in the client's progress notes, "Will switch medications from the older medications to a newer GABAergic anticonvulsant to treat client's instability of mood, transient mood crashes, and inappropriate and intense outbursts of anger." Which medication should the nurse consider when reviewing the HCP's new prescriptions?

1. Lithium
2. Gabapentin
3. Valproic acid
4. Carbamazepine

**2215.** MoC PHARM The nurse is checking the MAR illustrated for the client newly admitted to a behavioral health unit. Place an X on the medication that the nurse should question with the HCP.

| Client: 75-year-old | | Allergies: None | |
|---|---|---|---|
| **Medication** | **0001–0759** | **0800–1559** | **1600–2400** |
| Risperidone oral 1 mg bid on day 1; 2 mg bid on day 2; 3 mg bid on day 3 | | 0900___  2 mg | |
| Fluoxetine 10 mg oral daily | | 0900___ | |
| Carbamazepine 200 mg oral bid | | 0900___ | 2100___ |
| Docusate sodium 100 mg oral daily | | 0900 | |

**2216.** **PHARM** The client with a BPD is prescribed phenelzine for decreasing impulsivity and self-destructive acts. The nurse teaches the client to avoid foods high in tyramine when taking phenelzine to prevent what effect?

1. A hypotensive crisis
2. A hypertensive crisis
3. Poor absorption of tyramine
4. Cardiac rhythm abnormalities

**2217.** The nurse teaches the communication triad to the client to manage his or her feelings. Which components should the nurse include? **Select all that apply.**

1. Use an "I" statement to identify the present feeling.
2. Use a "you" statement to identify the cause of the feeling.
3. Make a nonjudgmental statement about an emotional trigger.
4. Identify with the client what would restore comfort to the situation.
5. Use a "they" statement to examine the effect of the client's feelings on others.

**2218.** **MoC** The client has antisocial personality disorder. What is the nurse's **best** rationale for including milieu therapy in the client's treatment plan?

1. Sets limits on the client's unacceptable behavior
2. Provides a very structured setting that helps the client learn how to behave
3. Simulates a social community where the client can learn to interact with peers
4. Provides one-on-one interaction and reality orientation with client and nursing personnel

## SOMATIC SYMPTOM AND DISSOCIATIVE DISORDERS

**2219.** The nurse is assessing the client diagnosed with pseudocyesis. Which statement from the client is consistent with pseudocyesis?

1. "These bruises are from falling when I black out and faint."
2. "Everyone tells me that I just 'glow' now that I am pregnant."
3. "I can't even smell the lilacs even though their scent is strong."
4. "The doctor says I'm not having a seizure with these staring spells."

**2220.** The nurse is caring for the client diagnosed with psychogenic fugue. Which information in the client's medical record should indicate to the nurse that the diagnosis is correct? **Select all that apply.**

1. The client demonstrates having more than one distinct personality.
2. The client recently forgot all personal information following an accident.
3. The client left home and assumed a new identity following the loss of a child.
4. The client claims to have superhero qualities following a recent suicide attempt.
5. The client resides in a homeless shelter after being physically abused by his or her spouse.

**2221.** The nurse is treating the client diagnosed with dissociative identity disorder (DID). Which actions should the nurse take when working with this client? **Select all that apply.**

1. Focus on long-term goals.
2. Actively listen to each identity state.
3. Maintain a calm, reassuring environment.
4. Document changes in the client's behavior
5. Observe for signs of suicidal thoughts or behavior.

**2222.** The client diagnosed with dissociative amnesia is increasingly frustrated and begins to threaten to commit suicide. Which technique should the nurse use to establish a rapid working relationship with the client?

1. Instruct the client to remain calm.
2. Bargain with the main personality.
3. Attend to the client's medical needs.
4. Actively listen to the personality speaking.

**2223.** The client with a dissociative identity disorder (DID) has amnesia. Which intervention should the nurse **initially** implement?

1. Inform the client about all information gathered about the client's past life.
2. Have the client keep a diary of duration and intensity of physical symptoms.
3. Focus on developing a trusting relationship with only the original personality.
4. Expose the client to smells associated with the client's past enjoyable activities.

# DISRUPTIVE, IMPULSE-CONTROL, AND CONDUCT DISORDERS

**2224.** The nurse is assessing the client who reports that setting and watching fires helps relieve anxiety. The client states, "After I watch something burn, I feel so much better." Which mental health disorder should the nurse associate with the client's behavior?

1. Pyromania
2. Kleptomania
3. Conduct disorder
4. Antisocial personality disorder

**2225.** The adolescent with a conduct disorder is yelling and having temper tantrums in the psychiatric unit's common area. Which nursing intervention is **most** appropriate for reducing the client's outbursts?

1. Mimic the client's behavior.
2. Instruct the client to stop yelling.
3. Ignore initial yelling and tantrums.
4. Guide the client for a walk away from the area.

**2226.** MoC The nurse determines that the client with major depressive disorder is suffering from suicidal ideation and is at risk for committing suicide. The client states, "Death is better than living with depression." Which nursing intervention is **priority**?

1. Talk with the client about reasons to live and instill positive affirmations.
2. Educate the client on medical and psychological treatments for depression.
3. Alert the appropriate authorities and monitor the client's behavior frequently.
4. Assess the surroundings for harmful substances or methods to commit suicide.

**2227.** The psychiatric nurse observes the client becoming increasingly agitated and threatening, and is concerned that a crisis situation could occur. What should be the nurse's **primary** goal at this time?

1. Eliminate and/or resolve present conflicts.
2. Help to reconstruct the client's thought process.
3. Secure an HCP's order for restraints.
4. Have the client talk about the feelings that led to the situation.

**2228.** MoC The nurse manager is discussing management of the aggressive client. Which statement **best** stresses important information about the use of physical restraints?

1. "The hospital administration is reluctant to have staff rely on physical restraints for legal reasons."
2. "The use of physical restraints has a highly negative emotional impact on the client and should be avoided if possible."
3. "Physical restraints can be used only after other de-escalating strategies have failed to control the behavior."
4. "We use physical restraints when the client is disinterested or unwilling to control his or her aggressive behavior."

**2229.** The nurse is caring for four clients in the ED. Which client has the greatest potential for demonstrating violent behavior toward the staff?

1. The young adult in severe pain after a motorcycle accident
2. The inebriated client who has frostbite after falling asleep in the park
3. The teenager being treated for injuries received in a gang-related fight
4. The client who has schizophrenia and requires stitches to a forearm cut

**2230.** MoC During the orientation to the mental health unit, the nurse states, "I'm not sure how I'll react when faced with a violent client." Which response by the nurse manager would enhance the nurse's self-awareness?

1. "How would you go about de-escalating a violent individual?"
2. "Have you had a negative experience with a violent individual?"
3. "Describe what you would do when the client becomes aggressive."
4. "Think about how you usually respond to angry or aggressive people."

**2231.** The nurse is assessing the client with a history of aggressive behavior toward others. Which client behavior requires immediate nursing intervention?

1. Refusing to attend a mandatory group session on the unit.
2. Stating, "The guy over there needs to sit down and shut up."
3. Petitioning the staff to extend recreation time by 30 minutes.
4. Crying while talking on the telephone with a family member.

**2232.** The nurse is caring for multiple clients with unpredictable and often dangerous behaviors in a mental health unit. Which is the nurse's **best** method for managing the safety of multiple clients?

1. Monitor client medication effectiveness.
2. Develop a trusting relationship with clients.
3. Document client behavior that is disturbing.
4. Keep clients separated as much as possible.

**2233.** MoC The nurse observes the client, who has a history of aggressive behavior toward others, swearing and kicking the furniture. Based on the client's behavior, what should be the nurse's **priority**?

1. De-escalate the client's agitation.
2. Eliminate the source of agitation.
3. Assess the client's agitation level.
4. Provide for a safe, therapeutic milieu.

## SEXUAL DISORDERS

**2234.** The client diagnosed with paraphilia has been advised to participate in psychoanalytical therapy and asks the nurse about the therapy. Which statement by the nurse is correct?

1. "Psychoanalytical therapy focuses on achieving satiation."
2. "Psychoanalytical therapy focuses on aversion techniques."
3. "Psychoanalytical therapy focuses on resolving early conflicts."
4. "Psychoanalytical therapy focuses on reducing the level of circulating androgens."

**2235.** The nurse is assessing the client who claims to have sexual fantasies that recur daily. The nurse should consider paraphilia when the client describes which sexual fantasy?

1. Repetitive sexual activity in public places
2. Repetitive sexual activity with numerous partners
3. Repetitive sexual activity with members of the same sex
4. Repetitive sexual activity involving suffering or humiliation

**2236.** The nurse is assessing the client who reports symptoms descriptive of hypoactive sexual desire disorder. Which information identified in the client's history may predispose the client to hypoactive sexual desire disorder?

1. Past sexual abuse
2. Chronic alcohol use
3. Sexual identity conflicts
4. Decreased serum prolactin level

## SCHIZOPHRENIA SPECTRUM AND OTHER PSYCHOTIC DISORDERS

**2237.** The client diagnosed with schizophrenia is refusing to take a prescribed psychotropic medication. The nurse attempts to persuade the client to comply with the HCP's orders. Under which circumstance could the client be forced to take medication?

1. If the client claims to be God and here to save the world
2. If the client threatens to leave the hospital immediately
3. If the client talks about a suicide attempt that occurred last week
4. If the client claims to be a vampire and threatens to kill the nurse

**2238.** The nurse is discussing discharge plans with the client who is homeless and diagnosed with paranoid schizophrenia. What is the **primary** factor that will affect developing the discharge plan for this client?

1. The identification of a support system for the client
2. The nurse's ability to work effectively with the client
3. The client's ability to comply with the discharge plan
4. The existence of resources such as homeless shelters

**2239.** MoC The mental health NA is assigned to work with the client who has delusions. Which action by the NA requires the nurse's **most** immediate attention?

1. Reassuring the client by saying, "I'll eat the food if you do."
2. Attempting to convince the client that the food here isn't poisoned
3. Asking the nurse what to do because the client says, "I'm being poisoned."
4. Asking another NA to change assignments to avoid working with this client

**2240.** MoC The client diagnosed with schizoaffective disorder was recently treated for a major depressive episode. Following a 72-hour involuntary commitment, the client is stable, no longer displaying suicidal ideation, and asking to leave the hospital. Which client right should the nurse consider while deciding if the client can be discharged?

1. Right to refuse treatment
2. Right to freedom from restraint
3. Right to least-restrictive treatment
4. Right to an appropriate service plan

**2241.** MoC PHARM The client due for a dose of antipsychotic medication begins to exhibit severe parkinsonian muscle rigidity, a temperature of 105°F (40.6°C), P 130 bpm, and diaphoresis. Prioritize the steps that the nurse should take to respond to this situation.

1. Notify the HCP of the assessment findings and obtain the order for a medication to counteract the effects of neuroleptic malignant syndrome (NMS).
2. Withhold all doses of antipsychotic medication.
3. Assess level of consciousness.
4. Give bromocriptine as prescribed by the HCP STAT.
5. Assess degree of muscle rigidity.
6. Retake vital signs.

Answer: _____

**2242.** The nurse is educating the client with schizophrenia. Which interventions should the nurse encourage the client to use to help prevent the relapse of schizophrenic symptoms? **Select all that apply.**

1. Ignore auditory hallucinations.
2. Engage in regular physical exercise.
3. Report changes in sleeping patterns.
4. Enroll in stress-management classes.
5. Avoid employment that is demanding.

**2243.** The nurse is reviewing the discharge plan with the father of the adolescent recently diagnosed with paranoid schizophrenia. Which statement made by the father indicates understanding of the client's diagnosis?

1. "My wife and I will need to watch for signs of depression."
2. "He won't get worse if he continues to take his medication."
3. "He has a good chance that this'll be his only hospitalization."
4. "We'll keep him at home so we can monitor his illness closely."

**2244.** The client is admitted to the psychiatric unit with a diagnosis of paranoid schizophrenia. Two days after admission, the client's mother tells the nurse, "He's still talking about how the government is controlling his thoughts." What is the nurse's **most** accurate evaluation of the mother's statement?

1. The mother's expectations about her son are realistic.
2. The mother should request a medication adjustment.
3. The mother thinks her son has an issue with the government.
4. The mother requires further education regarding the client's diagnosis.

**2245.** PHARM The nurse is caring for the client prescribed the traditional antipsychotic drug haloperidol for the treatment of schizophrenia. Which medication should the nurse plan to administer if extrapyramidal side effects develop?

1. Olanzapine
2. Benztropine
3. Chlorpromazine
4. Escitalopram oxalate

**2246.** The client admitted to a behavioral medicine unit with a diagnosis of catatonic schizophrenia is constantly rearranging furniture and appears to be responding to internal stimuli. In addition to being free of physical injury during phases of hyperactivity, which short-term goal is appropriate for this client?

1. The client will sleep at least 6 hours per night.
2. The client will consume adequate food and fluid per day.
3. The client will engage in at least one client-to-client interaction daily.
4. The client will show decreased activity within 24 hours of onset of hyperactivity.

**2247.** The nurse includes the problem of *Disturbed thought processes secondary to paranoia* in the care plan for the newly admitted client with schizophrenia. Which nursing intervention is **most** appropriate for this client?

1. Avoid laughing or whispering in front of the client.
2. Have the client sign a written release of information form.
3. Encourage the client to interact with the others on the unit.
4. Help the client to identify social supports in the community.

**2248.** The nurse is evaluating the client with paranoid schizophrenia who reports hearing a voice say, "Do not remove your hat because they will be able to read your mind." Which response by the nurse is therapeutic?

1. "Who are the 'they' that can read your mind?"
2. "Why would someone want to read your mind?"
3. "I do not believe that anyone can read another person's mind."
4. "It must be frightening to believe that someone can read your mind."

**2249.** **PHARM** The client, who has a history of paranoid schizophrenia and chronic alcohol abuse, has been taking olanzapine for 2 weeks and has not consumed alcohol in the last 5 days. The client reports, "I am having trouble sleeping. My hands shake, and I have nightmares. Could olanzapine be causing this?" Which is the nurse's **most** therapeutic response?

1. "Don't worry; these are not typical side effects for olanzapine."
2. "Just ignore the symptoms. These will go away in just a few days."
3. "These symptoms are more likely from not drinking alcohol for 5 days."
4. "It's possible that olanzapine is the cause; it should not be taken with alcohol."

**2250.** The nurse is evaluating the client experiencing paranoid delusions. The client states, "Two men wearing gray shirts keep coming into the dayroom and watching me." Which response by the nurse is **most** therapeutic?

1. "What makes you think they are interested in you?"
2. "Are you sure they are looking at you and not someone else?"
3. "Ignore them, and let's select a movie to watch after dinner."
4. "Those are maintenance personnel discussing the room remodeling."

**2251.** The client experiencing paranoid delusions states "Turn off the TV. It's controlling my thoughts." Which nursing intervention is **most** appropriate?

1. Refuse the request in order to show control over the client.
2. Comply with the request in order to lessen the client's concerns.
3. Comply with the request to show an understanding of the client's concerns.
4. Show empathy but refuse the request to avoid supporting the client's delusions.

**2252.** The nurse observes that the client with a history of violent command hallucinations mumbles erratically while making threatening gestures directed toward a staff member. Which nursing intervention is **most** appropriate?

1. Ask the client to explain the cause of the anger.
2. Observe the client for signs of escalating agitation.
3. Place the client in seclusion to help de-escalate anger.
4. Inform the client of the use of restraints if the behavior does not subside.

**2253.** The client with paranoid schizophrenia is being discharged. The family member asks, "What should I do if the voices come back again?" Which nurse response is **most** appropriate?

1. "Be sure that all follow-up appointments are kept."
2. "I will give you a list of emergency crisis centers."
3. "Stay with the client and use the distracting techniques we discussed."
4. "Here is the behavioral unit's telephone number; call if there is a problem."

**2254.** **MoC** The nurse is evaluating the client who threatens suicide. Which nursing intervention is **most** effective in establishing a safe environment for the client?

1. Place the client in a seclusion room designed to minimize stimulation.
2. Remove all potential items that could assist the client in committing suicide.
3. Assign a staff member to stay with the client and provide constant observation.
4. Keep the client involved in structured activities with others who are being observed.

**2255.** The client is experiencing paranoid delusions. While the nurse is attempting to explain the need for obtaining blood for lab tests, the client shouts, "You all just want to drain my blood. Get away from me!" Which response by the nurse is **most** therapeutic?

1. "I'll leave and come back later when you are calmer."
2. "What makes you think that I want to drain your blood?"
3. "You know I am not going to hurt you; I am here to help you!"
4. "It must be extremely frightening to think others want to hurt you."

**2256.** The client experiencing paranoid delusions tells the nurse that "the foreigner who lives next to me wants to kill me." Which nursing response is **most** therapeutic to assist the client experiencing paranoid delusions?

1. "Do you feel afraid that people are trying to hurt you?"
2. "That's not true. I'm sure your neighbor is a nice person."
3. "What makes you think your neighbor wants to kill you?"
4. "You believe that your foreign neighbor wants to kill you?"

**2257.** MoC PHARM The client recently prescribed haloperidol is experiencing severe muscle pain. Assessment findings include an HR of 104 bpm, BP of 172/92 mm Hg, and an oral temperature of 101.2°F (38.4°C). What should the nurse do **next**?

1. Question the client concerning known cardiovascular health status.
2. Assure the client that the symptoms are unrelated to the new medication.
3. Immediately notify the HCP of the assessment findings and medication given.
4. Gather information about the possibility that the client has developed an infection.

**2258.** The nurse is observing the client in a catatonic state. The client is lying on the bed in a fetal position. Which nursing interventions are appropriate? **Select all that apply.**

1. Sit quietly beside the client's bed.
2. Move the client into the dayroom.
3. Ask occasional open-ended questions.
4. Encourage client-to-client interaction.
5. Leave alone, but assess every 15 minutes.
6. Assign staff to attempt social communication.

**2259.** The client has a history of hallucinations and is at risk to harm self or others. In preparing the client for discharge, the nurse provides instructions regarding interventions directed toward managing hallucinations and anxiety. Which statement indicates that the client has an appropriate understanding of the instructions?

1. "Anxiety is not a typical side effect of any of my medications."
2. "I should call my therapist when I'm experiencing hallucinations."
3. "I'll learn a lot about my condition by meeting with my support group."
4. "If I eat well and get enough sleep, I will be less likely to hear the voices."

**2260.** The nurse completes teaching with the client diagnosed with schizophreniform disorder. Which statement made by the client demonstrates an understanding of the disorder?

1. "My prognosis is good if I don't get worse over the next 6 months."
2. "This disorder will eventually affect even my ability to hold down a job."
3. "Schizophreniform disorder shares many similarities with schizophrenia."
4. "I understand that I will have full-blown schizophrenia within 3 months."

**2261.** The nurse is administering medications to various clients on the mental health unit. The nurse should most definitely complete a variance report if which medication is found in the secured drawer on the unit for the client's prescribed medications?

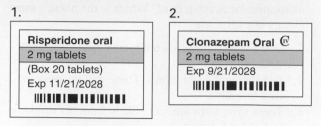

1.

| Risperidone oral |
|---|
| 2 mg tablets |
| (Box 20 tablets) |
| Exp 11/21/2028 |

2.

| Clonazepam Oral Ⓒ |
|---|
| 2 mg tablets |
| Exp 9/21/2028 |

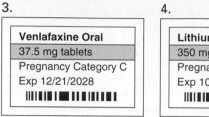

3.

| Venlafaxine Oral |
|---|
| 37.5 mg tablets |
| Pregnancy Category C |
| Exp 12/21/2028 |

4.

| Lithium Carbonate |
|---|
| 350 mg Capsules |
| Pregnancy Category D |
| Exp 10/21/2028 |

**2262.** The client is diagnosed with paranoid hallucinations. The nurse concludes that the client is having a stage IV reaction to hallucinations when observing which behavior?

1. Eyes are darting around the room
2. Reports "my heart is really pounding"
3. Pounding fists against the dayroom table
4. Ignores request to "come with me to your room"

**2263.** MoC The nurse in an inpatient mental health unit is aware of the importance of managing sexual behavior among clients. Which statement is accurate regarding the standard protocol of managing sexual behavior on adult psychiatric inpatient units?

1. Sexual behavior is strictly prohibited in inpatient units.
2. Sexual behavior can be therapeutic and speed recovery.
3. Sexual behavior is governed by least-restrictive legal policies.
4. Sexual behavior is helpful for clients diagnosed with personality disorders.

# NEUROCOGNITIVE DISORDERS

**2264.** The nurse is performing health assessments on several clients. Which individuals should the nurse identify as at risk for developing dementia? **Select all that apply.**

1. The toddler who was physically abused and had two concussions
2. The teenager who has a history of "huffing" paint thinner
3. The middle-aged adult being treated for hyperthyroidism
4. The young adult with type 1 DM for 5 years
5. The older adult receiving treatment for PD

**2265.** The nurse engages the older adult client by describing the weather as "raining cats and dogs." The client looks bewildered and shows concern for the "animals." Which response by the nurse is **most** therapeutic?

1. Assure the client that the animals are not being hurt in any way.
2. Explain to the client that it is a way of saying it is raining heavily.
3. Alert the staff to the client's inability to understand abstract concepts.
4. Document the client's response to the conversation as concrete thinking.

**2266.** The nurse is assessing the older adult postoperative client who is displaying signs of delirium. The nurse observes that the client is convinced that it is 1954 and is complaining about "the bugs in this hotel." Which should be the nurse's **priority** intervention?

1. Request that the HCP prescribe prn haloperidol.
2. Move the client to a room by the nurse's station.
3. Call the spouse to come and stay with the client.
4. Arrange for the NA to stay with the client.

**2267.** During a home visit to the client with Alzheimer's disease, the nurse assesses the stress level of the client's spouse, the primary caregiver. Which question is **most** appropriate for assessing the spouse's stress level?

1. "So, what is a typical day like for you?"
2. "What do you do to relieve stress for yourself?"
3. "May I arrange for some part-time help for you?"
4. "Being a full-time caregiver must be very stressful, isn't it?"

**2268.** The hospitalized client is diagnosed with delirium. Which statements by the nurse to the family demonstrate an understanding of the condition? **Select all that apply.**

1. "With proper treatment the prognosis for delirium is good."
2. "The emotional swings you see are common with delirium."
3. "Symptoms of delirium are usually short-term and reversible."
4. "Do you have a history of Alzheimer's disease in your family?"
5. "The short-term memory loss will continue for a few months."

**2269.** The nurse is assessing the client with dementia and moderate cognitive decline. Which statements would the client have difficulty understanding? **Select all that apply.**

1. "Only cross the street when it is safe."
2. "Red sky tonight means sailor's delight."
3. "Tell me a story about when you were growing up."
4. "Put on your good clothes; your grandson is visiting today."
5. "You were a baker for 40 years; I bet you could tell me how to bake cookies."

**2270.** MoC The NA is assigned to provide care for the severely disoriented older adult client who has been restrained for client safety after least-restrictive methods have been tried. Which statement made by the NA indicates the **most** immediate need for education regarding safe client care?

1. "I'll remove the restraints when the client falls asleep."
2. "I am careful to check in on the client every 15 minutes."
3. "If the client doesn't want to take a drink, there is nothing I can do about it."
4. "He pulled on the restraints, and his wrists are bruised, but he's not really hurt."

**2271.** The nurse is assessing the client recently admitted into a psychiatric unit for observation. Which client behavior is indicative of impaired cognition?

1. Mumbling and rambling speech
2. Asking repeatedly, "How did I get here?"
3. Spending hours staring out of the window
4. Discussing "the voices" with another client

**2272.** MoC The nurse is developing the plan of care for the client who has behaviors associated with dementia and a self-care deficit. Which goals should be included? **Select all that apply.**

1. The client will be provided with unlimited time to care for personal needs independently.
2. The client will function at the highest possible level of self-independence.
3. The client will consistently complete all daily hygiene needs independently.
4. The client will have all daily hygiene needs met by the ancillary or nursing staff.
5. The client's family will receive instructions on supporting the client's independence.

**2273.** PHARM The nurse has been discussing the medication therapy prescribed for the client newly diagnosed with Alzheimer's disease. Which statement by the client's wife **best** demonstrates an understanding of the treatment goals of anticholinesterase medications?

1. "I'm so thankful we were able to get him on these pills now instead of later."
2. "With these medications, his memory loss will likely be no worse than it is now."
3. "We have the greatest faith that these medications will improve his quality of life."
4. "These medications will at least give us a chance of slowing down his memory loss."

**2274.** The cognitively impaired nursing home resident is beginning to show physical signs of agitation. Which activity would be **most** therapeutic to de-escalate the client's agitation?

1. Playing bingo with other residents
2. Spending time alone in the client's room
3. Taking a walk outside with ancillary staff
4. Watching television in the presence of staff

**2275.** The client is displaying behaviors consistent with middle stage Alzheimer's disease. The client can no longer recognize family members and requires assistance with personal hygiene and dressing. The client is frequently incontinent of both urine and feces and displays violent outbursts during these times. Which nursing problem should be the nurse's **priority**?

1. Violence: directed at self or others
2. Incontinence: both bowel and bladder
3. Self-care deficient: hygiene, dressing, toileting
4. Altered thought processes with impaired memory

**2276.** MoC During a home visit to the client with Alzheimer's disease, the nurse attempts to determine whether the client's daughter understands her father's prognosis. Which question by the daughter **best** indicates an understanding of the prognosis of Alzheimer's disease?

1. "What types of support services are available?"
2. "What can we do to improve our father's memory?"
3. "How long does it take for his medication to help?"
4. "Which local hospital has the best treatment program?"

# EATING DISORDERS

**2277.** The father of the teenager diagnosed with an eating disorder states to the nurse, "My wife was always too protective; that's the reason our child has this problem now." The nurse should realize that the father's statement is indicative of what?

1. A possible indication of the couple's marital discord
2. A correct interpretation of the result of the protective tendencies
3. A misconception regarding the cause of the child's eating disorder
4. An attempt to deflect personal responsibility for his child's eating disorder

**2278.** The mother of the teenager diagnosed with anorexia nervosa confides in the nurse that she has always been very protective and is concerned her overprotectiveness is the reason her child developed the eating disorder. Which statement is the **most** therapeutic response by the nurse?

1. "Does your child feel that being overprotected as a child contributed to the problem?"
2. "What makes you feel that your overprotective tendencies caused the eating disorder?"
3. "Don't worry. The cause of the eating disorder is more likely the stress of adolescence."
4. "There is no research to confirm that overprotective parenting results in an eating disorder."

**2279.** The young adult is diagnosed with anorexia nervosa. The nurse should plan to include which physiological health topics in the client's education plan? **Select all that apply.**

1. Special skin and hair hygiene measures
2. The need for effective oral and dental hygiene
3. The dangers associated with weight loss products
4. Safety measures to avoid falls related to dizziness
5. Recognizing early symptoms of electrolyte imbalance

**2280.** The nurse is completing the health history and an assessment for the client diagnosed with anorexia nervosa. Which findings should the nurse expect? **Select all that apply.**

1. Refusal to eat foods
2. Age of onset 25 years old
3. Heavy bleeding during menses
4. Intense fear of getting fat despite being underweight
5. Weighs less than 85% of expected weight for body size and age

**2281.** The nurse is reviewing the care plan for the client newly diagnosed with anorexia nervosa who is receiving inpatient treatment. Which outcome should the nurse establish as the **priority?**

1. Achieves minimum normal weight
2. Resumes a normal menstrual cycle
3. Perceives body weight and shape as normal and acceptable
4. Consumes adequate calories for age, height, and metabolic needs

**2282.** **MoC** The nurse is developing a care plan for the client newly diagnosed with bulimia nervosa who is receiving inpatient treatment. Place the outcomes in the order of priority from the most urgent to the least urgent.

1. Demonstrates more effective coping skills to deal with conflicts
2. Ceases binge/purge episodes while in inpatient setting
3. Maintains normal fluid and electrolyte levels
4. Perceives body shape and weight as normal and acceptable
5. Consumes adequate calories for age, height, and metabolic need

Answer: _____

**2283.** **PHARM** The nurse assesses that the client with an eating disorder is taking 20 laxative products daily, diuretics twice daily, and is self-inducing vomiting. What should the nurse do **next**?

1. Notify the HCP.
2. Auscultate the client's apical pulse.
3. Ask the client to state the products taken.
4. Ask about the consistency and frequency of stools.

**2284.** The 13-year-old is being discharged from a behavioral health unit with a diagnosis of bulimia nervosa. Which statement should the nurse include when completing the discharge teaching with the parent and child?

1. "Because the cycle of eating disorder behaviors is life-threatening and must be interrupted, continue to monitor your child for at least 1 hour after eating."
2. "The behavior-modification program easily changed your child's eating disorder behavior, but you need to continue to offer nourishing foods."
3. "Discourage your child from discussing insights from group and individual therapy because of the potential adverse effects on the entire family."
4. "Continue to prepare separate meals to encourage your child to eat nourishing foods, and offer foods that your child desires and will eat."

**2285.** The nurse is evaluating the attainment of outcomes for the adolescent client diagnosed with bulimia nervosa. Which behavior indicates that the client is meeting an expected outcome for the disorder?

1. Gains 1 pound after being in treatment for 3 weeks
2. Engages staff in conversations that center on eating food
3. Decreases self-purging frequency from daily to twice weekly
4. Draws to express feelings about body image and to deal with conflicts

## SLEEP DISORDERS

**2286.** The nurse is completing a health history for the client with narcolepsy. Which finding should the nurse anticipate when completing the assessment?

1. Sudden loss of muscle tone
2. Inability to speak 1 hour before a sleep attack
3. Falling asleep at inappropriate times during the day
4. Sudden loss of muscle tone after taking a narcotic analgesic

**2287.** **MoC** The client diagnosed with major depressive disorder has insomnia. Which statements are **most** appropriate for the nurse to include in the client's plan of care? **Select all that apply.**

1. Reinforce reality thinking.
2. Record and limit caffeinated foods and drinks.
3. Discourage sleeping during the day.
4. Teach progressive muscle relaxation.
5. Identify sleep patterns prior to hospitalization.

**2288.** **MoC** The nurse reads in the 12-year-old client's medical record, "Fractured left leg from a fall during an episode of somnambulism." Which nursing intervention is **most** important to add to the client's plan of care?

1. Restrict visitors to immediate family only.
2. Ensure that the bed exit alarm is turned on.
3. Teach to turn on the call light for help when getting out of bed.
4. Avoid shadows and whispering, and monitor for hallucinations.

**2289.** The client states to the nurse, "I can't sleep. I'm getting only a few hours of sleep at night. I started a new job, and I can't do my best without getting enough sleep." The client's history includes a recent breakup with a long-term companion. Which should be the nurse's **initial** statement?

1. "Describe what you feel are major stressors in your life."
2. "New jobs can be stressful, and stress can certainly affect sleep."
3. "Tell me more about your past and current number of hours sleeping."
4. "Do you think your breakup has something to do with your problem?"

**2290.** The nurse is overheard responding to the client who reports sleeping only 3 hours at night. Which statement by the nurse is inappropriate?

1. "You sound worried that you may lose your job."
2. "How much sleep did you usually get each night?"
3. "Sleep disorders are common among people who are depressed."
4. "Do you think stress may be interfering with your ability to sleep?"

**2291.** The nurse is assessing the client. Which statement made by the client **best** indicates the possibility of a sleep disorder?

1. "I realize now that I've never needed more than 5 hours of sleep at night."
2. "I'm waking up about every 3 hours because I need to go to the bathroom."
3. "I used to sleep 8 hours at night; now I get about 6 and feel tired when I get up."
4. "Before I received treatment for hyperthyroidism, I was awake most of the night."

## *Answers and Rationales*

## ANXIETY AND MOOD DISORDERS
### 2153. ANSWER: 2

1. Denial is the refusal to accept a painful reality by pretending it did not happen.
2. **Sublimation involves redirecting unacceptable feelings or drives into an acceptable channel.**
3. Identification involves taking on attributes and characteristics of someone admired.
4. Intellectualization involves excessive focus on reasoning to avoid feelings associated with a situation.

♦ *Test-taking Tip: Narrow the options by eliminating those that include avoidance.*

Content Area: Mental Health; Concept: Grief and Loss; Stress; Integrated Processes: Nursing Process: Analysis; Client Needs: Psychosocial Integrity; Cognitive Level: Comprehension [Understanding]

### 2154. ANSWER: 4

1. Anticipatory grief is grief before a loss occurs.
2. In uncomplicated grief, the client's self-esteem remains intact with symptom resolution.
3. Delayed grief reaction is the absence of the expression of grief during situations when a grief reaction is expected.
4. **The nurse's focus for counseling should be directed toward the client's distorted grief reaction. The symptoms reported by the client are exaggerated and prolonged.**

♦ *Test-taking Tip: Narrow the options by focusing on the "5 years" stated in the stem; then think about whether this is a usual response after 5 years.*

Content Area: Mental Health; Concept: Grief and Loss; Stress; Integrated Processes: Nursing Process: Analysis; Client Needs: Psychosocial Integrity; Safe and Effective Care Environment: Safety and Infection Control; Cognitive Level: Analysis [Analyzing]

### 2155. ANSWER: 3

1. How suicide was initially attempted would have been addressed during the initial assessment and does not determine future coping.
2. Asking the client a "why" question is not helpful and conveys a judgmental attitude.
3. **Asking the client directly what skills he or she could utilize if similar problems occurred in the future, provides the client with an opportunity to reflect on learned behaviors and to determine a plan for future prevention.**
4. Although asking the client if the suicide prevention center number is known would be helpful, the question does not determine learned coping strategies.

♦ *Test-taking Tip: Focus on using therapeutic communication techniques, and eliminate any options that include communication barriers. The key word is "future." Look for related words in the options.*

**Content Area:** Mental Health; **Concept:** Mood; Stress; Assessment; Communication; **Integrated Processes:** Nursing Process: Assessment; **Client Needs:** Psychosocial Integrity; **Cognitive Level:** Application [Applying]

## 2156. ANSWER: 2

1. The presence of powerlessness is concerning but does not take priority over the suicide.
2. **The potential for suicidal behavior is priority for the client with a major depressive disorder who previously attempted suicide.**
3. Anticipatory grieving is concerning because it may be the cause of the major depressive disorder, but it is not the priority.
4. The presence of a disturbed sleep pattern is concerning and should be addressed, but it is not the priority.

▶ **Test-taking Tip:** *Use Maslow's Hierarchy of Needs theory to identify the priority. Safety is priority, because attempting suicide could result in life-threatening injury.*

**Content Area:** Mental Health; **Concept:** Safety; Mood; Self; **Integrated Processes:** Nursing Process: Analysis; **Client Needs:** Safe and Effective Care Environment: Safety and Infection Control; Psychosocial Integrity; **Cognitive Level:** Application [Applying]

## 2157. MoC ANSWER: 2

1. There is no indication that the client sustained injuries that require hospitalization on an acute care unit.
2. **The client with a history of suicidal behavior and current suicidal ideation is at risk for self-harm and in need of hospitalization. The most appropriate setting is an inpatient mental health unit that is equipped to handle the safety issues of risky behaviors.**
3. An outpatient mental health clinic does not provide the level of safety required for the client reporting suicidal ideation.
4. There is no indication that the client's attempted suicide was due to drug or alcohol intoxication.

▶ **Test-taking Tip:** *The key words are "suicidal ideation." Focus on the safest environment for the client and eliminate other less safe options.*

**Content Area:** Mental Health; **Concept:** Safety; Stress; Mood; **Integrated Processes:** Nursing Process: Planning; **Client Needs:** Safe and Effective Care Environment: Management of Care; **Cognitive Level:** Application [Applying]

## 2158. MoC ANSWER: 2, 3, 4, 5

1. Feeling sad can be a normal mood variation and is not considered a warning sign of suicide.
2. **Hopelessness is a warning sign for suicide. Statements about problems never resolving or about feelings of giving up indicate hopelessness.**
3. **Feeling trapped as if there is no way out is a warning sign of suicide.**
4. **Severe anxiety or agitation and recklessness can be an indication of suicide risk.**
5. **Increasing drug or alcohol use can be indicative of suicide risk.**

▶ **Test-taking Tip:** *Use the process of elimination to eliminate any option pertaining to normal mood variation.*

**Content Area:** Mental Health; **Concept:** Mood; Safety; **Integrated Processes:** Nursing Process: Planning; **Client Needs:** Safe and Effective Care Environment: Management of Care; Psychosocial Integrity; **Cognitive Level:** Application [Applying]

## 2159. PHARM ANSWER: 2

1. Having the client fast is unnecessary prior to initiating treatment with lithium carbonate.
2. **Because lithium carbonate (Lithobid) is excreted by the kidneys, a baseline evaluation of normal kidney function should be completed before treatment begins.**
3. Room seclusion is used as a last resort and is unrelated to medication administration.
4. Benzodiazepines are often used in treatment during the initiation phase to aid in controlling mania, because it can take up to a week for lithium to become effective.

▶ **Test-taking Tip:** *Think about how lithium carbonate is excreted.*

**Content Area:** Mental Health; **Concept:** Medication; Mood; **Integrated Processes:** Nursing Process: Planning; **Client Needs:** Physiological Integrity: Pharmacological and Parenteral Therapies; Psychosocial Integrity; **Cognitive Level:** Application [Applying]

## 2160. PHARM ANSWER: 3

1. Increasing fluids is important because both drugs are eliminated in the urine, but this is not the most important action.
2. Tramadol hydrochloride (Ultram) intensifies the action of fluoxetine (Prozac); the dose may need to be reduced, not increased.
3. **Tramadol hydrochloride (Ultram), a centrally acting analgesic, and fluoxetine (Prozac), an SSRI, both inhibit the reuptake of serotonin in the CNS. This combination can result in serotonin syndrome, a life-threatening event.**
4. Although it is best to take tramadol hydrochloride (Ultram) with food because it can irritate the stomach, this is not the most important nursing action.

▶ **Test-taking Tip:** *Focus on the issue: the actions of tramadol and fluoxetine individually and then when combined. Recall that both medications inhibit the reuptake of serotonin in the CNS.*

**Content Area:** Mental Health; **Concept:** Medication; Comfort; Mood; **Integrated Processes:** Nursing Process: Evaluation; **Client Needs:** Physiological Integrity: Pharmacological and Parenteral Therapies; **Cognitive Level:** Evaluation [Evaluating]

## 2161. PHARM ANSWER: 2

1. The Dilantin level is within the normal range (10–20 mcg/mL).
2. **Symptoms of lithium toxicity appear at levels greater than 1.5 mEq/L. At a level greater than 3.5 mEq/L, the symptoms of toxicity include coma, nystagmus, seizures, and cardiovascular collapse.**

3. The serum sodium is WNL (135–145 mEq/L). The WBCs are low (normal = 4500–11,000/microL or /mm$^3$). Lithium can cause an increase in WBCs.
4. Serum creatinine and BUN are elevated (normal creatinine is 0.5–1.5 mg/dL; normal BUN values are 5–25 mg/dL), but at these levels they would not result in impaired consciousness, nystagmus, and seizures.

▶ **Test-taking Tip:** Narrow the options by eliminating lab values that are WNL. Of the remaining options, consider the client's diagnosis and the likely medication for treatment.

**Content Area:** Mental Health; **Concept:** Medication; Mood; **Integrated Processes:** Nursing Process: Evaluation; **Client Needs:** Physiological Integrity: Pharmacological and Parenteral Therapies; **Cognitive Level:** Evaluation [Evaluating]

## 2162. PHARM ANSWER: 1

1. **Evidence-based practice guidelines recommend continuing antidepressant medication for a minimum of 6 months after recovery following the first episode of depression in order to decrease the chance of relapse.**
2. Symptom improvement begins approximately 2 weeks after medication is initiated, and it often takes 6 to 8 weeks at a therapeutic dose to achieve significant remission of symptoms.
3. SSRI antidepressants are equally efficacious. The individual's personal and family history and specific cluster of symptoms guide medication selection.
4. Dry mouth, blurred vision, and urinary retention are anticholinergic side effects associated with a TCA, not an SSRI.

▶ **Test-taking Tip:** Relate information to what you know about medications; most medications should be continued until the prescription is gone.

**Content Area:** Mental Health; **Concept:** Medication; Mood; Nursing Roles; Evidence-based Practice; **Integrated Processes:** Teaching/Learning; **Client Needs:** Health Promotion and Maintenance; Physiological Integrity: Pharmacological and Parenteral Therapies; **Cognitive Level:** Evaluation [Evaluating]

## 2163. PHARM ANSWER: 4

1. Akathisia (unpleasant sensations of "inner" restlessness that results in an inability to sit still) is not a symptom associated with MAOIs and food restrictions.
2. Agranulocytosis is not a symptom associated with MAOIs and food restrictions.
3. Hypertension, not hypotension, is a symptom associated with MAOIs and food restrictions.
4. **Explosive occipital headache is a symptom of hypertensive crisis, which is a major concern with the combination of an MAOI and certain foods (e.g., aged cheeses, overripe fruit, and sausage).**

▶ **Test-taking Tip:** Narrow the options by focusing on symptoms; some options are conditions.

**Content Area:** Mental Health; **Concept:** Medication; Perfusion; Nutrition; **Integrated Processes:** Teaching/Learning; **Client Needs:** Physiological Integrity: Pharmacological and Parenteral Therapies; **Cognitive Level:** Application [Applying]

## 2164. ANSWER: 1

1. **An effective therapeutic intervention for the client diagnosed with major depressive disorder is to sit with the client in silence. Nonverbal communication conveys respect, understanding, and interest.**
2. Lack of energy is a common symptom of depression.
3. Clients diagnosed with depression have a decreased attention span and concentration.
4. Clients diagnosed with depression are often indecisive and dependent.

▶ **Test-taking Tip:** Three options are similar, and one is different. Often the option that is different is the answer.

**Content Area:** Mental Health; **Concept:** Mood; Nursing Roles; **Integrated Processes:** Nursing Process: Implementation; **Client Needs:** Psychosocial Integrity; **Cognitive Level:** Application [Applying]

## 2165. PHARM ANSWER: 3

1. Both doxepin and amitriptyline are TCAs; there is no benefit in changing to a medication in the same drug classification.
2. Amitriptyline should not be taken before surgery because it can cause a hypertensive episode.
3. **Hypertensive episodes have occurred during surgery with TCAs such as amitriptyline (Elavil). For client safety, the dosage should be gradually decreased and discontinued several days prior to surgery.**
4. Although some oral medications should be continued on the day of surgery and taken with a minimum amount of water, amitriptyline is not one of these because it should be discontinued.

▶ **Test-taking Tip:** The key word is "safety." If unsure, think about which action would be the safest.

**Content Area:** Mental Health; **Concept:** Medication; Safety; **Integrated Processes:** Nursing Process: Planning; **Client Needs:** Physiological Integrity: Pharmacological and Parenteral Therapies; Physiological Integrity: Reduction of Risk Potential; **Cognitive Level:** Evaluation [Evaluating]

## 2166. PHARM ANSWER: 10

**The client's new dose is 30 mg daily. If the tablets are 20 mg, then the amount needed for one dose is 1.5 tablets:**

$$\frac{20 \text{ mg}}{1 \text{ tab}} = \frac{30 \text{ mg}}{X \text{ tab}} \text{ (cross multiply)} \quad 20X = 30; \ X = 1.5$$

**If there are 15 tablets remaining and the dose is 1.5 tablets, the tablets will last 10 days (15 ÷ 1.5 = 10).**

▶ **Test-taking Tip:** Be sure to carefully read what the question is asking. You need to calculate the number of tablets for the newly prescribed dose. Then, you need to determine the number of days that 15 tablets of citalopram (Celexa) will last at the new dose.

**Content Area:** Mental Health; **Concept:** Medication; Mood; **Integrated Processes:** Nursing Process: Planning; **Client Needs:** Physiological Integrity: Pharmacological and Parenteral Therapies; **Cognitive Level:** Application [Applying]

## 2167. ANSWER: 4

1. Gestalt therapy emphasizes self-expression, self-exploration, and self-awareness in the present, and is not an evidenced-based practice for the treatment and management of depression.
2. Client-centered therapy is a humanistic approach that emphasizes expression of feelings through reflection and clarification, and is not an evidenced-based practice for the treatment and management of depression.
3. Therapeutic touch is used to reduce pain and anxiety and to promote relaxation; it is not an approach for treating depression.
4. **Cognitive behavioral therapy is a research-supported treatment for depression that focuses on patterns of thinking that are maladaptive and the beliefs that underlie such thinking. The aim of therapy is to influence and change disturbed thinking patterns and the messages that the client gleans.**

♦ *Test-taking Tip: Select the therapy that will influence and change disturbed thinking patterns.*

Content Area: Mental Health; Concept: Pregnancy; Medication; Mood; Evidence-based Practice; Integrated Processes: Nursing Process: Planning; Client Needs: Psychosocial Integrity; Cognitive Level: Application [Applying]

## 2168. ANSWER: 1, 2, 3, 4, 5

1. **Impaired concentration nearly daily for 2 weeks is a criterion for major depressive disorder.**
2. **Feelings of worthlessness nearly daily is a criterion for major depressive disorder.**
3. **Depressed mood nearly daily for at least 2 weeks is a criterion for major depressive disorder.**
4. **Loss of interest or pleasure for at least 2 weeks meets the diagnostic criteria for major depressive disorder.**
5. **Psychomotor retardation or agitation for at least 2 weeks is one criterion for major depressive disorder.**
6. Rapid, pressured speech is a diagnostic criterion for bipolar disorder and not major depressive disorder.

♦ *Test-taking Tip: Determine the commonalities in the options and eliminate the one option that is different.*

Content Area: Mental Health; Concept: Mood; Assessment; Integrated Processes: Nursing Process: Assessment; Client Needs: Psychosocial Integrity; Cognitive Level: Application [Applying]

## 2169. ANSWER: 1

1. **Light therapy (phototherapy) is exposure to light that is brighter than indoor light but less bright than sunlight. This intervention has proven effectiveness compared to psychopharmacological treatments in various placebo controls.**
2. Quetiapine (Seroquel) is an atypical antipsychotic used for treatment of schizophrenia.
3. Lithium carbonate is used to treat bipolar disorder and not seasonal affective disorder.

4. Although there may be situations in which a person with seasonal affective disorder could seek therapy with a psychologist, it is not a first-line treatment.

♦ *Test-taking Tip: The key word is "first-line." Select the option that would require minimal cost.*

Content Area: Mental Health; Concept: Mood; Promoting Health; Evidence-based Practice; Integrated Processes: Nursing Process: Implementation; Client Needs: Physiological Integrity: Basic Care and Comfort; Psychosocial Integrity; Cognitive Level: Application [Applying]

## 2170. ANSWER: 3

1. A 2-week duration of feelings of sadness and emptiness is associated with a major depressive disorder.
2. Decreased concentration is a neurovegetative symptom most commonly associated with a major depressive disorder.
3. **Individuals diagnosed with dysthymia (chronic depressive disorder) describe their mood as sad or "down in the dumps" more days than not for at least 2 years. The depressive symptoms are chronic but less severe and may not be easily distinguished from the person's usual functioning.**
4. Recurrent thoughts of death, suicidal ideation, and attempted suicide are neurovegetative symptoms associated with a major depressive disorder.

♦ *Test-taking Tip: Narrow the options by eliminating those associated with a shorter time frame.*

Content Area: Mental Health; Concept: Mood; Assessment; Integrated Processes: Nursing Process: Assessment; Client Needs: Psychosocial Integrity; Physiological Integrity: Physiological Adaptation; Cognitive Level: Application [Applying]

## 2171. MoC ANSWER: 2, 5, 3, 1, 4

2. **Determine the client's risk for suicide by direct questioning and showing concern (asking about suicide intent and plan). The client's safety is priority.**
5. **Initiate suicide precautions as needed, according to policy and standards of care. Implementing a plan for suicide prevention occurs after an assessment and analysis of the client's risk for suicide.**
3. **Assist the client in maintaining nutritional needs, hygiene, and grooming and in meeting other physical needs. The physical needs of the client should be addressed before psychosocial needs.**
1. **Initiate prescribed psychosocial treatment plans. Once the immediate physical needs are met, the client's psychosocial needs can be addressed.**
4. **Contact the client's support system in collaboration with case manager and/or social services. The immediate needs of the client should be addressed before involving family.**

♦ *Test-taking Tip: Anhedonia and feelings of hopelessness are significant risk factors for suicide. Focus on the goal of suicide prevention. Use Maslow's Hierarchy of Needs and the nursing process to place items in the correct sequence.*

**Content Area:** Mental Health; **Concept:** Mood; Safety; **Integrated Processes:** Nursing Process: Analysis; **Client Needs:** Safe and Effective Care Environment: Management of Care; **Cognitive Level:** Synthesis [Creating]

## 2172. ANSWER: 1, 3

1. **Sadness is associated with depression and not delirium.**
2. A labile affect (mood swings or emotions inconsistent with the situation) is associated with both delirium and depression.
3. **Lack of motivation is associated with depression and not delirium.**
4. Presence of hallucinations is associated with delirium, not depression.
5. Disturbance in sleep patterns is associated with both delirium and depression.

▶ *Test-taking Tip:* The key word is "unique." You should eliminate the symptoms that are associated with both delirium and depression.

**Content Area:** Mental Health; **Concept:** Mood; Assessment; **Integrated Processes:** Nursing Process: Analysis; **Client Needs:** Psychosocial Integrity; **Cognitive Level:** Analysis [Analyzing]

## 2173. ANSWER: 4

1. This statement projects a judgmental attitude and is not a helpful comment; there is no indication that the spouse left after the client received a DUI.
2. Any client with possible depression should be screened for suicide risk, but this statement elicits only a "yes" or "no" response, or it may cause the client to become defensive.
3. This statement fails to acknowledge that both chemical dependency and depression are considered primary and need simultaneous treatment.
4. **Stating concern and referring the client to someone specializing in chemical dependency is the most therapeutic statement. The client needs to be assessed for substance abuse/dependence.**

▶ *Test-taking Tip:* The key words are "most therapeutic." Eliminate options that elicit a "yes" or "no" response. Of the two remaining options, select the option that conveys concern and is most direct.

**Content Area:** Mental Health; **Concept:** Addiction; Mood; Stress; Communication; **Integrated Processes:** Caring; Communication and Documentation; **Client Needs:** Psychosocial Integrity; Physiological Integrity: Physiological Adaptation; **Cognitive Level:** Analysis [Analyzing]

## 2174. MoC ANSWER: 2, 3, 4

1. Fluctuating mood is characteristic of bipolar disorder and not depression.
2. **Children in all age groups can become depressed.**
3. **The rate of depression rises after puberty to the late teenage years.**
4. **The reasons for increased susceptibility in women are unclear but may include stress, lifestyle, and hormonal factors.**

5. Perfectionism and rigid thought patterns are characteristic of OCD, not depression.

▶ *Test-taking Tip:* Carefully review the options and find the commonalities of age and gender for three options and behaviors for two options. Carefully consider that the behaviors are not associated with depression and eliminate these.

**Content Area:** Mental Health; **Concept:** Mood; Nursing Roles; **Integrated Processes:** Teaching/Learning; **Client Needs:** Safe and Effective Care Environment: Management of Care; Psychosocial Integrity; **Cognitive Level:** Application [Applying]

## 2175. ANSWER: 4

1. Secluding the client is unnecessary.
2. Rather than confront the client, it is more effective to redirect the client, because clients with mania are easily distracted.
3. Rather than acknowledge the provocative comment, it is more effective to redirect the client, because clients with mania are easily distracted.
4. **The most therapeutic response by the nurse is to redirect the client. Hypersexual behavior and impulsivity are symptoms of mania.**

▶ *Test-taking Tip:* Only one option redirects the client.

**Content Area:** Mental Health; **Concept:** Mood; Communication; **Integrated Processes:** Communication and Documentation; **Client Needs:** Psychosocial Integrity; **Cognitive Level:** Application [Applying]

## 2176. MoC ANSWER: 3

1. Being quiet one day and talking excessively the next day is a symptom of the client's bipolar disorder and not attention-seeking behavior.
2. Although asking the NA to refer to the client by name is an appropriate response, it is not the most helpful response.
3. **About one in six clients with bipolar disorder presents with a rapid-cycling pattern of quickly changing moods. Providing this information is most helpful because the nurse is teaching the NA about the client's illness.**
4. This response is likely to elicit defensiveness by the NA and is a missed teaching opportunity.

▶ *Test-taking Tip:* The most helpful response is one that focuses on the client's behavior and not the NA's behavior.

**Content Area:** Mental Health; **Concept:** Mood; Communication; **Integrated Processes:** Caring; Communication and Documentation; **Client Needs:** Safe and Effective Care Environment: Management of Care; Psychosocial Integrity; **Cognitive Level:** Analysis [Analyzing]

## 2177. ANSWER: 2

1. Group activities could increase level of stimuli and worsen agitation.
2. **Maintaining a low level of stimulation minimizes anxiety, agitation, and suspiciousness that is associated with acute mania.**

3. The client's behavior must be closely observed to ensure safety. The nurse should stay with the client, not leave the client alone.

4. The least-restrictive method for preventing harm to self or others should be used. Restraints should be used only if other interventions are unsuccessful and the client presents imminent risk of harm to self or others.

▶ *Test-taking Tip: When the client has acute mania, interventions should focus on decreasing stimuli.*

**Content Area:** Mental Health; **Concept:** Mood; Safety; **Integrated Processes:** Nursing Process: Planning; **Client Needs:** Safe and Effective Care Environment: Safety and Infection Control; **Cognitive Level:** Application [Applying]

## 2178. ANSWER: 3

1. The symptoms of confusion, loss of recent memory, and confabulation would be present in Korsakoff's psychosis.

2. Mood fluctuations would occur with bipolar disorder/mixed type.

3. **The symptoms of increased psychomotor activity with diminished need for sleep are associated with bipolar disorder of the manic type.**

4. With OCD, the client would report recurrent and persistent thoughts or impulses.

▶ *Test-taking Tip: You should find a term similar to "energy" in the stem in one of the options.*

**Content Area:** Mental Health; **Concept:** Mood; Assessment; Sleep, Rest, and Activity; **Integrated Processes:** Nursing Process: Analysis; Communication and Documentation; **Client Needs:** Psychosocial Integrity; **Cognitive Level:** Application [Applying]

## 2179. ANSWER: 4

1. Antidepressant medication takes 3 to 4 weeks to reach therapeutic effectiveness, not 2 days.

2. Treatment in a mental health setting would be longer than a few days.

3. There is no information about how familiar the client is with the unit.

4. **The clinical presentation of unipolar and bipolar depression can be similar. The client can have a manic episode precipitated if a bipolar disorder exists and the client receives only an antidepressant without a concurrent mood stabilizer.**

▶ *Test-taking Tip: The nurse's observation of the client's behavior can assist in making a correct diagnosis.*

**Content Area:** Mental Health; **Concept:** Mood; **Integrated Processes:** Nursing Process: Analysis; **Client Needs:** Psychosocial Integrity; Physiological Integrity: Physiological Adaptation; **Cognitive Level:** Analysis [Analyzing]

## 2180. ANSWER: 2

1. Conversations should be brief while the client is hypomanic or manic to minimize confusion and frustration.

2. **The nurse should plan to provide finger foods because nutritional status may be compromised due to hyperactive behaviors and the client being too distracted to sit down for a meal.**

3. Teaching the client and family about community resources should be completed, but it is not appropriate when the client is experiencing acute mania.

4. The client's anger is likely to be transitory and will improve as mania subsides. Family should avoid sensitive or volatile topics while the client is in a manic phase.

▶ *Test-taking Tip: You should eliminate options that will increase the client's mania.*

**Content Area:** Mental Health; **Concept:** Mood; Nutrition; **Integrated Processes:** Nursing Process: Planning; **Client Needs:** Safe and Effective Care Environment: Safety and Infection Control; **Cognitive Level:** Synthesis [Creating]

## 2181. PHARM ANSWER: 3

1. Limiting fluids would worsen lithium toxicity.

2. The nurse should not continue to administer lithium because the lithium level is toxic.

3. **The nurse should withhold the lithium (Lithobid) and notify the HCP. Lithium is at a toxic level. A therapeutic lithium level is 0.8 to 1.2 mEq/L.**

4. Coarse hand tremor is a symptom of lithium toxicity, and once the level is normalized the tremors should subside.

▶ *Test-taking Tip: Focus on the symptoms of lithium toxicity to select the correct option.*

**Content Area:** Mental Health; **Concept:** Mood; Medication; **Integrated Processes:** Nursing Process: Implementation; **Client Needs:** Physiological Integrity: Pharmacological and Parenteral Therapies; **Cognitive Level:** Analysis [Analyzing]

## 2182. ANSWER: 1, 2, 4

1. **The client with anxiety develops a sense of security when in the presence of a calm staff member.**

2. **The client's anxiety level may increase in a stimulating environment, so the environment should have low stimulation.**

3. Reinforcing reality is a strategy used with a thought disorder, not anxiety.

4. **The client with anxiety has a decreased attention span and a diminished level of concentration, so class time and amount of information should be limited.**

5. Self-harming behavior in the client with mild to moderate anxiety is usually not a concern.

▶ *Test-taking Tip: Examine options for a similar theme, and eliminate options with more intrusive strategies.*

**Content Area:** Mental Health; **Concept:** Stress; Nursing Roles; **Integrated Processes:** Teaching/Learning; Nursing Process: Planning; **Client Needs:** Health Promotion and Maintenance; **Cognitive Level:** Application [Applying]

**2183. ANSWER: 1, 2, 4, 5**

1. **Irritability is a criterion for generalized anxiety.**
2. **Muscle tension is a DSM-5 criterion for generalized anxiety.**
3. Expansive mood and pressured speech are symptoms of bipolar disorder, not generalized anxiety.
4. **Restlessness or feeling keyed up is a criterion for generalized anxiety.**
5. **Difficulty controlling anxiety is a criterion for generalized anxiety.**

▶ *Test-taking Tip: Use the process of elimination and identify the commonalities in options. One option is different and relates to bipolar disorder and not generalized anxiety disorder.*

**Content Area:** Mental Health; **Concept:** Stress; Assessment; **Integrated Processes:** Nursing Process: Assessment; **Client Needs:** Psychosocial Integrity; **Cognitive Level:** Application [Applying]

**2184. ANSWER: 3**

1. The client's symptoms meet diagnostic criteria for a psychopathological anxiety disorder.
2. Phobias can occur at any age. The disorder is diagnosed more often in women than in men.
3. **Marked fear due to the presence or anticipation of a specific object (e.g., dogs), recognition that the fear is excessive, and avoidance of the object/ situation are diagnostic criteria for a specific phobia.**
4. True phobias are common in the general population. Specific phobias frequently occur concurrently with other anxiety disorders.

▶ *Test-taking Tip: While phobias are common, people seldom seek treatment unless the phobia interferes with their ability to function.*

**Content Area:** Mental Health; **Concept:** Stress; Critical Thinking; **Integrated Processes:** Nursing Process: Analysis; **Client Needs:** Psychosocial Integrity; **Cognitive Level:** Analysis [Analyzing]

**2185. MoC ANSWER: 3**

1. Although reviewing policies may increase staff knowledge, a more active strategy has a greater likelihood of improving staff effectiveness.
2. Hearing from clients who experienced suicidal ideation may increase staff knowledge, but a more active strategy has a greater likelihood of improving staff effectiveness.
3. **Role-playing is an active strategy that has the greatest likelihood of improving staff effectiveness when caring for the client with possible suicidal ideation. Research supports that one of the primary barriers to effective suicidal ideation assessment is the level of discomfort regarding the phrases and questions that are most effective. Role-playing allows practice and the perfection of personal communication styles to ensure a naturally flowing conversation during the assessment for suicidal ideation.**

4. Hearing from experts about suicidal ideation may increase staff knowledge, but a more active strategy has a greater likelihood of improving staff effectiveness.

▶ *Test-taking Tip: Review the options to determine which option involves cognitive, affective, and psychomotor learning.*

**Content Area:** Mental Health; **Concept:** Safety; Communication; Stress; **Integrated Processes:** Nursing Process: Planning; Teaching/Learning; **Client Needs:** Safe and Effective Care Environment: Management of Care; Safe and Effective Care Environment: Safety and Infection Control; **Cognitive Level:** Analysis [Analyzing]

**2186. MoC ANSWER: 4**

1. Family systems therapy is a warranted intervention when the client's symptoms signal the presence of dysfunction within the whole family.
2. Psychoanalytic therapy focuses on repressed conflicts that are both conscious and unconscious.
3. ECT is primarily used as an intervention for major depression; medications are administered during ECT.
4. **CBT is a treatment that focuses on patterns of thinking that are maladaptive and would be an effective choice for the described symptoms.**

▶ *Test-taking Tip: The key words are "anxiety" and "crowds." Eliminate options that include multiple individuals.*

**Content Area:** Mental Health; **Concept:** Stress; Collaboration; **Integrated Processes:** Nursing Process: Implementation; **Client Needs:** Safe and Effective Care Environment: Management of Care; **Cognitive Level:** Application [Applying]

**2187. ANSWER: 4**

1. Sleep apnea may be a factor in insomnia.
2. A bath before bed may have a relaxing effect and promote sleep.
3. Insomnia can be a comorbid condition of depression.
4. **Black tea contains caffeine, a substance that should be avoided for several hours before bedtime.**

▶ *Test-taking Tip: Recall the factors that can contribute to dysfunctional sleep. Review the options and select the one that states a misconception or misuse of such a factor.*

**Content Area:** Mental Health; **Concept:** Nursing Roles; Sleep, Rest, and Activity; **Integrated Processes:** Nursing Process: Evaluation; **Client Needs:** Physiological Integrity: Basic Care and Comfort; **Cognitive Level:** Evaluation [Evaluating]

# TRAUMA- AND STRESSOR-RELATED DISORDERS

**2188. ANSWER: 2**

1. Narcolepsy is a disorder that produces excessive sleepiness; this client's symptoms suggest PTSD.
2. **The reported symptoms are consistent with PTSD and are often present with veterans who have been exposed to combat trauma. Asking about nightmares will help establish a diagnosis.**
3. Trichotillomania disorder is defined as the recurrent pulling out of one's own hair; this question is not helpful.

4. OCD is characterized by involuntary recurring thoughts but is not characterized by hypervigilance. This question is not helpful.

▶ **Test-taking Tip:** *Focus on the fact that the client is a recently discharged veteran and on the common disorder associated with trauma.*

**Content Area:** Mental Health; **Concept:** Stress; Assessment; **Integrated Processes:** Nursing Process: Assessment; **Client Needs:** Psychosocial Integrity; **Cognitive Level:** Application [Applying]

## 2189. ANSWER: 4

1. Asking the roommate to assume responsibility for the client is inappropriate and is a barrier to the establishment of the nurse-client relationship.
2. Redirecting the client so that evidence can be collected is inappropriate and a barrier to the establishment of the nurse-client relationship.
3. Encouraging the client to regain control of his or her emotions is a barrier to expressing the normal emotions.
4. **Feeling anger, rage, hopelessness, and disbelief are all normal emotional reactions to such a traumatic experience as a sexual assault. It is important to allow, even encourage, the victim to express these emotions in order to best initiate treatment.**

▶ **Test-taking Tip:** *Sexual assault generates strong emotions in the victim that must be expressed in a healthy manner. Review the options for the one that facilitates this expression in the healthiest way.*

**Content Area:** Mental Health; **Concept:** Communication; Stress; **Integrated Processes:** Nursing Process: Implementation; **Client Needs:** Psychosocial Integrity; **Cognitive Level:** Application [Applying]

## 2190. ANSWER: 4

1. This response makes a generalized comment and fails to provide any concrete information pertaining to the client.
2. Encouraging the client not to worry and giving an opinion are both nontherapeutic and appears to lessen the expressed concern.
3. This response conveys empathy, yet it is generalized and fails to provide any concrete information to address the client's concern.
4. **This response is best because it answers the client's question and addresses the goal of counseling. While crises do tend to be self-limiting (4 to 6 weeks), the way an individual recuperates can vary. The goal is to return to the precrisis level of function. This is best achieved through the use of effective coping skills, which are taught during counseling.**

▶ **Test-taking Tip:** *Focus on the key word "best" and review the options to determine which one best describes the most complete answer to the client's question.*

**Content Area:** Mental Health; **Concept:** Stress; Communication; **Integrated Processes:** Nursing Process: Implementation; **Client Needs:** Psychosocial Integrity; **Cognitive Level:** Analysis [Analyzing]

## 2191. MoC ANSWER: 1

1. **Asking the questions directly to the client allows the client and nurse to develop a relationship and allows the client to feel included in his or her plan of care.**
2. Asking the questions directly to the interpreter excludes the client and may make the client feel that his or her statements are unimportant.
3. The nurse should not ask the interpreter to step out of the room while doing a physical assessment because the nurse would need to ask the client questions and explain directions to the client. The client should also be allowed to ask questions during the physical assessment.
4. The interpreter should not be allowed to rephrase questions and responses as it may change the meanings of the response and may also provide inaccurate information.

▶ **Test-taking Tip:** *Eliminate the responses that decrease the client's ability to be active in the conversation.*

**Content Area:** Mental Health; **Concept:** Communication; **Integrated Processes:** Communication and Documentation; Culture and Spirituality; **Client Needs:** Safe and Effective Care Environment: Management of Care; Psychosocial Integrity; **Cognitive Level:** Application [Applying]

## 2192. ANSWER: 4

1. It is not practical or desired to have the child avoid all conflict, because conflict is a normal part of life.
2. Medication is not appropriate when nonpharmaceutical methods of managing this behavior have proven to be effective.
3. Although it is important for people to learn how to recognize and diffuse arguments effectively, this suggestion will not help to minimize the child's reaction to the assault.
4. **The flashbacks to the abuse are associated with the memories that may be now associated with a reluctance to obey an adult, especially a family member. The most effective tool to minimize this association is to discuss the memories on a regular basis. This will facilitate the child's ability to regain a sense of personal control.**

▶ **Test-taking Tip:** *Flashbacks are a result of traumatic memories. By evaluating each option's ability to impact the memory and then selecting the one most impactful, you will arrive at the correct option.*

**Content Area:** Mental Health; **Concept:** Stress; Critical Thinking; **Integrated Processes:** Nursing Process: Planning; **Client Needs:** Psychosocial Integrity; **Cognitive Level:** Application [Applying]

## 2193. ANSWER: 1

1. **The parents should tolerate the expression of anger with hair pulling until more acceptable behaviors to deal with anger can be introduced or until discussion of the emotion removes the need for the behavior.**

2. Ignoring the child's hair pulling and telling the child that abuse will never recur do not address the child's need to express the emotion of anger.

3. Distracting the child, even with a pleasurable experience, will not address the need to express the emotion of anger.

4. An explanation regarding why the behavior needs to stop will not address the child's underlying need.

▶ *Test-taking Tip: Abuse results in anger that is often repressed. Identifying the option that addresses the anger and its effective management will direct you to the correct option.*

Content Area: Mental Health; **Concept:** Stress; Self; **Integrated Processes:** Nursing Process: Implementation; **Client Needs:** Safe and Effective Care Environment: Safety and Infection Control; **Cognitive Level:** Application [Applying]

### 2194. ANSWER: 4

1. To state that the plan is ambitious and to question the wisdom of rebuilding in the same location are not as direct in determining the realistic nature of the client's statement.

2. Praising the client is not appropriate if the expectations are unrealistic.

3. This response is negative and not therapeutic.

4. **The client must be encouraged to set realistic goals. The initial step in this scenario is to have the client define the term a "few months" in order to determine whether it is possible to rebuild in that amount of time.**

▶ *Test-taking Tip: You need to focus on the term "rebuild," which is stated in both the stem of the question and the correct option.*

Content Area: Mental Health; **Concept:** Stress; Communication; **Integrated Processes:** Communication and Documentation; **Client Needs:** Psychosocial Integrity; **Cognitive Level:** Application [Applying]

### 2195. ANSWER: 2

1. Acknowledging the worth of therapy does not indicate the ability to regain control and move forward.

2. **A crisis is defined as an event that an individual is unprepared to deal with successfully. To be able to state that one is ready and able to move on with life regardless of the past event demonstrates successfully coping.**

3. Expressing that nothing could be worse than the previous experience fails to demonstrate the ability to function at a level equal to that of one before the event.

4. To state that one has gained self-awareness does not ensure effective function, which is the expected outcome of the therapy.

▶ *Test-taking Tip: The goal of crisis therapy is to promote the individual's ability to function effectively. Only one option reflects effective functioning.*

Content Area: Mental Health; **Concept:** Self; Communication; **Integrated Processes:** Nursing Process: Evaluation; **Client Needs:** Psychosocial Integrity; **Cognitive Level:** Evaluation [Evaluating]

# PERSONALITY DISORDERS

### 2196. ANSWER: 4

1. The individual with paranoid personality usually feels constant mistrust and suspicion toward others and is not able to trust those treating the client well.

2. Rather than seeing the good, the client with paranoid personality sees ill will in the actions of others when none exists.

3. Acting the opposite of what the client may be thinking or feeling is descriptive of reaction formation, a defense mechanism often used by persons with an OCD.

4. **The client with paranoid personality disorder exhibits mistrust and suspicion of others such that the behavior of others is analyzed to find hidden and threatening meanings.**

▶ *Test-taking Tip: Use the memory cue of the disorders by the clusters: **A** includes clients whose behavior is odd or eccentric; **B** includes clients who appear dramatic, emotional, or erratic; and **C** includes clients who appear anxious and fearful. Paranoid personality disorder is a cluster A disorder.*

Content Area: Mental Health; **Concept:** Self; Assessment; **Integrated Processes:** Nursing Process: Assessment; **Client Needs:** Psychosocial Integrity; **Cognitive Level:** Application [Applying]

### 2197. ANSWER: 1

1. **Individuals with paranoid personality disorder may have been subjected to parental antagonism and harassment. They served as scapegoats for displaced parental aggression and eventually gave up all hope of affection and approval.**

2. Lack of an empathetic upbringing and lack of nurturing are associated with schizoid personality disorder.

3. An early upbringing characterized by indifference is associated with schizotypal personality disorder.

4. The client likely received no recognition for accomplishments.

▶ *Test-taking Tip: Paranoid personality disorder involves mistrust of others and the fear that someone will harm them. This can be a result of lack of affection and lack of recognition of accomplishments in childhood.*

Content Area: Mental Health; **Concept:** Self; Assessment; **Integrated Processes:** Nursing Process: Analysis; **Client Needs:** Psychosocial Integrity; **Cognitive Level:** Application [Applying]

## 2198. ANSWER:

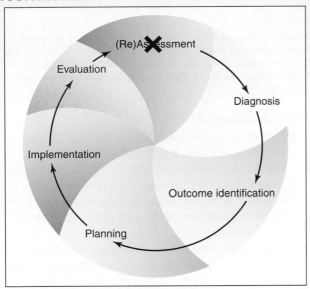

**The nurse is completing an assessment of the client by collecting information about the client's behavior.**

▶ *Test-taking Tip: When identifying that the client with antisocial personality disorder has poor judgment, emotional distance, aggression, and impulsivity, the nurse is collecting information about the client's behavior.*

Content Area: Mental Health; Concept: Self; Neurologic Regulation; Integrated Processes: Nursing Process: Assessment; Client Needs: Psychosocial Integrity; Cognitive Level: Application [Applying]

## 2199. ANSWER: 1

1. **Clients with paranoid personality disorder take everything seriously and are attuned to the actions and motivations of others. A businesslike approach with clear, concrete, and specific words keeps the intended message clear by decreasing ambiguity.**
2. Social conversation should be avoided because the client may read hidden, demeaning, or threatening meanings into benign remarks or events.
3. Jokes should not be included when working with the client with paranoid personality disorder, because the client may read hidden, demeaning, or threatening meanings into benign remarks or events.
4. Confrontation can be perceived as a threat and can precipitate client aggression and violence.

▶ *Test-taking Tip: Note that Options 2, 3, and 4 are similar and that Option 1 is different. Often the option that is different is the answer.*

Content Area: Mental Health; Concept: Self; Communication; Integrated Processes: Nursing Process: Implementation; Client Needs: Psychosocial Integrity; Cognitive Level: Application [Applying]

## 2200. ANSWER: 3

1. Psychotic episodes are not always associated with BPD; this is not descriptive of splitting.
2. An identity disturbance is a diagnostic criterion for BPD but does not describe splitting.

3. **Splitting is a primitive defense mechanism in which all objects, individuals, or situations are seen as good or bad. Individuals with BPD have an inability to accept and integrate positive and negative feelings.**
4. A pattern of unstable and intense interpersonal relationships is a diagnostic criterion for personality disorder and is not descriptive of splitting.

▶ *Test-taking Tip: Narrow the options by eliminating those that are descriptive of personality disorders.*

Content Area: Mental Health; Concept: Self; Nursing; Integrated Processes: Communication and Documentation; Nursing Process: Analysis; Client Needs: Psychosocial Integrity; Cognitive Level: Application [Applying]

## 2201. ANSWER: 1, 5

1. **The client with histrionic personality disorder requires constant affirmation of approval and acceptance from others and often uses physical appearance to gain attention and approval.**
2. Rather than apathy, the person with histrionic personality disorder shows self-dramatization and exaggerated emotional expression.
3. Lacking close friends or companions is associated with schizoid personality disorder.
4. Harboring suspicions is characteristic of paranoid personality disorder.
5. **Diagnostic criteria for histrionic personality disorder include discomfort in situations in which the client is not the center of attention. The client requires constant affirmation of approval and acceptance from others.**

▶ *Test-taking Tip: Narrow options to those that relate to excessive attention-seeking and emotion.*

Content Area: Mental Health; Concept: Self; Assessment; Integrated Processes: Nursing Process: Assessment; Client Needs: Psychosocial Integrity; Cognitive Level: Application [Applying]

## 2202. ANSWER: 1, 3, 5

1. **The nurse should question the dose of lithium because the lithium level of 1.5 mEq/L is nearing toxicity.**
2. Questioning the dose of fluoxetine (Prozac) is insufficient; the administration of fluoxetine should be questioned.
3. **The HCP should be notified. The lithium level of 1.5 mEq/L is nearing toxicity (therapeutic range is 0.6–1.2 mEq/L).**
4. Fluoxetine (Prozac) should not be administered. Fluoxetine will increase the risk of lithium toxicity.
5. **The nurse should question the addition of fluoxetine. Fluoxetine (Prozac) will increase the risk of lithium toxicity.**

▶ *Test-taking Tip: Lithium has a very narrow therapeutic range of 0.6 to 1.2 mEq/L and can easily cause toxicity, especially if used in combination with other medications.*

**Content Area:** Mental Health; **Concept:** Mood; Medication; Safety; **Integrated Processes:** Nursing Process: Evaluation; **Client Needs:** Physiological Integrity: Reduction of Risk Potential; **Cognitive Level:** Evaluation [Evaluating]

## 2203. ANSWER: 1

1. **Wanting to join others because of loneliness is a nonmanipulative behavior.**
2. Requesting cigarettes earlier than allowed is an attempt to manipulate the rules.
3. Telling the nurse that he or she is the best nurse is an attempt to influence the nurse by flattery.
4. Self-mutilation is a manipulative maneuver to avoid discharge.

▸ **Test-taking Tip:** *To manipulate is to influence another's behavior to serve one's own wishes. Focus on an option that does not involve influencing another's behavior.*

**Content Area:** Mental Health; **Concept:** Self; Safety; **Integrated Processes:** Nursing Process: Evaluation; **Client Needs:** Psychosocial Integrity; **Cognitive Level:** Evaluation [Evaluating]

## 2204. ANSWER: 3

1. Stating "hang in there" is making a stereotyped comment, and then the nurse's feelings are interjected.
2. Asking the name of the nurse uses probing, which is a barrier to therapeutic communication.
3. **The most therapeutic response is one in which the nurse avoids responding to the designation of favorite nurse and redirects the client to concentrate on the impending discharge.**
4. The nurse is giving approval to the client's statement when stating, "You are my favorite patient" and is conveying that the client will be missed. It is not therapeutic because the statements do not add to the interaction.

▸ **Test-taking Tip:** *Read each option carefully and eliminate the options that use barriers to a therapeutic interaction.*

**Content Area:** Mental Health; **Concept:** Self; Stress; Communication; **Integrated Processes:** Communication and Documentation; **Client Needs:** Psychosocial Integrity; **Cognitive Level:** Analysis [Analyzing]

## 2205. MoC PHARM ANSWER: 4

1. Combining SSRIs and MAOIs usually does not lower the BP.
2. Tension headache is not a side effect when carbamazepine (Carbatrol) and alprazolam (Xanax) are combined.
3. Even though suicide is a severe side effect of MAOIs, these are used in the treatment of BPD.
4. **Fluoxetine (Prozac) is an SSRI, and phenelzine (Nardil) is an MAOI. SSRIs and MAOIs should not be taken together because excessive release of serotonin (serotonin syndrome) may result with associated mental, CV, GI, and neuromuscular alterations.**

▸ **Test-taking Tip:** *You need to be aware of drug incompatibilities between psychiatric medications, especially those that affect the release of serotonin.*

**Content Area:** Mental Health; **Concept:** Self; Medication; **Integrated Processes:** Nursing Process: Analysis; **Client Needs:** Safe and Effective Care Environment: Management of Care; Physiological Integrity: Pharmacological and Parenteral Therapies; **Cognitive Level:** Analysis [Analyzing]

## 2206. ANSWER: 4

1. Paraphilia involves sexual fantasies or behaviors involving repetitive sexual activity with real or simulated suffering or humiliation. Paraphilias may include a sexual preference for a nonhuman object, as well as repetitive sexual activity with nonconsenting partners. There is no indication in the stem that this was a sexual assault.
2. Psychogenic amnesia is a neurocognitive disorder caused by an impact to the head or other mechanism that displaces the brain. Symptoms can include wandering, confusion, and disorientation. There is no mention of a head injury in the stem of the question.
3. A person with BPD will engage in self-injury before injuring others.
4. **Narcissistic personality disorder is characterized by the constant seeking of praise and attention; an egocentric attitude; and envy, rage, and violence when others are not supportive.**

▸ **Test-taking Tip:** *Read the options before the scenario and then focus on the characteristics of the different personality disorders and the client behaviors. Eliminate options as you read the behaviors.*

**Content Area:** Mental Health; **Concept:** Self; Safety; Stress; **Integrated Processes:** Nursing Process: Analysis; **Client Needs:** Psychosocial Integrity; **Cognitive Level:** Analysis [Analyzing]

## 2207. ANSWER: 3

1. Passive-aggressive personality disorder involves the resentment of responsibility and the expression of distaste; it does not include the behaviors exhibited by the client.
2. Histrionic personality disorders involve attention-seeking behavior; the accumulation of possessions would not be typical attention-seeking behavior.
3. **Hoarding behavior is associated with OCD and obsessive-compulsive personality disorder. It is due to fear and anxiety concerning loss of control over situations, objects, or people.**
4. BPDs involve fear of rejection in relationships and impulsivity, and not inattentiveness to their surroundings.

▸ **Test-taking Tip:** *Hoarding is a compulsive behavior done to excess.*

**Content Area:** Mental Health; **Concept:** Stress; Safety; **Integrated Processes:** Nursing Process: Analysis; **Client Needs:** Psychosocial Integrity; **Cognitive Level:** Analysis [Analyzing]

## 2208. MoC ANSWER: 4

1. Recognizing limits is an outcome for an individual with antisocial personality disorder.
2. The ability to cope and control emotions are outcomes for an individual with BPD.
3. Validating ideas before acting is an outcome for an individual with paranoid personality disorder.
4. **An outcome for the individual with schizoid personality disorder focuses on improving functioning within the community.**

▶ *Test-taking Tip: The person with a schizoid personality disorder has a profound defect in the ability to form personal relationships or to respond to others in any meaningful way. Three options pertain to self, and one pertains to community. Often the option that is different is the answer.*

**Content Area:** Mental Health; **Concept:** Self; **Integrated Processes:** Nursing Process: Planning; **Client Needs:** Safe and Effective Care Environment: Management of Care; Psychosocial Integrity; **Cognitive Level:** Synthesis [Creating]

## 2209. ANSWER: 1, 2, 3, 4

1. **Reframing is a cognitive behavioral technique where alternative points of view are examined to explain events and is used to enhance self-worth of the person with avoidant personality disorder.**
2. **Exploring positive aspects of self is used to enhance self-worth of the person with avoidant personality disorder.**
3. **Practicing social skills with the client in the safety of the nurse-client relationship will help the client reduce social fears and develop meaningful social contact and relationship skills.**
4. **Decatastrophizing is a method of learning to assess situations in a realistic manner instead of assuming a catastrophe will happen. Using this can enhance self-worth.**
5. Positive, not negative, responses from others should be explored.

▶ *Test-taking Tip: Because the individual with avoidant personality disorder is extremely sensitive to rejection and may lead a very socially withdrawn life, interventions should focus on enhancing self-worth and developing social skills.*

**Content Area:** Mental Health; **Concept:** Self; Nursing Roles; **Integrated Processes:** Nursing Process: Planning; **Client Needs:** Psychosocial Integrity; **Cognitive Level:** Application [Applying]

## 2210. ANSWER: 2

1. Using an inflexible and autocratic approach can induce anxiety.
2. **Persons with obsessive-compulsive personality disorder tend to maintain control by carefully and thoroughly following procedures. It is important to use a calm and nonconfrontational approach, as any request is likely to increase the client's anxiety level.**
3. A hurried approach will increase the client's anxiety level.

4. Using an uninterrupted and confrontational approach would likely induce anxiety.

▶ *Test-taking Tip: Note that Options 1, 3, and 4 are similar and that Option 2 is different. Often the option that is different is the answer.*

**Content Area:** Mental Health; **Concept:** Stress; Nursing Roles; **Integrated Processes:** Nursing Process: Implementation; **Client Needs:** Psychosocial Integrity; **Cognitive Level:** Application [Applying]

## 2211. MoC ANSWER: 1, 4

1. **The client has the right to refuse treatment; the client is competent.**
2. The nurse could be charged with assault if treatment is administered against the client's will.
3. The nurse cannot disclose confidential health information to family without the client's consent; the client is competent.
4. **The nurse should notify the client's HCP of the refusal for treatment, and acknowledge that the client is competent. A diagnosis of OCD does not indicate that the client is incompetent.**
5. The nurse should notify the client's HCP of the refusal for treatment, but the client is competent, not incompetent.

▶ *Test-taking Tip: First decide whether or not the client is competent and then review like options and use the process of elimination.*

**Content Area:** Mental Health; **Concept:** Self; Safety; **Integrated Processes:** Nursing Process: Implementation; **Client Needs:** Safe and Effective Care Environment: Management of Care; Psychosocial Integrity; **Cognitive Level:** Analysis [Analyzing]

## 2212. ANSWER: 1, 2, 5, 6

1. **Isolation is a defense mechanism to separate a thought or memory from the feelings or emotions associated with it.**
2. **Undoing is a defense mechanism to symbolically negate or cancel out a previous action or experience that is found to be intolerable.**
3. Projection is attributing to another person the feelings or impulses that are unacceptable to oneself.
4. Introjection is internalization of the beliefs and values of another person, and these symbolically become a part of the self to the extent that the feeling of separateness or distinctness is lost.
5. **Rationalization is the attempt to make excuses or formulate logical reasons to justify unacceptable feelings or behaviors.**
6. **Intellectualization is an attempt to avoid expressing actual emotions associated with a stressful situation by using the intellectual processes of logic, reasoning, and analysis.**

▶ *Test-taking Tip: Reaction formation involves developing conscious attitudes and behaviors and acting out behaviors opposite to what one really feels. Thus narrow the options by focusing on defense mechanisms that avoid expressing true feelings.*

Content Area: Mental Health; Concept: Stress; Self; Integrated Processes: Nursing Process: Planning; Client Needs: Psychosocial Integrity; Cognitive Level: Application [Applying]

## 2213. ANSWER: 1

1. **Projection is attributing feelings or impulses that are unacceptable to oneself onto another person. The person with antisocial personality disorder will exploit and manipulate others for personal gain.**
2. Sublimation is the channeling of unacceptable impulses, thoughts, and emotions into acceptable ones.
3. Compensation is a process of counterbalancing weaknesses with strengths. This is a more mature defense mechanism.
4. Rationalization is putting things into a different, acceptable perspective.

▶ *Test-taking Tip: Differentiate the more advanced defense mechanisms from the more primitive; individuals with personality disorders are more likely to use the more primitive defense mechanisms.*

Content Area: Mental Health; Concept: Stress; Self; Integrated Processes: Nursing Process: Planning; Client Needs: Psychosocial Integrity; Cognitive Level: Application [Applying]

## 2214. PHARM ANSWER: 2

1. Lithium (Lithobid) is an older medication used to control mood and has a greater number of side effects.
2. **GABA (γ-aminobutyric acid) is the main inhibitory neurotransmitter in the CNS. GABAergic anticonvulsants, such as gabapentin (Neurontin), appear to act by regulating neural firing in the mesolimbic area.**
3. Valproic acid (Depacon) is an older medication used to control mood and has a greater number of side effects.
4. Carbamazepine (Carbatrol) is an older medication used to control mood and has a greater number of side effects.

▶ *Test-taking Tip: If unsure, correlate "GABA" in the stem with the generic name of the medication. Be familiar with the use of off-label drugs when psychiatric medications are prescribed.*

Content Area: Mental Health; Concept: Medication; Communication; Integrated Processes: Communication and Documentation; Client Needs: Physiological Integrity: Pharmacological and Parenteral Therapies; Cognitive Level: Application [Applying]

## 2215. MoC PHARM ANSWER:

| Client: 75-year-old | | Allergies: None | |
| --- | --- | --- | --- |
| **Medication** | 0001–0759 | 0800–1559 | 1600–2400 |
| Risperidone oral **X** | | 0900___ | |
| 1 mg bid on day 1; 2 mg bid on day 2; 3 mg bid on day 3 | | 2 mg | |

Risperidone (Risperdal), an antipsychotic medication, is prescribed at the regular adult dose and is not at an appropriate dose for an older adult. Metabolism is slowed with aging, and adverse reactions can occur quickly in older adults.

▶ *Test-taking Tip: Be aware of the dosage differences for older adults taking antipsychotic medications.*

Content Area: Mental Health; Concept: Medication; Safety; Integrated Processes: Nursing Process: Implementation; Client Needs: Safe and Effective Care Environment: Management of Care; Physiological Integrity: Pharmacological and Parenteral Therapies; Cognitive Level: Application [Applying]

## 2216. PHARM ANSWER: 2

1. Eating foods high in tyramine while taking MAOIs causes hypertension, not hypotension.
2. **The combination of tyramine-containing foods and MAOIs, such as phenelzine (Nardil), can result in a hypertensive crisis.**
3. Foods high in tyramine do not delay absorption of MAOIs such as tyramine.
4. Although the hypertensive crisis state can cause cardiac rhythm abnormalities, this is not the primary reason to avoid foods high in tyramine.

▶ *Test-taking Tip: Examine options that are opposites first and eliminate one of these. Then consider that phenelzine is an MAOI to narrow the remaining options.*

Content Area: Mental Health; Concept: Self; Medication; Nutrition; Integrated Processes: Teaching/Learning; Client Needs: Physiological Integrity: Pharmacological and Parenteral Therapies; Physiological Integrity: Reduction of Risk Potential; Cognitive Level: Application [Applying]

## 2217. ANSWER: 1, 3, 4

1. **Using "I" statements helps to avoid judgment and is part of the communication triad.**
2. Using "you" statements to identify the cause is being judgmental and would not be included.
3. **Nonjudgmental statements are included in the communication triad to manage feelings.**
4. **A mechanism for restoring comfort is included in the communication triad to manage feelings.**
5. Using "they" statements can be judgmental and presumptuous and would not be included.

▶ *Test-taking Tip: The key word is "triad," so three options are right, and two are incorrect.*

Content Area: Mental Health; Concept: Nursing Roles; Communication; Integrated Processes: Teaching/Learning; Client Needs: Psychosocial Integrity; Cognitive Level: Application [Applying]

## 2218. MoC ANSWER: 3

1. Limit-setting is important for milieu therapy to be effective but is not the best reason.
2. A structured setting is a component of milieu therapy but is not the best reason for including it with this client.

3. **Milieu therapy helps the client with antisocial personality disorder learn to respond adaptively to feedback from peers. The democratic approach with specific rules and regulations, community meetings, and group therapy sessions simulates the societal situation in which the client must live.**

4. Reality orientation and one-on-one interaction are a part of milieu therapy but are not its most helpful aspects.

▶ *Test-taking Tip: Read each option and select the most global option that would be inclusive of the other options.*

Content Area: Mental Health; **Concept:** Self; Communication; **Integrated Processes:** Nursing Process: Analysis; **Client Needs:** Safe and Effective Care Environment: Management of Care; Psychosocial Integrity; **Cognitive Level:** Synthesis [Creating]

# SOMATIC SYMPTOM AND DISSOCIATIVE DISORDERS

## 2219. ANSWER: 2

1. Blacking out and fainting are not associated with pseudocyesis (false pregnancy).

2. **Pseudocyesis is a conversion symptom due to a strong desire to be pregnant, even though pregnancy has not occurred.**

3. An inability to smell is anosmia. Anosmia can be a symptom associated with a neurological disease or with a conversion symptom associated with severe trauma when no underlying disease has been found.

4. Seizures and staring spells are not associated with pseudocyesis (false pregnancy).

▶ *Test-taking Tip: Pseudocyesis is a false pregnancy.*

Content Area: Mental Health; **Concept:** Stress; Self; **Integrated Processes:** Nursing Process: Assessment; **Client Needs:** Psychosocial Integrity; **Cognitive Level:** Application [Applying]

## 2220. ANSWER: 2, 3

1. The demonstration of having more than one distinct personality is a sign of dissociative identity disorder, not psychogenic fugue.

2. **Forgetting previous personal information following a traumatic event or stressor is associated with psychogenic fugue.**

3. **The nurse should identify that the diagnosis of psychogenic fugue is based upon the client's symptoms of assuming a new identity.**

4. Claiming superhero qualities is not associated with a psychogenic fugue.

5. Residing in a homeless shelter after being physically abused is not associated with a psychogenic fugue.

▶ *Test-taking Tip: Associate the term "fugue" with forgetting to narrow the options.*

Content Area: Mental Health; **Concept:** Trauma; Stress; **Integrated Processes:** Nursing Process: Analysis; Communication and Documentation; **Client Needs:** Psychosocial Integrity; **Cognitive Level:** Application [Applying]

## 2221. ANSWER: 2, 3, 4, 5

1. The nurse should focus on short-term, not long-term, goals because this helps to create smaller successes for the client with DID and results in better personality integration.

2. **Because two or more personalities exist when a person has DID, the nurse should focus on actively listening to each alternate personality.**

3. **When working with the client diagnosed with DID, the nurse should maintain a calm environment because it is thought that a traumatic event may have triggered the alternate personalities.**

4. **The nurse should document any changes in behavior because they can help to identify each alternate personality.**

5. **It is important to observe for signs of suicide to protect the client from self-harm.**

▶ *Test-taking Tip: DID is characterized by the existence of two or more personalities in a single individual.*

Content Area: Mental Health; **Concept:** Stress; Self; Trauma; **Integrated Processes:** Nursing Process: Implementation; **Client Needs:** Psychosocial Integrity; **Cognitive Level:** Application [Applying]

## 2222. ANSWER: 4

1. Telling the client to remain calm may cause the client's behavior to escalate.

2. Bargaining with the client may create an attitude of distrust; it may not be the main personality speaking.

3. The nurse should attend to the client's immediate needs, including emotional needs and not just the medical needs.

4. **The nurse should use active listening to establish a relationship with the personality speaking.**

▶ *Test-taking Tip: Focus on using a therapeutic communication technique.*

Content Area: Mental Health; **Concept:** Violence; Self; **Integrated Processes:** Nursing Process: Implementation; **Client Needs:** Safe and Effective Care Environment: Safety and Infection Control; **Cognitive Level:** Application [Applying]

## 2223. ANSWER: 4

1. If exposed to painful information from which the amnesia is providing protection, the client may decompensate even further into a psychotic state.

2. A diary may be used in treating the client with a somatic symptom disorder and not dissociative disorder.

3. The nurse should develop a trusting relationship with the original personality and each of the subpersonalities because each personality views itself as a separate entity and should initially be treated as a separate entity.

4. **Smells associated with pleasant life experiences may stimulate recall. Only positive life experiences should be included initially to prevent the client from decompensating further into the psychotic state.**

▶ *Test-taking Tip: Options should be narrowed by associating them with what you know about DID (the existence of two or more personalities in a single individual) and amnesia (loss of memory), and eliminating options with absolute words.*

**Content Area:** Mental Health; **Concept:** Stress; Self; Trauma; **Integrated Processes:** Nursing Process: Implementation; **Client Needs:** Psychosocial Integrity; **Cognitive Level:** Application [Applying]

# DISRUPTIVE, IMPULSE-CONTROL, AND CONDUCT DISORDERS

## 2224. ANSWER: 1

1. **Pyromania is an impulse-control disorder in which a person sets fires to relieve tension.**
2. Kleptomania is an impulse control disorder characterized by stealing to relieve tension or to satisfy an uncontrollable urge.
3. Conduct disorder is not mainly explained through fire-setting behavior; however, some clients having this disorder have a history of setting fires.
4. Antisocial personality disorder is not mainly explained through fire-setting behavior; however, some clients having this disorder have a history of setting fires.

▶ *Test-taking Tip: The prefix "pyro-" pertains to fire.*

**Content Area:** Mental Health; **Concept:** Stress; Self; Assessment; **Integrated Processes:** Nursing Process: Assessment; **Client Needs:** Psychosocial Integrity; **Cognitive Level:** Knowledge [Remembering]

## 2225. ANSWER: 3

1. Mimicking the behavior would not be appropriate and would increase aggression.
2. Instructing the client to stop yelling might provoke aggression in the client.
3. **An appropriate nursing intervention is to ignore initial yelling and tantrums. The lack of feedback often eliminates the behavior. Ignoring the client should be therapeutic and not unintentional.**
4. Using a guided walk might provoke the client to become aggressive.

▶ *Test-taking Tip: Select the only option that eliminates giving positive feedback or attention to the client. Three options are similar, and one is different; often the option that is different is the answer.*

**Content Area:** Mental Health; **Concept:** Stress; Mood; **Integrated Processes:** Nursing Process: Implementation; **Client Needs:** Psychosocial Integrity; **Cognitive Level:** Application [Applying]

## 2226. MoC ANSWER: 3

1. Providing positive affirmation is important but is not priority.
2. Educating the client is an intervention when caring for the client, but client safety is priority.
3. **The most appropriate nursing intervention for the client experiencing suicidal ideation is to notify the appropriate authorities of the client's intent to harm. Nurses are obligated under the *Meier v. Ross General Hospital* case to report any suspicion of suicide among clients.**

4. Assessing the client's surroundings is an important intervention when caring for the client with major depressive disorder, but alerting the appropriate authorities is priority.

▶ *Test-taking Tip: The key word is "priority," which suggests that other options may be correct but that one option is more important than the other options. Look for the more global option that protects the client from harm.*

**Content Area:** Mental Health; **Concept:** Mood; Self; Safety; **Integrated Processes:** Nursing Process: Implementation; **Client Needs:** Safe and Effective Care Environment: Management of Care; Safe and Effective Care Environment: Safety and Infection Control; **Cognitive Level:** Analysis [Analyzing]

## 2227. ANSWER: 1

1. **The nurse's primary goal should be to resolve present conflicts and help the client return to the precrisis state.**
2. Helping to alter thought processes would occur during therapeutic intervention.
3. The client has shown no harmful behavior that would warrant physical restraint.
4. Encouraging the client to talk about feelings is an appropriate intervention but is not the primary goal.

▶ *Test-taking Tip: The key words are "primary goal." Use the process of elimination to eliminate options that are interventions.*

**Content Area:** Mental Health; **Concept:** Safety; Violence; Stress; **Integrated Processes:** Nursing Process: Implementation; **Client Needs:** Safe and Effective Care Environment: Safety and Infection; **Cognitive Level:** Application [Applying]

## 2228. MoC ANSWER: 2

1. It is true that the inappropriate use of physical restraints is a legal liability, but this option does not emphasize the most important information.
2. **Historically, use of physical restraints was viewed as an intervention to manage violent or self-destructive clients. Thus the most important information should be that the use of physical restraints has a highly negative emotional impact and should be avoided when possible.**
3. It is true that physical restraints are used only if all other strategies to manage the aggressive behavior have failed, but the most important information is the negative emotional impact that restraints have on the client.
4. In most cases the mentally ill client who is acting in an aggressive manner is unable (not unwilling) to control the behavior. Physical restraints should never be used as a form of punishment.

▶ *Test-taking Tip: Client safety, both physically and emotionally, is a primary concern. Only one option addresses the impact on the client.*

**Content Area:** Mental Health; **Concept:** Safety; **Integrated Processes:** Teaching/Learning; **Client Needs:** Safe and Effective Care Environment: Management of Care; Safe and Effective Care Environment: Safety and Infection Control; **Cognitive Level:** Application [Applying]

**2229. ANSWER: 2**
1. While pain is a stressor, it alone is not an indication that the client will become violent.
2. **Alcohol or drug intoxication is a predictor of violent behavior due to the individual's altered cognitive function.**
3. Gang affiliation, while suggestive of a violent environment, is not by itself an indicator of violent behavior in the ED setting.
4. While schizophrenia can result in paranoid delusions that can precipitate aggression, a diagnosis of schizophrenia alone is not a factor in violent behavior.

♦ *Test-taking Tip: Concentrate on the key words "greatest potential." Violence is predictable in situations where the individual is cognitively impaired and not capable of making rational decisions.*

Content Area: Mental Health; Concept: Violence; Addiction; Integrated Processes: Nursing Process: Analysis; Client Needs: Safe and Effective Care Environment: Safety and Infection Control; Cognitive Level: Analysis [Analyzing]

**2230.** **MoC** **ANSWER: 4**
1. Understanding and possessing effective de-escalating techniques is valuable but will not be effective until the person engages in self-reflection concerning personal responses to violence.
2. This question requires a "yes" or "no" response and adds little to the nurse's self-awareness.
3. Self-reflection into how one would react cannot effectively occur until one is aware of the emotions triggered when facing the situation.
4. **This statement best enhances the nurse's self-awareness. The nurse's ability to intervene safely with a violent client depends on self-awareness of strengths, needs, concerns, and vulnerabilities.**

♦ *Test-taking Tip: Self-awareness requires self-reflection. Only one option encourages self-reflection.*

Content Area: Mental Health; Concept: Self; Nursing Roles; Integrated Processes: Nursing Process: Implementation; Client Needs: Safe and Effective Care Environment: Management of Care; Psychosocial Integrity; Cognitive Level: Application [Applying]

**2231. ANSWER: 2**
1. While refusing to attend a mandatory group session requires the nurse's intervention, it is not the priority of the options.
2. **Making an overtly aggressive statement presents a risk to the safety of other clients and the unit milieu, and it requires immediate intervention by the nurse.**
3. Petitioning for a modification of a perceived unfair regulation is a healthy, socially acceptable attempt at change.
4. Crying is an expression of grief, not typically of aggression.

♦ *Test-taking Tip: The key word is "immediate." Note that one option is different from the others.*

Content Area: Mental Health; Concept: Safety; Assessment; Mood; Integrated Processes: Nursing Process: Assessment; Client Needs: Safe and Effective Care Environment: Safety and Infection Control; Cognitive Level: Analysis [Analyzing]

**2232. ANSWER: 2**
1. Monitoring medication effectiveness is important, but developing a trusting relationship is best.
2. **Developing a trusting relationship with clients enables the nurse to better predict and prevent dangerous behavior through early intervention. A trusting relationship allows the nurse to use psychological support to reduce risk.**
3. Proper documentation is a nursing task that should be completed but provides little help to promote unit safety.
4. Keeping clients separated is often not part of the therapeutic process, as the goal is to reintegrate clients into society.

♦ *Test-taking Tip: Narrow the options to an intervention with clients.*

Content Area: Mental Health; Concept: Safety; Violence; Integrated Processes: Nursing Process: Implementation; Client Needs: Safe and Effective Care Environment: Safety and Infection; Cognitive Level: Application [Applying]

**2233.** **MoC** **ANSWER: 4**
1. De-escalating the client's agitation only addresses the individual client's needs.
2. Eliminating the source of the client's agitation is client-centered and does not address the safety of others.
3. Assessing the client's agitation level does not address the safety of the environment and focuses solely on the client's needs.
4. **The safety of the client, staff, and others is a nursing priority when the client begins to show aggression.**

♦ *Test-taking Tip: Use Maslow's Hierarchy of Needs theory to prioritize the options. Three options focus on the client, whereas one option is different. Usually the option that is different is the answer.*

Content Area: Mental Health; Concept: Violence; Safety; Integrated Processes: Nursing Process: Implementation; Client Needs: Safe and Effective Care Environment: Management of Care; Psychosocial Integrity; Cognitive Level: Analysis [Analyzing]

# SEXUAL DISORDERS
**2234. ANSWER: 3**
1. Behavioral therapy focuses on achieving satiation to make the sexual fantasy less arousing or exciting.
2. Behavioral therapy focuses on aversion techniques to reduce undesirable behavior.
3. **Psychoanalytical therapy focuses on resolving unresolved conflicts and trauma from early childhood. The goal is to alleviate anxiety that prevents the client from forming appropriate sexual relationships.**

4. Biological treatment focuses on reducing the level of circulating androgens. The goal is to reduce libido by administering antiandrogenic medications that block testosterone synthesis or block androgen receptors.

▶ *Test-taking Tip: Narrow the options to think about which description fits best with behavioral therapy, biological therapy, or psychoanalytical therapy.*

**Content Area:** Mental Health; **Concept:** Trauma; Stress; **Integrated Processes:** Communication and Documentation; **Client Needs:** Psychosocial Integrity; **Cognitive Level:** Application [Applying]

### 2235. ANSWER: 4

1. Sexual activity in public places is not a criterion for paraphilia.
2. Sex with numerous partners does not classify as paraphilia.
3. Sexual activity with members of the same sex does not meet the criteria for paraphilia.
4. **The nurse should be aware that paraphilia involves sexual fantasies or behaviors involving repetitive sexual activity with real or simulated suffering or humiliation. Paraphilias may include a sexual preference for a nonhuman object as well as repetitive sexual activity with nonconsenting partners.**

▶ *Test-taking Tip: Apply knowledge of medical terminology. Select the option that is vastly different from the other options.*

**Content Area:** Mental Health; **Concept:** Sexuality; Stress; Trauma; **Integrated Processes:** Nursing Process: Analysis; **Client Needs:** Psychosocial Integrity; **Cognitive Level:** Application [Applying]

### 2236. ANSWER: 2

1. Past sexual abuse may be a factor in hypoactive sexual desire, but it is considered a psychosocial factor and not a biological factor.
2. **The nurse should identify that chronic alcohol use could predispose the client to hypoactive sexual desire disorder. Other substances that may contribute to this disorder are cocaine and antidepressant use.**
3. Sexual identity conflict may impact sexual desire; however, this is a psychosocial issue.
4. Elevated (not decreased) serum prolactin levels have been found for both men and women to be a biological factor contributing to hypoactive sexual desire disorder.

▶ *Test-taking Tip: Note that three options pertain to mental health disorders, whereas one option is different. Often the option that is different is the answer.*

**Content Area:** Mental Health; **Concept:** Sexuality; Addiction; Assessment; **Integrated Processes:** Nursing Process: Assessment; **Client Needs:** Health Promotion and Maintenance; **Cognitive Level:** Application [Applying]

# SCHIZOPHRENIA SPECTRUM AND OTHER PSYCHOTIC DISORDERS

### 2237. ANSWER: 4

1. Claiming to be God does not meet the criteria of being a danger to self or others.
2. Leaving the hospital does not meet the criteria of being a danger to self or others.
3. Talking about a previous suicide attempt does not meet the criteria of being a danger to self or others. Discussion of past suicidal behavior does indicate present state of mind.
4. **The client can be forced to take medication if dangerous behavior is exhibited to self or others. The client must also be judged incompetent, and the medication must have a reasonable chance of helping the client.**

▶ *Test-taking Tip: Note that three options pertain to self-harm, whereas one option pertains to harming others. Select the option that is different from the other options.*

**Content Area:** Mental Health; **Concept:** Medication; Cognition; Safety; **Integrated Processes:** Nursing Process: Implementation; **Client Needs:** Safe and Effective Care Environment: Safety and Infection Control; **Cognitive Level:** Application [Applying]

### 2238. ANSWER: 2

1. While a strong, effective support system is important to any client with similar needs, the development of a discharge plan is not solely dependent on it.
2. **Research has identified that the nurse-client relationship that is accepting, trusting, and mutually respectful is the most important factor in the therapeutic treatment of the homeless client. Compliance of the client with paranoid delusions is especially dependent on the ability to trust health care professionals and the information and services they provide.**
3. Although consideration needs to be given to the client's ability to comply with the discharge plan, the nurse's ability to work effectively with the homeless client is the primary factor when developing the plan.
4. While the availability of needed services and community acceptance is vital to discharge planning, it is not the primary factor in the development of an appropriate, effective discharge plan.

▶ *Test-taking Tip: The key term is "primary factor." Use the process of elimination to select the option that best indicates knowledge of the needs of the client who is homeless and diagnosed with paranoid schizophrenia.*

**Content Area:** Mental Health; **Concept:** Cognition; Collaboration; **Integrated Processes:** Caring; Nursing Process: Planning; **Client Needs:** Psychosocial Integrity; **Cognitive Level:** Synthesis [Creating]

### 2239. MoC ANSWER: 2

1. This statement is an inappropriate and ineffective means of working with a delusional client. However, this action does not require the most immediate attention because it is not likely to result in a safety issue.

2. Attempting to convince a delusional client and prove the client wrong is likely to increase the client's anxiety and result in acting out behavior that can be a risk to both the client and the milieu. The NA needs to be instructed immediately that such attempts to logically address the client's delusions are nontherapeutic and pose a concern for safety.
3. This statement requires follow-up when requested but is not likely to result in a safety issue.
4. Requesting a transfer to another client requires follow-up but is not likely to result in a safety issue.

▶ *Test-taking Tip: A safety issue would require the nurse's immediate attention. Narrow the options to the only two options where the assistant is providing care to the client.*

Content Area: Mental Health; Concept: Cognition; Management; Integrated Processes: Nursing Process: Evaluation; Client Needs: Safe and Effective Care Environment: Management of Care; Safe and Effective Care Environment: Safety and Infection Control; Cognitive Level: Evaluation [Evaluating]

**2240. MoC ANSWER: 3**
1. To refuse treatment is an important client right, but it does not directly affect the client's ability to be discharged from involuntary commitment.
2. Freedom from restraint is an important client right, but it does not directly affect the client's ability to be discharged from involuntary commitment.
3. **The nurse should consider the client's right to the least-restrictive environment. If the client has been stabilized and no longer displays suicidal ideation, it is possible to treat the client on an outpatient basis.**
4. The right to an appropriate service plan is an important client right but does not directly affect the client's ability to be discharged.

▶ *Test-taking Tip: Avoid reading into the question. The client is not refusing treatment but requesting to leave the hospital. Use the process of elimination to narrow the options.*

Content Area: Mental Health; Concept: Mood; Self; Safety; Integrated Processes: Nursing Process: Planning; Client Needs: Safe and Effective Care Environment: Management of Care; Psychosocial Integrity; Cognitive Level: Analysis [Analyzing]

**2241. MoC PHARM ANSWER: 2, 6, 3, 5, 1, 4**
2. **Withhold all doses of antipsychotic medication; the client is experiencing NMS, and these medications can worsen the client's condition.**
6. **Retake vital signs. Current information is needed before contacting the HCP.**
3. **Assess level of consciousness. Level of consciousness and muscle rigidity will fluctuate in that order of progression.**
5. **Assess degree of muscle rigidity. As the level of consciousness decreases, muscle rigidity increases.**
1. **Notify the HCP of the assessment findings and obtain the order for a medication to counteract the effects of NMS. A focused assessment should be complete before notifying the HCP.**

4. **Give bromocriptine (Parlodel) as prescribed by the HCP STAT; bromocriptine will counteract the effects of NMS.**

▶ *Test-taking Tip: Because this is a life-threatening concern, an action should be taken before completing the focused assessment. Then use the nursing process to prioritize the remaining assessments and actions.*

Content Area: Mental Health; Concept: Medication; Safety; Neurologic Regulation; Integrated Processes: Nursing Process: Implementation; Client Needs: Safe and Effective Care Environment: Management of Care; Physiological Integrity: Pharmacological and Parenteral Therapies; Cognitive Level: Synthesis [Creating]

**2242. ANSWER: 2, 3, 4**
1. The client will need intervention when hallucinations occur; they should not be ignored.
2. **The client should maintain good physical health through exercise to prevent relapse.**
3. **Adequate sleep is important in the prevention of a relapse of schizophrenic symptoms.**
4. **Stress-management is an important part of preventing a schizophrenic relapse.**
5. While the client will need to recognize and manage stress, there is no known therapeutic value in avoiding certain types of employment.

▶ *Test-taking Tip: Look for the key words in the options: "ignore," "engage," "report," "enroll," and "avoid," respectively. Select the options that are positive in nature.*

Content Area: Mental Health; Concept: Cognition; Nursing Roles; Integrated Processes: Nursing Process: Planning; Client Needs: Psychosocial Integrity; Cognitive Level: Analysis [Analyzing]

**2243. ANSWER: 1**
1. **Stating the need to watch for signs of depression indicates the father understands that the client's diagnosis of paranoid schizophrenia is associated with a high risk of depression. Clients diagnosed with schizophrenia are also at a higher risk for suicide when suffering from depression.**
2. While medication compliance is an important factor in managing paranoid schizophrenia, it does not guarantee that symptoms will not get worse.
3. Although there have been incidences of a sole schizophrenic episode resulting in hospitalization, the course of this condition typically includes both periods of exacerbation requiring further hospitalization and periods of remission of symptoms.
4. The client diagnosed with schizophrenia will function best with a treatment plan that encourages independence within the capabilities of the client. A lifestyle that is too restrictive is likely to result in rebellion and noncompliance.

▶ *Test-taking Tip: You need to focus on "diagnosis" in the stem and associated problems that can occur with paranoid schizophrenia.*

Content Area: Mental Health; Concept: Mood; Nursing Roles; Communication; Integrated Processes: Nursing Process: Evaluation; Client Needs: Safe and Effective Care Environment: Safety and Infection Control; Cognitive Level: Evaluation [Evaluating]

## 2244. ANSWER: 4

1. The mother's expectation is not a realistic expectation because medication does not improve symptoms associated with paranoid schizophrenia within 2 days.
2. A request for medication adjustment reflects a need to provide the mother with appropriate information related to her son's condition.
3. There is no information to suggest that the mother thinks her son has an issue with the government.
4. **Two days is insufficient time for the client to experience the therapeutic benefits of treatment for paranoid schizophrenia.**

▶ *Test-taking Tip: The key phrase is "two days after admission." With treatment, improvement of symptoms associated with paranoid schizophrenia usually occurs between 5 and 9 days.*

Content Area: Mental Health; Concept: Cognition; Nursing Roles; Integrated Processes: Nursing Process: Evaluation; Client Needs: Psychosocial Integrity; Cognitive Level: Evaluation [Evaluating]

## 2245. PHARM ANSWER: 2

1. Olanzapine (Zyprexa) is an atypical antipsychotic drug that can cause extrapyramidal side effects.
2. **Benztropine (Cogentin) is an anticholinergic drug that is the drug of choice to control the extrapyramidal side effects caused by traditional antipsychotic medications.**
3. Chlorpromazine (Thorazine) is an antipsychotic in the same drug classification as haloperidol.
4. Escitalopram oxalate (Lexapro) is an SSRI used to treat depression.

▶ *Test-taking Tip: Narrow the options by eliminating antipsychotic and SSRI medications.*

Content Area: Mental Health; Concept: Cognition; Medication; Integrated Processes: Nursing Process: Planning; Client Needs: Physiological Integrity: Pharmacological and Parenteral Therapies; Cognitive Level: Application [Applying]

## 2246. ANSWER: 2

1. Sleeping 6 hours a night may not be a realistic goal for the client.
2. **The excited phase of catatonic schizophrenia is marked by periods of extreme activity and potential violent behavior. The primary nursing focus for the client during this phase is to prevent both physical exhaustion and injury by providing adequate food and fluids and by maintaining a safe, low-stimulus environment.**
3. The client-to-client interaction each day may be unrealistic.
4. Showing decreased activity within 24 hours of the onset of hyperactivity may not be a realistic goal for the client.

▶ *Test-taking Tip: Use Maslow's Hierarchy of Needs theory to identify the correct responses. Physiological need should be the priority; only a single option addresses the most basic physiological need.*

Content Area: Mental Health; Concept: Safety; Nursing Roles; Cognition; Integrated Processes: Nursing Process: Analysis; Client Needs: Psychosocial Integrity; Cognitive Level: Analysis [Analyzing]

## 2247. ANSWER: 1

1. **The client is experiencing paranoia and is distrustful and suspicious of others. Laughing or whispering in front of the client would only serve to increase the client's suspicions.**
2. Having the client sign a release may not be appropriate due to the client's current level of awareness.
3. Asking the client to trust and to share personal information with strangers is unachievable at this time.
4. The client is not ready to identify information concerning community support.

▶ *Test-taking Tip: You need to focus on the nursing problem of paranoia to select the most appropriate intervention.*

Content Area: Mental Health; Concept: Safety; Cognition; Integrated Processes: Nursing Process: Planning; Communication and Documentation; Client Needs: Psychosocial Integrity; Cognitive Level: Application [Applying]

## 2248. ANSWER: 4

1. Discussion concerning the hallucination has no therapeutic value.
2. Asking a "why" question is not therapeutic and can initiate a defensive response.
3. Disagreeing may initiate a defensive response and hinder therapeutic communication.
4. **Empathizing with the client's experience is most therapeutic so that the true root of the client's concern can be addressed. The main characteristic of paranoid schizophrenia is the presence of persecutory or grandiose delusions and hallucinations.**

▶ *Test-taking Tip: The key phrase is "therapeutic." Only one option uses an approach that is not challenging the client.*

Content Area: Mental Health; Concept: Communication; Cognition; Sensory Perception; Integrated Processes: Nursing Process: Implementation; Client Needs: Psychosocial Integrity; Safe and Effective Care Environment: Safety and Infection Control; Cognitive Level: Application [Applying]

## 2249. PHARM ANSWER: 3

1. Dismissing the symptoms is not a therapeutic approach to the client's concerns.
2. Telling the client to ignore the symptoms is being insensitive to the client's concerns.
3. **Nightmares and tremors are common in alcohol withdrawal, but not as side effects of olanzapine. Olanzapine (Zyprexa) is more likely to cause sleeplessness, nausea, dizziness, constipation, weight gain, and headache.**

4. If the client were currently drinking alcohol, there might be an additive effect, but this is not true since the client has abstained for 5 days.

▸ **Test-taking Tip:** The key phrase is "most therapeutic." Narrow to those options providing information and eliminate options that give nontherapeutic responses.

Content Area: Mental Health; Concept: Cognition; Assessment; Addiction; Integrated Processes: Nursing Process: Implementation; Client Needs: Physiological Integrity: Pharmacological and Parenteral Therapies; Cognitive Level: Analysis [Analyzing]

## 2250. ANSWER: 4

1. This response supports the client's delusion and does not enforce reality.
2. This statement is challenging and can initiate defensiveness. It also supports the client's delusion.
3. Although this may refocus the client, this response does not provide an opportunity to discuss the root of the client's true fears.
4. **Telling the client who the men are and why they are in the room reinforces reality for the client with paranoid delusions.**

▸ **Test-taking Tip:** When the client has paranoid delusions, the primary intervention is directed toward therapeutic communication between the nurse and client that will help the client identify and express the reason(s) for anxiety while reinforcing reality.

Content Area: Mental Health; Concept: Cognition; Communication; Nursing Roles; Integrated Processes: Communication and Documentation; Client Needs: Psychosocial Integrity; Cognitive Level: Analysis [Analyzing]

## 2251. ANSWER: 4

1. The client's delusion does not pose any immediate threat to the nurse's ability to provide a safe setting. Therefore the nurse should not refuse the request to show control.
2. The nurse should not comply with the request, as it supports the delusion.
3. The nurse should show understanding, but avoid complying with the request as it supports the delusion.
4. **The most appropriate intervention is to empathize with the client's concerns/fear while making it clear that the nurse does not share the client's delusion by refusing to comply with the client's request.**

▸ **Test-taking Tip:** Examine options with duplicate information first (Options 1 and 4, and then 2 and 3). Eliminate one of each of these to narrow the options.

Content Area: Mental Health; Concept: Cognition; Communication; Integrated Processes: Caring; Nursing Process: Implementation; Client Needs: Psychosocial Integrity; Cognitive Level: Analysis [Analyzing]

## 2252. ANSWER: 1

1. **When dealing with the client who is hallucinating, the most appropriate intervention is for the nurse to empathize with the client's experience while engaging in therapeutic communication to discuss the root of the client's concern. Asking the client to explain the cause of the anger is client-centered and focuses on the behavior.**

2. Observation does nothing to control and/or de-escalate the situation.
3. Seclusion is used only as a last resort and in cases of client/milieu safety.
4. Threatening restraint use may cause the client to escalate the inappropriate behavior.

▸ **Test-taking Tip:** Only one option focuses on a continuing interaction with the client, and other options are different.

Content Area: Mental Health; Concept: Cognition; Safety; Violence; Integrated Processes: Nursing Process: Implementation; Client Needs: Safe and Effective Care Environment: Safety and Infection Control; Cognitive Level: Analysis [Analyzing]

## 2253. ANSWER: 2

1. A crisis may occur between appointments and require immediate professional counseling.
2. **The most appropriate response is for the nurse to provide a list of centers that are prepared to provide immediate crisis intervention for the client experiencing hallucinations.**
3. Distracting the client may only serve to exacerbate the hallucinations.
4. Providing the unit's telephone number does not guarantee immediate crisis intervention.

▸ **Test-taking Tip:** You need to consider the safe management of schizophrenic relapse to select the correct option.

Content Area: Mental Health; Concept: Cognition; Family; Nursing Roles; Integrated Processes: Nursing Process: Planning; Client Needs: Safe and Effective Care Environment: Safety and Infection Control; Health Promotion and Maintenance; Cognitive Level: Analysis [Analyzing]

## 2254. MoC ANSWER: 3

1. Seclusion should not be considered as an initial intervention because it is the most restrictive of the options.
2. Removing items that would aid in an act of self-harm does not provide the degree of safety that constant one-on-one observation provides.
3. **The most effective nursing intervention to ensure that the client is in a safe environment is for the nurse to assign a staff member to constantly observe the client.**
4. The client should not be involved in structured activities with others because undivided attention of staff is required in order to reduce/eliminate the risk of suicide.

▸ **Test-taking Tip:** You need to focus on the option most likely to result in the safest, least-restrictive environment for this client.

Content Area: Mental Health; Concept: Safety; Self; Cognition; Integrated Processes: Nursing Process: Planning; Client Needs: Safe and Effective Care Environment: Management of Care; Safe and Effective Care Environment: Safety and Infection Control; Cognitive Level: Analysis [Analyzing]

## 2255. ANSWER: 4

1. Leaving avoids the client's concerns.
2. Asking the client to provide a rationale for the fear does not foster a therapeutic relationship.

3. Being argumentative and avoiding the client's concerns are not examples of therapeutic communication techniques.

4. **It is most therapeutic for the nurse to empathize with the client's experience while engaging in therapeutic communication to discuss the true root of the client's concern.**

▶ **Test-taking Tip:** *Only one option shows empathy while not supporting the client's delusion.*

**Content Area:** Mental Health; **Concept:** Cognition; Communication; Safety; **Integrated Processes:** Communication and Documentation; **Client Needs:** Psychosocial Integrity; **Cognitive Level:** Analysis [Analyzing]

### 2256. ANSWER: 1

1. **When communicating with the client with paranoid delusions, the most appropriate response is for the nurse to empathize with the client's experience while engaging in therapeutic communication to discuss the true root of the client's concern. Asking if the client is afraid is client-centered and focuses on the client's fears.**

2. Disagreeing with the client may make the client more defensive and thus interfere with therapeutic communication.

3. Encouraging discussion only about the delusion is nontherapeutic.

4. Encouraging the client to discuss the delusion more is nontherapeutic.

▶ **Test-taking Tip:** *The key phrase is "most therapeutic." Eliminate options that focus on the delusion. Note that three options include the "neighbor," and one option is different. The option that is different is often the answer.*

**Content Area:** Mental Health; **Concept:** Cognition; Safety; Communication; **Integrated Processes:** Nursing Process: Implementation; Caring; **Client Needs:** Psychosocial Integrity; **Cognitive Level:** Analysis [Analyzing]

### 2257. MoC PHARM ANSWER: 3

1. While the symptoms would indicate a possible cardiac problem, questioning the client does not address the immediate seriousness of the potential problem and the need for intervention.

2. Assuring the client is inappropriate since neuroleptic malignant syndrome (NMS) is possible with the use of antipsychotic medication. The nurse should never ignore symptoms of tachycardia, hypertension, or hyperthermia.

3. **The nurse should immediately notify the HCP because severe muscle spasms, muscle rigidity, hypertension, fever, and tachycardia associated with the use of haloperidol (Haldol) suggest the possibility of the life-threatening condition of NMS.**

4. While an infection may result in some of the symptoms, it would not account for the hypertension and severe muscle pain.

▶ **Test-taking Tip:** *The key word is "next." When a life-threatening condition exists, immediate intervention is necessary.*

**Content Area:** Mental Health; **Concept:** Assessment; Medication; Safety; **Integrated Processes:** Nursing Process: Assessment; **Client Needs:** Safe and Effective Care Environment: Management of Care; Physiological Integrity: Pharmacological and Parenteral Therapies; **Cognitive Level:** Analysis [Analyzing]

### 2258. ANSWER: 1, 3

1. **The client experiencing a catatonic state may be immobile and mute, but the client still requires constant monitoring for safety. The nurse facilitates safety by sitting with the client.**

2. The client should not be moved into the dayroom, as safety evaluations could not be assured.

3. **Therapeutic communication with a withdrawn client should be maintained since it is believed that the client in a catatonic state is aware of surroundings. Communication with the client, occasionally asking open-ended questions, and pausing to provide opportunities for the client to respond are important.**

4. The client is not capable of the client-to-client interaction.

5. It is unsafe to leave the client alone.

6. Social communication is not possible while the client is in a catatonic state.

▶ **Test-taking Tip:** *Use the nursing process and eliminate assessments because the question is asking for interventions.*

**Content Area:** Mental Health; **Concept:** Safety; Communication; Cognition; **Integrated Processes:** Nursing Process: Implementation; **Client Needs:** Psychosocial Integrity; **Cognitive Level:** Application [Applying]

### 2259. ANSWER: 2

1. This statement does not demonstrate knowledge of interventions for anxiety; anxiety may be a side effect.

2. **The client should be aware of the importance of discussing hallucinations as they occur with the therapist. Calling the therapist is a specific agreement to seek help and evidences self-responsible commitment and control over the client's own behavior.**

3. Attending a support group does not provide any specific intervention for the management of hallucinations and/or anxiety.

4. Eating well and getting enough sleep does not provide any specific intervention for the management of hallucinations and/or anxiety.

▶ **Test-taking Tip:** *Use the process of elimination to select the only option that provides a specific intervention for hallucinations.*

**Content Area:** Mental Health; **Concept:** Stress; Safety; Nursing Roles; **Integrated Processes:** Nursing Process: Evaluation; **Client Needs:** Safe and Effective Care Environment: Safety and Infection Control; Health Promotion and Maintenance; **Cognitive Level:** Evaluation [Evaluating]

**2260. ANSWER: 1**

1. **The prognosis for clients diagnosed with schizophreniform disorder is good as long as they do not develop the characteristic behaviors of schizophrenia. The duration of this disorder is greater than 1 but less than 6 months.**
2. Impaired social or occupational functioning is not always apparent with schizophreniform disorder.
3. There are dissimilarities between schizophreniform disorder and schizophrenia.
4. It is not true that schizophreniform disorder always progresses to schizophrenia.

▶ *Test-taking Tip: Three options focus on negative aspects, and one focuses on the positive. Often the option that is different is the answer.*

Content Area: Mental Health; Concept: Cognition; Self; Nursing Roles; Integrated Processes: Nursing Process: Evaluation; Client Needs: Psychosocial Integrity; Cognitive Level: Evaluation [Evaluating]

**2261. ANSWER: 2**

1. Risperidone (Risperdal) is not a controlled substance. Some agencies may provide multidose medication packets. There is no need for the nurse to complete a variance report.
2. **The nurse should complete a variance report when finding a controlled substance in the client's medication box. The Ⓒ IV on the label indicates that clonazepam (Klonopin) is a controlled substance. Schedule IV medications must be secured differently than medications that are not controlled substances.**
3. There is no need for the nurse to complete a variance report when finding venlafaxine (Effexor) in the client's medication drawer. Pregnancy category C medications do not require additional security measures.
4. There is no need for the nurse to complete a variance report when finding lithium carbonate in the client's medication drawer. Pregnancy category D medications do not require additional security measures.

▶ *Test-taking Tip: Controlled substances have a categorization of schedule I to V, which indicates the potential for abuse. Schedule I controlled substances have the highest potential for abuse and are not acceptable for medical use (such as heroin). Controlled substances require additional security measures and must be counted and signed out from a specified location at the time of administration.*

Content Area: Mental Health; Concept: Cognition; Self; Nursing Roles; Integrated Processes: Nursing Process: Evaluation; Client Needs: Safe and Effective Care Environment: Safety and Infection Control; Cognitive Level: Evaluation [Evaluating]

**2262. ANSWER: 3**

1. The rapid eye movement is characteristic of stage I reaction to hallucination.
2. Increased HR is seen in stage II reaction to hallucination.
3. **The stage IV reaction to hallucinations includes violence and/or agitation as observed by the client's fist pounding.**
4. Failing to follow directions other than those provided by the hallucination is representative of stage III reaction to hallucination.

▶ *Test-taking Tip: Hallucination staging occurs in four stages, with the most severe symptoms occurring in stage IV.*

Content Area: Mental Health; Concept: Stress; Cognition; Assessment; Integrated Processes: Nursing Process: Assessment; Client Needs: Safe and Effective Care Environment: Safety and Infection Control; Cognitive Level: Application [Applying]

**2263. MoC ANSWER: 3**

1. Hospitals are restricted from prohibiting sexual behavior because they are governed by a least-restrictive policy.
2. Sexual behavior in inpatient units is not used as a therapeutic tool to speed recovery.
3. **Due to the legal case *Johnson v. The United States*, clients residing in adult inpatient psychiatric units should be governed by a "least restrictive" policy. This includes developing policies that least restrict the freedom of clients.**
4. Sexual behavior is not used to help those diagnosed with personality disorders.

▶ *Test-taking Tip: Relate words in the stem of the question with words in the options, such as "protocol" in the stem and "policy" in an option.*

Content Area: Mental Health; Concept: Sexuality; Safety; Ethics; Integrated Processes: Nursing Process: Evaluation; Client Needs: Safe and Effective Care Environment: Management of Care; Cognitive Level: Evaluation [Evaluating]

# NEUROCOGNITIVE DISORDERS

**2264. ANSWER: 1, 2, 5**

1. **Dementia is associated with having experienced head trauma during childhood.**
2. **Dementia is associated with inhalant abuse, especially as a teenager.**
3. While there is some evidence that hypothyroidism is a risk factor for dementia, there is none showing a relationship with hyperthyroidism.
4. There is no research to support that type 1 DM is a risk factor for dementia.
5. **Dementia is associated with degenerative brain disorders such as Parkinson's disease.**

▶ *Test-taking Tip: Narrow the options to those that affect brain function.*

Content Area: Mental Health; Concept: Cognition; Integrated Processes: Nursing Process: Analysis; Client Needs: Physiological Integrity: Reduction of Risk Potential; Cognitive Level: Knowledge [Remembering]

**2265. ANSWER: 2**

1. Even though this addresses the client's concern for the well-being of the animals, it does not clarify the statement of "raining cats and dogs." This response can falsely reinforce the idea that the cats and dogs are real.

2. The most therapeutic response is to explain to the client that "raining cats and dogs" is a way of saying that it is raining heavily. The client who continually gives literal translations to verbal communication is exhibiting concrete thinking. Due to the client's inability to think in the abstract, care must be taken to avoid conversations that include abstract concepts.

3. While the staff needs to be aware of the client's limitation in understanding the abstract, alerting the staff does not address the issue of presenting information for the client in an acceptable manner.

4. Documentation of the client's limitations is appropriate but does not address the issue of clarification of ideas and information.

▶ *Test-taking Tip: The key phrase is "most therapeutic." Only one option clarifies the nurse's statement.*

**Content Area:** Mental Health; **Concept:** Cognition; Communication; **Integrated Processes:** Communication and Documentation; **Client Needs:** Psychosocial Integrity; **Cognitive Level:** Application [Applying]

## 2266. ANSWER: 4

1. While medication may become appropriate, it should not be the first response to manage the client's behavior. It does not address the issue of observing the client for safety.

2. Transferring the client closer to the nurse's station does not provide the constant observation that is most appropriate for the client at this time.

3. Asking the client's spouse to stay may not be a realistic expectation.

4. The client's immediate safety is the primary concern, and constant observation is the best means of providing a safe environment for this client.

▶ *Test-taking Tip: Use Maslow's Hierarchy of Needs theory to determine the priority action. Client safety is priority.*

**Content Area:** Mental Health; **Concept:** Cognition; Safety; **Integrated Processes:** Nursing Process: Implementation; **Client Needs:** Safe and Effective Care Environment: Safety and Infection Control; **Cognitive Level:** Analysis [Analyzing]

## 2267. ANSWER: 1

1. **The nurse should ask the client's spouse to describe a typical day. Using an open-ended questioning technique provides the client's spouse with an opportunity to share information that the spouse feels is appropriate. Based on the information provided, the nurse can then ask questions that are more specific to the areas of concern.**

2. This question presumes that the client's spouse is experiencing stress and may cause the spouse to become defensive.

3. This is a closed-ended question that limits the discussion.

4. This question presumes that the spouse is experiencing stress and limits discussion, since it requires only a "yes" or "no" answer.

▶ *Test-taking Tip: Three options are similar, assuming that the client's spouse has stress, and one option is different. Often the option that is different is the answer.*

**Content Area:** Mental Health; **Concept:** Cognition; Stress; Assessment; Communication; **Integrated Processes:** Nursing Process: Assessment; **Client Needs:** Psychosocial Integrity; **Cognitive Level:** Application [Applying]

## 2268. ANSWER: 1, 2, 3

1. **Delirium is a condition that has a good prognosis when treatment is appropriate and initiated in a timely manner.**

2. **A delirious individual often demonstrates varied and rapid mood swings.**

3. **Delirium involves a rapid change in mental status often due to alcohol or sedative withdrawal, electrolyte imbalances, infection, surgery, change in medications, and other causes. It is usually short-term and reversible once the cause has been identified and treated.**

4. A family history of Alzheimer's disease is related to dementia rather than delirium.

5. Short-term memory loss usually resolves once the cause for the delirium has been identified and interventions initiated.

▶ *Test-taking Tip: Options 3 and 5 are opposites. Both cannot be correct.*

**Content Area:** Mental Health; **Concept:** Cognition; Nursing Roles; **Integrated Processes:** Teaching/Learning; **Client Needs:** Psychosocial Integrity; **Cognitive Level:** Application [Applying]

## 2269. ANSWER: 1, 2, 4

1. **Dementia affects an individual's ability to think abstractly. Crossing the street when it is safe requires abstract thinking.**

2. **"Red sky tonight means sailor's delight" requires an understanding of the phrase and the ability to think abstractly.**

3. The client with dementia will likely remember a story; some long-term memory is usually retained until dementia is in its final stages.

4. **To dress in "good" clothes is a judgment that would not likely be within the abilities of a person with dementia.**

5. Remembering how to perform a task that was repeated over the years will likely remain with the individual until the dementia is in its final stages.

▶ *Test-taking Tip: Cognitive effects commonly associated with dementia include decreased access to short-term memory, decreased ability to make solid judgments, and inability to think abstractly. Eliminate options related to long-term memory.*

**Content Area:** Mental Health; **Concept:** Cognition; **Integrated Processes:** Nursing Process: Assessment; **Client Needs:** Psychosocial Integrity; **Cognitive Level:** Analysis [Analyzing]

**2270.** **MoC** **ANSWER: 2**

1. Removing the restraints when the client sleeps may need clarification and teaching, but this is not the most immediate need.
2. **The immediate concern is client safety. A severely disoriented client should never be left alone while in restraints. The client's impaired judgment places him at high risk for injury.**
3. While this remark shows insensitive care by the NA, it is not the most immediate concern.
4. The bruising on the client's wrists requires follow-up because the restraints may be too tight and teaching may be needed, but leaving a severely disoriented client alone is more important.

▶ *Test-taking Tip: Note the key phrase "safe client care." Reviewing the options and selecting the one that addresses the greatest risk for client injury will direct you to the correct option.*

Content Area: Mental Health; **Concept:** Safety; Cognition; **Integrated Processes:** Nursing Process: Evaluation; **Client Needs:** Safe and Effective Care Environment: Management of Care; Safe and Effective Care Environment: Safety and Infection Control; **Cognitive Level:** Evaluation [Evaluating]

**2271. ANSWER: 2**

1. Mumbling is observed in clients with impaired cognition, but it can be a response to any number of situations, including anger, bewilderment, or experiencing hallucinations.
2. **The client's disorientation is indicative of impaired cognition. Cognitive impairment can affect an individual's orientation to person, place, or time, or memory of recent events.**
3. Staring is seen in clients with impaired cognition, but it can be a response to any number of situations, including fatigue and/or attempts at social isolation.
4. Clients experiencing impaired cognition do not typically experience auditory hallucinations.

▶ *Test-taking Tip: You need to relate "cognition" in the stem to orientation. Only one option focuses on orientation.*

Content Area: Mental Health; **Concept:** Cognition; Assessment; **Integrated Processes:** Nursing Process: Assessment; **Client Needs:** Psychosocial Integrity; **Cognitive Level:** Analysis [Analyzing]

**2272.** **MoC** **ANSWER: 2, 5**

1. While support in the form of sufficient time is appropriate, this response fails to address the fact that the client may never reach total independence.
2. **The client's goals should include being able to function at the highest level of self-independence.**
3. Assuming that the client with dementia and a self-care deficit will reach total independence may not be realistic.
4. Not allowing for client autonomy by assisting with daily needs is not directed toward the client's best interest.

5. **Supporting the family to encourage the client's independence contributes to the client's sense of control and well-being.**

▶ *Test-taking Tip: Options with absolute words such as "unlimited" or "all" are usually incorrect.*

Content Area: Mental Health; **Concept:** Cognition; Nursing Roles; **Integrated Processes:** Nursing Process: Planning; **Client Needs:** Safe and Effective Care Environment: Management of Care; Physiological Integrity: Basic Care and Comfort; Psychosocial Integrity; **Cognitive Level:** Synthesis [Creating]

**2273.** **PHARM** **ANSWER: 4**

1. This statement expresses the wife's gratitude for starting the anticholinesterase medication, but it does not show an understanding of the treatment goals for anticholinesterase medications.
2. Anticholinesterase medications have not been shown to be successful in stopping or reversing the loss of memory resulting from Alzheimer's disease.
3. While it is true that anticholinesterase medications may improve the quality of life, this statement does not address the treatment goals of such therapy as does the correct option.
4. **Drugs classified as anticholinesterase medications are prescribed for clients diagnosed with Alzheimer's disease because they have shown efficacy in slowing the rate of memory loss by interfering with the action of acetylcholinesterase.**

▶ *Test-taking Tip: You should associate Alzheimer's disease in the stem with memory loss in the options.*

Content Area: Mental Health; **Concept:** Nursing Roles; Cognition; **Integrated Processes:** Nursing Process: Evaluation; **Client Needs:** Physiological Integrity: Pharmacological and Parenteral Therapies; **Cognitive Level:** Evaluation [Evaluating]

**2274. ANSWER: 3**

1. Bingo is competitive, which may accelerate the client's agitation and thus place the client and the other residents in a potentially unsafe environment.
2. Spending time alone is not appropriate, as it is not a structured activity and does not promote de-escalation.
3. **The most therapeutic activity would be to take a walk with ancillary staff. Structured activities will provide the client with a release for physical tension as well as an opportunity to build a trusting relationship.**
4. Watching television does not provide a structured outlet for the client and does not promote de-escalation.

▶ *Test-taking Tip: The key phrase is "most therapeutic." Options 1 and 4 are similar in that they increase stimulation; Option 2 eliminates stimulation, and Option 3 has minimal stimulation. If uncertain, select the option with minimal stimulation.*

Content Area: Mental Health; **Concept:** Cognition; Safety; Stress; **Integrated Processes:** Nursing Process: Implementation; **Client Needs:** Safe and Effective Care Environment: Safety and Infection Control; **Cognitive Level:** Analysis [Analyzing]

**2275. ANSWER: 1**

1. **The nurse's priority should be directed at the client's violence. The client's memory loss and violent outbursts pose safety issues for both the client and others.**
2. Although addressing incontinence is important, it does not take priority over the safety of the client and others.
3. Self-care deficit is important to address but is not priority.
4. The nurse should address the client's altered thought processes and impaired memory, but this is not the priority over safety.

▸ **Test-taking Tip:** The key phrase is "priority." Use Maslow's Hierarchy of Needs theory to identify the priority item. Safety is a priority need.

**Content Area:** Mental Health; **Concept:** Cognition; Nursing Roles; Safety; **Integrated Processes:** Nursing Process: Analysis; **Client Needs:** Safe and Effective Care Environment: Safety and Infection Control; **Cognitive Level:** Analysis [Analyzing]

**2276.** **MoC** **ANSWER: 1**

1. **The daughter's question about support services indicates an understanding that her father will experience increased cognitive impairment that will require the support of outside personnel and/or agencies.**
2. While current drug therapy delays the progressive deterioration of cognitive function, there may not be any apparent improvement for this chronic, irreversible, progressive disease.
3. Asking about how long it will take for the medication to help does not demonstrate understanding; medication delays progression but does not necessarily offer improvement.
4. Being able to identify the best treatment program does not mean that the daughter understands the prognosis.

▸ **Test-taking Tip:** The key word is "best." Options 2, 3, and 4 focus on improvement, whereas Option 1 is different. Often the option that is different is the answer.

**Content Area:** Mental Health; **Concept:** Cognition; Nursing Roles; Communication; **Integrated Processes:** Nursing Process: Evaluation; **Client Needs:** Safe and Effective Care Environment: Management of Care; **Cognitive Level:** Evaluation [Evaluating]

# EATING DISORDERS

**2277. ANSWER: 3**

1. While there may be marital discord, the nurse should not make an assumption based solely on this statement. Eating disorders are likely the result of multiple factors.
2. There may be overprotective tendencies within the family, but no one issue is the likely cause.
3. **There is no clear agreement regarding the causes of eating disorders. Current research suggests an interaction of biological susceptibility, including genetic markers for both neurobiological vulnerability and personality traits, and environmental influences, including family, social, and cultural environments.**

4. The father may be experiencing ineffective coping, but the nurse should not assume this based solely on this one statement.

▸ **Test-taking Tip:** Options 2 and 3 are opposites, so both cannot be correct. Knowing that there are multiple factors involved in eating disorders should allow the elimination of all options except 3.

**Content Area:** Mental Health; **Concept:** Nutrition; Stress; Self; **Integrated Processes:** Nursing Process: Analysis; **Client Needs:** Psychosocial Integrity; **Cognitive Level:** Application [Applying]

**2278. ANSWER: 4**

1. While this question encourages discussion, it does not clarify the misconception.
2. This question, while encouraging discussion, does not clarify the misconception.
3. Telling the mother not to worry is a nontherapeutic response.
4. **Research has shown that overprotective parenting usually exists as a reaction to the eating disorder, not as a causative factor.**

▸ **Test-taking Tip:** The most therapeutic response is one that addresses the mother's concern.

**Content Area:** Mental Health; **Concept:** Nutrition; Communication; Stress; Self; **Integrated Processes:** Communication and Documentation; **Client Needs:** Psychosocial Integrity; **Cognitive Level:** Analysis [Analyzing]

**2279. ANSWER: 3, 4, 5**

1. While skin and hair can eventually be affected by poor nutrition, there is no particular need to include special hygiene measures.
2. Oral hygiene is relevant to an individual who purges, such as with bulimia.
3. **The anorexic client may attempt to manage weight with the ingestion of over-the-counter diet products or herbal supplements. These substances can often cause dangerous cardiovascular side effects.**
4. **Orthostatic hypotension can exist due to fluid and electrolyte imbalances, or dizziness can occur from lack of nutrients to the brain. These can result in falls.**
5. **The anorexic client is at risk for developing electrolyte imbalances due to poor food intake.**

▸ **Test-taking Tip:** Focus on the key words "physiological health" and then identify physical systems and functions that are affected by anorexia nervosa.

**Content Area:** Mental Health; **Concept:** Nutrition; Nursing Roles; **Integrated Processes:** Teaching/Learning; **Client Needs:** Physiological Integrity: Basic Care and Comfort; Health Promotion and Maintenance; **Cognitive Level:** Synthesis [Creating]

**2280. ANSWER: 1, 4, 5**

1. **Refusal to eat is associated with anorexia nervosa.**
2. The mean age of onset is between 11 and 18 years. While the onset of 25 years of age is atypical and not expected, this is possible.

3. Anorexia can lead to amenorrhea (absence of three consecutive menstrual cycles) rather than heavy bleeding during menses.

4. **An intense fear of getting fat despite being underweight is associated with anorexia nervosa.**

5. **Criteria for diagnosing anorexia nervosa include weight loss leading to maintaining a body weight less than 85% of the expected weight for body size and age.**

▶ *Test-taking Tip: Read each option carefully; some options are opposite of those seen with anorexia and should be eliminated. Consider that the age of onset can be as young as 8 years old.*

**Content Area:** Mental Health; **Concept:** Nutrition; Stress; Assessment; Self; **Integrated Processes:** Nursing Process: Assessment; **Client Needs:** Psychosocial Integrity; Physiological Integrity: Physiological Adaptation; **Cognitive Level:** Application [Applying]

## 2281. ANSWER: 4

1. Achieving a minimum normal weight is an appropriate outcome but will take time to achieve.

2. Resuming a normal menstrual cycle is an appropriate outcome but will take time to achieve.

3. The client's perception of body weight and shape as normal is a psychosocial outcome and, while appropriate, is not the most urgent.

4. **Consuming adequate calories for metabolic needs meets a basic physiological need and is priority.**

▶ *Test-taking Tip: Use Maslow's Hierarchy of Needs theory to establish a physiological need as the priority outcome to be achieved.*

**Content Area:** Mental Health; **Concept:** Nutrition; Self; **Integrated Processes:** Nursing Process: Analysis; **Client Needs:** Physiological Integrity: Basic Care and Comfort; **Cognitive Level:** Synthesis [Creating]

## 2282. MoC ANSWER: 3, 5, 2, 1, 4

3. **Maintains normal fluid and electrolyte levels. According to client needs, physiological needs should be the most urgent. Because the client has been purging, the outcome that the client will maintain normal fluid and electrolyte levels is priority.**

5. **Consumes adequate calories for age, height, and metabolic need. This also is a physiological need and is next in priority.**

2. **Ceases binge/purge episodes while in inpatient setting. This is a psychosocial outcome but is next because the remaining outcomes cannot be achieved until binging/purging ceases.**

1. **Demonstrates more effective coping skills to deal with conflicts. This is a psychosocial outcome that would come after meeting the client's physiological needs.**

4. **Perceives body shape and weight as normal and acceptable. According to Maslow's Hierarchy of Needs theory, self-actualization is the highest level. This level cannot be achieved until physiological and psychosocial needs have been met.**

▶ *Test-taking Tip: Use Maslow's Hierarchy of Needs theory to place items in the correct sequence. Remember that the basic physiological needs are priority, whereas self-actualization is the least urgent need.*

**Content Area:** Mental Health; **Concept:** Nutrition; Self; **Integrated Processes:** Communication and Documentation; **Client Needs:** Safe and Effective Care Environment: Management of Care; **Cognitive Level:** Synthesis [Creating]

## 2283. PHARM ANSWER: 2

1. Unless a life-threatening situation exists, the nurse should complete the assessment before notifying the HCP of the findings.

2. **By auscultating the client's apical pulse, the nurse can assess the client's HR and rhythm to assess whether an irregularity is present. Abuse of laxatives and diuretics and self-induced vomiting can lead to serious electrolyte imbalances that lead to cardiac dysrhythmias.**

3. Obtaining the names of the abused products is important but is not the next action.

4. Laxatives would produce diarrhea, so asking about the stool consistency and frequency is important but not the next action.

▶ *Test-taking Tip: Think about the effect of laxatives, diuretics, and self-induced vomiting on the client's fluid and electrolyte balance before selecting an option. Use the steps of the nursing process; assessment should be completed before initiating an action unless an initial observation indicates the situation is life-threatening.*

**Content Area:** Mental Health; **Concept:** Nutrition; Fluid and Electrolyte Balance; Safety; **Integrated Processes:** Nursing Process: Implementation; **Client Needs:** Physiological Integrity: Pharmacological and Parenteral Therapies; **Cognitive Level:** Analysis [Analyzing]

## 2284. ANSWER: 1

1. **The cycle of eating disorders must be interrupted because it is life-threatening. The client should be monitored for 1 hour or more after meals to discourage the child from purging.**

2. Eating disorder behaviors are hard (not easy) to change because gaining weight or stopping purging is terrifying to the client.

3. The child should be encouraged, not discouraged, to share what has been learned in group and individual therapy about the particular psychological issues relating to the eating disorder.

4. The child should be expected to follow family rules, including eating meals prepared for the family. The parent should stop preparing separate meals.

▶ *Test-taking Tip: Read each option carefully and examine key words and phrases that make an option incorrect, such as "easily changed," "discourage," and "separate meals." Think about the option that should reinforce the child's treatment for bulimia nervosa.*

**Content Area:** Mental Health; **Concept:** Nutrition; Self; Nursing Roles; **Integrated Processes:** Teaching/Learning; **Client Needs:** Safe and Effective Care Environment: Safety and Infection Control; **Cognitive Level:** Evaluation [Evaluating]

**2285. ANSWER: 4**

1. The expected amount of weight gain is 1 lb per week, not 1 lb in 3 weeks.
2. Engaging in conversations about eating food demonstrates that the client is still preoccupied with food. The expected outcome is absence of preoccupation with food.
3. The absence, not just a reduction, of purging is expected.
4. **Using art therapy demonstrates an ability to choose more effective coping skills to deal with conflicts other than preoccupation with food. Because a person diagnosed with bulimia has difficulty naming feelings or finding the words needed for "talk" therapy, art therapy or other expressive therapies allow for greater self-disclosure and exploration of issues.**

▶ *Test-taking Tip: When reviewing the options, consider the more global issues experienced by clients diagnosed with bulimia nervosa.*

Content Area: Mental Health; Concept: Nutrition; Self; Integrated Processes: Nursing Process: Evaluation; Client Needs: Physiological Integrity: Physiological Adaptation; Cognitive Level: Evaluation [Evaluating]

# SLEEP DISORDERS

**2286. ANSWER: 3**

1. Cataplexy is the sudden loss of muscle tone and voluntary muscle movement. Approximately 70% of persons with narcolepsy also experience cataplexy.
2. The inability to speak or move just before the onset of a brief sleep attack or upon awakening is sleep paralysis.
3. **Narcolepsy is a sleep disorder characterized by excessive daytime sleepiness and multiple sleep attacks during the client's normal period of wakefulness, typically taking place at inappropriate times.**
4. Narcolepsy is not associated with taking a narcotic analgesic medication.

▶ *Test-taking Tip: Three options deal with muscle tone, and one option is different. Often the option that is different is the answer.*

Content Area: Mental Health; Concept: Sleep, Rest, and Activity; Assessment; Integrated Processes: Nursing Process: Assessment; Client Needs: Physiological Integrity: Reduction of Risk Potential; Cognitive Level: Application [Applying]

**2287. MoC ANSWER: 2, 3, 4, 5**

1. Encouraging reality thinking would be an appropriate intervention for a thought, not sleeping, disorder.
2. **Caffeine is a stimulant that interferes with sleep patterns and should be limited.**
3. **Limiting daytime sleeping promotes nighttime sleep routines.**
4. **Measures such as muscle relaxation exercises or soft music may be helpful in promoting sleep.**
5. **Identifying past sleep patterns is important in determining what is normal for the client.**

▶ *Test-taking Tip: Focus on the issue, interventions to promote sleep. This should lead you to select all options except one.*

Content Area: Mental Health; Concept: Mood; Sleep, Rest, and Activity; Integrated Processes: Nursing Process: Planning; Client Needs: Safe and Effective Care Environment: Management of Care; Psychosocial Integrity; Cognitive Level: Synthesis [Creating]

**2288. MoC ANSWER: 2**

1. Somnambulism is not associated with visitors.
2. **Somnambulism is a sleepwalking disorder in which the individual will participate in complex activities, such as walking, dressing, and toileting, all while in a deep non-REM stage of sleep. A hospitalized client is at risk for a fall or wandering. The nurse should turn on the bed exit alarm to alert staff that the client is getting out of bed.**
3. Teaching the client on call light use will not help when sleepwalking; the client is unaware that he/she is sleepwalking.
4. Visual and auditory hallucinations are not associated with sleepwalking.

▶ *Test-taking Tip: Somnambulism is a sleepwalking disorder. Knowing this information should direct you to the correct option.*

Content Area: Mental Health; Concept: Sleep, Rest, and Activity; Safety; Integrated Processes: Nursing Process: Planning; Client Needs: Safe and Effective Care Environment: Management of Care; Cognitive Level: Synthesis [Creating]

**2289. ANSWER: 3**

1. Beginning to identify stressors that can affect sleep is important, but fully assessing the extent of the client's sleeping problem should occur first.
2. Although this statement provides information, it is not helpful in determining the extent of the client's sleep problem.
3. **The client should describe current and past sleeping patterns in order to assess the extent of the sleep problem and expectations about the normal sleep patterns for the client.**
4. Although a relationship breakup is a stressor that can affect sleep, this question does not fully assess the extent of the client's sleep problem.

▶ *Test-taking Tip: Three options are similar, and one is different. Often the option that is different is the answer.*

Content Area: Mental Health; Concept: Sleep, Rest, and Activity; Assessment; Integrated Processes: Nursing Process: Assessment; Client Needs: Physiological Integrity: Basic Care and Comfort; Cognitive Level: Analysis [Analyzing]

**2290. ANSWER: 3**

1. This statement is appropriate; it is using an open-ended statement to seek information that might be used to assess the client's sleep problem.
2. This statement is appropriate; it is seeking information to determine the extent of the client's sleeping problem.

3. **Telling the client that sleep disorders are common among people who are depressed prematurely informs the client that a sleep disorder has been confirmed or tells that client that he or she is depressed. The statement is inappropriate.**

4. Although this statement is closed-ended, allowing only for a "yes" or "no" response, it is appropriate in determining the underlying problem for the client's sleep disturbance.

▶ ***Test-taking Tip:*** *Read each option carefully, and select a statement in which the nurse is making a medical diagnosis of the client's possible problem.*

**Content Area:** Mental Health; **Concept:** Sleep, Rest, and Activity; Mood; Nursing Roles; **Integrated Processes:** Nursing Process: Assessment; **Client Needs:** Physiological Integrity: Basic Care and Comfort; **Cognitive Level:** Application [Applying]

## 2291. ANSWER: 3

1. While the average is 8 hours of sleep at night, the amount of sleep required to feel refreshed varies, and some people may need only 5 hours of sleep at night for optimal functioning.

2. Waking up frequently to urinate indicates a problem with elimination that is affecting sleep, not a sleep disorder. The elimination problem should be addressed.

3. **Sleeping 6 hours indicates a change in the client's sleep pattern and the resulting dysfunction it has created.**

4. Hyperthyroidism can result in hyperactivity, but a statement about its treatment indicates that the problem with sleep has been resolved.

▶ ***Test-taking Tip:*** *Note the key word "best." Use the process of elimination to select an option that indicates a disruption to the normal sleep pattern and to the amount of sleep obtained.*

**Content Area:** Mental Health; **Concept:** Sleep, Rest, and Activity; Assessment; **Integrated Processes:** Nursing Process: Analysis; **Client Needs:** Physiological Integrity: Basic Care and Comfort; **Cognitive Level:** Application [Applying]

## Chapter Fifty

# Pharmacological and Parenteral Therapies for Mental Health Disorders

**2292.** **PHARM** The client taking sertraline for treatment of depression reports feeling much better and wishes to discontinue the medication after 11 months. Which is the nurse's **most** appropriate response?

1. "Sertraline will need to be reduced gradually to prevent undesirable effects."
2. "You should not stop the medication without talking to your HCP first."
3. "Sertraline has worked very well. It should be safe to discontinue its use."
4. "You need sertraline indefinitely to prevent recurrence of depression."

**2293.** **PHARM** The client calls the clinic to discuss medications being taken and possible adverse effects. The nurse should conclude that the client is experiencing a common side effect of sertraline when the client provides which information?

1. States last bowel movement was 5 days ago
2. Feels palpitations and an irregular heartbeat
3. Glucose reading of 60 four hours after taking sertraline
4. States needing to drink fluids more often than usual

**2294.** **MoC** **PHARM** Two days ago, the client's evening dose of mirtazapine was increased from 15 mg to 30 mg. When the nurse is preparing to administer mirtazapine, the client reports insomnia, irritability, and panic attacks. What should the nurse do **next**?

1. Document the symptoms, hold the dose, and notify the HCP.
2. Telephone the HCP to request a PRN sedative to help the client sleep.
3. Have the client participate in a card game with other clients on the unit.
4. Reassure the client that these symptoms will subside after taking this dose.

**2295.** **PHARM** The client is started on citalopram for treatment of depression. Which information is **most** important for the nurse to include when teaching the client?

1. "Notify the HCP if it is not working; antidepressants are ineffective for some ethnic groups."
2. "If sexual side effects become bothersome, consult your health care provider."
3. "Taking St. John's wort with your citalopram can enhance its effectiveness."
4. "Take your blood pressure every morning and report any significant changes."

**2296.** **PHARM** The client taking imipramine is preparing for a summer vacation. Which information should the nurse include when planning client education regarding imipramine? **Select all that apply.**

1. Drink additional fluids and add extra fiber to the diet.
2. Stop imipramine if experiencing any unpleasant side effects.
3. Avoid alcohol, which can cause an additive depressant effect.
4. Request an "as needed" sleeping pill in the event of insomnia.
5. Wear sunglasses, protective clothing, and sunscreen while outdoors.

**2297.** **MoC** **PHARM** The male college-age student is diagnosed with ADHD and atomoxetine is prescribed. What information should the nurse include in teaching the client?

1. Expect improved attention within 1 to 2 days.
2. Take atomoxetine with food or at meals.
3. Side effects include changes in male sexual function.
4. Discontinue taking atomoxetine during summer breaks.

**2298.** The client taking paroxetine telephones the mental health clinic nurse and states, "Since I started taking St. John's wort, I have had a high fever and muscle stiffness, and I am sweating a lot." Which statement is **most** appropriate?

1. "You may have the flu; call your primary provider to make an appointment."
2. "Take ibuprofen, drink fluids, and rest; call tomorrow if the symptoms worsen."
3. "Could you have doubled up on your medication, taking more than prescribed?"
4. "You should be taken to the emergency department right away to be evaluated."

**2299.** MoC PHARM The nurse is assessing the client who has begun therapy with duloxetine. Which assessment parameter should be the nurse's **priority?**

1. Relief of neuropathic pain
2. Increase in anxiety or irritability
3. Liver function test (LFT) results
4. Suicidal ideations

**2300.** PHARM The client admitted for inpatient treatment of an anxiety disorder has been taking fluoxetine for the past 9 months. The HCP prescribes a new antianxiety medication and discontinues fluoxetine. What is the nurse's **most** appropriate intervention?

1. Monitor the client closely for dizziness and lethargy due to discontinuation syndrome.
2. Teach the client relaxation measures to use while adjusting to the new medication.
3. Call the HCP to question whether fluoxetine should be tapered rather than discontinued.
4. Reassure the client that there is little risk of adverse effects when discontinuing fluoxetine.

**2301.** PHARM The nurse is teaching the client newly started on propranolol for acute situational anxiety disorder. In addition to treating the client's anxiety, the nurse should inform the client that propranolol's use is effective in treating which associated problem?

1. Bradycardia
2. Hand tremors
3. Muscle spasms
4. Hypertensive crisis

**2302.** PHARM The client is placed on lorazepam for short-term treatment of anxiety. Which instruction by the nurse is **most** important with lorazepam use?

1. "Take a second tablet if your anxiety is not being adequately relieved."
2. "If lorazepam is less effective after a few weeks, notify your provider."
3. "Avoid caffeinated foods and beverages, including tea and chocolate."
4. "If you experience drowsiness or dizziness, notify your provider."

**2303.** PHARM The nurse is developing a teaching plan for the client prescribed nortriptyline. Which self-care aspects should be included to minimize medication side effects and prevent injury? **Select all that apply.**

1. Avoid processed meats, cheeses, and wines.
2. Suck on candy or ice chips to keep your mouth moist.
3. Run water in the bathroom to stimulate urination if needed.
4. Increase fluid and fiber in the diet to prevent constipation.
5. Avoid driving until vision is completely clear to prevent injury.
6. Increase exposure to sunlight to facilitate vitamin D absorption.

**2304.** PHARM The new nurse describes the action of TCAs as relieving symptoms of depression by inhibiting neuronal uptake of the neurotransmitters serotonin and norepinephrine. Place an X on the labeled site where the new nurse is stating that inhibition takes place.

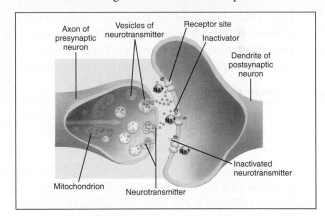

**2305.** **PHARM** The nurse is developing a teaching plan for the client who has been started on amitriptyline. Which information is **most** appropriate to include?

1. Discuss a calorie-controlled diet plan suitable to the client's preferences.
2. Inform about possible sexual dysfunction and be ready to provide support.
3. Instruct to stop amitriptyline immediately if there is a sudden elevation in BP.
4. Advise to take amitriptyline upon waking to mitigate the side effect of insomnia.

**2306.** **PHARM** The client taking tranylcypromine develops a list of possible meal plans. Which should the nurse identify as safe for the client? **Select all that apply.**

1. Pepperoni pizza, Caesar salad, 16 oz iced tea
2. Grilled pork loin, rice, green beans, 12 oz diet clear soda
3. Grilled salmon, steamed broccoli, 12 oz lemon-lime soda
4. Baked chicken, mashed potatoes and gravy, 8 oz 2% milk
5. Granola with raisins and almonds, low-fat yogurt, 8 oz coffee
6. Beef burritos with sour cream and guacamole topping, corn chips, 12 oz beer

**2307.** **MoC** **PHARM** The client taking sertraline and lithium for treatment of bipolar disorder reports symptoms of restlessness, tachycardia, tremors, and sweating. What should the nurse do **next?**

1. Give a PRN prescribed antihypertensive medication.
2. Notify the HCP regarding the client's symptoms.
3. Document the findings as expected side effects.
4. Give a PRN prescribed anticholinergic medication.

**2308.** **MoC** **PHARM** The nurse is reviewing medications prescribed for the client taking phenelzine. Which should prompt the nurse to notify the HCP about a potentially serious medication interaction?

1. Cefaclor 250 mg oral q8h
2. Glyburide 2.5 mg oral daily
3. Ibuprofen 200 mg, 1–2 tabs, oral, q4hr prn
4. Oxycodone 10 mg, 1–2 tabs, oral, q3-4hr prn

**2309.** **PHARM** The newly hospitalized client admits using heroin 8 hours ago. Which assessment findings, if observed in the client, should the nurse associate with heroin withdrawal?

1. Mental confusion, drowsiness, hypotension
2. Dysphoric mood, pupillary dilation, sweating
3. Pinpoint pupils, constipation, urinary retention
4. No withdrawal signs until 2 to 3 days have passed

**2310.** **PHARM** The nurse is reviewing client information for adverse effects of trazodone. Which finding should the nurse identify as an adverse effect unique to trazodone?

1. Priapism
2. Weight gain
3. Hepatic failure
4. Cardiac dysrhythmias

**2311.** **MoC** **PHARM** The client taking lithium for bipolar disorder participated in a recreational game of basketball in the mental health unit gym. The client now is feeling nauseated and shaky, has blurred vision, and is finding it hard to stand. Considering this information, which action should be taken by the nurse?

1. Instruct the client to sit and rest for a while in a cool place.
2. Call the HCP to request an order for a STAT serum lithium level.
3. Give the PRN prescribed antiemetic with a large glass of cold water.
4. Alert the emergency team for the client's impending cardiac arrest.

**2312.** **PHARM** At discharge, the nurse documents that the client taking lithium has an accurate understanding of self-care. On which client statement should the nurse base this judgment?

1. "I need to have my blood lithium level checked every 2 weeks."
2. "I should take my lithium on an empty stomach for best absorption."
3. "I know I need to restrict foods high in sugar while I'm taking lithium."
4. "I need to eat foods containing sodium and drink 2 to 3 liters of fluid daily."

**2313.** **PHARM** The mother asks why the anticonvulsant valproic acid is being prescribed for her adolescent who is beginning therapy for aggressive behaviors. The nurse's response is based on the fact that valproic acid is helpful in reducing manic and impulsive behavior by what mechanism of action?

1. Blocks the effects of dopamine at the postsynaptic neuron
2. Enhances the reuptake of norepinephrine and serotonin in the CNS
3. Alters sodium channels in the neurons, thus decreasing nerve impulse transmission
4. Increases gamma-aminobutyric acid (GABA) levels to inhibit CNS neurotransmission

**2314.** PHARM The nurse is reviewing a lithium toxicity chart to determine symptoms of significance for assessment. Place an X on the chart column that includes signs the client might have when the serum lithium level is 3.6 mEq/L.

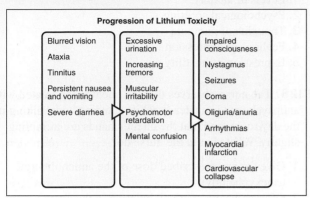

**Progression of Lithium Toxicity**

| Blurred vision | Excessive urination | Impaired consciousness |
| Ataxia | Increasing tremors | Nystagmus |
| Tinnitus | | Seizures |
| Persistent nausea and vomiting | Muscular irritability | Coma |
| Severe diarrhea | Psychomotor retardation | Oliguria/anuria |
| | Mental confusion | Arrhythmias |
| | | Myocardial infarction |
| | | Cardiovascular collapse |

**2315.** PHARM New medications are prescribed for the client taking lithium. Which medication should the nurse question with the HCP?

1. Isosorbide dinitrate by mouth TID
2. Prednisone 20 mg by mouth daily
3. Furosemide 80 mg by mouth daily
4. Insulin aspart 2 units subcut with meals

**2316.** PHARM The nurse is teaching the client taking alprazolam. Which substances should the client be instructed to avoid? **Select all that apply.**

1. Alcohol
2. Caffeine
3. Narcotics
4. Antioxidants
5. Antihistamines
6. Antidepressants

**2317.** PHARM The nurse telephones the HCP to request a prn anxiolytic medication order for a hospitalized client having occasional anxiety. Which medication, if prescribed, should the nurse question regarding its effectiveness for prn use?

1. Buspirone
2. Lorazepam
3. Clorazepate
4. Clonazepam

**2318.** PHARM The parent of the adolescent taking chlordiazepoxide for the past 2 months telephones the nurse requesting to have the dose increased. The parent states, "Chlordiazepoxide is being given as directed, but my child's anxiety is increasing." Which should be the nurse's **best** interpretation of this situation?

1. The client may be developing tolerance to chlordiazepoxide and needs the dose reevaluated.
2. The client may be skipping drug doses when not anxious and now needs the dose doubled.
3. The client is becoming resistant to the drug's effects, and an alternative medication is needed.
4. The client's anxiety may be hormone-related, and larger doses of chlordiazepoxide are needed.

**2319.** PHARM The nurse is reviewing medications for all assigned clients on an inpatient psychiatric unit. The nurse anticipates assessing for extrapyramidal symptoms (EPS) in clients taking which antipsychotic medication?

1. Clozapine
2. Risperidone
3. Haloperidol
4. Ziprasidone

**2320.** PHARM The nurse is assessing the client newly started on benztropine mesylate. Which findings indicate that the client is experiencing the most common side effects of benztropine mesylate?

1. Dizziness, headache, insomnia
2. Weight gain, tremors, sedation
3. Blurred vision, dry mouth, constipation
4. Headache, dry mouth, sexual dysfunction

**2321.** PHARM The nurse is discussing prescribed atypical antipsychotic medication therapy with the client who has schizophrenia. What information should the nurse include in this discussion? **Select all that apply.**

1. Atypical antipsychotic medications will reduce the client's hallucinations and inappropriate emotional responses.
2. Atypical antipsychotic medications are prescribed after other medications have proven ineffective in treating symptoms.
3. The greatest concern with taking atypical antipsychotic medications is that they produce extrapyramidal side effects.
4. Regular laboratory appointments must be scheduled to monitor the client's blood glucose levels.
5. The client may experience an increase in appetite and weight when taking an atypical antipsychotic medication.

**2322.** **PHARM** The HCP prescribes haloperidol 4 mg tid oral liquid for the client diagnosed with schizophrenia. How many mL should the nurse administer for each dose from a bottle labeled "haloperidol 2 mg/mL"?

_____ mL (Record a whole number.)

**2323.** **PHARM** The HCP prescribes risperidone to manage the hallucinations of the client diagnosed with paranoid schizophrenia. Which client statements reflect a need for further education regarding the medication's side effects? **Select all that apply.**

1. "Diarrhea may be a problem for me."
2. "I'll most likely develop high blood pressure."
3. "With long-term use, I could develop bizarre facial and tongue movements."
4. "I will need to watch what I eat so I won't gain weight."
5. "Getting up too quickly from a sitting position can make me dizzy."
6. "I will need to be careful driving because this can make me drowsy."

**2324.** **PHARM** Risperidone is prescribed for the client experiencing hallucinations. Which condition should the nurse assess for, considering the risk of this side effect of risperidone?

1. Asthma
2. Hypertension
3. Crohn's disease
4. Diabetes mellitus

**2325.** **PHARM** The nurse is educating the client concerning the possible side effects of a newly prescribed traditional antipsychotic medication. Which client statement reflects a need for further education regarding the side effects of this drug classification?

1. "I need to get up from bed slowly so I will not get dizzy."
2. "The medication can cause constipation, so I need to eat fiber."
3. "I may need a sleeping pill because insomnia is a possible side effect."
4. "I can't risk gaining weight, so I will need to add some exercise to my routine."

**2326.** **PHARM** The client is being treated with clozapine. Which findings during the nurse's assessment indicate that the client is experiencing adverse effects of the medication? **Select all that apply.**

1. Dehydration
2. Agranulocytosis
3. Increasing anxiety
4. Extreme salivation
5. Blood glucose 192 mg/dL

**2327.** **PHARM** The client diagnosed with BPD is taking olanzapine. The nurse evaluates that olanzapine is effective when observing a reduction in which behaviors? **Select all that apply.**

1. Levels of anxiety
2. Psychological splitting
3. Thoughts of paranoia
4. Feelings of depression
5. Expression of hostility

**2328.** The nurse observes that the client being treated with antipsychotics is unsteady while standing and walking in the day room, and that the client's hands are trembling slightly. What should the nurse do?

1. Give the prn prescribed dose of the anticholinergic trihexyphenidyl.
2. Offer assistance with ambulation to the client's room for rest.
3. Insist that the client remain seated, applying limb restraints if needed.
4. Call the HCP to report that early signs of tardive dyskinesia are present.

**2329.** **PHARM** The nurse is preparing to administer a prn dose of benztropine to the client with worsening akathisia. The client is prescribed benztropine 0.5 mg IM q4h prn. The vial contains 1 mg/mL. How many mL should the nurse administer?

_____ mL (Round to the nearest tenth.)

**2330.** **PHARM** The client is prescribed varenicline for smoking cessation. The nurse concludes that varenicline is being prescribed primarily for its antagonistic effect. Which statement describes this effect?

1. Gets readily absorbed into the bloodstream for rapid effectiveness
2. Demonstrates a high degree of attraction for a specific receptor
3. Blocks receptors in the brain that produce the pleasurable effects of smoking
4. Stimulates receptors activated by smoking, producing similar pleasurable effects

**2331.** PHARM The hospitalized adult is having difficulty falling and staying asleep. The nurse consults standing orders, which include medications in the table illustrated. Which hypnotic medication should the nurse administer to help the client sleep soundly throughout the night?

| Medication | Onset (hr) | Peak (hr) | Duration (hr) |
|---|---|---|---|
| Flurazepam | 0.5 | 0.5–1 | 7–8 |
| Triazolam | 0.5 | 6–8 | 10–12 |
| Zaleplon | 0.5 | 1 | 3–4 |
| Eszopiclone | Rapid | 1 | 6 |

1. Zaleplon
2. Triazolam
3. Flurazepam
4. Eszopiclone

**2332.** PHARM The nurse is working with the family whose child is taking atomoxetine for ADHD. Which instructions should the nurse include when teaching the parents? **Select all that apply.**

1. Provide stimulation because atomoxetine causes sedation.
2. Administer atomoxetine immediately after a meal.
3. Administer atomoxetine at least 6 hours before bedtime.
4. Weigh the child weekly to monitor for unintended weight loss.
5. Consult the prescriber before giving cold or allergy medication.

**2333.** PHARM The nurse is performing a health history on the child with ADHD who is being evaluated for treatment with psychostimulants. Which information is **most** critical to collect prior to treatment with psychostimulants?

1. Musculoskeletal history
2. Genitourinary history
3. Immunization history
4. Cardiovascular history

**2334.** PHARM The client has been prescribed clonidine for the unlabeled purpose of easing the discomfort associated with smoking cessation. Which body system should be the nurse's **initial** focus when completing the client's physical assessment?

1. Neurological
2. Cardiovascular
3. Gastrointestinal
4. Musculoskeletal

**2335.** PHARM The client is beginning treatment with bupropion for depression. After meeting with the HCP, the client tells the nurse, "I'm taking Zyban to help me stop smoking." Which is the **most** appropriate action for the nurse?

1. Encourage and support the client in following the smoking cessation regimen.
2. Notify the HCP to request an increased dose of bupropion due to drug interactions.
3. Instruct the client to report any allergic-type reactions after beginning the bupropion.
4. Inform the HCP that the client already is taking bupropion, but for smoking cessation.

**2336.** PHARM Six months after starting disulfiram for treatment of alcoholism, the client has serum laboratory tests performed (see exhibit). Place an X on each serum laboratory result that the nurse should report immediately to the HCP.

| Serum Laboratory Test | Client's Result |
|---|---|
| Potassium | 4.0 mEq/L |
| RBCs | $5.9 \times 10^6$ cells/microL |
| Hgb | 12.8 g/dL |
| Albumin | 2.8 g/dL |
| AST | 65 units/L |
| ALT | 60 units/L |
| Total bilirubin | 3.8 mg/dL |
| Alkaline phosphatase (ALP) | 160 units/L |

**2337.** PHARM The client being treated for opiate dependence is receiving a buprenorphine/naloxone combination. The nurse understands that the reason for adding naloxone to the buprenorphine is for what effect?

1. Prevent intoxication should the client abuse an opiate.
2. Replace essential nutrients due to malnutrition from drug abuse.
3. Reduce the incidence of adverse reactions to the buprenorphine.
4. Induce an adverse reaction if the client uses an opiate while on buprenorphine.

**2338.** **PHARM** The client seeking treatment for insomnia tells the nurse about researching complementary therapies promoting sleep. Which herbal sleep remedies might the client wish to discuss with the nurse?

1. Fennel and ginger tea
2. Chamomile tea and hops
3. Feverfew and peppermint
4. Echinacea and goldenseal

**2339.** **PHARM** The client admitted to the ED has drowsiness, clammy skin, and slow, shallow breathing. A friend states that the client took multiple oxycodone tablets. Which medication should the nurse plan to administer to this client?

1. Naloxone
2. Disulfiram
3. Flumazenil
4. Acetylcysteine

**2340.** **PHARM** The client is experiencing delirium from substance withdrawal. Which medication, if prescribed prn, should the nurse administer to help calm the client?

1.

| **Flumazenil Injection** |
| For IV use only |
| 0.5 mg/5 mL |
| Exp 12/21/2028 |

2.

| **Guaifenesin** |
| Oral solution |
| 100 mg/5 mL |
| Exp 12/28/2028 |

3.

| **Bupropion Oral** |
| 100 mg tablet |
| Exp 10/21/2028 |

4.

| **Lorazepam Injection** |
| For IV use only |
| 2 mg/1 mL |
| Exp 11/26/2028 |

**2341.** **PHARM** The client with schizophrenia has a history of nonadherence to prescribed medication regimens. Injectable antipsychotic agents are being considered for long-term use. Which medications, if prescribed by the HCP, should the nurse question? **Select all that apply.**

1. Olanzapine
2. Ziprasidone
3. Aripiprazole
4. Risperidone Consta
5. Fluphenazine decanoate

**2342.** **PHARM** The 30-year-old has been taking olanzapine for the past 5 years for treatment of schizophrenia. The client, who has a positive family history of DM, is now overweight but is not showing signs of hyperglycemia. When the client asks about the next steps for treatment, how should the nurse respond?

1. "You'll be started on an oral hyperglycemic agent."
2. "I will teach you how to self-administer insulin."
3. "You'll need to have a fasting blood glucose level drawn."
4. "Olanzapine will be discontinued and another drug started."

**2343.** **MoC** The adolescent is brought to the ED with wheezing, nystagmus, ataxia, and sensorimotor neuropathy after inhaling paint thinner by "bagging." Which nursing intervention is **priority?**

1. Monitor the client's cardiac rhythm.
2. Place the client on seizure precautions.
3. Apply oxygen via nasal cannula at 4 liters.
4. Notify lab to obtain a toxicology screen.

**2344.** **MoC** The nurse is leading a group session for clients with panic disorder. Which statement by the client indicates that further teaching is needed?

1. "I need to be able to identify triggers that escalate my anxiety to the point of panic."
2. "I will take the diazepam that was prescribed a year ago because it is nonaddictive."
3. "I plan to pray every day; praying can prevent recurrences of a panic attack."
4. "I can use guided imagery and meditation to effectively reduce my anxiety symptoms."

**2345.** **MoC** **PHARM** The nurse receives a shift report for five clients, and all are taking lithium. Place the clients in order of priority.

1. The client who has a dry mouth, headache, and thirst
2. The client who has a fever, rash, and the beginning of hives
3. The client who has blurred vision, ataxia, and tinnitus
4. The client who has mild hand tremors, nausea, and vomiting
5. The client who has increasing confusion and nystagmus and just had a seizure

Answer: _____

**2346.** `PHARM` The school-aged child taking guanfacine for ADHD is being seen by the nurse at school. The child is pale and diaphoretic and feels dizzy. What should the nurse do **first?**

1. Take the child's BP.
2. Obtain a capillary glucose level.
3. Telephone the parent about the child.
4. Put a cool cloth on the child's forehead.

**2347.** `PHARM` The client undergoing detoxification from chronic alcohol abuse is to receive phenobarbital 120 mg IM and promethazine 50 mg IM. Which explanation by the nurse about this medication combination is correct?

1. "Promethazine will prevent a potential allergic reaction to the phenobarbital."
2. "Combining promethazine and phenobarbital will have a greater sedative effect."
3. "Promethazine will decrease the nausea from phenobarbital when it is given IM."
4. "Combining these reduces sedative effects and prevents a 'hangover' feeling."

**2348.** `PHARM` The child diagnosed with ADHD is to receive a total of 20 mg of dextroamphetamine daily in two divided doses. The dextroamphetamine on hand is supplied in 5 mg tablets. How many tablet(s) should the nurse administer for the morning dose?

_____ tablet(s) (Record a whole number.)

**INSTRUCTIONS:** The nurse is reviewing information about four clients prior to administering medications. Use the information in the table to answer Questions 2349 and 2350.

| Client 1<br>**Dx:** Schizophrenia<br>**New Dx:** Type 2 DM | Client 2<br>**Dx:** Bipolar Mania;<br>hypertension | Client 3<br>**Dx:** Schizophrenia | Client 4<br>**Dx:** Psychosis |
|---|---|---|---|
| Taking aripiprazole for 3 months and metformin for 2 days | Taking risperidone and lisinopril for 5 years | Taking fluphenazine for 2 years | Taking haloperidol for 15 years |
| Has hand tremors, shuffling gait, and rigidity when walking across the room. | Unable to sit due to spasms of legs, arms, and neck. | Eyes rolling back and is very upset and agitated. | Lip smacking and has bizarre facial, tongue, and extremity movements. |

**2349.** CJ MoC PHARM Which four medications require notification of the HCP? Complete the following statements by choosing the number of the medication from the left column that would require notification of the HCP, and the letter for the correct reason for notifying the HCP from the right column. Place the number and letter of the correct answer in the blank lines that follow.

| The nurse should <u>notify the HCP regarding:</u> | Because: |
|---|---|
| 1. Aripiprazole | A. The client is showing signs of dystonia. |
| 2. Fluphenazine | B. The client is showing signs of tardive dyskinesia. |
| 3. Haloperidol | C. The client is showing signs of pseudoparkinsonism. |
| 4. Lisinopril | D. The client is showing signs of hypotension. |
| 5. Metformin | E. The client is showing signs of oculogyric crisis. |
| 6. Risperidone | F. The client is showing signs of hypoglycemia. |

Answer:

Medication number _____ Reason letter _____

Medication number _____ Reason letter _____

Medication number _____ Reason letter _____

Medication number _____ Reason letter _____

**2350.** MoC CJ PHARM Which client is the nurse's **priority** to withhold medication and immediately notify the HCP?

1. Client 1
2. Client 2
3. Client 3
4. Client 4

## Answers and Rationales

**2292.** PHARM **ANSWER: 1**

1. **Sertraline (Zoloft) is an SSRI antidepressant. Stopping it abruptly can cause withdrawal symptoms. The dose should be reduced gradually.**
2. Clients have the right to discontinue medication treatment, although it is advisable that the client should discuss this with the HCP and taper off rather than discontinue abruptly.
3. It should not be discontinued. Antidepressants should not be stopped abruptly because this can precipitate withdrawal symptoms.
4. Treatment with antidepressants may last for months to several years but should not be used indefinitely.

▸ *Test-taking Tip: Use Maslow's Hierarchy of Needs theory, focusing on physiological aspects of SSRI withdrawal. Select an option that should prevent withdrawal.*

Content Area: Mental Health; **Concept:** Medication; Mood; **Integrated Processes:** Communication and Documentation; **Client Needs:** Physiological Integrity: Pharmacological and Parenteral Therapies; Safe and Effective Care Environment: Safety and Infection Control; **Cognitive Level:** Application [Applying]

**2293.** PHARM **ANSWER: 4**

1. Diarrhea (not constipation) is a more common side effect of sertraline. Constipation is more commonly a side effect of both TCAs and MAOIs due to their anticholinergic side effects.
2. An irregular heart rhythm is more commonly a side effect of TCAs.
3. Sertraline has been associated with hyperglycema, not hypoglycemia.
4. **The nurse should consider that the client may have a dry mouth when the person states a need to drink fluids more often than usual. Dry mouth is a common side effect of sertraline (Zoloft).**

▸ *Test-taking Tip: The key word is "common." You should narrow the options to the two that would be considered less severe. Then, think about the action of sertraline, which is an SSRI.*

Content Area: Mental Health; **Concept:** Medication; Mood; **Integrated Processes:** Nursing Process: Evaluation; **Client Needs:** Physiological Integrity: Pharmacological and Parenteral Therapies; **Cognitive Level:** Evaluation [Evaluating]

**2294.** MoC PHARM **ANSWER: 1**

1. **Mirtazapine (Remeron) is an antidepressant. Adverse effects include insomnia, irritability, panic attacks, and suicidal ideation. A change in medication may be needed rather than a dosage increase.**
2. The nurse is ignoring the possible adverse effects of mirtazapine.
3. The client should be in a low-stimulus environment.
4. It can take 1 to 2 weeks before the desired therapeutic effects are observed, but the symptoms indicate that the client is experiencing an adverse effect.

▸ *Test-taking Tip: Mirtazapine (Remeron) is a tetracyclic antidepressant. You need to determine whether the symptoms are life-threatening.*

Content Area: Mental Health; **Concept:** Medication; Nursing Roles; **Integrated Processes:** Nursing Process: Implementation; **Client Needs:** Safe and Effective Care Environment: Management of Care; Physiological Integrity: Pharmacological and Parenteral Therapies; **Cognitive Level:** Application [Applying]

**2295.** PHARM **ANSWER: 2**

1. Studies have shown that there are no significant differences in ethnic responses to antidepressant medications.
2. **Sexual dysfunction is a common side effect associated with SSRIs. The client taking the SSRI citalopram (Celexa) should consult the HCP if experiencing bothersome sexual side effects.**
3. Taking St. John's wort with citalopram can cause serotonin syndrome.
4. Cardiovascular effects are associated with TCA use; there is no need to take the BP daily when taking citalopram an SSRI.

▸ *Test-taking Tip: Antidepressants ending in "-pram" are medications in the SSRI category. You can remember sexual dysfunction as a side effect by remembering the letter s, which is in both.*

Content Area: Mental Health; **Concept:** Medication; Mood; Nursing Roles; **Integrated Processes:** Teaching/Learning; Culture and Spirituality; **Client Needs:** Physiological Integrity: Pharmacological and Parenteral Therapies; **Cognitive Level:** Analysis [Analyzing]

**2296.** PHARM **ANSWER: 1, 3, 5**

1. **TCAs such as imipramine (Tofranil) may cause constipation. Increasing liquids and dietary fiber can reduce constipation.**
2. Clients should not abruptly stop taking any antidepressant medication.
3. **Alcohol combined with imipramine (Tofranil) can cause CNS depression.**
4. TCAs usually cause sedation and should not be combined with a sleeping agent.
5. **Wearing sunglasses, protective clothing, and sunscreen guards against photosensitivity, a concern with TCAs.**

▸ *Test-taking Tip: Think about the side effects and nursing implications of TCA medications.*

Content Area: Mental Health; **Concept:** Medication; Nursing Roles; **Integrated Processes:** Teaching/Learning; **Client Needs:** Health Promotion and Maintenance; Physiological Integrity: Pharmacological and Parenteral Therapies; **Cognitive Level:** Application [Applying]

**2297.** MoC PHARM **ANSWER: 3**

1. Therapeutic effects of atomoxetine are not seen for at least a week.
2. Atomoxetine can be administered without regard to food.
3. **Ejaculatory problems, decreased libido, and impotence are common side effects of atomoxetine (Strattera). The nurse should include this information when teaching the client.**
4. Daily doses should be taken to maintain therapeutic levels and should not be eliminated at any time.

▶ **Test-taking Tip:** When gender is included in the stem, look for the option related to gender. It likely is the answer if no other options are related to gender.

Content Area: Mental Health; Concept: Medication; Cognition; Integrated Processes: Nursing Process: Implementation; Teaching/Learning; Client Needs: Safe and Effective Care Environment: Management of Care; Physiological Integrity: Pharmacological and Parenteral Therapies; Cognitive Level: Application [Applying]

**2298. ANSWER: 4**

1. Making an appointment with another HCP delays appropriate treatment for the client; he or she may require hospitalization due to serotonin syndrome.
2. The client should not be instructed to call tomorrow. He or she should be assessed in the ED because serotonin syndrome is a possibility and can be life-threatening.
3. Asking whether the client doubled the dose of paroxetine is not a priority at this time.
4. **Fever, muscle stiffness (rigidity), and diaphoresis are symptoms of serotonin syndrome, a potentially fatal condition that may occur with concurrent use of St. John's wort and paroxetine (Paxil). The client should be taken to the ED.**

▶ **Test-taking Tip:** Use the ABC's to establish that this is an emergency situation. Serotonin syndrome may occur with concomitant use of paroxetine (Paxil) and St. John's wort.

Content Area: Mental Health; Concept: Medication; Nursing Roles; Integrated Processes: Nursing Process: Analysis; Client Needs: Physiological Integrity: Physiological Adaptation; Cognitive Level: Application [Applying]

**2299.** MoC PHARM **ANSWER: 4**

1. Duloxetine is used in relieving neuropathic pain, but assessing its effectiveness is of lesser importance than assessing for suicidal ideation.
2. In deciding whether the medication is effective, determining the level of increased anxiety or irritability is of lesser importance than assessing for suicidal ideation. Beneficial effects of duloxetine may not be felt for approximately 4 weeks.
3. Lab tests for liver function are not routinely prescribed. LFTs are completed to evaluate for complications if the client is experiencing abdominal pain or an enlarged liver.

4. **Duloxetine (Cymbalta) is a selective serotonin norepinephrine reuptake inhibitor (SSNRI) used in the treatment of major depression. Suicidal ideation is the most acute threat to life and should be assessed, especially when initiating duloxetine.**

▶ **Test-taking Tip:** Prioritize the parameters based on lethality and client acuity; client safety is always a priority.

Content Area: Mental Health; Concept: Medication; Assessment; Integrated Processes: Nursing Process: Assessment; Client Needs: Safe and Effective Care Environment: Management of Care; Safe and Effective Care Environment: Safety and Infection Control; Physiological Integrity: Pharmacological and Parenteral Therapies; Cognitive Level: Application [Applying]

**2300.** PHARM **ANSWER: 4**

1. While it is important to monitor the client when a medication is changed, the client should not experience discontinuation syndrome when fluoxetine is stopped.
2. Although teaching relaxation measures is important, the focus of the question is a change in medication. Fluoxetine has a long half-life. Reassuring the client is most appropriate.
3. Tapering of fluoxetine is unnecessary. Other antidepressants such as TCAs, SSRIs, norepinephrine reuptake inhibitors, and dopamine agonists should be tapered over a 2- to 4-week period to avoid discontinuation syndrome.
4. **Because of its long half-life, there is a relatively low risk of adverse effects when discontinuing fluoxetine (Prozac). The client should be reassured and taught about the change of antianxiety medication.**

▶ **Test-taking Tip:** Fluoxetine (Prozac) has a long half-life. Three of the options imply that the client will have to adjust to the change in medication. Often, the option that is different is the answer.

Content Area: Mental Health; Concept: Medication; Mood; Integrated Processes: Nursing Process: Implementation; Client Needs: Physiological Integrity: Pharmacological and Parenteral Therapies; Cognitive Level: Application [Applying]

**2301.** PHARM **ANSWER: 2**

1. Bradycardia is a side effect of propranolol.
2. **Propranolol (Inderal), a beta blocker, has been shown to be effective in ameliorating the somatic symptoms of anxiety such as hand tremor.**
3. Muscle spasms are extrapyramidal symptoms not associated with propranolol use.
4. Hypertensive crisis is an adverse effect of MAOIs and can be treated by phentolamine, not propranolol.

▶ **Test-taking Tip:** You need to think about situational anxiety and which symptom listed is most likely to occur with this.

Content Area: Mental Health; Concept: Medication; Mood; Nursing Roles; Integrated Processes: Nursing Process: Implementation; Client Needs: Physiological Integrity: Pharmacological and Parenteral Therapies; Cognitive Level: Application [Applying]

**2302.** PHARM **ANSWER: 2**

1. The nurse should instruct the client to use the medication exactly as prescribed and not take an additional dose.
2. **This instruction is the most important. Lorazepam (Ativan) is a benzodiazepine anxiolytic and sedative-hypnotic medication. If it becomes less effective after a few weeks, the client may be developing a tolerance to lorazepam, and the HCP should be notified of this.**
3. While excess caffeine can increase anxiety, this is not the most important instruction.
4. Drowsiness and dizziness are expected side effects and need not be reported to an HCP unless excessive.

▶ *Test-taking Tip: A key phrase is "lorazepam use." Although Option 3 is important information regarding anxiety reduction, only one option correctly pertains to lorazepam use.*

Content Area: Mental Health; Concept: Medication; Nursing Roles; Integrated Processes: Teaching/Learning; Client Needs: Physiological Integrity: Pharmacological and Parenteral Therapies; Cognitive Level: Application [Applying]

**2303.** PHARM **ANSWER: 2, 3, 4, 5**

1. Dietary restrictions are necessary with MAOIs, not TCAs.
2. **Dry mouth is a side effect of nortriptyline (Pamelor) and can be relieved with hard candy, ice, or water.**
3. **Urinary retention is a side effect of nortriptyline; running water stimulates urination.**
4. **Constipation is a side effect of nortriptyline; fluid and fiber help relieve constipation.**
5. **Blurred vision is a side effect of nortriptyline; driving is dangerous until vision is clear.**
6. TCAs cause photosensitivity; clients should use sun protection measures.

▶ *Test-taking Tip: Nortriptyline is a TCA antidepressant. Four major anticholinergic side effects of TCAs include blurred vision, urinary retention, dry mouth, and constipation. Think about nursing actions that address resolution of these side effects.*

Content Area: Mental Health; Concept: Medication; Safety; Nursing Roles; Integrated Processes: Nursing Process: Planning; Client Needs: Health Promotion and Maintenance; Physiological Integrity: Pharmacological and Parenteral Therapies; Cognitive Level: Synthesis [Creating]

**2304.** PHARM **ANSWER:**

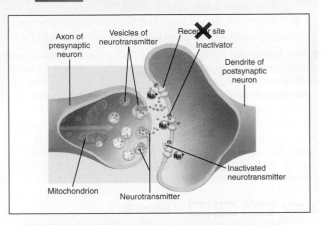

**Neuronal uptake of the neurotransmitters occurs at the receptor sites on the postsynaptic neuron.**

▶ *Test-taking Tip: To answer this question, focus on the illustration and description provided for the action of TCAs.*

Content Area: Mental Health; Concept: Medication; Nursing Roles; Integrated Processes: Nursing Process: Analysis; Client Needs: Physiological Integrity: Pharmacological and Parenteral Therapies; Cognitive Level: Comprehension [Understanding]

**2305.** PHARM **ANSWER: 1**

1. **Weight gain is often a major concern for clients taking TCAs such as amitriptyline (Elavil). A calorie-controlled diet plan will assist in avoiding weight gain.**
2. Sexual dysfunction is most commonly associated with the use of SSRIs, not TCAs.
3. Sudden hypertension results from food-medication interactions associated with MAOIs, not TCAs.
4. Antidepressants are more likely to cause sedation than stimulation and therefore are frequently taken at bedtime.

▶ *Test-taking Tip: Amitriptyline is a TCA. Associate the word "plan" in the stem of the question with "plan" in an option. Often, the option with the same word or a related one is the answer.*

Content Area: Mental Health; Concept: Mood; Medication; Nursing Roles; Integrated Processes: Nursing Process: Planning; Client Needs: Physiological Integrity: Pharmacological and Parenteral Therapies; Cognitive Level: Application [Applying]

**2306.** PHARM **ANSWER: 2, 3, 4**

1. Tyramine is found in the pepperoni and should not be eaten while taking an MAOI.
2. **The meal of grilled pork loin, rice, green beans, and a 12 oz diet clear soda does not include any items containing tyramine and is safe for the client.**
3. **The meal of grilled salmon, steamed broccoli, and a 12 oz lemon-lime soda is appropriate; it contains no tyramine and is safe for the client.**
4. **The meal of baked chicken, mashed potatoes and gravy, and an 8 oz 2% milk is appropriate because it contains no tyramine and is safe for the client.**

5. Raisins and yogurt both contain tyramine and should not be eaten while taking an MAOI.

6. Sour cream, avocadoes, and beer all contain tyramine and should not be ingested while taking an MAOI.

▶ *Test-taking Tip: Tranylcypromine (Parnate) is an MAOI, and foods containing tyramine should be eliminated. Most foods with tyramine are processed and aged or contain alcohol, chocolate, or caffeine. Use this information to eliminate options that have foods containing tyramine.*

Content Area: Mental Health; Concept: Medication; Nutrition; Nursing Roles; Integrated Processes: Nursing Process: Evaluation; Client Needs: Safe and Effective Care Environment: Safety and Infection Control; Physiological Integrity: Pharmacological and Parenteral Therapies; Cognitive Level: Evaluation [Evaluating]

### 2307. MoC PHARM ANSWER: 2

1. There is no indication that the client is hypertensive. A hypertensive crisis is associated with the combination of MAOIs and a diet high in tyramine.

2. **The client may experience increased effects of sertraline (Zoloft), an SSRI, when taken with lithium (Lithobid). Serotonin syndrome may occur when two medications that potentiate serotonergic neurotransmission are used concurrently. Symptoms of serotonin syndrome include restlessness, tachycardia, tremors, and sweating.**

3. Restlessness, tachycardia, tremors, and sweating are not expected side effects of SSRI or lithium therapy.

4. Anticholinergic medication is given to treat extrapyramidal side effects. These are associated with the use of some antipsychotic medications and include tremors and Parkinson-like symptoms.

▶ *Test-taking Tip: Focus on the client's symptoms. Consider that extrapyramidal side effects are motor-related and use the process of elimination.*

Content Area: Mental Health; Concept: Medication; Management; Integrated Processes: Nursing Process: Implementation; Client Needs: Safe and Effective Care Environment: Management of Care; Physiological Integrity: Pharmacological and Parenteral Therapies; Cognitive Level: Analysis [Analyzing]

### 2308. MoC PHARM ANSWER: 4

1. Cefaclor (Raniclor), a cephalosporin antibiotic, is safe when combined with MAOIs.

2. Glyburide (DiaBeta), a hypoglycemic agent, is safe when combined with MAOIs.

3. Ibuprofen (Motrin) is an NSAID medication and is safe when combined with MAOIs.

4. **Hypertension, hypotension, coma, or convulsions may occur with concurrent use of phenelzine (Nardil), an MAOI, with oxycodone (OxyContin), a narcotic analgesic. A large dose has been prescribed.**

▶ *Test-taking Tip: Phenelzine (Nardil) is an MAOI and has both food and medication interactions. It can be life-threatening when combined with a narcotic analgesic.*

Content Area: Mental Health; Concept: Medication; Integrated Processes: Nursing Process: Analysis; Client Needs: Safe and Effective Care Environment: Management of Care; Physiological Integrity: Pharmacological and Parenteral Therapies; Cognitive Level: Analysis [Analyzing]

### 2309. PHARM ANSWER: 2

1. Mental confusion, drowsiness, hypotension, and respiratory depression are signs of heroin overdose.

2. **Dysphoric mood, pupillary dilation, and sweating are signs of heroin withdrawal. Heroin is an opioid.**

3. Pinpoint pupils, constipation, and urinary retention are common signs of heroin (opioid) overdose.

4. Withdrawal symptoms from heroin, a short-acting drug, occur within 6 to 8 hours after the last dose, peak within 1 to 3 days, and gradually subside over 5 to 10 days.

▶ *Test-taking Tip: When asked to identify signs and symptoms of drug withdrawal or overdose, you first should identify the drug classification of the medication and then recall the common adverse effects associated with that classification. Heroin is an opioid.*

Content Area: Mental Health; Concept: Medication; Assessment; Integrated Processes: Nursing Process: Assessment; Client Needs: Physiological Integrity: Pharmacological and Parenteral Therapies; Cognitive Level: Analysis [Analyzing]

### 2310. PHARM ANSWER: 1

1. **Prolonged or inappropriate erection is a rare but problematic side effect of trazodone (Oleptro), a serotonin antagonist and reuptake inhibitor. If left untreated, it can lead to impotence.**

2. Weight gain is associated with many of the TCAs.

3. Hepatic failure is a life-threatening condition reported with the use of nefazodone (Serzone), an atypical antidepressant.

4. Cardiac dysrhythmias are associated with many of the TCAs.

▶ *Test-taking Tip: Trazodone is in the class of unique antidepressants and therefore is not likely to share common side effects with major classifications such as TCAs or SSRIs. Use the process of elimination to rule out side effects common to the major antidepressant categories.*

Content Area: Mental Health; Concept: Medication; Assessment; Safety; Integrated Processes: Nursing Process: Analysis; Client Needs: Physiological Integrity: Pharmacological and Parenteral Therapies; Cognitive Level: Knowledge [Remembering]

### 2311. MoC PHARM ANSWER: 2

1. Having the client rest will not resolve the symptoms if the serum lithium level is elevated.

2. **The client is showing signs of lithium (Lithane) toxicity, especially apparent after participating in high levels of physical activity. The HCP should be notified for a STAT lithium level and corrective action. The therapeutic range for maintenance of bipolar disorder is 0.6–1.2 mEq/L. Signs of toxicity are seen when the level is above 1.5 mEq/L.**

3. Administering an antiemetic will not resolve the symptoms if the serum lithium level is elevated.
4. The nurse is misinterpreting the symptoms if the emergency team is notified for an impending cardiac arrest.

▶ **Test-taking Tip:** *Use the nursing process to perform further assessment before appropriate interventions can be carried out.*

**Content Area:** Mental Health; **Concept:** Medication; Safety; Nursing Roles; **Integrated Processes:** Nursing Process: Implementation; **Client Needs:** Safe and Effective Care Environment: Management of Care; Physiological Integrity: Pharmacological and Parenteral Therapies; Physiological Integrity: Reduction of Risk Potential; **Cognitive Level:** Analysis [Analyzing]

## 2312. PHARM ANSWER: 4

1. Lithium levels should be checked every 1 to 2 months, not every 2 weeks.
2. Lithium often causes stomach upset and can be taken with food for better tolerance.
3. Sugary foods only should be avoided if weight gain becomes a problem.
4. **When taking lithium (Lithobid), the client must consume adequate dietary sodium and 2500 to 3000 mL of fluids per day to prevent dehydration that can lead to lithium toxicity.**

▶ **Test-taking Tip:** *Hyponatremia and dehydration will lead to lithium toxicity.*

**Content Area:** Mental Health; **Concept:** Medication; Fluid and Electrolyte Balance; Safety; **Integrated Processes:** Nursing Process: Evaluation; **Client Needs:** Physiological Integrity: Pharmacological and Parenteral Therapies; **Cognitive Level:** Evaluation [Evaluating]

## 2313. PHARM ANSWER: 4

1. Antipsychotics (not valproic acid) block the effects of dopamine at the postsynaptic neuron.
2. Lithium (not valproic acid) is thought to enhance reuptake of norepinephrine and serotonin in the CNS.
3. Another anticonvulsant such as carbamazepine (not valproic acid) alters sodium channels in neurons, thus decreasing synaptic transmission.
4. **Valproic acid (Depakote) increases levels of GABA, an inhibitory neurotransmitter in the CNS, thus decreasing manic and impulsive behavior.**

▶ **Test-taking Tip:** *You should note that "acid" appears in the stem and in only one option.*

**Content Area:** Mental Health; **Concept:** Medication; Mood; Violence; **Integrated Processes:** Nursing Process: Analysis; **Client Needs:** Physiological Integrity: Pharmacological and Parenteral Therapies; **Cognitive Level:** Comprehension [Understanding]

## 2314. PHARM ANSWER:

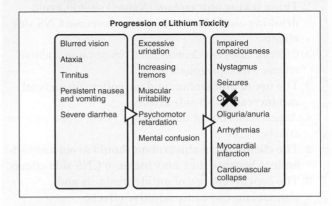

**Progression of Lithium Toxicity**

| Blurred vision | Excessive urination | Impaired consciousness |
| Ataxia | Increasing tremors | Nystagmus |
| Tinnitus | | Seizures |
| Persistent nausea and vomiting | Muscular irritability | ✗ Coma |
| Severe diarrhea | Psychomotor retardation | Oliguria/anuria |
| | Mental confusion | Arrhythmias |
| | | Myocardial infarction |
| | | Cardiovascular collapse |

**Symptoms of lithium (Lithane) toxicity begin to appear at blood levels greater than 1.5 mEq/L. The third column lists symptoms of lithium levels above 3.5 mEq/L, some of which include impaired consciousness, nystagmus, seizures, and arrhythmias. The first column lists symptoms of lithium levels between 1.5 and 2.0 mEq/L. The middle column lists symptoms of serum levels between 2.0 and 3.5 mEq/L.**

▶ **Test-taking Tip:** *Lithium levels above 3.5 mEq/L are extremely toxic. To remember the normal range, recall that the high value is double the low value. It is also similar to serum creatinine, except that serum creatinine is expressed in mg/dL. A toxic level is also the same as the low normal value for a serum potassium level of 3.5 mEq/L.*

**Content Area:** Mental Health; **Concept:** Medication; Safety; Assessment; **Integrated Processes:** Nursing Process: Assessment; **Client Needs:** Physiological Integrity: Pharmacological and Parenteral Therapies; Physiological Integrity: Reduction of Risk Potential; **Cognitive Level:** Analysis [Analyzing]

## 2315. PHARM ANSWER: 3

1. Isosorbide dinitrate (Isordil) does not interact with lithium.
2. Prednisone (Deltasone) does not interact with lithium.
3. **The nurse should question the use of furosemide (Lasix). It is a loop diuretic that promotes sodium loss and lithium (Lithane) retention. It can increase serum lithium levels, resulting in toxicity.**
4. Insulin aspart (NovoLog) does not interact with lithium, but lithium should be used cautiously in clients with DM.

▶ **Test-taking Tip:** *Lithium competes with various cations including Na+, K+, Ca+, and Mg+, thereby affecting cell membranes, body water, and neurotransmitters. As you review options, consider medications that also affect cations.*

**Content Area:** Mental Health; **Concept:** Medication; Safety; **Integrated Processes:** Nursing Process: Implementation; **Client Needs:** Safe and Effective Care Environment: Safety and Infection Control; Physiological Integrity: Pharmacological and Parenteral Therapies; **Cognitive Level:** Analysis [Analyzing]

**2316.** **PHARM** **ANSWER: 1, 3, 5, 6**

1. **Those taking alprazolam (Xanax) should avoid drinking alcohol because it may increase CNS side effects.**
2. Caffeine does not depress the CNS or cause additive effects with alprazolam.
3. **The use of alprazolam and narcotics concurrently can increase CNS side effects.**
4. Antioxidants do not depress the CNS or cause additive effects.
5. **The client taking alprazolam should avoid antihistamines because they may increase CNS side effects.**
6. **The concurrent use of antidepressants and alprazolam can cause additive effects.**

▶ *Test-taking Tip: Use the process of elimination. Alprazolam is a CNS depressant, and alcohol, narcotics, antihistamines, and antidepressants can further decrease CNS.*

**Content Area:** Mental Health; **Concept:** Medication; Stress; Safety; **Integrated Processes:** Teaching/Learning; **Client Needs:** Health Promotion and Maintenance; Physiological Integrity: Pharmacological and Parenteral Therapies; **Cognitive Level:** Application [Applying]

**2317.** **PHARM** **ANSWER: 1**

1. **Buspirone (BuSpar), an antianxiety agent in the azaspirodecanedione drug classification, is not recommended for prn use because of a 10- to 14-day delay in therapeutic onset. The nurse should question the order if prescribed for prn use.**
2. Lorazepam (Ativan) is a benzodiazepine. It has a rapid onset of therapeutic effectiveness and is appropriate for prn use.
3. Clorazepate (Tranxene) is a benzodiazepine. It has a rapid onset of therapeutic effectiveness and is appropriate for prn use.
4. Clonazepam (Klonopin) is a benzodiazepine. It has a rapid onset of therapeutic effectiveness and is appropriate for prn use.

▶ *Test-taking Tip: Although all the options are anxiolytics, two medications end in "-am," indicating that they are likely benzodiazepines. Since both cannot be correct, they should be eliminated. Of the remaining options, eliminate the medication that is a benzodiazepine but does not end in "-am."*

**Content Area:** Mental Health; **Concept:** Medication; Stress; **Integrated Processes:** Nursing Process: Evaluation; **Client Needs:** Physiological Integrity: Pharmacological and Parenteral Therapies; **Cognitive Level:** Evaluation [Evaluating]

**2318.** **PHARM** **ANSWER: 1**

1. **Physical and psychological dependence often are associated with the use of benzodiazepines such as chlordiazepoxide (Librium). The client is describing tolerance, a sign of dependence, and the dose needs reevaluated.**
2. Doses should not be doubled if medication is being skipped. Skipping chlordiazepoxide reduces its therapeutic effects.

3. Resistance is not the same as dependence; chlordiazepoxide will continue to exert its pharmacological effect with higher doses. Increasing the dosage is not indicated in the development of dependence.
4. Insufficient information is provided in the situation to determine if the client's anxiety is hormone-related.

▶ *Test-taking Tip: Think about precautions required with continued use of benzodiazepines. Remember that tolerance and/or withdrawal constitutes drug dependency. Eliminate any options in which there is insufficient information to make the judgment stated in the option.*

**Content Area:** Mental Health; **Concept:** Stress; Medication; Critical Thinking; **Integrated Processes:** Nursing Process: Analysis; **Client Needs:** Physiological Integrity: Pharmacological and Parenteral Therapies; **Cognitive Level:** Analysis [Analyzing]

**2319.** **PHARM** **ANSWER: 3**

1. Clozapine (Clozaril) is a member of the newer generation of antipsychotics with less potential for EPS.
2. Risperidone (Risperdal) is a member of the newer generation of antipsychotics with less potential for EPS.
3. **Haloperidol (Haldol), a conventional antipsychotic, is the only medication listed with a high probability of EPS.**
4. Ziprasidone (Geodon) is a member of the newer generation of antipsychotics with less potential for EPS.

▶ *Test-taking Tip: Place the medication in the typical and newer-generation atypical classes of antipsychotics. One option does not fit in the same classification as the others, and that is the answer.*

**Content Area:** Mental Health; **Concept:** Medication; Cognition; **Integrated Processes:** Nursing Process: Planning; **Client Needs:** Physiological Integrity: Pharmacological and Parenteral Therapies; **Cognitive Level:** Application [Applying]

**2320.** **PHARM** **ANSWER: 3**

1. Hypertension, dizziness, headache, and insomnia frequently are seen with the use of MAOIs.
2. Weight gain, tremors, and sedation are commonly associated with atypical antipsychotics.
3. **Blurred vision, dry mouth, and constipation are common side effects of anticholinergic agents such as benztropine mesylate (Cogentin). This medication counteracts the extrapyramidal symptoms secondary to the use of typical antipsychotics.**
4. Headache, dry mouth, and sexual dysfunction are associated with SSRIs.

▶ *Test-taking Tip: Think about the classification for benztropine mesylate and narrow the options to those associated with anticholinergic agents.*

**Content Area:** Mental Health; **Concept:** Medication; Assessment; **Integrated Processes:** Nursing Process: Assessment; **Client Needs:** Physiological Integrity: Pharmacological and Parenteral Therapies; **Cognitive Level:** Application [Applying]

**2321.** PHARM **ANSWER: 1, 4, 5**

1. **Atypical antipsychotic medications are designed to target both positive and negative symptoms, which include hallucinations and inappropriate emotional responses.**
2. Atypical antipsychotic medications generally are chosen as first-line treatments over conventional antipsychotics.
3. Atypical antipsychotic medications often are favored over conventional antipsychotic medications because they are less likely to cause anticholinergic and extrapyramidal side effects.
4. **Atypical antipsychotic medications can increase the risk of elevated blood glucose levels, so regular laboratory testing is performed.**
5. **Atypical antipsychotic medications can increase the risk of metabolic syndrome characterized by elevated blood glucose levels, increased appetite, and weight gain.**

♦ *Test-taking Tip: To narrow the options, consider that atypical antipsychotic medications often are prescribed because of their effectiveness and less-severe side effects.*

Content Area: Mental Health; Concept: Nursing Roles; Medication; Integrated Processes: Teaching/Learning; Client Needs: Physiological Integrity: Pharmacological and Parenteral Therapies; Cognitive Level: Application [Applying]

**2322.** PHARM **ANSWER: 2**

**Use the formula for calculating medication dosages. Formula:**

$$\frac{\text{Desired}}{\text{Have}} \times mL = mL \text{ per dose}; \frac{4 \text{ mg}}{2 \text{ mg}} \times 1 \text{ mL} = 2 \text{ mL}$$

**The nurse should administer 2 mL haloperidol (Haldol).**

♦ *Test-taking Tip: Focus on the information in the question and use a calculator. The key phrase is "for each dose." Verify your response, especially if it is an unusual amount.*

Content Area: Mental Health; Concept: Cognition; Medication; Safety; Integrated Processes: Nursing Process: Implementation; Client Needs: Physiological Integrity: Pharmacological and Parenteral Therapies; Cognitive Level: Application [Applying]

**2323.** PHARM **ANSWER: 1, 2**

1. **Constipation, not diarrhea, is a characteristic side effect of risperidone (Risperdal). The client needs additional teaching.**
2. **Hypotension, not hypertension, is a characteristic side effect of risperidone (Risperdal). The client needs additional teaching.**
3. Tardive dyskinesia involves bizarre facial and tongue movements, a stiff neck, and difficulty swallowing. It may occur as an adverse effect of long-term therapy with some antipsychotic medications, including risperidone (Risperdal).
4. Weight gain is a potential side effect of atypical antipsychotic medications.

5. Orthostatic hypotension is a side effect of an atypical antipsychotic medication.
6. Drowsiness is a potential side effect of an atypical antipsychotic medication.

♦ *Test-taking Tip: Use the process of elimination and focus on the side effects of atypical antipsychotic medications, especially risperidone.*

Content Area: Mental Health; Concept: Cognition; Medication; Integrated Processes: Nursing Process: Evaluation; Client Needs: Physiological Integrity: Pharmacological and Parenteral Therapies; Cognitive Level: Evaluation [Evaluating]

**2324.** PHARM **ANSWER: 4**

1. There is no known increased risk for the development of respiratory disease.
2. Hypotension rather than hypertension is a known potential side effect of antipsychotic medications.
3. There is no known increased risk for GI diseases.
4. **The use of the antipsychotic medication risperidone (Risperdal) appears to increase the risk of diabetes, especially in the first few months of drug therapy.**

♦ *Test-taking Tip: Use the process of elimination and focus on the side effects of atypical antipsychotic medications, especially risperidone.*

Content Area: Mental Health; Concept: Cognition; Metabolism; Assessment; Integrated Processes: Nursing Process: Assessment; Client Needs: Psychosocial Integrity; Physiological Integrity: Pharmacological and Parenteral Therapies; Physiological Integrity: Physiological Adaptation; Cognitive Level: Analysis [Analyzing]

**2325.** PHARM **ANSWER: 3**

1. Dizziness is a possible side effect of traditional antipsychotic medications.
2. Constipation is a possible side effect of traditional antipsychotic medications.
3. **Drowsiness, not insomnia, is a common side effect of traditional antipsychotic medications. This statement shows that the client needs further teaching.**
4. Weight gain is a possible side effect of traditional antipsychotic medications.

♦ *Test-taking Tip: Use the process of elimination and focus on the potential side effects of traditional antipsychotic medications.*

Content Area: Mental Health; Concept: Medication; Cognition; Nursing Roles; Integrated Processes: Nursing Process: Evaluation; Client Needs: Physiological Integrity: Pharmacological and Parenteral Therapies; Cognitive Level: Evaluation [Evaluating]

**2326.** PHARM **ANSWER: 2, 4, 5**

1. Dehydration is not an adverse effect of clozapine.
2. **Agranulocytosis (failure of the bone marrow to produce enough neutrophils) is an adverse effect of clozapine (Clozaril). About 20 percent of Jewish people develop agranulocytosis, which has been attributed to a specific genetic haplotype.**
3. Increasing anxiety is not an adverse effect of clozapine.

4. **Hypersalivation is an adverse effect of clozapine (Clozaril).**

5. **Hyperglycemia is an adverse effect of clozapine (Clozaril).**

▶ *Test-taking Tip: Clozapine is an atypical antipsychotic medication producing anticholinergic adverse effects. Select options that include anticholinergic effects.*

**Content Area:** Mental Health; **Concept:** Medication; Assessment; **Integrated Processes:** Nursing Process: Evaluation; **Client Needs:** Physiological Integrity: Pharmacological and Parenteral Therapies; **Cognitive Level:** Evaluation [Evaluating]

## 2327. PHARM ANSWER: 1, 3, 5

1. **With BPD, a reduction in the client's anxiety indicates olanzapine (Zyprexa) is effective.**

2. Cognitive restructuring techniques, rather than medications, are more likely to improve the overuse of psychological splitting. Psychological splitting is a defense mechanism. The person's thinking is either all-or-nothing or black-and-white. There is no gray area.

3. **With BPD, a reduction in the client's paranoia indicates olanzapine is effective.**

4. Olanzapine has not shown a more significant rate of improvement for depression over time than placebo.

5. **With BPD, a reduction in the client's hostility indicates olanzapine is effective.**

▶ *Test-taking Tip: Olanzapine is an atypical antipsychotic. When selecting options, consider its effects on cognitive improvement and controlled behavioral functioning.*

**Content Area:** Mental Health; **Concept:** Mood; Medication; **Integrated Processes:** Nursing Process: Evaluation; **Client Needs:** Physiological Integrity: Pharmacological and Parenteral Therapies; **Cognitive Level:** Evaluation [Evaluating]

## 2328. ANSWER: 1

1. **Because the client is experiencing extrapyramidal symptoms (EPS) of pseudoparkinsonism, akinesia, and akathisia, the nurse should administer an antiparkinsonian agent to restore the natural balance of acetylcholine and dopamine in the CNS.**

2. Escorting the client to his or her room is not the least-restrictive intervention. The client should be able to sit while in the day room, or have assistance with walking.

3. Using limb restraints is not the least-restrictive intervention appropriate for this client.

4. The assessment reveals EPS, not tardive dyskinesia.

▶ *Test-taking Tip: Focus on using the least-restrictive intervention and identify the side effects described in the stem.*

**Content Area:** Mental Health; **Concept:** Medication; Assessment; **Integrated Processes:** Nursing Process: Implementation; **Client Needs:** Physiological Integrity: Physiological Adaptation; **Cognitive Level:** Application [Applying]

## 2329. PHARM ANSWER: 0.5

Use a proportion formula to calculate the dosage. Then multiply the extremes (outside values) and the means (inside values) and solve for $X$.

$1 \text{ mg} : 1 \text{ mL} :: 0.5 \text{ mg} : X \text{ mL}$
$X = 0.5 \text{ mL}$

▶ *Test-taking Tip: Focus on the information in the question and use a calculator. Verify your response, especially if it is an unusual amount.*

**Content Area:** Mental Health; **Concept:** Medication; Neurologic Regulation; **Integrated Processes:** Nursing Process: Implementation; **Client Needs:** Physiological Integrity: Pharmacological and Parenteral Therapies; **Cognitive Level:** Application [Applying]

## 2330. PHARM ANSWER: 3

1. *Absorption* refers to the rate at which the medication enters the bloodstream.

2. *Affinity* is how strongly a medication binds to a specific receptor.

3. **Varenicline (Chantix) functions as an antagonist. These drugs cause receptor blockade, thereby resulting in a reduction in transmission and decreased neurotransmitter activity.**

4. *Agonists* increase neurotransmitter activity by direct stimulation of specific receptors; varenicline is not an agonist.

▶ *Test-taking Tip: Look for a word related to "antagonist" in the options.*

**Content Area:** Mental Health; **Concept:** Medication; Addiction; **Integrated Processes:** Nursing Process: Analysis; **Client Needs:** Physiological Integrity: Pharmacological and Parenteral Therapies; **Cognitive Level:** Application [Applying]

## 2331. PHARM ANSWER: 2

1. Zaleplon (Sonata) has a 30-minute onset, peak concentration at 1 hour, and a 3- to 4-hour duration.

2. **The peak effectiveness point of triazolam (Halcion) is much later than that of the other medications listed in the table. It has a slightly longer duration of action. Triazolam will have the greatest effect, helping the client fall asleep and stay asleep longer.**

3. Flurazepam has an onset of 30 minutes, peak effect of 30 minutes to 1 hour, and duration of 7 to 8 hours. Because it reaches peak effect sooner than zaleplon (Sonata), the client may have difficulty staying asleep.

4. Eszopiclone (Lunesta) has a rapid to 30-minute onset, a peak concentration 1 hour after administration, and a 6-hour duration. Because it reaches peak effect sooner than zaleplon, the client may have difficulty staying asleep.

▶ *Test-taking Tip: Look for information in the chart that stands out as different, such as the peak and duration of triazolam.*

**Content Area:** Mental Health; **Concept:** Medication; Sleep, Rest, and Activity; **Integrated Processes:** Nursing Process: Analysis; **Client Needs:** Physiological Integrity: Pharmacological and Parenteral Therapies; **Cognitive Level:** Application [Applying]

**2332. PHARM ANSWER: 2, 3, 4, 5**

1. For a child with ADHD, stimuli should be low and the environment kept as quiet as possible.
2. **The atomoxetine (Strattera) should be administered after meals to reduce anorexia.**
3. **To prevent insomnia, the dose should be administered at least 6 hours before bedtime.**
4. **Weekly weights are indicated due to potential anorexia, weight loss and temporary interruption of growth and development.**
5. **OTC cold and allergy medications should be avoided because many contain sympathomimetic agents that could compound the drug's effect.**

▶ *Test-taking Tip: Atomoxetine (Strattera) is a selective norepinephrine reuptake inhibitor with an end effect of increasing adrenergic neurotransmission. Use this information to narrow the options.*

Content Area: Mental Health; Concept: Development; Medication; Nursing Roles; Integrated Processes: Teaching/Learning; Client Needs: Physiological Integrity: Pharmacological and Parenteral Therapies; Cognitive Level: Application [Applying]

**2333. PHARM ANSWER: 4**

1. There are no significant musculoskeletal effects associated with the use of stimulant medications in a child with ADHD.
2. There are no significant genitourinary effects associated with the use of stimulant medications in a child with ADHD.
3. There are no significant immunological side effects associated with the use of stimulant medications in a child with ADHD.
4. **The most critical information to collect on the child with ADHD is the cardiovascular (CV) history. Certain CV conditions contraindicate the use of psychostimulants.**

▶ *Test-taking Tip: Use the ABC's to determine a priority body system. ADHD is treated with CNS stimulants, which could have adverse effects on the client with cardiovascular disease.*

Content Area: Mental Health; Concept: Development; Medication; Safety; Integrated Processes: Nursing Process: Assessment; Client Needs: Physiological Integrity: Pharmacological and Parenteral Therapies; Cognitive Level: Analysis [Analyzing]

**2334. PHARM ANSWER: 2**

1. The neurological system should be assessed because dizziness and drowsiness may occur as adverse effects, but these are of less importance than the cardiovascular system.
2. **The nurse should focus the initial assessment on the cardiovascular (CV) system because the sympathetic activity of clonidine (Catapres) can cause hypotension and bradycardia.**
3. Dry mouth is a side effect of clonidine, so the GI system should be assessed, but it is of less importance than the CV system.
4. Because there are no anticipated musculoskeletal reactions to clonidine, an assessment of the musculoskeletal system is the least important.

▶ *Test-taking Tip: Clonidine is prescribed often to treat hypertension. Use the ABC's to determine the system that should be priority.*

Content Area: Mental Health; Concept: Perfusion; Medication; Safety; Integrated Processes: Nursing Process: Assessment; Client Needs: Physiological Integrity: Pharmacological and Parenteral Therapies; Cognitive Level: Application [Applying]

**2335. PHARM ANSWER: 4**

1. Encouraging smoking cessation is important but does not advocate for client safety in this situation.
2. Bupropion is the generic name for Zyban, which the client is already taking. Requesting a dose increase will be harmful.
3. Overdose is more of a concern than allergic reaction because the client already has been taking bupropion.
4. **Bupropion is the generic name for Zyban. The medication should not be used to treat more than one condition at a time. Additive doses can increase the risk of seizures.**

▶ *Test-taking Tip: Be familiar with both generic and trade names. Recognize that medication duplication is occurring. This can lead to overmedication if not addressed.*

Content Area: Mental Health; Concept: Safety; Medication; Nursing Roles; Integrated Processes: Nursing Process: Implementation; Caring; Client Needs: Physiological Integrity: Pharmacological and Parenteral Therapies; Cognitive Level: Application [Applying]

**2336. PHARM ANSWER:**

| Serum Laboratory Test | Client's Result |
|---|---|
| Albumin (3.2–4.6 g/dL) | 2.8 g/dL X |
| AST (15–40 units/L) | 65 units/L X |
| ALT (10–40 units/L) | 60 units/L X |
| Total bilirubin (0.2–1.3 mg/dL) | 3.8 mg/dL X |
| Alkaline phosphatase (ALP) (35–142 units/L) | 160 units/L X |

**The liver function tests (LFTs) are abnormal. Albumin is low and AST, ALT, total bilirubin, and ALP are elevated (see normal values in the answer table). Disulfiram (Antabuse) can affect the liver. Potassium, RBCs, and Hgb are normal. The normal potassium range is 3.5 to 5.5 mEq/L. Normal RBCs are male: 5.21–5.81×10^6 cells/microL and female: 3.91–5.11×10^6 cells/microL. The normal Hgb is male: 13.5–17.3 g/dL and female: 11.7–15.5 g/dL.**

▶ *Test-taking Tip:* A method for remembering the LFTs is to think of Alcoholics Anonymous (AA) and use the initials as a memory cue for the four LFTs that begin with the letter A (albumin, AST, ALT, ALP). Then, to remember bilirubin, recall that there are five LFTs and that the letter B follows A.

**Content Area:** Mental Health; **Concept:** Safety; Medication; Nursing Roles; **Integrated Processes:** Nursing Process: Implementation; **Client Needs:** Physiological Integrity: Pharmacological and Parenteral Therapies; Physiological Integrity: Reduction of Risk Potential; **Cognitive Level:** Application [Applying]

## 2337. **PHARM** ANSWER: 1

1. **The buprenorphine/naloxone combination (Suboxone) has both agonistic and antagonistic effects. Buprenorphine is an agonist, enabling opioid-addicted individuals to discontinue opioid misuse without experiencing withdrawal. The antagonist naloxone is added to decrease the potential for opiate abuse by blocking receptor sites targeted by opiates, thus preventing feelings of pleasure or euphoria.**
2. Naloxone (Narcan) is an opiate antagonist, not a nutritional supplement.
3. Naloxone does not minimize the opiate-like side effects of buprenorphine.
4. Since naloxone is given with buprenorphine, it does not induce an adverse reaction when given in combination.

▶ *Test-taking Tip:* The question is focusing on naloxone, not buprenorphine. Draw on knowledge of narcotic antagonists that begin with "Na-" (Narcan, naltrexone, naloxone, nalmefene) and apply their actions.

**Content Area:** Mental Health; **Concept:** Medication; **Integrated Processes:** Nursing Process: Analysis; **Client Needs:** Physiological Integrity: Pharmacological and Parenteral Therapies; **Cognitive Level:** Comprehension [Understanding]

## 2338. **PHARM** ANSWER: 2

1. Fennel and ginger ease stomachaches.
2. **Chamomile tea and hops are believed to relieve insomnia.**
3. Feverfew and peppermint are thought to be helpful in treating headaches.
4. Echinacea is used to boost immunity, and goldenseal is used as an antibiotic, antiseptic, and anti-inflammatory agent.

▶ *Test-taking Tip:* Knowledge of herbal remedies is necessary to answer this question. To narrow the choices, you should relate the options to something you already know.

**Content Area:** Mental Health; **Concept:** Sleep, Rest, and Activity; Medication; **Integrated Processes:** Nursing Process: Planning; **Client Needs:** Physiological Integrity: Pharmacological and Parenteral Therapies; Physiological Integrity: Basic Care and Comfort; **Cognitive Level:** Application [Applying]

## 2339. **PHARM** ANSWER: 1

1. **Naloxone (Narcan) is indicated for the reversal of CNS and respiratory depression due to suspected opioid overdose.**

2. Disulfiram (Antabuse) is used for aversion therapy in recovery from alcohol dependency.
3. Flumazenil (Romazicon) reverses the action of a benzodiazepine.
4. Acetylcysteine (Acetadote) injection is an IV antidote for the treatment of acetaminophen overdose.

▶ *Test-taking Tip:* Note the similarity in the medication name naloxone to its use as a narcotic agonist. Eliminate the other options.

**Content Area:** Mental Health; **Concept:** Medication; Addiction; **Integrated Processes:** Nursing Process: Planning; **Client Needs:** Physiological Integrity: Pharmacological and Parenteral Therapies; **Cognitive Level:** Analysis [Analyzing]

## 2340. **PHARM** ANSWER: 4

1. Flumazenil (Romazicon) reverses the action of a benzodiazepine on the CNS, including sedation, recall impairment, and psychomotor impairment. It is given to treat benzodiazepine toxicity or overdose and would not be used to calm the client during substance withdrawal.
2. Guaifenesin (Mucinex) reduces the viscosity of tenacious secretions by increasing respiratory tract fluid, and it would not be used to calm the client during substance withdrawal.
3. Bupropion (Zyban) is an antidepressant that decreases neuronal reuptake of dopamine in the CNS; it also is used for smoking cessation. Nicotine withdrawal does not typically produce delirium.
4. **Lorazepam (Ativan) is a benzodiazepine that depresses the CNS, probably by potentiating GABA, the anti-inhibitory neurotransmitter, thereby decreasing anxiety. This medication will help calm the client.**

▶ *Test-taking Tip:* Use the suffix "-pam" to identify a benzodiazepine that can be used to control anxiety.

**Content Area:** Mental Health; **Concept:** Cognition; Safety; Stress; **Integrated Processes:** Nursing Process: Implementation; **Client Needs:** Psychosocial Integrity; Physiological Integrity: Pharmacological and Parenteral Therapies; **Cognitive Level:** Analysis [Analyzing]

## 2341. **PHARM** ANSWER: 1, 2, 3

1. **The nurse should question orders for olanzapine (Zyprexa) because injections of the drug are indicated for short-term (not long-term) use in acute symptom management.**
2. **Ziprasidone (Geodon) injections are intended for short-term use to manage acute symptoms.**
3. **The antipsychotic aripiprazole (Abilify) is not available in injectable form.**
4. Risperidone Consta is a sustained-release injectable antipsychotic. With a duration of 2 weeks, it is appropriate for long-term use.
5. Fluphenazine decanoate is a sustained-release injectable form of antipsychotic. With a duration of 1 to 6 weeks, it is appropriate for long-term use.

▶ **Test-taking Tip:** *Sustained-release forms for long-term use have two-word names; thus, eliminate these options. This is a false-response option, so you should select the options that are not appropriate for long-term use in treating schizophrenia.*

**Content Area:** Mental Health; **Concept:** Medication; Cognition; Safety; **Integrated Processes:** Nursing Process: Implementation; **Client Needs:** Physiological Integrity: Pharmacological and Parenteral Therapies; **Cognitive Level:** Analysis [Analyzing]

## 2342. PHARM ANSWER: 3

1. Blood glucose testing would need to be performed before an oral hyperglycemic agent would be indicated. Antidiabetic agents are indicated only if blood glucose testing reveals hyperglycemia.
2. Insulin is indicated only if blood glucose testing reveals hyperglycemia that cannot be controlled with oral hyperglycemic agents.
3. **Atypical antipsychotics such as olanzapine (Zyprexa) are associated with treatment-related hyperglycemia. Because the client has a risk factor for DM and is overweight, blood glucose testing should be completed to determine whether medication therapy is indicated.**
4. Olanzapine is indicated for control of schizophrenia; it is not necessary to discontinue it and start another medication.

▶ **Test-taking Tip:** *You need to avoid reading into the situation and reaching the conclusion that the client also has DM. You need to assess the client for the common side effect of the medication.*

**Content Area:** Mental Health; **Concept:** Medication; Communication; **Integrated Processes:** Communication and Documentation; **Client Needs:** Physiological Integrity: Pharmacological and Parenteral Therapies; **Cognitive Level:** Analysis [Analyzing]

## 2343. MoC ANSWER: 3

1. The client's cardiac rhythm should be monitored for dysrhythmias that can occur with inhalant use; however, this is not the priority.
2. Because the CNS is affected and can be permanently damaged by inhalant use, seizure precautions may be warranted, but this is not the priority.
3. **The nurse's priority is to apply oxygen. Wheezing indicates that the airways are narrowed due to inflammation or an allergic response. When the chemical solvent paint thinner is inhaled, it replaces the oxygen in the client's system.**
4. A toxicology screen should be obtained to determine the chemicals in the client's system, but first the nurse should give oxygen.

▶ **Test-taking Tip:** *Use the ABC's to determine the priority.*

**Content Area:** Mental Health; **Concept:** Medication; Critical Thinking; **Integrated Processes:** Nursing Process: Implementation; **Client Needs:** Safe and Effective Care Environment: Management of Care; Physiological Integrity: Physiological Adaptation; **Cognitive Level:** Application [Applying]

## 2344. MoC ANSWER: 2

1. This statement is correct; the client can learn to identify triggers that can heighten anxiety.
2. **This statement indicates that the client needs further teaching. Buspirone (BuSpar) and not diazepam (Valium) is the long-term medication of choice because of its nonaddictive quality. Valium is highly addictive.**
3. Research has shown that clients who give a high importance to religious practices have improved panic symptoms and fewer recurrences.
4. Guided imagery and meditation have been shown to effectively reduce anxiety symptoms.

▶ **Test-taking Tip:** *This is a false-response item; you need to select the statement that is incorrect.*

**Content Area:** Mental Health; **Concept:** Medication; Stress; Nursing Roles; Promoting Health; **Integrated Processes:** Nursing Process: Evaluation; **Client Needs:** Safe and Effective Care Environment: Management of Care; Health Promotion and Maintenance; **Cognitive Level:** Application [Applying]

## 2345. MoC PHARM ANSWER: 5, 3, 2, 4, 1

5. **The client who has had increasing confusion and nystagmus and just had a seizure may have severe lithium toxicity and is the nurse's priority. These symptoms occur when the serum lithium level is above 3.5 mEq/L.**
3. **The client who has blurred vision, ataxia, and tinnitus is the nurse's next priority. This client is experiencing signs of lithium toxicity and requires immediate intervention. Blurred vision, ataxia, and tinnitus occur when the serum lithium level is 1.5 to 2.0 mEq/L.**
2. **The client who has a fever, rash, and the beginning of hives is the third priority. The client likely is experiencing an allergic reaction that could worsen.**
4. **The client who has mild hand tremors, nausea, and vomiting is the nurse's next priority. The client's symptoms need to be evaluated, and the client needs an antiemetic medication. The client is experiencing side effects from lithium and may need treatment for this.**
1. **The client who has a dry mouth, headache, and thirst can be addressed last. The client is experiencing side effects that can be minimized by teaching the client appropriate interventions such as sucking on an ice cube or gumdrop and relieving headache with acetaminophen.**

▶ **Test-taking Tip:** *Use the ABC's to establish priority. You need to think about the symptoms associated with lithium (Lithane) toxicity when prioritizing the clients. Place the clients in order from the most severe reactions to the least severe.*

**Content Area:** Mental Health; **Concept:** Medication; Critical Thinking; Nursing Roles; Management; **Integrated Processes:** Nursing Process: Assessment; **Client Needs:** Safe and Effective Care Environment: Management of Care; Physiological Integrity: Pharmacological and Parenteral Therapies; **Cognitive Level:** Synthesis [Creating]

**2346.** PHARM **ANSWER: 1**

1. **Guanfacine (Tenex) is used to target ADHD symptoms through central alpha-2 receptor activity in the prefrontal cortex. However, because guanfacine is a central-acting antihypertensive agent, the nurse should take the child's BP first.**
2. The child does not have DM, and guanfacine does not cause hypoglycemia. Equipment would not be available to check the glucose level. The HCP must prescribe the glucose check.
3. Although the parent should be telephoned about the child's symptoms, this is not the first action.
4. A cool cloth may feel comforting but is not the first action.

▸ **Test-taking Tip:** Use the nursing process; assessment is the first step. Invasive procedures are not performed in a school setting without being prescribed by an HCP.

**Content Area:** Mental Health; **Concept:** Assessment; Safety; Medication; **Integrated Processes:** Nursing Process: Assessment; **Client Needs:** Physiological Integrity: Pharmacological and Parenteral Therapies; **Cognitive Level:** Application [Applying]

**2347.** PHARM **ANSWER: 2**

1. Although promethazine is used to treat an allergic reaction, this is not the primary indication for combining it with phenobarbital during detoxification.
2. **Promethazine (Phenergan) will potentiate the CNS depression of the phenobarbital, producing a greater sedative effect to reduce withdrawal symptoms. Both promethazine and phenobarbital are CNS depressants.**
3. Although promethazine is used to treat nausea, there is no increased incidence of nausea when given IM.
4. The combination of promethazine and phenobarbital will produce sedation and a hangover effect.

▸ **Test-taking Tip:** Note that Options 2 and 4 are opposites. Eliminate one or both of these. Then eliminate options that address actions of promethazine that may be correct but are not indicated in this situation (prevents allergic reactions and decreases nausea).

**Content Area:** Mental Health; **Concept:** Medication; Nursing Roles; **Integrated Processes:** Nursing Process: Evaluation; **Client Needs:** Physiological Integrity: Pharmacological and Parenteral Therapies; **Cognitive Level:** Evaluation [Evaluating]

**2348.** PHARM **ANSWER: 2**

**First, determine the number of tablets for the total daily dose:**

**5 mg : 1 tablet :: 20 mg : $X$ tablets; $5X = 20$; $X = 20 \div 5$; $X = 4$ tablets.**

**The total daily dose of 20 mg would be 4 tablets of dextroamphetamine (Adderall). Next, determine just the number of morning tablets to administer ($4 \div 2 = 2$). The nurse should administer 2 tablets for the morning dose.**

▸ **Test-taking Tip:** First, determine the total dosage for the day and then divide the total dose by 2 to determine the amount of each dose.

**Content Area:** Mental Health; **Concept:** Medication; **Integrated Processes:** Nursing Process: Implementation; **Client Needs:** Physiological Integrity: Pharmacological and Parenteral Therapies; **Cognitive Level:** Application [Applying]

**2349.** CJ MoC PHARM **ANSWER: 1C, 2E, 3B, 6A**

1. **Aripiprazole (Abilify) is an atypical antipsychotic. Tremors, shuffling gait, and rigidity are signs of pseudoparkinsonism, a side effect of aripiprazole (Reason C). The HCP should be notified. This client's symptoms are reversible if treated with benztropine, an anticholinergic medication.**
2. **Fluphenazine (Prolixin) is an antipsychotic medication. Involuntary deviation and fixation of the eyeballs, usually in the upward position, suggests oculogyric crisis (Reason E). This is an extrapyramidal side effect of some antipsychotic medications. The HCP should be notified because the dose may need adjustment or a different medication may be prescribed.**
3. **Haloperidol (Haldol), a first-generation antipsychotic medication, blocks postsynaptic dopamine receptors and increases dopamine turnover. Lip smacking and uncontrolled rhythmic movement of the mouth, face, and extremities suggest tardive dyskinesia (Reason B). The HCP should be notified.**
4. Lisinopril (Prinivil) is an ACE inhibitor. There is no reason to contact the HCP regarding this medication. The client's assessment findings are related to risperidone and not lisinopril.
5. A side effect of aripiprazole (Abilify) is hyperglycemia and the development of DM. Metformin (Glucophage) may be prescribed for the hyperglycemia associated with aripiprazole use. The client's assessment findings are related to aripiprazole use and not metformin.
6. **Risperidone (Risperdal) is an atypical antipsychotic. The involuntary muscular movements indicate that this client is experiencing dystonia (Reason A). The HCP should be notified because the dose may need adjustment or a different medication may be prescribed.**

▸ **Test-taking Tip:** This type of question requires careful analysis of the information. You need to carefully consider medication side effects and drug interactions. On the NCLEX-RN exam, the medications and reasons may appear as drop-down menus so you can select the medication and then the reason.

**Content Area:** Mental Health; **Concept:** Medication; Safety; **Integrated Processes:** Nursing Process: Assessment, Communication and Documentation; **Client Needs:** Safe and Effective Care Environment: Management of Care; Physiological Integrity: Pharmacological and Parenteral Therapies; **Cognitive Level:** Application [Applying]

**2350.** MoC CJ PHARM **ANSWER: 4**

1. Although the HCP should be notified about the client's pseudoparkinsonism, this client's symptoms are reversible with benztropine, an anticholinergic medication.
2. The HCP should be notified about the client's dystonia because the dose may need adjustment or a different medication may need to be prescribed, but this client is not priority.
3. The HCP should be notified about the extrapyramidal side effect because the dose may need adjustment or a different medication may be prescribed. But this client is not priority.
4. **This client is priority. When the person has signs of tardive dyskinesia, the medication should be immediately withheld and the HCP notified because these symptoms may be irreversible.**

▶ *Test-taking Tip: Although the HCP may be notified if the client's symptoms are observed for the first time, you need to decide which symptoms would be irreversible if the medication were not withheld and discontinued.*

**Content Area:** Mental Health; **Concept:** Medication; Safety; **Integrated Processes:** Nursing Process: Assessment, Communication and Documentation; **Client Needs:** Safe and Effective Care Environment: Management of Care; Physiological Integrity: Pharmacological and Parenteral Therapies; **Cognitive Level:** Application [Applying]

# Comprehensive Tests

## Chapter Fifty-One

# Comprehensive Exam 1

1. **MoC** The former wife of the hospitalized client telephones to ask the nurse for a status report on the client's condition. Which statement by the nurse is **most** appropriate?

   1. "He has been comfortable throughout the day. He'll be discharged tomorrow."
   2. "I'm sorry; I can neither confirm nor deny whether this person is at the hospital."
   3. "You may contact your ex-husband. Here is the room's telephone number."
   4. "Due to confidentiality laws, I need to know your name before I can give you information."

2. The nurse is preparing medications. The nurse should wear gloves when giving which medications? **Select all that apply.**

   1. Chlorothiazide 250 mg orally
   2. Phytonadione 10 mg intramuscularly
   3. Tamoxifen 15 mg oral supplied in 10 mg tablets
   4. Hydrocortisone 0.5% topically to skin lesions
   5. Azithromycin 500 mg by IVPB

3. **MoC** **PHARM** The client's laboratory report following surgery shows WBCs 18,000/mm$^3$, SCr 2.2 mg/dL, K 3.5 mEq/L, and Hgb 6.8 mg/dL. The nurse reports the findings to the HCP, who prescribes interventions. As directed, the nurse removes the subclavian venous access device and sends the tip for culture. Place the remaining interventions in the order they should be performed by the nurse.

   1. Start infusing cephazolin sodium 1 g IV.
   2. Administer 1 unit packed RBCs.
   3. Prime the blood tubing with 0.9% NaCl.
   4. Insert a new IV access device.
   5. Send ancillary personnel to obtain the blood from the blood bank according to agency policy.
   6. With another nurse, verify the client's identification and complete the checks for safe administration of the packed RBCs.

   Answer: _____

4. The client is admitted to a facility for treatment of alcohol dependence and admits to drinking 12 beers a day for 7 years. Which information, collected during the admission interview, is **most** significant in planning care during the initial stages of treatment?

   1. Malnourished
   2. Tongue tremors
   3. Family discord
   4. High school graduate

5. The nurse admits the client who has cool, pale extremities, HR 110 bpm, BP 100/55 mm Hg, RR 34, restlessness, diaphoresis, and a low urine output. Prioritize the nurse's actions by placing the interventions in the order they should be performed.

   1. Administer intravenous fluids.
   2. Apply oxygen per nasal cannula.
   3. Provide warm blankets.
   4. Initiate cardiac monitoring.

   Answer: _____

6. The client with type 2 DM has made lifestyle changes to control elevated blood glucose levels. Which finding supports the nurse's conclusion that the client's efforts to control the elevated levels have been highly effective over the last 3 months?

   1. Hemoglobin A$_{1c}$ level at 5%
   2. Absence of ketones in the urine
   3. No occurrence of diabetic ketoacidosis
   4. Negative oral glucose tolerance test

7. **PHARM** Hydrocortisone 2.5 mg/kg IV q12h is prescribed for a pediatric client experiencing dyspnea and wheezing from an asthma episode. The child weighs 25 kg. The medication vial is labeled 100 mg/2 mL. How many mL of medication should the nurse administer?

   _____ mL (Round to hundredths.)

**8.** MoC The OR nurse is preparing for the client's procedure. How should the nurse ensure that the correct procedure is being performed on the correct client?

1. Ask the client to state his or her first and last name.
2. Check the medical record for the name and date of birth.
3. Apply the universal protocol and perform a "timeout."
4. Make sure that the operative site is marked with an "X."

**9.** MoC The nurse is planning a room assignment for the client diagnosed with hepatitis C. Which room type and precautions should the nurse assign?

1. Semiprivate room and standard precautions
2. Private room and droplet isolation precautions
3. Private room and airborne isolation precautions
4. Semiprivate room and contact isolation precautions

**10.** MoC The nurse has been assigned to care for four newborns. Which one should the nurse assess **first?**

1. Baby A, who is large for gestational age (LGA)
2. Baby B, who was born through meconium-stained fluid
3. Baby C, who is at 35 weeks gestation with stable VS
4. Baby D, who had an Apgar score of 3 at 1 minute and 5 at 5 minutes

**11.** PHARM The client with severe depression asks the nurse about taking St. John's wort as an alternative to prescription antidepressants. Which is the **best** response by the nurse?

1. "I would suggest you discuss the possibility of using St. John's wort with your doctor."
2. "Two doses of St. John's wort are equivalent to one dose of a prescription antidepressant."
3. "There is insufficient evidence indicating St. John's wort is effective for treating depression."
4. "Since St. John's wort is an herbal therapy, it is a safe alternative to using an antidepressant."

**12.** PHARM The nurse in the presurgical holding area is caring for the client who has a WBC count of 2.8 K/mm$^3$. Which action is **most** important for the nurse to plan prior to initiating an IV access?

1. Request an order for prophylactic antibiotics.
2. Perform hand hygiene with an alcohol-based rub.
3. Use antibacterial soap to cleanse the client's arm.
4. Initiate respiratory isolation precautions.

**13.** PHARM The nurse is preparing to initiate TPN in a central venous line for the client with acute pancreatitis. The nurse has properly identified the client and verified the container of TPN solution with the HCP's order. Prioritize the remaining steps the nurse should take to initiate the TPN.

1. Purge the IV tubing with the TPN solution.
2. Check patency of the central line by injecting with 10 mL of saline, then connect the tubing to the client's central line port.
3. Assess the client's knowledge of TPN and educate as needed.
4. Set the infusion pump at the prescribed rate and start the infusion.
5. Select the appropriate tubing and filter.
6. Place the tubing in a volume control IV pump.

Answer: _____

**14.** PHARM The mother of the toddler with type 1 DM asks the nurse if her child would benefit from an insulin infusion pump. Which statement should be the basis for the nurse's response?

1. The child newly diagnosed with type 1 DM produces decreasing amounts of insulin for about 1 year, then insulin production stops.
2. Toddlers are too young to have an insulin pump due to the risk of hyper- or hypoglycemia and concerns about keeping the tubing patent.
3. The toddler receives only a small amount of insulin in one injection; an insulin pump is not needed until larger amounts of insulin are required.
4. Parents must be willing to check blood sugar levels every 3 to 4 hours and adjust the child's insulin, food, and/or physical activity based on the results.

**15.** The nurse is calculating the obstetrical history of the client who is pregnant. The client reports having one miscarriage at 10 weeks and one child born at 39 weeks. What number should the nurse document on the client's medical record for gravida?

_____ Gravida (Record your answer as a whole number.)

**16.** PHARM The client is taking gabapentin. The nurse evaluates that gabapentin is effective when obtaining which assessment findings?

1. Less muscle weakness and decreased spasticity
2. Decrease in chronic pain intensity and seizures
3. Increased WBC count and increased hemoglobin
4. Improvement in mobility and cognitive function

**17.** `MoC` `PHARM` While reviewing the MAR of the client with depression, the nurse finds that the HCP prescribed sertraline but the dose is unclear. What is the nurse's **best** action?

1. Contact the HCP to clarify the dose and frequency.
2. Call the pharmacist to verify the dose prescribed.
3. Consult the drug book to determine normal doses.
4. Discuss the prescribed dose with the charge nurse.

**18.** The client states to the nurse, "I am thinking about not continuing chemotherapy. I only had the last round to please my family and oncologist." Which nursing intervention is the **most** appropriate?

1. Listen carefully and encourage the client to express his or her feelings and concerns.
2. Notify the oncologist about the client's decision and request a referral to hospice care.
3. Use therapeutic communication skills to speak to the client's family about these wishes.
4. Ask whether the client has searched the Internet or library for the newest treatment options.

**19.** `MoC` The nurse notes illustrated skin changes on the arm of the client who is 19 days post-autologous peripheral blood stem-cell transplantation (PBSCT) for treatment of NHL. The nurse notifies the HCP, concerned that the client is most likely experiencing which problem?

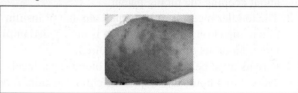

1. Herpes zoster infection
2. An allergic reaction to a new drug
3. Graft versus host disease (GVHD)
4. An infection from the PICC line

**20.** The client who had a transurethral resection of the prostate (TURP) 8 weeks ago tells the clinic nurse that he no longer ejaculates during sexual intercourse and asks if this is expected. Which statement should be the basis for the nurse's response?

1. Retrograde ejaculation can occur after a TURP, but it usually is resolved within 2 weeks.
2. Physical problems are rare after a TURP; this client may have another problem.
3. The client is describing an unusual symptom that needs thorough evaluation by an HCP.
4. The most common long-term side effect following TURP is retrograde ejaculation.

**21.** The nurse is evaluating the client's ability to perform active ROM. Which action is the client performing when the nurse makes the observation illustrated?

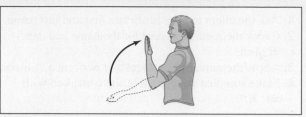

1. Internal rotation
2. Elbow flexion
3. Shoulder adduction
4. Pronation

**22.** The nurse is evaluating the client's understanding of care for a sigmoid colostomy. The nurse recognizes the need for additional teaching when the client makes which statement?

1. "I may not always need to wear a collection bag if I do colostomy irrigations."
2. "I will examine the skin around the stoma every time I change the appliance."
3. "If I injure the stoma during irrigation, I will know because it will be painful."
4. "The colostomy should be odor-free if the pouch is properly applied and sealed."

**23.** The parent of the 4-year-old boy is concerned about nocturnal enuresis. What information should the nurse include when educating the parent?

1. Proper hand washing will help prevent nocturnal enuresis episodes.
2. Antipyretics may be administered every 4 hours around the clock.
3. The incidence of nocturnal enuresis will increase as the child matures.
4. Bedwetting should not be considered a problem until 6 years of age.

**24.** `MoC` The nurse conducts an admission interview of the hospitalized client. Which approach would best assess the client's cultural needs?

1. During introductions, address the cultural backgrounds of both the client and nurse.
2. Ask with which specific culture the client identifies and if there are any cultural needs.
3. Ask if the client needs any of the available culture-specific services offered by the facility.
4. Determine where the client lives and if he or she has any social and religious affiliations.

**25.** The nurse is completing discharge teaching for the 18-year-old client hospitalized for treatment of anorexia nervosa. Which statement should the nurse include?

1. "Now that you have learned to eat again, you are likely to feel hungry often and should eat."
2. "Expect that you might feel fat and uncomfortable; this is characteristic of an eating disorder."
3. "You should have your parents prepare the foods you like to eat so you can regain weight you lost."
4. "Isn't it nice to feel that you are in control of your life now? You'll do fine with your meal plan."

**26.** The nurse is discharging the client who had an MI with stent placement and subsequent four-vessel coronary artery bypass graft surgery. The client has a BMI of 30 and a history of hypertension, smokes 1 pack per day (PPD) of cigarettes, and has prescriptions for aspirin, clopidogrel bisulfate, atenolol, and atorvastatin. Which discharge instructions are **most** appropriate? **Select all that apply.**

1. "Discontinue the use of your compression stockings when at home."
2. "Use a soft toothbrush and electric razor; you may bleed easily."
3. "Minimize alcohol intake; atorvastatin and alcohol affect the liver."
4. "Maintain your present weight; you need the calorie intake for healing."
5. "Begin smoking cessation once your incision is completely healed."
6. "Discontinue the atenolol when your heart rate is less than 60 bpm."

**27.** **PHARM** The client weighing 50 kg with a vascular leg ulcer requires a continuous IV infusion of heparin 15 units/kg/hr. To administer the correct dose, the nurse should prepare the infusion pump to deliver how many units of heparin per hour?

_____ units (Record a whole number.)

**28.** A pediatric voiding cystourethrography is prescribed for the 4-year-old who had four UTIs during the past year. When preparing the child and parents for the procedure, which statement by the nurse is **most** accurate?

1. "Your child will need an overnight hospital stay while this test is being performed."
2. "You will need to stay outside your child's room because radiation is used for the test."
3. "For the test, a catheter with contrast solution will be inserted into your child's bladder."
4. "The procedure is painless, so your child will not need to receive any medication."

**29.** **MoC** At 0700 hours, the HCP writes medication orders for the newly admitted client:

- Clopidogrel bisulfate 75 mg oral daily
- Aspirin 325 mg oral daily
- Piperacillin/tazobactam 3.37 g IVPB q6h
- Potassium chloride 40 mEq oral tid

At 0800, the nurse is validating the prescribed medications on the client's electronic MAR prior to administration. Place an X on the prescribed medication that was entered incorrectly by the pharmacist.

| Scheduled Medications | 0001-0759 | 0800-1559 | 1600-2400 |
|---|---|---|---|
| Clopidogrel bisulfate 75 mg oral daily | | 0800 _____ | |
| Aspirin 325 mg oral daily | | 0800 _____ | |
| Piperacillin/tazobactam 3.37 g q4h IV Mixed in 100 mL NS | 0200 _____ | 0800 _____ 1400 _____ | 2000_____ |
| Potassium chloride 40 mEq tid oral | | 0800 _____ 1200 _____ | 1700_____ |

**30.** The nurse is assisting the 32-year-old new mother who is struggling with breastfeeding her 1-day-old newborn. The mother starts crying and states, "I don't know why I can't get the baby to nurse. Maybe I am not ready to be a mother." Which is the **best** response by the nurse?

1. "Of course you are ready to be a mother; you are 32 years old."
2. "Maybe you should try giving the baby a bottle during the night."
3. "Do you know anyone who has been successful with breastfeeding?"
4. "Tell me what makes you feel like you're not ready to be a mother."

**31.** **PHARM** The client is not adhering to the HCP's advice about dietary modifications and taking lovastatin as prescribed. The nurse completes additional teaching. Based on the results of the client's serum laboratory results at follow-up, which conclusion by the nurse is accurate?

| Lipid Profile | Client's Results |
| --- | --- |
| Total Cholesterol | 170 mg/dL |
| Triglycerides | 100 mg/dL |
| HDL | 60 mg/dL |
| LDL | 100 mg/dL |

1. The teaching or lovastatin is ineffective; the LDL level is elevated.
2. The teaching or lovastatin is ineffective; the total cholesterol is elevated.
3. The teaching and lovastatin are effective; the HDL and triglyceride levels are normal.
4. The teaching and lovastatin are effective; the LDL is normal, and the HDL is elevated.

**32.** The client who is unresponsive and has sepsis develops hyperthermia. Which interventions should the nurse plan to treat the client's hyperthermia? **Select all that apply.**

1. Administer a bath with tepid water.
2. Place the client on a water-cooling blanket.
3. Place covered ice packs to axilla and groin.
4. Give belladonna and opium (B&O) rectally.
5. Give acetaminophen 500 mg rectal suppository.
6. Irrigate the client's NG tube with iced saline.

**33.** **MoC** The nurse is responding to the NA's call for help and brings the AED to the child's room. It appears to the nurse that the child is not breathing. The NA is standing by the child. What should the nurse do **now?**

1. Tell the NA to open the child's airway and give 2 breaths.
2. Direct the nursing assistant to check the child for a pulse.
3. Quickly set up the AED and apply the conduction pads.
4. Begin CPR; tell the next person arriving to set up the AED.

**34.** The 82-year-old who has had fatigue, ataxia, and confusion is brought to the clinic by a daughter. The client's laboratory report shows an Hgb of 7.0 g/dL. What additional information about the client is **most** important for the nurse to collect?

1. Recent exposure to toxic chemicals
2. Food and fluid intake and medication use
3. Ability to provide self-care following treatment
4. Amount of alcohol consumed daily and time of last drink

**35.** The nurse instructs the 13-year-old diagnosed with asthma about using a peak expiratory flow meter. Which **immediate** action should the nurse recommend if a reading falls below 50% of the client's normal personal best?

1. Go to the ED.
2. Telephone the HCP.
3. Self-administer a nebulizer treatment.
4. Use the "as needed" inhaler medication.

**36.** The nurse in the ED is admitting an agitated young adult who tried to jump from a bridge after taking a hallucinogenic drug at a party. What should be the nurse's **initial** action?

1. Call the mental health unit to arrange for inpatient treatment.
2. Give medications to reverse the effects of the hallucinogenic drug.
3. Stay with the client to prevent self-harm until relieved.
4. Call hospital security to protect staff from injury.

**37.** **PHARM** The client is hospitalized in preterm labor at 30 weeks gestation. Testing showed that the lecithin to sphingomyelin (L/S) ratio was less than 2:1. Which interventions, if prescribed, should the nurse plan to implement? **Select all that apply.**

1. Administer hydralazine.
2. Maintain the client on bedrest.
3. Prepare the client for a nonstress test.
4. Administer betamethasone.
5. Administer metronidazole.

**38.** The parent provides the following food diary for a 2-year-old to the clinic nurse. Which meal should the nurse address with the parent because the foods are unsafe for the toddler?

| Food Diary for a 2-Year-Old | | |
| --- | --- | --- |
| **Breakfast** | **Lunch** | **Dinner** |
| ½ c whole milk<br>½ c iron-fortified cereal<br>½ c orange juice | ½ c whole milk<br>½ c vegetables<br>1 egg<br>½ c noodles | ½ c whole milk<br>2 oz hot dog slices<br>¼ c rice<br>½ c vegetables<br>¼ c whole cherries |
| **Morning Snack** | **Afternoon Snack** | **Evening Snack** |
| ½ c yogurt<br>½ c fruit | ½ c whole milk<br>½ slice toast<br>1 Tbs apple butter | ½ c whole milk<br>½ slice buttered toast |

1. Breakfast
2. Lunch
3. Dinner
4. Evening snack

**39.** **MoC** The nurse is caring for clients with multiple mental health diagnoses with the aid of an NA. The nurse should caution the NA about which client due to the likelihood that the person will exhibit aggressive behavior toward other clients and hospital personnel?

1. The client diagnosed with major depressive disorder
2. The client diagnosed with intermittent explosive disorder
3. The client diagnosed with histrionic personality disorder
4. The client diagnosed with oppositional defiant disorder

**40.** **PHARM** The adolescent client with hydronephrosis receives furosemide during diuretic renography. The nurse should monitor for which adverse effects of furosemide? **Select all that apply.**

1. Ototoxicity
2. Hypertension
3. Hypoglycemia
4. Electrolyte abnormalities
5. Orthostatic hypotension

**41.** The nurse is teaching clients during a health seminar. In addition to advanced age, which factors associated with the formation of cataracts should the nurse address during the session? **Select all that apply.**

1. Truncal obesity
2. Exposure to radiation
3. History of hypertension
4. History of diabetes mellitus
5. Chronic corticosteroid use
6. Chronic exposure to sunlight

**42.** The nurse observes the rhythm illustrated on the client's cardiac monitor. What should the nurse do?

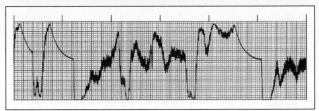

1. Call for help and activate the emergency response system used at that facility.
2. Continue to monitor the client; the rhythm is showing artifact from movement.
3. Check the client's electrodes, ECG pads, and cords plugged into electrical outlets.
4. Apply automated external defibrillator (AED) pads to interpret the client's rhythm.

**43.** The 77-year-old client has an AAA measuring 3.5 cm discovered on a routine health physical. The client has a 30-year history of cigarette smoking. Which learning need should the nurse identify as **most** important for the client?

1. Understand the importance of smoking cessation and quit smoking.
2. Understand and follow a reduced sodium and low saturated fat diet.
3. Keep medical appointments to monitor the size of the aneurysm.
4. Verbalize postoperative care following surgical repair of the aneurysm.

**44.** The client has degenerative joint disease of the left knee, which is to be treated conservatively. The nurse should include which information when planning teaching for the client? **Select all that apply.**

1. Begin a progressive walking program.
2. Modify the diet for weight reduction.
3. Apply cold or heat to the knee joint.
4. Perform rapid flexion and extension of the knee joint daily.
5. Request a prescription for narcotic analgesics for pain control.
6. Avoid prolonged standing, kneeling, squatting, and stair climbing.

**45.** The nurse is assessing the 7-month-old who has pneumonia. Which signs and symptoms should the nurse associate with pneumonia? **Select all that apply.**

1. Excessive crying
2. Rhonchi and tachypnea
3. Subnormal temperature
4. Dullness on lung percussion
5. Excessive sputum with cough

**46.** **PHARM** The nurse is educating the client on necessary dietary modifications while taking phenelzine sulfate. Which food is safe for the client to eat while taking phenelzine sulfate?

1. Bananas
2. Pepperoni
3. Wheat breads
4. Cheddar cheese

**47.** **MoC** The uninsured client arrives at the ED. The resident physician states to the client, "Since you don't have insurance, you need to go to another hospital." How should the nurse respond to the client?

1. "You can go to the hospital nearby. They will take good care of you there."
2. "I will try to find another doctor who is willing to provide the care you need."
3. "You have the right to be treated at this hospital. I will talk to the resident."
4. "I'll ask for something for your pain. I'm sorry; we can't do anything more."

**48.** **PHARM** The postpartum client asks whether she can take ibuprofen for severe afterpains due to breastfeeding. Which statement should be the basis for the nurse's response?

1. Naproxen is the NSAID of choice for mothers who are breastfeeding.
2. No analgesics should be taken when a postpartum woman is breastfeeding.
3. Acetaminophen is the only analgesic that should be avoided when breastfeeding.
4. Ibuprofen is the preferred analgesic because it has poor transfer into breast milk.

**49.** The nurse is caring for clients in an inpatient psychiatric unit. Which client behavior should the nurse identify as posing a high risk for sexual behavior?

1. Aggression
2. Visual hallucinations
3. Feelings of superiority
4. Need for independence

**50.** The client receiving hospice care has oxygen at 4L/NC. Which interventions should the nurse implement when the client develops increased respiratory effort, copious secretions, and increasing respiratory distress? **Select all that apply.**

1. Increase the dosage of morphine sulfate.
2. Raise the head of the bed to 60 degrees.
3. Administer hyoscyamine as prescribed.
4. Administer an expectorant medication.
5. Obtain a fan to circulate air in the room.

**51.** **MoC** The group of clients is assigned to a team consisting of an RN and an LPN. Which client should the RN assign to the LPN to provide client care and administer medications?

1. The 14-year-old client with CRF who will need a subcutaneous injection of epoetin
2. The 6-year-old client with hemophilia A who has been admitted for a blood transfusion
3. The 12-year-old who received a recent stem cell transplant and is to have a bone marrow aspiration
4. The 4-year-old with chemotherapy-induced neutropenia who has an elevated oral temperature

**52.** **MoC** The client who had a colon resection for removal of diverticula has comorbidities of DM and COPD. The team of HCPs includes a surgeon, hospitalist, endocrinologist, and pulmonologist. Which plan by the case manager should provide individualized client care?

1. Coordinate communication, plans, and goals from the various HCPs.
2. Plan a multidisciplinary care conference with all of the HCPs present.
3. Direct the nurse providing care to document about the HCP's plan of care.
4. Recommend to each HCP that the hospitalist should direct the plan of care.

**53.** **MoC** The client had a D&C for an incomplete spontaneous abortion. Which statements should the nurse include when preparing the client for discharge the same day? **Select all that apply.**

1. "Return for a blood transfusion if bleeding continues to be dark red."
2. "Intravenous antibiotics will be prescribed every 8 hours for 2 days."
3. "I can make a referral to a pregnancy loss support group if you like."
4. "You need to use contraceptives to avoid getting pregnant for 1 year."
5. "Someone should remain with you at home for the first 12 to 24 hours."

**54.** The nurse is assessing the client who has meningitis. Which illustration indicates that the client has decorticate posturing in response to pain?

**1.**

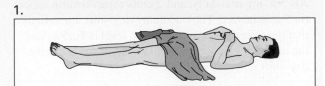

**2.**

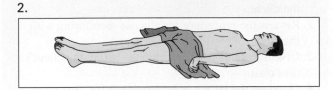

**3.**

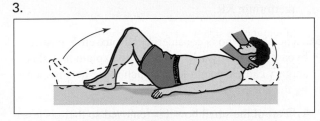

**4.**

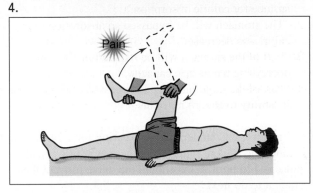

**55.** The client diagnosed with PD is noted to be at high risk for falls. Which intervention by the nurse would be **most** effective in fall prevention?

1. Assess the client more frequently than usual.
2. Apply a vest restraint to keep the client in bed.
3. Ask family to stay with the client at all times.
4. Instruct the NA to check the client more often.

**56.** The nurse is caring for the toddler who is sitting on the potty chair with a book. Based on this information, at which level of Erikson's Stages of Development should the nurse place the toddler?

1. Trust versus Mistrust
2. Initiative versus Guilt
3. Autonomy versus Guilt
4. Autonomy versus Shame and Doubt

**57.** MoC The nurse identifies the following outcome for the newly delivered full-term infant: *Area around umbilical cord will remain dry and free of erythema.* To accomplish this outcome, which intervention should the nurse include in the plan of care?

1. Cover the cord with a transparent dressing.
2. Apply a lubricating lotion to the cord twice daily.
3. Only give sponge baths until the cord falls off.
4. Rotate the cord in a circle with each diaper change.

**58.** The mother of the child is devastated and crying. She was just informed that the only chance for her child to live is to have a bone marrow transplant, and the only compatible donor is her other child. Which nursing intervention is **most** appropriate at this time?

1. Call a crisis counselor to come see the mother.
2. Listen quietly while the mother talks and cries.
3. Question the mother about her fears and concerns.
4. Describe how the bone marrow will be obtained.

**59.** The home-care nurse is visiting the client with Alzheimer's disease. Which question by the nurse is **most** appropriate when attempting to assess the level of depression that the client's spouse is experiencing as the primary caregiver?

1. "Do you feel that caring for your spouse is stressful?"
2. "What do you do when you have spare time to yourself?"
3. "Do you need someone in your home part-time to help?"
4. "Caregiving must keep you from doing the things you enjoy."

**60.** The 52-year-old client tells the nurse that she has not had a menstrual period for 15 months. The client wonders if she still needs to be concerned about an unplanned pregnancy. Which is the nurse's **best** response?

1. "The risk of pregnancy is reduced at your age, but it is still possible."
2. "As long as a female is having sexual intercourse, pregnancy is possible."
3. "Becoming pregnant at age 52 increases the risk of a spontaneous abortion."
4. "Since you have not had a menstrual period for so long, a pregnancy is unlikely."

**61.** The 4-year-old is crying and hugging a teddy bear while being admitted to the pediatric unit. Which response by the nurse is **best**?

1. "Hello, my name is Chris. Come with me; I am going to show you to your new room."
2. "I see that you are crying. Let's go to the playroom, where you can meet other children."
3. "Hi. You're likely afraid. I see that you have your teddy bear. What's your bear's name?"
4. "Can I hold you and your teddy bear to take you to the room? You can put teddy to bed."

**62.** **MoC** The hospitalized adolescent states, "It's difficult for me to fall asleep; I worry about my schoolwork." Which response by the LPN requires immediate follow-up by the nurse?

1. "You sound worried about your schoolwork, and it's affecting your sleep."
2. "When at home, how long does it usually take you to fall asleep at night?"
3. "Sleep problems are common among people who drink too much caffeine."
4. "Tell me more about the stressors or concerns that you are feeling right now."

**63.** **PHARM** The client being seen in the ED has a purulent forearm cut caused by a rusty piece of metal. The client has a temperature of 102.8°F (39.3°C) and neck stiffness. The client's last tetanus booster was 6 years ago. Which medications, if prescribed by the HCP, should the nurse administer at this time?

1. Fentanyl and metronidazole
2. Diazepam and penicillin G
3. Morphine sulfate and vecuronium
4. Tetanus and diphtheria toxoid (Td) booster and tetanus immune globulin (TIG)

**64.** **PHARM** The client has a serum potassium level of 3.3 mEq/L prior to surgery. The HCP prescribes KCL 20 mEq IV. Which intervention is the nurse's **priority**?

1. Wait to start the medication until the client is asleep during surgery.
2. Administer the medication as soon as obtained through IV bolus.
3. Apply a warm towel to the client's arm to prevent vein irritation.
4. Ensure that KCL is diluted in 100 mL of saline and given over an hour.

**65.** **PHARM** The client with type 2 DM is hospitalized during the night with an infected foot ulcer. The HCP prescribes capillary glucose qid a.c. and h.s., metformin XR 500 mg oral daily, and 2 units aspart insulin subcut tid 5 minutes a.c. The oncoming day-shift nurse finds that the client's glycosylated Hgb level is 10.5%, and the morning glucose level is 184 mg/dL. What is the day-shift nurse's **priority**?

1. Initiate a consult for the diabetic educator to see the client.
2. Review the procedure for glucose monitoring with the client.
3. Give the aspart insulin 5 minutes before the client's breakfast.
4. Question the HCP's order for aspart insulin and metformin XR.

**66.** The client who is considering a Roux-en-Y gastric bypass for obesity asks the nurse to explain how this surgery causes weight loss. Which is the **best** response by the nurse?

1. "Part of the small bowel is removed so there is less surface for calorie absorption."
2. "The stomach will be bypassed so absorption of calories is decreased."
3. "Part of the stomach will be reduced in size, thus decreasing the gastric capacity."
4. "Part of the large intestine is bypassed, thus decreasing its ability to absorb nutrients."

**67.** The nurse and student nurse is caring for a 24-hour-old infant. The student reports that the newborn's apical pulse is 146 bpm. What should the nurse instruct the student to do **next**?

1. Monitor the pulse again in 1 hour.
2. Place an oximeter on the newborn.
3. Document the apical pulse rate.
4. Call the HCP to report the high rate.

**68.** **PHARM** The older adult client is admitted to the ED after a fall. Which medications, if taken by the client, should the nurse identify as psychotropic drugs that may have contributed to the fall? **Select all that apply.**

1. Alprazolam 1 mg daily
2. Docusate sodium 100 mg daily
3. Hydrochlorothiazide 25 mg daily
4. Potassium chloride 10 mEq bid
5. Zolpidem tartrate 10 mg daily at h.s.
6. Lisinopril 10 mg daily

**69.** The 4-year-old is hospitalized with dehydration secondary to diarrhea and emesis from a norovirus infection. Which type of isolation precautions should the nurse initiate?

1. Contact
2. Droplet
3. Airborne
4. Protective

**70.** MoC The nurse manager's review of clients' medical records indicates that nurses are giving the prescribed presurgical antibiotics 2 hours prior to incision time rather than 1 hour as indicated by best practice. What approach should the nurse manager use to **best** ensure that the antibiotics are given according to best practice?

1. Tell nurses not to give the antibiotics too early.
2. Complete a variance on staff giving these too early.
3. Require mandatory education about the best practice.
4. Tell the pharmacist that the antibiotic cannot be delivered early.

**71.** PHARM The nurse is caring for the client who is receiving IV oxytocin for labor induction. The nurse determines that the appropriate dose of oxytocin is being given when what situation occurs?

1. The nurse assesses that the client's cervix is dilated to 5 cm.
2. The client expresses discomfort when there are uterine contractions.
3. The client has 60- to 90-second uterine contractions every 2 minutes.
4. The client has three 40- to 60-second uterine contractions every 10 minutes.

**72.** MoC The nurse is assessing the 76-year-old female client. Which findings require consultation with the HCP? **Select all that apply.**

1. Increased hair thinning
2. Warty growth on the vulva
3. Presence of actinic lentigo
4. Port-wine angioma on the arm
5. 2+ pitting edema of lower extremities
6. 6-mm asymmetric dark lesion on the perineum

**73.** The nurse is performing an admission assessment on the client with a history of trigeminal neuralgia (tic douloureux). What is the **best** method for the nurse to assess the severity of trigeminal neuralgia?

1. Count the number of times the client blinks within a minute.
2. Ask the client about factors that precipitate an episode of facial pain.
3. Gently palpate the areas under the cheekbones and assess for swelling.
4. Have the client stand, shut both eyes, and alternate hands to touch the nose.

**74.** PHARM The 76-year-old client hospitalized for cancer treatment has an emergency resection for a bowel obstruction. Four hours postoperatively, the client is experiencing pain. Which medication, if prescribed, should the nurse initially select to treat the client's postoperative pain?

1. Meperidine 75 mg IM
2. Fentanyl transdermal patch 50 mcg/hr
3. Morphine sulfate 4 mg IV push q3–4h prn
4. Hydromorphone continuous infusion 15 to 30 mg/hr

**75.** MoC The nurse is reviewing the chart of a client admitted for treatment of a PE. Based on the chart information, which conclusions by the nurse are correct? **Select all that apply.**

| Tab 1: Admitting History & Physical | Tab 2: Diagnostic and Serum Laboratory Data | Tab 3: Medications & Treatments |
|---|---|---|
| • Allergies: Latex and sulfonamides<br>• Had been on bedrest at home due to influenza; treated with antibiotics<br>• Severe abdominal cramping and diarrhea<br>• Chest pain with inhalation<br>• Dyspneic<br>• Hemoptysis<br>• Lung sounds: Pleural friction rub | • aPTT: 31 seconds<br>• INR: 1.2<br>• Hgb: 12.5 g/dL<br>• Hct: 37%<br>• K: 3.2 mEq/L<br>• SCr: 0.7 mg/dL<br>• WBCs: 18.9 K/mm³<br>• Stool culture positive for *Clostridium difficile*<br>• Lung scan: High ventilation perfusion (V/Q) ratio | • 0.9% NaCl at 100 mL/hr<br>• KCL 10 mEq IV now<br>• Metronidazole 500 mg IV q6h<br>• Initiate heparin IV infusion per protocol<br>• Contact isolation precautions<br>• Oxygen 2–4 liters by simple facemask |

1. Contact isolation will help prevent an allergic reaction to latex.
2. The prescribed metronidazole should be questioned with the HCP.
3. KCL was prescribed to treat the client's low serum potassium level.
4. *Clostridium difficile* may be from the antibiotics used to treat influenza.
5. The prescribed IV heparin infusion should be questioned with the HCP.
6. The oxygen as prescribed by mask should be questioned with the HCP.

## Answers and Rationales

1. MoC **ANSWER: 2**
   1. Telling the former wife about the status of the client is a breach of confidentiality.
   2. **HIPAA requires nurses to comply with privacy standards, including implementing measures to ensure privacy. If there is no permission for release of information, it may not be shared with anyone.**
   3. Providing the telephone number for the client's room still acknowledges that the client is hospitalized.
   4. Obtaining the divorced spouse's name and then providing information is a breach of client confidentiality.

   ♦ *Test-taking Tip: This is a positive-event question, so select an option that "supports" the HIPAA law.*

   Content Area: Management of Care; Concept: Legal; Communication; Integrated Processes: Communication and Documentation; Client Needs: Safe and Effective Care Environment: Management of Care; Cognitive Level: Application [Applying]

2. **ANSWER: 2, 3, 4**
   1. The nurse does not need to wear gloves when administering chlorothiazide (Diuril) unless contact with the client's mucous membranes is anticipated or the medication is hazardous.
   2. **With IM injections like phytonadione (Aquamephyton), there is potential for contact with bodily fluids.**
   3. **Tamoxifen (Tamofen) is an antiestrogen, antineoplastic agent. The nurse should wear two pairs of gloves when handling this biohazard medication. One tablet will need to be cut in half.**
   4. **Hydrocortisone (Cortaid) can be absorbed through the skin when large amounts are applied. There is the potential for contact with body fluids if skin lesions are exudative.**

5. Gloves do not need to be worn when preparing an antibiotic such as azithromycin (Zithromax) by IVPB.

▶ *Test-taking Tip: Use universal precautions when answering this question. Gloves should be worn when handling biohazard medications.*

Content Area: Fundamentals; Concept: Medication; Safety; Infection; Integrated Processes: Nursing Process: Implementation; Client Needs: Safe and Effective Care Environment: Safety and Infection Control; Cognitive Level: Application [Applying]

3. MoC PHARM **ANSWER: 4, 1, 5, 3, 6, 2**

4. **Insert a new IV access device. This will be needed to administer the antibiotics and blood transfusion.**

1. **Start infusing cephazolin sodium (Ancef) 1 g IV second. It will take about 20 minutes to infuse. This will be completed in about the time it takes to obtain the blood from the blood bank and prime the blood tubing.**

5. **Send ancillary personnel to obtain the blood from the blood bank according to agency policy. Obtaining blood can be delegated to ancillary personnel while the nurse assesses and prepares the client and readies the tubing for infusion. Blood should be started within 30 minutes of obtaining it from the blood bank. It should be obtained close to the time it is to be infused.**

3. **Prime the blood tubing with 0.9% NaCl. This is performed after delegating the obtaining of the blood. The nurse should be ready when the blood arrives because it will need to be returned to the blood bank for further refrigeration if out for more than 30 minutes.**

6. **With another nurse, verify the client's identification and complete the checks for safe administration of the packed RBCs. Verification with another nurse helps to ensure that the right client is receiving the right blood type.**

2. **Administer 1 unit packed RBCs. This is the last of the options because steps need to be taken first to ensure client safety.**

▶ *Test-taking Tip: When establishing priorities, determine the amount of time each action will take. Remember blood must be started within 30 minutes of retrieval from the blood bank, and medication administration with the blood is contraindicated.*

Content Area: Adult; Concept: Infection; Assessment; Management; Medication; Integrated Processes: Nursing Process: Implementation; Client Needs: Safe and Effective Care Environment: Management of Care; Physiological Integrity: Pharmacological and Parenteral Therapies; Cognitive Level: Synthesis [Creating]

4. **ANSWER: 2**

1. Nutritional status is important to address, but only after ensuring client safety.

2. **A tongue tremor is one sign of delirium tremens (DTs) and is most significant because of the concern for the client's safety during withdrawal.**

3. Family discord is important to address, but it does not take precedence over the client's safety.

4. Educational level is important information to include in appropriate care during the rehabilitation phase of treatment following a safe detoxification from alcohol, but it is not the most significant information.

▶ *Test-taking Tip: Use Maslow's Hierarchy of Needs theory. Physiological problems are priority. Consider which finding indicates a possible problem that may affect client safety.*

Content Area: Mental Health; Concept: Addiction; Assessment; Safety; Integrated Processes: Nursing Process: Analysis; Client Needs: Safe and Effective Care Environment: Safety and Infection Control; Cognitive Level: Analysis [Analyzing]

5. **ANSWER: 2, 4, 3, 1**

2. **Apply oxygen per nasal cannula. Oxygen is priority because it will help decrease the workload of the heart.**

4. **Initiate cardiac monitoring next. The symptoms suggest a possible cardiovascular problem, and more information is needed to initiate appropriate interventions.**

3. **Provide warm blankets next to increase client comfort and avoid hypothermia. Shivering increases oxygen demand, and warm blankets can be applied quickly. They also can promote peripheral vasodilation and make IV catheter insertion easier.**

1. **Administer IV fluids after placement of an IV access device. Fluids will increase intravascular volume, the client's BP, and urine output.**

▶ *Test-taking Tip: Use the ABC's and the nursing process to establish priority. Cardiac monitoring is an assessment and should be performed first. Next, consider the actions that could be performed more quickly than the remaining ones.*

Content Area: Adult; Concept: Perfusion; Safety; Critical Thinking; Integrated Processes: Nursing Process: Implementation; Client Needs: Physiological Integrity: Physiological Adaptation; Cognitive Level: Synthesis [Creating]

6. **ANSWER: 1**

1. **Hgb $A_{1c}$ shows the amount of glucose attached to the Hgb molecules. This remains attached to the RBC for the life of the RBC (about 120 days). According to the American Diabetes Association, an ideal Hgb $A_{1c}$ is 7% or less for individuals with DM.**

2. The absence of ketones in the urine is not the best measure of effective blood glucose control because ketosis may not occur with elevated blood glucose levels. This is because enough insulin may be produced to prevent DKA.

3. The absence of complications such as DKA is not the best measure of effective blood glucose control. Persons with type 2 DM are more prone to hyperosmolar hyperglycemic syndrome (HHS) because their bodies can produce enough insulin to prevent DKA, but not enough to prevent severe hyperglycemia.

4. The oral glucose tolerance test (OGTT) is used to diagnose DM, not to monitor effective glucose control.

▶ *Test-taking Tip: Think about the 120 days of RBC life when answering this question.*

**Content Area:** Adult; **Concept:** Metabolism; Assessment; **Integrated Processes:** Nursing Process: Evaluation; **Client Needs:** Physiological Integrity: Physiological Adaptation; **Cognitive Level:** Evaluation [Evaluating]

### 7. PHARM ANSWER: 1.25

**First, use a proportion formula to determine the dose. Multiply the means (inside values) and extremes (outside values) and solve for *X*:**

**2.5 mg : 1 kg :: *X* mg : 25 kg; *X* = 2.5 × 25; *X* = 62.5 mg**

**Next, calculate the amount with the proportion formula:**

**100 mg : 2 mL :: 62.5 mg : *X* mL; 100*X* = 125; *X* = 125 ÷ 100; *X* = 1.25 mL. The nurse should administer 1.25 mL of hydrocortisone (Solu-Cortef).**

▶ *Test-taking Tip: Focus on the information in the question, noting that first the child's dose should be calculated based on the weight, then the amount to administer should be determined.*

**Content Area:** Child; **Concept:** Medication; Oxygenation; **Integrated Processes:** Nursing Process: Implementation; **Client Needs:** Physiological Integrity: Pharmacological and Parenteral Therapies; **Cognitive Level:** Application [Applying]

### 8. MoC ANSWER: 3

1. Asking the client to state his or her name is not enough information to verify the correct client. A second unique identifier such as birth date or medical record number also must be used.

2. Checking the medical record alone does not ensure that it is for the client in the room.

3. **The Joint Commission's universal protocol for preventing wrong-site, wrong-procedure, and wrong-person surgery and the Institute for Clinical Systems Improvement safe-site protocol include performing a "timeout" to verify that the correct procedure is being performed on the correct site and the correct client. The "timeout" is a verbal confirmation of these measures by the surgical team.**

4. Marking the operative site will not validate whether the correct client is present for surgery.

▶ *Test-taking Tip: Apply knowledge of The Joint Commission's universal protocol. The key words are "correct procedure" on the "correct client." A timeout is needed to do additional checks.*

**Content Area:** Management of Care; **Concept:** Safety; Assessment; Perioperative; **Integrated Processes:** Nursing Process: Assessment; **Client Needs:** Safe and Effective Care Environment: Management of Care; **Cognitive Level:** Application [Applying]

### 9. MoC ANSWER: 1

1. **The client can be admitted to a semiprivate room with standard precautions that include appropriate needle disposal. Hepatitis C (HCV) is transmitted percutaneously through needle sharing and needlestick accidents. It also may be transmitted via blood transfusions. Twenty percent of HCV cases are the result of high-risk sexual behavior.**

2. The client does not need to be placed on droplet isolation in a private room because HCV is not transmitted through droplets.

3. The client does not need to be placed on airborne precautions, as HCV is not transmitted through the air.

4. The client does not need to be placed on contact precautions because HCV is not transmitted in this manner.

▶ *Test-taking Tip: The focus of this question is the mode of transmission of HCV. Knowing this would allow elimination of Options 2, 3, and 4.*

**Content Area:** Adult; **Concept:** Infection; Safety; Management; **Integrated Processes:** Nursing Process: Planning; **Client Needs:** Safe and Effective Care Environment: Management of Care; **Cognitive Level:** Analysis [Analyzing]

### 10. MoC ANSWER: 4

1. The LGA baby is at increased risk for birth trauma; however, the child is of lesser priority than the infant with a low Apgar score.

2. The newborn born through meconium-stained fluid is at risk for meconium aspiration; however, the baby is of lesser priority than the infant with a low Apgar score.

3. The preterm infant is at risk for many health concerns but at present has stable VS. Thus, assessment of this infant could be delayed until the nurse has been assured that the infant with a low Apgar score is stable.

4. **An Apgar score below 4 indicates the need for newborn resuscitation. The nurse should assess this infant first to determine if the baby is currently in stable condition.**

▶ *Test-taking Tip: Prioritize using the ABC's. Select the newborn most likely to have concerns in one or all of these areas.*

Content Area: Management of Care; Concept: Pregnancy; Assessment; Integrated Processes: Nursing Process: Assessment; Client Needs: Safe and Effective Care Environment: Management of Care; Cognitive Level: Analysis [Analyzing]

## 11. PHARM ANSWER: 3

1. The nurse should provide information about the client's questions rather than simply refer the person to the HCP.
2. The nurse cannot equate dosages of St. John's wort with antidepressant medications.
3. **For patients with major depression, there is insufficient evidence to recommend hypericum (St. John's wort) as a treatment alternative. Standard therapy may be of greater benefit for moderate to severe depression.**
4. The nurse cannot recommend St. John's wort as a safe alternative to an antidepressant.

▸ *Test-taking Tip: Three options suggest the possible use of St. John's wort for depression, and one option is different. Often, the option that is different is the answer.*

Content Area: Mental Health; Concept: Mood; Medication; Integrated Processes: Communication and Documentation; Teaching/Learning; Client Needs: Physiological Integrity: Pharmacological and Parenteral Therapies; Cognitive Level: Application [Applying]

## 12. PHARM ANSWER: 2

1. No information is known about the surgical procedure; the client may or may not require prophylactic antibiotics.
2. **Hand washing is most important because the client's WBC count is low (normal WBC is 3.9 to 11.9 K/mm³ [3900 to 11,900/mm³]) and the client is at risk for infection. Hand washing and aseptic technique help prevent the introduction of microorganisms.**
3. The IV insertion site should be cleansed with an alcoholic chlorhexidine solution containing a concentration of chlorhexidine gluconate greater than 0.5%.
4. There is no information to suggest that respiratory isolation is needed. If the client is neutropenic, the appropriate precautions should be used.

▸ *Test-taking Tip: Knowing the ranges for significant laboratory values is required when taking the NCLEX-RN examination. Remember that "K" as a unit of measure represents one thousand (10³) and that 1 mm³ is equivalent to a microliter.*

Content Area: Adult; Concept: Infection; Safety; Integrated Processes: Nursing Process: Planning; Client Needs: Physiological Integrity: Pharmacological and Parenteral Therapies; Cognitive Level: Application [Applying]

## 13. PHARM ANSWER: 3, 5, 1, 6, 2, 4

3. **Assess the client's knowledge of TPN and educate as needed. Client education is essential before new procedures to assist with coping, anxiety reduction, and promoting client cooperation.**

5. **Select the appropriate tubing and filter. TPN must be administered through tubing with an in-line filter to prevent contamination.**
1. **Purge the IV tubing with the TPN solution. Purging will remove air from the tubing. If it is not removed, an air embolus can occur.**
6. **Place the tubing in a volume control IV pump. An electronic infusion device prevents fluid overload and ensures an accurate administration rate.**
2. **Check patency of the central line by injecting with 10 mL of saline, then connect the tubing to the client's central line port. The TPN must be administered via central venous access because it is a highly osmotic solution.**
4. **Set the infusion pump at the prescribed rate and start the pump. If TPN is administered too rapidly, hyperglycemia and diuresis can result.**

▸ *Test-taking Tip: Visualize the steps for administering a medication via IV infusion. The steps are the same with the exception of using filtered tubing and central venous access.*

Content Area: Fundamentals; Concept: Inflammation; Safety; Nutrition; Integrated Processes: Nursing Process: Implementation; Client Needs: Safe and Effective Care Environment: Safety and Infection Control; Physiological Integrity: Pharmacological and Parenteral Therapies; Cognitive Level: Synthesis [Creating]

## 14. PHARM ANSWER: 4

1. Toddlers do produce decreasing amounts of insulin for up to 1 year. It is very difficult to adjust the basal rate for active toddlers when insulin is being produced, but they are still candidates for insulin pumps.
2. Toddlers are not too young and are candidates for insulin pumps. Measures can be taken to ensure that the tubing remains patent and that complications are prevented.
3. It is true that toddlers receive very small amounts of insulin, but that is not an issue affecting whether the child can have an insulin pump.
4. **Insulin pumps are becoming more common in children, including toddlers. Checking blood sugars, adjusting the insulin, getting the child to eat the appropriate amount of food, and maintaining a healthy activity level require parental diligence.**

▸ *Test-taking Tip: Options 1 and 3 relate to insulin production, Option 2 relates to age, and Option 4 relates to parental responsibility. You need to think about the parental responsibilities associated with a toddler.*

Content Area: Child; Concept: Metabolism; Safety; Nursing Roles; Integrated Processes: Caring; Nursing Process: Analysis; Client Needs: Safe and Effective Care Environment: Safety and Infection Control; Physiological Integrity: Pharmacological and Parenteral Therapies; Cognitive Level: Analysis [Analyzing]

## 15. ANSWER: 3

Gravidity indicates the number of times the client has been pregnant, regardless of the outcome. The first pregnancy ended in miscarriage, the second resulted in a live birth at 39 weeks, and the woman is now pregnant for the third time, so gravida = 3.

▶ *Test-taking Tip: It is essential to know the definitions of gravidity and parity.*

**Content Area:** Childbearing; **Concept:** Pregnancy; **Integrated Processes:** Nursing Process: Assessment; **Client Needs:** Health Promotion and Maintenance; **Cognitive Level:** Application [Applying]

## 16. PHARM ANSWER: 2

1. Weakness is a side effect of gabapentin; antiepileptic medications such as this do not decrease spasticity.
2. **Gabapentin (Neurontin) is an adjunct antiepileptic medication used in treating partial or mixed seizures. It also has unlabeled uses in preventing headaches and controlling chronic pain.**
3. Gabapentin may cause leukopenia (a reduction of WBCs), but it has no effect on RBCs and Hgb.
4. Antiepileptic medications do not improve mobility or cognitive function.

▶ *Test-taking Tip: Gabapentin is an antiepileptic medication that can be used for chronic pain control. Eliminate options that do not pertain to these uses.*

**Content Area:** Adult; **Concept:** Medication; Neurologic Regulation; Comfort; **Integrated Processes:** Nursing Process: Evaluation; **Client Needs:** Physiological Integrity: Pharmacological and Parenteral Therapies; **Cognitive Level:** Evaluation [Evaluating]

## 17. MoC PHARM ANSWER: 1

1. **The nurse's best action is to clarify the order for sertraline (Zoloft) with the HCP to prevent an error in administering the medication.**
2. The prescribing HCP should clarify the order, not the pharmacist.
3. Medication literature guides the nurse in verifying safe dosages but does not clarify what the client's actual dose should be.
4. The prescribing HCP should verify the order, not the charge nurse.

▶ *Test-taking Tip: Review the rights of safe medication administration. Never administer any medication if the order is unclear or unsafe.*

**Content Area:** Mental Health; **Concept:** Medication; Safety; Communication; **Integrated Processes:** Communication and Documentation; **Client Needs:** Safe and Effective Care Environment: Management of Care; Physiological Integrity: Pharmacological and Parenteral Therapies; **Cognitive Level:** Application [Applying]

## 18. ANSWER: 1

1. **The nurse should support the client in working through the decision to stop chemotherapy treatments by carefully listening to and encouraging the client's expression of feelings and concerns.**
2. The client is "thinking about" terminating chemotherapy. It is premature to notify the oncologist and initiate hospice care. There is no indication that her cancer is terminal.
3. The client is not asking for assistance to discuss the issue with family members.
4. The client is not asking for help to determine whether other treatment options exist.

▶ *Test-taking Tip: Read the scenario in the stem carefully. Only one option focuses on the client.*

**Content Area:** Adult; **Concept:** Communication; Grief and Loss; Nursing Roles; **Integrated Processes:** Communication and Documentation; Caring; **Client Needs:** Psychosocial Integrity; **Cognitive Level:** Application [Applying]

## 19. MoC ANSWER: 3

1. Herpes zoster lesions are more commonly noted on the anterior or posterior trunk and face. The vesicles and pustules of herpes zoster are grouped unilaterally, following the pathway of a spinal or cranial nerve (dermatomal distribution); they rupture, weep, and crust and are very painful.
2. An allergic reaction to a medication is a possibility, but typically the rash appears first on the trunk or back.
3. **Acute GVHD initially may appear as a pruritic or painful skin rash. Lesions are red to violet and typically appear first on the palms, soles of the feet, cheeks, neck, ears, and upper trunk. They can progress to involve the whole body. The median onset is post-transplantation day 19, with a range of 5 to 47 days.**
4. There is no indication that this client had a PICC line in place.

▶ *Test-taking Tip: Note the key phrase "most likely." Focus on the situation, "19 days postautologous peripheral blood stem-cell transplantation." Think about complications that can occur following transplantation.*

**Content Area:** Adult; **Concept:** Skin Integrity; Hematologic Regulation; Cellular Regulation; **Integrated Processes:** Nursing Process: Analysis; **Client Needs:** Safe and Effective Care Environment: Management of Care; **Cognitive Level:** Analysis [Analyzing]

## 20. ANSWER: 4

1. Absence of ejaculation will not resolve within 2 weeks of the TURP surgery.
2. Absence of ejaculation after a TURP is not related to another problem but due to physiological changes that occur with surgery.

3. Absence of ejaculation is a common side effect of a TURP procedure, not an unusual symptom.
4. **During a TURP, the urinary sphincter mechanism is partially resected. This causes muscle weakness along the bladder outlet. When the individual ejaculates, the sphincter cannot keep the bladder adequately closed, and the ejaculate goes backward into the bladder (retrograde ejaculation) rather than forward out of the penis.**

▸ *Test-taking Tip: Focus on the anatomical alterations that result in retrograde ejaculation.*

**Content Area:** Adult; **Concept:** Male Reproduction; Nursing Roles; **Integrated Processes:** Nursing Process: Analysis; **Client Needs:** Physiological Integrity: Physiological Adaptation; **Cognitive Level:** Application [Applying]

## 21. ANSWER: 2

1. Internal rotation is flexing the elbow and rotating the shoulder by moving the arm until the thumb is turned inward.
2. **Flexion is bending at the elbow such that the lower arm moves toward its shoulder joint, decreasing the elbow angle.**
3. Shoulder adduction is moving an extended lower arm sideways and across the body as far as possible.
4. Pronation is turning the lower arm so that the palm is down.

▸ *Test-taking Tip: Use the arrow as a cue to the correct option.*

**Content Area:** Fundamentals; **Concept:** Mobility; Assessment; **Integrated Processes:** Nursing Process: Evaluation; **Client Needs:** Physiological Integrity: Basic Care and Comfort; **Cognitive Level:** Knowledge [Remembering]

## 22. ANSWER: 3

1. By performing colostomy irrigations at the same time each day, the client may be able to predict the time of evacuation and thus eliminate the need for a continuous collection device.
2. The client should inspect the peristomal skin with each pouch change.
3. **The bowel has no sensory nerve endings for pain, so the client would not experience pain if the stoma were injured. This statement indicates that additional teaching is needed.**
4. There should not be an odor if the pouch is properly applied and sealed.

▸ *Test-taking Tip: "The need for additional teaching" indicates a false-response item. Look for the incorrect statement.*

**Content Area:** Adult; **Concept:** Bowel Elimination; Comfort; Safety; **Integrated Processes:** Nursing Process: Evaluation; Teaching/Learning; **Client Needs:** Safe and Effective Care Environment: Safety and Infection Control; **Cognitive Level:** Evaluation [Evaluating]

## 23. ANSWER: 4

1. Hand washing is unrelated to nocturnal enuresis.
2. The use of antipyretics is unrelated to nocturnal enuresis.
3. The incidence of bedwetting at night will decline (not increase) as the child matures.
4. **Nocturnal enuresis, or bedwetting at night, should not be considered a problem until after age 6 because the child is still developing. Bladder control is involuntary and requires the coordinated action of the muscles, nerves, spinal cord, and brain.**

▸ *Test-taking Tip: Apply knowledge about developmental milestones. Enuresis is bedwetting.*

**Content Area:** Child; **Concept:** Urinary Elimination; Development; Nursing Roles; **Integrated Processes:** Teaching/Learning; **Client Needs:** Physiological Integrity: Basic Care and Comfort; **Cognitive Level:** Application [Applying]

## 24. MoC ANSWER: 2

1. The self-disclosure of the nurse is inappropriate and unnecessary.
2. **The best approach is to ask the person an open-ended question that allows him or her to elaborate on cultural needs.**
3. Asking the client if culture-specific services are needed does not allow for open communication and can be a block to therapeutic communication because the client can give a yes or no response.
4. Determining where the client lives and whether the person has any social or religious affiliations may not reflect the client's cultural identification but rather the nurse's interpretation.

▸ *Test-taking Tip: Focus on therapeutic communication techniques when assessing the client's cultural heritage and needs.*

**Content Area:** Management of Care; **Concept:** Diversity; Communication; **Integrated Processes:** Communication and Documentation; Culture and Spirituality; **Client Needs:** Safe and Effective Care Environment: Management of Care; **Cognitive Level:** Application [Applying]

## 25. ANSWER: 2

1. Because of starvation or purging, the client may not feel hungry but should follow the meal plan despite feeling full.
2. **Feeling fat and uncomfortable is associated with the distorted thinking that accompanies anorexia nervosa, and the client should be prepared to expect this feeling.**
3. Enmeshment should be decreased for the person with anorexia nervosa by not preparing separate or special meals for the client. The client should be expected to follow the prescribed meal plan.
4. Telling the client that it is nice to feel in control of his or her life provides false reassurance. The cycle of eating disorder behaviors is life-threatening and must be interrupted.

▸ *Test-taking Tip:* *Focus on the option that provides the client insight into the eating disorder, and eliminate the other options.*

**Content Area:** Mental Health; **Concept:** Nutrition; Self; Communication; **Integrated Processes:** Teaching/Learning; **Client Needs:** Psychosocial Integrity; **Cognitive Level:** Analysis [Analyzing]

### 26. ANSWER: 2, 3

1. Compression stockings help decrease edema in the leg from which the saphenous vein was removed. Edema tends to increase with activity. These stockings should not be discontinued.
2. **Clopidogrel (Plavix) and aspirin prevent platelet aggregation and increase the risk for bleeding. Using bleeding precautions decreases the risk.**
3. **Alcohol affects the liver, and atorvastatin (Lipitor) is metabolized by the liver and can increase liver enzymes. Alcohol consumption also increases caloric intake. A BMI of 30 indicates the client is overweight.**
4. A healthy diet for weight reduction can be initiated during the healing process.
5. Interventions for smoking cessation should begin immediately, not after healing has occurred. Smoking causes a delay in healing. People who quit smoking after cardiac surgery reduce their risk of death by at least one-third.
6. Atenolol (Tenormin) should not be discontinued without consulting the HCP. Atenolol is used for treating hypertension and decreasing cardiac irritability after an MI and cardiac surgery. For a low HR, the client should consult with the HCP and not discontinue the atenolol.

▸ *Test-taking Tip:* *Focus on the client's risk factors, surgical procedure, and prescribed medications to determine appropriate teaching. Eliminate options that increase the potential for complications (1, 4, 5, and 6).*

**Content Area:** Adult; **Concept:** Medication; Nutrition; Perfusion; Nursing Roles; **Integrated Processes:** Teaching/Learning; **Client Needs:** Physiological Integrity/Integrity: Physiological Adaptation; **Cognitive Level:** Analysis [Analyzing]

### 27. PHARM ANSWER: 750

**Use a proportion formula to determine the dose. Multiply the means (inside values) and extremes (outside values) and solve for $X$.**

**15 units : 1 kg :: $X$ units : 50 kg; $X = 15 \times 50$; $X = 750$**

▸ *Test-taking Tip:* *Focus on the information in the question and use the on-screen calculator. Dimensional analysis or another drug calculation formula also can be used to arrive at the answer.*

**Content Area:** Adult; **Concept:** Medication; Skin Integrity; **Integrated Processes:** Nursing Process: Implementation; **Client Needs:** Physiological Integrity: Pharmacological and Parenteral Therapies; **Cognitive Level:** Analysis [Analyzing]

### 28. ANSWER: 3

1. The test is performed on an outpatient basis.
2. A parent is allowed to remain in the room with the child during the procedure if the parent wears a lead apron to prevent exposure of vital organs to radiation.
3. **The contrast solution allows for fluoroscopic monitor visualization of the bladder while it is being filled to determine if liquid flows backward into one or both ureters, a condition known as vesicoureteral (VU) reflux.**
4. While analgesics may not be needed, midazolam (Versed) may be given to ease the child's anxiety.

▸ *Test-taking Tip:* *Relate terms in the stem to a term in the options. "Cysto-" pertains to the bladder. Select the option that includes the word "bladder."*

**Content Area:** Child; **Concept:** Urinary Elimination; Nursing Roles; Communication; **Integrated Processes:** Teaching/Learning; **Client Needs:** Physiological Integrity: Reduction of Risk Potential; **Cognitive Level:** Application [Applying]

### 29. MoC ANSWER:

| Piperacillin/tazobactam 3.37 g q4h IV mixed in 100 mL NS X | 0200 _____ | 0800 _____ 1400 _____ | 2000 _____ |
|---|---|---|---|

**The medication frequency for piperacillin/tazobactam (Zosyn) was entered as every 4 hours instead of every 6 hours. Although the times are correct, the frequency is incorrect and could result in a medication error.**

▸ *Test-taking Tip:* *Carefully read the prescribed medications and compare these to the MAR. To ensure safety, all parts of a prescribed medication must be transcribed correctly onto the client's MAR.*

**Content Area:** Management of Care; **Concept:** Medication; Safety; Communication; **Integrated Processes:** Communication and Documentation; **Client Needs:** Safe and Effective Care Environment: Management of Care; **Cognitive Level:** Analysis [Analyzing]

**30. ANSWER: 4**

1. Making a statement about the client's age does not promote a therapeutic relationship and good communication. This statement gives the message that the new mother's feelings are trivial.
2. Telling the mother to give the baby a bottle does not address her feelings about parenting; it also does not facilitate communication between nurse and client and may add to the mother's feelings of inadequacy.
3. Asking the mother a yes/no question can put an end to the conversation quickly and does not address the mother's feelings.
4. **An open-ended statement that allows the client and nurse to work together to discuss the mother's issues is best.**

▸ *Test-taking Tip: Focus on selecting a response that encourages communication. A mother's feelings and emotions can affect attachment.*

Content Area: Management of Care; Concept: Communication; Pregnancy; Integrated Processes: Communication and Documentation; Client Needs: Psychosocial Integrity; Cognitive Level: Application [Applying]

**31. PHARM ANSWER: 4**

1. The LDL cholesterol of 100 mg/dL is normal (normal is less than 130 mg/dL).
2. The total serum cholesterol of 170 mg/dL is normal (normal is less than 200 mg/dL).
3. The HDL is above normal; lovastatin does not have an effect on triglycerides.
4. **HMG-CoA reductase inhibitors (statins such as lovastatin [Mevacor]) reduce LDL cholesterol and increase HDL cholesterol levels. The normal value of LDL cholesterol is less than 130 mg/dL. The goal is to raise HDL cholesterol to 50 mg/dL or higher with statin antilipidemics such as lovastatin.**

▸ *Test-taking Tip: HMG-CoA reductase inhibitors (statins) have an effect on the LDL and HDL cholesterol and not triglycerides. Use this information to narrow the options.*

Content Area: Adult; Concept: Medication; Perfusion; Nutrition; Integrated Processes: Nursing Process: Evaluation; Client Needs: Physiological Integrity: Pharmacological and Parenteral Therapies; Cognitive Level: Evaluation [Evaluating]

**32. ANSWER: 1, 2, 3, 5**

1. **A tepid bath increases heat loss through conduction.**
2. **A water-cooling blanket increases heat loss and reduces body temperature.**
3. **Nonpharmacological measures such as ice packs increase heat loss through conduction, reducing body temperature.**
4. A B&O suppository is used for bladder spasms and does not lower temperature.
5. **Interventions to reduce fever in clients with neurological alterations include pharmacological measures (administration of acetaminophen [Tylenol]).**

6. Iced saline lavage may be used to constrict blood vessels for bleeding esophageal varices. It is not a treatment for hyperthermia.

▸ *Test-taking Tip: The prefix "hyper-" means excessive; "-thermia" refers to temperature.*

Content Area: Adult; Concept: Neurologic Regulation; Thermo-regulation; Integrated Processes: Nursing Process: Planning; Client Needs: Physiological Integrity: Reduction of Risk Potential; Cognitive Level: Application [Applying]

**33. MoC ANSWER: 2**

1. The child's airway should be opened, but this occurs after checking for a pulse. CPR guidelines changed in 2010.
2. **The nurse should tell the NA to check for a pulse. The initial shock of seeing an unresponsive child for the first time can immobilize a person, but directions from another will help the NA act accordingly.**
3. The nurse should set up the AED while telling the NA to assess the child's pulse and begin CPR if needed.
4. When defibrillation is required, every minute of delay worsens the child's prognosis. The nurse can set up the AED while the NA performs CPR.

▸ *Test-taking Tip: Use the nursing process. The nurse should delegate appropriate actions that can be performed by the NA.*

Content Area: Child; Concept: Safety; Critical Thinking; Oxygenation; Perfusion; Integrated Processes: Nursing Process: Implementation; Client Needs: Safe and Effective Care Environment: Management of Care; Physiological Integrity: Physiological Adaptation; Cognitive Level: Application [Applying]

**34. ANSWER: 2**

1. Exposure to chemical toxins is less common than nutritional deficiencies as a cause of anemia in older adults.
2. **Fatigue, ataxia, confusion, and an Hgb level of 7.0 g/dL suggest anemia. This condition in older adults usually is due to nutritional deficiencies and medication use for chronic conditions.**
3. The symptoms of ataxia and confusion can occur because of inadequate tissue oxygenation from the low Hgb. The symptoms are likely to resolve with blood replacement.
4. Although alcohol consumption can cause ataxia and confusion and falls could cause bleeding, the situation does not indicate that the client has bruising or has been bleeding.

▸ *Test-taking Tip: Think about the major causes of anemia in older adults prior to answering the question.*

Content Area: Adult; Concept: Hematologic Regulation; Assessment; Integrated Processes: Nursing Process: Assessment; Client Needs: Physiological Integrity: Physiological Adaptation; Cognitive Level: Analysis [Analyzing]

## 35. ANSWER: 4

1. The child should go to the ED if the peak expiratory flow does not return and stay in the yellow range (50% to 79% of personal best) and the HCP is not seen.
2. If the peak expiratory flow rate does not return immediately and stay in the yellow range (50% to 79% of personal best), the HCP should be notified.
3. Preparing for a nebulizer treatment will delay intervention.
4. **When the peak flow rate is less than 50% of the personal best, the nurse should recommend immediately taking the "as needed" medication for asthma, which should be a short-acting bronchodilator. Severe airway narrowing may be occurring.**

▶ *Test-taking Tip: A peak expiratory flow of less than 50% of the person's personal best indicates respiratory distress, and immediate intervention is needed.*

**Content Area:** Child; **Concept:** Oxygenation; Nursing Roles; **Integrated Processes:** Teaching/Learning; **Client Needs:** Physiological Integrity: Physiological Adaptation; **Cognitive Level:** Application [Applying]

## 36. ANSWER: 3

1. Inpatient treatment may be prescribed, but this is not the initial action.
2. There are no reversal agents for hallucinogenic drugs. Medications can be administered to decrease agitation.
3. **Hallucinogenic drugs alter perception; the client should not be left unattended.**
4. The client is agitated, and there is no evidence of violence against others, but the potential still exists.

▶ *Test-taking Tip: Note that three options are similar and one is different. Often, the option that is different is the answer.*

**Content Area:** Mental Health; **Concept:** Safety; Stress; Addiction; **Integrated Processes:** Nursing Process: Implementation; **Client Needs:** Psychosocial Integrity; Physiological Integrity: Physiological Adaptation; **Cognitive Level:** Application [Applying]

## 37. PHARM ANSWER: 2, 3, 4

1. Hydralazine (Apresoline), an antihypertensive agent, is administered to clients experiencing preeclampsia, not preterm labor.
2. **Bedrest will maximize placental oxygenation while fetal lung maturity progresses.**
3. **The client should be prepared for a nonstress test. This is used to monitor for uterine contractions. Labor needs to be stopped until the fetal lungs are more fully developed.**
4. **Betamethasone (Celestone Soluspan), a corticosteroid, is given to stimulate fetal lung maturity.**
5. Metronidazole (Flagyl) is an antiprotozoal and antibacterial agent used to treat a vaginal infection; there is no indication that the client has a vaginal infection.

▶ *Test-taking Tip: The essential information in the question is "preterm labor" and L/S ratio of "less than 2:1," which indicates that the fetal lungs are not mature. The client needs to be treated until fetal lung maturity advances.*

**Content Area:** Childbearing; **Concept:** Pregnancy; Medication; **Integrated Processes:** Nursing Process: Planning; **Client Needs:** Physiological Integrity: Pharmacological and Parenteral Therapies; Physiological Integrity: Physiological Adaptation; **Cognitive Level:** Application [Applying]

## 38. ANSWER: 3

1. Safe foods are offered for breakfast.
2. Safe foods are offered for lunch. Eggs are introduced when the child is 1 year of age; the child should be monitored for an egg allergy.
3. **Infants and young children should not have hot dogs or cherries because these pose a choking risk. Hot dogs expand in the child's airway, and the fibrous skins of both hot dogs and cherries make sufficient chewing of these difficult.**
4. Safe foods are offered for the evening snack.

▶ *Test-taking Tip: The key word is "unsafe." Think about the ABC's. Examine each meal to determine if any food could compromise the airway of a 2-year-old.*

**Content Area:** Child; **Concept:** Safety; Nutrition; Assessment; **Integrated Processes:** Nursing Process: Evaluation; **Client Needs:** Physiological Integrity: Reduction of Risk Potential; **Cognitive Level:** Evaluation [Evaluating]

## 39. MoC ANSWER: 2

1. Major depressive disorder is not characterized by aggression.
2. **This client is most likely to exhibit aggressive behavior. Intermittent explosive disorder is characterized by a history of aggressive behavior to others and destruction of property.**
3. Histrionic personality disorder is not characterized by aggressive behavior.
4. Oppositional defiant disorder is more typically diagnosed in adolescents and is not typically characterized by aggression.

▶ *Test-taking Tip: The key words are "aggressive behavior." Look for similar words between the stem and one of the options.*

**Content Area:** Management of Care; **Concept:** Mood; Safety; **Integrated Processes:** Nursing Process: Analysis; **Client Needs:** Safe and Effective Care Environment: Management of Care; Safe and Effective Care Environment: Safety and Infection Control; **Cognitive Level:** Application [Applying]

## 40. PHARM ANSWER: 1, 4, 5

1. **Ototoxicity is a side effect of loop diuretics, such as furosemide (Lasix).**
2. Diuretics are used for treatment of hypertension.
3. Hyperglycemia, not hypoglycemia, and glycosuria are side effects of loop diuretics, such as furosemide (Lasix).

4. Electrolyte abnormalities can occur with the use of loop diuretics, such as furosemide (Lasix), due to potassium and sodium excretion.
5. **Orthostatic hypotension is a common side effect of loop diuretic therapy, such as furosemide (Lasix), due to fluid volume loss with diuresis.**

▸ *Test-taking Tip: Note that Options 2 and 5 are opposites, so one of these is likely to be incorrect. Furosemide (Lasix) is a loop diuretic. Think about the adverse effects of furosemide when reviewing the options.*

**Content Area:** Child; **Concept:** Medication; Safety; Assessment; **Integrated Processes:** Nursing Process: Implementation; **Client Needs:** Physiological Integrity: Pharmacological and Parenteral Therapies; **Cognitive Level:** Application [Applying]

## 41. ANSWER: 2, 4, 5, 6

1. Obesity is not related to cataract formation.
2. **Cataracts form under conditions that promote water loss and increase density of the lens. Exposure to toxic agents such as radiation damages the lens.**
3. Hypertension is not related to cataract formation.
4. **Complications of DM can lead to damage of the lens.**
5. **Corticosteroid use can damage the lens.**
6. **UV light from the sun can damage the lens.**

▸ *Test-taking Tip: Toxic agents, medications, some health conditions, and aging pose a risk of cataract formation.*

**Content Area:** Adult; **Concept:** Nursing Roles; Sensory Perception; **Integrated Processes:** Nursing Process: Analysis; **Client Needs:** Physiological Integrity: Reduction of Risk Potential; **Cognitive Level:** Knowledge [Remembering]

## 42. ANSWER: 3

1. The nurse first should assess the client to determine if activating the emergency response system is necessary.
2. The artifact indicates the leads are loose. Accurate rhythm interpretation is difficult if artifact is present.
3. **Movement or loose leads can cause the illustrated artifact (a distortion of the ECG baseline and waveforms from factors other than the heart's electrical activity). The electrodes should be removed and securely replaced in areas less affected by movement.**
4. Applying an AED is premature. The nurse should assess the client first.

▸ *Test-taking Tip: Always check the client first. Though you may not initially recognize the rhythm, the information provided in the options may assist in interpreting it.*

**Content Area:** Adult; **Concept:** Perfusion; Safety; Assessment; **Integrated Processes:** Nursing Process: Implementation; **Client Needs:** Physiological Integrity: Physiological Adaptation; **Cognitive Level:** Analysis [Analyzing]

## 43. ANSWER: 3

1. Smoking cessation is important, but it is not the most important learning need.
2. Following a diet that lowers the risk of arteriosclerosis is indicated, but it is not the most important learning need.

3. **The client's most important educational need is learning to keep medical appointments. With a 3.5-cm aneurysm, continued medical surveillance is indicated, including frequent CT exams to monitor the size of the aneurysm and risk for rupture.**
4. Asymptomatic AAAs less than 6 cm in older adults usually are managed nonsurgically.

▸ *Test-taking Tip: The age of the client and size of the aneurysm are cues to the correct option in the stem. The words "most important" are key words that indicate the need to prioritize. Note that some options address surgical management and others medical management.*

**Content Area:** Adult; **Concept:** Perfusion; Safety; Nursing Roles; **Integrated Processes:** Teaching/Learning; **Client Needs:** Physiological Integrity: Physiological Adaptation; **Cognitive Level:** Analysis [Analyzing]

## 44. ANSWER: 1, 2, 3, 6

1. **Progressive walking strengthens bone and muscle and helps reduce obesity. Walking should be of a duration that is well tolerated initially, then it can be increased gradually to 30 to 60 minutes, 5 to 7 days per week.**
2. **Weight reduction decreases stress on the joints.**
3. **Cold reduces swelling and inflammation; heat increases comfort and circulation to the area.**
4. Vigorous activities that produce prolonged pain and inflammation should be avoided because these stress the joint.
5. First-line medications include acetaminophen; if not effective, then an NSAID is recommended before taking narcotic analgesics.
6. **Avoiding prolonged standing, kneeling, squatting, and stair climbing will protect the knee joint.**

▸ *Test-taking Tip: Focus on initial measures to protect the knee joint, reduce pain, and increase activity tolerance.*

**Content Area:** Adult; **Concept:** Mobility; Nursing Roles; **Integrated Processes:** Nursing Process: Planning; **Client Needs:** Health Promotion and Maintenance; Physiological Integrity: Physiological Adaptation; **Cognitive Level:** Application [Applying]

## 45. ANSWER: 2, 4, 5

1. Excessive crying usually is not noted; children are lethargic and listless.
2. **Mucus in the airways causes scattered rhonchi throughout the lung fields, and the blocked airways increase respiratory effort (tachypnea).**
3. Children with pneumonia usually have high fever (not subnormal temperature) and are warm to the touch.
4. **Consolidation in the lungs causes dullness on percussion.**
5. **Coughing is due to excessive sputum production from the inflammation that occurs with pneumonia.**

▸ *Test-taking Tip: "Pneumo-" refers to lungs. Identify the options associated with the lungs.*

**Content Area:** Child; **Concept:** Infection; Assessment; Oxygenation; **Integrated Processes:** Nursing Process: Assessment; **Client Needs:** Physiological Integrity: Reduction of Risk Potential; **Cognitive Level:** Comprehension [Understanding]

## 46. PHARM ANSWER: 3

1. Bananas contain moderate to high levels of tyramine and should be avoided during MAOI therapy.
2. Pepperoni should be avoided during MAOI therapy due to the levels of tyramine in the food.
3. **Foods high in tyramine should be avoided when taking phenelzine sulfate (Nardil), an MAOI. Wheat bread is allowed because it is low in tyramine.**
4. Cheddar cheese has moderate to high levels of tyramine and should be avoided during MAOI therapy.

▶ **Test-taking Tip:** *Those taking MAOIs should avoid foods containing high amounts of tyramine.*

**Content Area:** Mental Health; **Concept:** Nutrition; Medication; Safety; **Integrated Processes:** Teaching/Learning; **Client Needs:** Physiological Integrity: Pharmacological and Parenteral Therapies; **Cognitive Level:** Application [Applying]

## 47. MoC ANSWER: 3

1. Sending the client to another hospital violates the person's right to care.
2. The HCP is required to see the client even if the client is uninsured.
3. **The nurse should inform the client of his or her rights. EMTALA ensures public access to emergency services regardless of ability to pay.**
4. Providing an analgesic is insufficient; the client has a right to emergency services.

▶ **Test-taking Tip:** *Note that three options deny care, whereas one is different. Often the option that is different is the answer.*

**Content Area:** Management of Care; **Concept:** Ethics; Nursing Roles; **Integrated Processes:** Caring; **Client Needs:** Safe and Effective Care Environment: Management of Care; **Cognitive Level:** Analysis [Analyzing]

## 48. PHARM ANSWER: 4

1. Naproxen (Naprosyn) can accumulate in the infant's system with prolonged use due to its long half-life.
2. Breastfeeding mothers do not need to avoid all analgesics. The infant's medication exposure can be limited by using topical or oral analgesics that are poorly absorbed, and by avoiding breastfeeding during the time of peak maternal serum drug concentration.
3. Acetaminophen (Tylenol) can be used safely in breastfeeding women.
4. **Of the NSAIDs, ibuprofen (Motrin) is the preferred analgesic because it has poor transfer to milk and has been well studied in children.**

▶ **Test-taking Tip:** *Often, options with absolute words such as "no" are incorrect.*

**Content Area:** Childbearing; **Concept:** Medication; Pregnancy; Comfort; **Integrated Processes:** Communication and Documentation; **Client Needs:** Physiological Integrity: Pharmacological and Parenteral Therapies; **Cognitive Level:** Analysis [Analyzing]

## 49. ANSWER: 1

1. **The nurse should identify that aggression is associated with the potential for increased sexual behavior.**
2. Auditory hallucinations and not visual hallucinations are associated with high risk for sexual behavior.
3. Perception of inferiority, not superiority, is associated with high risk for sexual behavior.
4. Deep dependency needs, and not independence needs, are associated with high risk for sexual behavior.

▶ **Test-taking Tip:** *Three options are behaviors opposite of those expected for the client with high risk for sexual behavior. These options should be eliminated.*

**Content Area:** Mental Health; **Concept:** Safety; Sexuality; Assessment; **Integrated Processes:** Nursing Process: Assessment; **Client Needs:** Psychosocial Integrity; **Cognitive Level:** Application [Applying]

## 50. ANSWER: 1, 2, 3, 5

1. **Dyspnea in hospice clients is treated with morphine sulfate to decrease venous return and to ease the effort of breathing.**
2. **Raising the head of the bed improves lung expansion.**
3. **Hyoscyamine (Levsin) is an anticholinergic medication that dries respiratory secretions.**
4. An expectorant thins secretions and may increase coughing.
5. **Circulating air from the fan often reduces the effort the client must put into breathing.**

▶ **Test-taking Tip:** *Read the scenario in the stem carefully to recognize that this client is receiving hospice care. Evaluate each option in terms of easing respiratory effort or decreasing respiratory secretions.*

**Content Area:** Fundamentals; Adult; **Concept:** Oxygenation; Grief and Loss; **Integrated Processes:** Nursing Process: Implementation; **Client Needs:** Physiological Integrity: Basic Care and Comfort; **Cognitive Level:** Analysis [Analyzing]

## 51. MoC ANSWER: 1

1. **The client with CRF is the most stable. Subcutaneous administration of epoetin (Procrit) is within the LPN scope of practice.**
2. The child with hemophilia is a more complex case; some facilities permit only RNs to administer blood transfusions.
3. The child who recently had a stem cell transplant and is to have a bone marrow aspiration is more complex and requires reverse isolation.
4. The client with chemotherapy-induced neutropenia and an elevated temperature needs careful monitoring and complex care.

▶ **Test-taking Tip:** *Think about the LPN scope of practice. Eliminate options that require complex skills or assessments, or that involve a client whose condition may be unstable.*

**Content Area:** Management of Care; **Concept:** Safety; Medication; Critical Thinking; **Integrated Processes:** Nursing Process: Planning; **Client Needs:** Safe and Effective Care Environment: Management of Care; **Cognitive Level:** Application [Applying]

**52.** MoC **ANSWER: 1**

1. **Coordination of care is a primary function of case managers. Overseeing services and resources to avoid duplication and breakdowns in quality is important in this role.**
2. Planning a conference with all HCPs may be difficult due to scheduling constraints. The conference also excludes the client and family, which would be inappropriate.
3. Documenting the HCPs' plan of care will not ensure that the client receives individualized care.
4. It would be inappropriate for the nurse to recommend that one HCP direct the plan of care.

▶ *Test-taking Tip: The key words include "case manager." You need to think about the role of the case manager and select the most global option.*

Content Area: Management of Care; Concept: Collaboration; Communication; Safety; Integrated Processes: Nursing Process: Planning; Client Needs: Safe and Effective Care Environment: Management of Care; Cognitive Level: Analysis [Analyzing]

**53.** MoC **ANSWER: 3, 5**

1. Dark red blood does not necessarily indicate the need for a transfusion; it could be old blood. The client should notify the HCP if experiencing heavy bleeding following the D&C.
2. A D&C to treat incomplete spontaneous abortion does not require the routine administration of IV antibiotics.
3. **The client who had an incomplete spontaneous abortion may experience grief and loss. The nurse should offer a referral to a pregnancy loss support group to provide ongoing support after hospital discharge.**
4. There is no medical need for the client who had a spontaneous abortion to avoid pregnancy for 1 year.
5. **A D&C usually is performed on an outpatient basis if there are no complications, and the client can return home a few hours after the procedure. Someone should remain with the client to ensure that she is safe and no complications develop.**

▶ *Test-taking Tip: When reviewing the options, consider that the client is being discharged on the same day as the D&C. You should eliminate options that would be considered extreme interventions.*

Content Area: Childbearing; Concept: Nursing Roles; Pregnancy; Grief and Loss; Management; Integrated Processes: Caring; Communication and Documentation; Client Needs: Safe and Effective Care Environment: Management of Care; Psychosocial Integrity; Physiological Integrity: Physiological Adaptation; Cognitive Level: Application [Applying]

**54. ANSWER: 1**

1. **Decorticate posturing is abnormal posturing indicative of severe brain damage. The client's arm is stiff and bent with the fist clenched and the arm flexed across the chest. The leg is held straight with the foot plantar flexed. This can occur on one or both sides of the body.**

2. This shows decerebrate posturing with arms extended and forearms pronated, wrists and fingers flexed, and feet plantar flexed.
3. This shows a positive Brudzinski's sign; the hips flex in response to neck flexion.
4. This shows a positive Kernig's sign. The person lies flat on the back, the thigh is flexed at a right angle to the trunk, and the leg is completely extended. Kernig's sign occurs if the leg cannot be completely extended due to pain.

▶ *Test-taking Tip: You can remember decorticate posturing by thinking about being in love and courting; when you are in love, someone is close to your heart. In decorticate posturing, the hands are drawn up to the chest near the heart.*

Content Area: Adult; Concept: Assessment; Neurologic Regulation; Integrated Processes: Nursing Process: Analysis; Client Needs: Physiological Integrity: Reduction of Risk Potential; Cognitive Level: Analysis [Analyzing]

**55. ANSWER: 1**

1. **Assessing the client more frequently is the most effective of the options provided.**
2. Restraints should be applied only if the client demonstrates noncompliance and the least-restrictive interventions have been attempted first. The nurse must contact the HCP before applying any restraint.
3. Family members may not be able to prevent a fall.
4. Instructing the NA to check the client more often may be helpful; however, the delegation lacks specific time frequency.

▶ *Test-taking Tip: The nursing process should be used to answer this question. Assessment is the first step in the nursing process.*

Content Area: Management of Care; Fundamentals; Concept: Safety; Mobility; Integrated Processes: Nursing Process: Implementation; Client Needs: Safe and Effective Care Environment: Safety and Infection Control; Cognitive Level: Application [Applying]

**56. ANSWER: 4**

1. Trust versus Mistrust is the stage for an infant.
2. Initiative versus Guilt is the stage for a preschooler.
3. Autonomy versus Guilt is not a stage.
4. **The toddler stage of development based on Erikson's developmental theory is Autonomy versus Shame and Doubt.**

▶ *Test-taking Tip: Apply knowledge of Erikson's Stages of Development. Examine options that have some of the same terms and use the process of elimination to rule out one or both of these.*

Content Area: Child; Concept: Development; Assessment; Integrated Processes: Nursing Process: Assessment; Client Needs: Health Promotion and Maintenance; Cognitive Level: Analysis [Analyzing]

**57.** MoC **ANSWER: 3**

1. The cord should be uncovered to promote drying and the diaper placed such that urine does not come in contact with the cord.

2. Use of lotions near the cord should be discouraged because this can decrease drying and predispose the area to infection.

3. **Until the umbilical cord falls off, it should be kept dry. Therefore, the infant should be given sponge baths rather than immersed in a tub of water.**

4. The cord should not be moved, as manipulation can cause infection to develop.

▶ *Test-taking Tip: Focus on the action that would best promote drying of the cord, and eliminate options that increase cord moistness or injury.*

**Content Area:** Childbearing; **Concept:** Pregnancy; Promoting Health; Skin Integrity; **Integrated Processes:** Nursing Process: Analysis; **Client Needs:** Safe and Effective Care Environment: Management of Care; **Cognitive Level:** Synthesis [Creating]

## 58. ANSWER: 2

1. A crisis counselor may be helpful, but what is needed at this time is the nurse's presence.

2. **Because the mother just received devastating news, the nurse's presence acknowledges the mother's feelings. The nurse is needed for support as the mother begins to cope with the news.**

3. Questioning the mother about her fears is a barrier to therapeutic communication.

4. While information is helpful in coping, the timing is inappropriate. What is needed at this time is listening and caring.

▶ *Test-taking Tip: Focus on selecting the option that best demonstrates caring.*

**Content Area:** Child; **Concept:** Hematologic Regulation; Cellular Regulation; Nursing Roles: Communication; **Integrated Processes:** Caring; Communication and Documentation; **Client Needs:** Psychosocial Integrity; **Cognitive Level:** Application [Applying]

## 59. ANSWER: 2

1. The nurse should not presume that the client is experiencing stress; this may cause the client's spouse to become defensive.

2. **The nurse should use an open-ended questioning technique that provides the client's spouse with an opportunity to share information deemed appropriate. The answers allow the nurse a chance to ask questions that are more specific to areas of concern.**

3. Closed-ended questions require only a "yes" or "no" answer and limit communication.

4. Using language that implies that caregiving is a burden may cause the client's spouse to become defensive.

▶ *Test-taking Tip: Key words are "most appropriate." Use the process of elimination and focus on therapeutic communication techniques as well as the needs of caregivers.*

**Content Area:** Mental Health; **Concept:** Stress; Mood; Assessment; Communication; **Integrated Processes:** Nursing Process: Assessment; **Client Needs:** Psychosocial Integrity; **Cognitive Level:** Analysis [Analyzing]

## 60. ANSWER: 4

1. The cessation of menses and not age will determine whether a pregnancy is possible.

2. The cessation of menses and not whether the female engages in sexual intercourse will determine whether a pregnancy is possible.

3. Although this statement may be true, the focus of the question is whether the client can become pregnant.

4. **Menopause is the physiological cessation of menses associated with declining ovarian function. It is usually considered complete after 1 year of amenorrhea. Once menopause is complete, reproductive function ends.**

▶ *Test-taking Tip: Recall the relationship between menopause and reproduction. Once a female is menopausal, pregnancy is not physiologically possible.*

**Content Area:** Adult; **Concept:** Pregnancy; Nursing Roles; Female Reproduction; **Integrated Processes:** Teaching/Learning; **Client Needs:** Health Promotion and Maintenance; **Cognitive Level:** Application [Applying]

## 61. ANSWER: 3

1. The nurse's introduction and directions to the child do not acknowledge his or her feelings and are an attempt to control the child.

2. Diverting the child's attention by taking him or her to the playroom will not alleviate fear and anxiety.

3. **Stating that the child is likely afraid and making a reference to the stuffed animal will acknowledge the child's feelings and direct focus to a familiar object of security.**

4. Asking the child questions that allow for a yes/no response is closed-ended questioning and, because of the child's fear and anxiety, likely will get a "no" response. The child is afraid. Holding the child could increase the child's fear.

▶ *Test-taking Tip: Select an option that will decrease fear and anxiety for the child.*

**Content Area:** Child; **Concept:** Development; Communication; Safety; **Integrated Processes:** Communication and Documentation; **Client Needs:** Psychosocial Integrity; **Cognitive Level:** Analysis [Analyzing]

## 62. MoC ANSWER: 3

1. Restating the concerns focuses on the client's problem and is appropriate.

2. Asking how long it takes for the client to fall asleep is appropriate as it further addresses the issue of difficulty sleeping.

3. **This statement prematurely informs the client that a sleep disorder has been confirmed and/or makes assumptions about the client's caffeine intake. The LPN needs to be remediated regarding the discussion of unconfirmed presumptions with the client.**

4. Asking about the stressors or concerns is an attempt to acquire additional information and does not need immediate follow-up by the nurse manager.

▶ **Test-taking Tip:** Note the key words "requires immediate follow-up." This is a false-response option. You need to select the inappropriate statement.

**Content Area:** Mental Health; **Concept:** Sleep, Rest, and Activity; Assessment; **Integrated Processes:** Nursing Process: Evaluation; **Client Needs:** Safe and Effective Care Environment: Management of Care; Physiological Integrity: Basic Care and Comfort; **Cognitive Level:** Evaluation [Evaluating]

63. **PHARM** **ANSWER: 4**
1. Fentanyl (Sublimaze), a sedative and narcotic analgesic, is for severe pain control and is not indicated at this time. Metronidazole (Flagyl), an anti-infective, antiprotozoal agent, is an alternative to penicillin G and would be appropriate.
2. Diazepam (Valium) is used for skeletal muscle relaxation to control spasms (which the client is not exhibiting). Penicillin (Pfizerpen) is appropriate and given to inhibit further growth of *Clostridium tetani*.
3. Morphine sulfate, a narcotic analgesic, is given for pain control, which is appropriate at this time. Vecuronium (Norcuron) is a neuromuscular blocking agent for severe cases of muscle spasm, which the client is not exhibiting at this time.
4. **Both Td and TIG should be administered at this time at different sites to neutralize circulating toxins.**

▶ **Test-taking Tip:** For the option to be a correct answer, both medications must be appropriate for the client at this time. Avoid reading into the question.

**Content Area:** Adult; **Concept:** Immunity; Safety; Infection; **Integrated Processes:** Nursing Process: Planning; **Client Needs:** Physiological Integrity: Pharmacological and Parenteral Therapies; **Cognitive Level:** Analysis [Analyzing]

64. **PHARM** **ANSWER: 4**
1. The client's serum potassium level should be within normal range prior to surgery. Waiting to administer KCL delays the benefits of the medication.
2. Administration of concentrated potassium chloride can cause cardiac dysrhythmias or arrest. A low serum potassium level increases the client's risk of dysrhythmias during anesthesia administration.
3. Hot packing may provide comfort since KCL is irritating to the veins, but ensuring that KCL is diluted before administration is more important.
4. **The nurse's priority is to ensure that KCL is diluted prior to administration. If given in a concentrated dose or too rapidly, it can cause hyperkalemia, cardiac arrhythmias, or arrest.**

▶ **Test-taking Tip:** Although the HCP may prescribe a dose of medication, the nurse must know how to safely administer it. If KCL is administered IV undiluted, it can be lethal.

**Content Area:** Adult; **Concept:** Medication; Fluid and Electrolyte Balance; **Integrated Processes:** Nursing Process: Planning; **Client Needs:** Physiological Integrity: Pharmacological and Parenteral Therapies; **Cognitive Level:** Application [Applying]

65. **PHARM** **ANSWER: 3**
1. The nurse should initiate a consult because the client already has developed a complication (foot ulcer), but this is not priority.
2. The procedure for glucose monitoring may need to be taught or reviewed with the client, but this is not priority.
3. **Aspart insulin (NovoLog) is rapid-acting. When given 5 minutes before a meal, it quickly reduces the blood glucose level. The use of insulin in a person with uncontrolled type 2 DM has been shown to decrease the Hgb $A_{1c}$ level and help prevent complications.**
4. Questioning the order is unnecessary. The order is correct.

▶ **Test-taking Tip:** Use Maslow's Hierarchy of Needs to determine the priority. Decide which intervention must be completed first by the oncoming day-shift nurse.

**Content Area:** Adult; **Concept:** Metabolism; Medication; **Integrated Processes:** Nursing Process: Implementation; **Client Needs:** Physiological Integrity: Pharmacological and Parenteral Therapies; **Cognitive Level:** Analysis [Analyzing]

66. **ANSWER: 3**
1. None of the small bowel is removed in a Roux-en-Y gastric surgery.
2. The stomach is not bypassed in a Roux-en-Y gastric surgery.
3. **A Roux-en-Y gastric bypass reduces the size of the upper part of the stomach to approximately 20 to 30 mL.**
4. The large intestine is not bypassed in a Roux-en-Y gastric surgery.

▶ **Test-taking Tip:** Eliminate options that do not address "gastric." Of the remaining two options, visualize the procedure to select the best one.

**Content Area:** Adult; **Concept:** Nutrition; Nursing Roles; **Integrated Processes:** Teaching/Learning; **Client Needs:** Physiological Integrity: Reduction of Risk Potential; **Cognitive Level:** Application [Applying]

67. **ANSWER: 3**
1. There is no need to recheck the pulse in 1 hour because 146 bpm is in the expected range.
2. There is no indication that oxygenation is affected.
3. **Because this apical rate is 146 bpm and within the normal range of 100 to 160 bpm, the student should document the findings without further action.**
4. There is no need to notify the HCP; if it was necessary, it would be completed by the nurse and not the student nurse.

▶ **Test-taking Tip:** The expected range for the newborn's apical pulse is 100 to 160 bpm.

Content Area: Childbearing; Concept: Assessment; Communication; Integrated Processes: Nursing Process: Implementation; Client Needs: Physiological Integrity: Reduction of Risk Potential; Cognitive Level: Application [Applying]

## 68. PHARM ANSWER: 1, 5

1. **A psychotropic medication is one that affects the mind, emotions, or behavior. Research has shown that psychotropic medications are associated with risk of falls in older adult clients. Alprazolam (Xanax XR), a benzodiazepine prescribed to control anxiety, can contribute to a fall.**
2. Docusate sodium (Colace) is a stool softener.
3. Hydrochlorothiazide (Hydrodiuril) is a diuretic. Although it can contribute to a fall due to loss of fluid volume, it is not a psychotropic medication.
4. Potassium chloride (Micro K) is a potassium supplement.
5. **Zolpidem tartrate (Ambien), a hypnotic prescribed for short-term insomnia, is considered a psychotropic medication. Its use can contribute to risk for a fall.**
6. Lisinopril (Zestril) is an ACE inhibitor that blocks the conversion of angiotensin I to the vasoconstrictor angiotensin II. It is used to treat hypertension. Its action in lowering BP can contribute to the risk of a fall, but it is not a psychotropic medication.

♦ Test-taking Tip: Determine the classification of each medication. Eliminate options that are not psychotropic medications, even if their drug classification is known to increase the risk of falls.

Content Area: Adult; Concept: Medication; Safety; Integrated Processes: Nursing Process: Evaluation; Client Needs: Physiological Integrity: Pharmacological and Parenteral Therapies; Cognitive Level: Evaluation [Evaluating]

## 69. ANSWER: 1

1. **Noroviruses are transmitted through the fecal-oral route, either by direct person-to-person contact or through food, water, or hand transfer of the virus to the oral mucosa after contact with an object contaminated with feces or vomitus. Contact isolation is necessary, and masks should be worn if vomiting is expected.**
2. Although norovirus can be spread via the droplet route from vomitus, the CDC recommends using contact precautions and wearing a mask if vomiting is expected.
3. A high-efficiency particulate (HEPA) mask or N-95 mask and a negative-airflow room are used in airborne precautions, and are unnecessary.
4. Those coming in contact with the client need self-protection measures; there is no indication that the client has immunodeficiency requiring protective isolation precautions.

♦ Test-taking Tip: Noroviruses are present in stool and emesis.

Content Area: Child; Concept: Fluid and Electrolyte Balance; Infection; Integrated Processes: Nursing Process: Implementation; Client Needs: Safe and Effective Care Environment: Safety and Infection Control; Physiological Integrity: Physiological Adaptation; Cognitive Level: Application [Applying]

## 70. MoC ANSWER: 3

1. Telling nurses not to give the antibiotics too early does not provide clear expectations or a rationale for the time period.
2. Completing a variance takes a negative approach to behavior change and can hinder morale on the unit.
3. **Staff education is important in establishing expectations and ensuring consistency in timing of antibiotic administration. Staff members are likely to be more compliant once they understand the rationale for the practice.**
4. The time to incision may vary due to unforeseen circumstances; some facilities keep a supply of antibiotics on the unit. This is not the best approach for changing nursing practice.

♦ Test-taking Tip: Three options use a negative approach, whereas one is different.

Content Area: Management of Care; Concept: Infection; Safety; Medication; Management; Integrated Processes: Teaching/Learning; Client Needs: Safe and Effective Care Environment: Management of Care; Cognitive Level: Application [Applying]

## 71. PHARM ANSWER: 4

1. Cervical dilation is not part of the criteria determining whether the goal of induction has been met.
2. Reports of client discomfort are not part of the criteria that determine if the induction goal has been achieved.
3. Contractions lasting 60 to 90 seconds and occurring every 2 minutes represent a pattern that exceeds the criteria limits.
4. **The goal of IV oxytocin (Pitocin) administration for labor induction is to achieve a contraction pattern of three 40- to 60-second uterine contractions over a 10-minute period. When this occurs, the appropriate dose is being given.**

♦ Test-taking Tip: Oxytocin causes the uterus to contract. Eliminate options that do not address the process of uterine contractions.

Content Area: Childbearing; Concept: Pregnancy; Medication; Integrated Processes: Nursing Process: Evaluation; Client Needs: Physiological Integrity: Pharmacological and Parenteral Therapies; Cognitive Level: Evaluation [Evaluating]

## 72. MoC ANSWER: 2, 5, 6

1. Increased hair thinning is a normal finding in the older adult population.
2. **The warty growth on the vulva could be a sign of HPV infection. The HCP should be consulted.**
3. Lentigo (sun freckles or age spots) often is found in the older adult population.

4. Port-wine angioma is a benign vascular tumor that involves the skin and subcutaneous tissues that are present at birth, usually persisting indefinitely.

5. **Pitting edema can be a sign of fluid volume overload due to a cardiac, renal, endocrine, medication-related, or other problem. The HCP should be consulted.**

6. **The 6 mm, dark, asymmetric lesion is a hallmark of cancer. The HCP should be consulted.**

▶ *Test-taking Tip: Eliminate normal age-related changes and any options occurring at birth that are considered normal findings.*

Content Area: Adult; Concept: Collaboration; Communication; Assessment; Integrated Processes: Nursing Process: Assessment; Client Needs: Safe and Effective Care Environment: Management of Care; Health Promotion and Maintenance; Cognitive Level: Analysis [Analyzing]

## 73. ANSWER: 2

1. The trigeminal nerve functions as part of the blink reflex, but counting the blinks is not a useful assessment.

2. **The nurse should ask the client about factors that trigger pain before proceeding to an examination. Pain associated with trigeminal neuralgia is very severe and occurs in spasms. Clients are often fearful of initiating an episode of facial pain.**

3. Palpating the face may trigger a pain episode that would prevent additional assessment of the client's symptoms.

4. This tests cerebellar function and is not indicated. This action may trigger facial pain in the client with trigeminal neuralgia.

▶ *Test-taking Tip: Neuralgia is a painful nerve condition (suffix "-algia" indicates pain). Consider that the nurse should be careful in performing any assessment that would initiate a pain episode.*

Content Area: Adult; Concept: Assessment; Neurologic Regulation; Comfort; Integrated Processes: Nursing Process: Assessment; Client Needs: Health Promotion and Maintenance; Cognitive Level: Analysis [Analyzing]

## 74. PHARM ANSWER: 3

1. Meperidine (Demerol) has been reported to cause delirium in the elderly; older adults are at increased risk for meperidine toxicity.

2. Fentanyl (Duragesic) is recommended for moderate to severe chronic pain requiring continuous opioid analgesic therapy.

3. **Morphine sulfate (Duramorph) is recommended for severe, acute pain. It alters the client's perception of and response to painful stimuli while producing generalized CNS depression.**

4. Hydromorphone (Dilaudid) takes additional time to prepare, and the dose is higher than the recommended range for older adult clients.

▶ *Test-taking Tip: Knowledge of analgesics for older adults is necessary to answer this question. If unsure, use the process of elimination, excluding Options 2 and 4 because of the longer onset time and because the client is in acute pain.*

Content Area: Fundamentals; Adult; Concept: Medication; Critical Thinking; Medication; Integrated Processes: Nursing Process: Evaluation; Client Needs: Physiological Integrity: Pharmacological and Parenteral Therapies; Cognitive Level: Evaluation [Evaluating]

## 75. MoC ANSWER: 3, 4, 6

1. A latex allergy requires appropriate precautions, which include the use of latex-free items.

2. Metronidazole (Flagyl) is an antiprotozoal anti-infective medication and is safe to use for clients with latex and sulfonamide allergies. It is used to treat *Clostridium difficile* infection.

3. **Normal serum potassium levels are 3.5 to 5.5 mEq/L. KCL is an appropriate treatment.**

4. *Clostridium difficile* **infection causes mild to severe diarrhea and abdominal cramping and can be associated with antibiotic treatment, which destroys the natural GI flora.**

5. While the aPTT is within normal range (24 to 33 seconds), the therapeutic range for dosing heparin would be 1.5 to 2.5 times the normal aPTT. The heparin infusion as prescribed is appropriate for anticoagulant treatment for the PE. Additional information may be needed based on the heparin infusion protocol.

6. **The oxygen flow should be questioned; a flow rate of at least 5 L per minute is needed to prevent accumulation of expired air in the mask.**

▶ *Test-taking Tip: Careful analysis of the chart information is needed to answer this question. The best strategy is to read the options first and then review the chart. Focus on verifying the appropriateness and/or accuracy of the treatments prescribed against the information presented.*

Content Area: Management of Care; Concept: Infection; Medication; Oxygenation; Legal; Integrated Processes: Nursing Process: Analysis; Client Needs: Safe and Effective Care Environment: Management of Care; Safe and Effective Care Environment: Safety and Infection Control; Cognitive Level: Analysis [Analyzing]

## Chapter Fifty-Two

# Comprehensive Exam 2

**1.** **PHARM** The nurse is preparing to administer medications to the adult client. Which medication may be given without first verifying it with the HCP?

1. Digoxin 2.5 mg IV now
2. Levofloxacin 500 mg daily
3. Heparin sodium 5000 U subq bid
4. Timolol 0.5% 2 drops right eye bid

**2.** The nurse is assessing the 2-month-old with suspected pyloric stenosis. Which findings should the nurse expect if pyloric stenosis is present?

1. Projectile vomiting, diarrhea, poor weight gain, low urine output
2. Bile-colored vomiting, diarrhea, signs of dehydration, weight loss
3. Nonbilious vomiting, hunger after vomiting, lethargy, weight loss
4. Vomiting related to feeding position, diarrhea, marasmus, weight loss

**3.** **PHARM** The nurse is to administer glycopyrrolate 0.2 mg through a single-lumen PICC that has 0.9% NaCl infusing at 60 mL/hr. After explaining the procedure, the nurse gathers supplies, performs hand hygiene, applies gloves, and assesses the site. Prioritize the nurse's remaining interventions by placing each step in the order it should be performed.

1. Cleanse the injection port with an antiseptic swab and allow the port to dry.
2. Select the IV injection port closest to the client.
3. Pinch (clamp) the IV line and inject glycopyrrolate over 1 to 2 min; the IV line can be unpinched at intervals to allow dilution of the medication.
4. Remove the syringe, ensure that the IV is infusing, and recheck the IV infusion rate.
5. Connect a 10 mL large-barrel syringe of medication to the injection port.

Answer: _____

**4.** **MoC** Two NAs are helping the client with left-sided weakness transfer from the chair to the bed. Based on the illustration provided, which action by the nurse observing this transfer is **best**?

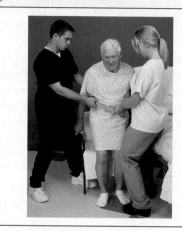

1. Intervene; the chair is incorrectly placed for transferring the client back to bed.
2. Compliment the female NA because she is supporting the client's weaker side.
3. Compliment the male NA because he is using a wide base of support to transfer.
4. Praise the client for using his hand for support on the chair to help prevent a fall.

**5.** The client with prerenal failure caused by severe hypotension receives a fluid bolus. Which finding should prompt the nurse to evaluate that the fluid bolus was **most** effective for treating the prerenal failure?

1. BP is 140/72 mm Hg
2. Mean arterial pressure is 55
3. Urine output is 70 mL/hr
4. HR is 120 bpm

6. **MoC** The new nurse is to obtain a urine specimen from a 12-month-old girl using a collection bag. Which action requires the mentor to intervene?

1. Cleans the perineal-genital area gently from front to back with alcohol wipes
2. Places the collection bag over the perineum, covering the meatus and vagina
3. Applies a diaper loosely to help hold the collection bag in place
4. Empties collected urine into a container and puts the container in a biohazard bag

7. **MoC** Two nurses are having a conflict about whose turn it is to float to a unit outside their usual assigned one. Which statement by one of the nurses indicates negotiation toward conflict resolution?

1. "I know it's not my turn to float, so you should go. I will take my turn next time."
2. "I'm willing to float today if you could come in 15 minutes early for me tomorrow."
3. "If you don't float today, I will end up floating 2 days in a row, and that's not fair."
4. "We all float too much, so neither of us should float. Let's talk with our nurse manager."

8. **MoC** The hospitalized client experienced a seizure. What information should the nurse document when describing the client's postictal period?

1. Whether it looked like the client had an "aura"
2. What the client was doing preceding the seizure
3. The client's condition immediately after the seizure
4. Where tonic-clonic activity started and duration

9. The community nurse is teaching mothers with children between the ages of 1 and 4 years about measures to prevent the most common cause of death in children this age. Which nurse's statement is **best?**

1. "Be sure that your children receive the vaccine to prevent pneumonia."
2. "Avoid physical punishment of children to prevent unintentional homicide."
3. "Apply sunscreen before taking your children outdoors to prevent skin cancer."
4. "Place medications and knives in locked cabinets to prevent unintentional injury."

10. **PHARM** The child is admitted to a hospital in hyperglycemic crisis. Which **initial** IV fluid, if prescribed, should the nurse prepare to administer?

1. 0.9% NaCl at 20 mL/kg/hr for the first hour
2. Ringer's lactate at 20 mL/kg/hr for the first hour
3. $D_5W$ with 20 mEq KCL at 50 mL/kg for 4 hrs
4. $D_{10}W$ and 0.45% NaCl 10 mL/kg for 4 hrs

11. The newly delivered full-term newborn is placed on the mother's chest. The mother asks about the periodic pauses she sees in her baby's breathing. Which statement should be the basis for the nurse's response?

1. Pauses cause skin color changes; the nurse should prepare the mother for this.
2. Periodic pauses are expected as the newborn transitions to life outside the uterus.
3. Newborn respirations should be regular; this pausing warrants further investigation.
4. Pauses suggest decreased surfactant production in the term newborn.

12. **MoC** The client reports continued but improving insomnia, anorexia, and crying episodes following the death of the client's spouse 1 month ago. Which is the **most** appropriate problem for the nurse to add to the client's plan of care?

1. Ineffective coping
2. Impaired adjustment
3. Dysfunctional grieving
4. Family processes, interrupted

13. The hospitalized client, experiencing chronic abdominal pain, desires to include guided imagery as an intervention to lessen pain. Which would be the **best** method for the nurse to evaluate the effectiveness of guided imagery in controlling the client's pain?

1. Check the BP and pulse rate before and after guided imagery.
2. Ask the client to describe and rate the pain after guided imagery.
3. Ask the client's significant other to describe changes in the client's behavior.
4. Monitor the client's facial expression before and after guided imagery.

14. A bridging strategy is planned to ensure that the client who is homeless and has a history of violent behavior will have positive outcomes after discharge. Which statement made by the client **best** shows the need for further teaching about using the bridging strategy?

1. "I want to thank you for giving me a list of places where I can go to get help."
2. "I want to get better; I plan to get help from one of the places you recommended."
3. "I will keep the list of outpatient services' telephone numbers where I won't lose it."
4. "I'll go to one of the recommended places when I no longer can stay healthy and be safe."

**15.** **PHARM** Immediately after the delivery of the client's placenta, the HCP prescribes an IV infusion of oxytocin at 20 milliunits/minute. The nurse should evaluate that the medication was effective when noting which finding?

1. Systolic BP is above 100 mm Hg
2. The amount of lochia flow is small
3. The mother reports feeling no afterpains
4. Uterine fundus is found to be firm

**16.** The nurse is reviewing the serum laboratory report of the 7-year-old who has been rehydrated following acute vomiting and diarrhea. Which lab value change should the nurse expect with successful rehydration?

1. Hematocrit was 31%; now 37%
2. Hemoglobin was 9.5 mg/dL; now 12.5 mg/dL
3. Blood urea nitrogen was 28 mg/dL; now 16 mg/dL
4. Serum creatinine was 1.2 mg/dL; now 0.9 mg/dL

**17.** The nurse is caring for the client following a left tibial osteotomy with bone graft from the left hip and cast application to the left lower leg. Which assessment finding is **priority** and requires the nurse to intervene immediately?

1. Experiencing nausea
2. Has not voided for 6 hours
3. Numbness and tingling of the left toes
4. Left hip dressing saturated with serosanguineous drainage

**18.** The nurse is caring for the client immediately following a TURP. Which nursing action is **most** important?

1. Monitor the urinary catheter to ensure that urine is flowing.
2. Have the client sit at the side of the bed as soon as possible.
3. Monitor the abdominal dressing for blood or urine drainage.
4. Alert the surgeon if blood clots are noted in the urinary drainage bag.

**19.** The client who had an MI is transferred from acute care to a step-down unit. The client calls the nurse often to check the rhythm on the ECG monitor and questions whether activity is appropriate so soon after an MI. The nurse should document that the client is displaying signs of which behavioral response?

1. Anger
2. Denial
3. Depression
4. Dependency

**20.** Two nurses are approaching the client to begin CPR. One nurse goes to the right side to check the client's pulse. In which location should the other nurse be positioned for rescue breathing with a mask?

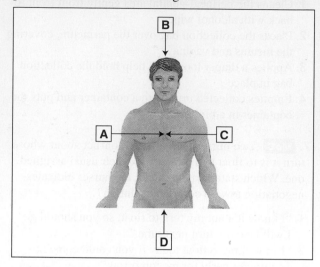

1. Location A
2. Location B
3. Location C
4. Location D

**21.** **MoC** The nurse plans to include the family in the treatment of the client who abuses substances. What should be the nurse's primary rationale for including family members?

1. Help the family learn ways to protect the client from additional harm.
2. Assist the family in ways that reduce the client's temptations for substances.
3. Reduce distress in family relationships to lessen the client's risk for relapse.
4. Help the family confront the client about the harm caused by substance abuse.

**22.** **PHARM** A powdered chemotherapy medication spills on a hard surface in a clinical area. Which required safety practice, in addition to wearing a protective gown and gloves, should the nurse use to clean the spill?

1. Wear goggles and head covering and use double-bag clean-up pads.
2. Wear a face shield and foot coverings and use single-bag clean-up pads.
3. Wear a face shield and head covering and use single-bag clean-up pads.
4. Wear goggles and a respirator mask and use double-bag clean-up pads.

23. **MoC** The charge nurse needs to assign a newly admitted client who is experiencing acute rejection following a liver transplant. Multiple IV medications have been prescribed. Which nurse is **most** appropriate for the charge nurse to assign to care for this client?

1. The RN who works in intensive care (ICU) but was floated to the medical unit
2. The licensed practice nurse (LPN) who has worked on the medical unit for 5 years
3. The newly licensed RN on the medical unit who needs experience with IV medications
4. The RN who has worked on the medical unit for 10 years and is working a double shift

24. **PHARM** The client with a URI is being given guaifenesin 400 mg orally q4hr. Which client statement indicates that the nurse should teach the person about guaifenesin use?

1. "I'll take guaifenesin with meals and at bedtime with a snack."
2. "I should drink water and increase my fluids to 3000 mL/day."
3. "I'll take acetaminophen if I get a headache from guaifenesin."
4. "Chewing sugarless gum should help relieve throat discomfort."

25. The nurse is teaching the woman who is 8 weeks pregnant and had a Roux-en-Y gastric bypass surgical procedure 19 months ago. The woman's BMI is now 30.3%, down from 39.5%. Which nutritional issues associated with gastric bypass should the nurse address with this client? **Select all that apply.**

1. Iron deficiency
2. Vitamin B$_{12}$ deficiency
3. Vitamin C deficiency
4. Vitamin A deficiency
5. Protein deficiency
6. Folate excess

26. **MoC** The multiparous client in her 42nd week of gestation is experiencing contractions upon arrival at the ED. The nurse determines that the client is in the second stage of labor. Which nursing action is **priority?**

1. Transfer the client to the delivery room.
2. Time the frequency of her contractions.
3. Notify the HCP and prepare for delivery.
4. Check the FHR with a fetoscope.

27. **MoC** The client states, "My illness is a cold disease, and I need to eat hot food in order to get healthy." Based on this information, which intervention should the nurse implement?

1. Monitor the client's temperature and lung sounds at least every 8 hours.
2. Direct the nursing assistant to warm the client's food before delivery.
3. Obtain extra spices from the cafeteria for the client's use with meals.
4. Initiate a referral to a dietitian to obtain specific foods for the client.

28. The nurse is assessing the client for possible scabies. Which common site should the nurse check **first?** Place an X in the circle indicating where the nurse should assess first for scabies.

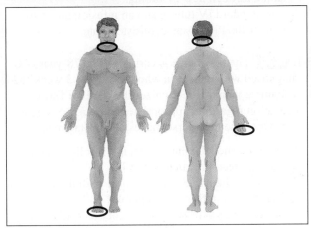

29. The parents of the toddler with CP express concern about their child's weight. The nurse advises the parents about enhancing the child's nutritional intake. On a subsequent home visit, which observation by the nurse indicates further teaching is needed?

1. Gives small, frequent feedings
2. Provides solid foods at mealtimes
3. Includes a high-calorie supplement
4. Offers large-handled, padded silverware

30. The nurse is receiving the client in the OR. Which action should the nurse perform **first?**

1. Assess the client's level of anxiety.
2. Confirm that the operative consent is signed.
3. Verify the correct operative site with the client.
4. Check the name band and ask the client's name.

**31.** The client receives radiation therapy for pharyngeal cancer. Which assessment findings should prompt the nurse to implement interventions for oral mucositis?

1. Gingivitis, plaque, halitosis
2. Oral erythema, pain, dysgeusia
3. Candidiasis, inflammation, cheilitis
4. Oral ulceration, caries, leukoplakia

**32.** **PHARM** The nurse is to administer a unit of PRBCs to the client. Which safety measure should the nurse implement when giving the blood transfusion?

1. Take VS q30 min during the transfusion to detect complications early.
2. Give PRBCs slowly over 5 hours to prevent a transfusion reaction.
3. Stop the transfusion if a reaction occurs and give saline through new IV tubing.
4. Use standard IV tubing and an infusion pump to deliver the PRBCs at a consistent rate.

**33.** **MoC** The new nurse is caring for the 78-year-old diagnosed with dementia who had a CVA 3 weeks ago. The nurse manager recognizes the need for further education regarding appropriate delegation of client care when the new nurse makes which statement?

1. "I've watched the nurse aide, and I believe the nurse aide can feed the client safely."
2. "I'll have the nurse aide reinforce with the client that swearing at staff is unacceptable."
3. "The client's skin needs to be checked; the nurse aide can do that when showering the client."
4. "The nurse aide can show the family when they visit that the client needs new slippers."

**34.** **PHARM** The client with depression and fibromyalgia is started on a TCA. Which common side effects of TCAs should the nurse address with the client? **Select all that apply.**

1. Diarrhea
2. Dry mouth
3. Agranulocytosis
4. Unintentional tremor
5. Urinary retention

**35.** The client develops thrombocytopenia. What should the nurse do when caring for the client?

1. Encourage the use of dental floss with oral care.
2. Keep the client on bedrest to prevent injury.
3. Assess for blurred vision or mental status changes.
4. Give aspirin for fever of 102°F (39°C) or greater.

**36.** **PHARM** The nurse gives an IV push medication through a port on a PICC. When the nurse removes the syringe, the port adheres to the syringe, which then leaves the catheter open to air. The nurse considers that air may have entered the PICC. What should the nurse do? **Select all that apply.**

1. Notify the HCP about the situation.
2. Close the clamp on the central line catheter if one is present.
3. Flush the PICC with 0.9% NaCl after absence of air in the line has been determined.
4. Turn the client onto the right side with the feet higher than the head.
5. Attach a 10 mL large-barrel syringe to the catheter and aspirate for blood return.

**37.** The nurse completes measurements for ECG monitor rhythm strips for four different clients. Following analysis of the ECG rhythms, the nurse determines that one of the clients requires an immediate intervention. Which measurement findings warrant the **most** immediate intervention?

1. PRI = 0.24 sec; QRS = 0.10 sec; QT = 0.44 sec; ventricular rate = 58 bpm
2. PRI = 0.20 sec; QRS = 0.10 sec; QT = 0.38 sec; ventricular rate = 102 bpm
3. P waves fibrillatory; PRI and QT unmeasurable; QRS = 0.08 sec; ventricular rate = 90 bpm
4. PRI varies; P and QRS unrelated; QRS = 0.14 sec; rate: atrial = 60 bpm, ventricular = 30 bpm

**38.** The nurse is assessing the mental status of the client with bipolar disorder. Which client behavior is the nurse **most** likely to assess during a manic episode?

1. Flight of ideas
2. Social withdrawal
3. Trembling or shaking
4. Somatic-type delusions

**39.** **MoC** **PHARM** The nurse is assisting the HCP who is placing a PICC. The nurse observes that the catheter tip touches a hair that has fallen from the client's head onto the sterile field. What should the nurse do?

1. Do nothing; the hair that fell in the sterile field is from the client's head.
2. Tell the HCP of the break in sterile technique and obtain replacement supplies.
3. Inform the HCP that the catheter touched a hair and let the HCP decide what to do.
4. Obtain an antiseptic solution for the HCP to cleanse the catheter tip before insertion.

40. [MoC] The client returns to a clinic for a follow-up visit and is diagnosed as positive for HIV. The client expresses fear related to lack of finances, social avoidance, and hopelessness. Which nursing intervention provides the **most** client support?

1. Refer to a community-based HIV clinic.
2. Refer to the local public health department.
3. Refer to an HCP who specializes in infectious diseases.
4. Recommend that the client disclose the diagnosis to family.

41. [MoC] The nurse assesses the 29-year-old client 30 minutes after a vaginal delivery and obtains the information illustrated. Which intervention should the nurse initiate **first**?

| Vital Signs | **BP:** 120/80 mm Hg; **P:** 70 bpm; **Respirations:** 20 breaths/min. |
|---|---|
| **Pain** | **Perineal:** 6 (0 to 10 scale) |
| **Assessment** | **Fundus:** soft and boggy; **Lochia:** large rubra; **Perineum:** bruised and swollen |

1. Provide perineal care.
2. Apply ice to the perineum.
3. Administer an analgesic.
4. Massage the fundus until it is firm.

42. The nurse is teaching the 8-year-old with precocious puberty about the child's physiological changes. Which statement would be **most** helpful in facilitating a positive body image for this child?

1. "You may want to dress like a teenager now that you are going through puberty."
2. "The medication you are receiving will decrease the size of your breasts."
3. "The changes in your body are normal but occurring at an earlier age. Your friends will eventually have the same changes."
4. "You look older. Tell others your age so they don't ask you to do things that you are not ready to do."

43. [MoC] The nurse is assessing the child with DM. Which findings support the nurse's immediate notification of an HCP to report the development of DKA? **Select all that apply.**

1. Kussmaul respirations
2. Slowing of the HR
3. Foul-smelling breath odor
4. Lethargic and unarousable
5. Blood glucose level 350 mg/dL

44. [MoC] Prehospital admission medications for the older adult client include warfarin and atenolol. Which statement made by the client should prompt the nurse to initiate a referral to a social worker?

1. "I crush my medications and take them with applesauce because they are hard to swallow."
2. "I stopped taking my blood pressure pill; I can't afford it, and my blood pressure is normal."
3. "I feel more alert after starting ginkgo, but I forgot to ask my doctor if this is okay."
4. "I have my daughter set up my medications for two weeks at a time in a medication bar."

45. The client is receiving negative-pressure wound therapy (vacuum-assisted closure) for a large pressure sore on the sacrum. The nurse should plan to monitor the client for which problem associated with negative-pressure wound therapy?

1. Air leaks
2. Air bubbles
3. Drainage of fluids
4. Saturated dressings

46. The nurse in the PACU is caring for the client who received general anesthesia. Which interventions should the nurse implement? **Select all that apply.**

1. Teach the client how to use an incentive spirometer.
2. Move the client into a lateral position to protect the airway.
3. Give morphine sulfate by the IV route for pain control.
4. Protect IV lines to prevent dislodgement during emergence delirium.
5. Repeat orientation explanations until the amnesic anesthesia wears off.

47. [MoC] The nurse contacts the HCP to obtain admission orders for the client hospitalized with community-acquired pneumonia. Which interventions should the nurse anticipate? **Select all that apply.**

1. An antipyretic such as acetaminophen
2. Peramivir 600 mg IV infused over 15-30 minutes
3. 0.9% NaCl per IV infusion and oral fluids as able
4. Physical therapy consult for limb exercises
5. Oxygen 2-4L/NC prn; keep SpO$_2$ above 92%

48. The clinic nurse assesses that the 9-year-old boy has a BP of 112/72 mm Hg. What should the nurse do about this finding?

1. Refer the child to have a work-up for hypertension.
2. Document the BP as a normal finding.
3. Discuss antihypertensive therapy with the HCP.
4. Teach about a low-sodium diet and exercise.

**49.** The nurse is assessing the client on a mental health unit. Which **initial** behavior demonstrates that the client is beginning to assume responsibility for anger management?

1. The client develops a plan on how to react when feeling stressed.
2. The client states plans for a regular exercise program to "work off anger."
3. The client identifies stressors that have led to violent outbursts in the past.
4. The client apologizes to those at whom he or she has directed the anger.

**50.** The client on a mental health unit is exhibiting dangerous and physically abusive behavior. After attempting other interventions, the nurse decides to place the client in seclusion. Which factor should the nurse consider when placing the client in seclusion?

1. A standing order may be used to place the client in seclusion.
2. The client should be removed from seclusion as soon as possible.
3. It is illegal to place the client in seclusion on a mental health unit.
4. Clients in seclusion should be monitored at least every 2 hours.

**51.** The nurse is planning to use an otoscope to view the tympanic membrane of the 12-month-old infant. Which actions should the nurse include when performing the examination? **Select all that apply.**

1. Rest the otoscope on the child's head.
2. Note the color of the tympanic membrane.
3. Pull the pinna up and back to properly align the ear canal.
4. Pull the pinna down and back to properly align the ear canal.
5. Select the smallest otoscope tip that will allow for visualization.

**52.** The nurse is caring for the young client scheduled for cystectomy with urinary diversion for treatment of bladder cancer. The client states to the nurse, "With all the smokers around, why couldn't one of them get bladder cancer instead of me? I've never smoked in my life!" Which is the **best** response by the nurse?

1. "It seems unfair that you developed cancer."
2. "Smoking isn't the only cause of bladder cancer."
3. "With your upcoming surgery, I can understand why you are afraid."
4. "You're angry; you really don't mean to wish this on someone else."

**53.** **PHARM** The home-care nurse visits the client who lives alone. The client is receiving palliative care for progressive cancer. Which nursing intervention **best** ensures that the client is receiving adequate pain control?

1. Assist in recognizing anxiety and employing relaxation techniques as soon as possible.
2. Schedule opioid medications at bedtime to ensure the client can sleep through the night.
3. Instruct on ample fluids and high-fiber foods to prevent constipation from narcotic use.
4. Teach about keeping a pain diary; contact the nurse if breakthrough pain occurs more than three times in 24 hours.

**54.** The nurse is calculating 24-hour carbohydrate intake for the client with type 1 DM. Based on the client's food intake record illustrated, the nurse should calculate that the client consumed how many grams of carbohydrate in the last 24 hours?

| 24-Hour Food Intake | | |
|---|---|---|
| **Breakfast** | **Lunch** | **Dinner** |
| 1 c whole milk (1 CHO*) | 1 c whole milk (1 CHO) | 1 c whole milk (1 CHO) |
| ½ c cooked oatmeal (1 CHO) | Carrot sticks | 3 oz beef patty |
| 1 c apple juice (1 CHO) | 3 oz tuna | ½ c corn (1 CHO) |
| 1 slice bacon | 2 slices bread (2 CHO) | ⅓ c pasta |
| | | 1 c orange juice (2 CHO) |

| | **Afternoon Snack** | **Evening Snack** |
|---|---|---|
| | 1 slice toast (1 CHO) | 1 small banana (1 CHO) |
| | 1 Tbs apple butter | |

| ***1 CHO = 15 g carbohydrate** |
|---|

_____ g (Record a whole number.)

**55.** **PHARM** Allopurinol 400 mg IV is prescribed for the client with tumor lysis syndrome. The medication vial contains 500 mg/25 mL. How many mL of medication should the nurse plan to prepare?

_____ mL (Record a whole number.)

**56.** **PHARM** The client who has a personality disorder is hospitalized on a medical unit. The psychiatrist prescribes mirtazapine to be continued. Prior to giving a dose, the nurse reviews the client's lab results illustrated. Based on the report, what should the nurse do?

| Serum Laboratory Test | Client's Value | Normal Values |
|---|---|---|
| Total cholesterol | 240 | 0–200 mg/dL |
| Triglycerides | 300 | 30–150 mg/dL |
| HDL | 28 | 35 mg/dL or greater |
| LDL | 160 | Less than 130 mg/dL |
| Albumin | 4.9 | 3.2–4.6 g/dL |
| AST | 52 | 15–40 units/L |
| ALT | 48 | 10–40 units/L |
| Total bilirubin | 1.6 | 0.2–1.3 mg/dL |
| Alkaline phosphatase | 144 | 35–142 units/L |

1. Administer the mirtazapine as prescribed by the psychiatrist.
2. Consult with the psychiatrist regarding increasing the dose of mirtazapine.
3. Consult with the psychiatrist regarding decreasing the dose of mirtazapine.
4. Consult with the general practitioner regarding additional lab tests.

**57.** **PHARM** The nurse is preparing to administer ondansetron 4 mg IV to the client with postoperative nausea. Ondansetron 2 mg/mL is available. How many mL of the medication should the nurse prepare to administer?

_____ mL (Record your answer as a whole number.)

**58.** **PHARM** The 70-year-old arrives at a clinic to receive an influenza vaccination. The client informs the nurse about having DM and CAD, states receiving an influenza vaccination last year, and denies having allergies. What is the nurse's **best** action?

1. Administer the vaccination as requested with live, attenuated influenza vaccine (LAIV).
2. Administer the vaccination as requested with trivalent inactivated influenza vaccine (TIV).
3. Counsel that the client is not a candidate for the vaccination due to heart disease and DM.
4. Inform the client that the influenza vaccination is good for 5 years and is not needed now.

**59.** **PHARM** The client has BPH and is questioning the need for prescribed tamsulosin. Which explanation about tamsulosin by the nurse is correct?

1. Reduces the prostate gland's size to relieve obstructive symptoms
2. Decreases inflammation caused by prostatic enlargement
3. Relaxes the smooth muscle in the prostate to facilitate urine flow
4. Decreases urine specific gravity, thus decreasing the risk of UTI

**60.** The first-time pregnant woman informs the obstetrics nurse that she wants to breastfeed her infant but is concerned about her ability to successfully do so. Which intervention should the nurse plan to implement immediately after delivery to promote successful breastfeeding?

1. Have the mother rest for 1 to 2 hours after delivery before attempting to breastfeed.
2. Provide privacy by allowing the mother and infant to be alone during the first feeding.
3. Place the infant on the mother's chest so there is skin-to-skin contact between them.
4. Feed the newborn a bottle of formula to stimulate bowel peristalsis before breastfeeding.

**61.** The orthopedic nurse is caring for the client who is being discharged to home following the repair of a leg fracture. Which orthopedic device is being used in the illustration, and which nursing intervention is required to maintain this device?

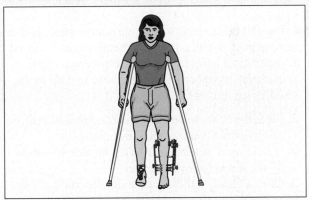

1. Internal fixation device, which requires daily pin care with hydrogen peroxide and saline
2. Buck's traction, which should be removed when the client is placed in bed for the night
3. Brace cast, which requires reminding the client to be non-weight-bearing on the affected leg
4. External fixation device, which requires daily inspection of the surrounding skin for redness

**62.** The nurse finds four prescribed medications with the labels illustrated below in a hospitalized client's locked medication drawer in the person's room. The nurse should complete a variance report after finding which medication in the client's medication box?

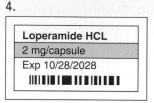

1.

| **Codeine** Ⓒ |
|---|
| 30 mg oral |
| Exp 12/28/2028 |
| ‖‖‖‖‖‖‖‖‖‖ |

2.

| **Phenytoin sodium** |
|---|
| 100 mg oral capsule |
| Exp 10/28/2028 |
| ‖‖‖‖‖‖‖‖‖‖ |

3.

| **Acetaminophen** |
|---|
| 325 mg oral |
| Exp 12/28/2028 |
| ‖‖‖‖‖‖‖‖‖‖ |

4.

| **Loperamide HCL** |
|---|
| 2 mg/capsule |
| Exp 10/28/2028 |
| ‖‖‖‖‖‖‖‖‖‖ |

**63.** **MoC** **PHARM** The nurse educator is observing the new nurse, who is applying topical triamcinolone 0.025% cream to a toddler's skin areas affected by dermatitis. Which action should be corrected by the nurse educator?

1. Inspects skin for erythema and purulent exudate, then assesses for increased pain to touch
2. Uses alcohol-based wash for hand hygiene and then puts on exam gloves to apply the cream
3. Spreads cream over the toddler's buttock and affected areas and applies an occlusive dressing
4. Asks the mother to hold the toddler while applying cream to affected areas on the child's back

**64.** The child diagnosed with acute nonlymphoid leukemia is hospitalized with a fever and neutropenia. To avoid complications associated with neutropenia, which nursing interventions should the nurse include in the child's plan of care?

1. Place the child in a private room, restrict ill visitors, and use strict hand washing techniques.
2. Encourage a well-balanced diet, include iron-rich foods, and avoid overexertion.
3. Offer a bland, soft diet, use toothettes for oral care, and provide saline mouthwashes often.
4. Avoid rectal temperatures and injections; apply pressure for 10 minutes after a venipuncture.

**65.** The female client, who was abused and sexually assaulted for the second time by her estranged husband, is being treated in an ED. The client is distraught and states, "The police can't keep him away, and I am afraid I might get pregnant." Which interventions should the nurse plan in treating this client? **Select all that apply.**

1. Administer a douche if prescribed by the HCP.
2. Obtain specimens of the woman's vaginal secretions for analysis.
3. Offer emergency contraception if pregnancy test results are negative.
4. Ask the client about making arrangements to stay at a women's shelter.
5. Keep the door open when out of the room so the woman does not feel alone.

**66.** The client who has HF tells the nurse, "I don't know why my ankles are so fat." What is the most appropriate **initial** response by the nurse?

1. "Tell me about your activity level."
2. "What have you eaten in the last 24 hours?"
3. "Has your weight gone up since yesterday?"
4. "How different are your ankles from yesterday?"

**67.** **MoC** The nurse observes the NA preparing a food tray for the 4-year-old who recently underwent a bone marrow transplant. Which food item should the nurse direct the NA to remove from the child's tray?

1. Orange juice
2. Apple slices
3. Slice of bread
4. Soft fried egg

**68.** **PHARM** The client with bipolar disorder is in an acute manic state. The nursing staff is unable to verbally de-escalate the situation, and the HCP orders a STAT dose of aripiprazole IM. Which client behavior indicates that aripiprazole has been effective?

1. The client becomes sedated.
2. The client's excitability is reduced.
3. The client's psychotic symptoms are alleviated.
4. The client's extrapyramidal symptoms are reduced.

**69.** The parish nurse is monitoring BPs at a screening clinic. The client who just finished smoking a cigarette asks the nurse for a BP check. Which is the nurse's **best** action?

1. Take the client's BP immediately as requested.
2. Ask the client not to smoke and then return in 30 minutes for the check.
3. Ask the client to refrain from smoking for a day and return for the check.
4. Ask what the client knows about the effects of smoking and heart disease.

70. The nurse working in a college health center receives a call from the student life office on campus. The client has had flu-like symptoms with neck stiffness for the past 4 hours. Which question by the nurse is **most** important?

   1. "Have you been able to drink anything?"
   2. "Do you have an elevated temperature?"
   3. "What do you mean by 'flu-like symptoms'?"
   4. "Do you have a rash anywhere on your body?"

71. The client who has worn contacts for more than 15 years asks the nurse about LASIK surgery. The nurse explains that this procedure corrects refraction errors through what mechanism?

   1. Reshaping the cornea
   2. Flattening of the retina
   3. Decreasing density of the lens
   4. Enhancing the outflow of aqueous humor

72. The nurse is preparing to apply the client's sequential compression device (SCD) for the first time to the lower extremities. The nurse explains the purpose, expected outcome, and procedure. Prioritize the nurse's remaining actions.

   1. Assess baseline color, temperature, and presence of peripheral pulses in the client's lower extremities.
   2. Monitor the client during treatment, including skin assessment and CMS.
   3. Apply the SCD sleeves, connect the sleeve cord to the device cord, set the control device at the prescribed pressure, and turn on the device.
   4. Document the placement of the SCD sleeves.
   5. Measure the size of the client's leg and obtain appropriate-sized SCD sleeves.

   Answer: _____

73. **MoC** While documenting in the client's EMR, Nurse A is called away and quickly leaves the computer. Seeing a free computer, Nurse B selects a different client. Nurse B is then called away. Nurse A returns, completes documentation on Nurse B's client's record, and logs off. Which actions should have prevented the incorrect EMR entry? **Select all that apply.**

   1. Log out of the computer before walking away from it.
   2. Log in with own user ID whenever accessing a client's medical record.
   3. Check that the correct client is selected before beginning documentation.
   4. Tell Nurse B to make sure to select the right client before documenting.
   5. Ask another nurse to complete documentation so the nurse can log off.
   6. Use the assigned user ID and created password to document in an EMR.

74. The client with normal lung function is receiving 40% oxygen by mask immediately following a surgical procedure. The nurse assesses that the client's SpO$_2$ is 90%. What should the nurse do?

   1. Place the client on room air.
   2. Leave the oxygen level at 40%.
   3. Increase the oxygen level to 50%.
   4. Decrease the oxygen level to 30%.

75. The nurse is performing chest physiotherapy on the child with cystic fibrosis. Which is the best client position for the nurse to perform middle lobe chest physiotherapy (chest percussion)?

   1.

   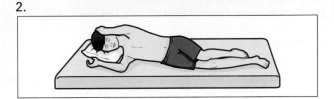

   2.

   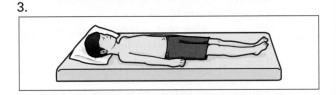

   3.

   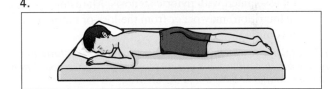

   4.

   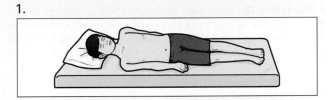

## Answers and Rationales

52 Comprehensive Exam 2 Answers and Rationales

### 1. PHARM ANSWER: 4

1. The digoxin (Lanoxin) dose is too high and can cause a lethal rhythm if given at this dose. The usual initial digitalizing dose is 0.25 to 0.5 mg.
2. The route for administering levofloxacin (Levaquin) is missing.
3. The U is an unacceptable abbreviation noted on The Joint Commission's "Do Not Use" List.
4. **Timolol, the generic name for Timoptic, is prescribed with the concentration, the dose, the route, and the frequency.**

▶ *Test-taking Tip: Read each option carefully to determine if essential parts of the medication order are noted and whether acceptable doses and abbreviations are being used. Eliminate options where components are missing or the dose is excessive.*

**Content Area:** Fundamentals; **Concept:** Medication; Safety; **Integrated Processes:** Communication and Documentation; **Client Needs:** Physiological Integrity: Pharmacological and Parenteral Therapies; **Cognitive Level:** Analysis [Analyzing]

### 2. ANSWER: 3

1. Diarrhea is not characteristic of pyloric stenosis.
2. Diarrhea and bile-colored vomiting are not symptoms of pyloric stenosis. If gastritis or a Mallory-Weiss tear develops, the emesis may become brown or coffee-colored due to blood.
3. **Nonbilious vomiting (not associated with nausea and not bile-colored), weight loss, hunger after vomiting, and lethargy are characteristic of pyloric stenosis.**
4. Vomiting unrelated to feeding position and diarrhea is not associated with pyloric stenosis. Marasmus (severe malnutrition) may occur from the loss of nutrients due to vomiting.

▶ *Test-taking Tip: Examine options with duplicate information first. Note that all options except No. 3 include diarrhea. Often, the option that is different is the answer.*

**Content Area:** Child; **Concept:** Nutrition; Assessment; **Integrated Processes:** Nursing Process: Assessment; **Client Needs:** Physiological Integrity: Physiological Adaptation; **Cognitive Level:** Application [Applying]

### 3. PHARM ANSWER: 2, 1, 5, 3, 4

2. **Select the IV injection port closest to the client. Using the closest port ensures that the medication is delivered when administered.**
1. **Cleanse the injection port with an antiseptic swab and allow the port to dry. Cleansing the port before attaching the syringe minimizes the introduction of microorganisms.**
5. **Connect a 10 mL large-barrel syringe of medication to the injection port. A large-barrel syringe is required when injecting medications into a PICC line because too much pressure is exerted by smaller syringes, and this can damage the catheter.**
3. **Pinch (clamp) the IV line and inject glycopyrrolate (Robinul) over 1 to 2 min; the IV line can be unpinched at intervals during administration to allow dilution of the medication. Administering it at the correct rate will prevent adverse effects.**
4. **Remove the syringe, ensure that the IV is infusing, and recheck the IV infusion rate. These safety checks are completed last to ensure that the client is receiving the prescribed fluids.**

▶ *Test-taking Tip: Use visualization to focus on the data in the question and then visualize the remaining steps of the procedure. Prioritizing means placing items in the correct sequence.*

**Content Area:** Management of Care; **Concept:** Medication; **Integrated Processes:** Nursing Process: Implementation; **Client Needs:** Physiological Integrity: Pharmacological and Parenteral Therapies; **Cognitive Level:** Synthesis [Creating]

### 4. MoC ANSWER: 1

1. **The nurse needs to intervene to correct the position of the chair. When transferring the client with left-sided weakness back to bed, the nurse should ensure that the client's strong side (not the weak side) is toward the bed.**
2. Although the female NA is supporting the client's weak side, complimenting the NA is not the best option.
3. Although the male NA is using a wide base of support, a compliment or praise will not protect the client from injury.
4. The client is using the strong side to push from the chair, but complimenting and praising are not the best actions to protect the client from injury.

▶ *Test-taking Tip: Select the option that uses ergonomic principles in transferring the client safely. Three options are similar (complimentary), and one is different. Often the option that is different is the answer.*

**Content Area:** Fundamentals; **Concept:** Mobility; Safety; **Integrated Processes:** Nursing Process: Implementation; **Client Needs:** Safe and Effective Care Environment: Management of Care; Safe and Effective Care Environment: Safety and Infection Control; Physiological Integrity: Basic Care and Comfort; **Cognitive Level:** Analysis [Analyzing]

### 5. ANSWER: 3

1. Although improvement is noted in the BP, the focus of the question is on treating the prerenal failure and not the BP.
2. An MAP of 55 is low, indicating decreased tissue perfusion exists.
3. **A common clinical finding in prerenal failure is decreased urine output. A urine output of greater than 30 mL/hr indicates that the fluid challenge is effective.**
4. Tachycardia is a manifestation of prerenal failure. If treatment is effective, the client's HR should be 60 to 100 bpm.

▶ *Test-taking Tip: Focus on the key words "for treating the prerenal failure." Eliminate Options 1, 2, and 4 because they do not evaluate kidney function.*

**Content Area:** Adult; **Concept:** Fluid and Electrolyte Balance; Urinary Elimination; **Integrated Processes:** Nursing Process: Evaluation; **Client Needs:** Physiological Integrity: Reduction of Risk Potential; **Cognitive Level:** Evaluation [Evaluating]

**6.** MoC **ANSWER: 1**

1. **Alcohol wipes will cause burning and irritation if used to cleanse the perineal-genital area. Either baby wipes or those supplied with the collection kits should be used. The nurse should intervene.**
2. Both the meatus and vagina are covered with a urine collection bag. The area is too small to just cover the meatus.
3. A diaper should be loosely applied; if too tight, it can cause reflux of urine or bag leakage.
4. The specimen container should have a client identification label that includes the specimen collected, date, and time. Body fluids can be infectious; urine should be transported in a biohazard bag.

▶ *Test-taking Tip: The key words are "most definitely," indicating that more than one option could be incorrect, but one is more important than the others. Client safety is priority.*

**Content Area:** Fundamentals; Child; **Concept:** Urinary Elimination; Management; **Integrated Processes:** Nursing Process: Evaluation; **Client Needs:** Safe and Effective Care Environment: Management of Care; **Cognitive Level:** Evaluation [Evaluating]

**7.** MoC **ANSWER: 2**

1. A response such as "not my turn" does not lead to conflict resolution.
2. **Generating possible solutions is an important step in conflict resolution.**
3. A response such as "that's not fair" will not promote conflict resolution.
4. The response that the nurses "all float too much" does not offer steps toward conflict resolution.

▶ *Test-taking Tip: Focus on the option that demonstrates conflict resolution first and then negotiation.*

**Content Area:** Management of Care; **Concept:** Collaboration; Communication; **Integrated Processes:** Nursing Process: Analysis; **Client Needs:** Safe and Effective Care Environment: Management of Care; **Cognitive Level:** Application [Applying]

**8.** MoC **ANSWER: 3**

1. If an aura is present, it appears before the onset of the seizure, not after the seizure.
2. The prefix "post" indicates that it follows, or comes after; therefore, the word "preceding" makes this option incorrect.
3. **The nurse should document the condition of the client immediately following the seizure. The "postictal" period pertains to the time following a seizure.**

4. Tonic-clonic activity occurs during a grand mal seizure and does not describe the postictal period.

▶ *Test-taking Tip: The option that uses words similar or related to those used in the stem is often the answer.*

**Content Area:** Adult; **Concept:** Neurologic Regulation; Safety; Communication; **Integrated Processes:** Communication and Documentation; Nursing Process: Assessment; **Client Needs:** Safe and Effective Care Environment: Management of Care; Physiological Integrity: Physiological Adaptation; **Cognitive Level:** Application [Applying]

**9. ANSWER: 4**

1. Pneumonia is not the most common cause of death.
2. Homicide is not the leading cause of death in children 1 to 4 years of age.
3. Cancer is not the leading cause of death in this age group.
4. **Over the last decade, unintentional injury has been the leading cause of death in children 1 to 4 years of age.**

▶ *Test-taking Tip: The key words are "most common." Focus on the age group and the leading cause of death.*

**Content Area:** Fundamentals; **Concept:** Safety; Communication; Nursing Roles; **Integrated Processes:** Teaching/Learning; **Client Needs:** Safe and Effective Care Environment: Safety and Infection Control; Health Promotion and Maintenance; **Cognitive Level:** Application [Applying]

**10.** PHARM **ANSWER: 1**

1. **Initial fluid therapy is directed toward expansion of the intravascular and extravascular volume and restoration of renal profusion. The usual rate is 10 to 20 mL/kg. This fluid is then continued at 1.5 times the 24-hour maintenance rate or replaced with 0.45% sodium chloride at the same rate.**
2. Ringer's lactate is not an isotonic solution.
3. Potassium is not added to the IV fluids until renal function is ensured, and then 20 to 40 mEq potassium is added. $D_5W$ also is not an isotonic solution.
4. $D_{10}W$ is not an isotonic solution.

▶ *Test-taking Tip: Only one IV solution is isotonic. Focus on eliminating the solutions with glucose because the child is already hyperglycemic. Of the remaining options, focus on whether potassium should be administered in the early phases of hyperglycemic crisis.*

**Content Area:** Child: **Concept:** Metabolism; Fluid and Electrolyte Balance; **Integrated Processes:** Nursing Process: Planning; **Client Needs:** Physiological Integrity: Pharmacological and Parenteral Therapies; **Cognitive Level:** Analysis [Analyzing]

**11. ANSWER: 2**

1. Periodic breathing is rarely associated with changes in skin color.
2. **Periodic pauses of up to 15 seconds in newborn respirations are expected during early newborn life. Rapid eye movement sleep, gross motor activity, sucking, and crying will increase the frequency of the pauses.**
3. Intermittent respiratory pauses up to 15 seconds are expected after birth.

4. Healthy term newborns are not lacking in surfactant. At 35 weeks' gestation, surfactant production is adequate to maintain good respiratory gas exchange in the majority of newborn infants.

▶ **Test-taking Tip:** *Three options focus on abnormalities, whereas one option is different. Often the option that is different is the answer.*

**Content Area:** Childbearing: **Concept:** Development; Pregnancy; Oxygenation; **Integrated Processes:** Nursing Process: Analysis; **Client Needs:** Health Promotion and Maintenance; **Cognitive Level:** Application [Applying]

**12.** **MoC** **ANSWER: 4**

1. Ineffective coping is the inability to form a valid appraisal of stressors, inadequate choices of practical response, and/or inability to use available resources.
2. Impaired adjustment is the inability to modify behavior in a manner consistent with a change in health status.
3. Dysfunctional grieving is the risk for extended, unsuccessful use of intellectual and emotional responses by which individuals, families, and communities attempt to work through the process of modifying self-concept based upon the perception of loss.
4. **The most appropriate problem is** *Family processes, interrupted.* **This option is the only one that supports uncomplicated grief. It is an emotional state following the death of a loved one that affects the client's physical and emotional well-being with impairment of functioning lasting for days, weeks, or months.**

▶ **Test-taking Tip:** *The key word in the stem is "improving." Three options include a maladaptive grief response, and one option is different.*

**Content Area:** Mental Health; **Concept:** Grief and Loss; Stress; Mood: **Integrated Processes:** Nursing Process: Analysis; **Client Needs:** Safe and Effective Care Environment: Management of Care; Psychosocial Integrity; **Cognitive Level:** Synthesis [Creating]

**13. ANSWER: 2**

1. Clients with chronic pain are less likely to have physiological changes because the ANS adapts to the pain.
2. **The single most important indicator of pain and its intensity is the client's report of pain, whether treatment includes medication, nonpharmacological interventions, or both.**
3. Asking the client's significant other's opinion is not as reliable as asking the client directly.
4. Assessing client facial expression is not as reliable as asking the client about pain.

▶ **Test-taking Tip:** *Read the scenario in the stem carefully. Determine that the question is asking the best method to evaluate pain. Consider which option focuses directly on the client's individual pain experience.*

**Content Area:** Fundamentals; **Concept:** Comfort; Medication; **Integrated Processes:** Nursing Process: Evaluation; **Client Needs:** Physiological Integrity: Basic Care and Comfort; **Cognitive Level:** Evaluation [Evaluating]

**14. ANSWER: 4**

1. Thanking the staff for information about sources of help provides some indication of an understanding of the importance of outpatient services.
2. Acknowledging that a service has been contacted shows an understanding of the importance of a bridging strategy.
3. Keeping a list of outpatient services' telephone numbers available shows an understanding of the importance of a bridging strategy.
4. **The statement about accessing services when the client no longer can get the things needed to be healthy and safe shows a lack of understanding of the need to access these services before breakdown of the plan of care occurs.**

▶ **Test-taking Tip:** *The key words are "need for further teaching." This is a false-response question. Select the option that demonstrates that the client would use a service only as a last resort.*

**Content Area:** Mental Health; **Concept:** Stress; Safety; Collaboration; Nursing Roles; **Integrated Processes:** Teaching/Learning; **Client Needs:** Health Promotion and Maintenance; **Cognitive Level:** Evaluation [Evaluating]

**15.** **PHARM** **ANSWER: 4**

1. A side effect of oxytocin is mild transient hypertension. Thus, a systolic BP above 100 mm Hg would be expected.
2. The purpose of the oxytocin is to contract the uterus. In response, the lochia flow should be moderate to small unless the client experienced a perineal laceration.
3. If the oxytocin causes continuous uterine contraction, the client will not experience afterpains. However, if the uterus contracts and relaxes, as sometimes happens with multigravidas, the client may feel afterpains when the oxytocin is infusing.
4. **Prevention of postpartum hemorrhage (PPH) involves the routine administration of oxytocin (Pitocin) immediately following delivery of the placenta to promote uterine contraction and vasoconstriction, thus preventing the uterus from becoming atonic. A firm fundus would indicate that the oxytocin was effective.**

▶ **Test-taking Tip:** *Recall that the action of oxytocin is to contract the uterus. Select the option that best describes that action.*

**Content Area:** Childbearing: **Concept:** Pregnancy; Medication; Assessment; **Integrated Processes:** Nursing Process: Evaluation; **Client Needs:** Physiological Integrity: Pharmacological and Parenteral Therapies; **Cognitive Level:** Evaluation [Evaluating]

**16. ANSWER: 3**

1. Before rehydration, it is likely that the Hct will be elevated due to hemoconcentration from loss of fluids, not reduced. Normal Hct is 35% to 45%.

2. Normal Hgb is 11.5 to 15.5 g/dL and likely would be elevated with hemoconcentration. It should normalize with rehydration.

**3. The nurse should expect blood urea nitrogen (BUN) to be elevated with dehydration and normalize when the child is rehydrated. A normal BUN for a child is 4 to 17 mg/dL.**

4. A normal serum creatinine (SCr) for a 7-year old is 0.3 to 0.7 mg/dL. The SCr is still elevated.

▶ *Test-taking Tip: Hgb, Hct, BUN, and creatinine elevate with acute diarrhea and normalize with rehydration. Narrow the options by eliminating values that are below normal before rehydration.*

Content Area: Child: Concept: Fluid and Electrolyte Balance; Integrated Processes: Nursing Process: Evaluation; Client Needs: Physiological Integrity: Reduction of Risk Potential; Cognitive Level: Evaluation [Evaluating]

## 17. ANSWER: 3

1. Nausea should be addressed but is not the priority.
2. Inability to void should be addressed but is not the priority.
**3. The nurse's priority is the client's numbness and tingling. This suggests circulatory impairment from compartment syndrome.**
4. Dressing saturation should be addressed because it increases the client's risk for an infection but it is not the priority.

▶ *Test-taking Tip: Use the ABC's to establish priority.*

Content Area: Adult; Concept: Perfusion; Safety; Integrated Processes: Nursing Process: Analysis; Client Needs: Physiological Integrity: Physiological Adaptation; Cognitive Level: Analysis [Analyzing]

## 18. ANSWER: 1

**1. During the first 24 to 48 hours after prostatectomy, it is critical that the patency of the catheter be assessed and maintained. The risk of blood clots forming and obstructing the flow of urine is greatest during this period.**
2. Activities that increase abdominal pressure, such as sitting, should be avoided as this predisposes the client to increased bleeding.
3. There is no abdominal incision or abdominal dressing with a TURP. Parts of the prostate gland are removed through a scope inserted into the urethra.
4. Blood clots in the urinary drainage bag are expected after prostate surgery for the first 24 to 36 hours; there is no need to notify the surgeon of this.

▶ *Test-taking Tip: The key phrase is "immediately following a TURP." Recall that bleeding is a major concern in the early postoperative period. Select the option that decreases bleeding or its complications.*

Content Area: Adult; Concept: Male Reproduction; Safety; Assessment; Integrated Processes: Nursing Process: Implementation; Client Needs: Physiological Integrity: Physiological Adaptation; Cognitive Level: Application [Applying]

## 19. ANSWER: 4

1. Anger is often manifested by antagonistic behaviors that may be directed at family, staff, or the medical regimen.
2. Denial is a defense mechanism that allows minimization of a threat. It may be manifested by minimizing the severity of the medical condition, ignoring activity restrictions, or avoiding the discussion of illness or its significance.
3. Depression is usually manifested by symptoms of withdrawal, crying, or apathy. These behaviors are not noted in the situation.
**4. The nurse should document that the client is showing signs of dependency. This is a state of reliance on another and can be a behavioral response to an MI.**

▶ *Test-taking Tip: Focusing on the client's behaviors of "frequently calls" and "questions" will direct you to Option 4.*

Content Area: Adult; Concept: Stress; Perfusion; Integrated Processes: Communication and Documentation; Client Needs: Psychosocial Integrity; Cognitive Level: Analysis [Analyzing]

## 20. ANSWER: 3

1. The person checking the pulse is on the right side of the bed. Two nurses would not be on the same side of the bed (Location A).
2. A person doing rescue breathing with a bag-mask resuscitator might be positioned at the head of the bed (Location B).
**3. If the person checking the pulse and performing compressions is on the right side of the client, then the person performing rescue breathing with a mask should be on the left side of the client (Location C).**
4. Location D is only assumed for abdominal thrusts on an unresponsive choking victim.

▶ *Test-taking Tip: Read the scenario carefully and visualize the position of the rescue breather.*

Content Area: Adult; Concept: Oxygenation; Safety; Perfusion; Integrated Processes: Nursing Process: Implementation; Client Needs: Physiological Integrity: Physiological Adaptation; Cognitive Level: Application [Applying]

## 21. MoC ANSWER: 3

1. The family is not responsible for protecting the client from the consequences of his or her actions.
2. The family is not responsible for reducing the client's temptation to use substances.
**3. Studies show that reducing relationship distress lessens the client's risk of relapse. Goals of therapy include helping families become aware of their own needs, working to shift power to the parental figures in a family, and improving communication.**
4. The family is not responsible for confronting the client about the harm caused by substance abuse.

♦ **Test-taking Tip:** *Note that Option 3 focuses on the family's needs, whereas the other options focus on the client's needs. Often the option that is different is the answer.*

**Content Area:** Mental Health; **Concept:** Addiction; Family; **Integrated Processes:** Nursing Process: Planning; Caring; **Client Needs:** Safe and Effective Care Environment: Management of Care; Psychosocial Integrity; **Cognitive Level:** Analysis [Analyzing]

## 22. PHARM ANSWER: 4

1. Because the chemotherapy agent is in powder form, a respirator mask should be worn.
2. Because the chemotherapy agent is in powder form, a respirator mask should be worn. Double- and not single-bag clean-up pads are needed.
3. If the spill involves liquid chemotherapy drugs, the nurse would need a protective gown, gloves, and goggles only, but still should double-bag the spilled waste; this is a spill of a powdered chemotherapy agent.
4. **Wearing a protective gown, gloves, goggles, and a respirator mask and using double-bag clean-up pads with open waste disposal bags provides protection when cleaning up powder chemotherapy spills. The respirator mask is needed to prevent the agent from being inhaled.**

♦ **Test-taking Tip:** *The key word is "powdered." Only one option will protect from inhalation of the powder.*

**Content Area:** Adult; **Concept:** Safety; Medication; **Integrated Processes:** Nursing Process: Implementation; **Client Needs:** Safe and Effective Care Environment: Safety and Infection Control; Physiological Integrity: Pharmacological and Parenteral Therapies; **Cognitive Level:** Application [Applying]

## 23. MoC ANSWER: 1

1. **The RN from ICU would have the most experience in monitoring the client and preparing IV medications for administration.**
2. The LPN's scope of practice may not include the administration of prescribed IV medications to treat liver transplant rejection.
3. The newly licensed RN may not have the experience needed to prepare the IV medications. The nurse's inexperience could cause delays in administering the prescribed medications.
4. Fatigue increases risk for errors. This client is critically ill and may require rapid interventions.

♦ **Test-taking Tip:** *You need to think about which nurse is best equipped to handle multiple medications quickly.*

**Content Area:** Management of Care; **Concept:** Medication; Safety; Management; **Integrated Processes:** Nursing Process: Planning; **Client Needs:** Safe and Effective Care Environment: Management of Care; **Cognitive Level:** Application [Applying]

## 24. PHARM ANSWER: 1

1. **This statement indicates that the client needs additional teaching. Guaifenesin (Robitussin) aids in expectoration by reducing adhesiveness and surface tension of secretions. It should be taken with a full glass of water, not with food.**

2. Increasing fluids helps to liquefy secretions.
3. Side effects of guaifenesin include headache, which can be relieved with acetaminophen.
4. Sugarless gum or hard candy will alleviate the throat discomfort caused by a nonproductive cough.

♦ **Test-taking Tip:** *Recall that guaifenesin is an expectorant. The key word is "teach." Select the option that is incorrect.*

**Content Area:** Adult; **Concept:** Medication; Infection; **Integrated Processes:** Nursing Process: Assessment; **Client Needs:** Physiological Integrity: Pharmacological and Parenteral Therapies; **Cognitive Level:** Analysis [Analyzing]

## 25. ANSWER: 1, 2, 4, 5

1. **The nurse should address iron deficiency that can occur after gastric bypass surgery due to malabsorption.**
2. **The nurse should address vitamin $B_{12}$ deficiency that can occur from reduced intrinsic factor production secondary to parietal cell loss and malabsorption after a gastric bypass.**
3. Vitamin C deficiency has not been associated with Roux-en-Y gastric bypass.
4. **The nurse should address vitamin A deficiency because the duodenum (where vitamin A is primarily absorbed) was bypassed.**
5. **The nurse should address protein deficiency due to reduced intake after a gastric bypass procedure.**
6. Folate deficiency, rather than excess, occurs due to reduced intake after a gastric bypass procedure.

♦ **Test-taking Tip:** *Consider which nutrients are absorbed in the stomach and which have the highest potential to be malabsorbed after Roux-en-Y gastric bypass.*

**Content Area:** Childbearing; Adult; **Concept:** Nutrition; Pregnancy; **Integrated Processes:** Nursing Process: Analysis; **Client Needs:** Physiological Integrity: Basic Care and Comfort; **Cognitive Level:** Analysis [Analyzing]

## 26. MoC ANSWER: 3

1. Birth may be imminent, and the client should not be transferred.
2. Timing contractions is not the primary responsibility at this time because birth is imminent.
3. **In the second stage of labor, the cervix is fully dilated and 100% effaced, and the infant descends into the birth canal and may crown. The nurse should notify the HCP and prepare for delivery.**
4. The primary responsibility in the second stage of labor is to support the infant's head and apply slight pressure to control the delivery, not to check the FHR with a fetoscope.

♦ **Test-taking Tip:** *In the second stage of labor, birth is imminent.*

**Content Area:** Childbearing: **Concept:** Safety; Pregnancy; **Integrated Processes:** Nursing Process: Implementation; Caring; **Client Needs:** Safe and Effective Care Environment: Management of Care; **Cognitive Level:** Analysis [Analyzing]

**27.** **MoC** **ANSWER: 4**
1. The nurse already should be monitoring the client's temperature and lung sounds.
2. Warming the food will not satisfy the client's request for "hot foods."
3. Extra spices will not satisfy the client's request for "hot foods."
4. **The client believes that certain foods and diseases are hot or cold. This belief is common to folk medicine in several cultures. The nurse should initiate a dietitian referral for a client with specific dietary needs such as this. Usually opposite foods and diseases have a therapeutic effect.**

▸ *Test-taking Tip: The client believes in the hot/cold theory of treating illness. Eliminate options dealing with the actual temperature or spiciness of the foods.*

Content Area: Management of Care; Concept: Diversity; Management; Integrated Processes: Nursing Process: Implementation; Culture and Spirituality; Client Needs: Safe and Effective Care Environment: Management of Care; Cognitive Level: Application [Applying]

**28. ANSWER:**

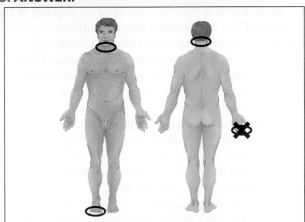

**Scabies lesions tend to be concentrated in the web spaces of the fingers. The neck, hairline, and toes are not common sites for scabies to be seen.**

▸ *Test-taking Tip: Focus on the key phrase "check first." Recall that the papules of scabies appear most frequently in finer webs, axillae, wrist folds, umbilicus, groin, and genitals.*

Content Area: Adult; Concept: Infection; Assessment; Integrated Processes: Nursing Process: Assessment; Client Needs: Physiological Integrity: Physiological Adaptation; Cognitive Level: Application [Applying]

**29. ANSWER: 2**
1. Small, frequent feedings help the child consume adequate calories without feeling tired after large meals.
2. **Soft foods (not solid foods) should be provided because soft ones require less energy use with mastication. CP increases the work of breathing due to thick, tenacious secretions that clog the airways. An increase in energy use will increase the RR, making it more difficult to breathe.**

3. High-calorie supplements provide additional calories.
4. Utensils with large, padded handles help the child engage in self-feeding when possible.

▸ *Test-taking Tip: Select an option that would increase energy expenditure.*

Content Area: Child: Concept: Nutrition; Safety; Nursing Roles; Integrated Processes: Nursing Process: Evaluation; Teaching/ Learning; Client Needs: Physiological Integrity: Basic Care and Comfort; Physiological Integrity: Reduction of Risk Potential; Cognitive Level: Evaluation [Evaluating]

**30. ANSWER: 4**
1. Although the client's level of anxiety is important, ensuring client safety is first.
2. Before checking the medical record, the nurse should determine if the correct client has been brought into the OR.
3. Before verifying the correct operative site, the nurse must admit the correct client.
4. **To protect the client from unintentional harm, the nurse first should confirm the person's identity.**

▸ *Test-taking Tip: Use Maslow's Hierarchy of Needs theory to eliminate options. Safety is priority.*

Content Area: Adult; Concept: Safety; Assessment; Legal; Integrated Processes: Nursing Process: Implementation; Client Needs: Safe and Effective Care Environment: Safety and Infection Control; Cognitive Level: Application [Applying]

**31. ANSWER: 2**
1. Gingivitis, plaque, and halitosis (bad breath) are not signs of oral mucositis.
2. **Oral erythema, pain, and dysgeusia (taste changes) commonly occur with oral mucositis; other findings include inflammation and ulceration.**
3. Candidiasis and cheilitis (lip inflammation) are not signs of oral mucositis.
4. Leukoplakia (white oral lesions) and caries (dental cavities) are not signs of mucositis.

▸ *Test-taking Tip: Eliminate options associated with the teeth and lips.*

Content Area: Adult; Concept: Assessment; Comfort; Cellular Regulation; Integrated Processes: Nursing Process: Assessment; Client Needs: Physiological Integrity: Reduction of Risk Potential; Cognitive Level: Analysis [Analyzing]

**32.** **PHARM** **ANSWER: 3**
1. VS are assessed before the transfusion begins, 15 minutes after it is started, and then hourly until the transfusion is finished. Upon completion, VS are taken and then repeated an hour later.
2. PRBCs should infuse in 4 hours or less to avoid the risk of septicemia.
3. **If the client experiences symptoms of a transfusion reaction, the transfusion should be stopped immediately. The line should be kept open for emergency medications, using saline (0.9% NaCl). Saline should not be given through the existing blood tubing because the client will receive the blood remaining in the tubing.**

4. Special tubing with a filter (not standard tubing) is used to administer blood.

▶ **Test-taking Tip:** *Three options are similar, and one is different (complications). Often the option that is different is the correct answer.*

**Content Area:** Adult; **Concept:** Safety; Hematologic Regulation; **Integrated Processes:** Nursing Process: Implementation; **Client Needs:** Safe and Effective Care Environment: Safety and Infection Control; Physiological Integrity: Pharmacological and Parenteral Therapies; **Cognitive Level:** Application [Applying]

## 33. MoC ANSWER: 3

1. The scope of practice for ancillary staff includes feeding the client if the nurse determines that it is appropriate.
2. Ancillary staff can reinforce information if the nurse determines that it is appropriate.
3. **The scope of practice for ancillary staff does not include assessment. Assessing the client's skin is not a responsibility the RN can delegate to the ancillary staff.**
4. The scope of practice for ancillary staff includes securing supplies.

▶ **Test-taking Tip:** *The key phrase "needs further education" indicates this is a false-response item. Select the option that indicates incorrect delegation, which includes assessment, planning, evaluation, or teaching; these are responsibilities the RN cannot delegate.*

**Content Area:** Management of Care; **Concept:** Management; Safety; Regulations; **Integrated Processes:** Nursing Process: Planning; Caring; **Client Needs:** Safe and Effective Care Environment: Management of Care; **Cognitive Level:** Application [Applying]

## 34. PHARM ANSWER: 2, 5

1. Diarrhea is a common side effect of SSRIs, a different class of antidepressant medications.
2. **TCAs block acetylcholine receptors, causing anticholinergic effects including dry mouth, blurred vision, constipation, and urinary retention.**
3. Agranulocytosis is a rare, serious and potentially fatal side effect of traditional antipsychotic medications.
4. Unintentional tremor is a common side effect with SSRIs, a different class of antidepressant medications.
5. **TCAs block acetylcholine receptors, causing anticholinergic effects including urinary retention, dry mouth, blurred vision, and constipation.**

▶ **Test-taking Tip:** *TCAs block acetylcholine receptors. Think about the side effects associated with this action.*

**Content Area:** Mental Health; **Concept:** Medication; Mood; Safety; **Integrated Processes:** Teaching/Learning; **Client Needs:** Physiological Integrity: Pharmacological and Parenteral Therapies; **Cognitive Level:** Knowledge [Remembering]

## 35. ANSWER: 3

1. Because the client is prone to bleeding, dental flossing is contraindicated.
2. The client should be ambulated with assistance and not remain on bedrest.

3. **The nurse should assess for signs of bleeding, which can occur with low platelet levels (usually less than 50,000/mm³ or 50 K/microL). Blurred vision and mental status changes can be signs of intracranial bleeding.**
4. The client is prone to bleeding, so aspirin, which inhibits platelet aggregation, is contraindicated.

▶ **Test-taking Tip:** *Apply knowledge of bleeding precautions to select the answer. If uncertain, select the option that uses the first step of the nursing process.*

**Content Area:** Adult; **Concept:** Clotting; Hematologic Regulation; **Integrated Processes:** Nursing Process: Implementation; **Client Needs:** Physiological Integrity: Reduction of Risk Potential; **Cognitive Level:** Application [Applying]

## 36. PHARM ANSWER: 1, 2, 3, 5

1. **The HCP should be notified; the client should be assessed by the HCP, and an echocardiogram may be needed to determine the presence of air.**
2. **The clamp, if present, should be closed to prevent additional air from entering the line.**
3. **After the aspiration of blood, the line should be flushed with 0.9% NaCl to maintain patency of the central line and prevent it from clotting.**
4. The client should be placed on the left side, not the right, with the feet higher than the head. This position traps air in the right atrium, which then can be removed directly by intracardiac aspiration if necessary.
5. **Attaching a syringe and aspirating until blood returns may prevent air in the line from entering the central circulation. The 10 mL syringe with a larger barrel should be used when injecting into or aspirating from central lines.**

▶ **Test-taking Tip:** *Visualize each option, recalling that the goals are to prevent air from entering the central circulation or to trap the air in the right atrium. Remember that air rises, so the client should be positioned on the left side.*

**Content Area:** Management of Care; **Concept:** Infection; Medication; **Integrated Processes:** Nursing Process: Implementation; **Client Needs:** Physiological Integrity: Pharmacological and Parenteral Therapies; **Cognitive Level:** Application [Applying]

## 37. ANSWER: 4

1. This is sinus bradycardia with a first-degree AV block (PRI is greater than 0.20 sec).
2. This is sinus tachycardia. A normal PRI = 0.12 to 0.20 sec; QRS = 0.06 to 0.10 sec; QT is rate dependent, and ventricular rate is 60 to 100 bmp. A ventricular rate greater than 100 bmp is tachycardia.
3. This is atrial fibrillation (P is fibrillatory, and PRI is not measurable).
4. **The measurements suggest complete heart block, a life-threatening dysrhythmia. There is no association between the P waves and QRS complexes; the atrial rate is normal, but the ventricular rate is very slow.**

▶ *Test-taking Tip: Read each option carefully. If unsure of normal waveform measurements, eliminate Options 1 and 2 because these have waveforms that are measurable. Of Options 3 and 4, note that Option 4 has more abnormal waveforms than Option 3.*

**Content Area:** Adult; **Concept:** Perfusion; Assessment; **Integrated Processes:** Nursing Process: Analysis; **Client Needs:** Physiological Integrity: Physiological Adaptation; **Cognitive Level:** Analysis [Analyzing]

## 38. ANSWER: 1

1. **The client experiencing a manic episode may say whatever comes to mind and rapidly change topics (flight of ideas).**
2. Social withdrawal is a symptom of a major depressive episode.
3. Trembling or shaking is more likely to be observed in the client with panic disorder.
4. Somatic-type delusions are associated with a major depressive episode with psychosis.

▶ *Test-taking Tip: Relate "manic" in the stem with a similar word in one of the options.*

**Content Area:** Mental Health; **Concept:** Mood; Assessment; **Integrated Processes:** Nursing Process: Assessment; **Client Needs:** Psychosocial Integrity; **Cognitive Level:** Analysis [Analyzing]

## 39. MoC PHARM ANSWER: 2

1. The hair in the sterile field contaminates the sterile field because it is not sterile. The nurse has an ethical and legal responsibility to protect the client from injury.
2. **The nurse should inform the HCP when contamination of a sterile field occurs and should obtain new supplies. Contaminated supplies should never be used for a sterile procedure.**
3. Allowing the HCP to decide is a breach of duty to the client.
4. An antiseptic agent is one that inhibits the growth of some microorganisms, but it does not render an object sterile.

▶ *Test-taking Tip: Implement principles of sterile technique when answering this question.*

**Content Area:** Adult; **Concept:** Infection; Safety; **Integrated Processes:** Nursing Process: Implementation; **Client Needs:** Safe and Effective Care Environment: Safety and Infection Control; Safe and Effective Care Environment: Management of Care; Physiological Integrity: Pharmacological and Parenteral Therapies; **Cognitive Level:** Application [Applying]

## 40. MoC ANSWER: 1

1. **A specialty clinic with experience in management of clients with newly diagnosed HIV will provide the most support for the type of concerns expressed by the client.**
2. The local public health department may be able to provide resources; however, it is likely that the specialty clinic is better prepared to deal with the holistic needs of the client.

3. Referral to the HCP who specializes in infectious diseases may not address the client's psychosocial needs.
4. Disclosure of the diagnosis to the family may not address the client's psychosocial needs.

▶ *Test-taking Tip: The key phrase is "most client support." Focus on what each option can provide in fulfilling client requirements according to Maslow's Hierarchy of Needs theory, including the need for love and belonging.*

**Content Area:** Management of Care; **Concept:** Stress; Infection; Collaboration; **Integrated Processes:** Nursing Process: Implementation; **Client Needs:** Safe and Effective Care Environment: Management of Care; **Cognitive Level:** Application [Applying]

## 41. MoC ANSWER: 4

1. Providing perineal care would be the lowest priority.
2. Applying ice to reduce pain is important but should be addressed after the fundus is firm.
3. Providing pain control with medication is important and should be addressed after the fundus is firm.
4. **The nurse should first massage the soft, boggy fundus until it is firm. Uterine atony is the most common cause of postpartum hemorrhage, which can be life-threatening.**

▶ *Test-taking Tip: Apply Maslow's Hierarchy of Needs theory and address the potentially life-threatening concern first.*

**Content Area:** Childbearing; **Concept:** Pregnancy; Safety; **Integrated Processes:** Nursing Process: Implementation; **Client Needs:** Safe and Effective Care Environment: Management of Care; **Cognitive Level:** Analysis [Analyzing]

## 42. ANSWER: 3

1. Dressing as a teenager reinforces that the child is different from peers the same age.
2. Gonadotropin-releasing hormone (GnRH) agonists can arrest the progression of, and in some cases reduce the size of, the breasts. But if there is no reduction in breast size, this information could negatively impact the child's body image.
3. **Reassuring the child that pubertal changes are normal, and that the child's friends eventually will develop the same characteristics, should be helpful in facilitating a positive body image.**
4. Encouraging the child to inform others of his or her age reinforces that the child is different from peers the same age.

▶ *Test-taking Tip: Three options are similar, and one is different; often, the option that is different is the correct answer.*

**Content Area:** Child; **Concept:** Development; Female Reproduction; **Integrated Processes:** Communication and Documentation; **Client Needs:** Psychosocial Integrity; **Cognitive Level:** Application [Applying]

## 43. MoC ANSWER: 1, 4, 5

1. **Kussmaul respirations occur in DKA due to metabolic acidosis from the breakdown of fats into ketones and the body's attempts to compensate for the acidosis by increasing RR and depth to eliminate excess carbon dioxide.**

2. The HR would be increased in DKA, not decreased.

3. In DKA the breath odor would be sweet-smelling, not foul-smelling.

4. **A change in consciousness occurs in DKA due to metabolic acidosis and the hyperglycemic state.**

5. **In DKA, blood glucose levels will be elevated (greater than 330 mg/dL).**

♦ *Test-taking Tip: This is an alternate-type question with more than one correct answer. Be sure to read all options to determine which ones are associated with DKA.*

**Content Area:** Management of Care; Child; **Concept:** Metabolism; Assessment; **Integrated Processes:** Nursing Process: Assessment; **Client Needs:** Safe and Effective Care Environment: Management of Care; Physiological Integrity: Physiological Adaptation; **Cognitive Level:** Analysis [Analyzing]

**44.** MoC **ANSWER: 2**

1. The client may need a referral to a dietitian, not a social worker, if experiencing swallowing difficulties.

2. **Responsibilities of a social worker include assisting the client with financial concerns. The social worker may help the client identify less costly alternatives for obtaining medications. Stopping atenolol (Tenormin), the BP medication, can precipitate a hypertensive crisis.**

3. Ginkgo can increase the effects of warfarin (Coumadin). The nurse should notify the HCP.

4. If medications and dosages will be changing, setting up medications for 2 weeks at a time could result in the wrong dose or the wrong medication. The nurse should address this concern with both the client and daughter.

♦ *Test-taking Tip: A social worker's responsibilities include addressing the client's financial concerns and identifying resources for financial assistance with medications.*

**Content Area:** Management of Care; **Concept:** Safety; Medication; **Integrated Processes:** Nursing Process: Analysis; **Client Needs:** Safe and Effective Care Environment: Management of Care; **Cognitive Level:** Analysis [Analyzing]

**45. ANSWER: 1**

1. **Maintaining an airtight seal is often a problem during negative-pressure wound therapy.**

2. Air bubbles are not a problem with negative-pressure wound therapy.

3. The negative pressure removes fluid drainage; this is not a problem.

4. The negative pressure prevents dressings from becoming saturated.

♦ *Test-taking Tip: Focus on the key words "negative-pressure wound therapy." Use association to select an option that would suggest inadequate pressure.*

**Content Area:** Adult; **Concept:** Skin Integrity; Safety; Infection; **Integrated Processes:** Nursing Process: Planning; **Client Needs:** Safe and Effective Care Environment: Safety and Infection Control; **Cognitive Level:** Application [Applying]

**46. ANSWER: 2, 3, 4, 5**

1. The client would not be alert enough to comprehend using the IS and would not be ready to sit up to use it.

2. **Unless contraindicated, the side-lying position will prevent aspiration of secretions. Turning also will mobilize secretions.**

3. **Analgesics are administered IV in the PACU for pain control in a rapid onset.**

4. **The nurse should protect the client from injury. Some clients emerge from anesthesia in an agitated state (emergence delirium) for a short period.**

5. **General anesthesia causes a temporary loss of memory. Repeat explanations such as, "Mr. Brown, surgery is over; you are in the recovery room."**

♦ *Test-taking Tip: Visualize the client recovering from anesthesia and use the ABC's and Maslow's Hierarchy of Needs theory to assist in identifying appropriate interventions.*

**Content Area:** Adult; **Concept:** Safety; Medication; Nursing Roles; **Integrated Processes:** Nursing Process: Implementation; Caring; **Client Needs:** Physiological Integrity: Reduction of Risk Potential; **Cognitive Level:** Application [Applying]

**47.** MoC **ANSWER: 1, 3, 5**

1. **Acetaminophen (Tylenol) is an antipyretic. These should be prescribed for an elevated temperature.**

2. The situation does not state whether the source of the infection is viral or bacterial. Peramivir (Rapivab) is an antiviral medication and is not appropriate if the client has a bacterial infection.

3. **An isotonic solution may be needed for fluid replacement. Oral fluids will help liquefy secretions.**

4. The client should rest during the acute phase of the illness.

5. **Oxygenation may be impaired due to the lung infection, and oxygen therapy may be needed.**

♦ *Test-taking Tip: Do not assume information that is not supplied. Community-acquired pneumonia can be viral or bacterial.*

**Content Area:** Adult; **Concept:** Infection: Oxygenation; **Integrated Processes:** Nursing Process: Planning; **Client Needs:** Safe and Effective Care Environment: Management of Care; **Cognitive Level:** Evaluation [Evaluating]

**48. ANSWER: 2**

1. The child with a normal BP does not need a referral for a hypertension work-up. The client should be rescreened periodically as per the guidelines set by age.

2. **The nurse should document the findings. The systolic BP of 112 is at 25% of the client's age and the diastolic of 72 is at 10%. No intervention is necessary.**

3. The child does not need antihypertensive therapy.

4. There is no need to begin teaching on measures to reduce the BP when the BP is appropriate for the child's age.

▶ *Test-taking Tip: Note that Options 1, 3, and 4 are related to treating hypertension, whereas Option 2 is the only one that considers the BP reading a normal finding. Often the option that is different is the answer.*

Content Area: Child; Concept: Assessment; Safety; Communication; Integrated Processes: Nursing Process: Implementation; Client Needs: Physiological Integrity: Reduction of Risk Potential; Cognitive Level: Application [Applying]

## 49. ANSWER: 3

1. The stressors must be identified before a plan can be addressed.
2. The client must identify precipitating factors before coping skills can be addressed.
3. **This initial behavior demonstrates that the client is assuming responsibility for anger management. The client must identify stressors before acting on the anger they create.**
4. Apologizing for past behavior does not indicate a change in the client's current behavior.

▶ *Test-taking Tip: Note the key word "initial." Focus on the use of the nursing process. Assessment should be completed prior to planning.*

Content Area: Mental Health; Concept: Assessment; Stress; Integrated Processes: Nursing Process: Evaluation; Client Needs: Psychosocial Integrity; Cognitive Level: Evaluation [Evaluating]

## 50. ANSWER: 2

1. Standing orders cannot be used for seclusion or restraints. The HCP must be contacted as soon as possible, in accordance with hospital policy.
2. **Alternative interventions such as negotiating or diversion should be attempted to remove the client from seclusion as soon as possible. Negative psychological effects of seclusion should be minimized by reducing the time spent there.**
3. Clients demonstrating harm to themselves or others legally can be restrained or secluded.
4. Clients in seclusion are at risk of death due to their uncontrollable behavior. Minimum monitoring must be every 15 minutes.

▶ *Test-taking Tip: Three options include information about placing the client in seclusion, and one is different (removal). Often the option that is different is the answer.*

Content Area: Management of Care; Mental Health Concept: Safety; Stress; Integrated Processes: Nursing Process: Analysis; Client Needs: Safe and Effective Care Environment: Safety and Infection Control; Cognitive Level: Analysis [Analyzing]

## 51. ANSWER: 2, 4, 5

1. Resting the otoscope on the child's head may lead to injury.
2. **Noting the color of the tympanic membrane is important in an ear assessment.**
3. Pulling the pinna up and back is performed to visualize the tympanic membrane in children 3 years and older, and in adults.

4. **Pulling the pinna down and back properly aligns the ear canal to visualize the tympanic membrane in children younger than 3 years.**
5. **Otoscope tips are available in different sizes, and using the smallest tip decreases the chance of injury.**

▶ *Test-taking Tip: Note the child's age. First, review options that are similar but opposite, and eliminate one of each of these. Eliminate options that could lead to injury.*

Content Area: Child; Concept: Assessment; Sensory Perception; Integrated Processes: Nursing Process: Assessment; Client Needs: Health Promotion and Maintenance; Cognitive Level: Application [Applying]

## 52. ANSWER: 1

1. **The client is in the "why me" stage of acceptance. Clarifying encourages communication and allows the client to express feelings and move toward acceptance.**
2. Telling the client that smoking is not the only cause of bladder cancer ignores the person's feelings and blocks communication.
3. Telling the client his or her feelings are understood belittles the person's feelings and blocks communication.
4. Telling the client that he or she is angry and doesn't mean to wish cancer on another is making a conclusion without enough data. This is also a judgmental response that blocks therapeutic communication.

▶ *Test-taking Tip: Note the key word "best." Eliminate responses that do not address the client's concerns and promote therapeutic communication.*

Content Area: Adult; Concept: Communication; Assessment; Integrated Processes: Communication and Documentation; Caring; Client Needs: Psychosocial Integrity; Cognitive Level: Analysis [Analyzing]

## 53. PHARM ANSWER: 4

1. Using relaxation techniques is an appropriate intervention but does not ensure pain control.
2. Opioid medications for palliative pain control should be administered around the clock.
3. Dietary practices to avoid constipation are appropriate but do not ensure pain control.
4. **For able clients, maintaining a pain diary is an effective way to monitor pain control. The client must know how to determine when pain is no longer adequately controlled and which action to take. This will ensure that the client is receiving adequate pain control.**

▶ *Test-taking Tip: Only one option gives the client control over requesting additional pain medication if needed.*

Content Area: Adult; Fundamentals; Concept: Comfort; Assessment; Safety; Integrated Processes: Nursing Process: Implementation; Client Needs: Physiological Integrity: Pharmacological and Parenteral Therapies; Cognitive Level: Analysis [Analyzing]

## 54. ANSWER: 180

**To determine the 24-hour grams of carbohydrate (CHO) intake, add the CHO choices (12 total CHO choices). Multiply the 12 CHO choices and the 15 g of carbohydrate per choice to obtain the total of 180 g of carbohydrates.**

▶ *Test-taking Tip: Read the question carefully. It is asking for grams of carbohydrates and not carbohydrate choices. This question requires a calculation.*

**Content Area:** Adult; **Concept:** Nutrition; Metabolism; **Integrated Processes:** Nursing Process: Assessment; **Client Needs:** Physiological Integrity: Basic Care and Comfort; **Cognitive Level:** Analysis [Analyzing]

## 55. PHARM ANSWER: 20

**Use the proportion method to calculate the correct dosage:**

$$\frac{400 \text{ mg}}{X \text{ mL}} = \frac{500 \text{ mg}}{25 \text{ mL}} = \text{(Cross multiply)} \frac{400 \text{ mg} \times 25 \text{ mL}}{500 \text{ mg} \times X \text{ mL}} = \frac{10,000}{500} = 20 \text{ mL}$$

**The nurse should prepare 20 mL of allopurinol (Zyloprim).**

▶ *Test-taking Tip: There are a number of different dosage calculation formulas; you should use the one you were taught and then check your answer against the book's answer.*

**Content Area:** Fundamentals; **Concept:** Medication; Cellular Regulation; **Integrated Processes:** Nursing Process: Planning; **Client Needs:** Physiological Integrity: Pharmacological and Parenteral Therapies; **Cognitive Level:** Application [Applying]

## 56. PHARM ANSWER: 3

1. Mirtazapine (Remeron) should not be administered without consulting with the psychiatrist.
2. An increased dose will cause toxic effects because the current dose cannot be metabolized when the liver is impaired.
3. **The client's serum lipid level and liver function tests are elevated. A reduced dose is warranted with hepatic impairment because mirtazapine is metabolized in the liver.**
4. The psychiatrist ordering the medication should be consulted because he or she has expertise in psychiatric conditions, whereas a general practitioner does not.

▶ *Test-taking Tip: First, focus on the two options that are opposite, then eliminate one of these. Then, examine the other options.*

**Content Area:** Mental Health; **Concept:** Medication; Self; **Integrated Processes:** Nursing Process: Analysis; **Client Needs:** Physiological Integrity: Pharmacological and Parenteral Therapies; **Cognitive Level:** Analysis [Analyzing]

## 57. PHARM ANSWER: 2

**Use a formula for calculating medication dosages.**
*Ratio-Proportion Formula:*
**2 mg : 1 mL :: 4 mg : X mL**
**Multiply the outside and inside values and solve for X.**
**2X = 4; X = 4 ÷ 2; X = 2; The nurse should administer 2 mL of ondansetron (Zofran).**

▶ *Test-taking Tip: Focus on the information in the question and use the on-screen calculator. Verify your response, especially if it seems like an unusual amount.*

**Content Area:** Adult; **Concept:** Medication; **Integrated Processes:** Nursing Process: Implementation; **Client Needs:** Physiological Integrity: Pharmacological and Parenteral Therapies; **Cognitive Level:** Application [Applying]

## 58. PHARM ANSWER: 2

1. LAIV is used in vaccinating healthy, nonpregnant persons aged 5 to 49 years.
2. **The nurse should administer the TIV. This is recommended for persons who are at increased risk for severe complications from influenza, such as those with a chronic illness. TIV should not be administered to persons known to have anaphylactic hypersensitivity to eggs or to other components of the influenza vaccine.**
3. TIV is recommended for persons with chronic health conditions such as DM and CAD.
4. The influenza vaccine is repeated annually. It is developed from representative influenza viruses anticipated to circulate in the United States during that year's season.

▶ *Test-taking Tip: Read each option carefully. Eliminate options that include administering live, attenuated vaccines because these are only administered to healthy individuals.*

**Content Area:** Adult; **Concept:** Immunity; Infection; Promoting Health; **Integrated Processes:** Nursing Process: Implementation; **Client Needs:** Health Promotion and Maintenance; Physiological Integrity: Pharmacological and Parenteral Therapies; **Cognitive Level:** Analysis [Analyzing]

## 59. PHARM ANSWER: 3

1. Tamsulosin does not decrease the size of the prostate.
2. Tamsulosin does not have anti-inflammatory actions.
3. **Tamsulosin (Flomax) is an alpha-adrenergic receptor blocker that relaxes the smooth muscle in the prostate. This ultimately facilitates urinary flow through the urethra.**
4. Urine specific gravity will not be altered by tamsulosin.

▶ *Test-taking Tip: Note that Options 1, 2, and 4 are similar (reduce, decrease, and decrease, respectively) and Option 3 is different.*

**Content Area:** Adult; **Concept:** Medication; Male Reproduction; **Integrated Processes:** Teaching/Learning; **Client Needs:** Physiological Integrity: Pharmacological and Parenteral Therapies; **Cognitive Level:** Application [Applying]

## 60. ANSWER: 3

1. Allowing the mother to rest for 1 to 2 hours immediately after delivery would bypass the initial period of newborn activity. Thirty minutes after birth, newborn activity begins to decrease, and the newborn enters a period of deep sleep.

2. Rather than privacy, most women appreciate having an experienced nurse with them for a first feeding to offer support and advice. Leaving the mother and infant alone during the first feeding does not promote successful breastfeeding.
3. **Skin-to-skin contact after birth leads to an eight-fold increase in spontaneous nursing and may be a critical component in breastfeeding success. For the first 30 minutes to 1 hour after birth, the infant is usually active, alert, and ready to breastfeed.**
4. Supplemental bottle feedings are not recommended for normal, healthy, breastfeeding newborns as they may lead to nipple confusion and decrease infant stimulation of the mother's breasts.

▶ *Test-taking Tip: Select an option that also will promote infant bonding.*

Content Area: Childbearing; Concept: Pregnancy; Promoting Health; Integrated Processes: Nursing Process: Planning; Client Needs: Physiological Integrity: Basic Care and Comfort; Cognitive Level: Application [Applying]

## 61. ANSWER: 4

1. An internal fixation involves the use of metal pins, screws, rods, or plates to immobilize the fracture. They are internal and inserted during open surgery.
2. Buck's traction is applied to the skin to immobilize the lower extremity after a hip fracture.
3. A brace cast is a patellar weight-bearing cast used with midshaft or distal fracture of the femur.
4. **The diagram shows an external fixation device that is placed percutaneously after the fracture has been reduced. A potential complication, pin-tract infection, necessitates daily inspection of the skin for redness and drainage at the pin sites.**

▶ *Test-taking Tip: Narrow the options by first examining the ones that have opposite information (Options 1 and 4).*

Content Area: Fundamentals; Concept: Mobility; Skin Integrity; Infection; Integrated Processes: Nursing Process: Analysis; Client Needs: Physiological Integrity: Basic Care and Comfort; Cognitive Level: Analysis [Analyzing]

## 62. ANSWER: 1

1. **The label indicates that codeine, an analgesic, is a controlled substance. The categorization of schedule I to V indicates the potential for abuse. Schedule II medications have a high potential for abuse. Controlled substances must be signed out from a double-locked drawer or box at the time of administration.**
2. Phenytoin sodium (Dilantin), an anticonvulsant, is not a controlled substance that requires signing out from a double-locked drawer before administration.

3. Acetaminophen (Tylenol), an analgesic and antipyretic, is not a controlled substance that requires signing out from a double-locked drawer before administration.
4. Loperamide (Imodium), an antidiarrheal, is not a controlled substance that requires signing out from a double-locked drawer before administration.

▶ *Test-taking Tip: You should look for the information that is different on the medication labels and select the correct option.*

Content Area: Fundamentals; Concept: Medication; Safety; Integrated Processes: Nursing Process: Analysis; Client Needs: Safe and Effective Care Environment: Safety and Infection Control; Cognitive Level: Application [Applying]

## 63. MoC PHARM ANSWER: 3

1. Erythema, purulent exudate, and increased pain are signs of infection; the medication should be withheld if signs of infection are present.
2. Creams should be applied to skin surfaces with gloved fingers. The gloves do not need to be sterile.
3. **Triamcinolone (Kenalog) is a corticosteroid. Covering the area with an occlusive dressing can result in systemic absorption. The nurse educator should correct this intervention.**
4. The mother can help by holding the toddler to ensure that the cream is applied to all affected areas.

▶ *Test-taking Tip: To select the correct option, you need to think about the process for applying topical creams and ointments as well as the action of the medication.*

Content Area: Management of Care; Fundamentals; Concept: Medication; Safety; Integrated Processes: Nursing Process: Evaluation; Client Needs: Safe and Effective Care Environment: Management of Care; Physiological Integrity: Pharmacological and Parenteral Therapies; Cognitive Level: Evaluation [Evaluating]

## 64. ANSWER: 1

1. **Induction with myelosuppressant therapy lowers the neutrophil count and the ability to fight infection; these measures will help prevent it. Children with leukemia often die of infection.**
2. A well-balanced diet, iron-rich foods, and avoiding overexertion are appropriate for treating anemia.
3. A soft diet, toothettes, and frequent saline mouthwashes can help treat stomatitis.
4. Avoiding rectal temperatures and injections and applying direct, prolonged pressure are more appropriate in preventing hemorrhage from thrombocytopenia.

▶ *Test-taking Tip: Neutropenia increases the client's risk for infection. Select an option that decreases this risk.*

Content Area: Child; Concept: Infection; Safety; Integrated Processes: Nursing Process: Implementation; Client Needs: Safe and Effective Care Environment: Safety and Infection Control; Cognitive Level: Synthesis [Creating]

**65. ANSWER: 1, 2, 3, 4**

1. **A douche may then be ordered to cleanse the vagina.**
2. **Multiple specimens should be collected to examine for sperm, semen, and STIs.**
3. **Emergency contraception is an oral contraceptive medication containing levonorgestrel and ethinyl estradiol and can prevent unwanted pregnancy if taken within 72 hours after intercourse.**
4. **A women's shelter can help maintain the woman's safety and provide support.**
5. The woman should never be left alone in the room. If available in the community, a volunteer from the Rape Victim Companion Program should be called.

♦ *Test-taking Tip: Focus on the goals of treating the client of sexual assault: sympathetic support, reducing emotional trauma, gathering evidence, and managing problems.*

**Content Area:** Mental Health; Adult; **Concept:** Violence; Pregnancy; Safety; **Integrated Processes:** Nursing Process: Planning; **Client Needs:** Physiological Integrity: Physiological Adaptation; **Cognitive Level:** Application [Applying]

**66. ANSWER: 3**

1. Asking about activity level is an appropriate assessment and will direct necessary client education, but asking about the client's weight is the most appropriate initial question.
2. Asking about foods eaten to determine salt content is an appropriate assessment, but asking about the client's weight is the most appropriate question.
3. **Weight is a critical indicator of fluid loss or gain. Clients with HF are taught to monitor weight daily at the same time using the same scale.**
4. Asking about whether the client's ankles are different in appearance from the previous day is an appropriate assessment, but asking about the client's weight is the most appropriate initial question.

♦ *Test-taking Tip: The key word is "initial." Remember that 1 kg (2.2 lb) is equivalent to 1000 mL of fluid gain.*

**Content Area:** Adult; **Concept:** Fluid and Electrolyte Balance; Perfusion; **Integrated Processes:** Nursing Process: Assessment; **Client Needs:** Physiological Integrity: Physiological Adaptation; **Cognitive Level:** Analysis [Analyzing]

**67.** MoC **ANSWER: 4**

1. Orange juice contains vitamins and is safe for this child to consume.
2. Apple slices are acceptable as long as the fruit has been washed before cutting and the fruit slices show no signs of spoiling.
3. Bread is nutritious and a safe food for this child.
4. **A soft egg is undercooked. It should be well cooked and firm. The egg should be removed from the food tray because the child has a weakened immune system and the egg may harbor microorganisms.**

♦ *Test-taking Tip: The child has undergone a bone marrow transplant and has a weakened immune system, which increases the risk for infection. Measures are taken to prevent the introduction of microorganisms.*

**Content Area:** Management of Care; Child; **Concept:** Hematologic Regulation; Immunity; **Integrated Processes:** Nursing Process: Evaluation; **Client Needs:** Safe and Effective Care Environment: Management of Care; **Cognitive Level:** Application [Applying]

**68.** PHARM **ANSWER: 2**

1. Aripiprazole (Abilify) is not given to produce sedation, but that is one of its side effects.
2. **Aripiprazole (Abilify) is an atypical psychotropic medication that has receptor antagonism at dopamine $D_2$ and serotonin 5-$HT_{18}$ receptors and alpha-2 adrenergic blocking activity. The desired outcome of aripiprazole is a reduction in excitable or paranoid behavior.**
3. This is no indication that the client has psychotic symptoms such as delusions, hallucinations, disorganized speech patterns, or bizarre or catatonic behaviors.
4. Extrapyramidal symptoms are a side effect of aripiprazole (Abilify).

♦ *Test-taking Tip: Narrow the options by noting that there is no information in the question suggesting the client has psychosis.*

**Content Area:** Mental Health; **Concept:** Mood; Medication; **Integrated Processes:** Nursing Process: Evaluation; **Client Needs:** Physiological Integrity: Pharmacological and Parenteral Therapies; **Cognitive Level:** Evaluation [Evaluating]

**69. ANSWER: 2**

1. If the BP is taken immediately, the effects of nicotine will increase the reading.
2. **The nurse should ask the client to refrain from smoking, then return after 30 minutes for a BP check. The nicotine's effects no longer will alter the BP reading.**
3. The nurse does not need to delay the BP reading for more than 30 minutes; the effects of nicotine will have worn off.
4. Although it is important to assess the client's knowledge, the situation is about when to best obtain BP in the client who smokes.

♦ *Test-taking Tip: Read the scenario in the stem carefully. One distractor does not fit the scenario and should be eliminated.*

**Content Area:** Fundamentals; **Concept:** Assessment; Communication; Promoting Health; **Integrated Processes:** Nursing Process: Planning; **Client Needs:** Physiological Integrity: Reduction of Risk Potential; **Cognitive Level:** Application [Applying]

## 70. ANSWER: 4

1. Asking about liquid intake is not the most important question.
2. Asking about a fever is not the most important question.
3. Asking the client to explain the symptoms is appropriate but not the most important question.
4. **Meningococcal meningitis presents as flu-like symptoms that last a short time with the subsequent development of a petechial rash. Nuchal rigidity is a significant sign of meningeal irritation. The condition becomes critical 12 to 48 hours after onset; thus, asking if the client has a rash is priority.**

▶ **Test-taking Tip:** *Decide which question would be most helpful in determining the severity of the student's illness. Consider that this is a college student.*

**Content Area:** Adult; **Concept:** Infection; Safety; Assessment; **Integrated Processes:** Nursing Process: Assessment; **Client Needs:** Physiological Integrity: Reduction of Risk Potential; **Cognitive Level:** Application [Applying]

## 71. ANSWER: 1

1. **LASIK surgery corrects the shape of the cornea in clients with refraction errors from myopia, hyperopia, and astigmatism.**
2. LASIK surgery does not include the retina.
3. LASIK surgery does not include the lens.
4. LASIK surgery does not include the aqueous humor.

▶ **Test-taking Tip:** *The issue is to define what area of the eye is involved with LASIK (laser in-situ keratomileusis) surgery. To narrow the options, recall that the prefix "kerato" refers to the cornea.*

**Content Area:** Adult; **Concept:** Sensory Perception; Nursing Roles; **Integrated Processes:** Teaching/Learning; **Client Needs:** Physiological Integrity: Reduction of Risk Potential; **Cognitive Level:** Comprehension [Understanding]

## 72. ANSWER: 1, 5, 3, 4, 2

1. **Assess baseline color, temperature, and presence of peripheral pulses in the client's lower extremities. Assessment should come first because if the client has abnormal findings such as DVT, the SCD should not be applied and the HCP should be notified.**
5. **Measure the size of the client's leg and obtain appropriate-sized SCD sleeves. Sleeves that are too large or small could result in uneven pressure distribution.**
3. **Apply the SCD sleeves, connect the sleeve cord to the device cord, set the control device at the prescribed pressure, and turn on the device. Assembly and activation of the device may vary by manufacturer.**
4. **Document the placement of the SCD sleeves. The nurse should document when the SCD is on or off. Sleeves should be removed when getting the client out of bed because they impair movement and could cause injury.**
2. **Monitor the client during treatment, including skin assessment and CMS. The sleeves should be removed to perform a skin reassessment. Evaluation is the last step of the nursing process.**

▶ **Test-taking Tip:** *Use the steps of the nursing process to place actions in the correct sequence.*

**Content Area:** Adult; **Concept:** Fluid and Electrolyte Balance; Safety; **Integrated Processes:** Nursing Process: Implementation; **Client Needs:** Safe and Effective Care Environment: Safety and Infection Control; Physiological Integrity: Reduction of Risk Potential; **Cognitive Level:** Synthesis [Creating]

## 73. MoC ANSWER: 1, 2, 3, 6

1. **To prevent errors, nurses always should log out before walking away from a computer. This ensures that client information remains confidential.**
2. **To prevent errors, nurses should log in with a personal user ID and password, and always log out before leaving the computer.**
3. **To prevent errors, the nurse should make sure the correct client is selected.**
4. Nurse B did select the correct client. However, Nurse B was documenting under the login for Nurse A; Nurse B also did not log out.
5. The nurse should never have another nurse finish incomplete documentation.
6. **To prevent an error, nurses should access the computer using the assigned user ID and created password.**

▶ **Test-taking Tip:** *Read each option carefully and think about actions that would prevent inappropriate documentation in an EMR. Apply knowledge of information technology for accurate documentation.*

**Content Area:** Management of Care; **Concept:** Medication; Safety; **Integrated Processes:** Communication and Documentation; **Client Needs:** Safe and Effective Care Environment: Management of Care; **Cognitive Level:** Application [Applying]

## 74. ANSWER: 3

1. Removing the oxygen may expose the client to tissue hypoxia and inhibit the normal healing process after surgery.
2. Leaving the client at the same oxygen level is unsafe, as it may lead to tissue hypoxia and inhibit normal healing.
3. **The oxygen saturation level, 90%, is below a normal level of greater than 95% for the client with normal lung function. The nurse should increase the oxygen level to 50%.**

4. Decreasing the oxygen level is unsafe, as it may expose the client to tissue hypoxia and inhibit the normal healing process after surgery.

◗ *Test-taking Tip: Remember that normal oxygen saturation (SpO₂) for the client with normal lung function should be greater than 95%. Use this information to eliminate options.*

Content Area: Adult; Concept: Oxygenation; Safety; **Integrated Processes:** Nursing Process: Analysis; **Client Needs:** Physiological Integrity: Reduction of Risk Potential; **Cognitive Level:** Analysis [Analyzing]

## 75. ANSWER: 2

1. The left lung has an upper and lower lobe only. Placing the client on the right side and exposing the left lateral chest wall would not be effective for middle lobe physiotherapy.

2. **The right lung has three lobes. Placing the client on the left side with the right arm rotated forward and supported will allow the nurse to perform middle lobe physiotherapy.**

3. Placing the client supine with the head of the bed flat is not helpful because a flat position does not promote drainage.

4. Placing the client prone with the head of the bed flat is not helpful because a flat position does not promote drainage.

◗ *Test-taking Tip: Study the illustration carefully to identify the location of the middle lung lobe.*

Content Area: Child; Concept: Oxygenation; **Integrated Processes:** Nursing Process: Implementation; **Client Needs:** Physiological Integrity: Reduction of Risk Potential; **Cognitive Level:** Analysis [Analyzing]

# Appendix

# Common Abbreviations

| | |
|---|---|
| A & P repair | anterior and posterior repair |
| a.c. or ac | before meals |
| AA/NA | Alcoholics Anonymous/Narcotics Anonymous |
| AAA | abdominal aortic aneurysm |
| ABCs | airway, breathing, circulation |
| ABG | arterial blood gas |
| ACE | angiotensin-converting enzyme inhibitor |
| ACLS | advanced cardiac life support |
| ACS | acute coronary syndrome |
| ACTH | adrenocorticotropic hormone |
| ADH | antidiuretic hormone |
| ADHD | attention-deficit hyperactivity disorder |
| ADLs | activities of daily living |
| AED | automated external defibrillator |
| AGN | acute glomerulonephritis |
| AIDS | acquired immunodeficiency syndrome |
| AKA | above-the-knee amputation |
| ALL | acute lymphocytic leukemia |
| ALP | alkaline phosphatase |
| ALS | amyotrophic lateral sclerosis |
| ALT | alanine aminotransferase |
| AMA | against medical advice |
| ANS | autonomic nervous system |
| aPTT | activated partial thromboplastin time |
| ARB | angiotensin receptor blockers |
| ARDS | acute respiratory distress syndrome |
| ARF | acute renal failure |
| ART | acute response team |
| ASAP | as soon as possible |
| ASD | atrial septal defect |
| AST | aspartate aminotransferase |
| bid | two times daily |
| BKA | below-the-knee amputation |
| BMI | body mass index |
| BNP | B-type natriuretic peptide |
| BP | blood pressure |
| BPD | borderline personality disorder |
| BPH | benign prostatic hyperplasia |
| BPH | benign prostatic hypertrophy |
| bpm | beats per minute |
| BSO | bilateral salpingo-oophorectomy |
| BUN | blood urea nitrogen |
| CAD | coronary artery disease |
| CAT scan | computerized axial tomography scan |
| CBC | complete blood count |
| CBI | continuous bladder irrigation |
| CDC | Centers for Disease Control and Prevention |
| CF | cystic fibrosis |
| CHF | congestive heart failure |
| CKD | chronic kidney disease |
| CMS | circulation, motion, and sensation |
| CMV | cytomegalovirus |
| CNS | central nervous system |
| COPD | chronic obstructive pulmonary disease |
| CP | cerebral palsy |
| CPAP | continuous positive airway pressure |
| CPM | continuous passive motion |
| CPR | cardiopulmonary resuscitation |
| CRF | chronic renal failure |
| CRT | capillary refill time |
| CSF | cerebrospinal fluid |
| CT | computed tomography |
| CVA | cerebrovascular accident |
| CXR | chest x-ray |
| D&C | dilation and curettage of the uterus |
| DASH | dietary approaches to hypertension |
| DI | diabetes insipidus |
| DIC | disseminated intravascular coagulation |
| DKA | diabetic ketoacidosis |
| DM | diabetes mellitus |
| DNA | deoxyribonucleic acid |
| DNR | do not resuscitate |
| DTaP | diphtheria, tetanus, and pertussis |
| DVT | deep vein thrombosis |
| ECG or EKG | electrocardiogram |
| ECT | electroconvulsive therapy |
| ED | emergency department |
| EEG | electroencephalogram |
| EGD | esophagogastroduodenoscopy |
| ELISA | enzyme-linked immunosorbent assay |
| EMG | electromyogram |
| EMR | electronic medical record |
| EMS | emergency medical services |
| EMTALA | Emergency Medical Treatment and Labor Act of 1986 |

| | | | |
|---|---|---|---|
| ERCP | endoscopic retrograde cholangiopancreatogram | LPM | liters per minute |
| ESR | erythrocyte sedimentation rate | LPN | licensed practical nurse |
| ESRD | end-stage renal disease | LTB | laryngotracheobronchitis |
| ET | endotracheal | MAOI | monoamine oxidase inhibitor |
| FAS | fetal alcohol syndrome | MAP | mean arterial pressure |
| FHR | fetal heart rate | MAR | medication administration record |
| FHT | fetal heart tones | MDI | metered dose inhaler |
| g | gram | mg | milligram |
| GERD | gastroesophageal reflux disease | MG | myasthenia gravis |
| GFR | glomerular filtration rate | MI | myocardial infarction |
| GH | growth hormone | mL | milliliter |
| GI | gastrointestinal | mm Hg | millimeters mercury |
| GVHD | graft versus host disease | MMR | measles, mumps, rubella |
| gtt | drops (IV flow rate) | MRI | magnetic resonance imaging |
| h.s. or hs | at bedtime | MRSA | methicillin-resistant staphylococcus aureus |
| HCD | health care directive | MS | multiple sclerosis |
| $HCO_3$ | bicarbonate | MVA | motor vehicle accident |
| HCP | health care provider | NA | nursing assistant |
| Hct | hematocrit | NATO | North Atlantic Treaty Organization |
| HDL | high-density lipoprotein | NEC | necrotizing enterocolitis |
| HF | heart failure | NFPA | National Fire Protection Association |
| Hgb | hemoglobin | NG | nasogastric |
| Hgb $A_{1c}$ | glycosylated hemoglobin | NHL | non-Hodgkin's lymphoma |
| HHNS | hyperosmolar hyperglycemic nonketotic syndrome | NPO | nothing by mouth |
| HIPAA | Health Insurance Portability and Accountability Act | NS | normal saline |
| | | NSAID | nonsteroidal anti-inflammatory drug |
| HIV | human immunodeficiency virus | NST | non-stress test |
| HOB | head of bed | OA | osteoarthritis |
| HPV | human papillomavirus | OCD | obsessive-compulsive disorder |
| HR | heart rate | OCPD | obsessive-compulsive personality disorder |
| HRT | hormone replacement therapy | OR | operating room |
| I&D | incision and drainage | OTC | over-the-counter |
| I&O | intake and output | P | pulse |
| IBD | inflammatory bowel disease | $PaCO_2$ | partial pressure of carbon dioxide |
| IBS | irritable bowel syndrome | PACU | post-anesthesia care unit |
| ICD | implantable cardioverter defibrillator | PAD | peripheral artery disease |
| ICP | intracranial pressure | $PaO_2$ | arterial partial pressure of oxygen |
| ICU | intensive care unit | PCA | patient-controlled analgesia |
| IM | intramuscular | PD | Parkinson's disease |
| INR | international normalized ratio | PDA | patent ductus arteriosus |
| IS | incentive spirometer | PE | pulmonary embolus |
| ITP | idiopathic thrombocytopenic purpura | PEARLA | pupils equal and reactive to light and accommodation |
| IUD | intrauterine device | PEG | percutaneous endoscopic gastrostomy |
| IV | intravenous | | |
| IV push | intravenous push | pH | hydrogen ion concentration |
| IVP | intravenous pyelogram | PICC | peripherally inserted central catheter |
| IVPB | intravenous piggyback | PICU | pediatric intensive care unit |
| JRA | juvenile rheumatoid arthritis | PID | pelvic inflammatory disease |
| JVD | jugular vein distention | PKU | phenylketonuria |
| KCL | potassium chloride | PPE | personal protective equipment |
| kg | kilogram | PPI | proton pump inhibitor |
| LASIK | laser-assisted in situ keratomileusis | PRBCs | packed red blood cells |
| lb | pound | prn | when required, as needed |
| LDL | low-density lipoprotein | PSA | prostate-specific antigen |
| | | PT | prothrombin time |

| | | | |
|---|---|---|---|
| PTCA | percutaneous transluminal coronary angioplasty | SVR | systemic vascular resistance |
| PTSD | post-traumatic stress disorder | SVT | supraventricular tachycardia |
| PTT | partial thromboplastin time | T | temperature |
| PUD | peptic ulcer disease | t.i.d. or tid | three times a day |
| PVC | premature ventricular contraction | TAH | total abdominal hysterectomy |
| PVD | peripheral vascular disease | TB | tuberculosis |
| q.i.d. or qid | four times daily | TBI | traumatic brain injury |
| R/O | rule out | TCA | tricyclic antidepressant |
| RBC | red blood cell | TENS | transcutaneous electrical nerve stimulation |
| RF | rheumatic fever | THR | total hip replacement |
| RhoGAM | Rh immune globulin | TIA | transient ischemic attack |
| RN | registered nurse | TKR | total knee replacement |
| ROM | range of motion | TPN | total parenteral nutrition |
| RR | respiratory rate | TSH | thyroid-stimulating hormone |
| RSV | respiratory syncytial virus | TURP | transurethral resection of the prostate |
| SARS | severe acute respiratory syndrome | U.S. | United States |
| SBAR | Situation Background Assessment Recommendation | UA | urinalysis |
| | | UAP | unlicensed assistive personnel |
| SCI | spinal cord injury | URI | upper respiratory infection |
| SIADH | syndrome of inappropriate antidiuretic hormone | UTI | urinary tract infection |
| | | UV | ultraviolet |
| SIDS | sudden infant death syndrome | V/Q | ventilation/perfusion quotient |
| SLE | systemic lupus erythematosus | VCUG | voiding cystourethrogram |
| SPF | sun protection factor | VRE | vancomycin-resistant enterococci |
| SSRI | selective serotonin reuptake inhibitor | VS | vital signs |
| STAT | immediately | VSD | ventricular septal defect |
| STI | sexually transmitted infection | WBC | white blood cell |
| | | WNL | within normal limits |

Note: Unless cited below, credits appear within the text.

## CHAPTER 12

Unnumbered Figure 12.6: From Agency for Toxic Substances and Disease Registry. 1998. *Hazardous Materials Classification Systems* (Appendix A). Retrieved from www.atsdr.cdc.gov/MHMI/mhmi-v1-a.pdf

## CHAPTER 17

Unnumbered Figure 17.1: From Centers for Disease Control.

## CHAPTER 23

Unnumbered Figures 23.3 and 23.4: Courtesy of MCP–Hahnemann University Department of Dermatology, Philadelphia, PA.

Unnumbered Table 23.2: Rubenstein, LZ, et al. (2001). Screening for undernutrition in geriatric practice: Developing the short-form mini-nutritional assessment (MNA-SF). *J Gerontol A Biol Sci Med Sci, 56*(6):M366–372.

## CHAPTER 24

Unnumbered Figure 24.6: From Armstrong Medical Industries, Inc., Lincolnshire, IL.

## CHAPTER 26

Unnumbered Figure 26.6: Used with permission from Medtronic.

## CHAPTER 27

Unnumbered Figure 27.6: From Pittsburgh Poison Center.

## CHAPTER 34

Unnumbered Figure 34.1: Courtesy of Wills Eye Hospital, Philadelphia, PA.

Unnumbered Figure 34.7: From Welch Allyn. (2004). *A guide to the use of diagnostic instruments in eye and ear examinations.* Skaneateles Falls, NY: Welch Allyn, Inc., with permission.

## CHAPTER 37

Unnumbered Figures 37.3 through 37.6: From Jones, S. A. (2007). Author's personal collection. In Jones, S. A. *ECG success: Exercises in ECG interpretation.* Philadelphia, PA: F. A. Davis.

## CHAPTER 41

Unnumbered Figure 41.1: From Centers for Disease Control.

## CHAPTER 46

Unnumbered Figures 46.1 through 46.4: From Welch Allyn. (2004). *A guide to the use of diagnostic instruments in eye and ear examinations.* Skaneateles Falls, NY: Welch Allyn, Inc., with permission.

Unnumbered Figure 46.6: Used with permission from Pfizer, Inc.

## CHAPTER 51

Unnumbered Figure 51.1: Courtesy of Romeo Mandanas, MD.

Unnumbered Figure 51.3: From Armstrong Medical Industries, Inc., Lincolnshire, IL.

# SECTION I: PREPARING FOR THE NCLEX-RN®

American Nurses Association. (2016). *Foreign educated nurses.* Retrieved from www.nursingworld.org/MainMenuCategories/ThePracticeof ProfessionalNursing/workforce/ForeignNurses

Anderson, L. W., & Krathwohl, D. R. (Eds.). (2001). *A taxonomy for learning, teaching, and assessing. A revision of Bloom's taxonomy of educational objectives.* New York: Addison Wesley Longman.

Aucoin, J., & Treas, L. (2005). Assumptions and realities of the NCLEX-RN. *Nursing Education Perspectives, 26,* 268–271.

Berman, A., Snyder, S., & Frandsen, G. (2016). *Kozier & Erb's fundamentals of nursing* (10th ed.). Upper Saddle River, NJ: Pearson Education.

Billings, D. (2017). *Lippincott's Q&A review for NCLEX-RN®* (12th ed.). Philadelphia, PA: Lippincott Williams & Wilkins.

*Bonis, S., Taft, L., & Wendler, M. (2007). Strategies to promote success on the NCLEX-RN: An evidence-based approach using the ACE Star Model of Knowledge Transformation. *Nursing Education Perspectives, 28*(2), 82–87.

Bristol, T. (2012). The National Council Licensure Examination across the curriculum: Low-tech learning strategies for student success. *Teaching and Learning in Nursing, 7*(2), 80–84.

Canadian Nursing Students' Association. (2015). *Position statement. The transitional NCLEX-RN® examination for Canadian candidates.* Retrieved from aeic.ca/files/files/2015/NA-Position%20Statement%20 The%20Transitional%20NCLEX-RN%20Examination%20for%20 Canadian%20Candidates%20(2).pdf

Commission on Graduates of Foreign Nursing Schools (CGFNS International). (2018). *Credentials Evaluation, Authentication and Verification, and Certification.* Retrieved from www.cgfns.org/

Dickison, P., & Tillman, C. (2017). Nursing clinical judgement and its cognitive processes. NCLEX Conference Presentation, September 25, 2017, Rosemont, IL.

Dickison, P., Luo, X., Kim, D., Woo, A., Muntean, W., & Bergstrom, B. (2016). Assessing higher-order cognitive constructs by using an information-processing framework. *Journal of Applied Testing Technology, 17*(1), 1-19.

Geist, M., & Catlette, M. (2014). Tap into NCLEX® success. *Teaching and Learning in Nursing, 9*(3), 115–119.

Immigration Direct: U.S. Immigration & Citizenship Form Services. (2018). *Home Page.* Retrieved from www.immigrationdirect.com/

Lavin, J., & Rosario-Sim, M. (2013). Understanding the NCLEX: How to increase success on the revised 2013 examination. *Nursing Education Perspective, 34*(3), 196-198.

McDowell, B. (2008). KATTS: A framework for maximizing NCLEX-RN performance. *Journal of Nursing Education, 47*(4), 183–186.

National Council of State Boards of Nursing. (2014). 2013 Canadian RN practice analysis: Applicability of the 2013 NCLEX-RN® Test Plan to the Canadian testing population. Retrieved from www.ncsbn.org/ 3973.htm

*National Council of State Boards of Nursing. (2018). 2017 RN Practice Analysis: Linking the NCLEX-RN to Examination and Practice U.S. and Canada. Volume 72. Retrieved from https://www.ncsbn.org/12095.htm

*National Council of State Boards of Nursing. (2018). Strategic Practice Analysis. *NCSBN Research Brief, 71,* January 2018.

National Council of State Boards of Nursing. (2018). Strategic Practice Analysis Executive Summary. Chicago, IL. Retrieved from https:// www.ncsbn.org/11995.htm

National Council of State Boards of Nursing. (2018). Next Generation NCLEX® News in Summer, 2018, 1-2.

National Council of State Boards of Nursing. (2015). 2016 *NCLEX-RN® Test Plan Overview* Retrieved from www.ncsbn. org/8507.htm

National Council of State Boards of Nursing. (2018). *NCLEX Candidate FAQs.* Retrieved from www.ncsbn.org/nclex-faqs.htm

National Council of State Boards of Nursing. (2018). *NCLEX-RN® Examination Candidate Bulletin 2018.* Retrieved from www.ncsbn. org/1213.htm

National Council of State Boards of Nursing. (2016). *NCLEX-RN® Examination: Test Plan for the National Council Licensure Examination for Registered Nurses, Effective April 2016.* Retrieved from www.ncsbn.org/testplans.htm

National Council of State Boards of Nursing. (2016). *Canadian Educators & Students FAQs.* Retrieved from www.ncsbn.org/ 4702.htm

National Council of State Boards of Nursing. (2018). *Home Page.* Retrieved from www.ncsbn.org

National Council of State Boards of Nursing. (2018). NCLEX and Other Exams. Retrieved from www.ncsbn.org/nclex.htm

National Council of State Boards of Nursing. (2018). NCLEX-RN Program Reports: Subscription. Retrieved from www.ncsbn.org/3807.htm

National Council of State Boards of Nursing. (2016). *NCLEX-RN® Detailed Test Plan Effective April 2016. Candidate Version.* Retrieved from www.ncsbn.org/2016_RN_Test_Plan_Candidate.pdf

National Council of State Boards of Nursing. (2018). *U.S. nursing licensure for internationally educated nurses.* Retrieved from www.ncsbn.org/ 171.htm

Nugent, P., & Vitale, B. (2015). *Fundamentals success: A Q&A review: Applying critical thinking to test taking* (4th ed.). Philadelphia, PA: F.A. Davis.

Nugent, P., & Vitale, B. (2018). *Test success: Test-taking techniques for beginning nursing students* (8th ed.). Philadelphia, PA: F.A. Davis.

Muntean, W. J. (2017). Nursing clinical decision-making: A literature review. Exam Statistics and Publications. Retrieved from https://www. ncsbn.org/11507.htm

Ohman, K. A. (2010). *Davis's Q&A for the NCLEX-RN® examination.* Philadelphia, PA: F.A. Davis.

Pearson Vue. (2017). *Online tutorial for NCLEX examinations.* Retrieved from www.pearsonvue.com/nclex/

Pearson Vue. (2017). *The NCLEX examinations.* Retrieved from www. pearsonvue.com/nclex/

U.S. Citizenship and Immigration Services. (2018). *Home Page.* Retrieved from www.uscis.gov/

Van Leeuwen, A. M., & Bladh, M. L. (2019). *Davis's comprehensive handbook of laboratory and diagnostic tests with nursing implications* (8th ed.). Philadelphia, PA: F.A. Davis.

Ward, S. L., & Hisley, S. M. (2015). *Maternal-child nursing care (2nd ed.).* Philadelphia, PA: F.A. Davis.

Wendt, A., & Harmes, C. (2009). Evaluating innovative items for the NCLEX-RN®, Part I: Usability and pilot testing. *Nurse Educator, 34*(2), 56-59.

Wendt, A., & Kenny, L. (2009). Alternate item types: Continuing the quest for authentic testing. *Journal of Nursing Education, 48*(3), 150-156.

Wilkinson, J. M., & Treas, L. S. (2015). *Fundamentals of nursing: Theory, concepts, & application* (3rd ed.). Philadelphia, PA: F.A. Davis.

Yoho, M. J. (2018). Overview of next generation NCLEX (NGN) test items. A presentation at the Texas Deans and Directors Meeting February 2, 2018, Austin, TX.

---

*Evidence-based Reference

# SECTION II: PRACTICE TESTS
## Unit 1: Management of Care

Adams, M., Holland, L., & Urban, L. (2017). *Pharmacology for nurses: A pathophysiologic approach* (5th ed.). Upper Saddle River, NJ: Prentice Hall.

American Nurses Association. (2015). *Code of ethics for nurses.* Retrieved from nursingworld.org/ethics/code/protected_nwcoe813.htm

American Nurses Association. (2015). *Code of ethics for nurses with interpretive statements.* Silver Spring, Maryland: Nursesbooks.org

American Nurses Association. (2015). *Nursing: Scope and standards of practice* (3rd ed.). Silver Spring, Maryland: Nursesbooks.org

American Nurses Association. (2010). *The nurse's role in ethics and human rights: Protecting and promoting individual worth, dignity, and human rights in practice settings.* Silver Spring, Maryland: Nursesbooks.org

American Nurses Association. (2018). *Nursing quality.* Retrieved from www.nursingworld.org/MainMenuCategories/ThePracticeof ProfessionalNursing/PatientSafetyQuality

Austin, S. (2011). What does EMTALA mean for you? *Nursing 2011, 41*(6), 55-59.

*Bakken, S. (2006). Informatics for patient safety: A nursing research perspective. *Annual Review of Nursing Research*, 24, 219–254.

Ball, J., Bindler, R., & Cowen, K. J. (2012). *Clinical skills manual for principles of pediatric nursing: Caring for children.* Upper Saddle River, NJ: Pearson Education.

Ball, J. W., Bindler, R. C., & Cowen, K. J. (2017). *Principles of pediatric nursing: Caring for children* (7th ed.). Upper Saddle River, NJ: Pearson Education.

Barnard, A. (2007). Providing psychiatric-mental health care for Native Americans. *The Journal of Psychosocial Nursing, 45*(5), 30-35.

Berman, A., & Snyder, S. (2016). *Kozier & Erb's fundamentals of nursing* (10th ed.). Upper Saddle River, NJ: Pearson Education.

Berman, A., Snyder, S., Kozier, B., & Frandsen, G. (2016). *Kozier & Erb's fundamentals of nursing: Concepts, process, and practice* (10th ed.). Upper Saddle River, NJ: Pearson Education.

Berman, A., Snyder, S., & McKinney, D. (2011). *Nursing basics for clinical practice.* Upper Saddle River, NJ: Pearson Education.

Black, B. (2017). *Professional nursing: Concepts and challenges* (8th ed.). St. Louis, MO: Saunders.

Boltz, M., Capezuti, E. Fulmer, T., & Zwicker, D. (2016). *Evidence-based geriatric nursing protocols for best practice* (5th ed.). New York: Springer.

Boyd, M. A. (2017). *Psychiatric nursing: Contemporary practice* (6th ed.). Philadelphia, PA: Lippincott Williams & Wilkins.

Burton, M. A., & Ludwig, L. J. M. (2015). *Fundamentals of nursing care: Concepts, connections & skills* (2nd ed.). Philadelphia, PA: F.A. Davis.

Catalano, J. (2015). *Nursing now! Today's issues, tomorrow's trends* (7th ed.). Philadelphia, PA: F.A. Davis.

*Centers for Disease Control and Prevention. (2017). Excerpt from *Guideline for isolation precautions: Preventing transmission of infectious agents in healthcare settings.* Retrieved from www. cdc.gov/infectioncontrol/guidelines/isolation/index.html

Chitty, K., & Black, B. (2011). *Professional nursing: Challenges and concepts* (6th ed.). St. Louis, MO: Saunders.

Craven, R. F., Hirnle, C. H., & Jensen, S. (2016). *Fundamentals of nursing: Human health and function* (8th ed.). Philadelphia, PA: Lippincott Williams & Wilkins.

Davidson, M., London, M., & Ladewig, P. (2016). *Olds' maternal-newborn nursing & women's health across the lifespan* (10th ed.). Upper Saddle River, NJ: Prentice Hall Health.

Doenges, M., Moorhouse, M., & Murr, A. (2014). *Nursing care plans: Guidelines for individualizing client care across the life span* (9th ed.). Philadelphia, PA: F.A. Davis.

Doenges, M., Moorhouse, M., & Murr, A. (2016). *Nursing diagnosis manual: Planning, individualizing, and documenting client care* (5th ed.). Philadelphia, PA: F.A. Davis.

Finkelman, A., & Kenner, C. (2016). *Professional nursing concepts: Competencies for quality leadership* (3rd ed.). Sudbury, MA: Jones & Bartlett Learning.

Fitzpatrick, J., Stone, P., & Walker, P. (2006). *Annual review of nursing research, focus on patient safety* (pp. 33, 40). New York: Springer.

Frandsen, G., & Pennington, S. (2018). *Abrams' clinical drug therapy: Rationales for nursing practice* (11th ed.). Philadelphia, PA: Lippincott Williams & Wilkins.

Fortinash, K., & Holoday Worret, P. (2015). *Psychiatric mental health nursing-revised reprint* (5th ed.). St. Louis, MO: Mosby/Elsevier.

Guido, G. W. (2014). *Legal and ethical issues in nursing* (6th ed.). Upper Saddle River, NJ: Pearson Education.

Hadaway, L. (2006). Best-practice interventions: Keeping central line infection at bay. *Nursing 2006, 36*(4), 58–63.

Halter, M. J. (2014). V*arcarolis' foundations of psychiatric mental health nursing* (7th ed.). St. Louis, MO: Saunders/Elsevier.

Harkreader, H., Hogan, M. A., & Thobaben, M. (2007). *Fundamentals of nursing* (3rd ed.). St. Louis, MO: Elsevier/Saunders.

*Hawthorne, K., Robles, Y., Cannings, J. R., & Edwards, A. G. K. (2010). Culturally appropriate health education for type 2 diabetes in ethnic minority groups: A systematic and narrative review of randomized controlled trials. *Diabetic Medicine, 27*(6), 613-623. doi:10.1111/ j.1464-5491.2010.02954.x

Hebda, T., & Czar, P. (2013). *Handbook of informatics for nurses & healthcare professionals* (5th ed.). Upper Saddle River, NJ: Pearson-Prentice Hall.

Hinkle, J. L., & Cheever, K. H. (2017). Brunner & Suddarth's textbook of medical-surgical nursing (14th ed.). Philadelphia, PA: Lippincott Williams & Wilkins.

Hockenberry, M. J., & Wilson, D. (2019). *Wong's nursing care of infants and children* (11th ed.). St. Louis, MO: Elsevier.

Huston, C. J. (2016). *Professional issues in nursing: Challenges & opportunities* (4th ed.). Philadelphia, PA: Wolters Kluwer Health/Lippincott Williams & Wilkins.

Ignatavicius, D. D., & Workman, M. L. (2018). *Medical-surgical nursing: Patient-centered collaborative care* (9th ed.). St. Louis, MO: Elsevier/ Saunders.

*Institute for Clinical Systems Improvement. (2018). *Palliative Care.* Available at: www.icsi.org/about_icsi/legacy_work/palliative_care/

*Institute for Healthcare Improvement. (2018). *Surgical Care Improvement Project.* Available at: www.ihi.org/resources/Pages/OtherWebsites/ SurgicalCareImprovementProject.aspx

*Institute for Healthcare Improvement. (2018). *Patient Safety.* Available at: www.ihi.org/Topics/PatientSafety/Pages/default.aspx

*Institute for Healthcare Improvement. (2018). *Rapid Response Teams.* Available at: www.ihi.org/Topics/RapidResponseTeams/Pages/ default.aspx

*Institute for Safe Medication Practices. (2007). *Action Needed to Prevent Dangerous Heparin-Insulin Confusion.* Available at: www.ismp.org/ resources/action-needed-prevent-dangerous-heparin-insulin-confusion

*Institute for Safe Medication Practices. (2014). *Still outside the bull's eye: 2014-2015 Targeted Medication Safety Best Practices (Baseline survey results).* Available at: www.ismp.org/resources/still-outside-bulls-eye-2014-2015-targeted-medication-safety-best-practices-baseline

Jones, R. (2007). *Nursing leadership and management: Theories, processes and practice.* Philadelphia, PA: F.A. Davis.

Killion, S., & Dempski, K. (2006). *Quick look nursing: Legal and ethical issues* (p. 71). Sudbury, MA: Jones and Bartlett.

Kunz Howard, P., & Steinmann, R. A. (Eds.). (2010). *Sheehy's emergency nursing: Principles and practice* (6th ed.). St. Louis, MO: Mosby Elsevier.

LaCharity, L., Kumagai, C., & Bartz, B. (2018). *Prioritization, delegation, assignment: Practice exercises for medical-surgical nursing* (4th ed.). St. Louis, MO: Mosby.

Lewis, S. L., Dirksen, S. R., Heitkemper, M. M., & Bucher, L. (2014). *Medical-surgical nursing: Assessment and management of clinical problems* (9th ed.). St. Louis, MO: Elsevier/Mosby.

Marquis, B. L., & Huston, C. J. (2017). *Leadership roles and management functions in nursing* (9th ed.). Philadelphia, PA: Wolters Kluwer Heath/Lippincott Williams & Wilkins.

Montalvo, I. (2007). The National Database of Nursing Quality Indicators® (NDNQI®). The *On-line Journal of Issues in Nursing, 12*(7), available at: www.nursingworld.org/MainMenuCategories/ANAMarketplace/ANAPeriodicals/OJIN/TableofContents/Volume122007/No3Sept07/NursingQualityIndicators.html

Motacki, K., & Burke, K. (2017). *Nursing delegation and management of patient care* (2nd ed.). St. Louis, MO: Mosby/Elsevier.

National Council of State Boards of Nursing. (2005). *Working with others: A Position Paper.* Available at: www.ncsbn.org/working_with_others.pdf

*National Council on Interpreting in Health Care. (2005). *National Standards of Practice for Interpreters in Health Care.* Santa Rosa, CA: National Council on Interpreting in Health Care. Available at: www.ncihc.org/assets/documents/publications/NCIHC%20National%20Standards%20of%20Practice.pdf

Neumann, T. (2010). Delegation—better safe than sorry. *AAOHN Journal, 58*(8), 321–322.

Pellico, L. H. (2013). *Focus on adult health medical-surgical nursing.* Philadelphia, PA: Wolters Kluwer Health/Lippincott Williams & Wilkins.

Pillitteri, A. (2017). *Maternal & child health nursing: Care of the child-bearing & childrearing family* (8th ed.). Philadelphia, PA: Lippincott Williams & Wilkins.

Potter, P. A., Perry, A. G., Stockert, P., & Hall, A. (2017). *Fundamentals of nursing* (9th ed.). St. Louis, MO: Mosby/Elsevier.

Purnell, L. (2013). *Transcultural health care: A culturally competent approach* (4th ed.). Philadelphia, PA: F.A. Davis.

Purnell, L. (2014). *Guide to culturally competent health care* (3rd ed.). Philadelphia, PA: F.A. Davis.

Salman, K., & Zoucha, R. (2010). Considering a faith within culture when caring for the terminally ill Muslim patient and family. *Journal of Hospice and Palliative Nursing, 12*(3), 156-163.

Sharpnack, P., Griffin, M., Benders, A., Fitzpatrick, J. (2010). Spiritual and alternative healthcare practices of the Amish. *Holistic Nursing Practice, 24*(2), 64-72.

Spector, R. (2016). *Cultural diversity in health and illness* (9th ed.). Upper Saddle River, NJ: Pearson Education.

Standing, T., & Anthony, M. (2008). Delegation: What it means to acute care nurses. *Applied Nursing Research, 21*(1), 8–14.

Stuart, G. (2013). *Principles and practice of psychiatric nursing* (10th ed.). St. Louis, MO: Elsevier/Mosby.

Taylor, C. R., Lillis, C., & Lynn, P. (2014). *Fundamentals of nursing: The art and science of nursing care* (8th ed.). Philadelphia, PA: Lippincott Williams & Wilkins.

*The Joint Commission (2018). *2018 National Patient Safety Goals.* Available at: www.jointcommission.org/standards_information/npsgs.aspx

*The Joint Commission. (2014). Managing risk during transition to new ISO tubing connector standards. Sentinel Event Alert Issue #53. Available at: www.jointcommission.org/sea_issue_53/

The National Coordinating Council for Medication Error Reporting and Prevention. (2018). Available at: www.nccmerp.org/

Townsend, M. (2018). *Psychiatric mental health nursing; Concepts of care in evidence-based practice* (9th ed.). Philadelphia: F.A. Davis.

Treas, L. S., & Wilkinson, J. M. (2018). *Basic nursing: Concepts, skills, and reasoning* (2nd ed.). Philadelphia, PA: F.A. Davis.

U.S. Department of Health & Human Services Office for Civil Rights. (ND). *Your Health Information Privacy Rights.* Available at: www.hhs.gov/sites/default/files/ocr/privacy/hipaa/understanding/consumers/consumer_rights.pdf

U.S. Department of Health and Human Services. (2012). *Center for Medicare and Medicaid Services: EMTALA.* Retrieved from www.cms.gov/Regulations-and-Guidance/Legislation/EMTALA/index.html?redirect=/emtala/

Videbeck, S. (2016). *Psychiatric-mental health nursing* (7th ed.). Philadelphia, PA: Wolters Kluwer/Lippincott Williams & Wilkins.

Wachter, R. M. (2007). *Understanding patient safety* (3rd ed.). New York: McGraw-Hill.

Weiss, S. A., & Tappen, R. M. (2015). *Essentials of nursing leadership and management* (6th ed.). Philadelphia, PA: F.A. Davis.

Wilkinson, J. M., & Treas, L. S. (2015). *Fundamentals of nursing: Theory, concepts, & application* (3rd ed.). Philadelphia, PA: F.A. Davis.

Wilson, B. A., Shannon, M. T., & Shields, K. M. (2014). Pearson nurse's drug guide 2014. Upper Saddle River, NJ: Pearson Education.

Yoder-Wise, P. (2015). *Leading and managing in nursing* (6th ed.). St. Louis, MO: Mosby/Elsevier.

Zerwekh, J., & Garneau, A. Z. (2018). *Nursing today: Transition and trends* (9th ed.). St. Louis, MO: Elsevier/Saunders.

---

*Evidence-based Reference

## Unit 2: Fundamentals of Nursing

*American Heart Association. (2010). *Highlights of the 2010 American Heart Association Guidelines for CPR.* Available at: www.heart.org/idc/groups/heart-public/@wcm/@ecc/documents/downloadable/ucm_317350.pdf

Ball, J. W., Bindler, R. C., & Cowen, K. J. (2017). *Principles of pediatric nursing: Caring for children* (7th ed.). Upper Saddle River, NJ: Pearson Education.

Bender, B., Ozuah, P., & Crain, E. (2007). Oral rehydration therapy: Is anyone drinking? *Pediatric Emergency Care, 23*(9), 624-626.

*Berg, R. H., Hemphill, R., Abella, B. S., Aufderheide, T. P., Cave, D. M., Hazinski, M. F., Swor, R.A. (2017). 2010 American Heart Association Guidelines for Cardiopulmonary Resuscitation and Emergency Cardiovascular Care Science, Part 5: Adult Basic Life Support. Available at: eccguidelines.heart.org/index.php/circulation/cpr-ecc-guidelines-2/part-5-adult-basic-life-support-and-cardiopulmonary-resuscitation-quality/

Berman, A., & Snyder, S. (2016). *Skills in clinical nursing* (8th ed.). Upper Saddle River, NJ: Prentice Hall.

Berman, A., Snyder, S., & Frandsen, G. (2016). *Kozier & Erb's fundamentals of nursing* (10th ed.). Upper Saddle River, NJ: Pearson Education.

*Boyd, A. E., DeFord, L. L., Mares, J. E., Leary, C. C., Garris, J. L., Dagohoy, C. G., Boving, V. G., Brook, J. P., Phan, A., & Yao, J. C. (2013). Improving the success rate of gluteal intramuscular injections. *Pancreas, 42*(5), 878-882. doi:10.1097/MPA.0b013e318279d552

Callahan, B. (2019). *Clinical nursing skills: A concept-based approach, volume III* (3rd ed.). Upper Saddle River, NJ: Pearson Education.

*Carlton G. (2006). Medication-related errors: A literature review of incidence and antecedents. *Annual Review of Nursing Research, 24,* 19–38.

*Centers for Disease Control and Prevention. (2017). *Smallpox bioterrorism response planning.* Available at: www.cdc.gov/smallpox/bioterrorism-response-planning/index.html

*Centers for Disease Control and Prevention. (2017). *Emergency preparedness and response: Questions and answers about infection control and isolation of smallpox patients.* Available at: www.cdc.gov/smallpox/bioterrorism-response-planning/healthcare-facility/prevent-spread-disease.html

*Centers for Disease Control and Prevention. (2015). *Emergency preparedness and response.* Available at: emergency.cdc.gov/

*Centers for Disease Control and Prevention. (2017). *Guideline for isolation precautions: Preventing transmission of infectious agents in healthcare settings.* Available at: www.cdc.gov/hicpac/2007IP/2007ip_appendA.html

*Centers for Disease Control and Prevention. (2014). *Recommended immunization schedules for persons aged 0 through 18 years United States, 2014.* Available at: www.cdc.gov/vaccines/schedules/downloads/child/0-18yrs-child-combined-schedule.pdf

*Centers for Disease Control and Prevention. (2014). *Shingles (herpes zoster).* Available at: www.cdc.gov/shingles/hcp/clinical-overview.html

*Centers for Disease Control and Prevention. (2015). *National Notifiable Diseases Surveillance System (NNDSS)*. Available at: www.cdc.gov/nndss/

Berg, R. A., Hemphill R., Abella, B. S., Aufderheide, T. P., Cave, D. M., Hazinski, M. F., Lerner, E. B., Rea, T. D., Sayre, M. R., Swor, R. A. (2010) Part 5: Adult basic life support: 2010 American Heart Association guidelines for cardiopulmonary resuscitation and emergency cardiovascular care. *Circulation*, 122, pp. S685-S705. Available at: American Heart Association circ.ahajournals.org/content/122/18_suppl_3/S685.full

Craven, R. F., Hirnle, C. H., & Henshaw, C. M. (2016). *Fundamentals of nursing: Human health and function* (8th ed.). Philadelphia, PA: Lippincott Williams & Wilkins.

Craven, R. F., Hirnle, C. H., & Jensen, S. (2013). *Fundamentals of nursing: Human health and function* (7th ed.). Philadelphia, PA: Lippincott Williams & Wilkins.

*Critchell, C., & Marik, P. (2007). Should family members be present during cardiopulmonary resuscitation? A review of the literature. *American Journal of Hospice and Palliative Medicine*, 24(4), 311–317.

*Department of Health and Human Services. Centers for Disease Control and Prevention. (2015). *Ebola Virus Disease. Guidance on Personal Protective Equipment To Be Used by Healthcare Workers During Management of Patients with Ebola Virus Disease in U.S. Hospitals, Including Procedures for Putting On (Donning) and Removing (Doffing)*. Available at: www.cdc.gov/vhf/ebola/hcp/procedures-for-ppe.html

*Department of Health and Human Services. Centers for Disease Control and Prevention. (2018). *Meningococcal Disease*. Available at: www.cdc.gov/meningitis/index.html

*Drug Enforcement Administration. (2010). *Controlled Substances Act*. Available at: www.dea.gov/controlled-substances-act

Dudek, S. (2017). *Nutrition essentials for nursing practice* (8th ed.). Philadelphia, PA: Lippincott Williams & Wilkins.

*Dumville, J. C., McFarlane, E., Edwards, P., Lipp, A., & Holmes, A. (2013). Preoperative skin antiseptics for preventing surgical wound infections after clean surgery. *The Cochrane Collaboration*. doi:10.1002/14651858.CD003949.pub3. Available at: onlinelibrary.wiley.com/doi/10.1002/14651858.CD003949.pub3/full

*Dupras, D., Bluhm, J., Felty, C., Hansen, C., Johnson, T., Lim, K., Maddali, S., Marshall, P., Messner, P., & Skeik, N. (2009). Venous thromboembolism diagnosis and treatment. *Institute for Clinical Systems Improvement*. Available at: lnx.mednemo.it/wp-content/uploads/2008/10/icsi652.pdf

Federal Emergency Management Agency. (2014). *FEMA are you ready guide*. Available at: www.fema.gov/pdf/areyouready/areyouready_full.pdf

Federal Emergency Management Agency. (2014). *Resources*. Available at: www.fema.gov/

*Flint, A., McIntosh, D., & Davies, M. (2005). Continuous infusion versus intermittent flushing to prevent loss of function of peripheral intravenous catheters used for drug administration in newborn infants. *Cochrane Database of Systematic Reviews*, Issue 4, Art. No. CD004593. doi:10.1002/14651858.CD004593.pub2. Available at: www.cochrane.org/reviews/en/ab004593.html

Fortinash, K., & Holoday Worret, P. (2015). Psychiatric mental health nursing-Revised Reprint (5th ed.). St. Louis, MO: Mosby/Elsevier.

Guido, G. W. (2014). *Legal and ethical issues in nursing* (6th ed.). Upper Saddle River, NJ: Pearson Education.

*Harding, L., & Petrick, T. (2008). Nursing student medication errors: A retrospective review. *Journal of Nursing Education*, 47(1), 43–47.

Harkness, G. A., & DeMarco, R. F. (2016). *Community and public health nursing: Evidence for practice* (2nd ed.). Philadelphia, PA: Wolters Kluwer.

Hinkle, J. L., & Cheever, K. H. (2017). *Brunner & Suddarth's textbook of medical-surgical nursing* (14th ed.). Philadelphia, PA: Lippincott Williams & Wilkins.

Hockenberry, M. J., & Wilson, D. (2019). *Wong's nursing care of infants and children* (11th ed.). St. Louis, MO: Elsevier.

Ignatavicius, D. D., & Workman, M. L. (2018). *Medical-surgical nursing: Patient-centered collaborative care* (9th ed.). St. Louis, MO: Elsevier/Saunders.

Insel, P., Ross, D., McMahon, K., & Bernstein, M. (2014). *Nutrition* (5th ed.). Sudbury, MA: Jones and Bartlett.

*Institute for Healthcare Improvement. (2018). *Surgical site infection*. Available at: www.ihi.org/topics/ssi/pages/default.aspx

*Jacobs, I., Sunde, K., Deakin, C. D., Hazinski, M., F., Kerber, R. E., Koster, R. W., Sayre, M. R. (2010). Part 6: Defibrillation, 2010 International consensus on cardiopulmonary resuscitation and emergency cardiovascular care science with treatment recommendations. *Circulation*, *122*, S325-S337. Available from American Heart Association circ.ahajournals.org/content/122/16_suppl_2/S325.full.pdf+html

Kee, J. L. (2014). *Laboratory and diagnostic tests with nursing implications* (9th ed.). Upper Saddle River, NJ: Pearson.

Kee, J. L., Hayes, E., & McCuistion, L. (2015). *Pharmacology: A nursing process approach* (8th ed.). St. Louis, MO: Elsevier.

*Kuhar, D. T., Henderson, D. K., Struble, K. A., Heneine, W., Thomas, V., Cheever, L.W., Gomaa, A., Panlilio, A. L., & U.S. Public Health Service Working Group (2013). Updated U.S. Public Health Service guidelines for the management of occupational exposures to human immunodeficiency virus and recommendations for postexposure prophylaxis. *Infection Control and Hospital Epidemiology*, *34*(9), 875-892. doi:10.1086/672271

LaMone, P., Burke, K. M., Bauldoff, G., & Gubrud, P. (2015). *Medical surgical nursing: Critical thinking in patient care* (6th ed.). Upper Saddle River, NJ: Pearson.

Lewis, S. L., Dirksen, S. R., Heitkemper, M. M., & Bucher, L. (2017). *Medical-surgical nursing: Assessment and management of clinical problems* (10th ed.). St. Louis, MO: Elsevier/Mosby.

*Link, M. S., Atkins, D. L., Passman, R. S., Halperin, H. R., Samson, R. A., White, R. D., Kerber, R. E. (2010). Part 6: Electrical therapies automated external defibrillators, defibrillation, cardioversion, and pacing, 2010 American Heart Association guidelines for cardiopulmonary resuscitation and emergency cardiovascular care. *Circulation*. 2010 Nov 2;122(18 Suppl 3):S706-19. doi:10.1161/CIRCULATIONAHA.110.970954

Lutz, C. A., Mazur, E. E., & Litch, N. A. (2015). *Nutrition and diet therapy* (6th ed.). Philadelphia, PA: F.A. Davis.

Lutz, C., & Przytulski, K. (2010). *Nutrition & diet therapy: Evidence-based applications* (5th ed.). Philadelphia, PA: F.A. Davis.

Maday, K. R. (2013). Understanding electrolytes: Important diagnostic clues to patient status. *Journal of the American Academy of Physician Assistants, 26*(1), 26-31.

*Michigan Quality Improvement Consortium. (2013). *Management of overweight and obesity in the adult*. Available at: www.mqic.org/pdf/mqic_management_of_overweight_and_obesity_in_the_adult_cpg.pdf

*Morrison, L. J., Kierzek, G., Diekema, D. S., Sayre, M. R., Silvers, S. M., Idris, A. H., & Mancini, M. E. (2010). 2010 American Heart Association guidelines for cardiopulmonary resuscitation and emergency cardiovascular care, Part 3: Ethics. *Circulation*, 122, S665-S675. Available at: circ.ahajournals.org/content/122/18_suppl_3/S665.full.pdf+html?sid=e609597f-0c01-44f5-929b-ddb87df46c1e

*Natal, B. L., & Doty, C. (2014). Venous air embolism treatment & management. *Medscape, Emedicine*. Retrieved from emedicine.medscape.com/article/761367-treatment#a1126

*National Institute for Clinical Excellence. (2012). *Infection control. Prevention of healthcare-associated infection in primary and community care*. Available at: www.ncbi.nlm.nih.gov/books/NBK115271/

*National Quality Forum. (2011). Serious reportable events: Fact sheet. Retrieved from www.qualityforum.org/Topics/SREs/SREs_Fact_Sheet.aspx

Pagana, K., Pagana, T., & Pagana, T. (2017). *Mosby's diagnostic and laboratory test reference* (13th ed.). St. Louis, MO: Elsevier.

*Perel, P., Roberts, I., & Kerr, K. (2013). Colloids versus crystalloids for fluid resuscitation in critically ill patients. *Cochrane Database Systematic Reviews* 2013, Issue 2. doi:10.1002/14651858.CD000567.pub6

Phillips, L. D., & Gorski, L. (2014). *Manual of I.V. therapeutics: Evidence-based practice for infusion therapy* (6th ed.). Philadelphia, PA: F.A. Davis.

Pickar, G. D., & Abernethy, A. P. (2013). *Dosage calculations* (9th ed.). Clifton Park, NY: Thomson Delmar Learning.

Pillitteri, A. (2017). *Maternal & child health nursing: Care of the childbearing and childrearing family* (8th ed.). Philadelphia, PA: Lippincott Williams & Wilkins.

Porth, C. M. (2015). *Essentials of pathophysiology* (4th ed.). Philadelphia, PA: Wolters Kluwer Health/Lippincott Williams & Wilkins.

Potter, P. A., Perry, A. G., Stockert, P., & Hall, A. (2017). *Fundamentals of nursing* (9th ed.). St. Louis, MO: Mosby/Elsevier.

*Registered Nurses Association of Ontario. (2007). *Assessment and management of stage I to IV pressure ulcers.* Available at: rnao.ca/sites/rnao-ca/files/Assessment__Management_of_Stage_I_to_IV_Pressure_Ulcers.pdf

*Registered Nurses Association of Ontario. (2013). Assessment and management of foot ulcers for people with diabetes (2nd ed.). Available at: rnao.ca/sites/rnao-ca/files/Assessment_and_Management_of_Foot_Ulcers_for_People_with_Diabetes_Second_Edition1.pdf

Resuscitation and Emergency Cardiovascular Care. *Circulation.* 122, S706-S719. Available at: American Heart Association: circ.ahajournals.org/content/122/18_suppl_3/S706.full.pdf+html

*Rogers, G. (2006). Reconciling medications at admission: Safe practice recommendations and implementation strategies. *Joint Commission Journal on Quality and Patient Safety,* 32(1), 37–50.

*Shang, J., Ma, C., Poghosyan, L., Dowding, D., & Stone, P. (2014). The prevalence of infections and patient risk factors in home health care: A systematic review. doi:dx.doi.org/10.1016/j.ajic.2013.12.018. *American Journal of Infection Control,* 42(5), 479–484.

Stanhope, M., & Lancaster, J. (2012). *Public health nursing - revised reprint: Population-centered health care in the community* (8th ed.). St. Louis, MO: Mosby.

*Stevens, D. L., Bisno, A. L., Chamber, H. G., Dellinger, E. P., Goldstein, E. J. C., Gorbach, S. L., Hirschmann, J. V., Kaplan, S. L., Montoya, J. G., & Wade, J. C. (2014). Practice guidelines for the diagnosis and management of skin and soft tissue infections: 2014 Update. *The Infectious Diseases Society of America.* Available at: cid.oxfordjournals.org/content/early/2014/06/14/cid.ciu296.full

*Surawicz, C. M., Brandt, L. J., Binion, D. G., Ananthakrishnan, A. N., Curry, S. R., Gilligan, P. H., McFarland, L. V., Mellow, M., & Zuckerbraun, B. S. (2013). Guidelines for diagnosis, treatment, and prevention of *Clostridium difficile* infections. *American Journal of Gastroenterology,* 108(4), 478-498.

*Tanner, J., Norrie, P., & Melen, K. (2011). Preoperative hair removal to reduce surgical site infection. *Cochrane Database of Systematic Reviews,* Nov 9(11):CD004122. doi:10.1002/14651858.CD004122.pub4. Available at: onlinelibrary.wiley.com/doi/10.1002/14651858.CD004122.pub4/full

Taylor, C. R., Lillis, C., & Lynn, P. (2014). *Fundamentals of nursing: The art and science of nursing care* (8th ed.). Philadelphia, PA: Lippincott Williams & Wilkins.

*The Joanna Briggs Institute. (2007). Preoperative hair removal to reduce surgical site infection. *Best Practice,* 11(6). Available at: connect.jbiconnectplus.org/ViewSourceFile.aspx?0=4347

*The Joint Commission. (2015). *National Patient Safety Goals.* Retrieved from www.jointcommission.org/assets/1/6/2015_HAP_NPSG_ER.pdf

*The Joint Commission. (2018). *Patient Do Not Use List.* Available at: www.jointcommission.org/assets/1/18/Do_Not_Use_List_9_14_18.pdf

*The Joint Commission. (2014). *Surgical Care Improvement Project.* Available at: manual.jointcommission.org/releases/archive/TJC2010B/SurgicalCareImprovementProject.html

*The Joint Commission. (2018). *2018 National Patient Safety Goals.* Available at: www.jointcommission.org/standards_information/npsgs.aspx

*The Joint Commission. (2016). *Facts about the Universal Protocol.* Available at: www.jointcommission.org/standards_information/up.aspx

*The Joint Commission. (2017). *Sentinel Event Policy and Procedures.* Available at: www.jointcommission.org/Sentinel_Event_Policy_and_Procedures/

*Thorson, D., Biewen, P., Bonte, B., Epstein, H., Haake, B., Hansen, C., Hooten, M., Hora, J., Johnson, C., Keeling, F., Kokayeff, A., Krebs, E., Myers, C., Nelson, B., Noonan, M.P., Reznikoff, C., Thiel, M., Trujillo, A., Van Pelt, S., Wainio, J. (2014). Acute pain assessment and opioid prescribing protocol. *Institute for Clinical Systems Improvement.* Available at: crh.arizona.edu/sites/default/files/u35/Opioids.pdf

Treas, L. S., & Wilkinson, J. M. (2018). *Basic nursing: Concepts, skills, and reasoning* (2nd ed.). Philadelphia, PA: F.A. Davis.

*U.S. Department of Agriculture. (2014). *ChooseMyPlate.gov.* Available at: www.choosemyplate.gov/food-groups/

Vallerand, A. H., Sanoski, C. A., & Deglin, J. H. (2019). *Davis's drug guide for nurses* (16th ed.). Philadelphia, PA: F.A. Davis.

Van Leeuwen, A. M., & Bladh, M. L. (2017). Davis's comprehensive handbook of laboratory and diagnostic tests with nursing implications (8th ed.). Philadelphia, PA: F.A. Davis.

Whitney, E., DeBruyne, L., Pinna, K., & Rolfes, S. (2017). *Nutrition for health and health care* (6th ed.). Belmont, CA: Thomson Learning.

Wilkinson, J. M., & Treas, L. S. (2015). *Fundamentals of nursing: Theory, concepts, & application* (3rd ed.). Philadelphia, PA: F.A. Davis.

Wilkinson, J., & Treas, L. (2011). *Fundamentals of nursing. Volume 2: Thinking, doing, and caring.* (2nd ed.). Philadelphia, PA: F.A. Davis.

---

*Evidence-based Reference

## Unit 3: Care of Childbearing Families

*American Academy of Pediatrics. (2010). Policy statement, hospital stay for healthy term newborns. *Pediatrics,* 125(2), 405-409. doi:10.1542/peds.2009-3119

*American College of Obstetricians and Gynecologists. (2013). Fetal growth restriction. Washington (DC): *American College of Obstetricians and Gynecologists.* Available at: www.ncbi.nlm.nih.gov/pubmed/23635765

*American College of Obstetricians and Gynecologists. (2012). Improving medication safety. *ACOG.* Available at: www.acog.org/-/media/Committee-Opinions/Committee-on-Patient-Safety-and-Quality-Improvement/co531.pdf?dmc=1&ts=20141019T0309039885

*American College of Obstetricians and Gynecologists. (2014). Multifetal gestations: twin, triplet, and higher-order multifetal pregnancies. Washington (DC): *American College of Obstetricians and Gynecologists.* Available at: www.ncbi.nlm.nih.gov/pubmed/24785876

Ball, J. W., Bindler, R. C., & Cowen, K. J. (2017). *Principles of pediatric nursing: Caring for children* (7th ed.). Upper Saddle River, NJ: Pearson Education.

*Benfield, R.D., Hortobagyi, T., Tanner, C.J., Swanson, M., Heitkemper, M. M., & Newton, E. R. (2010). The effects of hydrotherapy on anxiety, pain, neuroendocrine responses, and contraction dynamics during labor. *Biological Research for Nursing,* 12(1), 28-36.

*Brownfoot, F. C., Gagliardi, D. I., Bain, E., Middleton, P., & Crowther, C. A. (2013). Corticosteroid treatments before early birth for reducing death, lung problems and brain haemorrhage in babies. *Cochrane.* Available at: www.cochrane.org/CD006764/PREG_corticosteroid-treatments-before-early-birth-for-reducing-death-lung-problems-and-brain-haemorrhage-in-babies

Burchum, J., & Rosenthal, L. (2016). *Lehne's pharmacology for nursing care* (9th ed.). St. Louis, MO: Saunders Elsevier.

*Centers for Disease Control and Prevention. (2016). Vaccines and immunizations. Available at: www.cdc.gov/vaccines/vpd/hepb/index.html

*Centers for Disease Control and Prevention. (2018). *Recommended immunization schedule for persons aged 0 through 18 years United States.* Available at: www.cdc.gov/vaccines/schedules/hcp/imz/child-adolescent.html

*Chang, L. J., Chen, S. U., Tsai, Y. Y., Hung, C.-C., Fang, M.-Y., Su, Y.-N., & Yang, Y.-S. (2011). An update of preimplantation genetic diagnosis in gene diseases, chromosomal translocation, and aneuploidy screening. *Clinical & Experimental Reproductive Medicine,* 38(3), 126–134.

Craig, G. (2015). *Clinical calculations made easy: Solving problems using dimensional analysis* (6th ed.). Philadelphia, PA: Lippincott Williams & Wilkins.

Davidson, M., London, M., & Ladewig, P. A. (2016). *Olds' maternal-newborn nursing & women's health across the lifespan* (10th ed.). Upper Saddle River, NJ: Pearson Education.

Durham, R., & Chapman, L. (2019). *Maternal-newborn nursing: The critical components of nursing care* (3rd ed.). Philadelphia, PA: F.A. Davis.

*Euliano, T. Y., Nguyen, M., Darmanjian, S., McGorray, S., Euliano, N., Onkala, A., & Gregg, A. (2013). Monitoring uterine activity during labor: A comparison of 3 methods. *American Journal of Obstetrics & Gynecology, 208*(66), 1–6.

*Gartlehner, G., Patel, S.V., Viswanathan, M., Feltner, C., Palmieri Weber, R., Lee, R., Mullican, K., Boland, E., Lux, L., & Lohr, L. (2017). Hormone Therapy for the Primary Prevention of Chronic Conditions in Postmenopausal Women: An Evidence Review for the U.S. Preventive Services Task Force. Evidence Synthesis No 155. AHRQ Publication No. 15-05227-EF-1. Rockville, MD: *Agency for Healthcare Research and Quality.* Retrieved from https://www.ncbi.nlm.nih.gov/books/NBK488033/

Hockenberry, M. J., & Wilson, D. (2015). *Wong's nursing care of infants and children* (10th ed.). St. Louis, MO: Elsevier.

*Institute for Safe Medicine Practices (ISMP). (2015). ISMP's list of confused drug names. *ISMP.* Available at: www.ismp.org/tools/confuseddrugnames.pdf

*Jorgensen, J. S., Weile, L. K., & Lamont, R. F. (2014). Preterm labor: Current tocolytic options for the treatment of preterm labor. *Expert Opinion Pharmacotherapy, 15*(5), 585-588. doi:10.1517/14656566.2014.880110

*Joy, S. (2017). Postpartum depression. *Medscape.* Available at: reference.medscape.com/article/271662-overview

*Kluge, J., Hall, D., Louw, Q., Theron, G., & Grové, D. (2011). Specific exercises to treat pregnancy-related low back pain in a South African population. *International Journal of Gynaecology and Obstetrics, 113*(3), 187-191. doi:10.1016/j.ijgo.2010.10.030. Retrieved from www.sciencedirect.com/science/article/pii/S0020729211000816

Lowdermilk, D. L., Perry, S. E., Cashion, K., & Rhodes, K. (2016). *Maternity & women's health care* (11th ed.). St. Louis, MO: Elsevier/Mosby.

*Makic, M. B., VonRueden, K. T., Rauen, C. A., & Chadwick, J. (2011). Evidence-based practice habits: Putting more sacred cows out to pasture. *Critical Care Nurse, 31*(2), 38-62. doi:10/4037/ccn2011908. Retrieved from ccn.aacnjournals.org/content/31/2/38.full

Murray, S. S., & McKinney, E. S. (2014). *Foundations of maternal-newborn and women's health nursing* (6th ed.). Maryland Heights, MO: Saunders.

Nagtalon-Ramos, J. (2014). *Maternal-newborn nursing care: Best evidence-based practices.* Philadelphia, PA: F.A. Davis.

Perry, S. E., Hockenberry, M. J., Lowdermilk, D. L., & Wilson, D. (2014). *Maternal child nursing care* (5th ed.). St. Louis, MO: Elsevier/Mosby.

Pillitteri, A. (2017). *Maternal & child health nursing: Care of the childbearing and childrearing family* (8th ed.). Philadelphia, PA: Lippincott Williams & Wilkins.

Porth, C. M. (2015). *Essentials of pathophysiology* (4th ed.). Philadelphia, PA: Wolters Kluwer Health/Lippincott Williams & Wilkins.

*Public Health Service Task Force. (2014). *Recommendations For Use of Antiretroviral Medications in Pregnant HIV-1-Infected Women for Maternal Health and Interventions to Reduce HIV-1 Transmission in the United States.* Available at: aidsinfo.nih.gov/guidelines/html/3/perinatal-guidelines/0

Ricci, S. S. (2016). *Essentials of maternity, newborn, and women's health nursing* (4th ed.). Philadelphia, PA: Lippincott Williams and Wilkins, Wolters Kluwer Health.

*Seng, J. S., Sperlich, M., Low, L. K., Ronis, D. L., Muzik, M., & Liberzon, I. (2013). Childhood abuse history, posttraumatic stress disorder, postpartum mental health, and bonding: A prospective cohort study. *American College of Nurse-Midwives, 58*(1), 57–68.

*The Joint Commission. (2014). Facts about the official "Do Not Use" list of abbreviations. The Joint Commission. Available at: www.jointcommission.org/facts_about_the_official_/

Vallerand, A. H., Sanoski, C. A., & Deglin, J. H. (2019). *Davis's drug guide for nurses* (16th ed.). Philadelphia, PA: F.A. Davis.

*Verdurmen, K. M., Renckens, J., van Laar, J. O., & Oei, S. G. (2013). The influence of corticosteroids on fetal heart rate variability: A systematic review of the literature. *Obstetrical & Gynecological Survey, 68*, 811.

Ward, S. L., & Hisley, S. M. (2015). *Maternal-child nursing care (2nd ed.).* Philadelphia, PA: F.A. Davis.

Wilson, B. A., Shannon, M. T., & Shields, K. M. (2015). *Pearson nurse's drug guide 2015.* Upper Saddle River, NJ: Pearson Education.

*Yeo, S. (2010). Prenatal stretching exercise and autonomic responses: Preliminary data and a model for reducing preeclampsia. *Journal of Nursing Scholarship, 42*(2), 113-121. doi:10.1111/j.1547-5069.2010.01344.x

*Evidence-based Reference

# Unit 4: Care of Adults

Adams, M., Holland, L., & Urban, C. (2017). *Pharmacology for nurses: A pathophysiologic approach* (5th ed.). Upper Saddle River, NJ: Prentice Hall.

*American Academy of Ophthalmology Cataract and Anterior Segment Panel. (2016). *Cataract in the adult eye.* San Francisco, CA: American Academy of Ophthalmology (AAO). Available at: www.aao.org/Assets/5215127e-87b8-4ddc-af88-3d9d03c02fcb/636217263645470000/cataract-in-the-adult-eye-ppp-pdf

*American Academy of Ophthalmology Cornea/External Disease Panel. (2013). *Conjunctivitis. Limited revision.* San Francisco, CA: American Academy of Ophthalmology (AAO). Available at: www.aao.org/Assets/07524e1e-859e-4862-a32f-0235f076ede0/635200264565170000/conjunctivitis-ppp-pdf

*American Academy of Orthopaedic Surgeons. (2013). *American Academy of Orthopaedic Surgeons clinical practice guideline on treatment of osteoarthritis of the knee.* 2nd ed. Rosemont (IL): American Academy of Orthopaedic Surgeons. Available at: www.aaos.org/research/guidelines/treatmentofosteoarthritisofthekneeguideline.pdf

*American Association of Neuroscience Nurses. (2014). Care of the adult patient with a brain tumor. Chicago (IL): American Association of Neuroscience Nurses (AANN). Retrieved from aann.org/uploads/Membership/SFG/neurooncology/AANN14_ABT_Module_2016_update.pdf

*American Association of Neuroscience Nurses, Association of Rehabilitation Nurses. (2011). Care of the patient with mild traumatic brain injury. Glenview (IL): American Association of Neuroscience Nurses, Association of Rehabilitation Nurses. Retrieved from rehabnurse.org/uploads/about/AANN14_MildTBI.pdf

*American Diabetes Association. (2015). *Carbohydrate counting.* Available at: www.diabetes.org/food-and-fitness/food/what-can-i-eat/understanding-carbohydrates/carbohydrate-counting.html

Aschenbrenner, D. S., & Venable, S. J. (2013). *Drug therapy in nursing* (4th ed.). Philadelphia, PA: Lippincott Williams & Wilkins.

*Beithon, J., Gallenberg, M., Johnson, K., Kildahl, P., Krenik, J., Liebow, M., Linbo, L., Myers, C., Peterson, S., Schmidt, J., & Swanson, J. (2013). Diagnosis and treatment of headache. *Institute for Clinical Systems Improvement.* Available at:www.icsi.org/guidelines__more/catalog_guidelines_and_more/catalog_guidelines/catalog_neurological_guidelines/headache/

*Benbow, M. (2010). International pressure ulcer guidelines. *Journal of Community Nursing, 24*(6), 42-46.

*Bergman-Evans, B. (2012). Improving medication management for older adult clients. Iowa City (IA): University of Iowa College of Nursing, *John A. Harford Foundation Center of Geriatric Nursing Excellence.* Available at: //doi.org/10.3928/00989134-20130904-01

Berman, A., Snyder, S., & Frandsen, G. (2016). *Kozier & Erb's fundamentals of nursing* (10th ed.). Upper Saddle River, NJ: Pearson Education.

*Boltz, M., Capezuti, E., Fulmer, T., & Zwicker, D. (2016). *Evidence-based geriatric nursing protocols for best practice* (5th ed.). New York: Springer.

*Brandt, L. J., Chey, W. D., Foxx-Orenstein, A. E., Schiller, L. R., Schoenfeld, P. S., Spiegel, B. M., ... Moayyedi, P. (2009). An evidence-based systematic review on the management of irritable bowel syndrome. *American Journal of Gastroenterology*, 104:S1. Retrieved from acggi.net/wp-content/uploads/2011/07/media-releases-ajg2008122a.pdf

*Brink, D., Barlow, J., Bush, K., Chaudhary, N., Fareed, M., Hayes, R., Jafri, I., Nair, K., Retzer, K., & Rueter, K. (2012). Colorectal cancer screening. *Institute for Clinical Systems Improvement*. Available at: www.guideline.gov/content.aspx?id=37276

Burchum, J., & Rosenthal, L. (2016). *Lehne's pharmacology for nursing care* (9th ed.). St. Louis, MO: Saunders Elsevier.

Carpenito, L. J. (2016). *Handbook of nursing diagnosis* (15th ed.). Philadelphia, PA: Lippincott Williams & Wilkins.

*Centers for Disease Control and Prevention (CDC). (2011). Guide to contraindications and precautions to commonly used vaccines. *MMWR*, *60*(RR-2): 40-41. Available at: www.immunize.org/catg.d/p3072a.pdf

*Centers for Disease Control and Prevention (CDC). (2015). Life stages & specific populations. Available at: www.cdc.gov/features/lifestages.html

Craven, R. F., Hirnle, C. H., & Henshaw, C. M. (2016). *Fundamentals of nursing: Human health and function* (8th ed.). Philadelphia, PA: Lippincott Williams & Wilkins.

Craven, R. F., Hirnle, C. H., & Jensen, S. (2013). *Fundamentals of nursing: Human health and function* (7th ed.). Philadelphia, PA: Lippincott Williams & Wilkins.

*Department of Health and Human Services: Centers for Disease Control and Prevention. (2017). *Genital herpes-CDC fact sheet*. Available at: www.cdc.gov/std/Herpes/STDFact-Herpes.htm

Dillon, P. (2007). *Nursing health assessment: A critical thinking, case studies approach* (2nd ed., pp. 420–421). Philadelphia, PA: F.A. Davis.

*Donahue, K.E., Gartlehner, G., Schulman, E.R., Jonas, B., Coker-Schwimmer, E., Patel, S.V., Weber, R.P., Lohr, K.N., Bann, C., & Viswanathan, M. (2018). Drug Therapy for Early Rheumatoid Arthritis: A Systematic Review Update. Comparative Effectiveness Review No. 211. (Prepared by the RTI International–University of North Carolina at Chapel Hill Evidence-based Practice Center under Contract No. 290-2015-00011-I for AHRQ and PCORI.) AHRQ Publication No. 18-EHC015-EF. PCORI Publication No. 2018-SR-02. Rockville, MD: *Agency for Healthcare Research and Quality*; July 2018. Posted final reports are located on the Effective Healthcare Program. Retrieved from https://doi.org/10.23970/AHRQEPCCER211

*do Rego Furtado, L. C. (2010). Nutritional management after Roux-en-Y gastric bypass. *British Journal of Nursing, 19*(7), 428-436.

*Dupras, D., Bluhm, J., Felty, C., Hansen, C., Johnson, T., Lim, K., Maddali, S., Marshall, P., Messner, P., & Skeik, N. (2009). Venous thromboembolism diagnosis and treatment. Bloomington, MN: *Institute for Clinical Systems Improvement*. Available at: lnx.mednemo.it/wp-content/uploads/2008/10/icsi652.pdf

Eliopoulos, C. (2017). *Gerontological nursing* (9th ed.). Philadelphia, PA: Lippincott Williams and Wilkins/Wolters Kluwer Health.

Estes, M. E. Z. (2014). *Health assessment and physical examination* (5th ed.). Clifton Park, NY: Delmar, Cengage Learning.

Frandsen, G., & Pennington, S., (2018). *Abrams' clinical drug therapy: Rationales for nursing practice* (11th ed.). Philadelphia, PA: Lippincott Williams & Wilkins.

*Fulmer, T. (2012). Try this: Best practices in nursing care to older adults. *Fulmer SPICES: An Overall Assessment Tool for Older Adults*. New York University: Hartford Institute for Geriatric Nursing. Retrieved from consultgeri.org/try-this/general-assessment/issue-1.pdf

*Gardner, T. B., & Berk, B. S. (2014). Acute pancreatitis, acute. *E-Medicine Medscape*. Available at: emedicine.medscape.com/article/181364-overview

*Gaucher, S., Nicco, C., Jarraya, M., & Batteux, F. (2010). Viability and efficacy of coverage of cryopreserved human skin allografts in mice. *International Journal of Lower Extremity Wounds*, *9*(3),132-140.

*Goblirsch, G., Bershow, S., Cummings, K., Hayes, R., Kokoszka, M., Lu, Y., Sanders, D., & Zarling, K. (2013). Stable coronary artery disease. Bloomington, MN: Institute for Clinical Systems Improvement. Available at: citeseerx.ist.psu.edu/viewdoc/download?doi=10.1.1.658.3632&rep=rep1&type=pdf

*Goertz, M., Thorson, D., Bonsell, J., Bonte, B., Campbell, R., Haake, B., Johnson, K., Kramer, C., Mueller, B., Peterson, S., Setterlund, L., & Timming, R. (2012). Adult acute and subacute low back pain. *Institute for Clinical Systems Improvement*. Available At: www.icsi.org/_asset/bjvqrj/LBP.pdf

Guido, G. W. (2014). *Legal and ethical issues in nursing* (6th ed.). Upper Saddle River, NJ: Pearson Education.

*Hadley, M. N., Walters, B. C., Aarabi, B., Dhall, S. S., Gelb, D. E., Hurlbert, R. J., Rozzelle, C. J., Ryken, T. C., & Theodore, N. (2013). Clinical assessment following acute cervical spinal cord injury. In: Guidelines for the management of acute cervical spine and spinal cord injuries. *Neurosurgery, 72*(Suppl 2), 40-53. Retrieved from doi.org/10.1227/NEU.0b013e318276edda

Harkness, G. A., & DeMarco, R. F. (2016). *Community and public health nursing: Evidence for practice* (2nd ed.). Philadelphia, PA: Wolters Kluwer.

*Hauser, R. A. (2015). Diagnosis and management of Parkinson's disease. Retrieved from emedicine.medscape.com/article/1831191-overview

*Heart Failure Society of America. (2010). Evaluation and therapy for heart failure in the setting of ischemic heart disease: HFSA 2010 comprehensive heart failure practice guideline. Available at: www.hfsa.org/heart-failure-guidelines-2/

Hinkle, J. L., & Cheever, K. H. (2017). *Brunner & Suddarth's textbook of medical-surgical nursing* (14th ed.). Philadelphia, PA: Lippincott Williams & Wilkins.

*Hooten, W. M., Timming, R., Belgrade, M., Gaul, J., Goertz, M., Haake, B., Myers, C., Noonan, M. P., Owens, J., Saeger, L., Schweim, K., Shteyman, G., & Walker, N. (2017). Pain: assessment, non-opioid treatment approaches and opioid management. *Institute for Clinical Systems Improvement*. Available at: www.icsi.org/_asset/f8rj09/Pain.pdf

Huether, S. E., McCance, K. L., Brashers, V. L., & Rote, N. S. (2016). *Understanding pathophysiology* (6th ed.). St. Louis, MO: Elsevier/Mosby.

Ignatavicius, D. D., & Workman, M. L. (2018). *Medical-surgical nursing: Patient-centered collaborative care* (9th ed.). St. Louis, MO: Elsevier/Saunders.

Ignatavicius, D. D., & Workman, M. L. (2013). *Medical-surgical nursing: Patient-centered collaborative care* (7th ed.). St. Louis, MO: Elsevier/Saunders.

*Institute for Clinical Systems Improvement (2012). Pressure ulcer prevention and treatment protocol. Health care protocol. *Institute for Clinical Systems Improvement*. Available at: www.dhs.wisconsin.gov/regulations/training/c10-h03.pdf

*Institute for Clinical Systems Improvement (2016). Diagnosis and management of asthma. *Institute for Clinical Systems Improvement*. Available at: www.icsi.org/guidelines__more/catalog_guidelines_and_more/catalog_guidelines/catalog_respiratory_guidelines/asthma/

*Institute for Clinical Systems Improvement (2017). Pain: Assessment, non-opioid treatment approaches and opioid management. *Institute for Clinical Systems Improvement*. Available at: https://www.icsi.org/guidelines__more/catalog_guidelines_and_more/catalog_guidelines/catalog_neurological_guidelines/pain/

Jarvis, C. (2016). *Physical examination and health assessment* (7th ed.). St. Louis, MO: Elsevier Saunders.

*Jones, J., Nelson, E., & Al-Hity, A. (2013). Skin grafts to improve leg ulcer healing. *Cochrane Database of Systematic Reviews*, *3*. Available at: www.cochrane.org/CD001737/WOUNDS_skin-grafts-to-improve-leg-ulcer-healing

Karch, A. M. (2016). *Focus on nursing pharmacology* (7th ed.). Philadelphia, PA: Lippincott Williams & Wilkins.

Kee, J. L., Hayes, E., & McCuistion, L. (2015). *Pharmacology: A nursing process approach* (8th ed.). St. Louis, MO: Elsevier.

*Kidney Disease: Improving Global Outcomes (KDIGO) Glomerulonephritis Work Group. (2012). KDIGO clinical practice guideline for glomerulonephritis. *Kidney international. Supplement International Society of Nephrology, 2*(2), 139-274. Available at: kdigo.org/guidelines/gn/

*Kupas, D. F., & Miller, D. D. (2010). Out-of-hospital chest escharotomy: A case series and procedure review. *Prehospital Emergency Care, 14*(3), 349-354. ISSN: 1090-3127 PMID: 20397867

LaMone, P., Burke, K. M., Bauldoff, G., & Gubrud, P. (2015). *Medical surgical nursing: Critical thinking in patient care* (6th ed.). Upper Saddle River, NJ: Pearson.

*Leas, B.F., D'Anci, K.E., Apter, A.J., Bryant- Stephens, T., Schoelles, K., & Umscheid, C.A. (2018) Effectiveness of Indoor Allergen Reduction in Management of Asthma. Comparative Effectiveness Review No. 201. (Prepared by the ECRI Institute–Penn Medicine Evidence-based Practice Center under Contract No. 290-2015-0005-I.) AHRQ Publication No. 18-EHC002-EF. Rockville, MD: Agency for Healthcare Research and Quality; February 2018. Posted final reports are located on the Effective Health Care Program. http://doi.org/10.23970/AHRQEPCCER201

Lewis, S. L., Dirksen, S. R., Heitkemper, M. M., & Bucher, L. (2017). *Medical-surgical nursing: Assessment and management of clinical problems* (10th ed.). St. Louis, MO: Elsevier/Mosby.

*Loewenstein, A., Ferencz, J. R., Lang, Y., Yeshurun, I., Pollack, A., Siegal, R., Manor, Y. (2010). Toward earlier detection of choroidal neovascularization secondary to age-related macular degeneration: Multicenter evaluation of a preferential hyperacuity perimeter designed as a home device. *Retina, 30*(7), 1058-1064.

Lowdermilk, D. L., Perry, S. E., Casion, K., & Alden, K. R. (2016). *Maternity & women's health care* (11th ed.). St. Louis, MO: Elsevier/Mosby.

*Luque, S. (2011). Levofloxacin weight-adjusted dosing and pharmacokinetic disposition in a morbidly obese patient. *Journal of Antimicrobial Chemotherapy, 66*(7), 1653-1654.

Lutz, C. A., Mazur, E. E., & Litch, N. A. (2015). *Nutrition and diet therapy* (6th ed.). Philadelphia, PA: F.A. Davis.

Mauk, K. L. (2018). *Gerontological nursing: Competencies for care* (4th ed.). Sudbury, MA: Jones & Bartlett.

*McCusker, M., Ceronsky, L., Crone, C., Epstein, H., Greene, B., Halvorson, J., Kephart, K., Mallen, E., Nosan, B., Rohr, M., Rosenberg, E., Ruff, R., Schlecht, K., & Setterlund, L. (2013). Palliative care for adults. *Institute for Clinical Systems Improvement.* Available at: www.icsi.org/_asset/k056ab/PalliativeCare.pdf

*Michigan Quality Improvement Consortium. (2018). Management of uncomplicated acute bronchitis in adults. Southfield, MI: Michigan Quality Improvement Consortium. Available at: www.mqic.org/pdf/mqic_management_of_uncomplicated_acute_bronchitis_in_adults_cpg.pdf

*Michigan Quality Improvement Consortium. (2015). Adults with systolic heart failure. Southfield, MI: *Michigan Quality Improvement Consortium.* Available at: www.mqic.org/pdf/mqic_adults_with_systolic_heart_failure_cpg.pdf

*Michigan Quality Improvement Consortium. (2016). Diagnosis and management of adults with chronic kidney disease. Southfield, MI: *Michigan Quality Improvement Consortium.* Available at: mqic.org/pdf/mqic_diagnosis_and_management_of_adults_with_chronic_kidney_disease_cpg.pdf

Miller, C. (2018). *Nursing for wellness in older adults* (9th ed.). Philadelphia, PA: Lippincott Williams & Wilkins.

*Mulvey, M. R., Bagnall, A., Johnson, M., & Marchant, M. (2013). Transcutaneous electrical nerve stimulation (TENS) for phantom pain and stump pain following amputation in adults. *Cochrane Database of Systematic Reviews,* 2013, Issue 4. Available at: www.cochranelibrary.com/cdsr/doi/10.1002/14651858.CD007264.pub3/full

*National Cancer Institute. (2013). *Blood-forming stem cell transplants.* Available at: www.cancer.gov/cancertopics/factsheet/therapy/bone-marrow-transplant

*National Cancer Institute. (2018). *Pain (PDQ®). Pharmacologic Management.* Available at: www.cancer.gov/cancertopics/pdq/supportivecare/pain/HealthProfessional/page3

*National Institute of Neurological Disorders and Stroke. (NINDS). (2015). Multiple sclerosis: Hope through research. Retrieved from www.ninds.nih.gov/Disorders/Patient-Caregiver-Education/Hope-Through-Research/Multiple-Sclerosis-Hope-Through-Research

*Nieuwlaat, R., Wilczynski, N., Navarro, T., Hobson, N., Jeffery, R., Keepanasseril, A. ..... Haynes, R. B. (2014). Interventions for enhancing medication adherence. *The Cochrane Library* 2014, Issue 11. doi:10.1002/14651858.CD000011.pub4 Available at: www.cochranelibrary.com/cdsr/doi/10.1002/14651858.CD000011.pub4/full

*Olsson Ozanne, A. G., Strang, S., & Persson, L. I. (2011). Quality of life, anxiety and depression in ALS patients and their next of kin. *Journal of Clinical Nursing, 20*(1/2), 283–291. doi:10.1111/j.1365-2702.2010.03509

Osborn, K. S., Wraa, C. E., & Watson, A. (2014). *Medical-surgical nursing: Preparation for practice* (2nd ed.). Upper Saddle River, NJ: Pearson Education.

*Overdevest, G. M., Jacobs, W., Vleggeert-Lankamp, C., Thomé, C., Gunzburg, R., & Peul, W. (2015). Effectiveness of posterior decompression techniques compared with conventional laminectomy for lumbar stenosis. *Cochrane Database of Systematic Reviews,* Issue 3. Retrieved from www.cochranelibrary.com/cdsr/doi/10.1002/14651858.CD010036.pub2/full

*Parker, M., Livingstone, V., Clifton, R., & McKee, A. (2007). Closed suction surgical wound drainage after orthopedic surgery. *Cochrane Database of Systematic Reviews,* Issue 3, Art. No. CD001825. doi:10.1002/14651858.CD001825.pub2. Available at: www.cochrane.org/reviews/en/ab001825.html

Pickar, G. D., & Abernethy, A. P. (2013). *Dosage calculations* (9th ed.). Clifton Park, NY: Thomson Delmar Learning.

Pillitteri, A. (2017). *Maternal & child health nursing: Care of the childbearing and childrearing family* (8th ed.). Philadelphia, PA: Lippincott Williams & Wilkins.

*Pinkerman, C., Sander, P., Breeding, J. E., Brink, D., Curtis, R., Hayes, R., Ojha, A., Pandita, D., Raikar, S., Setterlund, L., Sule, O., & Turner, A. (2013). Heart failure in adults. Bloomington, MN: *Institute for Clinical Systems Improvement.* Available at: citeseerx.ist.psu.edu/viewdoc/download?doi=10.1.1.657.5616&rep=rep1&type=pdf

Porth, C. M. (2015). *Essentials of pathophysiology* (4th ed.). Philadelphia, PA: Wolters Kluwer Health/Lippincott Williams & Wilkins.

Potter, P. A., Perry, A. G., Stockert, P., & Hall, A. (2017). *Fundamentals of nursing* (9th ed.). St. Louis, MO: Mosby/Elsevier.

*Registered Nurses' Association of Ontario (RNAO). (2010). Nursing care of dyspnea: the 6th vital sign in individuals with chronic obstructive pulmonary disease (COPD) 2010 supplement. Toronto, ON: RNAO. Available at: rnao.ca/bpg/guidelines/dyspnea

*Registered Nurses Association of Ontario (RNAO). (2013). Assessment and management of pain. Toronto, ON: RNAO. Available at: rnao.ca/bpg/guidelines/assessment-and-management-pain

*Ross, H., Steele, S. R., Varma, M., Dykes, S., Cima, R., Buie, W. D., & Rafferty, J. (2014). Standards Practice Task Force of the American Society of Colon and Rectal Surgeons. Practice parameters for the surgical treatment of ulcerative colitis. *Diseases of the Colon & Rectum, 57*(1), 5-22. Available at: www.fascrs.org/sites/default/files/downloads/publication/practice_parameters_for_the_surgical_treatment_of.3.pdf

*Sanders, G.D., Lowenstern, A., Borre, E., Chatterjee, R., Goode, A., Sharan, L., Allen LaPointe N.M., Raitz, G., Shah, B., Yapa, R., Davis, J.K., Lallinger, K., Schmidt, R., Kosinski, & Al-Khatib S. (2018). Stroke prevention in patients with atrial fibrillation: A systematic review update. Comparative Effectiveness Review No. 214. (Prepared by the Duke Evidence-based Practice Center under Contract No. 290-2015-00004-I for AHRQ and PCORI.) AHRQ Publication No. 18(19)-EHC018-EF. PCORI Publication No. 2018-SR-04. Rockville, MD: Agency for Healthcare Research and Quality; October 2018. Posted final reports are located on the Effective Health Care Program. https://doi.org/10.23970/AHRQEPCCER214

*Sasser, S. M., Hunt, R. C., Faul, M., Sugerman, D., Pearson, W. S., Dulski, T., Wald, M. M., Jurkovich, G. J., Newgard, C. D., Lerner, E. B., Cooper, A., Wang, S. C., Henry, M. C., Salomone, J. P., & Galli, R. L.

Centers for Disease Control and Prevention. (2012). Guidelines for field triage of injured patients: recommendations of the National Expert Panel on Field Triage, 2011. *MMWR Recommendations and Reports, 61*(RR-1), 1-20.

*Seiter, K. (2017). Acute myelogenous leukemia. *E-Medicine*. Available at: emedicine.medscape.com/article/197802-overview

*Shahedi, K., & Chudasama, Y. N. (2017). Diverticulitis. *E-Medicine Medscape*. Available at: emedicine.medscape.com/article/173388-overview

*Skelly, A.C., Chou, R., Dettori, J.R., Turner, J.A., Friedly, J.L., Rundell, S.D., Fu, R., Brodt, E.D., Wasson, N., Winter, C., & Ferguson, A.J.R. (2018) Noninvasive Nonpharmacological Treatment for Chronic Pain: A Systematic Review. Comparative Effectiveness Review No. 209. (Prepared by the Pacific Northwest Evidence-based Practice Center under Contract No. 290-2015-00009-I.) AHRQ Publication No 18-EHC013-EF. Rockville, MD: Agency for Healthcare Research and Quality; June 2018. Posted final reports are located on the Effective Health Care Program search page. https://doi.org/10.23970/AHRQEPCCER209

*Society of American Gastrointestinal and Endoscopic Surgeons. (2013). Guidelines for the management of hiatal hernia. Los Angeles, CA: *Society of American Gastrointestinal and Endoscopic Surgeons* (SAGES). Available at: www.sages.org/publications/guidelines/guidelines-for-the-management-of-hiatal-hernia/

*Sveum, R., Bergstrom, J., Brottman, G., Hanson, M., Heiman, M., Johns, K., Malkiewicz, J., Manney, S., Moyer, L., Myers, C., Myers, N., O'Brien, M., Rethwill, M., Schaefer, K., & Uden, D. (2012). Diagnosis and management of asthma. Bloomington, MN: *Institute for Clinical Systems Improvement*. Available at: www.icsi.org/_asset/rsjvnd/Asthma.pdf

Tabloski, P. A., & Connell, W. F. (2014). *Gerontological nursing* (3rd ed.). Upper Saddle River, NJ: Pearson.

Taylor, C. R., Lillis, C., & Lynn, P. (2014). *Fundamentals of nursing: The art and science of nursing care* (8th ed.). Philadelphia, PA: Lippincott Williams & Wilkins.

*Tenner, S., Baillie, J., Dewitt, J., & Vege, S. S. (2013). American College of Gastroenterology guideline: management of acute pancreatitis. *American Journal Gastroenterology, 108*(9), 1400-1415. Available at: gi.org/guideline/acute-pancreatitis/

*Thomas, D., Elliott, E., & Naughton, G. (2006). Exercise for type 2 diabetes mellitus. *Cochrane Database of Systematic Reviews*, Issue 3, Art. No. CD002968. doi:10.1002/14651858.CD002968.pub2. Available at: www.cochranelibrary.com/cdsr/doi/10.1002/14651858.CD002968.pub2/epdf/full

*Thorson, D., Biewen, P., Bonte, B., Epstein, H., Haake, B., Hansen, C., Hooten, M., Hora, J., Johnson, C., Keeling, F., Kokayeff, A., Krebs, E., Myers, C., Nelson, B., Noonan, M.P., Reznikoff, C., Thiel, M., Trujillo, A., Van Pelt, S., Wainio, J. (2014). Acute pain assessment and opioid prescribing protocol. *Institute for Clinical Systems Improvement*. Available at: crh.arizona.edu/sites/default/files/u35/Opioids.pdf

Touhy, T. A., & Jett, K. F. (2018). *Ebersole and Hess' gerontological nursing and healthy aging* (5th ed.). St. Louis, MO: Mosby/Elsevier.

Treas, L. S., & Wilkinson, J. M. (2018). *Basic nursing: Concepts, skills, and reasoning* (2nd ed.). Philadelphia, PA: F.A. Davis.

*U.S. Department of Health and Human Services, Centers for Disease Control and Prevention. (2014). *National diabetes statistics report, 2014*. Available at: www.cdc.gov/diabetes/pdfs/data/2014-report-estimates-of-diabetes-and-its-burden-in-the-united-states.pdf

*U.S. Preventive Services Task Force. (2014). Behavioral counseling interventions to prevent sexually transmitted infections: U.S. Preventive Services Task Force recommendation statement. *Annals Internal Medicine. 161*(12):894-901.

*U.S. Preventive Services Task Force. (2014). Screening for chlamydia and gonorrhea: U.S. Preventive Services Task Force recommendation statement. *Annals Internal Medicine. 161*(12):902-910. Available at: www.uspreventiveservicestaskforce.org/Home/GetFile/1/1188/gonchlamfinalrec/pdf

*University of Michigan Health System. (2011). *Osteoporosis: Prevention and treatment*. Ann Arbor, MI: University of Michigan Health System. Available at: www.med.umich.edu/1info/FHP/practiceguides/osteoporosis/text.pdf

*University of Michigan Health System. (2013). *Allergic rhinitis*. Ann Arbor, MI: University of Michigan Health System. Available at: www.med.umich.edu/1info/FHP/practiceguides/allergic/allergic.pdf

*University of Michigan Health System. (2013). *Otitis media*. Ann Arbor, MI: University of Michigan Health System. Available at: ocpd.med.umich.edu/sites/default/files/guidelines/OM.pdf

Vallerand, A. H., Sanoski, C. A., & Deglin, J. H. (2019). *Davis's drug guide for nurses* (16th ed.). Philadelphia, PA: F.A. Davis.

Van Leeuwen, A. M., & Bladh, M. L. (2017). Davis's comprehensive handbook of laboratory and diagnostic tests with nursing implications (8th ed.). Philadelphia, PA: F.A. Davis.

Wilkinson, J., & Treas, L. (2011). *Fundamentals of nursing. Volume 2: Thinking, doing, and caring* (2nd ed.). Philadelphia, PA: F.A. Davis.

Wilkinson, J. M., & Treas, L. S. (2011). *Fundamentals of nursing: Theory, concepts, & application* (2nd ed.). Philadelphia, PA: F.A. Davis.

Wilson, B. A., Shannon, M. T., & Shields, K. M. (2015). *Pearson nurse's drug guide 2015*. Upper Saddle River, NJ: Pearson Education.

*Woolley, T., Canoniero, M., Conroy, W., Fareed, M., Groen, S., Helmrick, K., Kofron, P., Kottke, T., Leslie, S., Myers, C., Needham, R., O'Connor, P., Peters, J., Reddan, J., Sorge, L., & Zerr, B. (2017). Lipid management in adults. Bloomington, MN: *Institute for Clinical Systems Improvement*. Available at: www.icsi.org/_asset/qz5ydq/LipidMgmt.pdf

*World Health Organization. (2018). *Hepatitis B fact sheet*. Available at: www.who.int/mediacentre/factsheets/fs204/en/

*Young, K. A., Snell-Bergeon, J. K., Naik, R. G., Hokanson, J. E., Tarullo, D., & Gottlieb P. A., et al. (2011). Vitamin D deficiency and coronary artery calcification in subjects with type 1 diabetes. *Diabetes Care, 34*(2), 454-458.

---

*Evidence-based Reference

# Unit 5: Care of Children and Families

Adams, M., Holland, L., & Urban, C. (2017). *Pharmacology for nurses: A pathophysiologic approach* (5th ed.). Upper Saddle River, NJ: Prentice Hall.

*American Academy of Ophthalmology Pediatric Ophthalmology/Strabismus Panel. (2017). *Esotropia and exotropia*. San Francisco, CA: American Academy of Ophthalmology. Available at: www.aao.org/Assets/49451021-c413-437e-8e38-d975f9f563f6/636492808642570000/esotropia-and-exotropia-final-12-19-17-pdf

*American Diabetes Association, Clarke, W., Deeb, L. C., Jameson, P., Kaufman, F., Klingensmith, G., Schatz, D., Silverstein, J. H., & Siminerio, L. M. (2013). Diabetes care in the school and day care setting. *Diabetes Care, 36*(Suppl 1), S75-S79. Available at: www.ncbi.nlm.nih.gov/pmc/articles/PMC3006056/?report=reader

*American Diabetes Association. (2013). Standards of medical care in diabetes – 2013. *Diabetes Care, 36*(Suppl), S11-S66.

*American Heart Association. (2011). *BLS for healthcare providers manual*. United States of America: American Heart Association.

Aschenbrenner, D. S., & Venable, S. J. (2013). *Drug therapy in nursing* (4th ed.). Philadelphia, PA: Lippincott Williams & Wilkins.

Ball, J., Bindler, R., & Cowen, K. J. (2012). *Clinical skills manual for principles of pediatric nursing: Caring for children* (5th ed.). Upper Saddle River, NJ: Pearson Education.

Ball, J. W., Bindler, R. C., & Cowen, K. J. (2015). *Principles of pediatric nursing: Caring for children* (6th ed.). Upper Saddle River, NJ: Pearson Education.

Berman, A., Snyder, S., & Frandsen, G. (2016). *Kozier & Erb's fundamentals of nursing* (10th ed.). Upper Saddle River, NJ: Pearson Education.

*Bevan, A. L., & Reilly, S. M. (2011). Mothers' efforts to promote healthy nutrition and physical activity for their preschool children. *Journal of Pediatric Nursing*. doi:10.1016/j.pedn.2010.11.008

*Bonifant, C. M., Shevill, E., & Chang, A. B. (2014). The use of regular vitamin A preparations for children and adults with cystic fibrosis. *Cochrane Database of Systematic Reviews*, Issue 2, Art. No. CD006751. doi:10.1002/14651858.CD006751.pub4. Available at: www.cochrane.org/CD006751/CF_use-regular-vitamin-or-vitamin-preparations-children-and-adults-cystic-fibrosis

Bowden, V. R., Greenberg, C. S. (2013). *Children and their families: The continuum of care* (3rd ed.). Philadelphia, PA: Wolters Kluwer Lippincott Williams & Wilkins.

Burchum, J., & Rosenthal, L. (2016). *Lehne's pharmacology for nursing care* (9th ed.). St. Louis, MO: Saunders Elsevier.

*Centers for Disease Control and Prevention. (2018). *Vaccine storage and handling: Recommendations and guidelines*. Available at: www.cdc.gov/vaccines/recs/storage/default.htm; www.cdc.gov/vaccines/hcp/admin/storage/toolkit/storage-handling-toolkit.pdf

*Centers for Disease Control and Prevention. (2018). *Tuberculosis*. Available at: www.cdc.gov/tb/default.htm

*Centers for Disease Control and Prevention. (2018). *Vaccine information statements (VIS) meningococcal VIS*. Available at: www.cdc.gov/vaccines/hcp/vis/vis-statements/mening.html

*Centers for Disease Control and Prevention. (2012). *Top CDC recommendations to prevent healthcare-associated infections*. Available at: www.cdc.gov/HAI/pdfs/hai/top-cdc-recs-factsheet.pdf

*Centers for Disease Control and Prevention. (2018). *Human papillomavirus (HPV) vaccine*. Available at: www.cdc.gov/vaccinesafety/Vaccines/HPV/Index.html

*Centers for Disease Control and Prevention. (2017). *Human papillomavirus (HPV)*. Available at: www.cdc.gov/std/hpv/default.htm#vaccine

*Centers for Disease Control and Prevention. (2018). *Recommended immunization schedules for persons aged 0 through 18 years United States, 2015*. Available at: www.cdc.gov/vaccines/schedules/downloads/child/0-18yrs-child-combined-schedule.pdf

*Cincinnati Children's Hospital Medical Center. (2011). *Evidence-based care guideline for prevention and management of acute gastroenteritis (AGE) in children aged 2 months to 18 years*. Cincinnati, OH: Cincinnati Children's Hospital Medical Center. Available at: www.cincinnatichildrens.org/-/media/cincinnati%20childrens/home/service/j/anderson-center/evidence-based-care/recommendations/type/gastroenteritis-care-guideline

*Cincinnati Children's Hospital Medical Center. Best evidence statement. (2011). *Use of Lactobacillus rhamnosus GG in children with acute gastroenteritis*. Cincinnati, OH: Cincinnati Children's Hospital Medical Center. Available at: www.cincinnatichildrens.org/-/media/cincinnati%20childrens/home/professional/resources/physician-services/toolkit/section-g/section-g-accordion-probiotics—acute-gastroenteritis

*Committee on Infectious Diseases and Bronchiolitis: Guidelines Committee. (2014). Updated guidance for palivizumab prophylaxis among infants and young children at increased risk of hospitalization for respiratory syncytial virus infection. *Pediatrics, 134*(2), 415-420. doi:10.1542/peds.2014-1665.

Davidson, M., London, M., & Ladewig, P. A. (2016). *Olds' maternal-newborn nursing & women's health across the lifespan* (10th ed.). Upper Saddle River, NJ: Pearson Education.

*Department of Health and Human Services, Centers for Disease Control and Prevention (2018). *Recommended immunization schedule for persons aged 0 through 18 Years*. Available at: www.cdc.gov/vaccines/schedules/hcp/imz/child-adolescent.html

*Dupuis, L. L., Robinson, P. D., Boodhan, S., Holdsworth, M., Portwine, C., Gibson, P., Phillips, R., Maan, C., Stefin, N., & Sung, L. (2014). *Guideline for the prevention and treatment of anticipatory nausea and vomiting due to chemotherapy in pediatric cancer patients*. Toronto, ON: Pediatric Oncology Group of Ontario. Available at: doi.org/10.1002/pbc.25063

Frandsen, G., & Pennington, S., (2018). *Abrams' clinical drug therapy: Rationales for nursing practice* (11th ed.). Philadelphia, PA: Lippincott Williams & Wilkins.

*Griffin, G., & Flynn, C. A. (2011). Antihistamines and/or decongestants for otitis media with effusion (OME) in children. *Cochrane Database Syst Rev*, Sep 7. 9:CD003423.

*Guandalini, S., & Vallee, P. A. (2017). *Pediatric celiac disease*. Available at: emedicine.medscape.com/article/932104-overview

*Harris, D. J., Eilers, J., Harriman, A., Cashavelly, B. J., & Maxwell. C. (2014). Putting evidence into practice: Evidence-based interventions for the management of oral mucositis. Available at: cjon.ons.org/file/17456/download

Hockenberry, M. J., & Wilson, D. (2015). *Wong's nursing care of infants and children* (10th ed.). St. Louis, MO: Elsevier.

*Institute for Safe Medication Practices. (2018). *ISMP's list of high-alert medications in acute care settings*. Available at: www.ismp.org/Tools/highalertmedications.pdf

Karch, A. M. (2016). *Focus on nursing pharmacology* (7th ed.). Philadelphia, PA: Lippincott Williams & Wilkins.

Kee, J. L., Hayes, E., & McCuistion, L. (2014). *Pharmacology: A nursing process approach* (8th ed.). St. Louis, MO: Elsevier.

Kyle, T., & Carman, S. (2016). *Essentials of pediatric nursing* (3rd ed.). Philadelphia, PA: Wolters Kluwer Heath/Lippincott Williams & Wilkins.

*Lieberthal, A. S., Carroll, A. E., Chonmaitree, T., Ganiats, T. G., Hoberman, A., Jackson, M. A., Joffe, M. D., Miller, D. T., Rosenfeld, R. M., Sevilla, X. D., Schwartz, R. H., Thomas, P. A., & Tunkel, D. E. (2013). The diagnosis and management of acute otitis media. *Pediatrics, 131*(3):e964-e999.

McKee, C., & Bohannon, K. (2016). Exploring the reasons behind parental refusal of vaccines. Journal Pediatric Pharmacological Therapy, *21*(2), 104–109. doi:10.5863/1551-6776-21.2.104

*Michigan Quality Improvement Consortium Guideline. (2015). Acute pharyngitis in children 2-18 years old. Southfield, MI: *Michigan Quality Improvement Consortium Guideline*. Available at: www.mqic.org/pdf/mqic_acute_pharyngitis_in_children_2to18_years_old_cpg.pdf

*Michigan Quality Improvement Consortium. (2016). General principles for the diagnosis and management of asthma. Southfield, MI: *Michigan Quality Improvement Consortium*. Available at: www.mqic.org/pdf/mqic_general_principles_for_the_diagnosis_and_management_of_asthma_cpg.pdf

*Michigan Quality Improvement Consortium. (2017). Routine preventive services for children and adolescents (ages 2-21). Southfield, MI: *Michigan Quality Improvement Consortium*. Available at: mqic.org/pdf/mqic_routine_preventive_services_for_children_and_adolescents_ages_2_to_21_cpg.pdf

*National Heart, Lung, and Blood Institute. (2012). *Asthma care quick reference: Diagnosing and managing asthma*. Available at: www.nhlbi.nih.gov/health-pro/guidelines/current/asthma-guidelines/quick-reference

Perry, S. E., Hockenberry, M. J., Lowdermilk, D. L., & Wilson, D. (2014). *Maternal child nursing care* (5th ed.). St. Louis, MO: Elsevier/Mosby.

Pickar, G. D., & Abernethy, A. P. (2013). *Dosage calculations* (9th ed.). Clifton Park, NY: Thomson Delmar Learning.

Pillitteri, A. (2017). *Maternal & child health nursing: Care of the childbearing and childrearing family* (8th ed.). Philadelphia, PA: Lippincott Williams & Wilkins.

Porth, C. M. (2015). *Essentials of pathophysiology* (4th ed.). Philadelphia, PA: Wolters Kluwer Health/Lippincott Williams & Wilkins.

Potts, N. L., & Mandleco, B. L. (2012). *Pediatric nursing: Caring for children and their families*. Clifton Park, NY: Delmar/Cengage Learning.

*Ranmal, R., Prictor, M., & Scott, J. (2012). Ways of improving communication with children and adolescents about their cancer. *Cochrane*. Available at: www.cochrane.org/CD002969/COMMUN_ways-of-improving-communication-with-children-and-adolescents-about-their-cancer

*Reisfield, G., Salazar, E., & Bertholf, R. (2007). Rational use and interpretation of urine drug testing in chronic opioid therapy. *Annals of Clinical Laboratory Science, 37*(4), 301–314.

Ricci, S. S., Kyle, T., Carman, S. (2013). *Maternity and pediatric nursing* (2nd ed.). Philadelphia, PA: Wolters Kluwer Lippincott Williams & Wilkins.

*Simpson, S. A., Lewis, R., van der Voort, J., & Butler, C. C. Oral or topical nasal steroids for hearing loss associated with otitis media with effusion in children. *Cochrane Database Syst Rev.* 2011 May 11. CD001935.

*Snellman, L., Adams, W., Anderson, G., Godfrey, A., Gravley, A., Johnson, K., Marshall, P., Myers, C., Nesse, R., Short S. (2017). *Diagnosis and treatment of respiratory illness in children and adults.* Bloomington, MN: Institute for Clinical Systems Improvement. Available at: www.icsi.org/_asset/pwyrky/RespIllness.pdf

*Subcommittee on Urinary Tract Infection, Steering Committee on Quality. (2011). Urinary tract infection: Clinical practice guideline for the diagnosis and management of the initial UTI in febrile infants and children 2 to 24 months. *Pediatrics, 128*(3):595-610.

*Szajewska, H., Chmielewska, A., Piescik-Lech, M., Ivarsson, A., Kolacek, S., Koletzko, S., Auricchio, R., & Troncone, R. (2012). Systematic review: Early infant feeding and the prevention of coeliac disease. *Alimentary Pharmacology & Therapeutics, 36*(7):607-618.

Vallerand, A. H., Sanoski, C. A., & Deglin, J. H. (2019). *Davis's drug guide for nurses* (16th ed.). Philadelphia, PA: F.A. Davis.

Van Leeuwen, A. M., & Bladh, M. L. (2017). Davis's comprehensive handbook of laboratory and diagnostic tests with nursing implications (8th ed.). Philadelphia, PA: F.A. Davis.

Wilson, B. A., Shannon, M. T., & Shields, K. M. (2015). *Pearson nurse's drug guide 2015.* Upper Saddle River, NJ: Pearson Education.

---

*Evidence-based Reference

## Unit 6: Care of Individuals With Mental Health Disorders

Adams, M., Holland, L., & Urban, C. (2017). *Pharmacology for nurses: A pathophysiologic approach* (5th ed.). Upper Saddle River, NJ: Prentice Hall.

*American Psychiatric Association (2010). *Practice guideline for the treatment of patients with major depressive disorder* (3rd ed.). Arlington, VA: American Psychiatric Association (APA).

*Assessment and Management of Risk for Suicide Working Group. (2013). *VA/DoD clinical practice guideline for assessment and management of patients at risk for suicide.* Washington (DC): Department of Veterans Affairs, Department of Defense. Available at: www.healthquality. va.gov/guidelines/MH/srb/VADODCP_SuicideRisk_Full.pdf

Boyd, M. A. (2017). *Psychiatric nursing: Contemporary practice* (6th ed.). Philadelphia, PA: Lippincott Williams & Wilkins.

Burchum, J., & Rosenthal, L. (2016). *Lehne's pharmacology for nursing care* (9th ed.). St. Louis, MO: Saunders Elsevier.

*Butler, M., Urosevic, S., Desai, P., Sponheim, S.R., Popp, J., Nelson, V.A., Thao, V., & Sunderlin. B. (2018). Treatment for Bipolar Disorder in Adults: A Systematic Review. Comparative Effectiveness Review No. 208. (Prepared by the Minnesota Evidence-based Practice Center under Contract No. 290-2012-00016-I.) AHRQ Publication No. 18-EHC012-EF. Rockville, MD: *Agency for Healthcare Research and Quality*; August 2018. Posted final reports are located on the Effective Health Care Program. doi: https://doi.org/10.23970/AHRQEPCCER208

*Center for Behavior Health Statistics and Quality. (2015). Suicidal thoughts and behaviors among adults. Results from the 2014 National Survey on Drug Use and Health. Available at: www.samhsa.gov/data/sites/default/files/NSDUH-DR-FFR3-2015/NSDUH-DR-FFR3-2015.htm

*Department of Health and Human Services. (2013). Administration on Children, Youth, and Families. *Children Maltreatment.* Available at: www.acf.hhs.gov/sites/default/files/cb/cm2013.pdf

Fortinash, K., & Holoday Worret, P. (2015). *Psychiatric mental health nursing-Revised Reprint* (5th ed.). St. Louis, MO: Mosby/Elsevier.

*Hall, G. R., Gallagher, M., & Hoffmann-Snyder, C. (2013). *Bathing persons with dementia.* Iowa City (IA): University of Iowa College of Nursing, John A. Hartford Foundation Center of Geriatric Nursing Excellence. Available at: doi.org/10.3928/00989134-20131220-01

Halter, M. J. (2014). V*arcarolis' foundations of psychiatric mental health nursing* (7th ed.). St. Louis, MO: Saunders/Elsevier.

*Handford, C., Kahan, M., Srivastava, A., Cirone, S., Sanghera, S., Palda, V., Lester, M.D., Janecek, E., Franklyn, M., Cord, M., Selby, P., & Ordean, A. (2011). *Buprenorphine/naloxone for opioid dependence: Clinical practice guideline.* Toronto, ON: Centre for Addiction and Mental Health. Available at: www.cpso.on.ca/uploadedFiles/policies/guidelines/office/buprenorphine_naloxone_gdlns2011.pdf

*James, A. C., James, G., Cowdrey, F. A., Soler, A., & Choke, A. (2015). Cognitive behavioral therapy for anxiety disorders in children and adolescents. *Cochrane Database of Systematic Reviews.* doi:10.1002/14651858.CD004690.pub4. Available at: www.cochranelibrary.com/cdsr/doi/10.1002/14651858.CD004690.pub4/full

*Jones, J. D., Mogali, S., & Comer, S. D. (2012). Polydrug abuse: A review of opioid and benzodiazepine combination use. *Drug and Alcohol Dependence, 125*(1–2), 8–18.

Karch, A. M. (2016). *Focus on nursing pharmacology* (7th ed.). Philadelphia, PA: Lippincott Williams & Wilkins.

Lesser, I. M., Myers, H. F., Lin, K. M., Bingham, C. M., Joseph, N, T, Olmos, N. T., Phil, C., Schettino, J., & Poland, R. E. (2010). Ethnic differences in antidepressant response: a prospective multi site clinical trial. *Depression and Anxiety*, 27(1), 56–62. doi: 10.1002/da.20619

Meiner, S. E. (2015). *Gerontologic nursing* (5th ed.). St. Louis, MO: Mosby/Elsevier.

*Michigan Quality Improvement Consortium. (2013). *Screening, diagnosis and referral for substance use disorders.* Southfield, MI: Michigan Quality Improvement Consortium. Available at: www.guideline.gov/content.aspx?id=47911

*Michigan Quality Improvement Consortium. (2018). Primary care diagnosis and management of adults with depression. Southfield, MI: Michigan Quality Improvement Consortium. Available at: mqic.org/pdf/mqic_primary_care_diagnosis_and_management_of_adults_with_depression_cpg.pdf

Mohr, W. (2012). *Psychiatric mental health nursing: Evidence-based concepts, skills, and practices* (8th ed.). Philadelphia, PA: Lippincott Williams and Wilkins.

*Naegle, M. A. (2012). Try this: Best practices in nursing care to older adults. *Alcohol Use Screening and Assessment for Older Adults.* New York University: Hartford Institute for Geriatric Nursing. Available at: consultgeri.org/try-this/general-assessment/issue-17.pdf

O'Brien, P. G., Kennedy, W. Z., & Ballard, K. A. (2013). *Psychiatric mental health nursing: An introduction to theory and practice* (2nd ed.). Burlington, MA: Jones & Bartlett Learning.

Pickar, G. D., & Abernethy, A. P. (2013). *Dosage calculations* (9th ed.). Clifton Park, NY: Thomson Delmar Learning.

Shives, R. (2011). *Basic concepts of psychiatric—mental health nursing* (8th ed.). Philadelphia, PA: Wolters Kluwer /Lippincott Williams & Wilkins.

Stuart, G. (2013). *Principles and practice of psychiatric nursing* (10th ed.). St. Louis, MO: Elsevier/Mosby.

*Substance Abuse and Mental Health Administration. (2014). Benzodiazepines in combination with opioid pain relievers or alcohol: Greater risk of more serious ED visit outcomes. Available at: www.samhsa.gov/data/sites/default/files/DAWN-SR192-BenzoCombos-2014/DAWN-SR192-BenzoCombos-2014.pdf

*Substance Abuse and Mental Health Services Administration. (2011). Managing chronic pain in adults with or in recovery from substance use disorders. HHS publication no. (SMA) 12-4671. Rockville (MD): Substance Abuse and Mental Health Services Administration. Available at: www.ncbi.nlm.nih.gov/books/NBK92048/

Townsend, M. (2018). *Psychiatric mental health nursing; Concepts of care in evidence-based practice* (9th ed.). Philadelphia: F.A. Davis.

Townsend, M. C. (2017). *Essentials of psychiatric mental health nursing* (7th ed.). Philadelphia, PA: F.A. Davis.

*U.S. Department of Health and Human Services. Substance Abuse and Mental Health Services Administration. (2013). *Results from the 2013 National Survey on Drug Use and Health: Summary of national*

*findings.* Available at: www.samhsa.gov/data/sites/default/files/ NSDUHresultsPDFWHTML2013/Web/NSDUHresults2013.pdf

*U.S. Department of Justice, Drug Enforcement Agency. (2015). *Drug addiction in health care professionals.* Washington, DC. Available at: www.deadiversion.usdoj.gov/pubs/brochures/drug_hc.htm

*U.S. Preventive Services Task Force. (2013). Screening and behavioral counseling interventions in primary care to reduce alcohol misuse: U.S. Preventive Services Task Force recommendation statement. *Ann Intern Med, 159*(3):210-218. Available at: www.uspreventiveservicestaskforce. org/Page/Document/UpdateSummaryFinal/alcohol-misuse-screening- and-behavioral-counseling-interventions-in-primary-care

*U.S. Preventive Services Task Force. (2013). Primary care interventions to prevent child maltreatment: U.S. Preventive Services Task Force recommendation statement. *Ann Intern Med, 159*(4):289-295. Available at: annals.org/aim/fullarticle/1696071/primary-care-interventions- prevent-child-maltreatment-u-s-preventive-services

*U.S. Preventive Services Task Force. (2013). Screening for intimate partner violence and abuse of elderly and vulnerable adults: U.S. Preventive Services Task Force recommendation statement. *Ann Intern Med, 158*(6):478-486. Available at: annals.org/aim/fullarticle/1558517/ screening-intimate-partner-violence-abuse-elderly-vulnerable-adults-u-s

U.S. Preventive Services Task Force. (2014). Primary care behavioral inter- ventions to reduce illicit drug and nonmedical pharmaceutical use in children and adolescents: U.S. Preventive Services Task Force recom- mendation statement. *Ann Intern Med, 160*(9):634-639. Available at: annals.org/aim/fullarticle/1840850/primary-care-behavioral- interventions-reduce-illicit-drug-nonmedical-pharmaceutical-use

*University of Michigan Health System. (2011). *Depression.* Ann Arbor, MI: University of Michigan Health System. Available at: www. med.umich.edu/1info/FHP/practiceguides/depress/depress.pdf

*University of Michigan Health System. (2013). *Attention-deficit hyperactivity disorder.* Ann Arbor, MI: University of Michigan Health System. Available at: www.med.umich.edu/1info/FHP/ practiceguides/adhd/adhd.pdf

Vallerand, A. H., Sanoski, C. A., & Deglin, J. H. (2019). *Davis's drug guide for nurses* (16th ed.). Philadelphia, PA: F.A. Davis.

Videbeck, S. (2014). *Psychiatric–mental health nursing* (6th ed.). Philadelphia, PA: Wolters Kluwer/Lippincott Williams & Wilkins.

Wilson, B. A., Shannon, M. T., & Shields, K. M. (2015). *Pearson nurse's drug guide 2015.* Upper Saddle River, NJ: Pearson Education.

---

*Evidence-based Reference

# SECTION III: COMPREHENSIVE TESTS

*Academy of Nutrition and Dietetics. (2014). Prevention of type 2 diabetes evidence-based nutrition practice guideline. Chicago (IL): Academy of Nutrition and Dietetics. Available at: www.andeal.org/topic.cfm? menu=5344

*American Academy of Ophthalmology Pediatric Ophthalmology/ Strabismus Panel. (2017). Pediatric eye evaluations: I. Vision screening in the primary care and community setting. II. Comprehensive oph- thalmic examination. San Francisco, CA: American Academy of Ophthalmology. Available at: doi.org/10.1016/j.ophtha.2017.09.032

*American Academy of Orthopaedic Surgeons. (2014). American Academy of Orthopaedic Surgeons clinical practice guideline on management of hip fractures in the elderly. Rosemont (IL): American Academy of Orthopaedic Surgeons (AAOS). Available at: www.aaos.org/cc_files/ aaosorg/research/guidelines/hipfxguideline.pdf

*American Academy of Orthopaedic Surgeons. (2013). American Academy of Orthopaedic Surgeons appropriate use criteria for non-arthroplasty treatment of osteoarthritis of the knee. Rosemont (IL): AAOS. Available at: www.aaos.org/research/Appropriate_Use/oakaucfull.pdf

*American College of Obstetricians and Gynecologists. (2014). Improving medication safety. *ACOG.* Available at: www.acog.org/Clinical- Guidance-and-Publications/Committee-Opinions/Committee-on- Patient-Safety-and-Quality-Improvement/Improving-Medication- Safety

Aschenbrenner, D. S., & Venable, S. J. (2013). *Drug therapy in nursing* (4th ed.). Philadelphia, PA: Lippincott Williams & Wilkins.

Ball, J. W., Bindler, R. C., & Cowen, K. J. (2015). *Principles of pediatric nursing: Caring for children* (6th ed.). Upper Saddle River, NJ: Pearson Education.

Berman, A., Snyder, S., & Frandsen, G. (2016). *Kozier & Erb's fundamen- tals of nursing* (10th ed.). Upper Saddle River, NJ: Pearson Education.

Burchum, J., & Rosenthal, L. (2016). *Lehne's pharmacology for nursing care* (9th ed.). St. Louis, MO: Saunders Elsevier.

Catalano, J. T. (2015). *Nursing now! Today's issues, tomorrow's trends* (7th ed.). Philadelphia, PA: F.A. Davis.

*Centers for Disease Control and Prevention. (2015). *National Notifiable Diseases Surveillance System (NNDSS).* Available at: www.cdc.gov/ nndss/

*Committee on Substance Use, Prevention. Medication-Assisted Treatment of Adolescents with Opioid Use Disorders. *Pediatrics.* 2016 2016/9;138(3). doi:10.1542/peds.2016-1893

*Connor, T., & McDiarmid, M. (2009). Preventing occupational exposures to antineoplastic drugs in health care settings. Available at: onlinelibrary.wiley.com/doi/full/10.3322/canjclin.56.6.354

Craven, R. F., Hirnle, C. H., & Jensen, S. (2013). *Fundamentals of nursing: Human health and function* (7th ed.). Philadelphia, PA: Lippincott Williams & Wilkins.

Davidson, M., London, M., & Ladewig, P. A. (2016). *Olds' maternal- newborn nursing & women's health across the lifespan* (10th ed.). Upper Saddle River, NJ: Pearson Education.

*Department of Health and Human Services, Centers for Disease Control and Prevention (2018). *Recommended immunization schedule for persons aged 0 through 18 years.* Available at: www.cdc.gov/vaccines/ schedules/hcp/imz/child-adolescent.html

Doenges, M., Moorhouse, M., & Murr, A. (2014). *Nursing care plans: Guidelines for individualizing client care across the life span* (9th ed). Philadelphia, PA: F.A. Davis.

*Dumville, J.C., McFarlane, E., Edwards, P., Lipp, A., & Holmes, A. (2015). Preoperative skin antiseptics for preventing surgical wound infections after clean surgery. *The Cochrane Collaboration.* doi:10.1002/ 14651858.CD003949.pub3. Available at: www.cochranelibrary.com/ cdsr/doi/10.1002/14651858.CD003949.pub4/full

*Dupras, D., Bluhm, J., Felty, C., Hansen, C., Johnson, T., Lim, K., Maddali, S., Marshall, P., Messner, P., & Skeik, N. (2009). Venous thromboembolism diagnosis and treatment. *Institute for Clinical Systems Improvement.* Available at: lnx.mednemo.it/wp-content/ uploads/2008/10/icsi652.pdf

*Flint, A., New, K., & Davies, M. W. (2017). Cup feeding versus other forms of supplemental enteral feeding for newborn infants unable to fully breastfeed. *Cochrane Database of Systematic Reviews.* Available at: https://www.cochranelibrary.com/cdsr/doi/10.1002/14651858. CD005092.pub3/epdf/full

Fortinash, K., & Holoday Worret, P. (2015). *Psychiatric mental health nursing-Revised Reprint* (5th ed.). St. Louis, MO: Mosby/Elsevier.

*Goertz, M., Thorson, D., Bonsell, J., Bonte, B., Campbell, R., Haake, B., Johnson, K., Kramer, C., Mueller, B., Peterson, S., Setterlund, L., & Timming, R. (2012). Adult acute and subacute low back pain. *Institute for Clinical Systems Improvement.* Available at: www.healthpartners. com/ucm/groups/public/@hp/@public/documents/documents/cntrb_ 035022.pdf

Halter, M. J. (2014). *Varcarolis' foundations of psychiatric mental health nursing* (7th ed.). St. Louis, MO: Saunders/Elsevier.

Hinkle, J. L., & Cheever, K. H. (2017). *Brunner & Suddarth's textbook of medical-surgical nursing* (14th ed.). Philadelphia, PA: Lippincott Williams & Wilkins.

Hockenberry, M. J., & Wilson, D. (2019). *Wong's nursing care of infants and children* (11th ed.). St. Louis, MO: Elsevier.

Huether, S. E., McCance, K. L., Brashers, V. L., & Rote, N. S. (2016). *Un- derstanding pathophysiology* (6th ed.). St. Louis, MO: Elsevier/Mosby.

Ignatavicius, D. D., & Workman, M. L. (2018). *Medical-surgical nursing: Patient-centered collaborative care* (9th ed.). St. Louis, MO: Elsevier/ Saunders.

*Institute for Clinical Systems Improvement. (2013). *Palliative care.* Available at: www.icsi.org/_asset/k056ab/PalliativeCare.pdf

*Institute for Healthcare Improvement. (2018). Rapid response teams. Available at: www.ihi.org/Topics/RapidResponseTeams/Pages/default.aspx

*Institute for Safe Medicine Practices (ISMP). (2015). ISMP's List of Confused Drug Names. *ISMP.* Available at: www.ismp.org/tools/confuseddrugnames.pdf

Jones, S. A. (2008). *ECG success: Exercises in ECG interpretation.* Philadelphia, PA: F.A. Davis.

Karch, A. M. (2016). *Focus on nursing pharmacology* (7th ed.). Philadelphia, PA: Lippincott Williams & Wilkins.

Kyle, T., & Carman, S. (2016). *Essentials of pediatric nursing* (3rd ed.). Philadelphia, PA: Wolters Kluwer Heath/Lippincott Williams & Wilkins.

*Leucht, S., Helfer, B., Dold, M., Kissling, W., & McGrath, J. J. (2015). Lithium for schizophrenia. *Cochrane Database of Systematic Reviews.* doi:10.1002/14651858.CD003834.pub3. Available at: www.cochranelibrary.com/cdsr/doi/10.1002/14651858.CD003834.pub3/full

Lewis, S. L., Dirksen, S. R., Heitkemper, M. M., & Bucher, L. (2014). *Medical-surgical nursing: Assessment and management of clinical problems* (9th ed.). St. Louis, MO: Elsevier/Mosby.

*López Briz, E., Garcia, V.R., Cabello, J. B., Bort_Martí, S., Sanchis, R. C., & Burls, A. (2018). Heparin versus 0.9% sodium chloride locking for prevention of occlusion in central venous catheters in adults. *Cochrane Database of Systematic Reviews* Available at https://www.cochranelibrary.com/cdsr/doi/10.1002/14651858.CD008462.pub3/epdf/full

Lutz, C. A., Mazur, E. E., & Litch, N. A. (2019). *Nutrition and diet therapy* (7th ed.). Philadelphia, PA: F.A. Davis.

Mohr, W. (2012). *Psychiatric mental health nursing: Evidence-based concepts, skills, and practices* (8th ed.). Philadelphia, PA: Lippincott Williams and Wilkins.

*Moore E. R., Anderson, G. C., Bergman N., & Dowswell, T. (2012). Early skin-to-skin contact for mothers and their healthy newborn infants. *The Cochrane Collaboration, 2012,* 5. Available at: www.cochranelibrary.com/cdsr/doi/10.1002/14651858.CD003519.pub3/epdf/full

Pickar, G. D., & Abernethy, A. P. (2013). *Dosage calculations* (9th ed.). Clifton Park, NY: Thomson Delmar Learning.

Pillitteri, A. (2017). *Maternal & child health nursing: Care of the childbearing and childrearing family* (8th ed.). Philadelphia, PA: Lippincott Williams & Wilkins.

Potter, P. A., Perry, A. G., Stockert, P., & Hall, A. (2017). *Fundamentals of nursing* (9th ed.). St. Louis, MO: Mosby/Elsevier.

Stuart, G. (2013). *Principles and practice of psychiatric nursing* (10th ed.). St. Louis, MO: Elsevier/Mosby.

*Substance Abuse and Mental Health Services Administration. (2011). Addressing viral hepatitis in people with substance use disorders. HHS publication no. (SMA) 11-4656. Rockville (MD): Substance Abuse and Mental Health Services Administration. Available at: www.ncbi.nlm.nih.gov/books/NBK92036/

*Tabbers, M. M., DiLorenzo, C., Berger, M. Y., Faure, C., Langendam, M. W., Nurko, S., Staiano, A., Vandenplas, Y., & Benninga, M. A. (2014). Evaluation and treatment of functional constipation in infants and children: Evidence-based recommendations from ESPGHAN and NASPGHAN. *J Pediatr Gastroenterol Nutr, 58*(2):258-274.

*The Joint Commission. (2018). *National patient safety goals.* Retrieved from www.jointcommission.org/assets/1/6/2018_HAP_NPSG_goals_final.pdf

*The Joint Commission. (2018). Facts about the Official "Do Not Use" List of Abbreviations. The Joint Commission. Available at: www.jointcommission.org/facts_about_do_not_use_list/

*The National Coordinating Council for Medication Error Reporting and Prevention. (2018). Available at: www.nccmerp.org/

Townsend, M. C. (2017). *Essentials of psychiatric mental health nursing* (7th ed.). Philadelphia, PA: F.A. Davis.

Treas, L. S., & Wilkinson, J. M. (2018). *Basic nursing: Concepts, skills, and reasoning* (2nd ed.). Philadelphia, PA: F.A. Davis.

*U.S. Department of Health and Human Services, National Heart, Lung, and Blood Institute. (2014). Evidence-based management of sickle cell disease: Expert panel report, 2014 www.nhlbi.nih.gov/health-pro/guidelines/sickle-cell-disease-guidelines

*U.S. Department of Health and Human Services, National Heart, Lung, and Blood Institute. (2014). Management of blood cholesterol in adults: Systematic evidence review from the cholesterol expert panel. Available at: www.nhlbi.nih.gov/health-pro/guidelines/in-develop/cholesterol-in-adults

*University of Michigan Health System. (2011). *Osteoporosis: Prevention and treatment.* Ann Arbor, MI: University of Michigan Health System. Available at: www.med.umich.edu/1info/FHP/practiceguides/osteoporosis/text.pdf

Vallerand, A. H., Sanoski, C. A., & Deglin, J. H. (2019). *Davis's drug guide for nurses* (16th ed.). Philadelphia, PA: F.A. Davis.

Wachter, R. (2017). *Understanding patient safety* (3rd ed.). New York: McGraw-Hill.

Whitehead, D. K., Weiss, S. A., & Tappen, R. M. (2015). *Essentials of nursing leadership and management* (6th ed.). Philadelphia, PA: F.A. Davis.

Whitney, E., DeBruyne, L., Pinna, K., & Rolfes, S. (2013). *Nutrition for health and health care* (5th ed.). Belmont, CA: Thomson Learning.

Wilkinson, J. M., & Treas, L. S. (2011). *Fundamentals of nursing: Theory, concepts, & application* (2nd ed.). Philadelphia, PA: F.A. Davis.

Wilson, B. A., Shannon, M. T., & Shields, K. M. (2015). *Pearson nurse's drug guide 2015.* Upper Saddle River, NJ: Pearson Education.

Yoder-Wise, P. (2019). *Leading and managing in nursing* (7th ed.). St. Louis, MO: Mosby/Elsevier.

Zerwekh, J., & Garneau, A. Z. (2018). *Nursing today: Transition and trends* (9th ed., p. 302). St. Louis, MO: Elsevier/Saunders.

*Evidence-based Reference

Note: Page numbers followed by *f* refer to figures; page numbers followed by *t* refer to tables; page numbers followed by *b* refer to boxes.